HANDBOOK OF
MRI
PULSE SEQUENCES

HANDBOOK OF
MRI
PULSE SEQUENCES

MATT A. BERNSTEIN, PH.D.
*Department of Radiology, Mayo Clinic and
Mayo Clinic College of Medicine
Rochester, Minnesota*

KEVIN F. KING, PH.D.
*GE Healthcare
Waukesha, Wisconsin*

XIAOHONG JOE ZHOU, PH.D.
*University of Illinois Medical Center
Chicago, Illinois*

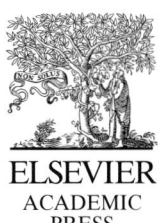

ELSEVIER
ACADEMIC
PRESS

*Amsterdam   Boston   Heidelberg   London   New York   Oxford
Paris   San Diego   San Francisco   Singapore   Sydney   Tokyo*

Nothing in this book implies endorsement by Mayo Foundation or University of Illinois of any medical equipment manufacturer.

Elsevier Academic Press
200 Wheeler Road, 6th Floor, Burlington, MA 01803, USA
525 B Street, Suite 1900, San Diego, California 92101-4495, USA
84 Theobald's Road, London WC1X 8RR, UK

This book is printed on acid-free paper. ∞

Library of Congress Cataloging-in-Publication Data
Application submitted

British Library Cataloguing in Publication Data
A catalogue record for this book is available from the British Library

ISBN-13: 978- 0-12-092861-3
ISBN-10:   0-12-092861-2

For all information on all Elsevier Academic Press publications
visit our Web site at www.books.elsevier.com

Printed in the United States of America
      06 07 08 09 9 8 7 6 5 4 3

To Rhoda, Juliet, Sara, and Lee
M.A.B.

To Sherry and our son Christopher
X.J.Z.

To Beth
K.F.K.

CONTENTS

PART I: BACKGROUND

CHAPTER 1

TOOLS

PART II: RADIOFREQUENCY PULSES

CHAPTER 2

RADIOFREQUENCY PULSE SHAPES

CHAPTER 3

BASIC RADIOFREQUENCY PULSE FUNCTIONS

CHAPTER 4

SPECTRAL RADIOFREQUENCY PULSES

CHAPTER 5

SPATIAL RADIOFREQUENCY PULSES

CHAPTER 6

ADIABATIC RADIOFREQUENCY PULSES

PART III: Gradients

PART IV: DATA ACQUISITION, K-SPACE SAMPLING, AND IMAGE RECONSTRUCTION

PART V: PULSE SEQUENCES

C H A P T E R 14
BASIC PULSE SEQUENCES

C H A P T E R 15
ANGIOGRAPHIC PULSE SEQUENCES

C H A P T E R 16
ECHO TRAIN PULSE SEQUENCES

C H A P T E R 17
ADVANCED PULSE SEQUENCE TECHNIQUES

FOREWORD

Magnetic resonance imaging is recognized as one of the most important medical advances of the century. It has opened new windows into the human body, revealing structure and function with a level of detail that would have been unimaginable only decades ago.

The award of the Nobel Prize in Medicine to Paul Lauterbur and Peter Mansfield is a wonderful recognition for their important contributions to the development of MRI. The award of the Nobel Prize in Medicine for work that is rooted in Physics and Engineering is also an important validation of these disciplines as important participants within the medical research community.

While the pioneering work of Lauterbur and Mansfield was critical to the early development of MRI, the amazingly wide range of its capabilities have resulted from the efforts of the many scientists and clinicians. Unlike other high-tech imaging modalities, a large proportion of the techniques currently used in state-of-the-art practice were *not* initially introduced by industry. Rather, these advances were made by investigators and physician specialists in academic centers and clinical imaging practices. In a very real way, MRI—one of the most important tools of modern medical practice—is a technology that was *invented by its users*!

The *Handbook of MRI Pulse Sequences* is a comprehensive and highly readable reference targeted squarely at those who want to understand the current state-of-the-art, as well as those who are committed to continuing the process of innovation. The authors have segmented the vast subject of MRI technology into five logical sections: Background Concepts, Radiofrequency

Pulses, Gradients, Data Acquisition, and Pulse Sequences. These sections contain carefully planned groups of chapters that systematically cover the field. The chapters use a modular building block approach that avoids repetition, allowing efficient presentation of a subject. Each of the main sections is self-contained, allowing the reader to go directly to any section without the need to review previous sections. Consistent nomenclature is used throughout.

Such disciplined and accessible coverage of the field would have been difficult if the book followed the model of chapters written by dozens of authors. Instead the *Handbook of MRI Pulse Sequences* is the product of three highly dedicated authors. Drs. Bernstein, King, and Zhou have all made significant contributions to the MRI field and have collective experience spanning from industry to academia. All three are highly accomplished in teaching the "nuts and bolts" of MRI technology.

Most chapters are accessible to readers with varying levels of expertise. The book should be useful to physicists and MRI radiologists alike. The chapters combine rigorous mathematical coverage of concepts to the level warranted by the subject matter, with qualitative descriptions wherever feasible.

This book is unique in the fact that it brings together in one reference many areas of MRI technology that are not well covered in other available references. Such areas include adiabatic fast passage radiofrequency pulses, stimulated echoes, ordered phase encoding, navigator echoes, and many others. The section on Gradients nicely clarifies the generally misunderstood terminology and purpose of the various types of correction gradients such as crushers, spoilers, and twisters.

Many scientists who are active in supervising MRI research by graduate and postdoctoral students have encountered, year after year, a relative paucity of comprehensive reference textbooks that can answer the recurring questions that arise. The *Handbook of MRI Pulse Sequences* will address this need in an outstanding fashion.

This book will become one of the classic texts in the field and will play a key role in helping the next generation of scientists and MRI clinicians to continue the process of invention.

Richard L. Ehman, M.D.
Professor of Radiology
Mayo Clinic

FOREWORD

MRI has now been developing for over 30 years. The first experiments did not use any technique that would ordinarily be called a "pulse sequence," employing CW applications of radiofrequency (RF) fields and static main magnetic fields and gradients, with iterative back projection reconstruction and T_1 discrimination by changing of RF intensity. It was soon realized, however, that time-dependent RF pulses and magnetic field gradients offered more flexibility in many applications, and the field of "pulse sequence" design opened. This book is the best evidence of its subsequent proliferation, both for the sake of novelty and to tailor instrument responses to a variety of applications. An unfortunate side effect has been that such efforts have introduced innumerable acronyms or near-acronyms in an effort to distinguish the various sequences, or fix credit for their designs. This book is the most valiant and successful attempt yet to provide a useful description of this "zoo," and to relate and classify the various denizens in it. Such a taxonomy can never be complete, as the inhabitants keep multiplying and providing new hybrids which must be classified to facilitate discourse among physicists, engineers, physicians, and others, and to help pulse sequence designers avoid inadvertent duplication of efforts. I believe that no MRI developer or user can read this book without learning more about the field, as I have.

But what does this suggest about future editions or successors? New applications will continue to become important, and new opportunities will continue to suggest themselves to creative pulse-sequence designers. Will we soon reach the limit of our ability to absorb, retain, and understand such innovations, which may include aspects of high-resolution solid-state spectroscopy and quantum computing? There is some evidence that we already have, as much MRI seems even now driven by habit, custom, and instrumental constraints rather than by medical and other needs. In the future, the functions that this book serves may be accomplished by interactive database programs that "understand" MRI physics, so that properly defined needs can be matched to the best sequences, and new sequences consistent with machine capabilities can be computer-developed as needed. I therefore look forward to the second edition of this book as a CD or equivalent, combined with a specialized search-engine. In the meantime, the first edition will well-repay careful study.

Paul C. Lauterbur, Ph.D.
Center for Advanced Study
Professor of Chemistry, Biophysics and
Computational Biology, and in the Bioengineering Program
Research Professor of Medical Information Sciences
College of Medicine at Urbana-Champaign
and Distinguished Professor, College of Medicine
University of Illinois at Chicago

PREFACE

Since its invention in the early 1970s, the development of magnetic resonance imaging (MRI) has been among the most active and exciting areas in science, technology, and medicine. Today, thousands of MRI scanners are operating throughout the world, providing crucial information in such diverse areas as material science, pharmaceutical development, and especially medical diagnosis.

MRI encompasses many areas of science and technology, including spin physics, biophysics, image reconstruction, and hardware design. Although each area performs a necessary function, it is the MRI pulse sequence that links many of the individual functions together and plays a pivotal role in data acquisition. Over the past 30 years, development of pulse sequences has been an extremely active area of MRI research. Many important concepts of MRI are realized through pulse sequence design, and virtually every imaging application is enabled by one or more pulse sequences. This book aims to help the reader gain a comprehensive understanding of many pulse sequences (and their associated techniques) in use today. The book is also intended to assist the reader to continue the innovation in pulse sequence design, and to carry MRI development into the future.

While this handbook focuses on MRI pulse sequences, it also covers the building blocks from which they are composed, as well as the related image reconstruction techniques and important mathematical tools that are helpful for understanding them. We have divided the book into five parts. Each part of the book is preceded by its own introduction, which provides an overview of its contents. Part I covers two basic mathematical tools: Fourier transforms and the rotating reference frame. Parts II through IV describe a variety of the basic building blocks and associated techniques of MRI pulse sequences: radiofrequency (RF) pulses, gradient waveforms, data acquisition strategies, and common image reconstruction methods. Part V describes how these components are integrated into some of the common pulse sequences. Selected applications of each pulse sequence are also discussed in Part V.

The five parts of the book are further subdivided into chapters. For example, Part III on Gradients contains chapters describing gradient lobe shapes, imaging gradients, motion-sensitizing gradients, and correction gradients. Each chapter in turn contains multiple sections that are usually arranged alphabetically. In all, there is a total of 65 sections. The sections in each chapter are independent, forming their own *self-contained* units. As such, the sections do not have to be read in any particular order. Each section contains an introduction to the subject and some qualitative description. Depending on the subject matter, mathematical analysis, practical implementation details, and/or descriptions of applications may also be included. At the end of each section, selected references are provided, and the related sections are listed.

It is also important to say what this book is *not*. This book is not meant to be an encyclopedia of pulse sequences. We have attempted to cover most of the MRI pulse sequences in common use today, but have made no attempt to describe every pulse sequence that has ever been published. We believe, however, that virtually every MRI pulse sequence that has ever been implemented (or even proposed) is composed, at least in part, of the building blocks described in detail in this handbook. We would also like to emphasize that exclusion of any particular sequence or technique is not meant to imply anything about its relative importance. The scope of this book encompasses MR imaging pulse sequences, but excludes purely spectroscopic pulse sequences, and only briefly touches on spectroscopic imaging. The physical description of spin dynamics (sometimes called spin "gymnastics") is limited to the classical picture, which is sufficient for the vast majority of the discussion throughout the book. Therefore, neither quantum mechanical formalism nor multiple-quantum phenomena are covered.

We make no rigorous attempt to provide an historical record of who invented or first published any particular pulse sequence or technique. Given the activity in the field of MRI, a thorough study of that subject could probably fill a large volume itself. The selected references at the end of each section are only intended to provide the reader with additional material to understand the subject matter, and do not necessarily correspond to the earliest work on that subject. The references are a collection of papers, review articles, conference abstracts, books, book chapters, and patents selected from those we have found instructive during our own study. The reader may also notice that some of the sections in Part V contain many more references than the earlier sections.

Perhaps this is an expression that there are many more ways to combine and permute the building blocks, compared to the number of building blocks themselves. Because of the breadth and depth of activity in MRI research, we realize that we have inevitably omitted some important references. We are eager to receive feedback about the book, so feel free to contact us if you would like to suggest additional references that should be included in future editions.

This book is written primarily for scientists and engineers working in the field of MRI. It can also serve as a supplementary textbook for a graduate course on medical imaging, medical physics, or biomedical engineering. Radiologists and other medical professionals interested in an in-depth understanding of various MRI pulse sequences will also benefit from the book. To cover the diverse background of the readership, both non-mathematical and mathematical descriptions are provided. Readers not interested in the mathematical description of a particular topic can skip over those portions of a section that contain complicated equations. It is our aim to provide those readers with sufficient qualitative description in text and figures to convey the gist of each section. The level of mathematical sophistication varies widely from section to section. This is because we have tried to tailor the mathematical level to the specific subject material, rather than to a specific readership. For example the mathematical level used in the sections describing SLR pulses (§2.3), gridding (§13.2), and parallel imaging reconstruction (§13.3) is considerably higher than that describing real-time imaging (§11.4). In general, however, the level of mathematical sophistication is at the first-year university level, with use of vectors, basic calculus, and linear algebra. A notable exception is the use of Fourier transforms, which are relied on extensively throughout the book. To help keep the book self-contained, §1.1 is entirely devoted to the properties of continuous and discrete Fourier transforms.

In writing this book, we have assumed that the reader has already acquired some basic knowledge of MRI physics. Although we provide discussion of a few essential physical concepts, such as the Bloch equations, gradients, and rotating reference frame, we encourage the reader to consult any of the excellent introductory MRI physics books, should there be a background concept that is unfamiliar. Similar to the level of mathematics, the level of physics is also tailored to individual sections. For example, §12.1 on cardiac triggering requires little background on spin physics, while to understand the adiabatic pulses described in Chapter 6 requires a somewhat deeper background in MRI physics. Many of the physical concepts used to understand adiabatic pulses, however, are described in that chapter, or in other sections of the book.

The idea of writing a handbook on MRI pulse sequences, with self-contained sections, was initiated by one of the authors (X.J.Z.) in the spring of 1999, but it was only through the effort of all three authors working in concert that the book took its current shape. Between 1999 and 2000, the three authors held numerous meetings and conference calls to define the scope. We focused on designing a book with three primary features, all aimed at helping the reader extract the maximal information with the minimal effort. First, as mentioned earlier, each section is self-contained so the reader can go straight to the material of interest without reading the preceding sections in sequential order. Second, also mentioned earlier, each subject in a section is discussed both qualitatively and quantitatively to serve readers with various backgrounds. Third, special attention is paid to maximizing consistency across all the sections. This frees the reader from having to make the mental adjustment for inconsistent notation, conventions, and terminology usually required when reading a set of original research papers, or an edited book that has many contributing authors. Many of the mathematical symbols, constants, abbreviations, and acronyms used across multiple sections of the book are listed in the appendices.

This handbook was written during a period from 2000 to early 2004. It is the product of three authors who contributed *equally*. The author names in various places are listed alphabetically and the order does not imply relative contribution to the book. Each step in the process was designed to ensure maximal consistency throughout while maintaining the breadth of coverage that three authors can provide. In this electronic era, being based in separate cities did not hamper this effort. A primary author drafted each section, and then sent it to one of the other authors for review. Based on the comments and additions received, the primary author revised the section and sent it to the third author for further review. The process was iterated as many times as necessary (in some cases, seven or eight iterations) until all authors were satisfied with the manuscript. To make the handbook as seamless as possible, the three authors participated in telephone conference calls at regular intervals. As a result, each author made substantial contributions to every section. In spite of our efforts, mistakes undoubtedly still exist. We encourage the reader to contact us, should she/he find any errors, omitted material, or any explanations that are not clear. Correspondence about a particular section can be addressed to the primary section author who is listed in the table of contents, and who will continue to manage the revisions of that section.

In addition to our own review process, we also asked a number of experts to review several sections of the manuscript. We are indebted to these guest reviewers who improved the quality of those sections with their insightful comments. Stephen Riederer, Ph.D. reviewed §11.4 on real-time imaging, and §15.3 on time-of-flight and contrast-enhanced MR angiography. James Glockner, M.D., Ph.D. reviewed §12.1 on cardiac triggering, as did Kiaran McGee, Ph.D. Heidi Ward, Ph.D. reviewed §12.2 on navigator echoes, and §14.1 on gradient echoes. Elisabeth Angelos, Ph.D. reviewed §13.3 on parallel imaging. Yihong Yang, Ph.D. reviewed §17.1 on arterial spin tagging. Sarah Patch,

Ph.D. reviewed §17.5 on projection acquisition. We greatly appreciate all of their help. Naturally, any errors remaining in those sections are solely ours.

We also thank the many contributors (Drs. Kimberly Amrami, Walter Block, Reed Busse, Kim Butts, Norbert Campeau, Bruce Daniel, J. Kevin DeMarco, Kevin Glaser, E. Mark Haacke, Romhild M. Hoogeveen, John Huston III, Emanuel Kanal, Chen Lin, Kiaran McGee, Paul McGough, Gary Miller, Koichi Oshio, Scott Reeder, Pr. Regent, Larry Tanenbaum, Heidi Ward, Qing-San Xiang, Yihong Yang, and Frank Q. Ye) who provided images for this handbook. Their contributions are individually acknowledged again in the figure captions.

We would also like to thank Linda Greene for her review of some of the page proofs, David Thomasson, Ph.D. for providing a glossary of MR terms used by Siemens Medical Solutions, and Tim Hiller for providing a list of acronyms used by Philips Medical Systems and other vendors. Our appreciation is also extended to Dr. K. Noelle Gracy, Anne Russum, Marcy Barnes-Henrie, Paul Gottehrer, and others at Elsevier who aided us during various stages of planning and writing the book.

Many other individuals also helped us in various ways to make this book possible. We would like to individually express our whole-hearted gratitude to them:

MAB: I am indebted to all my teachers and mentors. In the field of physics, the guidance from Drs. Bill Friedman, Gary Glover, and Norbert Pelc has been especially valued. Drs. John Huston III, Paul McGough, Patrick Turski, and many others have patiently taught me some of the clinical aspects of MRI. Larry Ploetz introduced me to the subtleties of pulse sequence programming. I am also indebted to my colleagues on the clinical MRI Physics team at the Mayo Clinic in Rochester, including Drs. Joel Felmlee, Chen Lin, and Kiaran McGee, as well as Diana Lanners and Renee Jonsgaard. Of course without the patience and support of my wife Rhoda Lichy, my contribution to this book would not have been possible.

KFK: Thanks to Paul Moran for introducing me to medical imaging and teaching me about magnetic resonance. Richard Kinsinger gave me career opportunities for which I will always be very grateful. The work of Gary Glover and Norbert Pelc has provided a standard by which I measure all of my own work. Thanks to the many colleagues at GE with whom I have had the privilege and pleasure to work. You have instructed, challenged, and inspired me. Special thanks to Carl Crawford, Alex Ganin, and Lisa Angelos. Without your collaboration, the work would not have been nearly as much fun.

XJZ: I would like to thank Professor Paul C. Lauterbur who introduced me to the field of MRI, shared his remarkable insight into MRI physics, and encouraged the idea of writing this book. I would also like to thank Drs. G. Allen Johnson, Keith R. Thulborn, and Richard E. Kinsinger who guided me, in various stages of my career, to acquire knowledge of pulse sequence design. My gratitude is owed to Drs. Norman E. Leeds, Edward F. Jackson, Haesun Choi, and Srikanth Mahankali for teaching me a great deal on the clinical aspects of MRI. Many colleagues, friends, and students also helped me in developing the materials that are included in the book. In particular, I am indebted to Dr. Fernando E. Boada, Gary P. Cofer, Dr. John D. Hazle, Dr. Christof Karmonik, Dr. Zhi-Pei Liang, Dr. James R. MacFall, Joseph K. Maier, Dr. Graeme C. McKinnon, Dr. Bryan J. Mock, Dr. Douglas C. Noll, Aziz H. Poonawalla, H. Glenn Reynolds, Dr. Gary X. Shen, Dr. R. Jason Stafford, Dr. S. Lalith Talagala, Dr. Qing-San Xiang, and Dr. Yihong Yang. Finally, my appreciation goes to Sherry Xia Yao who spent countless evenings and weekends taking care of our infant son during the period when the book was written.

The development of MRI pulse sequences over the last 30 years has been truly exciting. The process of writing this book has only enhanced our appreciation of the dedicated scientists, engineers, and clinicians who have advanced MRI into the essential tool that it has become. We hope you will enjoy this book, and find it to be a useful reference for continuing the advancement of this great field.

Matt A. Bernstein
Rochester, Minnesota
mbernstein@mayo.edu

Kevin F. King
Waukesha, Wisconsin
kevin.f.king@med.ge.com

Xiaohong Joe Zhou
Chicago, Illinois
xjzhou@uic.edu
May 2004

BACKGROUND

Introduction

Part I of this book contains selected background information that is used in many sections throughout the book. Chapter 1 (the only chapter in Part I) describes two mathematical tools that are universally used to analyze magnetic resonance imaging (MRI): the Fourier transform (Section 1.1), and the rotating reference frame (Section 1.2). Although neither of these tools is a pulse sequence (or pulse sequence element) itself, they are both described in considerable detail to establish the notation and conventions that are used throughout the book. A more extensive discussion of Fourier transform can be found in Bracewell (1978). A more thorough introduction to the rotating reference frame and other magnetic resonance (MR) physics concepts is contained in many references, for example, Slichter (1989).

Other mathematical tools (e.g., rotation matrices) used in specific applications are described in their own individual sections (e.g., Section 2.3), as needed. For additional general mathematical tools used in this book, the reader is encouraged to consult a mathematics handbook such as Arfken and Weber (2001).

SELECTED REFERENCES

Arfken, G. B., and Weber, H. J. 2001. *Mathematical methods for physicists. 5th ed.* San Diego: Academic Press.

Bracewell, R. N. 1978. *The Fourier transform and its applications.* New York: McGraw-Hill.

Slichter, C. P. 1989. *The principles of magnetic resonance. 3rd ed.* Berlin: Springer-Verlag.

1

TOOLS

1.1 Fourier Transforms

The *Fourier transform* (FT) is a mathematical operation that yields the spectral content of a signal (Bracewell 1978). It is named after the French mathematician Jean Baptiste Joseph Fourier (1768–1830). If a signal consists of oscillation at a single frequency (e.g., 163 Hz), then its FT will contain a peak at that frequency (Figure 1.1a). If the signal contains a superposition of tones at multiple frequencies, the FT operation essentially provides a histogram of that spectral content (Figure 1.1b). For example, consider the following physical analogy. Suppose several keys on a piano are struck simultaneously and the resultant sounds are sampled and digitized. The FT of that signal will provide information about which keys were struck and with what force.

Fourier transforms are ubiquitous in the practical reconstruction of MR data and also in the theoretical analysis of MR processes. This is because the physical evolution of the transverse magnetization is described very naturally by the FT. In Magnetic Resonance Imaging (MRI), we usually use *complex* Fourier transforms, which employ the complex exponential, rather than separate sine or cosine Fourier transforms. This choice is made because a complex exponential conveniently represents the precession of the magnetization vector. Table 1.1 reviews some basic properties of the complex exponential. Often a *magnitude* operation (i.e., $|Z|$) is used on a pixel-by-pixel basis to convert the complex output of the FT to positive real numbers that can be more conveniently displayed as pixel intensities.

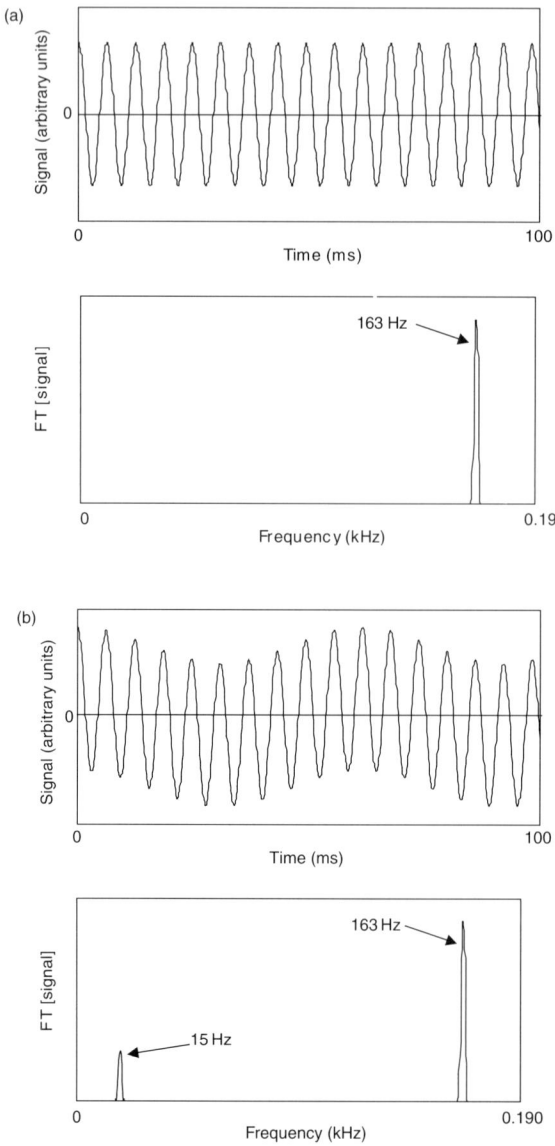

FIGURE 1.1 Schematic representations of the Fourier transform. (a) If a time domain signal contains a tone at a single frequency, its Fourier transform will contain a peak at that frequency, which in this case is 163 Hz. (b) If the signal contains a superposition of two tones, the Fourier transform displays a second peak. In the case shown, a 15-Hz tone with approximately one-quarter the amplitude is modulating the original tone.

TABLE 1.1
Properties of Complex Numbers

$i = \sqrt{-1} = e^{i\pi/2}$

$e^{i\theta} = \cos\theta + i\sin\theta$

$e^{i(a+b)} = e^{ia}\,e^{ib}$

$\cos\theta = \dfrac{e^{i\theta} + e^{-i\theta}}{2}$

$\sin\theta = \dfrac{e^{i\theta} - e^{-i\theta}}{2i}$

if $Z = \rho\,e^{i\theta}$,   then $|Z| = \rho$, $\arg(Z) = \angle Z = \theta$

if $Z = x + iy$,   then $|Z| = \sqrt{x^2 + y^2}$, $\arg(Z) = \tan^{-1}\left(\dfrac{y}{x}\right)$

$Z^* = x - iy = \rho e^{-i\theta}$ (complex conjugate of Z)

$Z_1 Z_2 = \rho_1 \rho_2 e^{i(\theta_1 + \theta_2)} = (x_1 x_2 - y_1 y_2) + i(x_1 y_2 + y_1 x_2)$

When we are provided with a function of a continuous variable, its FT is calculated by a process that includes integration. This continuous FT is widely used for theoretical work in MRI. The actual MRI signal that is measured, however, is sampled at a finite number of discrete time points, so instead a *discrete Fourier transform* (DFT) is used for practical image reconstruction. With the DFT, the integration operation of the FT is replaced by a finite summation. An important special case of the DFT is called the *fast Fourier transform* (FFT) (Cooley and Tukey 1965; Brigham 1988). The FFT is an algorithm that calculates the DFT of signals whose lengths are particular values (most typically equal to a power of 2, e.g., $256 = 2^8$). As its name implies, the FFT is computationally faster than the standard DFT.

1.1.1 THE CONTINUOUS FOURIER TRANSFORM AND ITS INVERSE

Let $g(x)$ be a function of the real variable x. The output of the function $g(x)$ can have complex values. The complex Fourier transform of $g(x)$ is another function, which we call $G(k)$:

$$\text{FT}[g(x)] = G(k) = \int_{-\infty}^{+\infty} g(x)e^{-2\pi ikx}dx \tag{1.1}$$

The two real variables x and k are known as Fourier *conjugates* and represent a pair of FT *domains*. Examples of domain pairs commonly used in MR are (time, frequency) and (distance, k-space). If the physical units of the pair of variables that represent the two domains are multiplied together, the result is always dimensionless. For example, with the time–frequency pair, the product:

$$1 \text{ millisecond} \times 1 \text{ kHz} = 1 \text{ (dimensionless)} \qquad (1.2)$$

The two functions $g(x)$ and $G(k)$ in Eq. (1.1) are called *Fourier transform pairs*. Knowledge about one of the pair is sufficient to reconstruct the other. If $G(k)$ is known, then $g(x)$ can be recovered by performing an *inverse Fourier transform* (IFT):

$$\text{FT}^{-1}[G(k)] = g(x) = \int_{-\infty}^{+\infty} G(k)\, e^{+2\pi i k x}\, dk \qquad (1.3)$$

The IFT undoes the effect of the FT, that is:

$$\text{FT}^{-1}\big[\text{FT}[g(x)]\big] = g(x) \qquad (1.4)$$

and vice versa:

$$\text{FT}\big[\text{FT}^{-1}[G(k)]\big] = G(k) \qquad (1.5)$$

Note that the right sides of Eqs. (1.4) and (1.5) are simply $g(x)$ and $G(k)$, respectively, and are not multiplied by any scaling factors. This is because the IFT definition in Eq. (1.3) is properly *normalized*. A further discussion of the normalization is given in subsection 1.1.10.

Note the factor of 2π that appears in the argument of the exponentials in Eqs. (1.1) and (1.3). If instead domain variables such as time and *angular* frequency (ω, measured in radians/second) are used, then the form of the FT appears somewhat differently. The FT and its inverse become:

$$G(t) = \frac{1}{2\pi} \int_{-\infty}^{+\infty} g(\omega)\, e^{-i\omega t}\, d\omega$$

$$g(\omega) = \int_{-\infty}^{+\infty} G(t)\, e^{i\omega t}\, dt \qquad (1.6)$$

Note the absence of the 2π factor in the exponential in Eq. (1.6) and the extra multiplicative normalization factor in front of the FT. Equation (1.6) could be recast into a more symmetric form by splitting the 2π into equal $\sqrt{(2\pi)}$ factors in the denominators of both the FT and IFT definitions. Alternatively, we can recast Eq. (1.6) by making the familiar substitution from angular frequency ω to standard frequency f (measured in cycles/second or hertz):

$$\omega = 2\pi f \qquad d\omega = 2\pi\, df \qquad (1.7)$$

Substituting Eq. (1.7) into Eq. (1.6) yields the symmetric FT pairs

$$G(t) = \int_{-\infty}^{+\infty} g(f)\, e^{-2\pi i f t} df \qquad (1.8)$$

and

$$g(f) = \int_{-\infty}^{+\infty} G(t)\, e^{2\pi i f t} dt \qquad (1.9)$$

In this book, we mainly use the form of the FT and IFT with the factor of 2π in the exponential, such as Eqs. (1.1) and (1.8).

1.1.2 MULTIDIMENSIONAL FOURIER TRANSFORMS, AND SEPARABILITY

Multidimensional FTs often arise in MRI. For example, the *two-dimensional FT* (2D-FT) of a function of two variables can be defined as:

$$FT[g(x, y)] = G(k_x, k_y) = \int_{-\infty}^{+\infty} \int_{-\infty}^{+\infty} g(x, y)\, e^{-2\pi i k_x x} e^{-2\pi i k_y y} dx\, dy$$

$$= \int_{-\infty}^{+\infty} \int_{-\infty}^{+\infty} g(x, y)\, e^{-2\pi i \vec{k}\cdot\vec{r}} dx\, dy \qquad (1.10)$$

where $\vec{r} = (x,\, y)$ and $\vec{k} = (k_x, k_y)$ are vectors. The inverse 2D-FT is given by:

$$FT^{-1}[G(k_x, k_y)] = g(x, y) = \int_{-\infty}^{+\infty} \int_{-\infty}^{+\infty} G(k_x, k_y)\, e^{+2\pi i \vec{k}\cdot\vec{r}} dk_x\, dk_y \qquad (1.11)$$

Eqs. (1.10) and (1.11) are readily generalized to three or more dimensions.

If the function g is *separable* in x and y:

$$g(x, y) = g_x(x) g_y(y) \tag{1.12}$$

then the FT is also separable:

$$FT[g(x, y)] = FT[g_x(x) g_y(y)] = G_x(k_x) G_y(k_y) \tag{1.13}$$

An example of a separable two-dimensional function is the Gaussian:

$$e^{\frac{-(x^2+y^2)}{2\sigma^2}} = e^{\frac{-x^2}{2\sigma^2}} e^{\frac{-y^2}{2\sigma^2}} \tag{1.14}$$

In contrast,

$$(x + y)^2 = x^2 + y^2 + 2xy \tag{1.15}$$

is not separable.

1.1.3 PROPERTIES OF THE FOURIER TRANSFORM

An important property of the FT is the *shift theorem*. A shift or offset of the coordinate in one domain results in a multiplication of the signal by a *linear phase ramp* in the other domain, and vice versa:

$$FT[g(x - a)] = \int_{-\infty}^{\infty} g(u) e^{-2\pi ik(u+a)} du = G(k) e^{-2\pi ika} \tag{1.16}$$

A second useful property of the FT is that *convolution* in one domain is equivalent to simple *multiplication* in the other. If $f(x)$ and $g(x)$ are two functions, then convolution is defined as:

$$f(x) \otimes g(x) = \int_{-\infty}^{+\infty} f(x - x') g(x') dx' \tag{1.17}$$

and

$$FT[f(x) \otimes g(x)] = F(k) G(k) \tag{1.18}$$

Parseval's theorem (named after Marc-Antoine Parseval des Chênes, 1755–1836, a French mathematician) is a third commonly used property of the FT. It states that if f and g are two functions with Fourier transforms F and G, respectively, then

$$\int_{-\infty}^{+\infty} f^*(x) g(x) dx = \int_{-\infty}^{+\infty} F^*(k) G(k) dk \tag{1.19}$$

where * denotes complex conjugation. Letting $g = f$ in Eq. (1.19) results in a useful special case, which shows that the FT operation conserves normalization:

$$\int_{-\infty}^{+\infty} |f(x)|^2 \, dx = \int_{-\infty}^{+\infty} |F(k)|^2 \, dk \tag{1.20}$$

Table 1.2 provides several 1D-FT pairs that are commonly used in MRI. These relationships can be applied to multidimensional FTs if the variables are separable.

1.1.4 THE DISCRETE FOURIER TRANSFORM AND ITS INVERSE

In MRI, the sampling process provides a finite number (e.g., 256) of complex data points, rather than a function of a continuous variable. Consequently, the MR image is normally reconstructed with a DFT. Given a string of N complex data points:

$$\{d\} = \{d_0, d_1, d_2, \ldots, d_{N-1}\} \tag{1.21}$$

the Jth element of DFT is defined as:

$$\mathrm{DFT}[\{d\}]_J = D_J = \sum_{K=0}^{N-1} d_K e^{\frac{-2\pi i J K}{N}}, \quad J = 0, 1, 2, \ldots, N - 1 \tag{1.22}$$

Note that the index $J = 0$ represents the DC, or zero-frequency element, of the DFT (DC is adopted from the abbreviation for direct current used in electrical engineering). The exponential factor in Eq. (1.22) is sometimes called a *twiddle factor*. The Kth element of the *inverse DFT* (IDFT) is defined as

$$\mathrm{DFT}^{-1}[\{D\}]_K = d_K = \frac{1}{N} \sum_{J'=0}^{N-1} D_{J'} e^{\frac{+2\pi i J' K}{N}}, \quad K = 0, 1, 2, \ldots, N - 1 \tag{1.23}$$

The factor of $1/N$ in Eq. (1.23) is required for normalization, so that

$$\mathrm{DFT}^{-1}\big[\mathrm{DFT}[\{d\}]\big] = \{d\}$$
$$\mathrm{DFT}\big[\mathrm{DFT}^{-1}[\{D\}]\big] = \{D\} \tag{1.24}$$

In analogy to the manipulation of the 2π-normalization factor of the complex FT described for Eqs. (1.6)–(1.9), the normalization factor of $1/N$ in Eq. (1.23) can be moved from the IDFT to the DFT. Alternatively, it is sometimes symmetrically distributed as equal $1/\sqrt{N}$ factors on both the DFT and IDFT. It is

TABLE 1.2

Fourier Transform Pairs Commonly Used in Magnetic Resonance Imaging

$g(x)$	$\mathrm{FT}[g(x)] = G(k) = \displaystyle\int_{-\infty}^{+\infty} g(x)e^{-2\pi ikx}\,dx$
$g(x)e^{2\pi ik_0 x}$	$G(k - k_0)$
$g(x - x_0)$	$G(k)e^{-2\pi ikx_0}$
$g\left(\dfrac{x}{\alpha}\right)$	$\lvert\alpha\rvert G(\alpha k)$
$g(-x)$	$G(-k)$
$\dfrac{dg(x)}{dx}$	$2\pi ik\,G(k)$
$g^*(x)$	$G^*(-k)$
$xg(x)$	$\dfrac{i}{2\pi}\dfrac{dG(k)}{dk}$
$af(x) + bg(x)$	$aF(k) + bG(k)$
$f(x) \otimes g(x)$	$F(k)G(k)$
$\delta(x) = \begin{cases} 0 & \text{if } x \neq 0 \\ \displaystyle\int_{-\infty}^{+\infty}\delta(x)\,dx = 1 \end{cases}$	1
1	$\delta(k)$
$e^{2\pi ik_0 x}$	$\delta(k - k_0)$
$\cos(2\pi k_0 x)$	$\dfrac{1}{2}[\delta(k - k_0) + \delta(k + k_0)]$
$\sin(2\pi k_0 x)$	$\dfrac{1}{2i}[\delta(k - k_0) - \delta(k + k_0)]$
$\cos^2(2\pi k_0 x)$	$\dfrac{1}{2}\left[\delta(k) + \dfrac{\delta(k - 2k_0) + \delta(k + 2k_0)}{2}\right]$
$\sin^2(2\pi k_0 x)$	$\dfrac{1}{2}\left[\delta(k) - \dfrac{\delta(k - 2k_0) + \delta(k + 2k_0)}{2}\right]$
$\cos^3(2\pi k_0 x)$	$\dfrac{1}{8}[3(\delta(k - k_0) + \delta(k + k_0)) + \delta(k - 3k_0) + \delta(k + 3k_0)]$
$\sin^3(2\pi k_0 x)$	$\dfrac{1}{8i}[3(\delta(k - k_0) - \delta(k + k_0)) - \delta(k - 3k_0) + \delta(k + 3k_0)]$

TABLE 1.2
Continued

$\displaystyle\sum_{n=-\infty}^{\infty} \delta(x - nx_0)$	$\displaystyle\frac{1}{x_0} \sum_{m=-\infty}^{\infty} \delta\left(k - \frac{m}{x_0}\right)$
$H(x) = \begin{cases} 1 & \text{if } x > 0 \\ 0 & \text{if } x < 0 \end{cases}$	$\displaystyle\frac{1}{2\pi}\left[\pi\delta(k) - i \text{ Principle part}\left(\frac{1}{k}\right)\right]$
$\text{RECT}\left(\dfrac{x}{x_0}\right) = \begin{cases} 1 & \text{if } |x| \le x_0 \\ 0 & \text{if } |x| > x_0 \end{cases}$	$2x_0\text{SINC}(u), \quad \text{SINC}(u) \equiv \dfrac{\sin(u)}{u}, \quad u = 2\pi kx_0$
$e^{-x^2/2\sigma^2}$	$\sigma\sqrt{2\pi}e^{-2\pi^2\sigma^2 k^2}, \qquad \sigma \text{ real}$
$e^{-\lambda|x|}$	$\dfrac{2\lambda}{\lambda^2 + (2\pi k)^2}, \qquad \text{Re } \lambda > 0$
$H(x)e^{-\lambda x}$	$\dfrac{1}{\lambda + 2\pi ik}, \qquad \text{Re } \lambda > 0$

best to check the documentation of the particular numerical routines that you use. The $1/N$ normalization factor is required (somewhere) for Eq. (1.24) to hold, because:

$$\sum_{K=0}^{N-1} e^{\frac{-2\pi i K(J'-J)}{N}} = \begin{cases} N, & J = J' \\ 0, & \text{otherwise} \end{cases} \tag{1.25}$$

Although the DFT is typically evaluated numerically, it does have some useful analytical properties, which are summarized in Table 1.3.

1.1.5 IDENTIFYING PHYSICAL UNITS WITH THE DISCRETE FOURIER TRANSFORM OUTPUT

In the complex Fourier transform of Eq. (1.1), it is easy to identify physical units with x (e.g., cm) and k (e.g., cm^{-1}). With the DFT of Eq. (1.22), however, J and K are simply dimensionless integer indices. When we perform a DFT on a signal that has physical meaning, such as MRI data, how do we associate physical units with the string of numbers that is the output of the computer? Consider a one-dimensional MR signal $S(k)$, which can be reconstructed with an IFT:

$$I(x) = \int_{-\infty}^{+\infty} S(k)e^{+2\pi ikx}dk \tag{1.26}$$

TABLE 1.3
Discrete Fourier Transform Pairs

d_K	$\mathrm{DFT}[\{d\}]_J = D_J = \displaystyle\sum_{K=0}^{N-1} d_K e^{\frac{-2\pi i JK}{N}}$
$a d_K + b c_K$	$a D_J + b C_J$
$d_K e^{\frac{-2\pi i K a}{N}}$	D_{J+a}
d_{K-a}	$D_J e^{-\frac{2\pi i J a}{N}}$
$(-1)^K d_K$	$D_{J+\frac{N}{2}}$
1	$\dfrac{1 - e^{-2\pi i J}}{1 - e^{\frac{-2\pi i J}{N}}}$
$d_{K \pm N}$	D_J
d_{N-1-K}	$D_{-J} e^{\frac{2\pi i J}{N}}$

In order to see how Eq. (1.26) relates to the DFT, first approximate the continuous variables x and k with their discrete representations:

$$
\begin{aligned}
x_J &= J \Delta x \\
k_M &= M \Delta k
\end{aligned}
\tag{1.27}
$$

Approximating the integral by a discrete summation and substituting Eq. (1.27) into Eq. (1.26) yields:

$$
I(J \Delta x) = C \sum_{M=-\infty}^{\infty} S(k_M) e^{+2\pi i J M (\Delta k \Delta x)}
\tag{1.28}
$$

where the constant C is determined by the normalization conditions; that is, it is equivalent to a factor of Δk that converts the integral to a sum. The important point is, comparing the exponentials in Eqs. (1.23) and (1.28), we conclude that:

$$
\Delta x \Delta k = \frac{1}{N}
\tag{1.29}
$$

Equation (1.29) provides the link between the step sizes of the input and output of the DFT operation and the number of complex points in the data string. It is a very useful relationship for MRI. For example, it tells us that the product of the pixel size and the step size in k-space is equal to the inverse of the number of sampled points. Equation (1.29) can be rearranged as:

$$N \Delta k = \frac{1}{\Delta x} \tag{1.30}$$

which says that the total extent in k-space is equal to the inverse of the spatial pixel size. Similarly, the field of view is the inverse of the step size in k-space.

Example 1.1 Suppose 256 complex points are sampled for a total duration of 8.192 ms. An image is reconstructed with a 256-point DFT. Find the bandwidth, and express it in two common forms: bandwidth per pixel $\Delta \nu_{pp}$ and the half-bandwidth $\pm \Delta \nu$.

Answer Applying Eq. (1.30) with the time–frequency domain pairs, the total bandwidth is:

$$N \Delta \nu_{pp} = 2 \Delta \nu = \frac{1}{\Delta t} = \frac{256}{8.192 \text{ ms}} = 31.25 \text{ kHz} \tag{1.31}$$

Thus $\Delta \nu = \pm 15.625$ kHz. The bandwidth in units of hertz per pixel is:

$$\Delta \nu_{pp} = \frac{1}{N \Delta t} = \frac{1}{8.192 \text{ ms}} = 122 \text{ Hz/pixel}$$

1.1.6 PROPERTIES OF THE DISCRETE FOURIER TRANSFORM

Like the continuous FT, the DFT obeys a shift theorem as well. Similar to Eq. (1.16), multiplying the data by a linearly increasing phase ramp results in the shift:

$$D_{J+a} = \sum_{K=0}^{N-1} d_K e^{\frac{-2\pi i (J+a)K}{N}} = \sum_{K=0}^{N-1} \left(d_K e^{\frac{-2\pi i a K}{N}} \right) e^{\frac{-2\pi i J K}{N}} \tag{1.32}$$

A common case is called the *half field of view* or *Nyquist shift* (named after Harry Nyquist, 1889–1976, a Swedish-born American engineer). Setting $a = N/2$, Eq. (1.32) becomes:

$$D_{J+\frac{N}{2}} = \sum_{K=0}^{N-1} \left(d_K e^{-\pi i K} \right) e^{\frac{-2\pi i J K}{N}} = \sum_{K=0}^{N-1} \left[d_K (-1)^K \right] e^{\frac{-2\pi i J K}{N}} \tag{1.33}$$

The Nyquist shift is used when we want the DC component of the DFT to be centered, instead of occurring at the zeroth point. Because this is typically the case in MR images, the two-dimensional raw data are multiplied by a

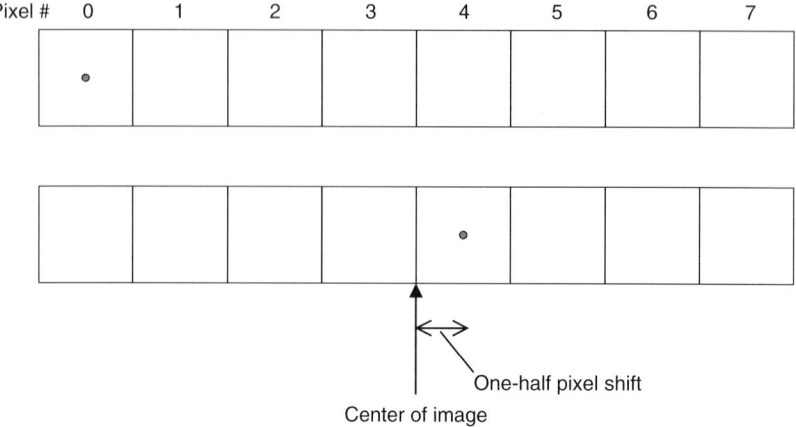

Pixel #   0   1   2   3   4   5   6   7

One-half pixel shift

Center of image

FIGURE 1.2 Demonstration of the one-half pixel shift that arises with the discrete FT. Here the DFT length is $N = 8$. The zero frequency, or DC, component of the DFT occupies the zeroth pixel, whose center is indicated with a dot. After a Nyquist shift, the DC signal occupies the fourth pixel. The center of the fourth pixel is shifted by one-half pixel compared to the image center.

checkerboard $[1, -1]$ pattern before reconstruction (see Section 13.1). Note that if N is an even integer and the $(-1)^K$ multiplier is used to center the DFT response, then the DC component will not be exactly centered but, rather, offset by one-half pixel. Figure 1.2 illustrates using an example with $N = 8$. The shift constant a in Eq. (1.32) need not necessarily be an integer, so shifts by fractions of a pixel can be accomplished with the appropriate linear phase ramp. This is sometimes used to correct the one-half pixel offset.

1.1.7 MULTIDIMENSIONAL DISCRETE FOURIER TRANSFORMS

The two-dimensional DFT can be defined as:

$$D_{JH} = \sum_{L=0}^{M-1} \sum_{K=0}^{N-1} d_{KL} e^{\frac{-2\pi i JK}{N}} e^{\frac{-2\pi i LH}{M}}, \quad J = 0, 1, 2, \ldots, N - 1,$$

$$H = 0, 1, 2, \ldots, M - 1$$

$$(1.34)$$

Three-dimensional (and higher) DFTs are defined analogously to Eq. (1.34). Note that the data input for the 2D-DFT is a rectilinear $N \times M$ matrix of complex numbers, d_{KL}. Because this matrix can be rearranged either as series of rows or columns, 2D-DFTs can be evaluated by performing either the row or column 1D-DFT first. Similarly, 3D (or higher dimensionality) DFTs can be evaluated by performing the 1D-DFTs in any order. This is a very useful property for partial Fourier reconstructions (Section 13.4), where it is necessary to perform the reconstruction along the partial Fourier direction last.

1.1.8 DISCRETENESS AND PERIODICITY

If the signal in one domain consists of discretely sampled points, then the FT (or IFT) in the other domain is *periodic*. In MRI, the signal is discretely sampled, so the image is periodic or consists of *replicates* that can lead to aliasing artifacts. (This is discussed in more detail in Section 11.1.)

To understand how this property of periodicity arises, consider the continuous signal $S(t)$, $-\infty < t < \infty$. In practice, the signal will be sampled over a finite time interval, $-T < t < T$. To represent the finite sampling interval, first we multiply the signal $S(t)$ by a rectangle (RECT) function, which is defined in Table 1.2 and which is zero for $|t| > T$. Next, the discreteness of the sampling process can be mathematically represented by multiplication by a sampling comb, which consists of a series of Dirac deltas (further described in Section 1.1.10). If the samples are separated in time by Δt, then the sampled signal becomes:

$$S'(t) = S(t)\text{RECT}\left(\frac{t}{T}\right) \sum_{n=-\infty}^{\infty} \delta(t - n\Delta t) \qquad (1.35)$$

According to the convolution theorem, the FT of product in Eq. (1.35) is the convolution of the FTs of the three factors. From Table 1.2, the FT of the RECT function is a sine x over x, or SINC function. Convolution with this factor gives rise to the shape of the point-spread function. The FT of the sampling comb is another series of deltas, this time spaced by $1/\Delta t$. Convolution with this comb gives rise to the periodic nature of the image. In order to avoid aliasing, the replicates must not overlap. This is accomplished by satisfying the *Nyquist criterion*—that is, the sampling rate $1/\Delta t$ must be at least twice the highest frequency contained in the signal. (These properties are further discussed in Section 11.1 on bandwidth and sampling.)

1.1.9 THE FAST FOURIER TRANSFORM

A modern MRI scanner must perform a large number of DFTs to reconstruct an image. Computational speed is an important issue. Consider the DFT from Eq. (1.22)

$$D_J = \sum_{K=0}^{N-1} d_K W_N^{JK}, \qquad J = 0, 1, 2, \ldots, N-1 \qquad (1.36)$$

where we have abbreviated the twiddle factor

$$W_N = e^{\frac{-2\pi i}{N}} \tag{1.37}$$

If the twiddle factors are precalculated and stored in a table of complex numbers, then it takes approximately N^2 complex multiplications to evaluate Eq. (1.36) for all values of J. The FFT algorithm reduces the number of operations and thereby increases the computational efficiency.

If N is even, then the signal can be split into two subsignals: its even-indexed elements and its odd-indexed elements. It can be shown that the DFT can be expressed as a linear combination of two half-length DFTs of the even- and odd-indexed signals. The total number of complex multiplications is then approximately $2(N/2)^2 = N^2/2$. If N is a power of 2 (1, 2, 4, 8, 16, 32, ...), then this process can be continued recursively all the way down to single-point DFTs. When the sub-FFTs are finally reassembled, the number of complex multiplications is on the order of $N \log_2 N$. For $N = 512 = 2^9$, this increases the speed by a factor of approximately $512/9 \approx 57$, which is very substantial. Clinical high-resolution MRI would not be feasible without the invention of the FFT.

Although 2 is by far the most common base, or *radix*, for the length of the FFT, some computational speed can be gained whenever N is not a prime number. Because of the wide availability and maximal computational efficiency of the radix-2 FFT, however, signals of arbitrary length are often extended to the next power of 2 by using zero filling (see Section 13.1.2) prior to reconstruction.

1.1.10 THE DIRAC DELTA AND NORMALIZATION OF THE FOURIER TRANSFORM

This section describes the Dirac delta function (named after Paul Adrien Maurice Dirac, 1902–1984, an English physicist and mathematician) and the normalization of the continuous FT. Those who are not interested in these mathematical properties can skip to the next section.

The Dirac delta function (Dirac 1957, 58–61) (or perhaps more properly the Dirac delta distribution) is zero everywhere except at the origin, yet has unit area:

$$\delta(x) = \begin{cases} 0 & \text{if } x \neq 0 \\ \int\limits_{-\infty}^{+\infty} \delta(x)\,dx = 1 \end{cases} \tag{1.38}$$

Thus, the $\delta(x)$ must not be finite at the origin. The Dirac delta has the property of picking out a single value of a function under multiplication and integration:

$$\int_{-\infty}^{+\infty} \delta(x - x') f(x) \, dx = f(x') \tag{1.39}$$

The normalization of continuous FTs, for example, Eqs. (1.1), (1.3), and (1.4), requires that:

$$g(x) = \int_{-\infty}^{+\infty} e^{2\pi ikx} \left[\int_{-\infty}^{+\infty} e^{-2\pi ikx'} g(x') \, dx' \right] dk \tag{1.40}$$

By rearranging Eq. (1.40):

$$g(x) = \int_{-\infty}^{+\infty} g(x') \, dx' \left[\int_{-\infty}^{+\infty} e^{2\pi ik(x-x')} dk \right] \tag{1.41}$$

and comparing this with Eq. (1.39), we conclude that the contents of the square brackets in Eq. (1.41) must be a representation of the Dirac delta:

$$\delta(x - x') = \int_{-\infty}^{+\infty} e^{2\pi ik(x-x')} dk \tag{1.42}$$

or, substituting $(x - x') = a$, and $2\pi k = u$:

$$\delta(a) = \frac{1}{2\pi} \int_{-\infty}^{+\infty} e^{iau} \, du \tag{1.43}$$

To show that Eq. (1.43) is true, it is useful to first state the result:

$$\int_{-\infty}^{+\infty} \frac{\sin u}{u} \, du = \pi \tag{1.44}$$

which can be demonstrated either with contour or numerical integration.

Then consider:

$$\int_{-\infty}^{+\infty} f(a) \left(\int_{-g}^{g} e^{iav} dv \right) da = \int_{-\infty}^{+\infty} f(a) \left[\frac{e^{iav}}{ia} \right]_{v=-g}^{g} da$$

$$= \int_{-\infty}^{+\infty} f(a) \frac{2 \sin ag}{ag} g \, da \qquad (1.45)$$

Letting $u = ag$, Eq. (1.45) becomes:

$$2 \int_{-\infty}^{+\infty} f\left(\frac{u}{g}\right) \frac{\sin u}{u} \, du \qquad (1.46)$$

Letting $g \rightarrow \infty$ and using the result from Eq. (1.44):

$$2 \int_{-\infty}^{+\infty} f\left(\frac{u}{g}\right) \frac{\sin u}{u} \, du \rightarrow 2f(0) \int_{-\infty}^{+\infty} \frac{\sin u}{u} \, du = 2\pi f(0) \qquad (1.47)$$

Combining Eqs. (1.45) and (1.47):

$$\int_{-\infty}^{+\infty} f(a) \left(\int_{-\infty}^{+\infty} e^{iau} du \right) da = 2\pi f(0) \qquad (1.48)$$

Thus, the integral of the complex exponential is a Dirac delta function. Specifically, Eq. (1.43) is verified, and the continuous FT and IFT pair of Eqs. (1.1) and (1.3) is properly normalized.

SELECTED REFERENCES

Bracewell, R. N. 1978. *The Fourier transform and its applications.* New York: McGraw-Hill.
Brigham, E. O. 1988. *The fast Fourier transform and its applications.* Englewood Cliffs, NJ: Prentice Hall.
Cooley, J. W., and Tukey, J. W. 1965. An algorithm for the machine calculation of complex Fourier series. *Mathematics of Computation* 19: 297–301.
Dirac, P. A. M. 1957. *The principles of quantum mechanics.* 4th ed. Oxford: Oxford, University Press.

RELATED SECTIONS

Section 11.1 Bandwidth and Sampling
Section 13.1 Fourier Reconstruction
Section 13.4 Partial Fourier Reconstruction

1.2 Rotating Reference Frame

The description of many physical quantities and processes requires a coordinate system, or *reference frame*. Depending on the choice of reference frame, the description of a physical process can be drastically different. For example, suppose a bicyclist is traveling east as viewed from a building's window. The same bicyclist will appear to be going west when viewed from a car traveling east at a higher speed. In this example, the building and the car are two different reference frames. They give entirely different descriptions of the same physical process.

Two reference frames, the *laboratory reference frame* and the *rotating reference frame*, are often employed to describe MRI phenomena. The laboratory reference frame is defined with respect to the scanner or the magnet. By convention, when discussing the rotating frame, the B_0-field direction is always chosen to be the z axis (also known as the *longitudinal axis*). (This is somewhat different from the definition of logical gradient axes in Section 7.3, in which z axis may or may not correspond to the B_0-field direction.) The x and y axes in the laboratory reference frame are selected as a pair of orthogonal vectors in a plane normal to the B_0-field (denoted by x' and y' in Figure 1.3a). In a horizontal magnet with a cylindrical bore, the y axis is usually chosen to be from floor to ceiling (or from down to up). When the z axis is pointing toward the viewer, the x axis is selected to be from left to right. These three axes conform to the right-hand rule, which states that if the fingers of the right hand are curled from the positive x axis to the positive y axis, the thumb points along the positive z axis. Such a coordinate system is called a *right-handed Cartesian coordinate system*, and the plane defined by the x and y axes is known as the *transverse plane*.

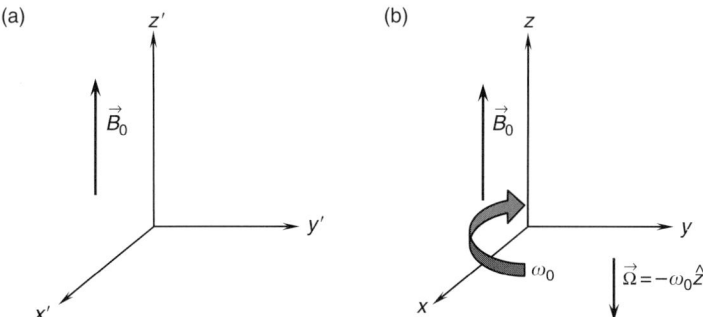

FIGURE 1.3 (a) The laboratory reference frame and (b) a rotating reference frame. These frames are related by a rotation about the z axis with an angular frequency ω_0.

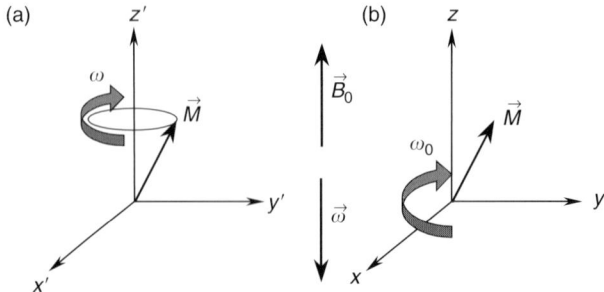

FIGURE 1.4 Spin precession as viewed from (a) the laboratory reference frame and (b) a rotating reference frame. The rotating reference frame slows down the precession. When the angular frequency of the rotating reference frame is equal to the spin precession frequency, the rotational motion of the spin is frozen. (Note that the angular frequency vector $\vec{\omega}$ follows the right-hand rule in the convention that we use.)

When the transverse plane of the laboratory reference frame rotates about the z axis with a nonzero angular frequency ω_0 (Figure 1.3b), a rotating reference frame results. Although ω_0 is usually a constant, it does not have to be.

The rotating reference frame greatly simplifies the description of many MRI phenomena. For example, in the laboratory reference frame, spins will precess about the magnetic field with their Larmor frequency ω (Figure 1.4a, named after Joseph Larmor, 1857–1942, an Irish physicist). In the reference frame rotating with the Larmor frequency, the precession of the spins appears stopped (Figure 1.4b). Using the rotating frame is analogous to stepping onto a moving merry-go-round. From that reference fram__, the rotation of the carousel also appears stopped. A mathematical description of this simplification is given in subsection 1.2.2. The concept of the rotating frame is widely used in analyzing and describing the precession and nutation of magnetization, the radiofrequency (RF) magnetic field (i.e., B_1 field), and, in particular, the interaction between spin systems and magnetic fields. Many examples can be found throughout this book (e.g., in Sections 3.1, 3.3, and 6.3).

1.2.1 MATHEMATICAL DESCRIPTION

Let x', y', and z' denote the three Cartesian axes in the laboratory reference frame, and x, y, and z denote the three axes in the corresponding rotating reference frame. Consider a time-dependent vector $\vec{p}(t)$ whose three components in the laboratory reference frame are $p_{x'}(t)$, $p_{y'}(t)$, and $p_{z'}(t)$, respectively:

$$\vec{p}'(t) = p_{x'}(t)\hat{x}' + p_{y'}(t)\hat{y}' + p_{z'}(t)\hat{z}' \tag{1.49}$$

(Recall that the symbol $^\wedge$ denotes a unit vector.) The same vector can also be expressed in the rotating reference frame:

$$\vec{p}(t) = p_x(t)\hat{x} + p_y(t)\hat{y} + p_z(t)\hat{z} \tag{1.50}$$

Because the reference frame rotates about the z axis, it can be readily seen that:

$$\hat{z}' = \hat{z} \tag{1.51}$$

The two sets of transverse axes are related to one another by a rotation:

$$x = x' \cos(\omega_0 t) - y' \sin(\omega_0 t) \tag{1.52}$$

$$y = x' \sin(\omega_0 t) + y' \cos(\omega_0 t) \tag{1.53}$$

where ω_0 is the angular frequency of the rotating frame.

In light of Eqs. (1.51–1.53), the three components of $\vec{p}(t)$ in the rotating frame are related to their laboratory-frame counterparts by:

$$\begin{bmatrix} p_x \\ p_y \\ p_z \end{bmatrix} = \begin{bmatrix} \cos \omega_0 t & -\sin \omega_0 t & 0 \\ \sin \omega_0 t & \cos \omega_0 t & 0 \\ 0 & 0 & 1 \end{bmatrix} \begin{bmatrix} p_{x'} \\ p_{y'} \\ p_{z'} \end{bmatrix} = \Re\,\vec{p}' \tag{1.54}$$

where $\Re$ is a rotation matrix. If the components in the rotating reference frame are known, the components in the laboratory frame can be determined from:

$$\begin{bmatrix} p_{x'} \\ p_{y'} \\ p_{z'} \end{bmatrix} = \begin{bmatrix} \cos \omega_0 t & \sin \omega_0 t & 0 \\ -\sin \omega_0 t & \cos \omega_0 t & 0 \\ 0 & 0 & 1 \end{bmatrix} \begin{bmatrix} p_x \\ p_y \\ p_z \end{bmatrix} = \Re^{-1}\vec{p} = \Re^T\vec{p} \tag{1.55}$$

where the inverse of the rotation matrix $\Re^{-1}$ equals its transpose $\Re^T$.

A useful relation between the rates of change of a vector in the two reference frames can be derived (Slichter 1989) by taking the time derivative of Eq. (1.49):

$$\left(\frac{d\vec{p}(t)}{dt}\right)_{\text{lab}} = \left(\frac{d\vec{p}(t)}{dt}\right)_{\text{rot}} + \vec{\Omega} \times \vec{p}(t) \tag{1.56}$$

$$\vec{\Omega} = -\omega_0\hat{z} \tag{1.57}$$

where, subscripts lab and rot represent laboratory and rotating reference frames, respectively, and $\vec{\Omega}$ is a rotational angular velocity vector. For a clockwise-rotating reference frame (as viewed from the positive z axis), $\vec{\Omega}$ points to the negative z axis as indicated in Eq. (1.57) and Figure 1.4. ($\vec{\Omega}$ follows a right-hand rule: If the fingers of the right hand curl in the direction of the rotation of the rotating frame, then the thumb points along $\vec{\Omega}$.) The relationships given by Eqs. (1.54) and (1.56) are often used to simplify the descriptions of MRI phenomena, some of which are detailed in the following subsection.

1.2.2 SIMPLIfiCATIONS PROVIDED BY THE ROTATING FRAME

Description of Spin Precession   Consider a group of spins precessing with the same phase in a static magnetic field B_0. The net magnetization of the spins, $\vec{M}$, will precess about the magnetic field direction (i.e., the z axis) with a Larmor frequency $\omega = \gamma B_0$ (where γ is the gyromagnetic ratio). In the laboratory reference frame, this rotational motion can be mathematically described by:

$$\left(\frac{d\vec{M}}{dt}\right)_{\text{lab}} = \vec{M} \times (\omega\hat{z}) \tag{1.58}$$

According to Eqs. (1.56) and (1.57), the rate of change of $\vec{M}$ in the rotating reference frame is:

$$\left(\frac{d\vec{M}}{dt}\right)_{\text{rot}} = \left(\frac{d\vec{M}}{dt}\right)_{\text{lab}} - \vec{\Omega} \times \vec{M} = (\omega - \omega_0)\vec{M} \times \hat{z} \tag{1.59}$$

(Note that we have used $\vec{\Omega} \times \vec{M} = -\vec{M} \times \vec{\Omega}$ to derive Eq. (1.59).) If we choose the angular frequency of the rotating frame to be equal to the Larmor frequency (i.e., $\omega_0 = \omega$), then the magnetization becomes a *stationary* vector, that is, $(d\vec{M}/dt)_{\text{rot}} = 0$. This example illustrates how the rotating reference frame simplifies the description of spin precession.

Radiofrequency Magnetic Field   In order to produce transverse magnetization that generates the MRI signal, a component of the RF magnetic field must be in the transverse plane. Suppose that the RF magnetic field $\vec{B}_1(t)$ is initially applied along the x axis and has a frequency of ω_{rf} (also known as the carrier frequency). In the laboratory frame, a *circularly polarized*, or *quadrature*, B_1 field can be expressed as:

$$\vec{B}_1(t) = \hat{x}' B_1(t) \cos \omega_{\text{rf}} t - \hat{y}' B_1(t) \sin \omega_{\text{rf}} t \tag{1.60}$$

Using Eq. (1.54), we can readily transform this B_1 field to the rotating frame:

$$\begin{bmatrix} B_{1,x}(t) \\ B_{1,y}(t) \\ B_{1,z}(t) \end{bmatrix}_{\text{rot}} = \begin{bmatrix} \cos \omega_0 t & -\sin \omega_0 t & 0 \\ \sin \omega_0 t & \cos \omega_0 t & 0 \\ 0 & 0 & 1 \end{bmatrix} \begin{bmatrix} B_1(t) \cos \omega_{\text{rf}} t \\ -B_1(t) \sin \omega_{\text{rf}} t \\ 0 \end{bmatrix} \tag{1.61}$$

If we set the rotating frame angular frequency ω_0 to be equal to the carrier frequency ω_{rf}, Eq. (1.61) then becomes:

$$\begin{bmatrix} B_{1,x}(t) \\ B_{1,y}(t) \\ B_{1,z}(t) \end{bmatrix}_{rot} = \begin{bmatrix} B_1(t) \\ 0 \\ 0 \end{bmatrix} \tag{1.62}$$

Clearly, the rotating frame has demodulated the RF oscillation and transformed the rapidly oscillating RF field into a much simpler form—the time-dependent envelope $B_1(t)$. This simplification is widely used in analyzing RF pulses throughout Part II of this book (see examples in Sections 3.1, 6.1, and 6.3).

Two-Dimensional Vectors and Their Complex Representation   Often two-dimensional vectors given by Eq. (1.63) are used to describe quantities in the transverse plane, such as the B_1 field or the magnetization. A two-dimensional vector precessing with an angular frequency ω can be expressed as:

$$\vec{p}(t) = \vec{p}_x(t) + \vec{p}_y(t)$$
$$= \hat{x}\, p(t)\, \cos \omega t - \hat{y}\, p(t)\, \sin \omega t \tag{1.63}$$

If the following identifications are made:

$$\hat{x} \Leftrightarrow 1, \qquad \hat{y} \Leftrightarrow i = \sqrt{-1} \tag{1.64}$$

then the two-dimensional vector $\vec{p}(t)$ in Eq. (1.63) is equivalent to a complex variable $p_c(t)$ given by:

$$p_c(t) = p(t) \cos \omega t - i p(t) \sin \omega t = p(t) e^{-i\omega t} \tag{1.65}$$

Equation (1.65) is called the *complex representation* of the two-dimensional vector $\vec{p}$. This representation is particularly convenient to work with because of properties of the complex exponential. For example, a straightforward multiplication can translate a vector from the laboratory frame to the rotating frame:

$$[p(t) e^{-i\omega t}]_{rot} = p(t) e^{-i\omega t} e^{i\omega_0 t} = p(t) e^{-i(\omega - \omega_0)t} \tag{1.66}$$

We can use this relationship to rederive the results in the earlier part of subsection 1.2.2 with a greater simplicity.

The complex representation is a natural way to describe the precessing transverse magnetization. The MRI signals induced by the precessing transverse magnetization are also often expressed in the complex form and simplified using Eq. (1.66). An example is provided in the following subsection.

The Bloch Equations The Bloch equations (1.67), named after Felix Bloch 1905–1983, a Swiss born American physicist, relate the time evolution of magnetization to the external magnetic fields, the relaxation times (T_1 and T_2), the molecular self-diffusion coefficient (D), and other parameters (Slichter 1989; Torrey 1956).

$$\frac{d\vec{M}}{dt} = \gamma \vec{M} \times \vec{B} - \frac{M_x \hat{x} + M_y \hat{y}}{T_2} + \frac{(M_0 - M_z)\hat{z}}{T_1} + D\nabla^2 \vec{M} \qquad (1.67)$$

If we apply a static B_0 field and the RF B_1 field given by Eq. (1.60) to a spin system, then the overall magnetic field becomes:

$$\vec{B} = \hat{x}\, B_1(t) \cos \omega_{rf} t - \hat{y}\, B_1(t) \sin \omega_{rf} t + \hat{z} B_0 \qquad (1.68)$$

Let us ignore the relaxation and diffusion processes for now. Then, Eq. (1.67) reduces to:

$$\frac{d\vec{M}}{dt} = \gamma \vec{M} \times (\hat{x}\, B_1(t) \cos \omega_{rf} t - \hat{y}\, B_1(t) \sin \omega_{rf} t + \hat{z} B_0) \qquad (1.69)$$

Next, we convert Eq. (1.69) from the laboratory reference frame into a rotating reference frame. Applying Eq. (1.56) to Eq. (1.69), we obtain:

$$\left(\frac{d\vec{M}}{dt}\right)_{rot} = \left(\frac{d\vec{M}}{dt}\right)_{lab} - \vec{\Omega} \times \vec{M} = \gamma \vec{M} \times \left(\hat{x}\, B_1(t) \cos \omega_{rf} t \right.$$

$$\left. - \hat{y}\, B_1(t) \sin \omega_{rf} t + \hat{z} B_0 + \frac{\vec{\Omega}}{\gamma} \right) \qquad (1.70)$$

This conversion, however, is not yet complete because the B_1 field is still in the laboratory frame. The components of the B_1 field in the rotating frame can be obtained from Eq. (1.61):

$$\begin{cases} B_{1,x,rot}(t) = B_1(t)(\cos \omega_0 t \cos \omega_{rf} t + \sin \omega_0 t \sin \omega_{rf} t) = B_1(t) \cos(\omega_0 - \omega_{rf})t \\ B_{1,y,rot}(t) = B_1(t)(\sin \omega_0 t \cos \omega_{rf} t - \cos \omega_0 t \sin \omega_{rf} t) = B_1(t) \sin(\omega_0 - \omega_{rf})t \\ B_{1,z,rot}(t) = 0 \end{cases}$$

$$(1.71)$$

Incorporating the B_1 field of Eq. (1.71) into Eq. (1.70) and explicitly expressing $\vec{\Omega}$ using Eq. (1.57), the rotating reference frame Bloch equation is derived:

$$\left(\frac{d\vec{M}}{dt}\right)_{rot} = \gamma \vec{M} \times \left[B_1(t)(\hat{x} \cos(\omega_{rf} - \omega_0)t - \hat{y} \sin(\omega_{rf} - \omega_0)t) + \hat{z}\left(B_0 - \frac{\omega_0}{\gamma} \right) \right]$$

$$(1.72)$$

The magnetic field in the square brackets is known as the *effective field*, $\vec{B}_{\text{eff}}$:

$$\vec{B}_{\text{eff}} = B_1(t)(\hat{x}\cos(\omega_{\text{rf}} - \omega_0)t - \hat{y}\sin(\omega_{\text{rf}} - \omega_0)t) + \hat{z}\left(B_0 - \frac{\omega_0}{\gamma}\right) \quad (1.73)$$

In the rotating reference frame, the magnetization always precesses about $\vec{B}_{\text{eff}}$. A special scenario occurs at resonance (i.e., $\omega = \omega_{\text{rf}} = \omega_0$), where the effective field reduces to $\hat{x}B_1(t)$ and the magnetization precesses about the applied B_1 field, as if there were no static magnetic field B_0 present. The concept of effective field is frequently used to describe the interactions between RF pulses and the spin systems (see, for example, Sections 6.1 and 6.2).

Equation (1.72) can be equivalently expressed as three scalar equations after explicitly carrying out the vector cross product:

$$\left(\frac{dM_x}{dt}\right)_{\text{rot}} = \gamma M_y\left(B_0 - \frac{\omega_0}{\gamma}\right) + \gamma M_z B_1(t)\sin(\omega_{\text{rf}} - \omega_0)t \quad (1.74)$$

$$\left(\frac{dM_y}{dt}\right)_{\text{rot}} = -\gamma M_x\left(B_0 - \frac{\omega_0}{\gamma}\right) + \gamma M_z B_1(t)\cos(\omega_{\text{rf}} - \omega_0)t \quad (1.75)$$

$$\left(\frac{dM_z}{dt}\right)_{\text{rot}} = -\gamma M_x B_1(t)\sin(\omega_{\text{rf}} - \omega_0)t - \gamma M_y B_1(t)\cos(\omega_{\text{rf}} - \omega_0)t$$

$$(1.76)$$

Let us define a complex quantity to represent the vector component of the magnetization in the transverse plane:

$$M_+ = M_x + iM_y \quad (1.77)$$

Using this complex quantity, we can derive Eq. (1.78) by multiplying Eq. (1.75) by i and adding the result to Eq. (1.74):

$$\left(\frac{dM_+}{dt}\right)_{\text{rot}} = -i\gamma M_+\left(B_0 - \frac{\omega_0}{\gamma}\right) + i\gamma M_z B_1(t)e^{-i(\omega_{\text{rf}} - \omega_0)t} \quad (1.78)$$

Equation (1.78) is particularly useful in solving for the transverse magnetization after an RF excitation pulse (see Section 3.1).

Finally, let us consider two special cases. In the first case, we set the rotating frame frequency to be identical to the carrier frequency of the RF field (i.e., $\omega_0 = \omega_{\text{rf}}$). Thus, Eq. (1.72) becomes:

$$\left(\frac{d\vec{M}}{dt}\right)_{\text{rot}} = \gamma\vec{M}\times\left[\hat{x}B_1(t) + \hat{z}\left(B_0 - \frac{\omega_{\text{rf}}}{\gamma}\right)\right] \quad (1.79)$$

This reference frame is sometimes referred to as the *RF reference frame* or B_1 *reference frame* because the B_1 field is stationary in this frame. Note that the B_1 field lies along the x axis because we have chosen a specific initial condition for $t = 0$, as implied by Eq. (1.60). In general, the $\hat{x} B_1$ term can be replaced by $(\hat{x} \cos \alpha + \hat{y} \sin \alpha) B_1$, where α is the angle between the initial B_1 vector and the x axis. Equation (1.79) shows that in a rotating reference frame with $\omega_0 = \omega_{rf}$, the B_1 field is demodulated and the main magnetic field is effectively reduced by ω_{rf}/γ. At resonance (i.e., $\omega_{rf} = \gamma B_0$), the z component of the effective magnetic field disappears and the magnetization will precess about the B_1 field.

In the second case, we can set the rotating frame frequency equal to the Larmor frequency (i.e., $\omega_0 = \omega$). Thus, Eq. (1.72) becomes:

$$\left(\frac{d\vec{M}}{dt}\right)_{rot} = \gamma \vec{M} \times [B_1(t)(\hat{x} \cos(\omega_{rf} - \omega)t - \hat{y} \sin(\omega_{rf} - \omega)t)] \quad (1.80)$$

This reference frame is known as the *Larmor reference frame* or B_0 *reference frame* because the B_0 field disappears in this reference frame. If we keep the RF field at a fixed frequency and sweep the B_0 field (i.e., changing ω), resonance can also occur when $\omega = \omega_0 = \omega_{rf}$.

SELECTED REFERENCES

Slichter, C. P. 1989. *Principles of magnetic resonance*. Berlin: Springer-Verlag.
Torrey, H. C. 1956. Bloch equations with diffusion terms. *Physical Review* 104: 563.

RELATED SECTIONS

Section 3.1 Excitation Pulses
Section 3.2 Inversion Pulses
Section 3.3 Refocusing Pulses
Section 4.1 Composite Pulses
Section 4.3 Spectrally Selective Pulses
Section 6.1 Adiabatic Excitation Pulses
Section 6.2 Adiabatic Inversion Pulses
Section 6.3 Adiabatic Refocusing Pulses

RADIOFREQUENCY PULSES

Introduction

Part II of this book describes radiofrequency (RF) pulses. Chapter 2 focuses on several commonly used RF pulse shapes including hard pulses (Section 2.1), SINC pulses (Section 2.2), and a family of tailored pulses generated with the Shinnar–Le Roux (SLR) algorithm (Section 2.3). The SLR section is more mathematically involved than many others in the book, and that section can be skipped unless the reader has a special interest in this topic. Some of the theoretical results from Section 2.3, however, have wider practical significance and reappear in other sections of Part II. For example, SLR analysis can be used to explain when and how an excitation pulse also can be used for refocusing. A discussion of variable-rate pulses (Section 2.4) completes Chapter 2. Variable rate is not a specific pulse shape but rather a method to modify the shape of any spatially selective RF pulse in order to reduce its RF power deposition. In addition to the basic pulse shapes covered in Chapter 2, other pulse shapes are used in MRI and several less commonly used pulse shapes are discussed in the other sections of the book (for example, a discussion of Gaussian and Fermi pulse shapes is provided in Section 4.2).

Chapter 3 discusses three basic RF pulse functions: excitation (Section 3.1), inversion (Section 3.2), and refocusing (Section 3.3) of the magnetization. These sections describe nonadiabatic RF pulses; the adiabatic pulses performing these same three functions are the focus of Chapter 6. The slice profile and nonlinearity of the Bloch equations are explored in Section 3.1; Section 3.3 introduces the formation of RF spin echoes. The relationship among the three RF pulse functions is explored in both Sections 3.2 and 3.3. All the sections in Chapter 3 examine the effect of spins being off-resonance on their respective functions.

Spectrally selective RF pulses (i.e., pulses that are played without a concurrent slice-selection gradient and affect spins only within a specific frequency range) are discussed in Chapter 4. Composite pulses (Section 4.1) are more widely used in magnetic resonance (MR) spectroscopy, but have found application to imaging as well. Magnetization transfer pulses (Section 4.2) are mainly used in 3D time-of-flight MR angiography. A general discussion of spectrally selective pulses is given in Section 4.3, which includes a discussion of lipid suppression with spectrally selective excitation and saturation, widely used in imaging applications.

Spatially selective RF pulses are the topic of Chapter 5. This chapter covers a number of RF pulses that are played along with a gradient pulse to affect the magnetization in a spatially dependent fashion. The pulses included in this chapter are multidimensional pulses (Section 5.1), ramp pulses, also known as tilted optimized non saturating excitation (TONE) pulses (Section 5.2); spatial saturation pulses (Section 5.3); spatial-spectral pulses (Section 5.4); and spatial tagging pulses (Section 5.5). Multidimensional pulses are selective in more than one spatial direction. Ramp pulses intentionally yield a nonuniform spatial profile and are used for MR angiography. Spatial saturation pulses attenuate signal from specified regions and are widely used in imaging applications to suppress artifacts from aliasing, flow, and motion. Spatial-spectral (SPSP) pulses are simultaneously selective in one spatial and the spectral dimension. (The placement of the spatial-spectral section in Chapter 5 rather than in Chapter 4 is somewhat arbitrary). The chapter concludes with a discussion of spatial tagging pulses, which are used to prepare the longitudinal magnetization with a set of stripes or grids prior to an imaging sequence. Unlike the other pulses described in Chapter 5, tagging pulses are not necessarily played with a concurrent slice-selection gradient but rather can be interleaved with a gradient pulse.

Chapter 6 revisits the basic RF pulse functions of excitation (Section 6.1), inversion (Section 6.2), and refocusing (Section 6.3) using adiabatic pulses. Adiabatic pulses are insensitive to variations in B_1-amplitude as long as a minimum amplitude threshold is met. These pulses are governed by a specific set of rules, known collectively as the adiabatic condition, discussed in Section 6.1. As such, the properties of adiabatic pulses and their interaction with the magnetization are quite different from their nonadiabatic counterparts. In clinical MR imaging, perhaps the most widely used adiabatic pulse is the hyperbolic secant inversion pulse, which is described in Section 6.2. That pulse can be made spatially selective by applying a concurrent slice-selection gradient. Other adiabatic pulses are less frequently used in imaging, mainly because of lack of robustness in spatial selectivity. They are quite useful in localized spectroscopy, however, especially when RF power deposition is not problematic.

It should be noted that the classification of RF pulses in Chapters 2–6 is somewhat arbitrary. The placement of a pulse in a particular category does not preclude it from belonging in other categories as well. For example, a SINC pulse can be used as spatial saturation pulse, a spectrally selective pulse, an excitation pulse, an inversion pulse, or a refocusing pulse. Thus, Chapters 3–6 focus on the general properties of any RF pulse used for that function rather than concentrating on specific pulse shapes.

Several physical quantities are used repeatedly throughout Part II to characterize RF pulses. The *RF envelope*, which we denote by $B_1(t)$ or $A(t)$, is typically measured in microteslas. The RF envelope is a (relatively) slowly varying function of time, with at most a few zero-crossings per millisecond. The RF pulse played at the physical RF coil is a sinusoidal *carrier* waveform that is modulated (i.e., multiplied) by the RF envelope. The RF carrier varies much more rapidly than the RF envelope; its frequency is typically set equal to Larmor frequency (e.g. 63.85 MHz at 1.5 T), plus (or minus) the frequency offset δf required for the desired slice location, as described in Section 4.3. (For spectrally selective pulses, the chemical shift rather than the spatial offset determines the carrier frequency, as described in Section 4.3.)

The duration of the RF pulse is called the *pulse width* (T) and is typically measured in seconds or milliseconds. The RF *bandwidth* Δf, specified in hertz or kilohertz, is a measure of the frequency content of the pulse and is typically given by the full width at half maximum (FWHM) of the frequency profile (Section 4.3). (Note that the RF bandwidth Δf differs from the receiver bandwidth Δv discussed in Section 11.1, and from the carrier frequency offset δf). The dimensionless *time-bandwidth product* $T \Delta f$ is a measure of the selectivity of the pulse and is determined by the pulse shape.

Another parameter that is commonly used to describe an RF pulse is its *flip angle* θ. The flip angle is measured in radians or degrees and describes the nutation angle produced by the pulse. For example, an excitation pulse that tips the longitudinal magnetization completely into the transverse plane has a flip angle of $90°$, or $\pi/2$ rad. As shown in Section 3.1, the flip angle (on-resonance) can be calculated by finding the area underneath the envelope of the RF pulse. This calculation, however, is not valid for adiabatic pulses.

RF pulses deposit RF energy that can cause unwanted heating of the patient. This heating is measured by the *specific absorption rate* (SAR) (in watts per kilogram). Clinical MRI scanners operate under regulatory guidelines for the maximal amount of SAR that can be deposited. In the United States, the Food and Drug Administration specifies nonsignificant risk guidelines for the maximal amount of SAR that can be deposited into the patient's head, whole body, torso, or extremities. Although typically the exact amount of SAR deposited must be empirically calibrated, several convenient scaling relationships exist. For example, in the clinical range of field strengths ($B_0 = 0.2$–3.0 T) SAR is proportional to the square of the Larmor frequency or, equivalently, the square of B_0. As discussed in Section 2.4, SAR is also proportional to the square of the B_1-amplitude. Thus, for a nonadiabatic pulse, the SAR is proportional to the flip angle squared, θ^2. Holding other parameters (i.e., the flip angle and pulse width) fixed, SAR is linearly proportional to the RF bandwidth. To summarize the scaling relationships:

$$\text{SAR} \propto B_0^2 \theta^2 \Delta f$$

It is interesting to note that in MRI, unlike computed tomography, the spatial distribution of the dose (i.e., the SAR) is not concentrated near the selected slice. Instead in MRI the deposited energy covers the entire sensitive region of the RF transmit coil. This is because the energy involved in tipping the spins is negligible compared to the energy dissipated as heat, which is nearly the same whether or not the spins are on-resonance. For a more complete discussion of SAR, the reader is referred to Bottomley et al. (1985).

SELECTED REFERENCES

Bottomley, P. A., Redington, R. W., Edelstein, W. A., and Schenck, J. F. 1985. Estimating radiofrequency power deposition in body NMR imaging. *Magn. Reson. Med.* 2: 336–349.

2

RADIOFREQUENCY PULSE SHAPES

2.1 Rectangular Pulses

A rectangular or hard pulse is simply a pulse shaped like a RECT function in the time domain (Figure 2.1). (In contrast, pulses that are time-varying or shaped are sometimes called soft pulses.) Hard pulses can be used when no spatial or spectral selection is required and are convenient because the pulse length can be very short. Like a spectrally selective pulse, a hard pulse is played without a concurrent gradient. The bandwidth of a hard pulse, however, is broad enough so that spins with a wide range of resonant frequencies are affected.

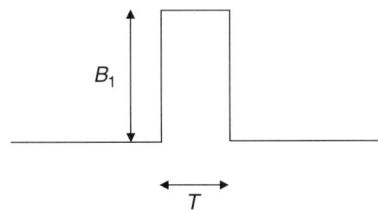

FIGURE 2.1 A rectangular or hard RF pulse.

In the small flip angle approximation, the frequency profile corresponding to a hard pulse is a SINC. Because the first zero-crossing of a SINC is the inverse of the corresponding RECT width, the narrow pulse width means that a hard pulse flips spins over a very wide bandwidth. The flip angle θ of a hard pulse is directly proportional to the amplitude (B_1) and the width (T) of the pulse:

$$\theta = \gamma B_1 T \tag{2.1}$$

Example 2.1 A commercial MR scanner generates a maximum B_1 field of $30\,\mu T$. What is the length T of a hard pulse that gives a 90° flip angle?

Answer

$$T = \frac{\pi/2}{\gamma B_1} = \frac{\pi/2}{(2\pi \times 42.57\,\text{MHz/T})(30\,\mu T)} = 1.96 \times 10^{-4}\,\text{s} = 196\,\mu s$$

2.1.1 RECTANGULAR PULSE USES

Because most imaging pulse sequences require RF pulses with spectral or spatial selectivity, hard pulses are very infrequently used. One exception is 3D acquisitions (Section 11.6), in which sometimes the imaging volume is sufficiently large to cover the entire sensitive region of the coil. Hard pulses can be grouped together to form composite pulses that are spectrally selective (see Section 4.1). Hard pulses are also used for magnetization transfer, but even there a small amount of windowing may be applied to the pulse (see Section 4.2), for example, to form a Fermi pulse. Hard pulses are also used in combination with gradients to create tagging pulses (see Section 5.5).

One problem with implementing a hard pulse is that it may be played with poor fidelity by some RF amplifiers because of the waveform discontinuities. In this case, a windowed hard pulse, such as a half-sine pulse, usually works better. Another option is to play a trapezoidal RF waveform. Table 2.1 lists some properties of rectangular and related pulse shapes. Hard pulses must have sufficiently high bandwidth (i.e., sufficiently short temporal duration) so that all the frequencies of interest are excited. From Table 2.1, we see that when the hard pulse duration is 100–500 μs, bandwidths on the order of 2–10 kHz result, which easily cover the range of resonant frequencies encountered in most imaging volumes in the absence of a gradient.

RELATED SECTIONS

Section 4.1 Composite Pulses
Section 4.2 Magnetization Transfer Pulses
Section 5.5 Tagging Pulses

TABLE 2.1
Properties of Rectangular Pulses and Related Pulse Shapes

Pulse Shape[a]	Fourier Transform	FWHM[b]
$\text{RECT}\left(\frac{t}{T/2}\right)$ $= \begin{cases} 1 & \text{if } \|t\| < \frac{T}{2} \\ 0 & \text{if } \|t\| > \frac{T}{2} \end{cases}$	$T\,\text{SINC}(\pi f T)$	$\frac{1.21}{T}$
$\text{HS}(t) = \cos\left(\frac{\pi t}{T}\right)\text{RECT}\left(\frac{t}{T/2}\right)$	$\frac{T}{2}\text{SINC}\left(\pi f T + \frac{\pi}{2}\right)$ $+ \frac{T}{2}\text{SINC}\left(\pi f T - \frac{\pi}{2}\right)$	$\frac{1.64}{T}$
$\text{TRAP}(t)$ $= \begin{cases} 0 & \text{if } \|t\| > \frac{T}{2} \\ \frac{(T/2+t)}{r} & \text{if } -\frac{T}{2} \le t \le -\frac{T}{2}+r \\ 1 & \text{if } -\frac{T}{2}+r < t < \frac{T}{2}-r \\ \frac{(T/2-t)}{r} & \text{if } \frac{T}{2}-r \le t \le \frac{T}{2} \end{cases}$	$\begin{array}{c}(T-r)\\ \times\text{SINC}\,(\pi f(T-r))\\ \text{SINC}\,(\pi f r)\end{array}$	$\frac{1.21}{T}\quad(r=0)$ $\frac{1.77}{T}\quad\left(r=\frac{T}{2}\right)$

[a] HS(t) is a half-sine pulse. TRAP(t) is a trapezoidal pulse with ramp time r and total width T.
[b] FWHM is the full width at half maximum in the frequency domain under the small flip angle approximation.

2.2 SINC Pulses

SINC pulses (Runge et al. 1988; MacFall et al. 1990) have been widely used for selective excitation, saturation, and refocusing. A SINC pulse consists of several adjacent lobes of alternating polarity. The central lobe has the highest amplitude and is also twice as wide as every other lobe. The amplitude of the lobes progressively decreases on either side of the central lobe, as their polarity alternates.

Under the conditions described in Section 3.1, the frequency profile produced by an RF excitation pulse is well approximated by the Fourier transform of its RF envelope. (The shapes of the frequency and slice profiles are equivalent when a slice-selection gradient is played during the RF pulse.) The Fourier transform of an infinitely long SINC pulse is the RECT function (see Chapter 1, Table 1.1); that is, it has the top-hat shape of the ideal slice profile. Consequently SINC pulses have been natural choices when a uniform slice profile is desired. A SINC pulse that can be generated in practice has a finite duration and is obtained by truncating all but the central lobe and a few of its neighbors, or side lobes. In general, the greater the number of lobes that are included in the SINC pulse, the better the approximation to the ideal frequency profile.

Adding more lobes increases the duration of the pulse. This can lead to a number of adverse effects, such as prolonging the minimum echo time (TE) and repetition time (TR) of the pulse sequence and increasing the sensitivity to flow and off-resonance effects. An apodizing window is usually applied to the SINC pulse to ease the effects caused by truncation and to smooth its slice profile.

An asymmetric or truncated SINC pulse (MacFall et al. 1990) is implemented by retaining an unequal number of side lobes to the left and to the right of the central lobe. Retaining fewer lobes to the right can be used to reduce the minimum TE.

On commercial MR scanners, tailored pulses, designed with methods such as the SLR algorithm (Section 2.3) have replaced many SINC pulses. For example, for a fixed product of the pulse duration and bandwidth (i.e., the dimensionless time-bandwidth product $T \Delta f$) minimum phase SLR pulses can generally produce a more desirable slice profile than an asymmetric SINC pulse. Still, SINC pulses, especially symmetric ones, are simple to implement and remain popular, especially for excitation with small flip angles.

2.2.1 MATHEMATICAL DESCRIPTION

SINC Formula   The time dependence of the RF envelope of a SINC pulse (without windowing) is given by:

$$B_1(t) = \begin{cases} A \text{ SINC} \left(\dfrac{\pi t}{t_0} \right) \equiv A t_0 \dfrac{\sin \left(\dfrac{\pi t}{t_0} \right)}{\pi t} & -N_L t_0 \leq t \leq N_R t_0 \quad (2.2) \\ 0 & \text{elsewhere} \end{cases}$$

where A is the peak RF amplitude occurring at $t = 0$, t_0 is one-half the width of the central lobe (which is equal to the full width of each side lobe), and N_L and N_R are the number of zero-crossings in the SINC pulse to the left and right of the central peak, respectively. If $N_L = N_R$, the SINC pulse is symmetric. To a good approximation, the bandwidth of the SINC pulse (FWHM of the slice profile) is given by:

$$\Delta f \approx \frac{1}{t_0} \tag{2.3}$$

The precise value of the bandwidth can be determined with Bloch equation analysis; some examples are given in Table 2.2. According to Eqs. (2.2) and (2.3), the dimensionless time-bandwidth product of a SINC pulse is given by:

$$T \Delta f = N_L + N_R \tag{2.4}$$

The time-bandwidth product of a SINC pulse also equals the number of zero-crossings of the RF envelope, including the start and end (i.e., the margins) of the pulse. Because, in practice, N_L and N_R are both finite (e.g., typically 1 to 4), the SINC pulse has a discontinuous first derivative at $N_L t_0$ and $N_R t_0$, which can lead to unwanted ringing in the slice profile. For a symmetric SINC with $N_L = N_R = N$, the discontinuity in the first derivative at the margins of the pulse is given by:

$$\left. \left| \frac{dB_1(t)}{dt} \right| \right|_{t=\pm N t_0} = \begin{cases} \dfrac{A}{N t_0} & \text{when } |t| \rightarrow (N t_0)_+ \\ 0 & \text{when } |t| \rightarrow (N t_0)_- \end{cases} \tag{2.5}$$

The problem of the discontinuous first derivative can be addressed by apodizing the SINC pulse. The apodization window gently tapers the RF amplitude, especially at the start and end of the pulse. Common apodization functions include the Hamming and Hanning windows. SINC pulses apodized by these windows are described by:

$$B_1(t) = \begin{cases} A t_0 \left[(1 - \alpha) + \alpha \cos\left(\dfrac{\pi t}{N t_0} \right) \right] \dfrac{\sin\left(\dfrac{\pi t}{t_0} \right)}{\pi t} & -N_L t_0 \leq t \leq N_R t_0 \\ 0 & \text{elsewhere} \end{cases} \tag{2.6}$$

where N is the larger of N_L and N_R. Setting the parameter $\alpha = 0.5$ yields the Hanning window, and setting $\alpha = 0.46$ yields the Hamming window. Equation (2.6) reduces to the unapodized SINC of Eq. (2.2) when $\alpha = 0$. The Hanning window ensures a continuous first derivative for a symmetric SINC, whereas the Hamming window reduces the first derivative at the margins of the symmetric pulse by a factor of 12.5. Figure 2.2 shows an $N = 2$ symmetric

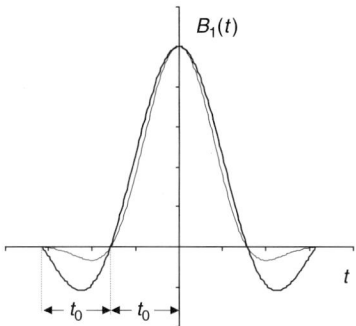

FIGURE 2.2 A symmetric $N = 2$ SINC pulse. The bold line shows the pulse without apodization; the thin line shows the pulse apodized with a Hamming window. The width of the central lobe is $2 \times t_0$, and the width of all the side lobes is t_0.

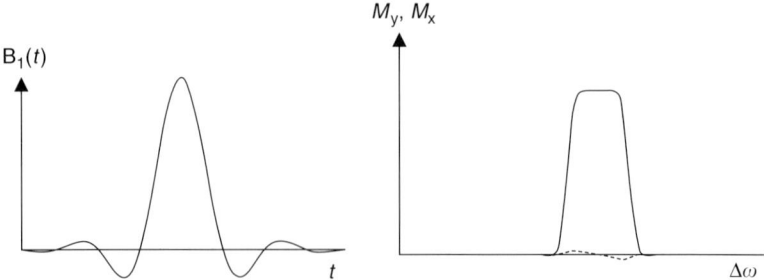

FIGURE 2.3 An $N = 4$ symmetric SINC pulse apodized with a Hamming window and the resultant frequency profile at a flip angle of 30°. The solid line indicates M_y, and the dotted line M_x. This frequency profile produced by the SINC pulse is a good approximation of the ideal profile.

SINC pulse with and without a Hamming apodization window. Figure 2.3 shows an $N = 4$ symmetric windowed SINC pulse and the resultant frequency (or slice) profile for a 30° flip angle calculated with the Bloch equations or a forward SLR transform.

Example 2.2 A SINC pulse has a total duration of 3.2 ms. The pulse is symmetric and has one negative lobe on each side of the central lobe. What is the approximate value of the bandwidth in hertz? What are the values of N and $T \Delta f$ for this pulse?

Answer Recalling that the central lobe is twice as broad as the other two, we can infer that:

$$t_0 = \frac{3.2 \text{ ms}}{1 + 2 + 1} = 0.8 \text{ ms}$$

Therefore the bandwidth is approximately:

$$\Delta f \approx \frac{1}{t_0} = 1250 \text{ Hz}$$

$N_L = N_R = N = 2$ for this pulse because there are two zero-crossings on each side of the central lobe. The time-bandwidth product can be calculated either directly, or with the use of Eq. (2.4):

$$T \Delta f = 3.2 \text{ ms} \times 1250 \text{ Hz} = 4.00$$

or

$$T \Delta f = N_L + N_R = 2 + 2 = 4$$

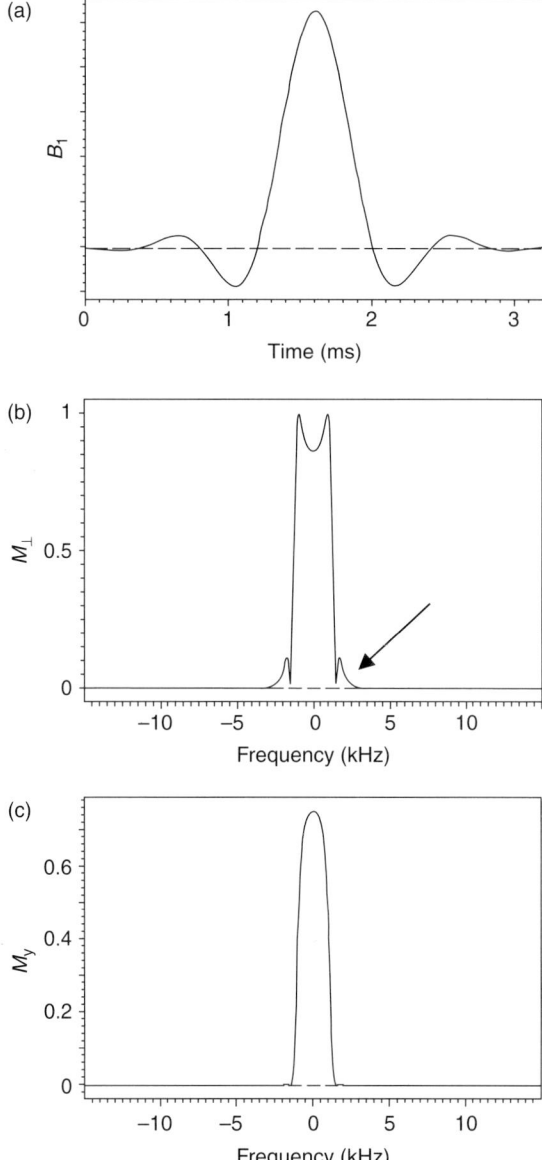

FIGURE 2.4 (a) An $N = 4$ symmetric SINC pulse apodized with a Hamming window. (b) When played as an excitation pulse at a flip angle of $120°$, prominent side lobes appear (arrow). (c) When played as a refocusing pulse (assuming crushers are used), the side lobes are suppressed and the bandwidth is narrowed.

SINC Refocusing Pulses   Given the severe nonlinearity of the Bloch equations for RF excitation with flip angles greater than 90° (see Section 3.1), it is somewhat surprising that SINC pulses can make effective refocusing pulses. (Refocusing pulses are normally played at a flip angle of 180°, but reduced flip angles, e.g., 130°, are sometimes used when SAR is a limiting factor, as discussed in Section 3.3.)

One reason that SINC pulses can be effectively used for refocusing pulses is that they are typically played with accompanying crusher gradients (see Section 10.2). It can be shown that the slice profile of a refocusing pulse with crushers is equal to the square of the small flip angle profile, which can be demonstrated with SLR analysis (Section 2.3). (Recall that the profile obtained at small flip angles is well approximated by the Fourier transform of the RF envelope and therefore does not contain nonlinearity introduced by the Bloch equations.) Figure 2.4 shows the responses of a SINC pulse with a 120° flip angle played as an excitation pulse and as a refocusing pulse (with crushers). Both responses were calculated with forward SLR transforms. The lack of side lobes in the refocusing pulse profile is a general result for this pulse and is valid even at a flip angle of 180°, as long as crushers accompany the pulse. Generally the effect of squaring any slice profile is to make it more sharply peaked, to suppress its side lobes, and to narrow it. Therefore, if SINC pulses that are identical (except in flip angle) are used for both excitation and refocusing in a spin echo pulse sequence, the amplitude of the slice-selection gradient of the refocusing SINC pulse is reduced by 25–40% to counteract the slice narrowing effect.

Table 2.2 gives some quantitative examples of the slice narrowing. When played as a small flip angle pulse ($\theta = 30°$), the values are nearly equal to unity, indicating that Eq. (2.3) holds to an excellent approximation. At $\theta = 90°$ the approximation is less accurate. When the SINC pulses are played as refocusing pulses, with crushers, the bandwidth is substantially lower, so that the amplitude of the slice-selection gradient must be reduced to obtain the expected slice thickness.

TABLE 2.2

RF Bandwidth[a], as Measured by the FWHM of the Slice Profile, for Two SINC Pulses Apodized with a Hamming Window

$\Delta f \times t_0$	$\theta = 30°$	$\theta = 90°$	$\theta = 180°$[b]
$N_L = N_R = N = 2$	1.01	1.09	0.67
$N_L = N_R = N = 4$	1.00	1.02	0.70

[a] In units of $1/t_0$. See Eq. (2.6).
[b] Refocus (with crushers).

SELECTED REFERENCES

MacFall, J. R., Charles, H. C., and Prost, R. 1990. Truncated SINC slice excitation for ^{31}P spectroscopic imaging. *Magn. Reson. Imaging* 8: 619–624.
Runge, V. M., Wood, M. L., Kaufman, D. M., and Silver, M. S. 1988. MR imaging section profile optimization: Improved contrast and detection of lesions. *Radiology* 167: 831–834.

RELATED SECTIONS

2.3 SLR Pulses

Given a slice-selective RF pulse and the initial orientation of the magnetization vector, the slice profile can be determined by solving the Bloch equations for M_x, M_y, and M_z (e.g., see Eq. 3.13 in Chapter 3). Although numerical methods are usually required, the process is straightforward and deterministic. The inverse problem, however, is much more difficult. Given the desired slice profile and the initial condition of the magnetization, what RF pulse should be applied? For small flip angles, the shape of an excitation pulse can be determined (to an excellent approximation) by inverse Fourier transformation of the slice profile (Section 3.1). This procedure begins to fail for pulses with larger flip angles (i.e., over the range 30–90°) due to the nonlinearity of the Bloch equations. In those cases, the RF pulse can be determined by iterative numerical optimization methods (for example, using optimal control theory), but this process is time-consuming and has limited flexibility for making trade-offs among pulse parameters. A summary of iterative and other RF pulse design methods can be found in Warren and Silver (1988, chap. 4).

The Shinnar–Le Roux (SLR) algorithm (Le Roux 1986; Shinnar, Eleff, et al. 1989; Shinnar, Bolinger, et al. 1989a, 1989b; Shinnar and Leigh 1989; Pauly et al. 1991) allows this inverse problem to be solved directly and efficiently, without iteration. Characteristics such as RF bandwidth, pulse duration, flip angle, percent ripple in the passband, and percent ripple in the stopband are specified, and the algorithm returns the exact RF pulse through a straightforward computational process. Moreover, the SLR algorithm allows the pulse designer to make trade-offs among these parameters before the pulse is even generated. Because of these advantages, the SLR algorithm has found widespread use for nonadiabatic pulse design in imaging and spectroscopy.

The SLR algorithm uses two key concepts: the two-dimensional mathematical representation of rotations known as SU(2), and the hard pulse approximation. Rotations in three-dimensional space can be described equally well by two distinct representations. The first representation uses the familiar 3×3 orthogonal rotation matrices and 3×1 vectors. This set of 3×3 rotation matrices is said to be the special orthogonal 3D group, or SO(3). The second representation uses 2×2 unitary matrices, and 2×1 complex vectors called *spinors* (Le Roux 1986; Shinnar and Leigh 1989; Pauly et al. 1991). The set of rotation 2×2 unitary matrices is said to be the special unitary 2D group, or SU(2). Both the SO(3) and SU(2) representations are equally valid to describe macroscopic rotations such as those experienced by the magnetization vector. The SU(2) representation for rotations is used in the SLR algorithm because it offers considerable mathematical simplification.

The second key concept of the SLR algorithm is the hard pulse approximation (Le Roux 1986; Shinnar, Eleff, et al. 1989), which is useful for nonadiabatic pulses and is depicted in Figure 2.5. The hard pulse approximation states that any shaped, or soft, pulse $B_1(t)$ can be approximated by a series of short hard pulses separated by periods of free precession. The approximation becomes progressively more accurate as the number of hard pulses increases and the duration of the free precession periods decreases. When rotations are described in the SU(2) representation and the hard pulse approximation is used, the effect of any soft pulse on the magnetization can be mathematically described by two polynomials with complex coefficients. The process that transforms from the RF pulse to the two polynomials is called the *forward SLR transform*. It is important that the *inverse SLR transform* also can be calculated. The inverse transform yields the RF pulse, given the two complex polynomials corresponding to the desired magnetization.

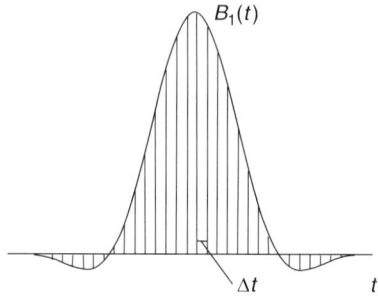

FIGURE 2.5 The hard pulse approximation. A selective or 'soft' RF pulse $B_1(t)$ can be approximated by a series of hard pulses, represented by the vertical lines. The hard pulses are separated by periods of free precession of duration Δt. As the number of hard pulses increases and Δt decreases, the accuracy of the hard pulse approximation improves.

In digital signal processing (DSP), these polynomials are filters for which there are well-established and powerful design tools available. In the SLR algorithm, the inverse SLR transform is used in conjunction with finite impulse response (FIR) filter design tools to design RF pulses directly (Shinnar, Bolinger, et al. 1989b; Pauly et al. 1991).

This section introduces the reader to the main concepts underlying the SLR algorithm. If the reader wants to actively engage in SLR pulse design, additional details beyond the scope of this section will be required and the reader is referred to Pauly et al. (1991) the DSP references therein. Several excellent commercial and shareware software packages for FIR filter design are also available. (We cannot recommend any particular package here, but if the reader enters key words such as *filter design*, *Remez*, and *Parks-McClellan* into an Internet search engine, several options will appear.)

2.3.1 MATHEMATICAL DESCRIPTION

Rotations   Rotations in three dimensions can be described equivalently by either the SO(3) or SU(2) representations. In the SO(3) representation, the familiar 3×3 rotation matrices have nine real matrix elements. The matrices are orthogonal and normalized (often called orthonormal):

$$\Re\Re^T = \Re^T\Re = \mathbb{I} \tag{2.7}$$

where $\Re^T$ represents the transpose of the matrix $\Re$ and $\mathbb{I}$ is the identity matrix. Because a general rotation can be completely specified by three free parameters (e.g., three Euler angles χ, ψ, and η), Eq. (2.7) represents $9 - 3 = 6$ constraints.

In the SU(2) representation, a general rotation matrix $\mathbb{Q}$ can be written:

$$\mathbb{Q} = \begin{bmatrix} \alpha & -\beta^* \\ \beta & \alpha^* \end{bmatrix} \tag{2.8}$$

where α and β are complex numbers known as the Cayley-Klein parameters and the asterisk represents complex conjugation. The matrix $\mathbb{Q}$ is unitary; that is:

$$\mathbb{Q}\mathbb{Q}^\dagger = \mathbb{Q}^\dagger\mathbb{Q} = \mathbb{I} \tag{2.9}$$

where $\mathbb{Q}^\dagger$ is the Hermitian conjugate or adjoint of $\mathbb{Q}$, which is obtained by transposing $\mathbb{Q}$ and taking the complex conjugate of each element. Note the product of unitary matrices is also a unitary matrix. Because the two complex Cayley-Klein parameters α and β contain a total of four real numbers, Eq. (2.9) contains only $4 - 3 = 1$ constraint. (Again recall that three free parameters are required to describe a general rotation.) From Eqs. (2.8) and (2.9), that single constraint is the normalization condition:

$$\alpha\alpha^* + \beta\beta^* = |\alpha|^2 + |\beta|^2 = 1 \tag{2.10}$$

The rotation matrix $\mathbb{Q}$ acts on 2×1 complex vectors (i.e., the spinors). In the SLR algorithm, the initial state of the spinor is taken to be:

$$s_0 = \begin{bmatrix} 1 \\ 0 \end{bmatrix} \tag{2.11}$$

Note that the effect of the unitary rotation matrix in Eq. (2.8) on the initial state of the spinor is

$$\mathbb{Q}s_0 = \begin{bmatrix} \alpha \\ \beta \end{bmatrix} \tag{2.12}$$

In other words the elements of the spinor are the Cayley-Klein parameters. Thus, the elements of the spinor satisfy the same normalization constraint that is given in Eq. (2.10).

The mathematical simplification afforded by the SU(2) representation is a consequence of the fewer number of constraints implicit in Eq. (2.9) versus Eq. (2.7) (i.e., one versus six). This situation is analogous to solving a system of linear equations, where it is nearly always easier to solve fewer equations with fewer constraints.

Given three Euler angles χ, ψ, and η, a two-dimensional unitary matrix can be written for the rotation (Goldstein 1980, Chap. 4):

$$\mathbb{Q} = \begin{bmatrix} e^{i(\chi+\psi)/2}\cos\dfrac{\eta}{2} & ie^{-i(\chi-\psi)/2}\sin\dfrac{\eta}{2} \\ ie^{i(\chi-\psi)/2}\sin\dfrac{\eta}{2} & e^{-i(\chi+\psi)/2}\cos\dfrac{\eta}{2} \end{bmatrix} \tag{2.13}$$

Note the appearance of the half values of the angles in Eq. (2.13), which is typical in the SU(2) representation. A rotation by 2π (i.e., $\eta \rightarrow \eta + 2\pi$) negates the matrix $\mathbb{Q}$, whereas the same rotation leaves the corresponding 3×3 orthogonal rotation matrix $\mathfrak{R}$ unchanged. Thus there is a one-to-one correspondence between elements of SO(3) and SU(2), that is, between $\mathfrak{R}$ and the pair $(-\mathbb{Q}, \mathbb{Q})$.

Although the SU(2) representation offers some mathematical simplification, ultimately the rotation of the magnetization vector occurs in real, three-dimensional space. A set of rules, or dictionary, that translates between the SU(2) and the SO(3) representations is required. Those rules were given by Jaynes (1955) and later adapted in Pauly et al. (1991). Defining the complex transverse magnetization in terms of the x and y components of the magnetization vector:

$$M_\perp = M_x + i M_y$$
$$M_\perp^* = M_x - i M_y \tag{2.14}$$

the magnetization before $(-)$ and after $(+)$ a rotation is given by:

$$\begin{bmatrix} M_\perp(+) \\ M_\perp^*(+) \\ M_z(+) \end{bmatrix} = \begin{bmatrix} (\alpha^*)^2 & -\beta^2 & 2\alpha^*\beta \\ -(\beta^*)^2 & \alpha^2 & 2\alpha\beta^* \\ -(\alpha\beta)^* & -\alpha\beta & \alpha\alpha^* - \beta\beta^* \end{bmatrix} \begin{bmatrix} M_\perp(-) \\ M_\perp^*(-) \\ M_z(-) \end{bmatrix} \tag{2.15}$$

where α and β are the Cayley-Klein parameters. Several important special cases (Pauly et al. 1991) can be extracted from Equation (2.15). For example, consider an inversion pulse. Prior to the application of the pulse, assume the magnetization is entirely aligned with the z axis and is assumed to have its maximal equilibrium value:

$$M_\perp(-) = 0$$
$$M_z(-) = M_0 \tag{2.16}$$

Substituting Eq. (2.16) into Eq. (2.15), and applying the normalization condition of Eq. (2.10) yields:

$$M_z(+) = M_0(\alpha\alpha^* - \beta\beta^*) = M_0(1 - 2|\beta|^2) \tag{2.17}$$

Note that the expression for the inversion slice profile in Eq. (2.17) is a real quantity, as it must be, even though the individual Cayley-Klein parameters are complex numbers. Table 2.3 gives several other special cases.

The Hard Pulse Approximation and the Forward SLR Transform   This subsection gives an overview of the hard pulse approximation and forward SLR transform. For more details, the reader is referred to Pauly et al. (1991); here we mainly follow the notation of that paper.

Recall that a selective, or soft, pulse can be approximated by a series of hard pulses, separated by periods of free precession (Fig. 2.5). In this way the net effect of the RF pulse can be approximated by a series of nutations and free precessions. Each nutation and each precession produces a rotation of the magnetization vector, which can be described by a unitary rotation matrix in the SU(2) representation. If relaxation effects are ignored, the net effect of all the nutations and precessions is a composite rotation that can be described by a

TABLE 2.3

Response of the Magnetization to Commonly used RF Pulse Types in Terms
of the Cayley-Klein Parameters

Pulse Type	Initial Condition (M_x, M_y, M_z)	Final State
Excitation or saturation	$(0, 0, M_0)$	$M_x = 2M_0\text{Re}(\alpha\beta^*)$ $M_y = 2M_0\text{Im}(\alpha\beta^*)$ $M_\perp = 2\alpha\beta^*$
Inversion	$(0, 0, M_0)$	$M_z = M_0(1 - 2|\beta|^2)$
Refocus (without crushers)	$(0, M_0, 0)$	$M_\perp = iM_0((\alpha^*)^2 + \beta^2)$
Refocus (with crushers, which dephase the $(\alpha^*)^2$ term giving a voxel average of 0)	$(0, M_0, 0)$	$M_\perp = iM_0\beta^2$

single unitary matrix obtained by multiplying the individual rotation matrices
in sequence.

As shown in Figure 2.5, the hard pulses are taken to be a series of spikes
(i.e., delta functions) with adjacent hard pulses separated by a time interval
Δt. So that the entire series of hard pulses produces the same flip angle as the
soft pulse, the incremental flip angle produced by the jth hard pulse must be

$$\theta_j = \gamma |B_{1,j}| \Delta t \tag{2.18}$$

(Equation 2.18 can be interpreted as approximating the integral under the soft
pulse by a series of rectangles.) The SLR algorithm does not require the RF
field to lie along a single direction in the rotating frame, so $B_{1,j}$ is represented
by a complex value, as discussed in Section 1.2 (hence the absolute value in
Eq. 2.18). If the phase of the RF field in the rotating frame is given by:

$$\varphi_j = \angle(B_{1,j}) = \arg(B_{1,j}), \tag{2.19}$$

then, θ_j and φ_j are related to the three Euler angles by $\eta = \theta_j$, $\chi = -\psi$ and
$\chi - \psi = 2\varphi_j$. The rationale behind choosing these values for the Euler angles
is explained in Figure 2.6. Equation (2.13) then provides the unitary matrix
that describes the jth nutation:

$$\mathbb{Q}_{\text{nutation},j} = \begin{bmatrix} \cos\dfrac{\theta_j}{2} & ie^{-i\varphi_j}\sin\dfrac{\theta_j}{2} \\ ie^{i\varphi_j}\sin\dfrac{\theta_j}{2} & \cos\dfrac{\theta_j}{2} \end{bmatrix} \tag{2.20}$$

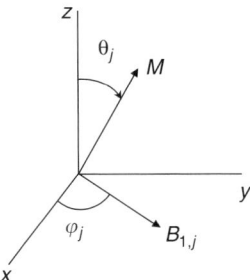

FIGURE 2.6 Nutation of the magnetization by the jth hard pulse. Because $B_{1,j}$ can be complex (i.e., can make any angle φ_j with respect to the x axis in the rotating frame) the nutation is described by three Euler angles. First, a rotation about z by the Euler angle $\psi = -\varphi_j$ aligns $B_{1,j}$ with the x axis. Then, a rotation about the x axis by $\eta = \theta_j$ accomplishes the nutation. Finally, $B_{1,j}$ is restored to its initial orientation with a rotation about the z axis by $\chi = +\varphi_j$.

Again using Eq. (2.13), and assuming both Δt and the resonant offset ω to be independent of the index j, the unitary rotation matrix describing any precession period is obtained by setting $\eta = \chi = 0$ and ψ equal to the precession angle:

$$\mathbb{Q}_{\text{precession}} = \begin{bmatrix} e^{i\psi/2} & 0 \\ 0 & e^{-i\psi/2} \end{bmatrix} = \begin{bmatrix} z^{1/2} & 0 \\ 0 & z^{-1/2} \end{bmatrix} = z^{1/2} \begin{bmatrix} 1 & 0 \\ 0 & z^{-1} \end{bmatrix} \quad (2.21)$$

The variable z is related to the resonant offset, which is determined by the gradient $\vec{G}$ and displacement $\vec{r}$ from isocenter:

$$z = \exp(i\psi) = \exp(i\omega\Delta t) = \exp(i2\pi f \Delta t) = \exp(i\gamma \vec{G} \cdot \vec{r} \Delta t) \quad (2.22)$$

(For spectrally selective pulses in Section 4.3, there is no slice-selection gradient, so the last term of Eq. 2.22 does not apply.) If, without loss of generality, it is assumed that the free precession precedes the nutation, then the effect of the first precession and nutation on the initial state given in Eq. (2.11) is:

$$s_1 = \mathbb{Q}_{\text{nutation},1}\,\mathbb{Q}_{\text{precession}}\,s_0 = z^{1/2} \begin{bmatrix} \cos\dfrac{\theta_1}{2} & ie^{-i\varphi_1}\sin\dfrac{\theta_1}{2} \\ ie^{i\varphi_1}\sin\dfrac{\theta_1}{2} & \cos\dfrac{\theta_1}{2} \end{bmatrix} \begin{bmatrix} 1 & 0 \\ 0 & z^{-1} \end{bmatrix} \begin{bmatrix} 1 \\ 0 \end{bmatrix}$$

$$= z^{1/2} \begin{bmatrix} \cos\dfrac{\theta_1}{2} \\ ie^{i\varphi_1}\sin\dfrac{\theta_1}{2} \end{bmatrix} \equiv z^{1/2} \begin{bmatrix} C_1 \\ S_1 \end{bmatrix} \quad (2.23)$$

Equation (2.23) contains the definition of C_1 and S_1, and C_j and S_j are defined analogously. The spinor state after the jth precession can be obtained by recursion:

$$s_j = \mathcal{Q}_{\text{nutation},\,j} \mathcal{Q}_{\text{precession}} s_{j-1} \tag{2.24}$$

For example,

$$s_2 = \mathcal{Q}_{\text{nutation},2} \mathcal{Q}_{\text{precession}} s_1$$

$$= z \begin{bmatrix} \cos\dfrac{\theta_2}{2} & ie^{-i\varphi_2}\sin\dfrac{\theta_2}{2} \\ ie^{i\varphi_2}\sin\dfrac{\theta_2}{2} & \cos\dfrac{\theta_2}{2} \end{bmatrix} \begin{bmatrix} 1 & 0 \\ 0 & z^{-1} \end{bmatrix} \begin{bmatrix} \cos\dfrac{\theta_1}{2} \\ ie^{i\varphi_1}\sin\dfrac{\theta_1}{2} \end{bmatrix}$$

$$= z \begin{bmatrix} C_2C_1 - S_1 S_2^* z^{-1} \\ C_1 S_2 + S_1 C_2 z^{-1} \end{bmatrix} \tag{2.25}$$

Defining the jth spinor state in terms of two complex polynomials:

$$s_j = z^{j/2} \begin{bmatrix} A_j(z) \\ B_j(z) \end{bmatrix} \tag{2.26}$$

it can be seen from Eqs. (2.24) and (2.25) that $A_j(z)$ and $B_j(z)$ are each polynomials of order $j-1$ in the variable z^{-1}. After the entire RF pulse has been approximated by N interleaved periods of free precession and hard pulses, we have:

$$s_N = z^{N/2} \begin{bmatrix} A_N(z) \\ B_N(z) \end{bmatrix} \tag{2.27}$$

Note that from Eq. (2.25), the constant term in the polynomial A_N is a product of the cosine terms:

$$A_{N,0} = C_N C_{N-1} C_{N-2} \cdots C_2 C_1 \tag{2.28}$$

All of the other terms in the polynomial A_N contain at least one factor of S_j, each of which is proportional to $\sin(\theta_j/2)$ and hence proportional to θ_j (because $\theta_j \ll 1$ rad). For small flip angles, all those terms are negligible in comparison to the constant term, so

$$A_N(z) \approx A_{N,0} = C_N C_{N-1} C_{N-2} \cdots C_2 C_1 \approx 1 \tag{2.29}$$

because C_j is equal to $\cos\left(\dfrac{\theta_j}{2}\right) \approx 1$.

From Eqs. (2.12) and (2.27), the two polynomials A_N and B_N are related to the Cayley-Klein parameters for the net rotation by:

$$A_N(z) = z^{-N/2}\alpha$$
$$B_N(z) = z^{-N/2}\beta \tag{2.30}$$

According to Eq. (2.22), $|z| = 1$, so the polynomials A_N and B_N satisfy the normalization constraint:

$$|A_N(z)|^2 + |B_N(z)|^2 = 1 \tag{2.31}$$

At this point, we have demonstrated the forward SLR transform from the RF pulse to the two polynomials in Eq. (2.27). The resulting magnetization is found from Eq. (2.30) and the relationships in Table 2.3.

Equation (2.29) provides further insight when used to interpret Table 2.3. For example, small flip angle excitation pulses satisfy $|\alpha| \approx 1$ because the cosines of all the hard pulse flip angles are approximately 1, and the sines are approximately 0. Because the small flip angle response is approximately proportional to the Fourier transform of the pulse, we can infer that $|\alpha\beta^*| \approx |\beta^*| = |\beta|$ must also be proportional to the magnitude of the Fourier transform of $B_1(t)$. Examining the result for the refocusing pulse (with crushers), we see that its slice profile is related to the square of the small flip angle excitation slice profile. This explains, for example, the narrowing of the slice profile of a SINC pulse used as a refocusing pulse (with crushers) compared to one used as an excitation pulse (Section 2.2).

The Inverse SLR Transform   The inverse SLR transform translates from the two polynomials $A_N(z)$ and $B_N(z)$ back to the jth RF pulse element $B_{1,j}$. Like the forward SLR transform, the inverse is calculated recursively. Inverting Eq. (2.24), and recalling the unitary property of the matrices (i.e., Eq. 2.9) yields:

$$s_{j-1} = z^{(j-1)/2}\begin{bmatrix} A_{j-1}(z) \\ B_{j-1}(z) \end{bmatrix} = \mathbb{Q}_{precession}^{-1}\mathbb{Q}_{nutation,j}^{-1}s_j$$
$$= \mathbb{Q}_{precession}^{\dagger}\mathbb{Q}_{nutation,j}^{\dagger}s_j \tag{2.32}$$

Because $A_j(z)$ and $B_j(z)$ are polynomials of order $j-1$ in z^{-1}, the constraint that their orders must decrease by one power of z^{-1} for each iteration provides sufficient information to calculate their coefficients. As described in detail in Pauly et al. (1991), that constraint allows the amplitude and phase of the hard pulse $B_{1,j}$ to be calculated with the relationship:

$$\gamma |B_{1,j}| \Delta t = 2 \arctan \left| \frac{B_{j,0}}{A_{j,0}} \right|$$

$$\angle(B_{1,j}) = \angle \left(-i \frac{B_{j,0}}{A_{j,0}} \right)$$

(2.33)

where $A_{j,0}$, and $B_{j,0}$ are the lowest order (i.e., constant) terms of the polynomials $A_j(z)$ and $B_j(z)$ (note that on the left-hand side of Eq. (2.33) $B_{1,j}$ is the RF field strength, not to be confused with the polynomial B.) By proceeding with the recursion, the entire hard pulse approximation can be recovered from the polynomials A and B. This provides the inverse SLR transform.

In practical calculations, for computational efficiency N is usually taken to be less than the number of the digital points used to ultimately represent the RF pulse on the MRI scanner. The final high-resolution digital representation of the pulse is obtained with interpolation (e.g., with cubic splines) of the hard pulse representation. If N is chosen too small, the hard pulse approximation begins to break down. Typically, N might be chosen to be 20–100, while the final digital resolution of the pulse can be 100–1000 or more, depending on its duration and on the details of the digital-to-analog converter (DAC) in the RF chain.

The Polynomials A and B   To design an RF pulse, the filter (i.e., polynomial) $B_N(z)$ is matched to the desired frequency response. This is done by a procedure described in Le Roux (1986) and Pauly et al. (1991) and outlined next. From Eqs. (2.8) and (2.13), we note that $|\beta| = |B_N| = \sin(\eta/2)$ where η is the net nutation angle of the pulse. First we generate up an ideal $B_N(z)$ polynomial that is equal to the sine of one-half the desired flip angle of the ideal profile. (Recall that z is related to the spatial coordinates by Eq. 2.22.) For example, to design a 90° pulse we set the ideal $B_N(z)$ equal to 0 in the stopband and equal to the constant value:

$$\sin \left(\frac{90°}{2} \right) \approx 0.707$$

(2.34)

in the passband. This ideal slice profile cannot be realized with a finite-length RF pulse, so a more realistic profile with a finite transition band and ripples is used instead. We can generate the realistic polynomial with the Parks-McClellan algorithm (Oppenheim and Schaeffer 1975, Chap. 5), which is also sometimes referred to as the Remez exchange algorithm. Figure 2.8a (later in this chapter) shows an example of the resulting $B_N(z)$ polynomial. Note that the finite-width transition band, the passband ripples, and the amplitude in the passband ($\sim$0.7) are consistent with Eq. (2.34).

To perform the inverse SLR transform we also need to determine the polynomial $A_N(z)$. There are many possible choices that satisfy the normalization constraint:

$$|A_N(z)| = \sqrt{1 - B_N(z)B_N^*(z)} \tag{2.35}$$

The problem of selecting the most physically meaningful filter $A_N(z)$ was solved by Le Roux (1986), who pointed out that minimum phase $A_N(z)$ yields the pulse that deposits the least amount of RF energy. That choice for the polynomial maximizes its constant term $A_{N,0}$, which from Eq. (2.29) is equivalent to minimizing all the flip angles of the hard pulses and hence the total RF power. Minimum phase polynomials have the property that all of their zeros (roots) lie within the unit circle; that is, if $A_N(z_R) = 0$, then $|z_R| < 1$. Once its magnitude has been determined as in Eq. (2.35), the complete polynomial, including its phase, can be calculated or retrieved with a mathematical tool called a Hilbert transform (named for David Hilbert, 1862–1943, a German mathematician), as explained in Pauly et al. (1991).

Once the minimum phase solution is selected for $A_N(z)$, there are still several inputs to be made to the SLR pulse design. The phase of the filter $B_N(z)$ dropped out of Eq. (2.35), but it is a design choice in the Parks-McClellan algorithm. Minimum, linear, and maximum phases are the most commonly used. In order to reduce the peak RF power, other phase choices (Shinnar 1994), including quadratic phase, can be used instead. The final RF pulse is often referred to according to the phase choice of the filter $B_N(z)$, for example, a minimum phase pulse. Note that the minimum phase solution is always used for $A_N(z)$, regardless of whether minimum, maximum, or linear phase solutions are used for $B_N(z)$.

2.3.2 Design Considerations

The time-bandwidth product (the product of the pulse duration T and the RF bandwidth Δf) is a dimensionless measure of the selectivity of the pulse. A highly selective pulse has an abrupt transition from its passband to its stopband. Because of requirements such as minimum TE or maximum RF power, the desired slice profile might not be attainable with the $T\Delta f$ product available for the pulse. Defining W to be the dimensionless width of the transition band of the response (i.e., $W \times \Delta f$ is the transition width in hertz), then W is determined by the relation (Pauly et al. 1991):

$$T\Delta f\, W = D_\infty \tag{2.36}$$

where D_∞ is a function of the pulse design parameters. Equation (2.36) allows the pulse designer to trade off parameters before the pulse is generated. In Eq. (2.36), D_∞ can be expressed by a simple function (Pauly et al. 1991) of the amount of ripple allowed in the passband and the stopband and of the phase type for the polynomial B. A more selective pulse has a smaller value of W, which can be accomplished either by increasing the time-bandwidth product $T \Delta f$ or by changing the pulse design to decrease D_∞. Increasing the percentage of ripple allowed, particularly in the stopband, is an effective way to decrease D_∞. Also, all other things being equal, minimum and maximum phase RF pulses have smaller values of D_∞ than linear phase pulses. For example, for an excitation pulse with $T \Delta f = 8$, 1.0% passband ripples, and 0.7% ripples in the stopband, $D_\infty = 2.037$ for the linear phase pulse and $D_\infty = 1.628$ for the minimum phase pulse. Therefore, the transition region W is 20% narrower for the minimum phase pulse.

Of the phase types discussed, only linear phase pulses produce a phase dispersion that can be completely rephased with a gradient rephasing lobe. Thus linear phase pulses are commonly used as spatial excitation pulses for 2D pulse sequences. The isodelay (see Section 3.1) of the linear phase pulse is equal to one-half its pulse width:

$$\Delta t_I = \frac{T}{2} \qquad \text{(linear phase)} \qquad (2.37)$$

Linear phase pulses also are widely used as slice refocusing pulses, because the phase dispersion accumulated during the first and second halves of the pulse cancel. Figure 2.7 shows an example of a linear phase pulse and its magnetization response.

Minimum phase pulses are useful in a number of applications because they have an isodelay that is less than one-half the pulse width:

$$\Delta t_I < \frac{T}{2} \qquad \text{(minimum phase)} \qquad (2.38)$$

and generally the inequality in Eq. (2.38) becomes more extreme as the time-bandwidth product increases. Minimum phase pulses are an excellent choice as excitation pulses for 3D volume gradient echo applications in which it is important to minimize TE. A drawback of minimum phase pulses is that their phase dispersion is a nonlinear function of frequency offset and cannot be completely rephased with a gradient lobe. For 3D acquisitions, however, this is not a serious problem because the phase dispersion of the slice profile is distributed across the entire 3D slab, while intravoxel dephasing is determined by the encoded slice width. In practice, intravoxel phase dispersion due to a minimum phase pulse will rarely result in more than a 1% signal loss if even a minimal number (e.g., 16) of slices are phase encoded. Figure 2.8 shows

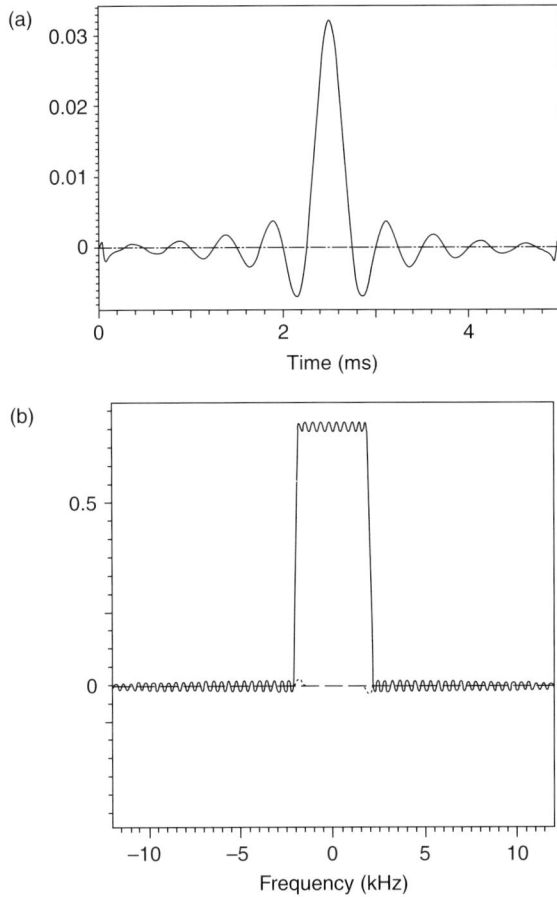

FIGURE 2.7 Linear phase excitation pulse with a time-bandwidth product of 20, a flip angle of 45°, and 2% ripple in both the passband (i.e., in-slice) and the stopband (i.e., out of slice). (a) RF amplitude versus time. (b) M_y and M_x (dotted line) responses. The plot assumes that the optimal rephasing gradient lobe has been applied. Note that M_x is nearly 0 (i.e., the phase across the slice is approximately constant), suggesting that the linear phase introduced during the pulse is effectively rephased by the rephasing gradient lobe.

an example of a minimum phase pulse that could be used as an excitation pulse for a 3D volume acquisition. Because minimum phase pulses have a reduced transition width W compared to linear phase pulses (holding T, Δf, and the ripple percentages constant), a minimum phase pulse also makes a good choice when the phase of the magnetization response is unimportant, such as for inversion pulses.

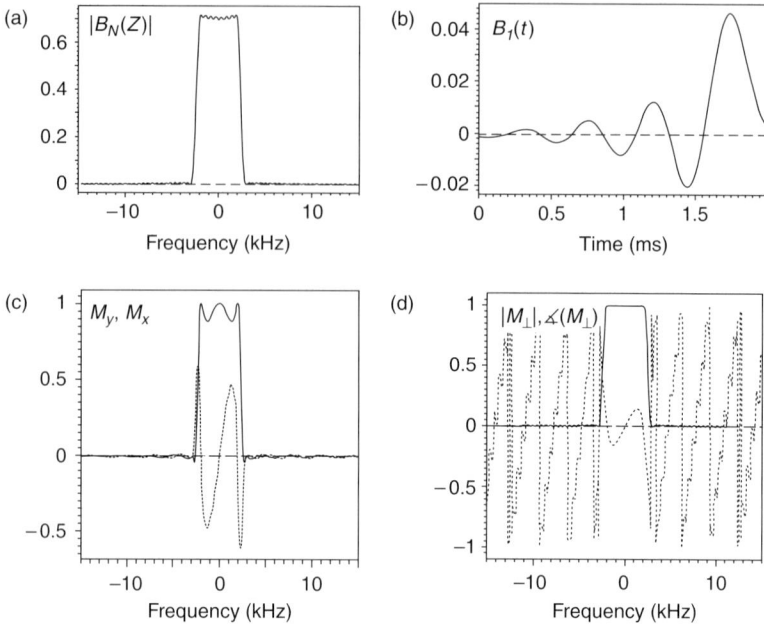

FIGURE 2.8 Minimum phase pulse with a time-bandwidth product of 10, a flip angle of 90°, and 0.5% ripple in the passband and the stopband. (a) The filter (polynomial) $B_N(z)$ plotted versus frequency. (b) The RF amplitude versus time. (c) The M_y and M_x (dotted line) response. (d) Plots of the same response as (c), but this time in terms of the polar instead of Cartesian components. Note from (b) that the isodelay is much less than one-half of the pulse duration ($T = 2$ ms and $\Delta t_I = 288\,\mu$s), and the nonlinear phase is apparent from (c) (real and imaginary) and (d) (modulus and phase). Also the ripples apparent on the filter passband are attenuated in the response (d) compared to (a) because the flip angle is 90°.

Maximum phase pulses can be thought of as time-reversed minimum phase pulses. Consequently their isodelay is greater than one-half their pulse width. Maximum phase pulses are sometimes used for spatial or spectral saturation, where signal dephasing is desirable instead of detrimental.

2.3.3 PRACTICAL CONSIDERATIONS

Pulses designed with the SLR algorithm account for the nonlinearity of the Bloch equations, but only at a single flip angle. For example, if an SLR excitation pulse is designed for a flip angle of 45° but played at a flip angle of 60°, then deviations from the designed profile will begin to emerge. If this is an important consideration, a set of pulses designed for different flip angles can be stored on the MR scanner. Alternatively, the SLR design could be done in real time when the operator selects the flip angle.

The amount of ripple that is tolerable for the filter $B_N(z)$ depends on the intended function of the pulse. For example, from Table 2.3, a small flip angle excitation pulse response is linearly related to the Cayley-Klein parameter β, and so from Eq. (2.30) it is also proportional to $B_N(z)$. Therefore the amount of ripple in the filter $B_N(z)$ is equal to the amount ripple in the slice profile. For a refocusing pulse with crushers, however, there is a quadratic relationship between β and the response. As shown in Pauly et al. (1991), this implies, for example, that the ripple in the passband of the magnetization response will be four times larger than the ripple in the passband of the filter. SLR pulses are always specified by the desired ripple in the magnetization response, and the corresponding ripple in the filter $B_N(z)$ is calculated according to the type of RF pulse being designed.

The intuitive basis for these types of relations between the ripple in the response and ripple in the filter can be appreciated by considering a 90° (i.e., $\pi/2$) excitation pulse. The magnetization response is proportional to the sine of the flip angle. Near 90°, the ripples in the passband are attenuated because the response is second-order in the ripple amplitude $\Delta\theta$:

$$|M_\perp| = M_0 \sin\left(\frac{\pi}{2} + \Delta\theta\right) = M_0 \cos\Delta\theta = M_0\left(1 - \frac{(\Delta\theta)^2}{2} + \cdots\right)$$

$$(2.39)$$

Consequently, higher amplitude ripples can be designed into the filter's passband. This effect is illustrated in Fig. 2.8. Quantitative relationships between filter ripple and response ripple for a variety of cases are given in Pauly et al. (1991). It should be noted, however, that if due to B_1 inhomogeneity a pulse intended to be played at 90° (and designed with higher passband ripples) is actually played at 45° over part of the subject, then the passband ripples can be unacceptable in that region.

The amount of stopband ripple that can be tolerated also depends on the specific use of the RF pulse. 3D volume excitation pulses tend to be less forgiving of stopband ripple because the phase encoding process in the slice direction can cause an unwanted signal from the stopband to alias into the desired slice locations (see Example 11.9). If, however, the main issue is whether or not the ripples in the stopband will disturb the z component of off-resonant magnetization (e.g., as with magnetization transfer, chemically selective, or some spatial saturation pulses), then the situation is much more forgiving. The amount of z magnetization that remains undisturbed is proportional to $\cos\Delta\theta$, which from Eq. (2.39) is second order in $\Delta\theta$.

SELECTED REFERENCES

Goldstein, H. 1980. *Classical mechanics*, 2nd ed. Reading: Addison-Wesley.

Jaynes, E. T. 1955. Matrix treatment of nuclear induction. *Phys. Rev.* 98: 1099–1105.

Le Roux, P. 1986. French patent 8610179.

Oppenheim, A. V., and Schaeffer, R. W. 1975. *Digital signal processing.* Englewood Cliffs: Prentice-Hall.

Pauly, J., Le Roux, P., Nishimura, D., and Makovski, A. 1991. Parameter relations for the Shinnar-Le Roux selective excitation pulse design algorithm. *IEEE Trans. Med. Imag.* 10: 53–65.

Shinnar, M. 1994. Reduced power selective excitation RF pulses. *Magn. Reson. Med.* 32: 658–660.

Shinnar, M., Bolinger, L., and Leigh, J. S. 1989a. The synthesis of soft pulses with a specified frequency response. *Magn. Reson. Med.* 12: 88–92.

Shinnar, M., Bolinger, L., and Leigh, J. S. 1989b. The use of finite impulse response filters in pulse design. *Magn. Reson. Med.* 12: 75–87.

Shinnar, M., Eleff, S., Subramanian, H., and Leigh, J. S. 1989. The synthesis of pulse sequences yielding arbitrary magnetization vectors. *Magn. Reson. Med.* 12: 74–80.

Shinnar, M., and Leigh, J. S. 1989. The application of spinors to pulse synthesis and analysis. *Magn. Reson. Med.* 12: 93–98.

Warren, W. S., and Silver, M. E. 1988. The art of pulse crafting: Applications to magnetic resonance and laser spectroscopy. In *Advances in magnetic resonance*, Vol. 12, edited by J. S. Waugh, pp. 247–384. New York: Academic Press.

RELATED SECTIONS

Section 3.1 Excitation Pulses
Section 3.2 Inversion Pulses
Section 3.3 Refocusing Pulses
Section 4.3 Spectrally Selective Pulses

2.4 Variable-Rate Pulses

A one-dimensional spatially selective RF pulse that is played concurrently with a time-varying gradient is called a *variable-rate* (VR) pulse (Conolly et al. 1988, 1991). VR pulses are also known as variable-rate gradient (VRG) pulses or variable-rate selective excitation (VERSE) pulses. One main application of VR pulses is to reduce RF power deposition to the patient, which is accomplished by decreasing the RF amplitude in the vicinity of the peak of the pulse. The peak of the pulse typically contributes the bulk of the power deposition because the contribution to the SAR from the pulse is proportional to the square of its B_1 amplitude. Another application of VR pulses is to play RF concurrently with the gradient ramps, as is commonly done with spatial subpulses in a spatial-spectral pulse (Section 5.4). Playing RF with the ramps makes efficient use of the entire time allotted for the slice-selection gradient lobe, which allows thinner slices or an improvement of the slice profile.

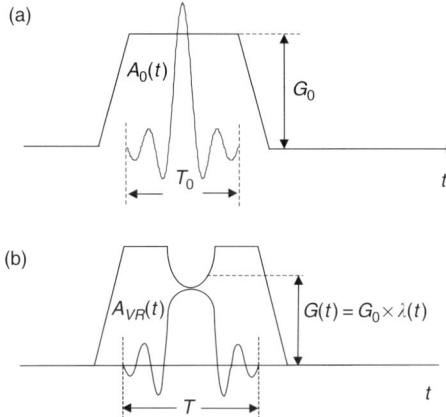

FIGURE 2.9 The variable-rate modification to a SINC RF pulse. The original RF envelope $A_0(t)$ is stretched and attenuated wherever the gradient amplitude is reduced. The gradient amplitude dips according to the function $\lambda(t)$.

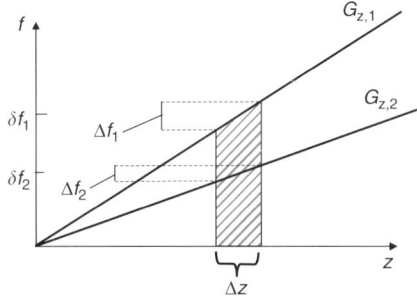

FIGURE 2.10 Whenever the gradient amplitude $G(t)$ is reduced, there is a proportionate reduction in the RF bandwidth Δf and frequency offset δf so that the same slice Δz is produced.

To maintain the nominal flip angle when the RF amplitude is reduced, the VR pulse is proportionately stretched, or time dilated. This in turn reduces the instantaneous RF bandwidth (defined later in Section 2.4) of any portion of the pulse that is stretched. To ensure that the entire VR pulse produces the desired slice profile, the slice-selection gradient amplitude must be proportionately reduced whenever the RF pulse is stretched in order to match the reduced RF bandwidth. Figure 2.9 shows an example of an original and a VR-modified SINC pulse with a concurrent gradient. Figure 2.10 illustrates how the reduced RF bandwidth and reduced gradient amplitude work in concert to maintain the same slice profile.

A VR-modified pulse is designed to produce exactly the same slice profile as the original pulse for on-resonance spins (e.g., water). The slice profile of off-resonance spins (e.g., lipids), however, will suffer distortion. This is because the pulse designer can dilate the RF and adjust the gradient, but has no control over the precession period of off-resonance spins. Off-resonance slice profile distortion often limits the degree of VR stretching that can be used in practice.

VR pulses are sometimes called the 10-speed bicycle of RF excitation because when the work gets strenuous (i.e., pedaling uphill or playing high-amplitude RF), the duration of the work is dilated (by using a lower gear or by stretching the RF pulse). VR pulses also can be thought of as a transmit analog of variable bandwidth reception described in Section 14.3 or data readout with ramp sampling described in Section 16.1. Both adiabatic and nonadiabatic pulses can be modified with the VR method.

2.4.1 QUANTITATIVE DESCRIPTION

Variable-Rate Stretching   Suppose the original envelope of an RF pulse is given by $A_0(t)$ and has pulse width T_0 (Fig. 2.9). Also, suppose that some or all of the RF pulse is stretched so that the new pulse width is $T > T_0$. To maintain the flip angle, the RF amplitude is attenuated by a dimensionless reduction factor, which we call $\lambda(t)$. For the example in Figure 2.9, $\lambda(t) = 1$, except in the region where the gradient amplitude is reduced, for which $\lambda(t) < 1$. The process of stretching and attenuating the pulse is described by the mathematical transformation:

$$A_{VR}(t) = \lambda(t) \times A_0(u) \tag{2.40}$$

where the variable u

$$u(t) = \int_0^t \lambda(t') \, dt' \tag{2.41}$$

can be interpreted as undilated time. The normalization of $A_{VR}(t)$ in Eq. (2.40) can be verified by comparing the flip angles produced by the original and VR pulses. We examine the important special case of a real, nonadiabatic pulse here; a more general derivation that covers the adiabatic pulses is given in Conolly et al. (1991). Also, to agree with the convention adopted for RF k-space stated in Section 5.4, we assume that the integrations begin at the end of the pulse T_{end}, which we set to $t = 0$, and then proceed to the left. The flip angle for the VR pulse for on-resonance spins is:

$$\gamma \int_0^T A_{VR}(t) \, dt = \gamma \int_0^{T_0} \lambda(t) \, A_0(u(t)) \, dt \tag{2.42}$$

Equation (2.41) implies $du = \lambda(t)dt$. Substituting this relationship into Eq. (2.42) demonstrates that the flip angles are equal:

$$\gamma \int_0^T A_{VR}(t)\, dt = \gamma \int_0^{T_0} A_0(u)\, du \tag{2.43}$$

The widths of the original and the VR pulses are related by:

$$T_0 = \int_0^T \lambda(t')\, dt' \quad \text{or} \quad T = \frac{T_0}{\langle \lambda(t) \rangle} \tag{2.44}$$

where $\langle \lambda(t) \rangle$ is the time average of the dimensionless reduction factor. Equation (2.43) indicates that the area underneath the RF envelope is conserved. This is true not only for the entire pulse, but also for any segment of the pulse. Whenever the RF pulse amplitude is reduced in the process of VR modification, the RF pulse width is stretched accordingly to maintain the same area.

The slice-selection gradient amplitude must also 'dip' by the reduction factor $\lambda(t)$ to account for the instantaneous variation of the RF bandwidth due to the stretching of the RF waveform. We can define instantaneous or time-varying bandwidth $\Delta f(t)$ to be the RF bandwidth that would result if the *entire* pulse were stretched by the value of the reduction factor at time t, $\lambda(t)$. Recall the RF bandwidth is inversely proportional to the duration of the pulse, so adapting Eq. (8.53) from Section 8.3 to account for the time-varying RF bandwidth $\Delta f(t)$:

$$G(t) = \frac{2\pi\, \Delta f(t)}{\gamma\, \Delta z} = \frac{2\pi\, \Delta f_0 \lambda(t)}{\gamma\, \Delta z} = G_0 \lambda(t) \tag{2.45}$$

where Δf_0 and G_0 are the bandwidth and slice-selection gradient amplitude of the original pulse, respectively, and Δz is the slice thickness.

RF k-Space Interpretation and Dwell Factor   The expression for the VR pulse in Eq. (2.40) has an elegant interpretation when the concept of the RF k-space is employed. As defined in Section 5.4 on spatial-spectral pulses, the RF k-space is related to the area under the slice-selection gradient by:

$$k(t) = \frac{\gamma}{2\pi} \int_0^t G(t')\, dt' \tag{2.46}$$

Substituting the time-varying gradient amplitude from Eq. (2.45) yields:

$$k(t) = \frac{\gamma G_0}{2\pi} \int_0^t \lambda(t')\, dt' \tag{2.47}$$

Using Eqs. (2.41) and (2.47) and recognizing that $k(t)$ is proportional $u(t)$, Eq. (2.40) can be recast as:

$$A_{VR}(t) = \frac{2\pi}{\gamma G_0} A_0(k) \frac{dk}{dt} \tag{2.48}$$

For small flip angle excitation pulses the slice profile is given by the Fourier transform of the RF envelope. Adapting Eq. (3.14) from the section on excitation pulses to account for the time-dependent slice-selection gradient $G(t)$, the slice profile for small flip angles is:

$$|M_\perp(z)| = \gamma M_0 \left| \int_0^t A_{VR}(t') e^{-i\gamma z \int_0^{t'} G(s)\, ds}\, dt' \right| \tag{2.49}$$

Substituting Eqs. (2.46) and (2.48) into Eq. (2.49) yields:

$$|M_\perp(z)| = \gamma M_0 \left| \int_0^t A_{VR}(t') e^{-i\gamma z \int_0^{t'} G(s)\, ds}\, dt' \right|$$

$$= \frac{2\pi M_0}{G_0} \left| \int_{k_{min}}^{k_{max}} A_0(k)\, e^{-2\pi i k z}\, dk \right| \tag{2.50}$$

Several inferences can be drawn from Eqs. (2.48) and (2.50). First, the factor $(dk/dt) \propto G(t)$ in Eq. (2.48) is a Jacobian required for the change of variables from t to $k(t)$. (Jacobians factors are named after the German mathematician Carl Gustav Jacob Jacobi, 1804–1851, and geometrically represent a ratio of differential lengths in 1D integrals, a ratio of areas in 2D integrals, etc.; Kreyszig 1998, 482.) Because Jacobian factors cannot change sign, we can infer that whenever $G(t) < 0$ (such as was encountered for spatial-spectral pulses) $|G(t)|$ must be used instead. Physically, $|dk/dt|$ is the dwell factor that is required to uniformly weight the RF k-space. When $|G(t)|$ is small, the traversal through k-space is slow, so the RF amplitude must be reduced in order to avoid overweighting that region. The analogous expression for traversal through a two-dimensional RF k-space is discussed in Section 5.1.

Second, comparing the integration expressions in Eq. (2.50) illustrates the value of the RF k-space concept. The integral on the upper line represents what is physically played, namely the VR pulse as a function of time. Note the very complicated functional dependence. The equivalent integral on the lower line represents a much simpler expression: the Fourier transform of the original RF pulse, which is known to yield the slice profile as originally designed.

The situation represented in Eq. (2.50) is analogous to variable bandwidth during signal reception (discussed in Sections 14.3 and 16.1)—although the raw data plotted versus time will be stretched or compressed depending on the value of the receiver bandwidth, the k-space representation of the data is independent of the bandwidth.

Off-Resonance Effects The design strategy represented by Eqs. (2.40) and (2.50) assumes on-resonance spins. In the presence of off-resonance effects, such as chemical shift f_{cs}, Eq. (2.50) becomes:

$$|M_\perp(z)| = \gamma M_0 \left| \int_0^t A_{VR}(t') e^{-i\left(2\pi f_{cs}t' + \gamma z \int_0^{t'} G(s)\,ds\right)} dt' \right| \qquad (2.51)$$

The additional term in the exponential of Eq. (2.51) means that the expression for the resulting slice profile is more complicated (i.e., it is the convolution of the desired profile with the Fourier transform of $e^{-i2\pi f_{cs}t(k)}$). This causes the slice profile to be distorted and the signal within the slice to be dephased. Conolly et al. (1991) show that the distortion tends to be lower for adiabatic pulses (which are typically both amplitude and phase modulated) than for pulses with only amplitude modulation.

Figure 2.11a shows the slice profile of a RF pulse with nominal bandwidth of 2 kHz for spins that are on-resonance. For spins that are 400 Hz below the resonant frequency (i.e., roughly the fat–water chemical shift at 3 T), the entire slice profile undergoes a bulk shift equal to 400 Hz/2000 Hz $= 0.2$, that is, one-fifth of the slice width (Figure 2.11b). If the RF pulse is a VR pulse, however, in addition to the bulk shift of the slice profile there is also distortion (Figure 2.11c). Figure 2.12 schematically illustrates the origin of the distortion.

VR to Minimize SAR For a given RF pulse width T, the RF power absorbed by the imaged object is given by:

$$SAR \propto \int_0^T B_1^2(t)\,dt \qquad (2.52)$$

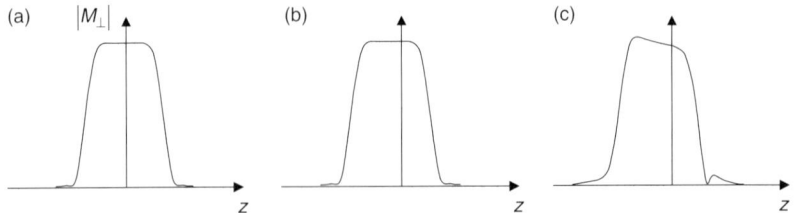

FIGURE 2.11 Bloch equation calculation of the slice profile of a VR SINC pulse with a bandwidth of $\Delta f = 2$ kHz, duration of $T = 4$ ms, and flip angle of $\theta = 45°$. (a) The on-resonance profile is identical to the profile that would have been produced by the original pulse. (b) The slice profile produced by the original pulse experiences a bulk chemical shift for spins that are 400 Hz below resonance. (c) The profile of the VR pulse experiences not only a bulk chemical shift, but also distortion for off-resonance spins.

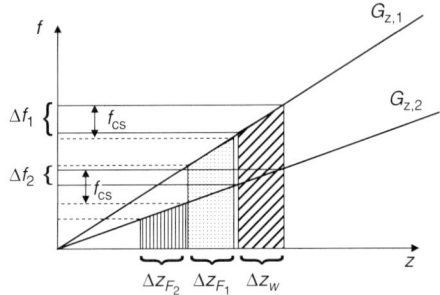

FIGURE 2.12 Schematic representation of the origin of the slice profile distortion calculated in Figure 2.11. As in Figure 2.10, the gradients, RF bandwidths, and frequency offsets are properly scaled to produce the same on-resonance slice, Δz_W (diagonal bar pattern). The pulse programmer, however, has no control over the chemical shift, f_{cs}, which is the same regardless of the gradient amplitude. Consequently, the two lipid slices Δz_{F1} (dotted pattern) and Δz_{F2} (vertical bar pattern) do not coincide. Note that Δz_{F2} is farther from Δz_W. In this diagram, the value of f_{cs} has been exaggerated so that the slice profiles do not overlap.

The SAR is minimized subject to the flip angle constraint:

$$\theta = \gamma \int_0^T B_1(t)\, dt \qquad (2.53)$$

when the RF envelope is a constant. The envelopes of most RF pulses (e.g., a SINC) have a single dominant peak, so they are hardly constant. The VR method, however, presents the opportunity to flatten out, or rectangularize, any

RF pulse so that it deposits the minimum possible SAR. With this strategy, $\lambda(t)$ is chosen to be approximately proportional to the inverse of the RF envelope; that is, $\lambda(t) < 1$ is used for the pulse peak, and $\lambda(t) > 1$ is used for the side lobes. (A ceiling value must be placed on $\lambda(t)$ so that it does not diverge at the zero-crossings of the RF pulse.) All the mathematical analysis of the previous subsections remains valid when $\lambda(t) > 1$.

Minimum power VR pulses have not been commonly used, however, mainly because their off-resonance profiles tend to be poor. More commonly, an additional constraint is added—namely, $\lambda(t)$ cannot differ from 1 by more than a predetermined amount. More design details are provided in Conolly et al. (1988).

Spatial Offset   The VR pulse given in Eq. (2.40) yields a slice centered at gradient isocenter, $z = 0$. Just as with spatial-spectral pulses, to offset the slice by a distance δz away from isocenter, the pulse is phase (or frequency) modulated by:

$$A_{VR}(t, \delta z) = e^{-i\gamma \delta z \int G(t')\, dt'} A_{VR}(t, \delta z = 0) = e^{-i\gamma G_0 \delta z \int \lambda(t')\, dt'} A_{VR}(t, \delta z = 0) \tag{2.54}$$

Figure 2.10 schematically illustrates why the time-dependent frequency offset is directly proportional to $G(t)$. Equation (2.54) also indicates that the frequency modulation must match the actual time-varying gradient. Any deviation will cause slice profile distortion and intraslice signal dephasing, resulting in a slice intensity that varies with slice offset δz. The offset slice profile also experiences the same slice distortion from chemical shift effects as depicted in Figure 2.11.

2.4.2 PRACTICAL CONSIDERATIONS

VR pulses can be generated by many methods. One procedure is to use the following steps.

1. Choose an original RF envelope $A_0(t)$ that has a duration T_0 and the desired slice profile.
2. Choose a function $\lambda(t)$ that dips near the peak of the RF pulse.
3. Calculate the pulse width T based on T_0 and $\lambda(t)$ using Eq. (2.44), and check that the calculated value of T is acceptable for the pulse sequence application (in terms of minimum TE, TR, or echo spacing). If T is too long, either go back to Step 1 and decrease T_0, or go back to Step 2 and make the dip in $\lambda(t)$ less severe.
4. Generate the pulse according to Eq. (2.40), using numerical integration and an interpolation method such as cubic splines.

5. Numerically calculate the slice profile of the pulse with the Bloch equations on-resonance and for various values of f_{cs} that might be encountered in practice (e.g., the lipid frequency shift at the field strength of interest.)
6. Increase or decrease the degree of the dip in $\lambda(t)$ depending on the results of Step 5.
7. Repeat Steps 2–6 until an acceptable $A_{VR}(t)$ is achieved.

Other more sophisticated design procedures are provided in Conolly et al. (1988, 1991).

The VR design principles are quite useful in reducing the RF power deposition of adiabatic pulses. For example, the adiabatic inversion pulse based on hyperbolic modulation functions (see Section 6.2) can be reshaped using the VR design to minimize the RF power deposition at the expense of prolonged pulse width. Conolly et al. (1991) describes an adiabatic inversion pulse with a bandwidth of 2.6 kHz and a pulse width of 5.376 ms.

Like spatial-spectral pulses, VR pulses are sensitive to system imperfections such as mismatches between the RF and gradient group delay, and gradient eddy currents, especially for slice locations far from isocenter. Similar correction methods can be applied. It should be noted that the performance and design strategies of VR pulses also depend on field strength. In the range of clinical field strengths (i.e., 0.2–3.0 T), the RF power deposition scales approximately as the square of the B_0 field. Thus, the need for VR pulses increases with increasing B_0. The chemical shift, f_{cs}, however, also increases linearly with B_0, so the VR design becomes more difficult.

SELECTED REFERENCES

Conolly, S., Glover, G., Nishimura, D., and Macovski, A. 1991. A reduced power selective adiabatic spin echo pulse sequence. *Magn. Res. Med.* 18: 28–38.

Conolly, S., Nishimura, D., Macovski, A., and Glover, G. 1988. Variable-rate selective excitation. *J. Magn. Reson.* 78: 440–458.

Kreyszig, E. 1998. *Advanced engineering mathematics*, 8th ed. New York: John Wiley & Sons.

RELATED SECTIONS

3

BASIC RADIOFREQUENCY PULSE FUNCTIONS

3.1 Excitation Pulses

Excitation pulses tip the magnetization vector away from the direction of the main magnetic field B_0 (Joseph et al. 1984; Hoult 1980; Pauly et al. 1991). Magnetization aligned with B_0 does not create any MR signal, but once a component of the magnetization lies in the transverse plane, an MR signal can be detected. Therefore every MR pulse sequence uses at least one excitation pulse. Excitation RF pulses can be applied either adiabatically (Section 6.1) or nonadiabatically. This section focuses on nonadiabatic excitation pulses.

The excitation pulse is implemented by switching on (i.e., pulsing) the RF field modulation envelope, denoted by $B_1(t)$, for a short time (typically $200 \, \mu s$ to 5 ms). This range is short enough so that T_1 and T_2 relaxation during the pulse typically can be neglected for proton MRI. Excitation pulses are characterized by their *tip angle*, or *flip angle*, which we denote by the Greek letter theta (θ). θ is the angle between the direction of the main magnetic field, and the magnetization vector immediately after the excitation pulse is terminated (Figure 3.1). With the exception of adiabatic excitation pulses, the flip angle for on-resonance spins can be calculated by finding the area under the envelope of the RF field. Typically a flip angle of $\theta = 90°$ is used for excitation pulses in spin echo pulse sequences, and a flip angle in the range of $\theta = 5–70°$ is used for gradient echo pulse sequences.

67

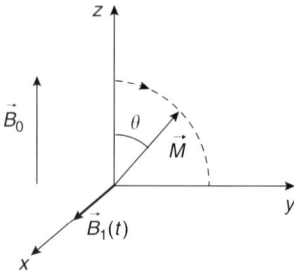

FIGURE 3.1 A representation of an excitation pulse in the rotating reference frame. The magnetization vector $\vec{M}$ is initially aligned with the main magnetic field $\vec{B}_0$, which lies in the z direction. An RF excitation pulse $B_1(t)$ is applied along the x axis. After the magnetization rotates in the yz plane by the flip angle θ, the RF excitation pulse is switched off.

Slice-selective excitation pulses are played concurrently with a slice-selection gradient (Section 8.3) to produce an excited section, or slice of magnetization. Hard pulses (Section 2.1) are short duration pulses, often rectangular in shape, that are played without an accompanying slice-selection gradient. A hard pulse typically excites all the magnetization that is coupled to the RF coil.

The flip angle produced by an excitation pulse can vary across the selected slice. This results in a distribution of transverse magnetization when plotted versus either position or frequency. This distribution is called the *slice profile*. The plot of the flip angle can also describe the slice profile because the flip angle and transverse magnetization are related as shown by Eq. (3.16) later in this chapter.

For small flip angles, the slice profile is approximated by the Fourier transform of the RF pulse. As illustrated in Figure 3.2, an ideal slice profile consists of a uniform flip angle within the desired slice (i.e., within the *passband*) and a flip angle of $\theta = 0°$ outside (i.e., in the *stopband*). The transition region between the passband and stopband of an ideal slice profile has infinitely narrow width. The ideal slice profile cannot be achieved in practice because it requires an excitation pulse of infinite duration. Several approximations to the ideal slice profile, however, can be achieved with a variety of shaped RF pulses such as SINC pulses (Section 2.2) and SLR pulses (Section 2.3).

3.1.1 MATHEMATICAL DESCRIPTION

Bloch Equations and Flip Angle On-Resonance   The flip angle produced on-resonance (i.e., when the RF frequency matches the Larmor

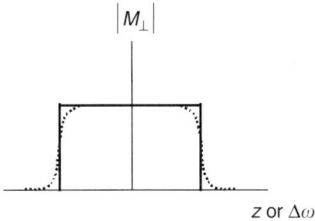

FIGURE 3.2 An ideal selective excitation pulse produces a uniform flip angle (and hence uniform transverse magnetization) within the passband of the pulse and a zero flip angle in the stopband (solid line). The width of the passband is equal to the slice thickness. The transition region of an ideal selective excitation pulse is infinitely narrow. Such an ideal slice profile cannot be produced in practice, but several effective approximations are available, which yield a nearly uniform flip angle profile (dotted line).

frequency) is:

$$\theta(t) = \gamma \int_{t'=0}^{t} B_1(t')dt' \qquad (3.1)$$

where γ is the gyromagnetic ratio in units of radians per second per tesla, and $B_1(t)$ is the RF modulation envelope, which is 0 prior to $t = 0$. By definition, the on-resonance condition is always met at the center of the slice profile (Note that chemical shift and magnetic susceptibility effects, which are neglected in Eq. 3.1., can shift the center of the slice). The integration in Eq. (3.1) is performed over the duration of the RF pulse, and the resulting flip angle is in radians.

Example 3.1 A hard RF pulse has a rectangular-shaped envelope. Its pulse width is 100 μs, and its flip angle (on-resonance) is 90°. What is its amplitude?

Answer A rectangular envelope has a constant $B_1(t)$ field. Recalling that $90° = \pi/2$ radians, substituting into Eq. (3.1) yields:

$$\theta = \frac{\pi}{2} = \gamma B_1 \times (100 \times 10^{-6} \text{ s})$$

$$B_1 = \frac{\pi}{2\gamma(100 \text{ μs})} = \frac{\pi \text{ (rad)}}{2 \times 2\pi \times 42.57 \times 10^6 (\text{rad/s} \cdot \text{T}) \times 100 \times 10^{-6}(\text{s})}$$

$$= 58.7 \text{ μT}$$

Equation (3.1) represents a linear relationship between the flip angle and the RF field. If $B_1(t)$ is scaled by a factor of 2, the flip angle θ also doubles. As is shown later in this section, the linear relationship between

$B_1(t)$ and θ holds only under one of the following two conditions: (1) for on-resonance excitation or (2) for small flip angles (i.e., $\theta \ll 1$ rad). In general, the response of the flip angle and the magnetization to RF excitation is quite nonlinear.

Equation (3.1) can be readily derived by considering the Bloch equations in the rotating reference frame. Equation (1.79) in Section 1.2 states that when relaxation effects are neglected and the angular frequency of the rotating frame is chosen to match the RF frequency, the Bloch equations for an RF pulse applied in the x direction become:

$$\left(\frac{d\vec{M}}{dt}\right)_{\text{rot}} = \gamma \vec{M} \times \left[\hat{x} B_1(t) + \hat{z}\left(B_0 - \frac{\omega_{\text{rf}}}{\gamma}\right)\right] \tag{3.2}$$

In this section, all of the analysis is carried out in that rotating frame, so the "rot" subscript is dropped. Defining an angular frequency offset,

$$\Delta\omega = \gamma B_0 - \omega_{\text{rf}} \tag{3.3}$$

Eq. (3.2), which is in vector form, can be expanded into three scalar equations:

$$\frac{dM_x}{dt} = \Delta\omega M_y$$

$$\frac{dM_y}{dt} = \gamma B_1(t) M_z - \Delta\omega M_x \tag{3.4}$$

$$\frac{dM_z}{dt} = -\gamma B_1(t) M_y$$

We note that Eq. (3.4) can equivalently be expressed in the vector-matrix form:

$$\frac{d\vec{M}}{dt} = \mathfrak{R}\vec{M} \qquad \mathfrak{R} = \begin{bmatrix} 0 & \Delta\omega & 0 \\ -\Delta\omega & 0 & \gamma B_1 \\ 0 & -\gamma B_1 & 0 \end{bmatrix} \tag{3.5}$$

which has the solution:

$$\vec{M}(t) = e^{\mathfrak{R}t}\vec{M}(t=0)$$

$$e^{\mathfrak{R}t} = \mathbb{I} + \mathfrak{R}t + \frac{1}{2}\mathfrak{R}^2 t^2 + \cdots \tag{3.6}$$

where $\mathbb{I}$ is the identity matrix. For analyzing excitation pulses, we generally choose the initial conditions $M_x = 0$, $M_y = 0$, and $M_z = M_0$ at $t = 0$ because the magnetization is initially aligned with the main magnetic field (i.e., the z direction). If Eq. (3.4) is further simplified by specifying that the

RF frequency matches the Larmor frequency (i.e., $\Delta\omega = 0$) the solution to the set of equations in (3.4) is:

$$M_x(t) = 0$$

$$M_y(t) = M_0 \sin\left\{\gamma \int_0^t B_1(t')dt'\right\}$$

$$M_z(t) = M_0 \cos\left\{\gamma \int_0^t B_1(t')dt'\right\} \tag{3.7}$$

Equation (3.7) simply states that, on-resonance, the magnetization precesses in the yz plane of the rotating frame (Figure 3.1), and the accumulated flip angle is given by Eq. (3.1). At the end of the pulse, Eq. (3.7) can be expressed, in terms of the flip angle θ, as:

$$M_x = 0$$
$$M_y = M_0 \sin\theta \tag{3.8}$$
$$M_z = M_0 \cos\theta$$

More generally, spherical coordinates can describe an arbitrary orientation of the magnetization vector. In that case the flip angle θ is the same as the polar angle, and ϕ represents the azimuthal angle that the transverse magnetization makes with the x axis:

$$M_x = M_0 \cos\phi \sin\theta$$
$$M_y = M_0 \sin\phi \sin\theta \tag{3.9}$$
$$M_z = M_0 \cos\theta$$

In general, $\phi \neq 90°$ except for the special case of on-resonance excitation ($\Delta\omega = 0$). Although we have assumed that the B_1 field is applied along the x axis in the rotating frame, similar results can also be obtained for B_1 field applied along other directions in the transverse plane. For example, when the B_1 field is applied along the y axis, the magnetization vector is rotated in the $(z, -x)$ plane and Eq. (3.9) becomes:

$$M_x = -M_0 \sin\phi' \sin\theta$$
$$M_y = M_0 \cos\phi' \sin\theta \tag{3.10}$$
$$M_z = M_0 \cos\theta$$

where ϕ' is the angle between the transverse magnetization and the y axis.

Fourier Transform Approximation   Except at the center of the selected slice profile, we cannot assume that the spins are exactly on-resonance. Therefore, in general, we cannot set $\Delta\omega = 0$ in Eq. (3.4). Instead, defining the complex transverse magnetization:

$$M_\perp = M_x + i M_y \qquad (3.11)$$

the first two equations in (3.4) can be reexpressed as:

$$\frac{dM_\perp}{dt} = -i \, \Delta\omega \, M_\perp + i\gamma B_1(t) M_z(t) \qquad (3.12)$$

With the initial condition $M_\perp = 0$ at $t = 0$, Eq. (3.12) has the solution (Joseph et al. 1984):

$$M_\perp(t) = i\gamma e^{-i\Delta\omega t} \int_0^t M_z(t') B_1(t') e^{i\Delta\omega t'} dt' \qquad (3.13)$$

Thus the complex transverse magnetization is proportional to the inverse Fourier transform of the product of the applied RF field and the z component of the magnetization. For practical calculations, Eq. (3.13) is not very helpful because $M_z(t)$ also changes throughout the RF pulse and is therefore not known. To a good approximation, however, for small flip angles $M_z(t) \approx M_0$, in which case:

$$M_\perp(t) \approx i\gamma M_0 e^{-i\Delta\omega t} \int_0^t B_1(t') e^{i\Delta\omega t'} dt' \qquad (3.14)$$

or

$$|M_\perp(t)| = \sqrt{M_x^2 + M_y^2} \approx \gamma M_0 \left| \int_0^t B_1(t') e^{i\Delta\omega t'} dt' \right| \qquad (3.15)$$

Combining Eqs. (3.9) and (3.15):

$$\sin\theta = \frac{\pm\sqrt{M_x^2 + M_y^2}}{M_0} = \frac{\pm|M_\perp(t)|}{M_0} \approx \pm\gamma \left| \int_0^t B_1(t') e^{i\Delta\omega t'} dt' \right| \qquad (3.16)$$

because $M_z(t) \approx M_0$, θ must be small and

$$\sin\theta \, (\Delta\omega) \approx \theta \, (\Delta\omega) \approx \pm\gamma \left| \int_0^t B_1(t') e^{i\Delta\omega t'} dt' \right| \qquad (3.17)$$

(Although mathematically θ and $\sin\theta$ can be either positive or negative, generally we chose the positive values because of the coordinate axis conventions that we have adopted.) Equation (3.17) states that, for small flip angles, the slice profile is approximately equal to the modulus of the inverse Fourier transform of the RF envelope. (Note the integration limits in Eq. 3.17 may be replaced by $-\infty$ to ∞ because $B_1(t)$ is 0 except during the pulse.) Equation (3.17) reduces to Eq. (3.1) on-resonance (i.e., when $\Delta\omega = 0$). The Fourier transform approximation (also called the *linear approximation* or the *small flip angle approximation*) given by Eqs. (3.16) and (3.17) generally holds quite well for flip angles up to $\theta = 30°$ and severely breaks down only when $\theta > 90°$. This robustness is due to the second-order dependence of $\cos\theta$ on θ, which is related to the key assumption in the Fourier transform approximation (i.e., $M_z \approx M_0$). That is, from Eq. (3.9):

$$M_z = M_0 \cos\theta = M_0 \left(1 - \frac{\theta^2}{2} + \cdots\right) \qquad (3.18)$$

Because the Fourier transform is a linear operation, deviations from Eq. (3.17) are known as *nonlinearity* in the Bloch equations.

For example, Figure 3.3 shows a windowed SINC (Section 2.2), which is a commonly used excitation pulse, along with its slice profile plotted versus frequency offset for three values of the flip angle. (The plots show the slice profiles for M_y (solid line) and M_x (dotted line), which are related to θ by Eq. 3.16.) At $\theta = 30°$ the magnetization response is essentially equal to the Fourier transform of the SINC excitation pulse. At the center of the slice profile $M_y(\Delta\omega = 0) = M_0 \sin 30° = 0.5\, M_0$, and $M_x = 0$, as predicted by Eq (3.7).

At $\theta = 90°$, some nonlinearity in the Bloch equation emerges. There is a side lobe (marked with an arrow) near the transition band of the response. Still, the slice profile is reasonably uniform. At the center of the slice $M_y(\Delta\omega = 0) = M_0 \sin(90°) = M_0$, which is twice as large as the $\theta = 30°$ case, and $M_x = 0$.

At $\theta = 150°$, nonlinearity in the Bloch equations is quite pronounced. The shape of the slice profile is severely distorted. Also, a substantial amount of the magnetization lies outside the yz plane, as illustrated by the relatively high amplitude of M_x, denoted by the dotted line. Despite this nonlinearity, at the center of the slice $M_y(\Delta\omega = 0) = M_0 \sin 150° = 0.5\, M_0$, and $M_x = 0$ as predicted by Eq. (3.7).

To summarize, θ is directly proportional to the amplitude $B_1(t)$ of a nonadiabatic pulse under two conditions: on-resonance excitation (i.e., at the center of the slice profile) and small flip angle excitation. On the other hand, the transverse magnetization $|M_\perp|$ is directly proportional to the amplitude of a nonadiabatic pulse only for small flip angles because $\sin\theta \approx \theta$ only when

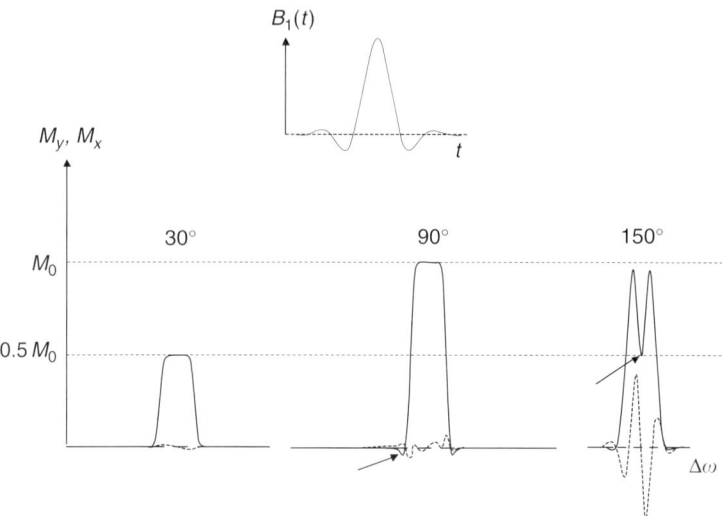

FIGURE 3.3 Nonlinearity of the Bloch equations. A windowed SINC excitation pulse is shown, along with the transverse magnetization responses (plotted versus angular frequency offset) at flip angles of $\theta = 30°$, $90°$, and $150°$. The solid line represents M_y, and the dotted line represents M_x. At $\theta = 30°$ the response is approximately equal to the inverse Fourier transform of the excitation pulse. At $90°$ the effects of nonlinearity are emerging, as illustrated by the side lobe (arrow). At $150°$, severe nonlinearity is apparent. At the center of the slice profile (on-resonance), the response is given by $M_x = 0$ and $M_y = M_0 \sin \theta$, even at $\theta = 150°$ (arrow).

$\theta \ll 1$ rad. Because of the Bloch equation nonlinearity, SLR (Section 2.3) or iterative numerical methods rather than Fourier methods are usually used for RF pulse design when high-quality slice profiles are needed.

Excitation as Resonance   The RF excitation process is a resonance phenomenon, which contributes the R to the acronyms NMR (nuclear magnetic resonance) and MRI. Mathematically, the resonance can be seen from Eq. (3.13). When the resonance offset $\Delta\omega$ is large (in units of γB_1), then the oscillation of the complex exponential in the integral causes cancellation, and hence zero $M_\perp$ and no MR signal. This same effect can be appreciated qualitatively by considering the precession of the B_1 field in relation to the precession of the magnetization. Only at or near resonance does B_1 precess at the same rate as the magnetization, so that the magnetization is efficiently tipped. Also, recall that in the rotating frame the magnetization precesses about the effective magnetic field (see Section 1.2, Eq. (1.73)). On-resonance, the effective field lies in the transverse plane and can effectively tip the magnetization away from the z axis. Far from resonance, however, the effective field is nearly aligned with the z axis and cannot create a large transverse component of the magnetization, regardless of the duration of the pulse. This property is exploited in adiabatic pulses to induce adiabatic excitation (Section 6.1).

3.1.2 Practical Implementation

Commonly used selective RF excitation pulses include SINC pulses (Section 2.2) and a variety of Shinnar–Le Roux (SLR) pulses (Section 2.3). Selective excitation pulses are used in conjunction with a slice-selection gradient (Section 8.3). Nonlinearity of the Bloch equations has an effect on the slice profiles of all of these pulses. SLR pulses account for that nonlinearity in their design, but it is important to remember that each SLR pulse is designed to be played at a specific flip angle and that if a different flip angle is selected the slice profile will deviate from its design. Short-duration rectangular hard pulses (Section 2.1) are also used when no slice-selection gradient is required, such as in some 3D volume acquisitions.

In addition to the flip angle and RF bandwidth (see Section 8.3 on slice selection), an important parameter of a selective excitation pulse is its *isodelay* Δt_I. After the selective RF pulse is played along the x axis, the transverse magnetization at different spatial locations will generally not lie exactly along the y axis in the rotating frame because of precession caused by the slice-selection gradient. Instead there will be phase dispersion (or variation of the azimuthal angle ϕ) across the slice. The isodelay is the effective precession or dephasing time that results in this phase dispersion. The purpose of the slice-rephasing gradient pulse is to refocus this slice dispersion to the maximal extent possible (Hutchinson et al. 1978). The isodelay parameter Δt_I is used to calculate the optimal area of the slice-rephasing gradient. The isodelay is therefore the amount of time, measured from the end of the pulse, to include in the refocusing calculation. For example, in Figure 3.4:

$$G_z \Delta t_I + \frac{G_z r_z}{2} = A_R \qquad (3.19)$$

where A_R is the area of the slice-rephasing lobe, including its ramps (shaded in Figure 3.4). Once the value of the area of the rephasing pulse is known, the details of its amplitude, plateau, and ramps can be determined using the methods of Section 7.1.

Generally the isodelay corresponds to the amount of time from the peak to the end of the RF excitation pulse. For SINC and linear-phase SLR pulses the

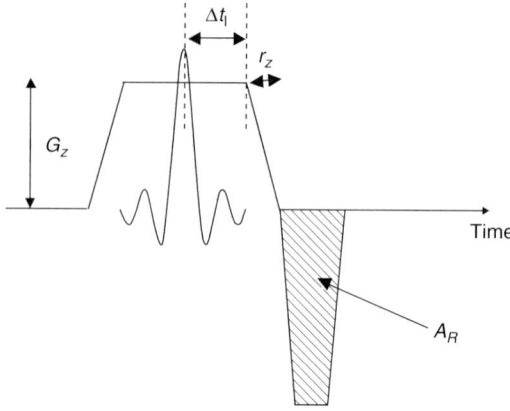

FIGURE 3.4 The isodelay Δt_I is a parameter of an RF excitation pulse that is used in Eq. (3.19) to calculate the optimal area of rephasing gradient lobe (shaded). The isodelay is approximately equal to the time from the peak to the end of the RF excitation pulse.

isodelay is nearly equal to one-half the RF pulse width. For minimum-phase SLR pulses the isodelay is much smaller than one-half the pulse width, which allows for shorter slice-rephasing lobes and hence reduced minimum TE. On the other hand, for maximum-phase SLR pulses the isodelay is greater than one-half the pulse width. Because of the nonlinearity of the Bloch equations, isodelay can depend on flip angle. Because the variation is typically only on the order of tens of microseconds, this dependence is often neglected.

SELECTED REFERENCES

Hoult, D. I. 1980. NMR imaging rotating frame selective pulses. *J. Magn. Reson.* 38: 369–374.

Hutchinson, J. M. S., Sutherland, R. J., and Mallard, J. R. 1978. NMR Imaging: Image recovery under magnetic fields with large non-uniformities. *J. Phys.* E.11: 217–221.

Joseph, P. M., Axel, L., and O'Donnell, M. 1984. Potential problems with selective pulses in NMR imaging systems. *Med. Phys.* 11: 772–777.

Pauly, J., Le Roux, P., Nishimura, D., and Macovski, A. 1991. Parameter relations for the Shinnar-LeRoux selective excitation pulse design algorithm. *IEEE Trans. Med. Imag.* 10: 53–65.

RELATED SECTIONS

3.2 Inversion Pulses

An inversion pulse nutates the magnetization vector from the direction of the main magnetic field $\vec{B}_0$ (i.e., the positive z axis by convention) to the negative $\vec{B}_0$ direction (Figure 3.5a). Although an inversion pulse nominally rotates the magnetization vector by 180° about an axis in the transverse plane (i.e., the xy plane), the flip angle can be slightly larger or smaller either by design or due to system imperfections. A non-180° pulse can still function as an inversion pulse, as long as it results in a magnetization vector whose z component is negative at the end of the pulse.

Inversion pulses can be categorized according to a variety of properties, such as pulse shape, spatial selectivity, spectral selectivity, and adiabaticity. These categories are not mutually exclusive. For example, a SINC-shaped inversion pulse can be used for spatial or spectral selection. Common inversion pulse shapes include SINC, minimum or linear phase SLR, rectangular, Gaussian, adiabatic hyperbolic secant, variable-rate, and composite. These pulse shapes are discussed individually in other sections of this book. The selectivity of an inversion pulse is determined by both its pulse shape and the pulse width. Inversion pulses with constant RF amplitude (i.e., rectangular or hard pulses) are typically nonselective, whereas amplitude modulated pulses are usually frequency selective. If a frequency selective inversion pulse

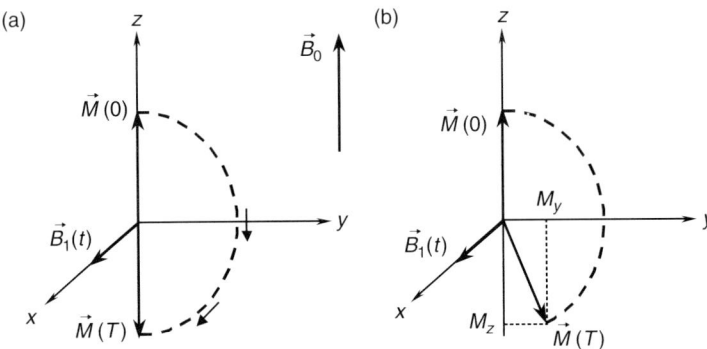

FIGURE 3.5 Time evolution of on-resonance magnetization during an inversion pulse in an RF rotating reference frame. The initial magnetization vector $\vec{M}(0)$ is aligned with the main magnetic field $\vec{B}_0$, which lies along the z axis. An RF inversion pulse $\vec{B}_1(t)$ that is applied along the x axis rotates the magnetization vector in the yz plane about the x axis. (a) At the end of the pulse (i.e., at time T), the magnetization $\vec{M}(T)$ is aligned along the negative z axis, provided that the flip angle is 180°. (b) When the flip angle deviates from 180°, the inversion is incomplete and a transverse magnetization M_y is produced.

is played out concurrently with a slice-selection gradient, then it becomes spatially selective; otherwise, it exhibits spectral selectivity. In this section, we focus primarily on nonadiabatic inversion pulses; a discussion of adiabatic inversion pulses is given in Section 6.2.

Inversion pulses share many properties with refocusing pulses; for example, their nominal flip angles are both 180°. Unlike the initial condition assumed for refocusing pulses, however, the magnetization vector is aligned along the z axis prior to an inversion pulse. Nonadiabatic, linear phase (e.g., SINC or linear phase SLR) inversion pulses and refocusing pulses are nearly interchangeable. For example, there is only a slight difference in frequency response between inversion and refocusing SLR pulses (Pauly et al. 1991). It is worth noting, however, that a refocusing pulse is typically accompanied by a crusher gradient pair (Section 10.2), whereas an inversion pulse is usually followed by a spoiler gradient to dephase any residual transverse magnetization (Section 10.5).

Inversion and excitation pulses share the same initial condition (i.e., the magnetization is initially aligned with the B_0 field). An excitation pulse, however, results in substantial transverse magnetization, whereas an ideal inversion pulse produces none (Figure 3.5a). A nonselective inversion pulse can be obtained by increasing the flip angle of a nonselective excitation pulse to 180°. A tailored selective inversion pulse (such an SLR pulse), on the other hand, usually cannot be obtained by simply increasing the flip angle of an excitation pulse.

3.2.1 MATHEMATICAL DESCRIPTION

Consider a magnetization vector $\vec{M}$ at equilibrium with a magnitude of M_0:

$$\vec{M}(0) = M_0 \begin{bmatrix} 0 \\ 0 \\ 1 \end{bmatrix} \tag{3.20}$$

According to Eq. (3.5), the time evolution of $\vec{M}$ during an RF pulse applied along the x axis can be calculated by solving the following Bloch equations in the rotating reference frame:

$$\begin{bmatrix} dM_x/dt \\ dM_y/dt \\ dM_z/dt \end{bmatrix} = \begin{bmatrix} 0 & \Delta\omega & 0 \\ -\Delta\omega & 0 & \gamma B_1 \\ 0 & -\gamma B_1 & 0 \end{bmatrix} \begin{bmatrix} M_x \\ M_y \\ M_z \end{bmatrix} \tag{3.21}$$

where $\Delta\omega$ is the off-resonant frequency and B_1 is the RF magnetic field of the pulse. In Eq. (3.21), we have neglected the relaxation effects, and assumed an RF rotating reference frame defined in Section 1.2.

As shown in Section 3.1, in the on-resonance case ($\Delta\omega = 0$) the magnetization simply precesses about the B_1 direction in the yz plane (Figure 3.5). The evolution of the magnetization can be described using the following equation:

$$\vec{M}(t) = M_0 \begin{bmatrix} 1 & 0 & 0 \\ 0 & \cos\theta(t) & \sin\theta(t) \\ 0 & -\sin\theta(t) & \cos\theta(t) \end{bmatrix} \begin{bmatrix} 0 \\ 0 \\ 1 \end{bmatrix} \qquad (3.22)$$

where:

$$\theta(t) = \gamma \int_0^t B_1(t')dt' \qquad (3.23)$$

The angle $\theta(t)$ is the instantaneous flip angle during the RF pulse and is directly proportional to the time integral of the B_1 field. At the end of an ideal inversion pulse (i.e., $t = T$), $\theta(T)$ equals π (or $180°$) and the magnetization is inverted. When the flip angle deviates from $180°$, the magnetization inversion is incomplete, resulting in nonzero transverse magnetization along the y axis (Figure 3.5b).

Equations (3.22) and (3.23) are valid only for spins exactly on-resonance. For off-resonance spins (i.e., $\Delta\omega \neq 0$), the evolution of the magnetization can be obtained by numerically solving the Bloch equations as outlined in Slichter (1989). With the off-resonance term, the time evolution of M_x now depends on M_y (i.e., $dM_x/dt = \Delta\omega M_y$, as implied by Eq. 3.21). Because M_y is not zero throughout the inversion pulse, a nonzero M_x component is inevitably produced. This reduces the magnitude of the longitudinal magnetization at the end of the pulse.

The off-resonant effect also can be graphically analyzed using the concept of effective magnetic field introduced in Section 1.2. With the off-resonance term, the effective magnetic field $\vec{B}_{\text{eff}}$ is tilted away from the x axis toward the z axis (Figure 3.6). The magnetization vector rotates about $\vec{B}_{\text{eff}}$, instead of the x axis, resulting in a nonzero M_x component (Figure 3.6). A nonzero M_y component is also produced unless the flip angle at the end of the pulse (i.e., $\gamma \int_0^T B_{\text{eff}}(t)dt$) is exactly $180°$.

The off-resonance term arises from a number of sources, including the slice-selection gradient, chemical shift, magnetic field inhomogeneity, and magnetic susceptibility variations. Although certain sources (e.g., magnetic field inhomogeneity) can be reduced through system calibration and compensation, sources such as the slice-selection gradient and chemical shift cannot be eliminated. Thus, the off-resonant effects should always be carefully examined when designing inversion pulses.

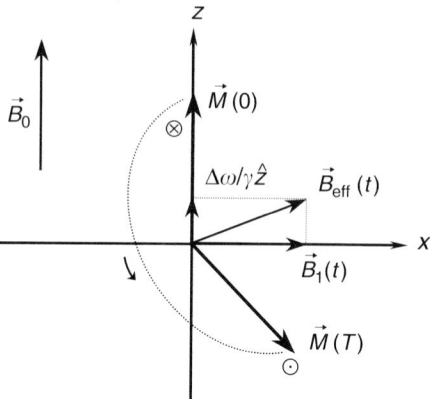

FIGURE 3.6 The effect of resonance offset on an inversion pulse. With the off-resonance term, $(\Delta\omega/\gamma)\hat{z}$ (where $\hat{z}$ is a unit vector long the z axis), the effective magnetic field becomes $\vec{B}_{\text{eff}}(t) = \vec{B}_1(t) + (\Delta\omega/\gamma)\hat{z}$. The magnetization vector rotates about $\vec{B}_{\text{eff}}(t)$, resulting in a transverse component along the x axis even with a 180° flip angle. The $\odot$ and $\otimes$ symbols schematically represent the head and tail of an arrow, respectively, to illustrate the path of the magnetization vector. These symbols indicate that the precession is such that the head of $\vec{M}(0)$ moves into the page and the head of $\vec{M}(T)$ moves out of the page.

3.2.2 PRACTICAL CONSIDERATIONS

Selective Inversion Pulses   The simplest approach to designing a selective inversion pulse is to choose the time-domain pulse shape as the Fourier transform of the desired spatial or spectral profile. For example, a SINC pulse (or a windowed SINC pulse as discussed in Section 2.2) together with a constant gradient can be used to approximate a rectangular slice profile. Due to the nonlinearity in the Bloch equations at large flip angles, however, the Fourier transform approximation produces errors in the targeted slice profile (Pauly et al. 1991). Although SINC inversion pulses are still used in some applications, they have been largely replaced by tailored RF pulses, such as SLR pulses (Pauly et al. 1991) and pulses generated using optimal control theory (Mao et al. 1986), or by selective adiabatic inversion pulses, such as the hyperbolic secant pulse (Silver et al. 1984).

SLR inversion pulses can considerably improve the quality of slice (or spectral) profile and allow trade-offs among a number of parameters, including the width of the transition regions, ripples within the slice, and ripples outside the slice. The details on how to design SLR pulses are given in Section 2.3 and Pauly et al. (1991). Once the pulse has been designed, the actual slice inversion profile can be obtained by numerically solving the Bloch equations

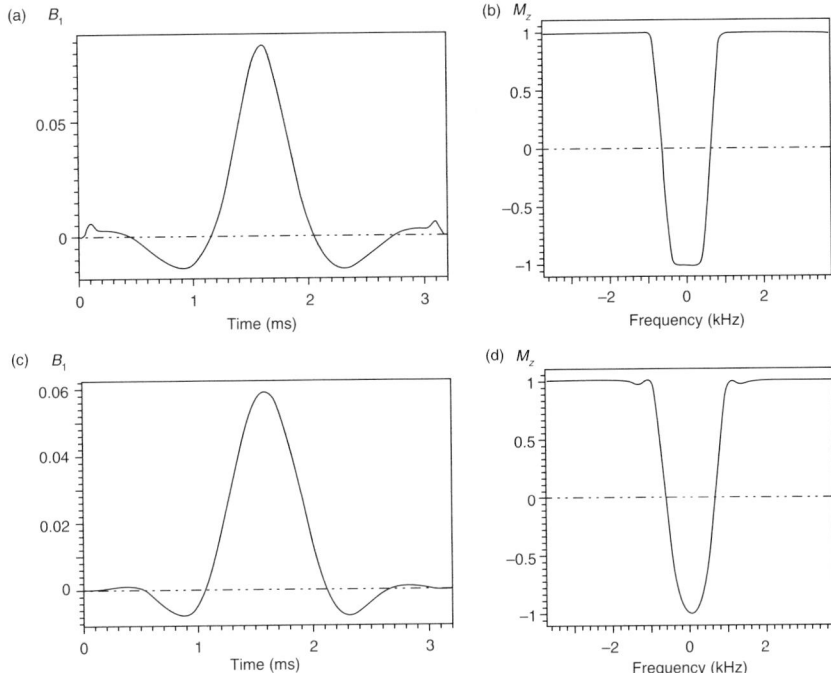

FIGURE 3.7 (a) A linear-phase SLR inversion pulse. (b) The frequency (or slice) profile of the SLR pulse. (c) A SINC inversion pulse with a symmetric Hamming window. (d) The frequency (or slice) profile of the SINC pulse. Both pulses have the same bandwidth of 1.28 kHz and the same pulse width of 3.2 ms. The SLR pulse is designed with passband ripple $= 0.5\%$ and stopband ripple $= 1\%$. The abscissa is displayed in kilohertz, but can be converted to distance (e.g., centimeters) if a slice-selection gradient with known amplitude is applied. The B_1 field is in arbitrary units, and the M_z axis is in units of M_0.

or by a forward SLR transform:

$$M_z(r) = M_0 \left(1 - 2\,|\beta|^2\right) \tag{3.24}$$

where β is one of the Cayley-Klein parameters defined in Section 2.3. An example of a linear-phase SLR inversion pulse and its slice profile is shown in Figure 3.7a–b. Its design parameters are pulse width $= 3.2$ ms, bandwidth $= 1.28$ kHz (full-width at $M_z = 0$), ripples in the passband $= 0.5\%$, ripples in the stopband $= 1\%$, and flip angle $= 180°$. Compared to a Hamming-windowed SINC inversion pulse with identical pulse width, bandwidth (also defined as full-width at $M_z = 0$), and flip angle (Figure 3.7c–d), the SLR inversion pulse clearly produces a more uniform slice profile.

The difference between the two pulses can be understood by recognizing that the SINC pulse is essentially the Fourier transform of an ideal rectangular profile. As such, the SINC pulse makes an effective excitation pulse because the slice profile in that case is proportional to $|\beta|$. (Note that $|\beta|$ is approximately proportional to the magnitude of the Fourier transform of an excitation RF pulse under the small flip angle approximation; Pauly et al. 1991.) The slice profile of an inversion pulse, however, is given by Eq. (3.24), which contains a $|\beta|^2$ term. The squaring operation tends to make the slice profile of the SINC more sharply peaked (i.e., pointy) as shown in Figure 3.7d. During the SLR design of an inversion pulse, however, the distortion of the profile due to squaring operation is accounted for in the design of β, so the final profile has a flatter response over the inverted spatial region as shown in Figure 3.7b.

Excellent slice profiles can also be obtained using a selective adiabatic inversion pulse. An example is the hyperbolic secant pulse discussed in Section 6.2. This pulse has a simple analytical form and exhibits a large degree of immunity to B_1 field variations. This is in sharp contrast to SLR inversion pulses designed only for specific flip angles.

Similar to selective excitation and refocusing pulses, the dimensionless time-bandwidth product $(T\Delta f)$ is an important parameter for designing selective inversion pulses. $T\Delta f$ is typically chosen between 2 and 8. Increasing $T\Delta f$ improves the spectral or spatial profile, but results in a longer pulse width (with bandwidth fixed). If an inversion pulse is used for spatial selection, the required gradient amplitude can be calculated as shown in Example 3.2.

Example 3.2 An SLR inversion pulse has a time-bandwidth product of 4 and a pulse width of 3.2 ms. If this pulse is used to invert a 5 mm slice, what is the amplitude of the slice-selection gradient?

Answer The bandwidth of the pulse is $\Delta f = 4/(3.2\,\mathrm{ms}) = 1.25\,\mathrm{kHz}$. The slice-selection gradient amplitude can be calculated using Eq. (8.52) (see Section 8.3):

$$G_{\text{slice}} = \frac{2\pi \Delta f}{\gamma \Delta z} = \frac{2\pi \times 1.25\,\mathrm{kHz}}{2\pi \times 42.57\,\mathrm{kHz/mT} \times 0.005\,\mathrm{m}} = 5.87\,\mathrm{mT/m}$$

Nonselective Inversion Pulses Nonselective inversion pulses, also known as hard pulses, are typically rectangular in shape with a short pulse width (e.g., from a few to several hundred microseconds) to ensure a broad frequency response. In practice, depending on the hardware, ramping up and ramping down periods for the RF pulse also might be required, as discussed in Section 2.1. Because the area of the inversion pulse must satisfy:

$$\gamma \int_0^T B_1(t)dt \simeq \pi \qquad (3.25)$$

a shorter pulse width requires a larger B_1 amplitude. The minimum pulse width is typically determined by the maximum power that an RF coil can receive and sustain. It is interesting to note that the shortest hard pulse width also depends on the type of nucleus to be inverted. For spins other than protons, such as ^{23}Na and ^{31}P, the gyromagnetic ratio is considerably smaller than that of ^{1}H. Thus, sodium or phosphorus imaging requires a longer pulse width to reach 180° inversion.

Example 3.3   An RF coil can produce a maximum B_1 field of 250 μT. What is the shortest pulse width for a rectangular nonselective pulse to invert proton and ^{23}Na magnetization, respectively? (Neglect RF ramps on the hard pulse.)

Answer   According to Eq. (3.25), the pulse width for a rectangular inversion pulse is $T = \pi/\gamma B_1$. For proton and ^{23}Na spins, $\gamma = 2\pi \times 0.04257$ kHz/μT and $\gamma = 2\pi \times 0.01126$ kHz/μT, respectively. Thus, the corresponding pulse widths are:

$$T_H = \pi/(2\pi \times 0.04257 \text{ kHz/μT} \times 250 \text{ μT}) = 47.0 \text{ μs}$$

$$T_{Na} = \pi/(2\pi \times 0.01126 \text{ kHz/μT} \times 250 \text{ μT}) = 178 \text{ μs}$$

3.2.3 APPLICATIONS

Inversion pulses have many applications in MRI. An inversion pulse followed by a delay time TI can be appended to the front of an excitation pulse to nullify a specific tissue with a distinct T_1 relaxation time. This approach is employed in short tau inversion recovery (STIR) (Bydder and Young, 1985) and spectral inversion at lipids (SPECIAL) (Foo et al. 1994) to suppress lipid signals and in fluid attenuated inversion recovery (FLAIR) (Hajnal et al. 1992) to eliminate hyperintense signals from cerebrospinal fluid. An inversion pulse can also be incorporated into a pulse sequence to alter the T_1 contrast in an image. This technique is sometimes referred to as inversion recovery preparation (IR-Prep) or magnetization preparation (MP) (Mugler and Brookeman 1990). In addition, inversion pulses are widely used in measuring the tissue T_1 relaxation times and in tissue perfusion as described in Section 17.1.

SELECTED REFERENCES

Bydder, G. M., and Young, I. R. 1985. MR imaging: clinical use of the inversion recovery sequence. *J. Comp. Assist. Tomogr.* 9: 659–675.

Foo, T. K. F., Sawyer, A. M., Faulkner, W. H., and Mills, D. G. 1994. Inversion in the steady-state—contrast optimization and reduced imaging time with fast 3-dimensional inversion-recovery–prepared GRE pulse sequences. *Radiology* 191: 85–90.

Hajnol, J. V., De Coene, B., Lewis, P. D., Baudouin, C. J., Cowan, F. M., Pennock, J. M., Young, I. R., and Bydder, G. M. 1992. High signal regions in normal white matter shown by heavily T2-weighted CSF nulled IR sequences. *J. Comp. Assist. Tomogr.* 16: 506–513.

Mao, J., Mareci, T. H., Scott, K. N., and Andrew, E. R. 1986. Selective inversion radio frequency pulses by optimal control theory. *J. Magn. Reson.* 70: 310–318.

Mugler, J. H., III, and Brookeman, J. R. 1990. Three-dimensional magnetization-prepared rapid gradient-echo imaging (3D MP-RAGE). *Magn. Reson. Med.* 15: 152–157.

Pauly, J., Le Roux, P., Nishimura, D., and Macovski, A. 1991. Parameter relations for the Shinnar-Le Roux selective excitation pulse design algorithm. *IEEE Trans. Med. Imag.* 10: 53–65.

Silver, M. S., Joseph, R. I., and Hoult, D. I. 1984. Highly selective $\pi/2$ and π pulse generation. *J. Magn. Reson.* 59: 347–351.

Slichter, C. P. 1989. *Principles of magnetic resonance.* Berlin: Springer-Verlag.

3.3 Refocusing Pulses

The transverse magnetization excited by an RF pulse usually consists of contributions from many spin isochromats. Due to applied imaging gradients, local magnetic field inhomogeneity, magnetic susceptibility variation, or chemical shift, these spin isochromats have a range of precession frequencies. Some precess faster than the average Larmor frequency, while others precess slower. This produces a *phase dispersion* (or fanning out) among the spin isochromats (Figure 3.8). A *refocusing RF pulse* rotates the dispersing spin isochromats about an axis in the transverse plane so that the magnetization vectors will rephase (or refocus) at a later time. The refocused magnetization is known as an *RF spin echo*, or simply a *spin echo* (Hahn 1950).

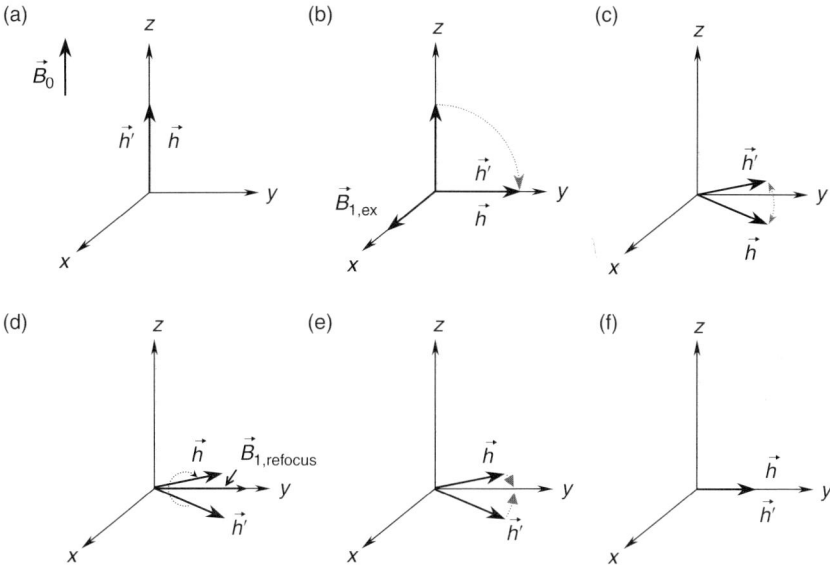

FIGURE 3.8 Time evolution of two spin isochromats $\vec{h}$ and $\vec{h}'$ in the rotating reference frame, demonstrating the effect of the refocusing pulse. (a) The initial magnetization vectors for both spin isochromats are aligned with the main magnetic field $\vec{B}_0$ (i.e., the z axis). (b) After an RF excitation pulse $B_{1,ex}(t)$ applied along the x axis, both magnetization vectors are rotated onto the y axis. (c) Because of off-resonance effects, $\vec{h}$ precesses faster than the frequency of the reference frame (i.e., clockwise rotation), while $\vec{h}'$ precesses slower (i.e., counter-clockwise rotation). (d) When a 180° refocusing pulse is applied, $\vec{h}$ and $\vec{h}'$ are rotated by 180° about the y axis. (e) Following the refocusing pulse, $\vec{h}$ and $\vec{h}'$ continue to precess as indicated by the arrows. (f) After a delay time, $\vec{h}$ and $\vec{h}'$ meet at the y axis, forming a spin echo. The transverse magnetization vectors are diminishing in size due to T_2 decay.

Refocusing RF pulses commonly have a flip angle of 180°. At this flip angle, the transverse magnetization is optimally refocused and the largest spin echo signal is produced. Pulses with flip angles other than 180° are also capable of refocusing the transverse magnetization vectors, although the refocusing is only partial. When multiple non-180° refocusing pulses are applied in a sequence, *stimulated echoes* can be produced. This phenomenon is described in Section 16.4.

Many types of pulses can be used for refocusing, including, but not limited to, rectangular (hard), SINC, SLR, composite, adiabatic, or variable-rate pulses. A refocusing pulse can be spatially selective, spectrally selective, or nonselective. Common spatially selective pulses include SINC pulses and SLR pulses, whereas nonselective pulses are almost exclusively rectangular in shape. These refocusing pulses are discussed later in this section. Adiabatic refocusing pulses belong to a special class of pulses that can provide excellent immunity to B_1 field variations, but require somewhat longer pulse widths (e.g., 8 ms) and typically deposit more RF power. They can be used as nonselective refocusing pulses, as detailed in Section 6.3.

3.3.1 QUALITATIVE DESCRIPTION

Figure 3.8a shows the magnetization vectors ($\vec{h}$ and $\vec{h}'$) associated with two spin isochromats. Immediately after a 90° excitation pulse, $\vec{h}$ and $\vec{h}'$ are both nutated to the y axis, as shown in Figure 3.8b. Consider the time evolution of $\vec{h}$ and $\vec{h}'$ in a rotating reference frame whose frequency is set to the average Larmor frequency of $\vec{h}$ and $\vec{h}'$. If $\vec{h}$ and $\vec{h}'$ both have the same Larmor frequency, they will appear stationary in this rotating frame. If, however, $\vec{h}$ precesses slightly faster and $\vec{h}'$ slightly slower than the average Larmor frequency, the two vectors will precess in opposite directions as viewed from the rotating frame (Figure 3.8c). When a 180° refocusing pulse $\vec{B}_1$ is applied along the y axis, both $\vec{h}$ and $\vec{h}'$ will be rotated about the y axis by 180° (Figure 3.8d). After the refocusing pulse is terminated, the two magnetization vectors continue to precess as before (Figure 3.8e) and rephase (or *refocus*) after a time delay as shown in Figure 3.8f. Therefore, an RF spin echo is produced.

This discussion assumes that the refocusing RF pulse is applied along the y axis and has a flip angle of 180° but refocusing pulses still function even if these assumptions are relaxed. For example, a refocusing pulse can be applied along the x axis, in which case the magnetization will be refocused along the negative y-axis instead. In fact, the refocusing pulse can be applied along any direction in the transverse plane as shown in Example 3.4. In addition, an RF spin echo can still be formed if the flip angle deviates from 180°, as quantitatively shown in the next subsection.

Example 3.4   Assuming that a 90° excitation and a 180° refocusing pulse make angles α_1 and α_2 with the positive x axis in the rotating reference frame, respectively, prove that magnetization is refocused along a direction at an angle $2\alpha_2 - \alpha_1 - 90°$ with respect to the x axis.

Answer   Let us consider the magnetization vectors and the B_1 field for the RF pulses in the transverse plane. Further, let us assume that both RF pulses are applied on resonance. At the end of the excitation pulse $\vec{B}_{1,ex}$, the magnetization vector $\vec{M}_{ex}$ is nutated to the transverse plane in a direction perpendicular to $\vec{B}_{1,ex}$, as shown in Figure 3.9a. Because $\vec{M}_{ex} \perp \vec{B}_{1,ex}$, the angle between $\vec{M}_{ex}$ and the y axis is also α_1. From Figure 3.9b, it can be seen that the angle

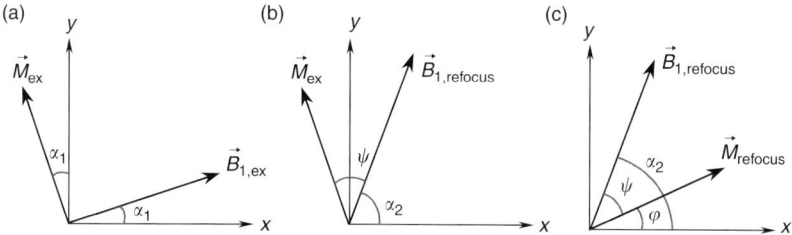

FIGURE 3.9 A top view of the transverse plane, showing the transverse magnetization and B_1 fields used in Example 3.4. (a) Magnetization vector $\vec{M}_{ex}$ after the 90° excitation pulse $\vec{B}_{1,ex}$. (b) The 180° refocusing pulse $\vec{B}_{1,refocus}$ in relation to the excited magnetization $\vec{M}_{ex}$. (c) The refocused magnetization $\vec{M}_{refocus}$ after the refocusing pulse.

between $\vec{M}_{ex}$ and the refocusing B_1 field $\vec{B}_{1,refocus}$ is:

$$\psi = \alpha_1 + (90° - \alpha_2) \tag{3.26}$$

At the end of the RF refocusing pulse, $\vec{M}_{ex}$ is rotated by 180° about $\vec{B}_{1,refocus}$ and the resultant magnetization vector becomes $\vec{M}_{refocus}$ (Figure 3.9c). The angle between $\vec{M}_{refocus}$ and the x axis is:

$$\varphi = \alpha_2 - \psi \tag{3.27}$$

Combining Eqs. (3.26) and (3.27), we obtain:

$$\varphi = 2\alpha_2 - \alpha_1 - 90° \tag{3.28}$$

3.3.2 MATHEMATICAL DESCRIPTION

Effects of a Refocusing Pulse on Magnetization   In this subsection we analyze an isochromat of transverse magnetization as it undergoes excitation, precession, refocusing, and finally formation of an RF spin echo. Suppose the isochromat has magnetization M_0 and resonance offset $\Delta\omega = \omega - \omega_{ref}$, where ω_{ref} is the angular frequency of the rotating frame. The magnetization M_0 can be expressed as:

$$M_0(\Delta\omega) = M_{0,total} \, f(\Delta\omega) \, d(\Delta\omega) \tag{3.29}$$

where $f(\Delta\omega)$ is the normalized distribution function of the off-resonant frequency $\Delta\omega$ (i.e., a spectrum of $\Delta\omega$) that satisfies:

$$\int_{-\infty}^{\infty} f(\Delta\omega) \, d(\Delta\omega) = 1 \tag{3.30}$$

and $M_{0,\text{total}}$ is the total magnetization. Immediately after an excitation pulse (flip angle $= \theta_1$) along the x axis, the magnetization of the spin isochromat can be described by:

$$\vec{M}(\Delta\omega, t = 0) = M_0 \begin{bmatrix} 0 \\ \sin\theta_1 \\ \cos\theta_1 \end{bmatrix} \tag{3.31}$$

(The argument of M_0 is dropped for simplicity.) In general, $\vec{M}$ can have a different Larmor frequency ω than the rotating frame frequency ω_{ref}, leading to nonzero values of $\Delta\omega$. Because of this resonance offset, $\vec{M}$ precesses about the z axis as described by:

$$\vec{M}(\Delta\omega, t) = M_0 \begin{bmatrix} e^{-t/T_2}\sin\theta_1\sin(\Delta\omega t) \\ e^{-t/T_2}\sin\theta_1\cos(\Delta\omega t) \\ e^{-t/T_1}\cos\theta_1 + (1 - e^{-t/T_1}) \end{bmatrix} \tag{3.32}$$

where the exponential terms account for the T_1 and T_2 relaxation effects (see Eq. 1.67). If a refocusing RF pulse with a flip angle of θ_2 and a duration $\ll T_2$ is applied along the y axis, the magnetization immediately before ($\vec{M}(\Delta\omega, \tau_-)$) and immediately after ($\vec{M}(\Delta\omega, \tau_+)$) the refocusing pulse are related by a rotation matrix $\Re_y(\theta_2)$:

$$\vec{M}(\Delta\omega, \tau_+) = \Re_y(\theta_2)\,\vec{M}(\Delta\omega, \tau_-) \tag{3.33}$$

where τ is the time between the isodelay points of the excitation and the refocusing pulses with subscripts $-$ and $+$ indicating immediately before and after reaching the isodelay point of the refocusing pulse, and $\Re_y(\theta_2)$ denotes a rotation about the y axis by θ_2 rad. Equation (3.33) can be equivalently expressed as:

$$\begin{bmatrix} M_x(\tau_+) \\ M_y(\tau_+) \\ M_z(\tau_+) \end{bmatrix} = \begin{bmatrix} \cos\theta_2 & 0 & -\sin\theta_2 \\ 0 & 1 & 0 \\ \sin\theta_2 & 0 & \cos\theta_2 \end{bmatrix} \begin{bmatrix} M_x(\tau_-) \\ M_y(\tau_-) \\ M_z(\tau_-) \end{bmatrix} \tag{3.34}$$

Using Eq.(3.32), we have:

$$\begin{bmatrix} M_x(\tau_-) \\ M_y(\tau_-) \\ M_z(\tau_-) \end{bmatrix} = M_0 \begin{bmatrix} e^{-\tau/T_2}\sin\theta_1\sin(\Delta\omega\tau) \\ e^{-\tau/T_2}\sin\theta_1\cos(\Delta\omega\tau) \\ e^{-\tau/T_1}\cos\theta_1 + (1 - e^{-\tau/T_1}) \end{bmatrix} \tag{3.35}$$

Because we are primarily interested in the transverse magnetization, let us define a complex quantity $M_\perp$ that includes both components of the transverse magnetization (see Section 1.2.):

$$M_\perp \equiv M_x + iM_y \tag{3.36}$$

Using Eqs. (3.34)–(3.36), $M_\perp$ at $t = \tau_+$ is found to be:

$$M_\perp(\Delta\omega, \tau_+) = i M_0 e^{-\tau/T_2} \sin\theta_1 \left(\cos^2(\theta_2/2) e^{-i\Delta\omega\tau} + \sin^2(\theta_2/2) e^{i\Delta\omega\tau} \right)$$
$$- M_0 \sin\theta_2 \left(1 - (1 - \cos\theta_1)e^{-\tau/T_1} \right) \tag{3.37}$$

After the refocusing pulse, the transverse magnetization will continue to precess about the z axis, as described by:

$$\vec{M}(\Delta\omega, t) =$$
$$\begin{bmatrix} e^{-(t-\tau)/T_2} \left(M_x(\tau_+) \cos(\Delta\omega(t-\tau)) + M_y(\tau_+) \sin(\Delta\omega(t-\tau)) \right) \\ e^{-(t-\tau)/T_2} \left(-M_x(\tau_+) \sin(\Delta\omega(t-\tau)) + M_y(\tau_+) \cos(\Delta\omega(t-\tau)) \right) \\ M_0(1 - e^{-(t-\tau)/T_1}) + M_z(\tau_+)e^{-(t-\tau)/T_1} \end{bmatrix}$$
$$\tag{3.38}$$

where t is the total time elapsed since the isodelay point of the excitation pulse. Equation (3.38) indicates that the transverse magnetization continuously experiences T_2 decay while freely precessing with a frequency $\Delta\omega$. This is equivalent to modulating $M_\perp(\Delta\omega, \tau_+)$ with an amplitude $e^{-(t-\tau)/T_2}$ and a phase $e^{-i\Delta\omega(t-\tau)}$:

$$M_\perp(\Delta\omega, t) = M_\perp(\Delta\omega, \tau_+)e^{-(t-\tau)/T_2}e^{-i\Delta\omega(t-\tau)}$$
$$= i M_0 e^{-t/T_2} \sin\theta_1 \cos^2(\theta_2/2) e^{-i\Delta\omega t}$$
$$+ i M_0 e^{-t/T_2} \sin\theta_1 \sin^2(\theta_2/2) e^{-i\Delta\omega(t-2\tau)}$$
$$- M_0 e^{-(t-\tau)/T_2} \left(1 - (1 - \cos\theta_1)e^{-\tau/T_1} \right) \sin\theta_2 e^{-i\Delta\omega(t-\tau)}$$
$$\tag{3.39}$$

Equation (3.39) has several implications. First, when $\theta_1 = 90°$ and $\theta_2 = 180°$, the transverse magnetization becomes:

$$M_\perp(\Delta\omega, t) \big|_{\theta_1=90°,\, \theta_2=180°} = i M_0 e^{-t/T_2} e^{-i\Delta\omega(t-2\tau)} \tag{3.40}$$

Thus, at $t = 2\tau$, all spin isochromats point along the y axis (i.e., the imaginary axis in the complex plane), irrespective of their off-resonance terms $\Delta\omega$. The magnetization is rephased, or refocused, to its initial orientation (see Eq. 3.31), with the only effect being the T_2 relaxation. This indicates that a 180° pulse can effectively refocus the transverse magnetization and form a spin echo. Second, even when the flip angle θ_2 is not 180°, refocusing can still occur at

$t = 2\tau$ as long as $\theta_2 \neq n \times 360° (n = 0, \pm 1, \pm 2, \ldots)$, as can be seen from the second term of Eq. (3.39). When a non-180° refocusing pulse is used, however, the magnetization is only partially refocused because of the weighting factor $\sin^2 (\theta_2/2)$. For example, if $\theta_2 = 90°$, a spin echo with 50% of the maximal amplitude is produced. Finally, the first term in Eq. (3.39) represents a free-induction decay (FID) signal following the initial excitation pulse, whereas the third term originates from the longitudinal magnetization excited by the refocusing pulse when the flip angle is not 180°.

Off-Resonance Effects   Although we have considered the off-resonance effect in magnetization dephasing and rephasing before and after the refocusing pulse, this effect has not been accounted for during the RF pulse itself. For off-resonance spins, the effective magnetic field $\vec{B}_{\text{eff}}$ (Section 1.2) is tilted away from the transverse plane towards the z axis (or the negative z axis, depending on the sign of the off-resonance term), as shown in Figure 3.10. In addition, the amplitude of the effective field $\left(\left| \vec{B}_{\text{eff}} \right| = \sqrt{B_1^2 + (\Delta\omega/\gamma)^2} \right)$ becomes larger

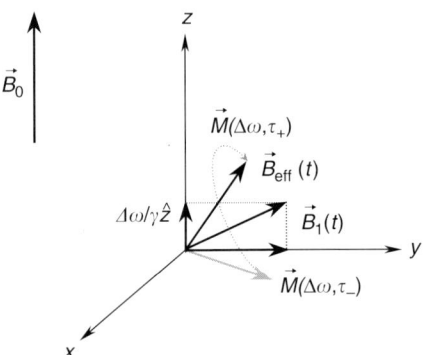

FIGURE 3.10 Off-resonance effects on a refocusing pulse. With the off-resonance term, $\Delta\omega/\gamma\hat{z}$ ($\hat{z}$ is a unit vector along the z axis), the effective magnetic field $\vec{B}_{\text{eff}}(t) = \vec{B}_1(t) + \Delta\omega/\gamma\hat{z}$ is tilted away from the transverse plane and its amplitude becomes larger than the applied B_1 field. The magnetization vector rotates about $\vec{B}_{\text{eff}}(t)$ by a flip angle θ, resulting in a longitudinal component even with $\theta = 180°$ flip angle. The gray vector labeled with $\vec{M}(\Delta\omega, \tau_-)$ represents an off-resonance spin isochromat immediately before the refocusing pulse, and the black vector labeled with $\vec{M}(\Delta\omega, \tau_+)$ shows the position of magnetization immediately after the pulse. Because the effective flip angle exceeds 180°, refocusing of the magnetization vector is in general incomplete.

than the applied B_1 field, increasing the flip angle to:

$$\theta = \gamma \int\limits_0^T \left| \vec{B}_{\mathrm{eff}}(t) \right| dt \tag{3.41}$$

Therefore, off-resonant isochromats in the transverse plane will be rotated about the $\vec{B}_{\mathrm{eff}}$ axis by a flip angle larger than that for on-resonance spins. Spin refocusing becomes incomplete and a longitudinal magnetization component is produced even when $\theta = 180°$ (Figure 3.10). For spatially selective refocusing RF pulses, the off-resonance effect can be particularly severe due to the presence of imaging gradients. This effect must be considered when designing slice-selective refocusing pulses. More discussion on this topic can be found in Section 2.3.

3.3.3 PRACTICAL CONSIDERATIONS

Spatially Selective Refocusing Pulses   A spatially selective refocusing pulse is accompanied by a slice-selection gradient so that only the spins within the selected slice experience the refocusing effect. A pair of crusher gradient pulses (Section 10.2) straddling the refocusing RF pulse is often included to improve the slice profile and to eliminate unwanted FID and stimulated echo signals caused by imperfections of the refocusing pulse.

Spatially selective refocusing pulses are almost always amplitude modulated to produce a desired frequency profile. The resulting frequency profile is converted to a spatial profile by a linear gradient. A simple, but nonoptimal, approach for designing a selective refocusing pulse is to choose the time-domain pulse shape as the Fourier transform (FT) of the targeted spatial profile. The actual slice profile, however, can deviate considerably from the FT due to nonlinearity in the Bloch equations at large flip angles (e.g., ~180°). This is demonstrated in Figure 3.11 for a SINC refocusing pulse with a Hamming window. The SINC pulse (Figure 3.11a) has a pulse width of 3.2 ms and a time-bandwidth product of 4.0. The difference between the FT and the actual slice profile is seen by comparing Figures 3.11b and 3.11c. The slice profile can be improved when a crusher gradient is added to each side of the pulse (Figure 3.11d), as discussed in Section 2.2. It should be noted that the crusher gradient causes narrowing in the slice profile. In practice, this effect can be compensated for by empirically reducing the slice-selection gradient amplitude. In Figure 3.11, we have assumed that all the magnetization is aligned along the $+y$ axis after an excitation pulse and the refocusing pulse is also along the $+y$ axis. Thus, the slice profiles are more meaningful when combined with the profile of specific excitation pulse.

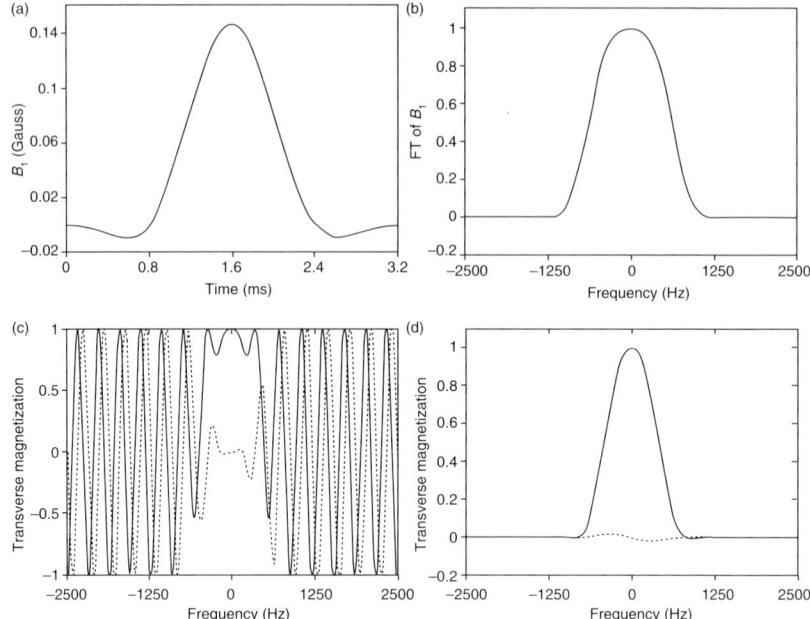

FIGURE 3.11 (a) A Hamming-windowed SINC pulse with time-bandwidth product $= 4$ and pulse width $= 3.2$ ms. (b) The Fourier transform of the RF pulse (only the magnitude is shown; the maximum amplitude is normalized to 1). (c) The slice profile without using crusher gradients (solid line: M_y; dashed line: M_x). (d) The slice profile with crusher gradients (solid line: M_y; dashed line: M_x). The y axes in (c) and (d) represent transverse magnetization in arbitrary units.

In many commercial MRI scanners, SINC refocusing pulses have been largely replaced by tailored RF pulses, such as those designed using the SLR algorithm (Pauly et al. 1991) or optimal control methods (Mao et al. 1988; Conolly et al. 1986). SLR refocusing pulses can considerably improve the quality of the slice profile and allow trade-offs among a number of parameters including the width of the transition regions and ripples within and outside the slice. The details on how to design SLR refocusing pulses are given in Section 2.3 and Pauly et al. (1991). Once the pulse is designed, the actual slice profile can be obtained by numerically solving the Bloch equations or by a forward SLR transform. For an initial magnetization along the y axis, the transverse magnetization after a refocusing pulse with and without crusher gradient, respectively, is given by:

$$M_\perp(r) = i M_0 \beta^2 \qquad \text{(with crusher gradient)} \qquad (3.42)$$

$$M_\perp(r) = i M_0 \left((\alpha^*)^2 + (\beta)^2 \right) \qquad \text{(without crusher gradient)} \qquad (3.43)$$

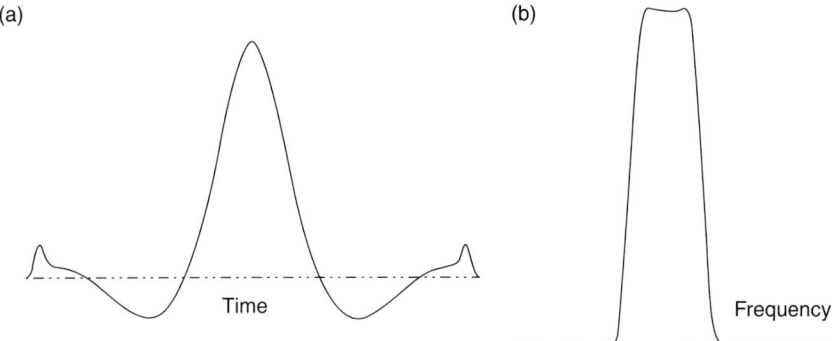

FIGURE 3.12 (a) An SLR refocusing pulse with time-bandwidth product = 4, pulse width = 3.2 ms, passband ripple = 1%, stopband ripple = 1%, and flip angle = 180°. (b) The slice profile of the SLR pulse with crusher gradient (solid line: M_y; dashed line: M_x).

where α and β are the Cayley-Klein parameters defined in Section 2.3. A representative SLR refocusing pulse with the following set of parameters is shown in Figure 3.12a: time-bandwidth product = 4, pulse width = 3.2 ms, passband ripple = 1%, stopband ripple = 1%, and flip angle = 180°. The transverse magnetization for this pulse with crusher gradients is shown in Figure 3.12b. The slice profile is noticeably improved compared to that in Figure 3.11d for the windowed SINC pulse with the same pulse width and time-bandwidth product.

A 180° SLR refocusing pulse is typically designed with linear phase. A linear phase refocusing pulse is interchangeable with a linear phase inversion pulse, as long as the flip angles are the same. When the same SLR pulse is used for refocusing and inversion, however, the corresponding slice profiles are not identical. The resulting ripple for the inversion profile is always less than that for the refocusing profile. In theory, the ratio of the ripple amplitude between the inversion and refocusing profiles is $1 : 2$ in the passband and $\sqrt{2} : 2$ in the stopband (Pauly et al. 1991).

Nonselective Refocusing Pulses   Nonselective refocusing pulses are typically rectangular in shape (i.e., a hard pulse; see Section 2.1), and have a much shorter pulse width (e.g., 100 µs) than their selective counterparts, whose pulse widths are typically in the range of 1–5 ms. The flip angle of a rectangular nonselective rectangular refocusing pulse is related to the pulse amplitude B_1 and pulse width T by a simple relationship:

$$\theta = \pi = \gamma B_1 T \tag{3.44}$$

Unlike selective SLR refocusing pulses, a rectangular refocusing pulse is scalable; a 180° refocusing pulse can be simply obtained by doubling the B_1 amplitude of a 90° hard excitation pulse. Alternatively, a 180° refocusing pulse can also be designed by doubling the pulse width of a hard 90° excitation pulse. This approach can be used when the maximum B_1 amplitude is limited by the available RF power delivered to or sustained by the coil. The pulse width difference means that the stretched refocusing pulses will have half the bandwidth of the hard excitation pulse. For most imaging applications, this will not cause a problem, as long as the bandwidth of the refocusing pulses is sufficiently large to encompass all of the Larmor frequencies contained in the imaged object.

There is virtually no difference in designing a nonselective refocusing pulse versus a nonselective inversion pulse with the same flip angle. The readers are referred to Section 3.2 for additional design details.

3.3.4 APPLICATIONS

Refocusing pulses are widely used in many imaging pulse sequences. Examples include conventional RF spin echo, rapid acquisition with relaxation enhancement (RARE) or fast spin echo, spin-echo echo planar imaging, and navigator echo generation. These applications of refocusing pulses are described in their respective sections in this book. Spatially selective refocusing pulses are most commonly employed in multislice 2D sequences. Single-slice 2D or single-slab 3D spin echo imaging can be performed with a spatially selective excitation pulse and a nonselective refocusing pulse, although spatially selective refocusing pulses may also be used to reduce artifacts. Spatially nonselective refocusing pulses are often employed in 3D acquisitions.

Another application of refocusing pulses is to measure the T_2 relaxation time of the imaged object (Breger et al. 1989). Because the magnetization at 2τ (i.e., the echo time TE) is given by $M_0 e^{-2\tau/T_2}$ with a $90 - \tau - 180 - \tau$ sequence (see Eq. 3.40), we can obtain a T_2 map by acquiring multiple images with various delay times (τ) and fitting the resulting intensities on a pixel-by-pixel basis to extract the T_2 value.

SELECTED REFERENCES

Breger, R. K., Rimm, A. A., and Fisher, M. E. 1989. T_1 and T_2 measurements on a 1.5-T commercial imager. *Radiology* 71: 273–276.

Conolly, S. M., Nishimura, D. G., and Macovski, A. 1986. Optimal control solutions to the magnetic resonance selective excitation problem. *IEEE Trans. Med. Imag.* MI-5: 106–115.

Hahn, E. L. 1950. Spin echoes. *Phys. Rev.* 80: 580–594.

Mao, J., Mareci, T. H., and Andrew, E. R. 1988. Experimental study of optimal selective 180° radiofrequency pulses. *J. Magn. Reson.* 79: 1–10.

Pauly, J., Le Roux, P., Nishimura, D., and Macovski, A. 1991. Parameter relations for the Shinnar-Le Roux selective excitation pulse design algorithm. *IEEE Trans. Med. Imag.* 10: 53–65.

RELATED SECTIONS

Section 1.2 Rotating Reference Frame
Section 2.1 Rectangular Pulses
Section 2.2 SINC Pulses
Section 2.3 Shinnar–Le Roux Pulses
Section 3.1 Excitation Pulses
Section 3.2 Inversion Pulses
Section 4.3 Spectrally Selective Pulses
Section 6.3 Adiabatic Inversion Pulses
Section 14.3 RF Spin Echo
Section 16.4 RARE

4

SPECTRAL RADIOFREQUENCY PULSES

4.1 Composite Radiofrequency Pulses

Composite RF pulses consist of simple RF pulses, or subpulses, that are concatenated to achieve improved excitation, refocusing, or inversion. When spatial selectivity is not required (e.g., with spectroscopic imaging, lipid suppression, or magnetization transfer), the primary goal is to obtain good frequency selectivity, that is, to uniformly flip all those spins that have precession frequencies within a desired range. Composite pulses can be used instead of the spectrally selective pulses described in Section 4.3 to perform frequency selection. Because B_0 and B_1 are not perfectly homogeneous over the imaged object, even with small-sample spectrometers, composite pulses have been designed to minimize sensitivity to B_0 and B_1 inhomogeneity (Levitt 1986). When spatial selectivity is desired, composite RF pulses can be combined with gradients, for example, in DANTE (Section 5.5) and spatial-spectral pulses (see Section 5.4). The subpulses that make up a composite pulse can be either hard or soft pulses, with flip angles, phases, and interpulse intervals that are adjusted to achieve the desired effect.

Any set of concatenated RF waveforms could be considered a composite pulse. A large number of composite pulses that have been developed for spectroscopy are outside the scope of this discussion, and the reader is referred to Levitt (1986) for a detailed discussion. In this section, we discuss composite pulses that are sometimes employed for imaging.

4.1.1 MATHEMATICAL DESCRIPTION

The composite pulses most frequently used for imaging are binomial pulses (Hore 1983). These are pulses for which the relative flip angles are coefficients of a binomial series, such as $q_{n,0}, q_{n,1}, \ldots, q_{n,n}$ in the following equation:

$$(a + b)^n = q_{n,0}a^n + q_{n,1}a^{n-1}b + \cdots + q_{n,m}a^{n-m}b^m$$
$$+ \cdots + q_{n,n-1}ab^{n-1} + q_{n,n}b^n \tag{4.1}$$

where the binomial coefficient (read as "n choose m") is:

$$q_{n,m} = \binom{n}{m} = \frac{n!}{(n-m)!m!} \tag{4.2}$$

Note that $q_{n,m} = q_{n,n-m}$ $(m = 0, 1, \ldots, n)$. The goal of these pulses is frequency selectivity, for example to excite only water and not fat. Binomial pulses that excite only spins near resonance are based on a frequency response:

$$S_n(f) = \cos^n(\pi f \tau) \tag{4.3}$$

where f is the frequency, τ is the time interval between the centers of two adjacent subpulses, and n is an integer. This function, shown in Figure 4.1 for several values of n, has nulls at frequencies that are (odd-integer) multiples of $1/(2\tau)$. In the small flip angle approximation (Section 3.1), the envelope of the RF pulse that produces $S_n(f)$ is approximately given by its Fourier transform. The Fourier transform of the frequency response of $S_n(f)$ is:

$$\text{FT}[S_n(f)] \propto \sum_{k=0}^{n} q_{n,k}\, \delta\left(t - \frac{n\tau}{2} + k\tau\right) \tag{4.4}$$

This can be shown recursively by noting that the Fourier transform of $\cos(\pi f \tau)$ is $\frac{1}{2}[\delta(t - \tau/2) + \delta(t + \tau/2)]$ followed by use of the convolution theorem (Section 1.1). The Fourier transform of $S_n(f)$ is also shown in Figure 4.1. The delta function amplitudes in that figure correspond to the binomial coefficients $q_{n,0}, q_{n,1}, \ldots, q_{n,n}$.

The effect of the binomial pulses can be understood more intuitively by considering a spin isochromat in the rotating reference frame exactly at resonance ($f = 0$) and another isochromat in the same rotating frame but slightly

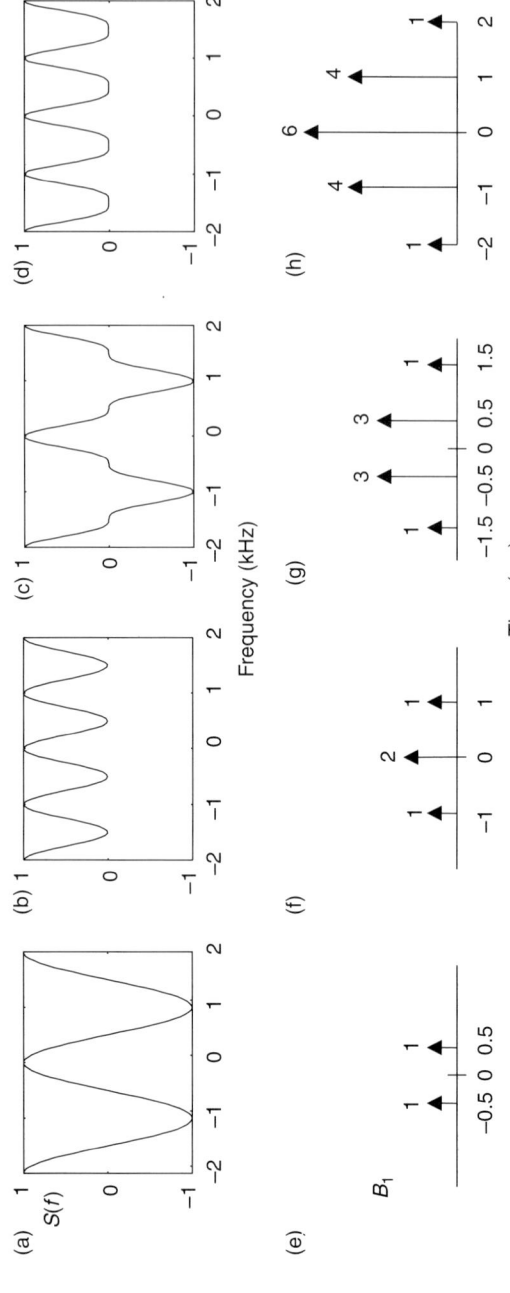

FIGURE 4.1 (a)–(d) are $S_1(f)$ through $S_4(f)$ (horizontal units in kilohertz) for $\tau = 1$ ms. (e)–(h) are their respective Fourier transforms (horizontal units in milliseconds). In plots (e)–(h), arrows represent delta functions, with relative amplitudes shown by accompanying numbers.

98

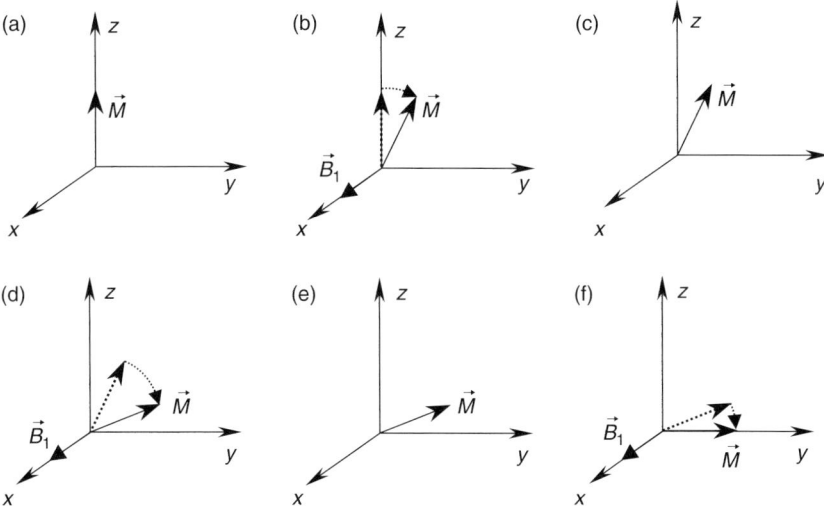

FIGURE 4.2 Magnetization vector in the rotating reference frame for a spin isochromat on resonance during application of a (121) pulse, assuming T_1 and T_2 are much longer than the interpulse interval τ. In (a) the magnetization is aligned along the z axis. In (b) the first RF subpulse nutates the magnetization by $\pi/8$. In (c) no precession takes place during the interpulse interval because the spin isochromat is exactly on-resonance. In (d) the second RF subpulse nutates the magnetization by $\pi/4$. In (e) no precession takes place in the interpulse interval. In (f) the third RF subpulse nutates the magnetization by $\pi/8$, placing it along the y axis.

off-resonance at frequency $f = 1/(2\tau)$ (Figures 4.2 and 4.3). In this example we assume T_1 and T_2 are both much longer than τ, so relaxation effects are negligible. If the RF pulses are delta functions, the nutation caused by the RF pulses is instantaneous and there is no precession during the pulses. The isochromat at resonance does not precess during the interpulse intervals, and after the last pulse in the series the total nutation angle is the sum of the nutation angles produced by each pulse. In Figure 4.2, the accumulative nutation angle is $\pi/2$. For the off-resonance isochromat, the precession angle (in radians) during each interpulse interval is

$$\psi = 2\pi f \tau = 2\pi[1/(2\tau)]\tau = \pi \qquad (4.5)$$

The nutation direction is therefore reversed for each successive pulse and consequently after the last pulse in the series, the net nutation angle is 0 (Figure 4.3). If the interpulse interval τ is chosen so that the off-resonance frequency $f = 1/(2\tau)$ coincides with the resonant frequency of a particular chemical species (e.g., lipids), those off-resonance spins will experience zero *net* excitation during excitation of the on-resonance spins (e.g., water).

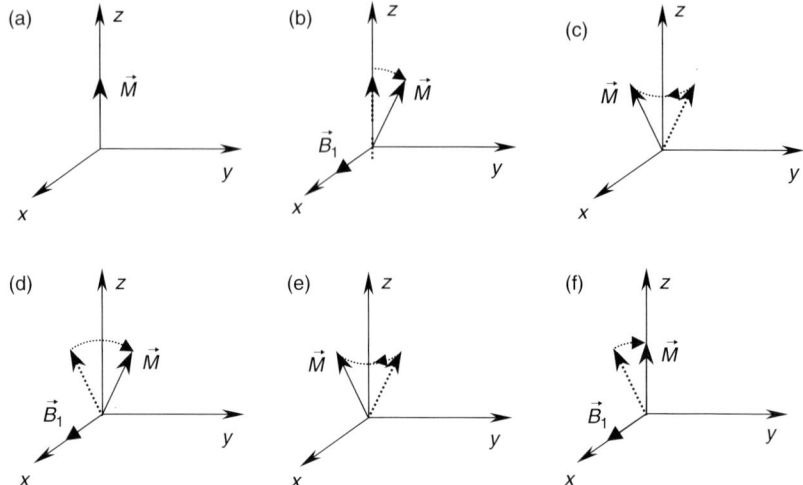

FIGURE 4.3 Magnetization vector in the rotating reference frame for a spin isochromat off-resonance by an amount $\delta f = 1/(2\tau)$ during application of a (121) pulse, assuming T_1 and T_2 are much longer than the interpulse interval τ. In (a) the magnetization is aligned along the z axis with the B_0 field. In (b) the first RF subpulse nutates the magnetization by $\pi/8$. In (c) the magnetization precesses through a phase angle of π. In (d) the second RF pulse nutates the magnetization by $\pi/4$. In (e) the magnetization again precesses through a phase angle of π. In (f) the third RF pulse nutates the magnetization by $\pi/8$, placing it back along the z axis.

4.1.2 IMPLEMENTATION

In practice, the delta function RF pulses are replaced by pulses of finite width, usually rectangular hard pulses (Section 2.1). The relative areas under the hard pulses are determined by the binomial coefficients. Binomial pulses are usually referred to by the coefficients of the series, for example (11), (121), (1331), and so forth. For a composite pulse designed for 90° excitation, the sum of the flip angles for all subpulses in the series is $\pi/2$. For finite-width pulses, the time between the centers of the pulses is τ. Figure 4.4 shows several examples that use pulses with the same amplitude and different widths. This design uses the smallest possible B_1. An alternative design to the one shown in Figure 4.4 is to use pulses having the same width and different amplitudes.

Binomial pulses can also be used to excite only off-resonance spins, for example, as a method of water suppression in spectroscopy or for fat suppression in imaging. A common application of off-resonant excitation in imaging is magnetization transfer (Graham and Henkelman 1997). For off-resonant excitation, the frequency spectrum is the same as for on-resonant excitation,

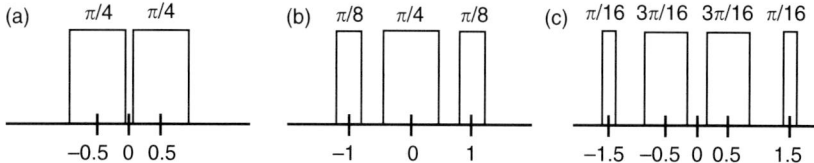

FIGURE 4.4 Rectangular (hard) pulses used to represent (a) (11), (b) (121), and (c) (1331) pulses with an interpulse interval $\tau = 1$ ms. Flip angles are given above the pulses. (The horizontal axis is in milliseconds.)

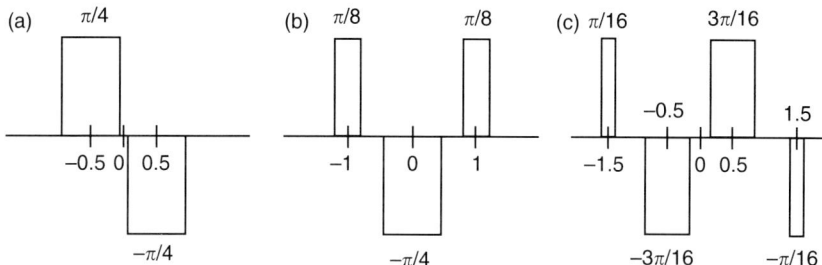

FIGURE 4.5 Rectangular (hard) pulses used to represent (a) $(1\bar{1})$, (b) $(1\bar{2}1)$, and (c) $(1\bar{3}3\bar{1})$ pulses with an interpulse interval $\tau = 1$ ms. Flip angles are given next to the pulses. (The horizontal axis is in milliseconds.)

except that it is shifted by $\delta f = 1/(2\tau)$ so that a null is placed at $f = 0$. Because a shift in the frequency domain is equivalent to a linear phase ramp in the time domain (Section 1.1), the RF pulses are multiplied by the function $e^{-i2\pi t \Delta f} = e^{-i\pi t/\tau}$. For delta function pulses spaced at time intervals $t = k\tau$, $e^{-i\pi t/\tau} = e^{-i\pi k} = (-1)^k$. In other words, every other RF pulse in the series is negated. Such off-resonant excitation pulses are usually referred to in the same way as on-resonant excitation pulses except that a bar denotes the inverted pulses, for example, $(1\bar{1})$, $(1\bar{2}1)$, $(1\bar{3}3\bar{1})$, and so forth. Examples are shown in Figure 4.5. It is straightforward to show that off-resonant binomial excitation pulses have the frequency response $S_n(f) = \sin^n(\pi f \tau)$, which has a Fourier transform:

$$\text{FT}[\sin^n(\pi f \tau)] \propto \sum_{k=0}^{n} (-1)^k q_{n,k}\, \delta\left(t - \frac{n\tau}{2} + k\tau\right) \tag{4.6}$$

Note that binomial pulses almost always use the first null for suppression of an off-resonant signal or the first maximum for excitation of an off-resonant signal. For a given frequency offset, the use of the higher-order nulls or maxima results in a shorter value of τ and therefore higher B_1. For most clinical whole-body scanners, the B_1 fields required to use the higher-order nulls or maxima are either not available or cause a considerable increase in specific absorption rate (SAR). Another consideration in favor of using the first null is that the larger the resonance offset is, the less accurate the Fourier approximation for the response becomes, due to nonlinearity of the Bloch equation. Thus Eq. (4.3) becomes progressively less accurate as f increases.

Unlike spectrally selective suppression pulses, which rely on applying a 90° flip to saturate spins at a given frequency offset, composite pulses rely on precession during the interpulse intervals to cause signal cancellation. This makes binomial pulses somewhat less sensitive to B_1 inhomogeneity than spectrally selective pulses. In addition, as long as the flip angle at a given spatial location follows the binomial pattern, the off-resonant spins will not be excited, irrespective of the local B_1-field strength. Examples of composite pulses that have reduced sensitivity to B_0 inhomogeneity can be found in Levitt (1986).

Binomial pulses can be made spatially selective, as well as spectrally selective (Schick et al. 1997). This is accomplished by using soft RF waveforms for the subpulses and employing a slice-selection gradient. For example, a series of SINC (Section 2.2) pulses can be played whose flip angle ratios are proportional to the binomial coefficients (Figure 4.6). Pulses such as the one in Figure 4.6 operate similarly to frequency-selective binomial pulses, except that each subpulse now flips only a selected slice of magnetization. Such pulses can be used for fat suppression and belong to the family of spatial-spectral pulses, which are discussed in Section 5.4.

Example 4.1   Find the interpulse interval τ for a binomial excitation pulse that places fat signals at the first null point. Assume a field strength of 1.5 T so that the fat–water frequency difference is approximately 210 Hz.

Answer   The first null is at a frequency $1/(2\tau)$, giving $\tau = 1/(2 \times 210\,\text{Hz}) = 2.38$ ms.

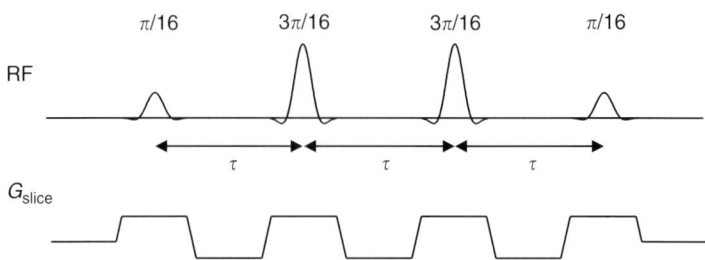

FIGURE 4.6 Example of a slice-selective (1331) binomial pulse. Flip angles are given above the RF pulses. RF pulse separation interval τ determines the location of the first null at $f = 1/(2\tau)$.

Example 4.2 A $1\bar{3}3\bar{1}$ pulse with rectangular hard pulses is used for magnetization transfer preparation. If the first maximum of the pulse spectrum is at 1 kHz, what is the minimum B_1 required for the pulse?

Answer

$$\tau = 1/(2 \times 1000\,\text{Hz}) = 500\,\mu\text{s}$$

The widest pulses are the second and third subpulses that have flip angles $(3/8)(\pi/2)$. The widths t_{pw} of these pulses must satisfy $\gamma B_1 t_{pw} = (3/8)(\pi/2)$. The minimum B_1 results when $t_{pw} = \tau$, giving:

$$B_1 = (3/8)(\pi/2)/(2\pi \times 42.57\,\text{MHz/T} \times 500\,\mu\text{s}) = 4.40 \times 10^{-6}\,\text{T} = 4.4\,\mu\text{T}$$

Some pulses use very high flip angles; for example, magnetization transfer pulses use flip angles as high as 1000–1500°. The actual B_1 for such pulses is usually several fold higher than the minimum value.

SELECTED REFERENCES

Graham, S. J., and Henkelman, R. M. 1997. Understanding pulsed magnetization transfer. *J. Magn. Reson. Imag.* 7: 903–912.

Hore, P. J. 1983. A new method for water suppression in the proton NMR spectra of aqueous solutions. *J. Magn. Reson.* 54: 539–542.

Levitt, M. H. 1986. Composite pulses. *Prog. NMR Spectrosc.* 18: 61–122.

Schick, F., Forster, J., Machann, J., Huppert, P., and Claussen, C. D. 1997. Highly selective water and fat imaging applying multislice sequences without sensitivity to B_1 field inhomogeneities. *Magn. Reson. Med.* 38: 269–274.

RELATED SECTIONS

4.2 Magnetization Transfer Pulses

A *magnetization transfer* (MT) or *magnetization transfer contrast* (MTC) pulse is a spectrally selective RF pulse that reduces the MR signal from some types of tissue while leaving other types virtually unaffected (Wolff and Balaban 1994; Balaban and Ceckler 1992; Henkelman et al. 1993, 2001;

Wang et al. 1997; Lin et al. 1993). Although MT pulses can only reduce MR signal, they can increase image contrast because their effect is tissue-specific.

The effect of MT pulses can be analyzed with a model that assumes some protons are bound to macromolecules or membranes, whereas others are not. Examples of protons bound to macromolecules are those in hydroxyl (i.e., —OH) groups in white matter lipids, and examples of unbound protons include those in free water molecules. This distinction defines two pools of protons in the body. The first pool is called the *restricted, semisolid,* or *macromolecular* pool, and the second is called the *free, mobile,* or *liquid* pool. The transverse relaxation time T_2 of the protons in the macromolecular pool is very short (less than 1 ms, often only tens of microseconds) due to their restricted mobility. Because of their short T_2, the signal from these protons is not visible in MR images obtained with conventional TE times. The signal that we see is generated instead entirely from protons in the liquid pool, which have longer T_2 (e.g., >10 ms) due to their mobility. The protons in the macromolecular pool have a much broader spectral width, because the full width at half maximum (FWHM) of a spectrum is inversely related to the transverse relaxation time:

$$FWHM \propto \frac{1}{T_2} \qquad (4.7)$$

The increase in T_2 (i.e., reduction in FWHM) that results from the averaging effects of motion is sometimes called motional narrowing.

As shown schematically in Figure 4.7, RF energy for MT is applied off-resonance, where it saturates some of the longitudinal magnetization in the macromolecular pool, while having hardly any direct effect on the protons in the liquid pool. The saturation of longitudinal magnetization of protons in the macromolecular pool is in turn transferred to the longitudinal magnetization of protons in the liquid pool by a process called *magnetization exchange.* Protons in some tissues such as blood, cerebral spinal fluid, and subcutaneous fat undergo almost no magnetization exchange with the macromolecular pool and hence display negligible MT attenuation. Protons in other tissues such as white matter, cartilage, muscle (including myocardium), and liver display stronger magnetization exchange, so their signal can be attenuated by 20–50% or more by adding an MT pulse to the sequence. The absolute amount of MT attenuation is not a fundamental property of the tissue but instead depends on the implementation details of the MT pulse and the pulse sequence.

One of the most widely accepted and widely used applications for MT is three-dimensional time-of-flight (3DTOF) MR angiography (Lin et al. 1993). In 3DTOF, MT is used to attenuate the MR signal from brain parenchyma, while leaving the signal from blood essentially unaffected. This increases the detectability of smaller vessels (Figure 4.8). Among the other applications of

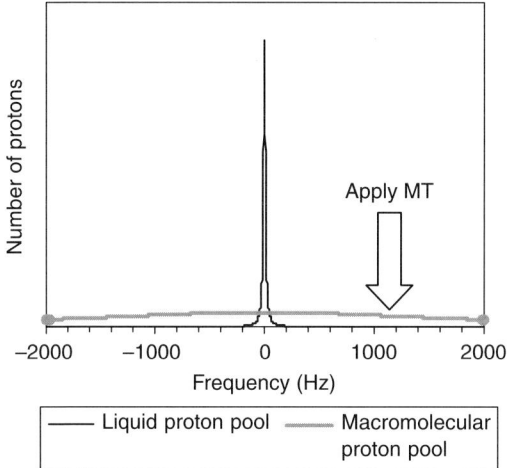

FIGURE 4.7 A schematic plot of the spectrum of two proton pools. Protons in the liquid pool have a narrow spectral width and generate the signal that produces MR images. Protons in the macromolecular pool have a broad spectral width and have a very short T_2 that dephases their MR signals. By applying off-resonance RF energy (arrow), some of the protons in the macromolecular pool can be saturated, with little direct effect on the protons in the liquid pool.

MT that are being actively developed are the study of white-matter diseases such as multiple sclerosis (Ge et al. 2002), breast imaging (Santyr et al. 1996), and cartilage imaging (Lattanzio 2000).

A mathematical model that describes the exchange of longitudinal magnetization between the macromolecular and liquid pools with the Bloch equations is beyond the scope of this book, as is a quantum mechanical analysis of the dipolar interactions that cause magnetization exchange. The interested reader is referred to Henkelman et al. (2001) for a review and a more complete set of references. Instead, this section presents some of the basic concepts and terminology used to describe MT and then focuses on implementation strategies.

4.2.1 MT Ratio and Direct Saturation

The aim of an MT pulse is to saturate the longitudinal magnetization of protons in the macromolecular pool. Some of this saturation is then transferred to selected protons in the liquid pool, thereby improving image contrast. Ideally, the MT pulse should not directly saturate any of the protons in the liquid pool

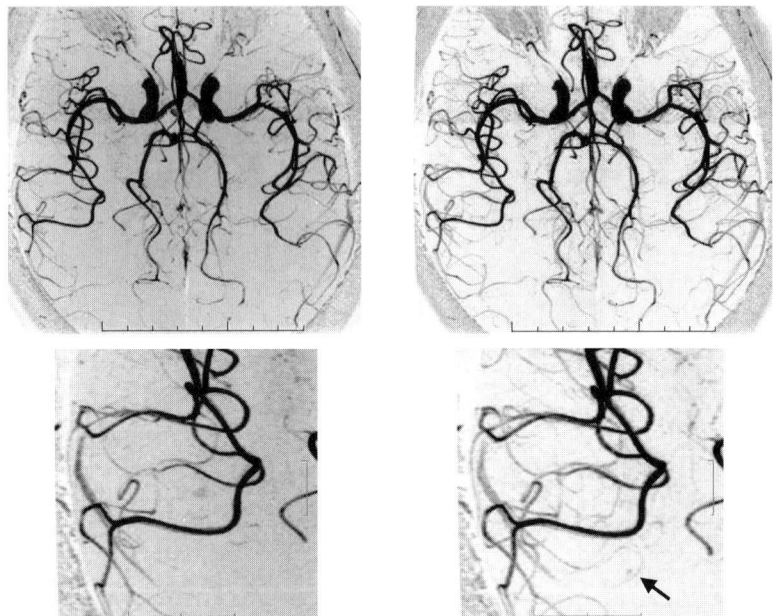

FIGURE 4.8 Axial MIP 3D time-of-flight images without (left) and with (right) MT. The images were acquired at 3.0 T, using an 8-ms Fermi pulse with a flip angle of 670°, applied only during the acquisition of the center of k-space. The bottom row shows a magnified portion of the right-posterior circulation. Note the suppression of brain parenchyma with MT, allowing the detection of smaller vessels (arrow). Also note that subcutaneous fat is hardly attenuated, so it appears more conspicuous.

because that would only reduce the overall image SNR. Although direct saturation cannot be avoided entirely, it can be held to a minimum with careful MT design. The quantities that we define next are used to analyze these effects.

Figure 4.9 shows a schematic plot of the longitudinal magnetization versus offset frequency Δf_{rf} of the applied RF for three classes of protons: a macromolecular pool, a liquid pool that experiences magnetization exchange, and a liquid pool that does not. For simplicity we assume that the equilibrium magnetization M_0 of all three classes of protons is equal. A magnetization level of $M_z = M_0$ in the plot indicates no saturation, whereas $M_z = 0$ indicates complete saturation. For all three classes indicated in Figure 4.9, the degree of saturation increases as the carrier frequency of the MT pulse is brought closer to the Larmor frequency ($\Delta f_{rf} = 0$). The saturation of protons in the macromolecular pool extends to higher frequencies because, according to Eq. (4.7), their spectrum is much broader.

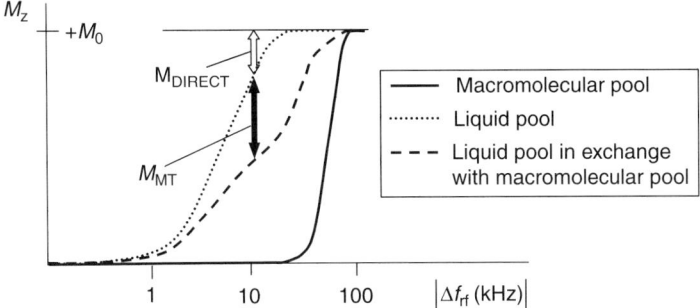

FIGURE 4.9 Schematic plot of the longitudinal magnetization plotted versus the logarithm of the offset frequency for three classes of proton. (Adapted from Henkelman et al. 2001, Fig. 5.)

The *direct* saturation M_{DIRECT} and the saturation due to the true MT effect M_{MT} are indicated by hollow and solid arrows, respectively, in Figure 4.9. It is customary to define the sum of the two as the total saturation:

$$M_{SAT} = M_{DIRECT} + M_{MT} \qquad (4.8)$$

A dimensionless quantity called the *MT ratio* (MTR) can be derived from M_{SAT} and the equilibrium magnetization:

$$MTR = \frac{M_0 - M_{SAT}}{M_0} \qquad (4.9)$$

With the RF pulse design we want to maximize M_{MT} while minimizing the direct saturation M_{DIRECT}. Note that a very low value of MTR is not necessarily desirable if it has a large contribution from M_{DIRECT}. From a practical point of view, the design of an MT pulse sequence can be simply stated: Maximize M_{MT} under the constraints that M_{DIRECT} is no more than 5–10% of M_0 and RF power limits are not exceeded.

4.2.2 IMPLEMENTATION STRATEGIES

General Considerations If an MR scanner is equipped with a second RF transmitter channel, then MT can be implemented by applying off-resonance RF energy continuously, which is called the *continuous wave* (CW) method. The CW method is preferred for some MT research where the complication of transient transverse magnetization is a concern. (By definition, the transients have decayed to zero when the CW is applied long enough for steady-state conditions to be reached). Clinical MRI systems, however, usually are equipped with only a single RF transmitter channel, so MT is nearly always implemented with finite-duration RF pulses interspersed in the image sequence. This is called the *pulsed* MT method. Pulsed MT methods generally deposit less RF power than CW methods. If the width of the MT pulse covers one-quarter of the TR interval (i.e., a duty cycle of 25%), then the power deposition from pulsed MT is reduced by approximately the same factor compared to its CW counterpart, provided that the RF amplitude is held constant.

Pulsed MT is implemented with long-duration RF pulses (e.g., pulse width $T = 5$–20 ms), followed by a spoiler gradient pulse that dephases any residual transverse magnetization. The RF pulse and spoiler gradient lobe together form an MT module, as depicted in Figure 4.10. MT pulses have relatively narrow RF bandwidths (on the order of a few hundred hertz), consistent with their long duration, and are applied off-resonance with $|\Delta f_{rf}| = 500$ to 1500 Hz (Figure 4.7). Because the RF pulse is applied off-resonance, it need not be very selective, and the RF envelopes used rarely have any zero-crossings (see Figure 4.11). As with other spectrally selective RF pulses (e.g., fat saturation), no gradient is applied during the MT pulse, although an exception to this general rule is discussed later in this section.

The amplitude of the MT pulse is set as high as possible without exceeding RF power limits because the degree of MT suppression increases monotonically with the applied RF power. Very high flip angles on the order of 1000–$1500°$ are typical, corresponding to peak RF amplitudes on the order of $10 \mu T$. The maximal RF power may be limited either by the hardware or by regulatory limits on the SAR (measured in watts per kilogram) delivered to the patient. Because RF power deposition is linearly proportional to bandwidth, the narrow bandwidth of MT pulses is helpful.

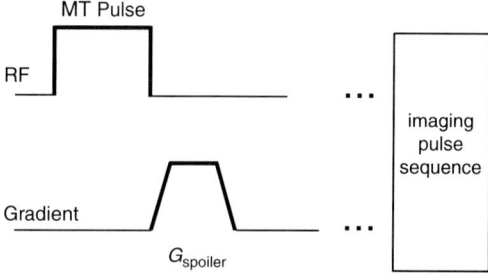

FIGURE 4.10 Schematic representation of an MT module, comprising an RF pulse and spoiler gradient. A rectangular RF pulse shape is shown here; more commonly used pulse shapes are shown in Figure 4.11.

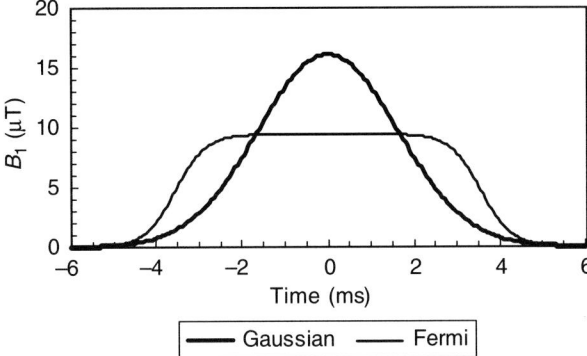

FIGURE 4.11 Plot of the RF envelopes versus time for the Gaussian and Fermi pulses derived in Example 4.3.

The MT module can be played either at the beginning or end of the imaging pulse sequence in a TR interval. Normally the MT module is played once during each TR interval, but in order to reduce the RF power deposition the MT module can be played less frequently. Because the image contrast is most strongly influenced by the central views in k-space, the MT module can be omitted at the periphery of k-space (Parker et al. (1995)) with minimal impact on image quality. This method of applying MT preferentially in the center of k-space is particularly effective if the regulatory limits for RF power deposition allow a higher value of SAR over short time durations (e.g., a higher SAR limit over a 10-s averaging time, compared to a 6-min averaging time).

In many pulse sequences, MT saturation is achieved unintentionally (Dixon et al. 1990; Santyr 1993), that is, without the application of a dedicated MT module. Whenever RF pulses are applied off-resonance, some MT effect will result. In standard interleaved multislice 2D imaging, RF excitation and refocusing pulses for slices adjacent (or near) to the imaging slice often function as effective MT pulses. Typical bandwidths for imaging pulses are on the order of 1–3 kHz, so adjacent slices have similar frequency offsets as custom-designed MT pulses. Pulse sequences in the RARE family, such as fast spin echo (FSE) and turbo spin echo (TSE), produce particularly strong unintentional MT suppression because of their large number of refocusing pulses. Another example is the perfusion pulse sequence used for arterial spin tagging. The RF pulse used to label spins at a location near the imaging slice can serve as an effective MT pulse. This effect can be compensated for using the techniques discussed in Section 17.1. Experimentally, the unintentional MT attenuation can be separated from confounding effects such as slice cross-talk with single and multislice acquisitions of a phantom that has both plain water and agar gel regions because agar gel displays MT attenuation while plain water does not.

4.2.3 RF PULSE SHAPES FOR MT

Many different RF pulse shapes have been used successfully for MT. The most important aspect of the pulse shape is that it produces negligible flip angle at the Larmor frequency of the liquid pool protons, so that direct saturation of water is kept minimal (e.g., <5–10%). Two commonly used RF pulse shapes are the Gaussian and Fermi, which are shown on Figure 4.11. (Both these functions were originally introduced for other purposes, but have been adopted as RF pulse shapes.) The rectangular (i.e., hard) and SINC pulses, which are described in Sections 2.1 and 2.2, respectively, as well as others can also be used. The Gaussian and Fermi pulse shapes are used less frequently in other imaging applications, so we describe them here.

The B_1 field for a Gaussian pulse (named for Carl Friedrich Gauss, 1777–1855, a German mathematician) in the rotating frame is given by the expression:

$$B_1(t) = A_G e^{-\frac{t^2}{2\sigma^2}} e^{i\Delta\omega_{rf}t} \quad \text{(Gaussian pulse centered at } t = 0) \quad (4.10)$$

where the angular frequency offset $\Delta\omega_{rf} = 2\pi\Delta f_{rf}$ produces the desired off-resonance irradiation. The envelope of the Gaussian pulse has two adjustable parameters: A_G is an overall scale factor (measured in microteslas), and σ is linearly proportional to the pulse width (measured in milliseconds). Although the Gaussian function theoretically is nonzero for all values of t, it falls off rapidly (for $t > \sigma$), and the RF pulse can be terminated when the magnitude of the B_1 field reaches a negligible level. For example at $t = \pm3.717\sigma$, the envelope of the RF field is $A_G/1000$, that is, a 60-dB attenuation. Thus, we estimate the pulse width of a Gaussian pulse to be approximately:

$$T_G \approx 2 \times 3.717\sigma = 7.434\sigma \quad (4.11)$$

The Fourier transform of a Gaussian pulse is another Gaussian function, and when the frequency offset is zero, from Table 1.2 in Section 1.1:

$$FT[B_1(t)] = A_G\sigma\sqrt{2\pi}e^{-2(\pi\sigma f)^2} \quad (4.12)$$

The rapid fall-off and the lack of side lobes in the frequency response of Eq. (4.12) are the main advantages of the Gaussian pulse. The FWHM of the frequency response is given by $\Delta f_G = 0.3748/\sigma$, which is a measure of the RF bandwidth. Thus, the dimensionless time-bandwidth product of any Gaussian is independent of σ and given by:

$$T_G\Delta f_G \approx 7.434\sigma \times \frac{0.3748}{\sigma} \approx 2.8 \quad (4.13)$$

Another popular RF shape used for MT irradiation is the Fermi pulse (named for Enrico Fermi, 1901–1954, an Italian and American physicist). The Fermi pulse is characterized by a flat central plateau straddled by exponentially decaying ramps. The B_1 field of the pulse is given by:

$$B_1(t) = \frac{A_F e^{i \Delta \omega_{rf} t}}{1 + \exp\left(\frac{|t| - t_0}{a}\right)} \qquad \text{(Fermi pulse centered at } t = 0) \qquad (4.14)$$

where A_F is B_1-field peak amplitude similar to A_G, and t_0 and a are two adjustable parameters having the dimension of time. The first parameter, t_0, is a measure of the pulse width, and the second parameter, a, is a measure of the transition width. Normally $t_0 \gg a$, so that $B_1(t = 0) = A_F$. As $a \to 0$, the Fermi pulse becomes a rectangular pulse with no ramps. Applying the same 60-dB standard that was used for the Gaussian, the width of the Fermi pulse is:

$$T_F = 2t_0 + 13.81a \qquad (4.15)$$

It is often useful to compare the relative SAR of two pulses when their flip angles, pulse widths, or both are equal. Assuming the pulse is real (i.e., zero imaginary part), the flip angle is obtained by integrating the RF envelope, as described in Section 3.1. When calculating the flip angle, we set $\Delta \omega_{rf} = 0$ because the flip angle is equal to the integral of the RF envelope only on resonance. Table 4.1 provides the results of the flip angle and relative SAR calculations for the Gaussian and Fermi pulses.

Example 4.3 Suppose we want to design an MT pulse with a flip angle $\theta = 1000°$ and a pulse width of $T = 12$ ms. (a) Determine the parameters for the Gaussian pulse envelope. (b) Determine the parameters for the Fermi pulse envelope, assuming that $t_0 = 10a$. (c) Suppose a pulse sequence with no MT module deposits 1.0 W/kg of SAR. With the Gaussian MT pulse from (a), the SAR is measured as 3.0 W/kg. What SAR deposition is expected if the Gaussian pulse is replaced with the Fermi pulse from (b)?

TABLE 4.1

Flip Angles and Relative Specific Absorption Rates for Gaussian and Fermi Radiofrequency Pulses Commonly Used for Magnetization Transfer

	Flip Angle (rad) $\gamma \int B_1(t)dt$	Relative SAR $\int |B_1(t)|^2 dt$
Gaussian	$\gamma A_G \sigma \sqrt{2\pi}$	$A_G^2 \sigma \sqrt{\pi}$
Fermi	$2\gamma A_F \left[t_0 + a \ln\left(e^{-t_0/a} + 1\right)\right]$	$2A_F^2 \left[t_0 + a \ln\left(e^{-t_0/a} + 1\right) - \frac{a}{1+e^{-t_0/a}}\right]$

Answer

(a) From Eq. (4.11), $\sigma = 12\,\text{ms}/7.434 = 1.614\,\text{ms}$. From Table 4.1:

$$A_G = \frac{\theta}{\gamma\sigma\sqrt{2\pi}}$$

$$= \frac{1000°(\pi\ \text{rad}/180°)}{2\pi\ \text{rad} \times 42.57\,\text{MHz/T}(1.614\,\text{ms})\sqrt{2\pi}} = 16.13\,\mu\text{T}$$

So the RF envelope for the Gaussian pulse is:

$$B_1(t) = \begin{cases} 16.13e^{-0.1919t^2}\,(\mu\text{T}) & -6\,\text{ms} \le t \le 6\,\text{ms} \\ 0 & |t| > 6\,\text{ms} \end{cases}$$

(b) Using Eq. (4.15) and the assumption that $t_0 = 10a$ yields $a = 0.3549\,\text{ms}$ and $t_0 = 3.549\,\text{ms}$. Table 4.1 gives:

$$A_F = \frac{\theta}{2\gamma\left[t_0 + a\ln\left(e^{-t_0/a} + 1\right)\right]}$$

$$= \frac{1000°(\pi\ \text{rad}/180°)}{2 \times 2\pi\ \text{rad} \times 42.57\,\text{MHz/T}\left[3.459\,\text{ms} + 0.3549\,\text{ms}\ln\left(e^{-10} + 1\right)\right]}$$

$$= 9.432\,\mu\text{T}$$

so that:

$$B_1(t) = \begin{cases} \dfrac{9.432}{1 + \exp\left(\dfrac{|t| - 3.459}{0.3459}\right)}\,(\mu\text{T}) & -6\,\text{ms} \le t \le 6\,\text{ms} \\ 0 & |t| > 6\,\text{ms} \end{cases}$$

The pulses derived in parts (a) and (b) are plotted in Figure 4.11.

(c) The Gaussian MT pulse is contributing $3.0 - 1.0 = 2.0\,\text{W/kg}$ to the SAR of the pulse sequence. According the parameters derived in (a) and (b) and from Table 4.1, the relative SAR of the Fermi pulse compared to the Gaussian pulse is:

$$\frac{\text{SAR}_F}{\text{SAR}_G} = \frac{2A_F^2\left[t_0 + a\ln\left(e^{-t_0/a} + 1\right) - \frac{a}{1+e^{-t_0/a}}\right]}{A_G^2\sigma\sqrt{\pi}} = 76.4\%$$

Therefore we expect the SAR with the Fermi pulse MT to be:

$$\text{SAR}_F = (1.0 + 2.0 \times 76.4\%)\,\text{W/kg} = 2.53\,\text{W/kg}$$

Pike, G. B., Glover, G. H., Hu, B. S., and Enzmann, D. R. 1993. Pulsed magnetization transfer spin-echo MR imaging. *J. Magn. Reson. Imag.* 3: 531–539.

Santyr, G. E. 1993. Magnetization transfer effects in multislice MR imaging. *Magn. Reson. Imag.* 11: 521–532, 1083.

Santyr, G. E., Kelcz, F., and Schneider, E. 1996. Pulsed magnetization transfer contrast for MR imaging with application to breast. *J. Magn. Reson. Imag.* 6: 203–212.

Wang, Y., Grist, T. M., and Mistretta, C. A. 1997. Dispersion in magnetization transfer contrast at a given specific absorption rate due to variations of RF pulse parameters in the magnetization transfer preparation. *Magn. Reson. Med.* 37: 957–962.

Wolff, S. D., and Balaban, R. S. 1994. Magnetization transfer imaging: Practical aspects and clinical applications. *Radiology* 192: 593–599.

RELATED SECTIONS

4.3 Spectrally Selective Pulses

Atomic nuclei are surrounded by electrons, which can shield the main magnetic field B_0 and reduce the net magnetic field experienced by nuclear spins. Due to this shielding, protons in different microscopic environments (i.e., different molecules or different locations in the same molecule) can resonate at slightly different frequencies. These frequency differences are known as *chemical shift*, which is quantitatively described by a dimensionless parameter δ. With chemical shift, the resonant frequency becomes:

$$f = \frac{\gamma}{2\pi} B_0 (1 - \delta) \qquad (4.16)$$

where γ is the gyromagnetic ratio, and B_0 is the externally applied magnetic field . By convention, zero chemical shift ($\delta = 0$) is arbitrarily assigned to the protons in tetramethyl silane, $Si(CH_3)_4$. The chemical shift of other protons is calculated from their resonant frequency f with:

$$\delta[\text{ppm}] = \frac{f - f_{\text{TMS}}}{f_{\text{TMS}}} \times 10^6 \qquad (4.17)$$

where f_{TMS} is the resonant frequency of tetramethyl silane, and ppm stands for parts per million.

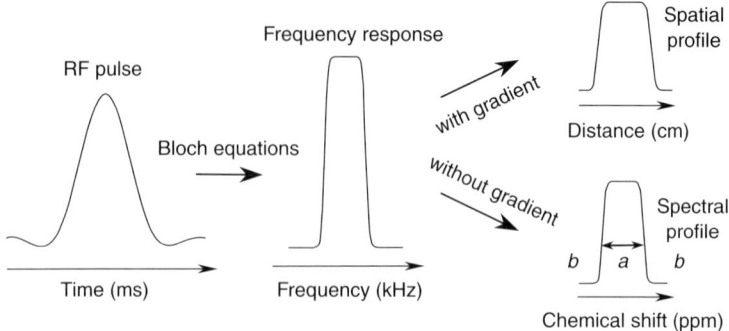

FIGURE 4.12 An RF pulse and its frequency response. In the presence of a gradient, the frequency response is linearly related to the slice profile; in the absence of a gradient during the RF pulse, the frequency response is referred to as a spectral profile. In the spectral profile, region *a* is called the passband, and region *b* is known as the stopband.

A plot of NMR signal intensity of an imaged object versus chemical shift δ constitutes a spectrum. RF pulses that are designed to selectively excite, refocus, or invert certain regions in the spectrum are called *spectrally* (or *chemically*) *selective pulses.*

Every RF pulse has a corresponding frequency response (Figure 4.12), which can be calculated by solving the Bloch equations or by performing a forward SLR transform (Section 2.3). For example, a SINC RF pulse (Section 2.2) yields approximately a rectangular frequency response. For a given pulse shape, the width of the frequency response (i.e., bandwidth in kilohertz) is inversely proportional to the RF pulse width (e.g., in milliseconds).

In the presence of a concurrently played gradient, the frequency response of an RF pulse is converted to a spatial profile (Figure 4.12), which is discussed in Section 8.3. With no concurrently played gradient, the frequency response is often referred to as a spectral profile. For spins whose resonant frequencies are inside the profile (i.e., the passband; region *a* in Figure 4.12), the pulse performs its designed functions, such as excitation, inversion, and refocusing. Outside the profile (i.e., the stopband; region *b* in Figure 4.12), the pulse has little or no effect on the spins.

SINC pulses and Gaussian pulses (Section 4.2) are often employed as spectrally selective pulses because of their simplicity. Tailored RF pulses, such as SLR pulses (Section 2.3) and band-selective, uniform-response, pure-phase (BURP) pulses (Geen and Freeman 1991), are also used on commercial MRI scanners for improved spectral profiles and more flexibility in the trade-off between parameters that define the profile quality (e.g., uniformity, phase variations, and transition width).

In MRI, spectrally selective pulses are primarily used for signal suppression. Examples include lipid suppression to increase the conspicuity of lesions in standard imaging, and water suppression in spectroscopic imaging. Spectrally selective pulses can also be used for chemically selective imaging, including imaging of lipids, water, or other chemical species (e.g., N-acetylaspartate and choline). Another application of spectrally selective pulses is magnetization transfer imaging (Section 4.2), in which a long RF pulse with a narrow spectral profile is applied off-resonance to saturate protons associated with macromolecules.

4.3.1 MATHEMATICAL DESCRIPTION

The vast majority of spectrally selective pulses are amplitude modulated with a fixed carrier frequency. Using complex notation (Section 1.2) these pulses can be expressed as:

$$B_1(t) = A(t)\, e^{-i\omega_{\mathrm{rf}}t} \tag{4.18}$$

where $A(t)$ is the amplitude modulation function (also known as the pulse waveform or envelope), and ω_{rf} is the carrier frequency in radians per second. $A(t)$ controls the shape of the spectral profile, and ω_{rf} determines the profile's central position. Some of the commonly used modulation functions are discussed in Sections 2.2, 2.3, and 4.2.

The spectral profiles of the pulses can be obtained by solving the Bloch equations. This is usually done in the RF rotating reference frame (Section 1.2), which rotates at the angular frequency ω_{rf}. Defining the frequency offset Δf_{cs}:

$$\Delta f_{\mathrm{cs}} = \frac{\Delta\omega}{2\pi} \tag{4.19}$$

where $\Delta\omega$ is the resonant frequency offset of a given chemical species relative to a reference. The spectral profile of the RF pulse given by Eq. (4.18) is calculated by solving the Bloch equations (Eq. (3.4)) over a predetermined range of frequency offsets Δf_{cs}:

$$\frac{dM_x}{dt} = 2\pi\,\Delta f_{\mathrm{cs}}\, M_y \tag{4.20}$$

$$\frac{dM_y}{dt} = \gamma\, M_z\, A(t) - 2\pi\,\Delta f_{\mathrm{cs}}\, M_x \tag{4.21}$$

$$\frac{dM_z}{dt} = -\gamma\, M_y\, A(t) \tag{4.22}$$

(Without loss of generality, Eqs. (4.20–4.22) assume that the RF pulse is applied along the x axis in the RF rotating reference frame.) For an excitation

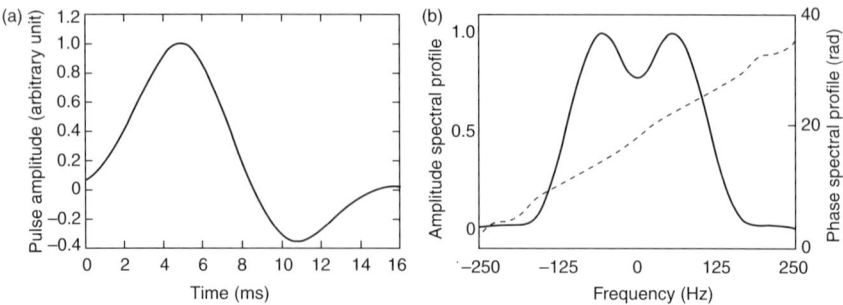

FIGURE 4.13 (a) An SLR maximum phase pulse and (b) its amplitude (solid line) and phase(dotted line) responses. The SLR pulse parameters are pulse width = 16 ms, time-bandwidth product = 4, flip angle = 90°, passband ripple = 5%, and stopband ripple = 1%. This pulse can be used for lipid suppression.

pulse, a plot of $\sqrt{M_x^2 + M_y^2}$ versus Δf_{cs} constitutes the amplitude response of the spectral profile, and a plot of $\arctan(M_x/M_y)$ gives the phase response. A method for solving Eqs. (4.20)–(4.22) can be found in Section 3.1 (keeping in mind that the quantity $2\pi \Delta f_{cs}$ corresponds to $\Delta\omega$ and $A(t)$ corresponds to $B_1(t)$ in that section). An example of the amplitude and the phase responses of an SLR pulse is shown in Figure 4.13. If a pulse is used for spectrally select-ive excitation (see next subsection), the phase dispersion within the passband must be minimized. If a pulse is used for signal suppression, however, maximal phase dispersion is desirable and the exact phase response becomes less import-ant. For spectrally selective excitation pulses with small flip angles (<90°), the spectral profile can be approximated by taking the Fourier transform of $A(t)$, as discussed in Sections 3.1 and 2.3.

4.3.2 APPLICATIONS

Signal Suppression The primary application of spectrally selective pulses is to suppress signals from nuclei with specified chemical shifts. For example, water signal can be suppressed in lipid imaging, and vice versa. Water suppression is also important in proton spectroscopic imaging because the con-centrations of N-acetylaspartate, citrate, creatine, choline, lactate, and other metabolites are 3–4 orders of magnitude lower than that of water protons. The prevailing application of spectrally selective pulses is to suppress lipid signals in imaging applications, as shown in Figure 4.14. We focus here on lipid suppression, with the understanding that the same principles are equally applicable to suppressing other chemically distinct signals, including water and silicone.

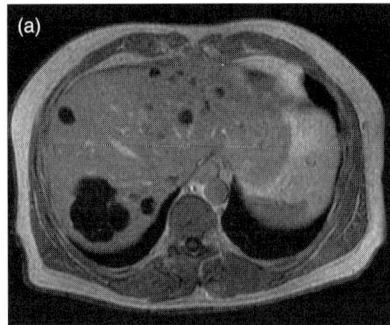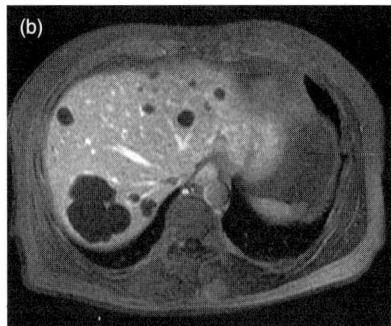

FIGURE 4.14 Postcontrast T_1-weighted images of the liver without (a) and with (b) lipid suppression using a spectrally selective RF pulse. Both images were acquired from the same patient using a gradient echo sequence with identical parameters except for lipid suppression. With lipid suppression, the contrast between liver and the other tissues has noticeably improved. The residual subcutaneous lipids at the lower right corner of the image can be caused by either B_0-field inhomogeneity, which alters the local lipid resonant frequency, or B_1-field nonuniformity.

Two dominant proton signals in the human body arise from water and triacylglycerol molecules. The latter forms lipids or fatty tissue. The lipid signals often appear bright in T_1-weighted and T_2-weighted RARE (or fast spin echo) images. Their signal can interfere considerably with the diagnosis of certain diseases, such as myeloma in the bone marrow, metastases in the vertebral body, and contrast-enhancing lesions throughout the body. Clinically, it is desirable to suppress the lipid signals for these applications.

Unlike water molecules in which the microscopic environment for the two protons are identical (i.e., the same chemical shift; $\delta = 4.7$ ppm), triacylglycerol consists of multiple groups of protons (CH_3, CH_2, $CH{=}CH$, etc.), each with a different chemical shift ranging from 0.9 to 5.7 ppm. The most abundant resonance (from the CH_2 group in the aliphatic chain) occurs at $\delta = 1.3$ ppm. The peak in the lipid spectrum is rather broad due to these multiple components. In practice, a chemical shift difference of 3.3–3.5 ppm is used between lipids ($\delta \approx 1.3$ ppm) and water ($\delta = 4.7$ ppm), with lipids resonating at a lower frequency. In many examples in this book we have used a chemical shift of 140 Hz/T, which corresponds to 3.3 ppm.

To suppress the signal from lipids, a spectrally selective pulse nutates the lipid magnetization to the transverse plane, while leaving the water magnetization unperturbed along the longitudinal axis (Figure 4.15). One or more spoiler or homospoil gradient pulses are subsequently applied to dephase (or spoil) the excited lipid signals (see Section 10.5). Because the water magnetization is stored along the longitudinal axis, the spoiler gradient has no effect on water

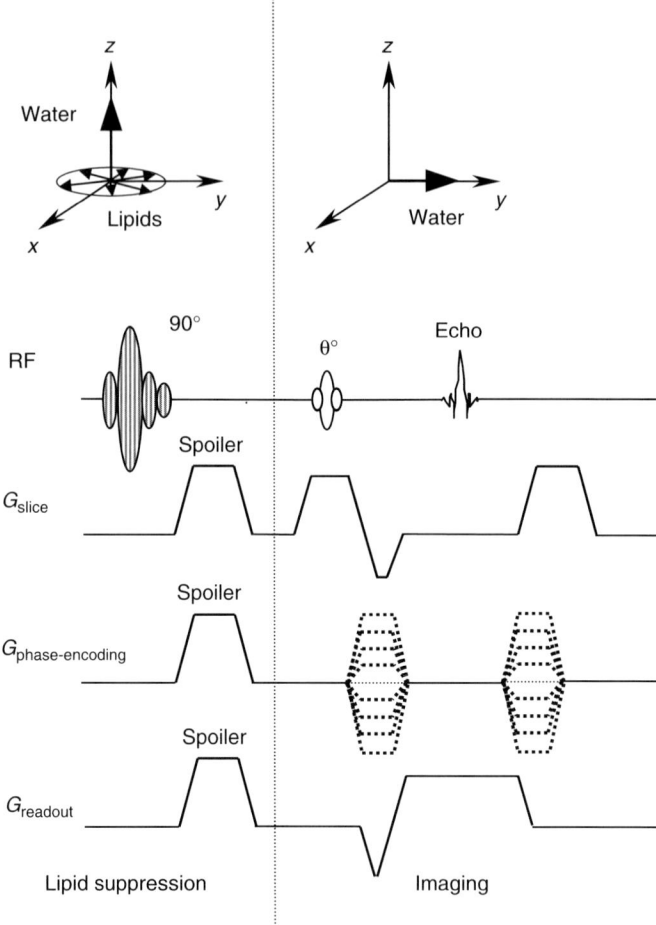

FIGURE 4.15 An example of using a spectrally selective pulse to suppress lipid signals in an imaging sequence. The 90° spectrally selective pulse (shaded area to denote the frequency offset), usually with maximal phase dispersion, is applied ∼217 Hz off-resonance with respect to the water resonant frequency to excite lipids at 1.5 T. The lipid signals are dephased by one or more spoiler gradients. After lipid suppression (portion to the left of the dotted vertical line), an imaging sequence is executed to excite water signals and form a water image (portion to the right of the dotted vertical line).

signals. This is analogous to the spoiler gradient following spatial saturation pulses. After the lipid magnetization is excited and dephased (it is said to be *saturated*), a standard imaging pulse sequence is executed to acquire an image with the fat signal substantially attenuated (Figures 4.14 and 4.15). For a pulse sequence with multiple repetitions, the spectrally selective pulse and the associated spoiling gradients are typically applied each TR period, unless the TR time is substantially shorter than the lipid T_1 relaxation time ($T_1 \approx 250\,\text{ms}$ for lipids at 1.5 T). Since the T_1 of the lipids is relatively short, longitudinal magnetization of the fatty tissue can regrow during a sequence. To offset the rapid lipid signal recovery, a flip angle larger than 90° (e.g., 110–150°) is often used in lipid suppression pulses.

To design a spectrally selective pulse for lipid suppression, the spectral profile must be broad enough to cover the majority of the lipid resonant frequencies, but not excessively broad to affect the water signal. At 1.5 T, the chemical shift difference between lipids and water ($\Delta\delta \approx 3.4\,\text{ppm}$) corresponds to a frequency separation of $\sim 217\,\text{Hz}$ as obtained from:

$$\Delta f_{cs} = \frac{\gamma B_0}{2\pi} \times \Delta\delta[\text{ppm}] \times 10^{-6} \qquad (4.23)$$

(In many other sections of the book we have used the abbreviated notation f_{cs} for the resonant frequency difference between lipids and water.) Thus, the width of the spectral profile is often chosen as $\sim 250\,\text{Hz}$. This bandwidth is considerably narrower than typically employed in spatially selective pulses. Consequently, the pulse width is much longer.

Example 4.4 A symmetric SINC pulse with a central lobe and a total of two side lobes (one on either side of the main lobe) is used for lipid suppression at 1.5 T. The water center frequency is found to be 63,858,470 Hz. What are the carrier frequency and pulse width for the SINC pulse?

Answer According to Eq. (4.23), the lipid resonant frequency is $\sim 217\,\text{Hz}$ below that of water at 1.5 T. To center the spectral profile at the lipid resonance, the carrier frequency of the SINC pulse must be set at $63,858,470 - 217 = 63,858,253\,\text{Hz}$. Because there are four zero-crossings, the time-bandwidth product $T\Delta f$ of the pulse is 4 (Section 2.2). To saturate the lipid signal without affecting the water signal, a spectral bandwidth of 250 Hz is typically used. Thus, the pulse width should be:

$$T = \frac{(T\Delta f)}{\Delta f_{cs}} = \frac{4}{250\,(\text{Hz})} = 16\,\text{ms} \qquad (4.24)$$

In addition to SINC pulses, many other pulses can be used for lipid suppression. Gaussian pulses feature a relatively short pulse width, but their spectral profile is not uniform (Gaussian in shape) and has a broad transition region between the passband and the stopband. SLR pulses can considerably improve the uniformity of the spectral profile as well as the transition region width with a reasonable pulse width (~ 8–16 ms at 1.5 T). SLR pulses with maximum or quadratic phase can also increase phase dispersion within the spectral profile, so that less gradient area might be required in the spoiler.

A variation of the aforementioned lipid suppression technique is to invert the lipid spins using a spectrally selective pulse without spoiling gradients. After a certain inversion time (e.g., $\sim$60 ms at 1.5 T), the lipid magnetization is considerably attenuated because of T_1 relaxation. When the lipid magnetization approaches the null (i.e., zero magnetization), multiple excitation RF pulses with a very short TR (e.g., a few milliseconds) are applied to acquire a number of k-space lines (e.g., 64), each with a different phase-encoding value. To maximize lipid-suppression efficiency, the central k-space lines are typically acquired when the lipid magnetization is nulled. This technique, known as SPECIAL (Foo et al. 1994), is used in some fast 3D gradient echo pulse sequences.

In the presence of B_0-field inhomogeneity, lipid and water resonant frequencies can be shifted at certain spatial locations, causing the lipid suppression pulse to saturate water signals while leaving the lipid signals intact. To avoid this problem, the B_0-field inhomogeneity must be considerably less than 3.4 ppm within the imaging volume. Because the B_0-field inhomogeneity can arise from the local magnetic susceptibility differences within the imaged object, good lipid suppression using a spectrally selective pulse can be difficult to achieve in some anatomic regions, such as the neck, or for patients with metallic implants. The use of resistive shimming that calibrates higher-order (e.g., z^2) shims on a per-patient basis can improve the performance of lipid suppression, especially at high magnetic fields.

The spectrally selective pulses for lipid suppression must be adjusted for different B_0-field strengths. At very high fields (e.g., 3.0 T), the frequency separation between lipid and water increases according to Eq. (4.23) and so does the range of the lipid resonant frequencies. Therefore, a broader spectral profile should be used. At an intermediate magnetic field (e.g., 0.7 T), the frequency separation between different spin species decreases, requiring a narrow spectral profile and a longer pulse width for lipid suppression. At low magnetic fields (e.g., 0.2 T) where the frequency separation between fat and water diminishes, lipid suppression using spectrally selective pulses becomes impractical. Other lipid suppression methods, such as STIR (Section 14.2) or Dixon's method (Section 17.3), are more suitable at low fields.

Selective Excitation Spectrally selective pulses can also be used to selectively excite certain spin species (fat, water, N-acetylaspartate, etc.) so that an image based only on the selected chemical species can be formed (Figure 4.16). This technique has been referred to as chemical shift selective (CHESS) imaging (Haase et al. 1985). Unlike the pulses for signal suppression,

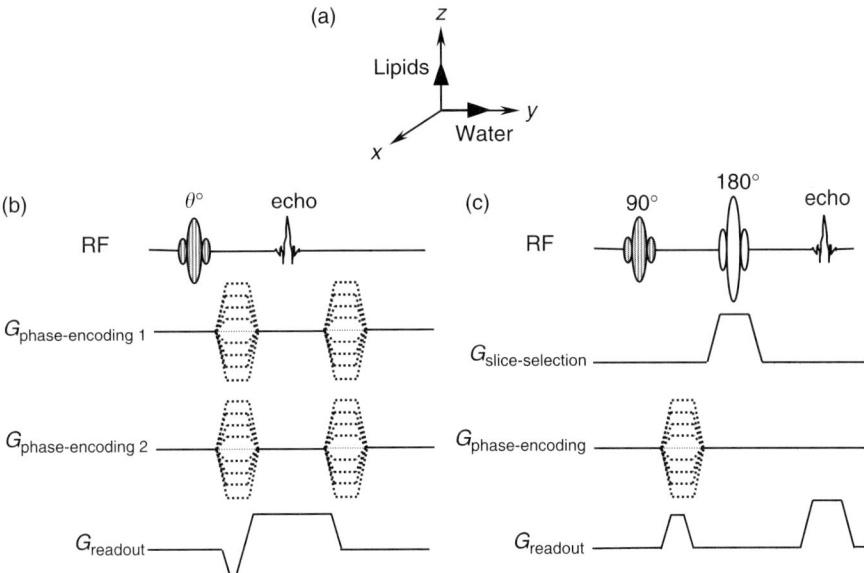

FIGURE 4.16 Spectrally selective pulses (shaded) used in (b) 3D and (c) 2D chemical shift selective imaging. In this example, the spectrally selective pulse selectively excites the water signal while leaving the lipid signal intact (a). Following the excitation, a 3D or 2D imaging sequence can be applied. In the 2D case, a 180° refocusing pulse is used to perform slice selection. (See Sections 14.1 and 14.3 for details on the imaging sequences.)

a spectrally selective pulse in CHESS requires minimal phase dispersion within the passband to avoid signal loss in the image. This can be accomplished using SLR pulses with minimum phase design (Section 2.3). Alternatively, we can employ BURP pulses with a somewhat longer pulse width.

In CHESS, the spectrally selective pulse excites all the spins within the selected frequency band irrespective of their spatial locations, making this technique well suited to 3D imaging. For 2D CHESS imaging, a slice-selective refocusing pulse can be applied after the spectrally selective excitation pulse to form a spin echo from the selected slice (Figure 4.16c). Two-dimensional spatial information can be encoded in the spin echo, as discussed in Section 14.3. Because the excitation pulse affects all the spins in the imaging volume, this 2D imaging technique is not compatible with the interleaved multislice imaging strategy (Section 11.5). When interleaved multislice imaging is required, spatial-spectral pulses (Section 5.4) can be employed instead.

Magnetization Transfer   Another application of spectrally selective pulses can be found in MT imaging, in which a pulse is applied $\sim$1.5 kHz away from the water resonant frequency to saturate protons associated with macromolecules in the tissue. The MT pulse is typically 5–20 ms in duration and has a single lobe (e.g., rectangular, Fermi, or Gaussian in shape). Thus the MT pulse has a very narrow spectral profile and essentially burns a hole in the broad spectrum of the macromolecules. Exchange between free water and water bonded to macromolecules provides a unique contrast mechanism. Details on this application can be found in Section 4.2.

SELECTED REFERENCES

Foo, T. K. F., Sawyer, A. M., Faulkner, W. H., and Mills, D. G. 1994. Inversion in the steady-state—contrast optimization and reduced imaging time with fast three-dimensional inversion-recovery–prepared GRE pulse sequences. *Radiology* 191: 85–90.

Geen, H., and Freeman, R. 1991. Band-selective radiofrequency pulses. *J. Magn. Reson.* 93: 93–141.

Haase, A., Frahm, J., Hanicke, W., Matthaei, D. 1985. ^{1}H NMR chemical shift selective (CHESS) imaging. *Phys. Med. Biol.* 30: 341.

RELATED SECTIONS

SPATIAL
RADIOFREQUENCY PULSES

5.1 Multidimensional Pulses

A *multidimensional RF pulse* (Bottomley and Hardy 1987; Hardy and Cline 1989) is spatially selective in more than one direction. Whereas the familiar 1D spatially selective RF pulse selects a planar slab of magnetization (i.e., a slice), a 2D RF pulse selects a long strip or cylinder (Figure 5.1). Similarly, 3D RF pulses are spatially selective in all three directions at once, so they affect a voxel of magnetization. Because of their long pulse duration, 3D RF pulses are less frequently used than their 2D counterparts. This section focuses on 2D pulses; additional information about 3D RF pulses can be found in Stenger et al. (2002).

Two-dimensional RF pulses are commonly used for excitation, but they can be used for other functions such as saturation, inversion, and refocusing as well (Bottomley and Hardy 1987; Pauly et al. 1993). A 2D spatially selective pulse requires that gradient waveforms be played on two independent gradient axes. The gradient waveforms played during the RF pulse usually resemble the readout gradient waveform of either echo planar imaging (EPI) or spirals, which are described in Sections 16.1 and 17.6, respectively. The design of 2D RF pulses with small flip angles is usually accomplished with k-space

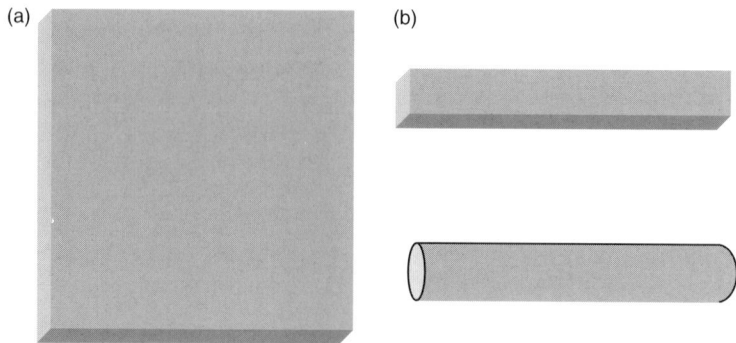

FIGURE 5.1 Representation of the spatial profile selected by RF pulses. (a) A standard, 1D spatially selective pulse excites a planar slab. (b) A 2D RF pulse excites either a long strip or a long cylinder. (Regardless of the dimensionality of the RF pulse, these are idealized shapes; the transition regions of the slice profile are never perfectly sharp.)

analysis (Pauly et al. 1989), which is described in the next subsection. Iterative (Bottomley and Hardy 1987) and SLR (Pauly et al. 1993) methods also can be used to design 2D RF pulses. These methods are particularly useful when the k-space method does not apply.

5.1.1 PULSE ANALYSIS AND DESIGN

RF k-Space Analysis   Two- (or three-) dimensional excitation pulses with small flip angles can be designed and analyzed with RF k-space methods. This procedure generally works well for flip angles as high as 90°. To generate a 2D pulse, at least one of the two selection gradients must oscillate so that a 2D k-space is traversed while the RF pulse is played. The spatial profile is then calculated with the 2D Fourier transform of the (suitably weighted) B_1 field applied during the traversal through the 2D k-space. The design considerations for a spatial selection gradient waveform are thus analogous to those for the readout gradient waveform in single-shot data collection in 2D imaging. Discussions of specific issues that are related to 2D RF excitation using echo planar and spiral trajectories are given in this subsection.

RF k-space analysis can be derived by generalizing the small flip angle approximation for the transverse magnetization generated by an excitation pulse with a constant gradient (i.e., Eq. 3.13):

$$M_\perp(t) \approx i\gamma M_0 e^{-i\Delta\omega t} \int_0^t B_1(t')e^{i\Delta\omega t'}\, dt' \qquad (5.1)$$

The phase $\Delta\phi$ accumulated by the transverse magnetization has contributions from off-resonance effects (which we denote f_{off}), which include contributions from gradient-induced fields, chemical shift (f_{cs}), susceptibility variations, and B_0-field inhomogeneity. The net phase accumulation is:

$$\Delta\phi(t) = 2\pi f_{\text{off}} t + \gamma \vec{r} \cdot \int_0^t \vec{G}(t')\, dt' \tag{5.2}$$

where the vector $\vec{r}$ denotes the spatial offset from gradient isocenter. In Eq. (5.2) the vector $\vec{G}$ represents the two applied gradients. Without loss of generality, we can write $\vec{G} = (G_x, G_y)$, although any two gradient axes can be used, including two oblique axes. To maximize the efficiency, the gradient axes are invariably chosen to be perpendicular to one another. The area under the slice selection waveform defines the RF k-space vector:

$$\vec{k}(t) = \frac{\gamma}{2\pi} \int_{T_{\text{end}}}^t \vec{G}(t')\, dt' = -\frac{\gamma}{2\pi} \int_t^{T_{\text{end}}} \vec{G}(t')\, dt' \tag{5.3}$$

As also mentioned in Section 5.4, it is a common convention to start the integration at the end of the RF pulse ($t = T_{\text{end}}$) as shown in Eq. (5.3) and then proceed to the left. Neglecting off-resonant effects for now, and substituting Eqs. (5.2) and (5.3) into Eq. (5.1):

$$M_{\perp}(T_{\text{end}}) \approx i\gamma M_0 e^{-2\pi i \vec{k}(T_{\text{end}}) \cdot \vec{r}} \int_0^{T_{\text{end}}} B_1(t') e^{2\pi i \vec{k}(t') \cdot \vec{r}}\, dt' \tag{5.4}$$

The exponential factor outside the integral is equal to unity because k-space variable is evaluated at T_{end}. Spiral trajectories that travel from the periphery to the center of k-space (i.e., spiral in) satisfy this condition and do not require a dedicated rephasing lobe. If the pulse is not self-rephased (like a 2D echo planar pulse) then we can choose T_{end} to be the end of the dedicated rephasing lobes, which again ensures that the peaks of the sub-pulses are played at the center of k-space. An example is shown in Figure 5.2.

The overall factor of $i = \sqrt{-1}$ in Eq. (5.4) indicates that, just like one-dimensional (nonadiabatic) pulses, for on-resonance spins there is 90° phase lag between the magnetization response and the applied B_1 field. For example, if a B_1 field is applied solely along the x axis in the rotating reference frame, the components of the rephased magnetization (close to resonance) will satisfy the relationship $M_x \ll M_y$ in that frame.

In order to design the 2D RF pulse, we specify a desired magnetization response $M_{\perp}(\vec{r})$ and the two selection gradient waveforms that define the

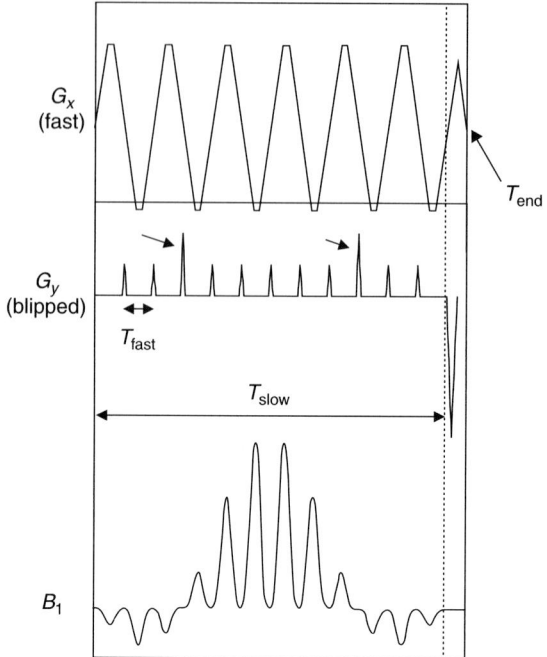

FIGURE 5.2 Gradient and RF waveforms for a 2D echo planar pulse. Two of the gradient blips (arrows) have twice as much area as the others because they are located near zero-crossings of the envelope pulse. It is often convenient to define T_{end} in Eq. (5.3) to occur at the end of the rephasing lobes (arrow).

k-space trajectory. Then, Eq. (5.4) is inverted to specify the B_1 field as a function of time. The inversion step requires a change of integration variables in Eq. (5.4) from time t to k-space. The path in k-space that is traced is defined by the vector $\vec{k}(t)$, which is parametrically defined in terms of the scalar t. As described in Pauly et al. (1989) and Hardy et al. (1990), the result of inverting Eq. (5.4) for the B_1 field is:

$$B_1(t) \propto \left\| \vec{G}(t) \right\| \left\| \Delta \vec{k}(t) \right\| \underbrace{\iint M_\perp(\vec{r}) e^{2\pi i \vec{k}(t) \cdot \vec{r}} \, dx \, dy}_{\text{2D spatial profile}} \qquad (5.5)$$

According to Eq. (5.5), the required RF field is the 2D Fourier transform of the desired spatial profile, weighted by two factors. The first weighting factor:

$$\left\| \vec{G}(t) \right\| = \sqrt{G_x^2(t) + G_y^2(t)} \propto \left\| \frac{d\vec{k}(t)}{dt} \right\| \qquad (5.6)$$

is the speed at which the RF k-space is traversed. The physical interpretation of this factor is, in order to produce uniform k-space weighting, the amplitude of the B_1 field must be reduced when the k-space traversal is slower. The factor $\|\vec{G}(t)\|$ is the multidimensional analog of the one-dimensional factor $|G(t)|$ that is discussed in Section 2.4 on variable-rate pulses.

The second factor $\|\Delta\vec{k}(t)\|$ in (5.5) is a correction for variable sampling density. This factor is analogous to the density compensation discussed in Section 13.2 on image reconstruction with gridding. If the RF k-space is sampled uniformly, then the sampling density term is a constant, and it can be dropped. If k-space is sampled nonuniformly, then $\|\Delta\vec{k}(t)\|$ is set equal to the distance in k-space between adjacent samples (Hardy et al. 1990). Note that the density compensation used in gridding includes both the $\|\vec{G}(t)\|$ and $\|\Delta\vec{k}(t)\|$ factors. In a simplification similar to that used in gridding, either factor can be omitted if it is constant over the RF k-space trajectory.

Example 5.1 Suppose you are designing a 2D RF pulse with a radial k-space trajectory. What is the variable sample density correction?

Answer With a radial k-space trajectory, the separation between adjacent radial spokes is proportional to the distance to the center of k-space. Therefore:

$$\left\|\Delta\vec{k}(t)\right\| = k_r = \sqrt{k_x^2 + k_y^2}$$

After substituting this factor into Eq. (5.5), note that the amplitude of the applied B_1 field at the exact center of the RF k-space is 0.

According to the shift theorem for Fourier transforms, the center of the spatial profile of a 2D RF pulse can be offset by an amount $\delta\vec{r}$ away from the gradient isocenter by modulating the B_1 field with a linear phase shift:

$$B_1(t, \delta\vec{r}) \propto \left\|\vec{G}(t)\right\| \left\|\Delta\vec{k}(t)\right\| e^{-2\pi i \vec{k}(t)\cdot\delta\vec{r}} \underbrace{\iint M_\perp(\vec{r})e^{2\pi i \vec{k}(t)\cdot\vec{r}}\,dxdy}_{\text{2D profile}}$$

$$(5.7)$$

In practice, the maximal amount of offset $\|\delta\vec{r}\|$ can be limited (e.g., to 15 cm or less) by spatial profile distortion introduced by phase errors from off-resonant effects. At large values of $\|\delta\vec{r}\|$, the dominant source of error is typically the concomitant magnetic field (see Section 10.1), which has quadratic spatial dependence in comparison to the linear spatial dependence of the desired gradients (Eq. 5.2).

Two-Dimensional Echo Planar Pulses Echo planar trajectories are popular for 2D RF pulses because the designs for the two directions conveniently separate, providing independent control over slice thickness in the two dimensions. Just like EPI readouts, 2D RF pulses that use echo planar trajectories employ an oscillating spatial selection gradient in the fast direction and a unipolar gradient in the slow, or blipped, direction. The oscillating, fast gradient waveform is similar to the sole gradient waveform used for spatial-spectral pulses (Section 5.4). Like the spatial-spectral gradient waveform, the oscillating waveform for an echo planar 2D pulse is usually composed of trapezoidal or triangular lobes of alternating polarity. This waveform produces a rapid back-and-forth traversal of k-space in the fast direction. Unlike spatial-spectral pulses, however, 2D RF pulses also apply a gradient along a second, perpendicular axis. This gradient can be either a weak constant gradient or blips. We assume the use of gradient blips here because they are more widely used. The purpose of the blipped gradient is to traverse k-space in the slow, or blipped, direction. The blips are played normally during the zero-crossings of the fast waveform, when the amplitude of the applied B_1 field is negligible. Figure 5.2 shows the gradient and RF waveforms for a typical 2D echo planar RF pulse. Twelve trapezoidal lobes of alternating polarity provide traversal through RF k-space in the fast direction. Eleven gradient blips, all of the same polarity, provide a single traversal through RF k-space in the slow direction.

A 2D echo planar pulse design is specified by its oscillatory and blipped gradient waveforms, which determine the k-space trajectory, and also a pair of one-dimensional RF pulses. We call the longer of the two pulses the *slow pulse* and denote its RF amplitude $A_{slow}(t)$. The slow pulse is analogous to the spectral envelope in a spatial-spectral pulse because it provides an overall modulation over the entire duration of the 2D RF pulse. In the example in Figure 5.2, the slow pulse is symmetric, so the RF waveform of the 2D pulse peaks near its center. If a minimum phase pulse were used instead, the 2D pulse would peak further to the right.

The shorter duration pulse, which we call the *fast pulse*, $A_{fast}(t)$, is analogous to the spatial kernel pulse in a spatial-spectral pulse, because it is played repeatedly, typically under each gradient lobe. The shapes of the fast and slow pulses can be chosen independently and can be SINC, SLR, Gaussians, or any other desired pulse shape. In Figure 5.2, the slow envelope pulse is a SINC (with a time-bandwidth product of 4.0) and the fast pulse is a Gaussian.

Echo planar pulses have two values of the isodelay (Section 3.1) that determine the area of the slice-rephasing gradient lobes. Referring again to Figure 5.2, the gradient lobes to the right of the dotted line provide rephasing. Because the fast pulse is symmetric in this case, the area of the rephasing lobe in the fast direction is equal to one-half the area of one of the trapezoidal lobes. The area of the rephasing lobe in the blipped direction is equal to one-half the total area of all the blips, because the slow pulse is also symmetric and its isodelay is one-half of its pulse width.

With the echo planar trajectory, the factor $\|\vec{G}(t)\|$ in Eq. (5.5) is important because the RF amplitude is typically nonzero during the ramps of the fast gradient waveform. The factor $\|\Delta\vec{k}(t)\|$ usually can be ignored, however, because the amount of RF played during the blips is negligible, so the k-space is filled in equally spaced lines. (Specifically, no $\|\Delta\vec{k}(t)\|$ correction is required for playing RF on the ramps of the fast gradient waveform because the variable sampling density correction is concerned with the spacing of the k-space lines, not the rate at which each line is traversed.) The B_1 amplitude is calculated by forming the product:

$$B_1(t) = C(\theta)A_{\text{slow}}(k_{\text{blip}}(t))A_{\text{fast}}(k_{\text{fast}}(t))\|\vec{G}(t)\| \qquad (5.8)$$

where $C(\theta)$ is a normalization factor that is used to set the flip angle θ. For more explanation of Eq. (5.8) and schematic diagrams illustrating the k-space filling procedure, see Pauly et al. (1989) and Hardy et al. (1990); for more on spatial-spectral pulses, see Section 5.4.

Suppose the fast and slow pulses have dimensionless time-bandwidth products $T_{\text{slow}}\Delta f_{\text{slow}}$ and $T_{\text{fast}}\Delta f_{\text{fast}}$, respectively. The pulse width T_{slow} is equal to the entire duration of the 2D RF pulse (not including the rephasing lobes), and T_{fast} is equal to the duration of a single fast gradient lobe (Figure 5.2). The thickness of the profile along the blipped direction is then given by (Alley et al. 1997):

$$\Delta y_{\text{blip}} = \frac{T_{\text{slow}}\Delta f_{\text{slow}}}{K_{\text{blip}}} \qquad (5.9)$$

where K_{blip} is the total extent of the RF k-space traversed along the blipped gradient direction. Similarly the thickness of the profile along the fast gradient direction is (Alley et al. 1997):

$$\Delta x_{\text{fast}} = \frac{T_{\text{fast}}\Delta f_{\text{fast}}}{K_{\text{fast}}} \qquad (5.10)$$

where K_{fast} is the total extent in k-space from a single fast gradient lobe.

Because the RF k-space is filled discretely in the blipped direction, the resulting slice profile is periodic in that direction. The center-to-center distance between the desired slice profile and the first replicates is the inverse of the separation of the lines in k-space:

$$\Delta y_{\text{replicate}} = \frac{N_{\text{blip}}}{K_{\text{blip}}} \qquad (5.11)$$

Because the blips are played in between each gradient lobe, the number of blips is related to the total number N of lobes in the fast gradient direction by $N_{\text{blip}} = N - 1$.

Example 5.2 Suppose a 2D echo planar pulse is 12 ms long and is composed of eight fast gradient lobes. If the slow pulse has a time-bandwidth product of 4, how much gradient area should each blip have if the desired thickness in the blipped direction is 5 cm? (Assume all the blips have equal area.)

Answer Because there are eight fast gradient lobes, there are $N_{blip} = 7$ blips spaced between them. From Eq. (5.9), the total extent in k-space produced by these 7 blips is:

$$K_{blip} = \frac{T_{slow}\Delta f_{slow}}{\Delta y_{blip}} = \frac{\gamma}{2\pi} a_{tot} = \frac{\gamma N_{blip}}{2\pi} a_{blip}$$

The gradient area under each blip a_{blip} is therefore:

$$a_{blip} = \frac{2\pi T_{slow}\Delta f_{slow}}{\gamma N_{blip}\Delta y_{blip}} = \frac{4}{(42.57\,\text{MHz/T})\,7(0.05\,\text{m})}$$

$$= 2.685 \times 10^{-4}\,\text{mTm}^{-1}\text{s}$$

   Two-dimensional RF pulses with echo planar trajectories are also prone to rather large chemical shift artifacts in the blipped direction. This is analogous to EPI readouts, in which the fat–water chemical shift can be a large fraction of a typical field of view. For the 2D RF pulse, the displacement in the blipped direction of the profile for fat relative to water is given by (Alley et al. 1997):

$$\Delta y_{cs} = \frac{N_{blip} f_{cs} T_{slow}}{K_{blip}} \tag{5.12}$$

where f_{cs} is the chemical shift in hertz. Using Eq. (5.9), we can recast this result into the form:

$$\Delta y_{cs} = \frac{N_{blip} f_{cs}}{\Delta f_{slow}} \Delta y_{blip} \tag{5.13}$$

Example 5.3 A 2D dimensional RF pulse with an echo planar k-space trajectory has a fast gradient waveform comprising 10 lobes. How big is the spatial offset of the fat profile at 3.0 T if the RF bandwidth of the slow pulse is 400 Hz and the profile thickness in the blipped direction is 1 cm.

Answer There are 10 fast gradient lobes, so $N_{blip} = 10 - 1 = 9$. At 3.0 T, the fat–water chemical shift is approximately 420 Hz. Therefore according to Eq. (5.13), the profile for fat is shifted by:

$$\Delta y_{cs} = \frac{N_{blip} f_{cs}}{\Delta f_{slow}} \Delta y_{blip} = \frac{(9)(420\,\text{Hz})}{400\,\text{Hz}}(1\,\text{cm}) = 9.45\,\text{cm}$$

Note that the chemical shift is much larger than thickness of the spatial profile.

Finally we note a common trick used in 2D echo planar pulse design. For a fixed time-bandwidth product, Eq. (5.9) states that in order to decrease the slice thickness Δy_{blip} the extent in k-space K_{blip} must be increased. This can be accomplished by increasing the number of blips, which increases the pulse duration, or by increasing the area under each blip, which has the drawback of decreasing the distance between replicated slice profiles $\Delta y_{\text{replicate}}$. Sometimes, however, the area under selected blips can be increased instead, without substantial penalty. If the slow pulse has zero-crossings, then from Eq. (5.8) the B_1 amplitude of the 2D RF pulse will be approximately zero at, and near, those times. Because the RF deposition for those lines in k-space is negligible, they can be skipped with little impact on the resulting spatial profile (Alley et al. 1997; Rieseberg et al. 2002). This is why the area under the blips is often doubled near the zero-crossing of the slow envelope pulse (Figure 5.2). (Also, to the extent that the RF weighting is zero for the skipped k-space lines, the variable sample density correction can be ignored. This is because we can imagine the missing k-space lines are present, but have zero weighting.) Note that this method of skipping k-space lines is unique to 2D RF echo planar pulses. It cannot be used with spatial-spectral pulses because k-space traversal in the frequency direction is accomplished by waiting a period of time. We cannot speed up time to increase the rate of k-space traversal during the zero-crossings of the spectral envelope. Similarly, this method cannot be used for data collection during EPI readout because we do not know a priori which lines of k-space (if any) will have zero signal associated with them.

Two-Dimensional Spiral Pulses Spiral (Hardy and Cline 1989; Pauly et al. 1989) is another popular k-space trajectory for 2D RF pulses. The spatial selection gradient waveform is a time-reversed version of the single-shot (i.e., one-interleaf) spiral readout described in Section 17.6. Because spiral trajectories use two oscillating gradients, they cover the 2D RF k-space very efficiently. Also, because the trajectory ends at the center of k-space (for an inward spiral), no dedicated rephasing lobe is required; that is, the value of the isodelay is zero. Also, the gradient moments are approximately nulled at the end of the pulse. The main drawback of spiral pulses is that off-resonant effects cause blurring (rather than a bulk shift) of the spatial profile.

Unlike echo planar, which uses a pair of 1D RF pulses in the design, 2D spiral RF pulse designs use only a single pulse. An example of a spiral RF pulse is shown in Figures 5.3 and 5.4. As illustrated in Figure 5.3a, often a half-Gaussian RF shape is used (Hardy and Cline 1989; Pauly et al. 1989). The resulting spatial profile is cylindrically symmetric, as illustrated in Figures 5.3c

(a)

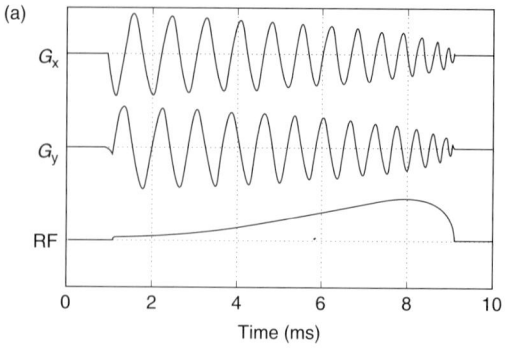

(b) Weighted k-space RF deposition

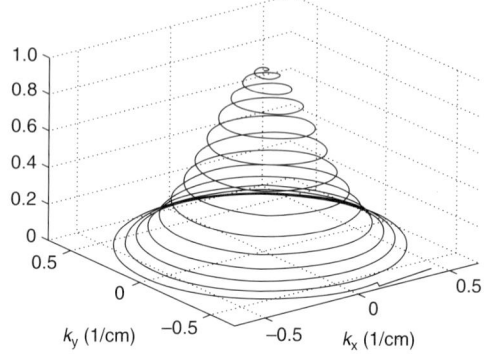

(c)   Theoretical selective excitation profile

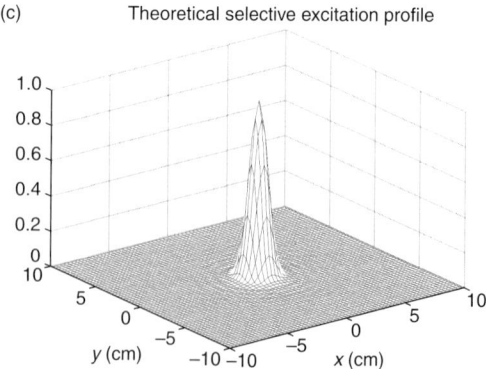

FIGURE 5.3 2D RF pulse using a spiral k-space trajectory. (a) Gradient and RF wave-forms. Note that no rephasing lobe is required. (b) Plot depicting the spiral trajectory in a 2D RF k-space and the deposited $B_1(t)/\|\vec{G}(t)\|$ (i.e., the quantity whose 2D Fourier transform is the slice profile, since the radial k-space sampling density is approximately uniform). (c) The calculated spatial profile (without variable sampling density correction). (Courtesy of Kevin Glaser, Ph.D., Mayo Clinic College of Medicine.)

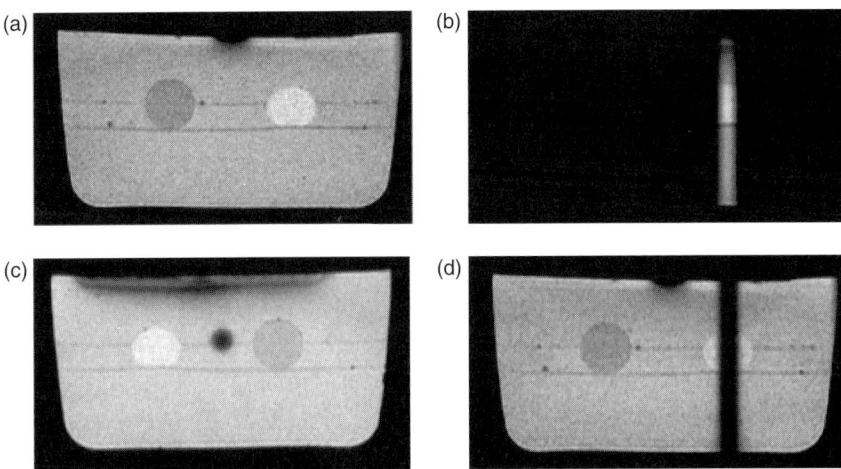

FIGURE 5.4 (a) MR image of a gel phantom. (b) Replacing the standard 1D excitation pulse with a 2D spiral pulse eliminates all the signal except that from a cylinder. The axis of the cylinder is up and down. (c) 2D-spiral RF pulse used for spatial saturation, with the axis of the cylinder in and out of the page, creating a dark spot. (d) 2D spiral RF pulse used for spatial saturation, with the axis of the cylinder up and down. (Courtesy of Kevin Glaser, Ph.D., Mayo Clinic College of Medicine.)

and 5.4. The half-Gaussian pulse shape peaks at the very end of the pulse, but when the factor $\|\vec{G}(t)\|$ in Eq. (5.5) is accounted for the peak is shifted slightly to the left (e.g., from $t = 9$ to 8 ms in Figure 5.3a.). Although most spiral trajectories produce a nearly uniform k-space weighting, sometimes the resulting profiles can benefit (Hardy et al. 1990) by the calculation and inclusion of the variable sampling density factor $\|\Delta \vec{k}(t)\|$ from Eq. (5.5).

The thickness d of the 2D profile (i.e., the diameter of the cylinder) can be expressed as the ratio of the dimensionless time-bandwidth product of the half-Gaussian pulse and the maximal k-space radius obtained by the trajectory:

$$d = \frac{T \Delta f}{2K_r} \qquad (5.14)$$

As shown in Section 4.2, the dimensionless time-bandwidth product of any Gaussian pulse is approximately 2.8. Because k-space is discretely sampled in the radial direction with the spiral trajectory, aliasing (i.e., undesired excitation) will occur at a spatial radius larger than:

$$r_{alias} > \frac{1}{\Delta k_r} \qquad (5.15)$$

where Δk_r is the largest radial spacing in the spiral trajectory as the angular variable is increased by 2π. With spiral RF pulses, the aliasing is cylindrical rather than a replication of the excited volume, as with echo planar pulses. As explained in Section 17.6, for most spiral trajectories, the largest value of Δk_r occurs at the edge of k-space, which corresponds to the beginning of the 2D spiral RF pulse.

It is interesting to note that a 2D spatial pulse can use echo planar, spiral, or virtually any other trajectory that covers the 2D k-space. Except for the blips, there is a strong resemblance between the RF and gradient waveforms for a 2D RF pulse that uses an echo planar trajectory and a spatial-spectral pulse (Section 5.4). A spatial-spectral pulse, however, limits the k-space coverage to one spatial dimension, while leaving the other dimension for time evolution. Therefore, the designer of a spatial-spectral pulse has limited choices and *must* use an oscillatory (i.e., such as the fast gradient in Figure 5.2) waveform for the one spatial dimension.

5.1.2 APPLICATIONS

If an application requires a 2D RF pulse, the designer must first choose the k-space trajectory. Although many choices are possible, the echo planar and spiral families described earlier are by far the most popular. Spiral pulses have excellent immunity to flow artifacts and provide shorter minimum TE and TR. They have been used for applications such as navigator pulses (Liu et al. 1993) and M-mode cardiac profiling (Cline et al. 1991 and see Section 11.4). Echo planar pulses, on the other hand, provide independent control of the thickness of the strip in two directions, and off-resonant spins produce a shifted (rather than blurred) profile. Echo planar pulses are ideal for restricted-field-of-view imaging, which has found application in MR angiography (MRA) (Alley et al. 1997) and reduced echo-train EPI (Rieseberg et al. 2002). We note, however, that since the publication of Alley et al. (1997), the advent of contrast-enhanced angiography has decreased the application importance of restricting the excited field of view in order to increase flow-related enhancement in MRA.

For 2D echo planar RF pulses, it would be convenient to align the blipped direction of the RF pulse with the frequency-encoded direction of the acquisition, so that the anti-alias filter can remove the replicates and chemically shifted regions. The main application of 2D echo planar RF pulses, however, has been to restricted-field-of-view imaging. With restricted-field-of-view imaging, the blipped direction corresponds to the phase-encoded direction of the acquisition, so other means must be used to remove the replicates, such as arranging them to fall outside the sensitive region of the coil. (Note that aligning the fast direction with the phase-encoded direction does not work very well either, because then the blipped direction corresponds to the slice direction and severe aliasing will usually result.)

As with any RF pulse, it is desirable to keep the duration of a multidimensional pulse shorter than the shortest T_2 component to be imaged. Also, as the pulse duration increases, so do the errors from off-resonant effects. For 2D pulses, it is quite practical to cover a 2D RF k-space with a single shot in 5–25 ms. To cover a 3D k-space often takes longer, so multishot excitation (Stenger et al. 2002) is used for that application.

Finally, let us consider the question of when a multidimensional pulse is needed and discuss alternative methods. Suppose a pulse sequence application requires the spatial localization of a strip of magnetization. If the pulse sequence uses two or more RF pulses to generate the MR signal (e.g., 90° and 180° RF pulses to form a spin echo), then the use of a dedicated 2D pulse might be unnecessary. Instead, the simplest and usually preferred method of obtaining a signal from a strip is to first select a plane with the 90° excitation pulse and then select a perpendicular plane with the 180° pulse by playing the slice-selection gradient on a different axis (Feinberg et al. 1985). The intersection of the two planes will be the desired strip (Figure 5.5). Similarly, if the pulse sequence employs three pulses to generate the signal, such as a stimulated echo pulse sequence that uses three 90° pulses, then three-dimensional localization is obtained if three different orthogonal gradient axes are used for the slice-selection gradients. This approach has been widely employed in localized *in vivo* spectroscopy. Therefore the main application of

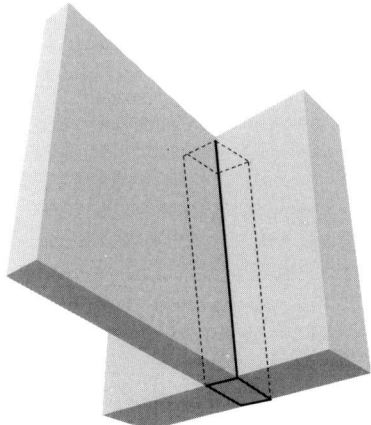

FIGURE 5.5 Drawing demonstrating that a strip of magnetization can be obtained from the intersection of two perpendicular planes, an alternative to using a 2D RF pulse in spin echo pulse sequences.

multidimensional pulses has been restricted to gradient echo pulse sequences, in which the MR signal results from the excitation pulse alone. If 3D localization is required in a spin echo pulse sequence, then an effective method is to use a 2D excitation pulse in conjunction with a slice-selective refocusing pulse.

SELECTED REFERENCES

Alley, M. T., Pauly, J. M., Sommer, G., and Pelc, N. J. 1997. Angiographic imaging with 2D RF pulses. *Magn. Res. Med.* 37: 260–267.

Bottomley, P. A., and Hardy, C. J. 1987. Two-dimensional spatially selective spin inversion and spin-echo refocusing with a single nuclear magnetic resonance pulse. *J. Appl. Phys.* 62: 4284–4290.

Cline, H. E., Hardy, C. J., and Pearlman, J. D. 1991. Fast cardiac profiling with two-dimensional selective pulses. *Magn. Res. Med.* 17: 390–401.

Feinberg, D. A., Hoenninger, J. C., Crooks, L. E., Kaufman, L., Watts, J. C., and Arakawa, M. 1985. Inner volume MR imaging: Technical concepts and their application. *Radiology* 156: 742–747.

Hardy, C. J., and Cline, H. E. 1989. Broadband nuclear magnetic resonance pulses with two-dimensional spatial selectivity. *J. Appl. Phys.* 66: 1513–1516.

Hardy, C. J., Cline, H. E., and Bottomley, P. A. 1990. Correcting for non-uniform k-space sampling in two-dimensional NMR selective excitation. *J. Magn. Reson.* 87: 639–645.

Liu, Y. L., Riederer, S. J., Rossman, P. J., Grimm, R. C., Debbins, J. P., and Ehman, R. L. 1993. A monitoring, feedback, and triggering system for reproducible breath-hold MR imaging. *Magn. Reson. Med.* 30: 507–511.

Pauly, J., Nishimura, D., and Macovski, A. 1989. A k-space analysis of small-tip-angle excitation. *J. Magn. Res.* 81: 43–56.

Pauly, J., Speilman, D., and Macovski, A. 1993. Echo-planar spin echo and inversion pulses. *Magn. Res. Med.* 29: 776–782.

Rieseberg, S., Frahm, J., and Finsterbusch, J. 2002. Two-dimensional spatially selective RF excitation pulses in echo planar imaging. *Magn. Res. Med.* 47: 1186–1193.

Stenger, V. A., Boada, F. E., and Noll, D. C. 2002. Multishot 3D slice-select tailored RF pulses for MRI. *Magn. Res. Med.* 48: 157–168.

RELATED SECTIONS

5.2 Ramp (TONE) Pulses

Ramp RF pulses (Atkinson et al. 1994; Priatna and Paschal 1995) have spatially varying flip angle profiles (Figure 5.6). They are also called tilted

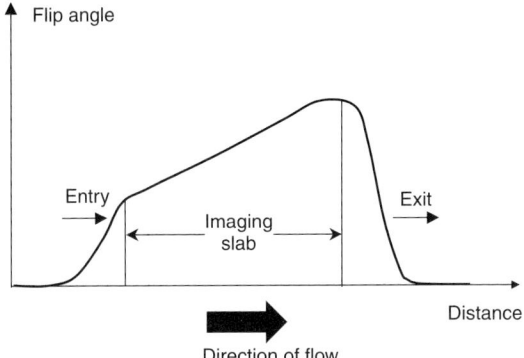

FIGURE 5.6 Schematic representation of a ramp pulse. The flip angle of the pulse increases as a function of distance in order to equalize the signal from flowing blood. The extent of the imaging slab (i.e., the entire set of encoded slices) is also indicated in the figure.

optimized nonsaturating excitation (TONE) pulses. Ramp pulses are used for RF excitation to equalize the signal produced by flowing blood as it traverses through a thick slab of slices. The most common application is to 3D time-of-flight (3DTOF) MR angiography. If a constant flip angle is used across the slab in 3DTOF, then flow-related enhancement causes blood to produce strong signal at the entry slices. Saturation (i.e., incomplete T_1 relaxation) of the longitudinal magnetization, however, then causes the signal to progressively fade as the blood experiences more RF pulses (Figure 5.7a). To counteract this uneven signal, the flip angle of a ramp pulse is set to a lower value (e.g., 15°) where the blood first enters the slab. The flip angle then progressively increases until it reaches its maximal value (e.g., 35°) where the blood exits the slab (Figure 5.7b).

The ratio of the exit-to-entrance flip angles (e.g., $40°/20° = 2:1$, or simply 2) is called the ramp or TONE ratio. By convention, the nominal flip angle of a ramp pulse is its flip angle on resonance, that is, at the center of the slab. The flip angle can vary either linearly or nonlinearly with spatial position, depending on the design of the pulse, but it always increases monotonically along the direction of flow. For a linear ramp pulse, the nominal flip angle is the average of the entry and exit values.

5.2.1 QUALITATIVE DESCRIPTION

Suppose you have $300 budgeted for the month of June. You could spend the money at a constant rate of $10 per day. If, however, there are other factors

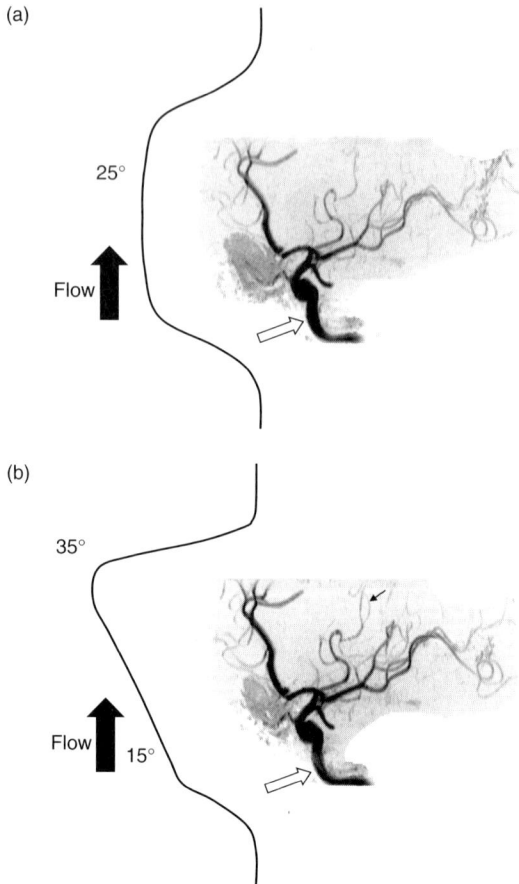

FIGURE 5.7 A sagittal targeted maximum-intensity projection view of the right-side intracranial circulation acquired with 3DTOF at 3.0 T. The 3D slab is composed of 64 1.4-mm slices, for a total thickness of 90 mm. (a) With a standard 25° flip angle excitation pulse the signal in the right internal carotid (hollow arrow) is strong, but the signal progressively fades due to saturation of the longitudinal magnetization. (b) With a ramp pulse (same acquisition parameters) note that some of the signal in the internal carotid artery is sacrificed but that the distal vessels are much better visualized (thin arrow).

that enter into the budget (e.g., interest is earned on any money that is not yet spent), then it might be advantageous to spend less than $10 per day in the beginning of the month and more toward the end. In this analogy (which is somewhat imperfect), the longitudinal magnetization corresponds to the unspent money, the flip angle of the excitation pulse corresponds to the rate of spending, and the MR signal corresponds to what is purchased. The higher the flip angle (assuming it is no greater than 90°), the greater the conversion from the longitudinal magnetization to the transverse magnetization that produces the MR signal.

In 3DTOF MR angiography, fresh blood that flows into the slab has longitudinal magnetization approximately equal to its maximum value, the equilibrium magnetization M_0. As blood flows through the slab, it experiences one RF pulse during each TR interval. The slower the blood flows through the slab, the more RF pulses the blood will experience before it exits the slab and the more saturated it will become. A ramp pulse is designed to preserve more of the longitudinal magnetization of the in-flowing blood by applying smaller flip angles at the entry slices, and the flip angle is progressively increased farther into the slab. Therefore, the slab profile of a ramp pulse is not spatially symmetric. The resultant signal response of flowing blood, however, is more uniform. To properly use a ramp pulse, the operator must specify the direction of flow. For the axial plane acquisitions that are commonly used for 3DTOF intracranial angiography, the ramp pulse slopes upward in the patient's foot-to-head direction, which is also called inferior-to-superior (I-to-S).

If a single known velocity characterizes the flow, then the optimized flip angle profile can be calculated, as illustrated in the next subsection. These flip angle profiles have slopes that progressively increase throughout the slab (Figure 5.8). As discussed in Section 5.2.3, however, often the vessels take tortuous paths through the slab, so the optimization calculation is not feasible.

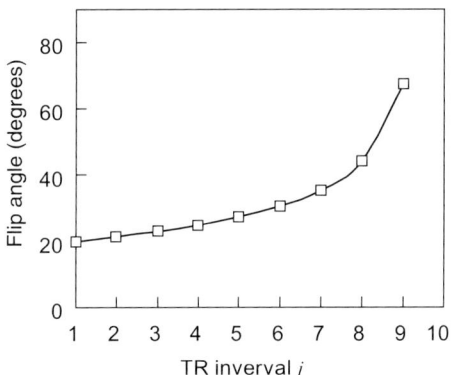

FIGURE 5.8 Plot of the optimized ramp pulse calculated in Example 5.4. The slope is nearly constant until the last few TR intervals. The iteration breaks down, and there is no solution for $j = 10$.

In that case a simple, linear ramp pulse can be used instead. A linear ramp pulse is not optimized for any particular flow geometry, but works well under a wide variety of flow conditions. Also, as shown on Figure 5.8, the linear ramp provides a good approximation to the optimized profile, except near the exit slices. Because they are more tolerant of patient-to-patient variations encountered in clinical imaging situations, linear ramp pulses are widely used. Although nonlinear ramp pulses are not as popular, the optimization process is instructive, and a simple example is presented next.

5.2.2 MATHEMATICAL DESCRIPTION

The concept of equalizing the MR signal from blood as it traverses a slab of slices can be quantified by setting up a recursion relationship for the MR signal in two adjacent TR intervals (Wang et al. 1991). This, in turn, provides a recursion relationship for the flip angles in those two TR intervals. Thus, we can calculate a series of flip angles that keeps the MR signal constant. Keep in mind, however, that for the actual ramp pulse we always repeat the same excitation pulse in each of the TR intervals, so the variation in the flip angle is implicitly caused by the flow of blood through the slab.

To simplify the analysis, assume that a spoiled gradient echo sequence (e.g., spoiled FLASH or SPGR, see Section 14.1) is used and that the excitation pulse is the only RF that the flowing blood experiences. There might be other RF pulses in the sequence (e.g., a magnetization transfer pulse), but if it is applied far off-resonance it will not affect the magnetization of the blood. As explained in Section 14.1, spoiled pulse sequences dephase any residual transverse magnetization at the end of each TR interval. The more complicated case in which the residual transverse magnetization is accounted for (e.g., in the true FISP sequence, see Section 14.1) is considered in Nagele et al.(1994, 1995).

For the spoiled gradient echo sequence, the MR signal produced in the jth TR interval is proportional to:

$$S_j = M_{z,j} \sin \theta_j \qquad j = 1, 2, 3, \ldots \qquad (5.16)$$

where $M_{z,j}$ is the longitudinal magnetization just before the RF pulse in the jth TR interval, and θ_j is the flip angle of the jth excitation pulse. The condition that the MR signal is equalized can be expressed by the simple relationship:

$$S_{j+1} = S_j \qquad j = 1, 2, 3, \ldots \qquad (5.17)$$

The longitudinal magnetization also undergoes T_1 relaxation between the RF pulses, which partially restores M_z. As described in Section 1.2, the Bloch equation for T_1 relaxation states:

$$\frac{dM_z}{dt} = \frac{M_0 - M_z}{T_1} \tag{5.18}$$

which has the solution:

$$M_z(t) = M_0 - \left[M_0 - M_z(0)\right] e^{-t/T_1} \tag{5.19}$$

In the context of our series of excitation pulses, the T_1 relaxation of Eq. (5.19) can be expressed as:

$$M_{z,j+1} = M_0 - \left(M_0 - M_{z,j} \cos\theta_j\right) e^{-\text{TR}/T_1} \tag{5.20}$$

because the z component of the magnetization remaining immediately after the jth RF pulse is $M_{z,j} \cos\theta_j$. Equation (5.20) also assumes that the spacing between RF pulses is TR, that is, that the pulse width of the excitation pulse can be neglected compared to TR. Combining Eqs. (5.16), (5.17), and (5.20) yields:

$$\theta_{j+1} = \arcsin\left(\frac{M_{z,j} \sin\theta_j}{M_0 - (M_0 - M_{z,j} \cos\theta_j)e^{-\text{TR}/T_1}}\right) \tag{5.21}$$

and

$$M_{z,j+1} = \frac{M_{z,j} \sin\theta_j}{\sin\theta_{j+1}} \tag{5.22}$$

Equations (5.21) and (5.22) provide a recursive approach for designing a ramp pulse. Fully magnetized blood (i.e., $M_z = M_0$) enters the slab and experiences a flip angle θ_1. Assuming that TR and T_1 are specified, Eqs (5.21) and (5.22) then provide the next flip angle in the series, θ_2, and so on. This iteration provides a flip angle series that monotonically increases, and both the first and second derivatives are positive.

Because typical repetition times of 3DTOF acquisitions are on the order of TR = 30 ms, and the T_1 of blood is approximately 1200 ms at 1.5 T, the exponential factor $e^{-\text{TR}/T_1} \approx 1$. Due to the small amount of longitudinal relaxation in each TR interval, the iterative process eventually breaks down and produces no valid solution as the flip angle approaches 90° and the longitudinal magnetization approaches 0. The eventual failure of the iteration can be inferred from Eq. (5.21), by recalling that $\cos 90° = 0$ and the arcsine function does not return a real angle when its argument is greater than 1. In practice, the maximal flip angle of a ramp pulse is normally designed to be much less than 90° (e.g., 40°), so that the instabilities in Eq. (5.21) are not a problem.

In order to apply the Eqs. (5.21) and (5.22) to the design of ramp pulse, we first estimate the total thickness $N_z \Delta z$ of the 3D slab of slices, where

N_z is the number of encoded slices, and Δz is the slice thickness. We also need to know the component of the blood velocity v in the slice direction. During each TR interval, the blood travels a distance $v \times$ TR, so that total number of pulses the blood experiences as it traverses the slab of slices is:

$$P = \text{Next highest integer} \left(\frac{N_z \Delta z}{v\text{TR}} \right) \tag{5.23}$$

The different values for initial flip angle θ_1 can be varied until the last flip angle in the series θ_P is a predetermined value less than $90°$ (e.g., $45°$).

Example 5.4 Suppose a 3DTOF acquisition is composed of a slab of 64 1.2-mm-thick slices. Assume the velocity of blood through the slab is $v = 40 \text{ cm/s}$, TR $= 30 \text{ ms}$, and $T_1 = 1200 \text{ ms}$. (a) How many TR intervals P does it take for the blood to traverse the slab? (b) If the magnetization is initially fully magnetized and the entry flip angle is $20°$, calculate the first P terms in the flip angle series. (c) What is the value of the constant product $S_j = M_{z,j} \sin \theta_j$, $j = 1, 2, 3, \ldots, P$?

Answer

(a) The blood travels a distance $v \times$ TR $= 12$ mm during each TR interval. The entire slab is 76.8 mm thick, so for $j = 6$ the blood is still in the slab and for $j = 7$ the blood is out of the slab. Therefore $P = 7$.

TABLE 5.1
Results for Example 5.4[a]

TR Interval Index j	$\dfrac{M_{z,j}}{M_0}$	θ_j (degrees)
1	1	20
2	0.941182	21.30879
3	0.879881	22.87437
4	0.815362	24.80113
5	0.746579	27.26564
6	0.671937	30.59768
7	0.588792	35.51278
8	0.49213	44.02552
9	0.369816	67.64387
10		Undefined

[a] The flip angle progressively increases, but after $j = 9$ the iteration fails.

(b) Using Eqs. (5.21) and (5.22) we can generate Table 5.1. The values for $j = 8$ and $j = 9$ are also provided to show the behavior of the flip angle just prior to the breakdown of the recursion relation. A plot of the flip angle θ_j versus j is shown in Figure 5.8.

(c) From Table 5.1, the constant value is $S_j = M_{z,j} \sin \theta_j = 0.34202 M_0$.

5.2.3 IMPLEMENTATION DETAILS

If the maximal flip angle in a ramp profile is on the order of $45°$ or less, then the nonlinearity in the Bloch equations can be neglected and the pulse can be designed with a Fourier transform method. First we start with a standard, nonramp excitation pulse such as a SINC or minimum-phase SLR pulse. Then the pulse is Fourier transformed (explained in Section 3.1) and provides the small flip angle slice profile. That profile is then multiplied by the desired ramp profile, and the product is then inverse Fourier transformed to yield the final ramp pulse. Thus the ramp pulse is the convolution of the original RF pulse and the inverse FT of the ramp function. The ramp pulse will always have both real and imaginary components in the time domain (i.e., it has nonzero phase) because its slice profile is asymmetric. A typical design procedure for a ramp pulse using the Fourier transform method is to start with a minimum phase pulse with a dimensionless time-bandwidth product of 10–20 and to apply a linear ramp with an exit-to-entrance ratio of 2:1. As described in Section 2.3 on SLR pulses, the relatively high value of the time-bandwidth product yields a sharper transition region in the profile, which in turn reduces wrap in the slice direction.

Ramp pulses can also be designed directly using the SLR method. The desired profile, including the ramp, is specified, converted into the appropriate polynomials, and then inverse SLR transformed to yield the desired RF pulse. This design method is not subject to the errors arising from nonlinearity in the Bloch equations and so is preferred for larger maximal flip angles.

5.2.4 APPLICATIONS AND RELATED PULSES

Ramp pulses are commonly used for 3DTOF angiography. The use of 3DTOF has been mainly supplanted by contrast-enhanced MR angiography, except for imaging the intracranial arteries, where the venous return time is nearly zero. Unlike the arteries of the neck and legs that take relatively straight paths, the vessels in the head tend to follow tortuous routes (Figure 5.7). Therefore, there is no single value for the perpendicular velocity component v that is valid for all the arteries. Moreover, there is a distribution of flow velocities (e.g., laminar) within each vessel that further complicates the problem. For these reasons, it is difficult to calculate an optimized ramp profile for intracranial 3DTOF. Instead, a linear ramp pulse is usually chosen because it performs well for a variety of velocity values. Typical ramp ratios range from 2:1 to 3:1, which could correspond to flip angle ranges of 40–20° or 30–10°, respectively.

Slower-flowing spins experience greater saturation by the time they exit the slab. Because the slowest flow tends to occur near the vessel wall, the use of a ramp pulse can sometimes appear to sharpen the vessel margins, as illustrated in Figure 5.7. Conversely, without the ramp pulse, the signal can become increasingly saturated near the vessel wall, sometimes giving the artery a blurred appearance. If the vessels are too tortuous, however, and the flow direction reverses (e.g., from superior to inferior), then the ramp pulse can increase signal saturation and be counterproductive.

Ramp pulses can be used with both single- and multiple-slab 3DTOF acquisitions. As explained in Section 15.3, multiple overlapping thin-slab acquisition (MOTSA) is used for the same purpose as ramp pulses—to reduce the signal saturation of blood as it traverses through a thick slab of slices. Using ramp pulses in conjunction with MOTSA may seem like unnecessary duplication, like wearing both a belt and suspenders. In practice, the combination of ramp pulses and MOTSA is quite useful because it allows each MOTSA slab to be somewhat thicker (e.g., 40 mm) without saturating the magnetization of the slower flowing blood. As a result, there is less time wasted in acquiring the overlapping slices. Figure 5.9 shows an example of a two-slab MOTSA acquisition, in which each slab uses its own ramp pulse. Note that the use of

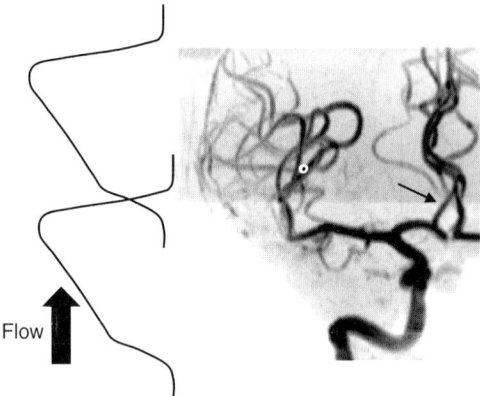

FIGURE 5.9 Example of a two-slab MOTSA acquisition in which each slab uses its own ramp excitation pulse. Each slab is composed of 32 1.4-mm slices. The use of the ramp pulse yields a very continuous vessel signal at the slab boundary (arrow), although there is enhanced discontinuity in the stationary tissue background signal.

the ramp pulse actually accentuates the discontinuity of the signal intensity of the stationary tissue background. More important, however, the vessel signal is quite uniform (arrow). Although it may initially look distracting, the venetian blind artifact in the stationary tissue background should not adversely affect the radiologist's diagnosis.

There are several pulse sequences that vary the RF flip angle in a way that is analogous to ramp pulses. A close analog is sometimes used to image hyperpolarized noble gases such as ^{3}He (Moller et al. 2002). Hyperpolarized gases achieve very high values of the longitudinal magnetization (e.g., 10^4–$10^5 \times M_0$) with optical pumping techniques. The hyperpolarized gas can then be inhaled and used to make images of the airways and bronchi. Unfortunately, any subsequent T_1 recovery is to M_0 rather than the hyperpolarized value of the longitudinal magnetization. For this reason, gradient recalled echo imaging with a series of excitation pulses that have progressively increasing flip angles has been proposed.

Other examples of varying the flip angle for a series of RF pulses in MRI include the echo stabilization that is used for the refocusing pulses in a RARE sequence and the half-angle catalyst pulse that is used in steady-state gradient echo sequences such as true FISP. These methods result in flip angle profiles that vary temporally but not spatially. These techniques are discussed in Sections 16.4 and 14.1, respectively.

SELECTED REFERENCES

Atkinson, D., Brant-Zawadzki, M., Gillan, G., Purdy, D., and Laub, G. 1994. Improved MR angiography with variable flip angle excitation and increased resolution. *Radiology* 190: 890–894.

Moller, H. E., Chen, X. J., Saam, B., Hagspiel, K. D., Johnson, G. A., Altes, T. A., De Lange, E. E., and Kauczor, H. U. 2002. MRI of the lungs using hyperpolarized noble gases. *Magn. Reson. Med.* 47: 1029–1051.

Nagele, T., Klose, U., Grodd, W., Nusslin, F., and Voigt, K. 1995. Non-linear excitation profiles for three-dimensional inflow MR angiography. *J. Magn. Reson. Imag.* 4: 416–420.

Nagele, T., Klose, U., Grodd, W., Petersen, D., and Tintera, J. 1994. The effects of linearly increasing flip angles on 3D inflow MR angiography. *Magn. Reson. Med.* 31: 561–566.

Priatna, A., and Paschal, C. B. 1995. Variable-angle uniform signal excitation (VUSE) for three-dimensional time-of-flight MR angiography. *J. Magn. Reson. Imag.* 4: 421–427.

Wang, S. J., Nishimura, D. G., and Macovski, A. 1991. Multiple-readout selective inversion recovery angiography. *Magn. Reson. Med.* 17: 244–251.

RELATED SECTIONS

5.3 Spatial Saturation Pulses

Spatial saturation or *presaturation* is a method for removing unwanted signals from a specified location (Felmlee and Ehman 1987; Edelman et al. 1988). It is especially useful for reducing respiratory artifacts arising from motion of the abdominal wall; for removing signals from spins flowing into a slice from a given direction, for example in 2DTOF imaging (see Section 15.3); or for reducing aliasing in the phase-encoded direction by attenuating the signal from outside the field of view.

The idea behind spatial saturation is to use a spatially selective 90° RF pulse to flip longitudinal magnetization into the transverse plane (i.e., saturate it) over one or more selected areas (saturation bands) as shown in Figure 5.10. Unlike excitation or refocusing RF pulses, spatial saturation pulses should result in as little transverse magnetization as possible. Therefore we intentionally create phase dispersion across the saturated band to dephase the transverse magnetization following the RF pulse. The RF pulse can be designed to produce maximal phase dispersion across the saturation band, and the gradient rephasing pulse normally used with selective excitation is omitted.

The RF pulse is followed instead by a gradient dephasing pulse (spoiler gradient pulse; see Section 10.5) to further eliminate signal from the saturation band (Figure 5.11). Because the magnetization is already partially dephased in the slice-selection direction following the spatial saturation RF pulse, placing the spoiler on the slice-selection axis sometime has limited benefit. Therefore the spoiler pulse is usually placed on a different gradient axis to give

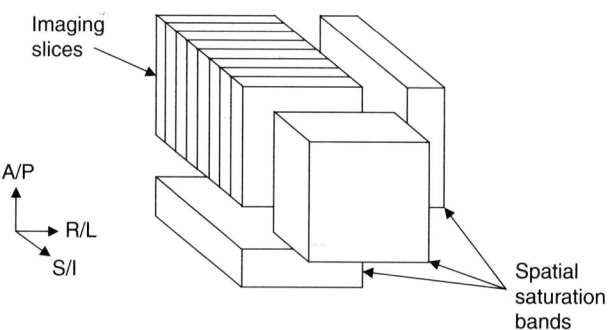

FIGURE 5.10 Spatial saturation bands placed to the superior, right, and posterior sides of the imaging slices. A/P, R/L, and S/I denote anterior/posterior, right/left, and superior/inferior, respectively.

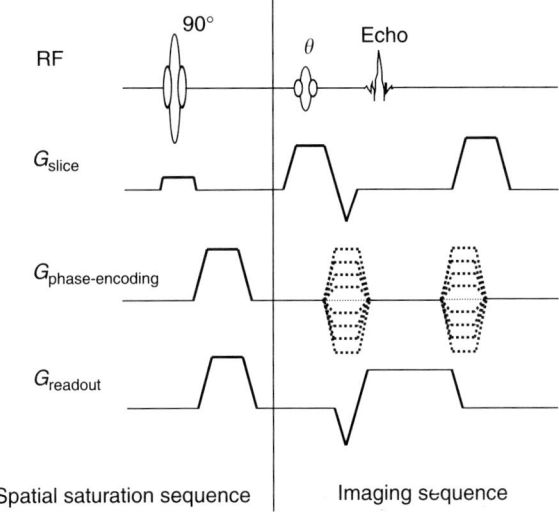

FIGURE 5.11 A spatial saturation sequence with spoilers followed by a gradient recalled-echo imaging sequence. In this example, the saturation band and imaging slices are parallel. The 90° saturation pulse has a different carrier frequency from the θ excitation pulse. The saturation pulse has spoilers on two of the gradient axes.

additional phase dispersion in an orthogonal direction. The spoiler is normally played at maximum amplitude to minimize the impact on imaging time.

Before the longitudinal magnetization has sufficient time to recover, the saturation pulse is followed by excitation and imaging of the desired area. The saturation pulse is typically played out for every TR of the pulse sequence, although for some fast gradient echo pulse sequences it can be played less frequently.

The imaged volume can intersect the saturated region or can be adjacent to it. The saturation region can have a different plane orientation than the imaging region. For example, in abdominal scanning the imaged slice could be axial with a coronal spatial saturation slice placed over the anterior part of the abdominal wall within the field of view.

5.3.1 IMPLEMENTATION

The thickness of the saturated band typically ranges from 10 to 80 mm. For imaging, the profile of the saturation band is somewhat less critical than for spectroscopy because in imaging its purpose is to reduce signal from a broad area rather than to localize a small voxel. Hence RF pulse design requirements are more demanding for spectroscopy than for imaging. Standard methods are typically applied to the design of spatial saturation RF pulses (as in Section 3.1, for example). Because the spatial saturation pulse is usually played once per TR interval, improving the slice profile of the pulse by increasing its pulse width can increase the minimum TR and hence impact imaging time or the maximal number of slices that can be acquired within a TR time. The pulse designer must therefore make a trade-off among the imaging time, saturation band profile, and number of slices within a TR.

Inadequate dephasing by the gradient spoiler can cause remnants of the FID from the saturation pulse to be superimposed on the imaging echo. If the FID becomes spatially encoded by the imaging gradients, the unwanted signal originating from the saturation band can overlay the image. Increasing the spoiler area usually eliminates the FID signal, although this can prolong the imaging time. If the spoiler area is too large, gradient coil or gradient amplifier heating limits can cause an unwanted increase in TR. The heating limits, which are less restrictive with modern hardware, can sometimes be overcome by moving the spoiler pulse to an axis with a lower gradient duty cycle.

An important application of spatial saturation is 2DTOF imaging. In this technique, the imaging slice and saturation band both lie in the same plane, which is usually chosen to be axial. The saturation band is slightly displaced from the imaging slice. The displacement direction depends on the type of flow to be saturated (Figure 5.12). For example, to saturate venous flow in the neck, the saturation volume is placed superior to the imaging slice. To saturate venous flow in the legs, the saturation volume is placed inferior to the imaging slice (i.e., in the caudal direction). The distance between the imaging and saturation slices (saturation gap) is typically 5–30 mm. The saturation gap is kept constant for all slices to ensure uniform flow suppression. A saturation

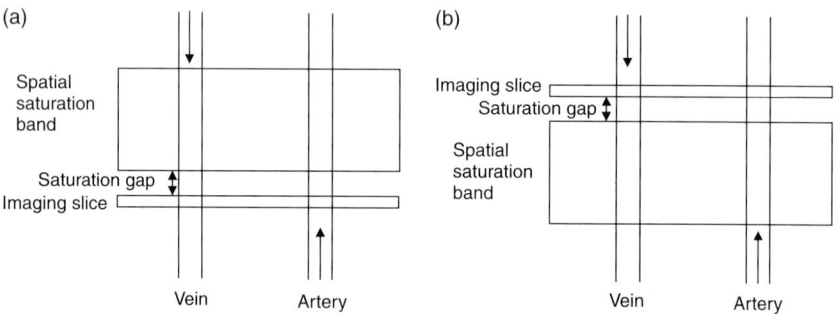

FIGURE 5.12 Spatial saturation band placement for (a) venous flow suppression and (b) arterial flow suppression. The arrows indicate the direction of blood flow.

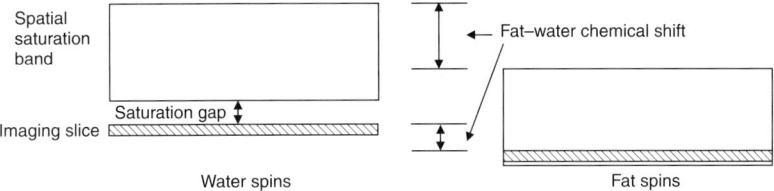

FIGURE 5.13 Spatial saturation for fat suppression. The fat spatial saturation band and imaging slice (hatched) are shifted with respect to water due to chemical shift in the slice direction. The saturation band shifts by a greater distance than the imaging slice mainly because the saturation band is much thicker than the imaging slice. The saturation gap is chosen so the fat spatial saturation band overlays the fat imaging slice. Distances are exaggerated for clarity.

pulse that moves to maintain a constant separation from the imaging slice is sometimes called a *traveling* or *concatenated* saturation pulse.

Spatial saturation can simultaneously suppress both unwanted flow and fat signals in 2DTOF. In a technique called spatially separated lipid presaturation (SLIP) (Doyle et al. 1991) the saturation gap and saturation pulse are chosen so that the chemical shift of fat causes the saturation pulse to saturate the fat spins in the imaging slice (Figure 5.13).

Example 5.5 A 2DTOF pulse sequence uses 1-mm-thick imaging slices and an excitation pulse with bandwidth 1.0 kHz. At 1.5 T, the chemical shift between fat and water is approximately 210 Hz. If the spatial saturation excitation pulse is chosen to have a bandwidth of 1.5 kHz and the slice-select gradient for the saturation pulse is chosen to give an 80-mm-thick saturation band, what is the maximum saturation gap that allows fat saturation of the imaging slice?

Answer The fat spins excited by the imaging pulse are shifted with respect to the water spins by 1 mm $\times$ (210 Hz/1000 Hz) = 0.21 mm. The fat spins excited by the saturation pulse are shifted with respect to the water spins by 80 mm $\times$ (210 Hz/1500 Hz) = 11.20 mm. Taking into account the 1-mm slice width and 0.21-mm slice shift, the saturation gap can be no more than $11.20 - 1.0 - 0.21 = 9.99$ mm.

Sometimes saturation bands are applied to two opposite sides of the acquisition volume. For example, to completely eliminate the blood flow signal from all in-flowing spins in axial slices, axial saturation bands are applied on both the superior and inferior sides of the imaging volume. If the bands have equal thickness, they can be conveniently generated with a single RF pulse by modulating the RF pulse by a cosine function, that is, by multiplying the RF pulse by $\cos 2\pi f_0 t$, where f_0 is chosen based on the saturation band separation.

This is sometimes known as *Hadamard* (after Jacques Salomon Hadamard, 1865–1963, a French mathematician) or *double-sideband modulation*. The cosine modulation function is used because its Fourier transform is two delta functions displaced symmetrically around DC by the cosine frequency f_0 (see Section 1.1):

$$FT[\cos 2\pi f_0 t] = \frac{[\delta(f - f_0) + \delta(f + f_0)]}{2} \tag{5.24}$$

The use of double-sideband saturation has the advantage that the total RF duration is only one-half that of playing two separate single-sideband pulses. The peak RF amplitude, however, doubles to compensate for the factor of 2 in the denominator in Eq. (5.24). Consequently, the average SAR also doubles compared to playing two separate single-sideband pulses, while the peak SAR quadruples. It should be noted that the double-sideband approach is valid only when the two saturation bands are parallel to one another. When two nonparallel saturation bands are required on either side of an imaged volume, two separate single saturation pulses must be employed.

Example 5.6 An RF excitation pulse $B_1(t)$ with bandwidth 1.0 kHz is to be used to saturate two identical axial slabs with thickness 80 mm surrounding the imaging volume. The slabs are centered at $z = -10$ cm and $z = +14$ cm, respectively. Using the small flip angle approximation (i.e., linear Bloch equation solution), calculate the cosine envelope modulation for the pulse and the necessary carrier frequency offset δf.

Answer The distance between the slabs is 24 cm. If the slabs were centered at $z = 0$, each slab would be offset by 12 cm. The corresponding cosine modulation frequency is given by $f_0 = (1000 \text{ Hz})(12 \text{ cm}/8 \text{ cm}) = 1500 \text{ Hz}$. To offset the two slabs to $z = -10$ cm and $z = +14$ cm, the center of mass is offset by 2 cm. The carrier frequency offset is therefore $\delta f = (1000 \text{ Hz})(2 \text{ cm})/(8 \text{ cm}) = 250 \text{ Hz}$.

SELECTED REFERENCES

Doyle, M., Matsuda, T., and Pohost, G. M. 1991. SLIP, a lipid suppression technique to improve image contrast in inflow angiography. *Magn. Reson. Med.* 21: 71–81.

Edelman, R. R., Atkinson, D. J., Silver, M. S., Loaiza, F. L., and Warren, W. S. 1988. FRODO pulse sequences: A new means of eliminating motion, flow, and wraparound artifacts. *Radiology* 166: 231–236.

Felmlee, J. P., and Ehman, R. L. 1987. Spatial presaturation: A method for suppressing flow artifacts and improving depiction of vascular anatomy in MR imaging. *Radiology* 164: 559–564.

5.4 Spatial-Spectral Pulses

Spatial-spectral (SPSP) *RF pulses* (Meyer et al. 1990; Block et al. 1997; Schick 1998; Zur 2000) (also known as *spectral-spatial pulses*) excite magnetization that has both a specified slice location and a specified spectral content. An SPSP pulse can be used to excite a slice of magnetization from one chemical species (e.g., water) while leaving the magnetization from another (e.g., lipids) virtually unaffected. A common application is to use a single SPSP pulse to replace the combination of a spectrally selective presaturation pulse (Section 4.3) and an excitation pulse (Section 3.1). SPSP pulses can also be used for other applications besides excitation, such as saturation (Zur 2000).

SPSP RF pulses have several advantages. First, the duration of the SPSP pulse is often shorter than the combined duration of the two pulses that it can replace. Second, and perhaps more important, SPSP pulses offer better tolerance to B_1 inhomogeneity than conventional fat-saturation pulses. This is because the signal from lipids is never excited, as opposed to being excited and then dephased. For example, suppose the nominal flip angles for a fat-saturation and excitation pulse are both $90°$, but due to B_1 inhomogeneity, a particular location experiences only $30°$ flip angles. In this case, the fraction of the lipid magnetization undisturbed by the fat-saturation pulse is $\cos(30°) = 87\%$. The excitation pulse will then excite $\sin(30°) = 50\%$ of the water magnetization, whereas $\sin(30°) \times \cos(30°) = 43\%$ of the lipid magnetization is excited. An SPSP pulse, however, is designed to provide only negligible excitation of lipids. Suppose a $90°$ SPSP pulse excites 4% of the lipid magnetization. In our example, only $\sin(30°) \times 4\% = 2\%$ of the lipid magnetization would be excited. The SPSP pulse therefore provides a 21-fold improvement in lipid suppression over conventional fat saturation in this example. Finally, not exciting lipids means that regrowth of their longitudinal magnetization due to T_1 relaxation is not a concern.

There are many variants of SPSP pulses, but all consist of multiple RF subpulses that are played under a broad RF envelope. The subpulses, together with a concurrent oscillating bipolar slice-selection gradient waveform (Figure 5.14), determine the spatial selectivity, whereas the RF envelope governs the spectral content. The spatial RF subpulses can be played under some, or all, of the gradient lobes. A time-varying gradient is required because

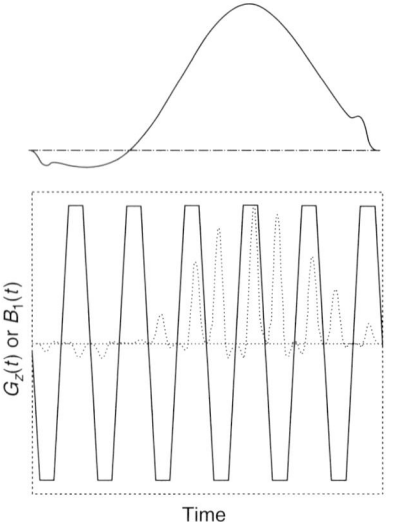

FIGURE 5.14 A spatial-spectral pulse. The oscillating gradient waveform (solid line) and RF waveform $B_{1,spsp}(t)$ (dotted line) are shown. The spectral RF envelope $A_{spec}(t)$ is shown (top) for reference. Note how the spectral envelope modulates the amplitudes of the spatial subpulses.

a constant slice-selection gradient produces identical (but spatially offset) replicates of the slice profiles for chemical species such as lipids and water. The oscillating gradient waveform can be sinusoidal in shape, but more commonly it is implemented with trapezoidal lobes of alternating polarity as in Figure 5.14. The trapezoid maximizes the area under the gradient lobes, which allows thinner slices.

5.4.1 MATHEMATICAL DESCRIPTION

Joint Spatial-Spectral RF k-Space   Just as the standard k-space is a useful concept for analyzing spatial encoding and data acquisition, a two-dimensional (2D) SPSP RF k-space (Meyer et al. 1990) is a useful tool for designing SPSP RF pulses. RF k-space is a valid construct for analyzing small-flip-angle RF excitation, in which the magnetization response is well approximated by the Fourier transform of the RF envelope. An RF k-space with two spatial dimensions is discussed in Section 5.1.

We denote spatial and spectral axes of the 2D RF k-space by k_z and k_f, respectively. As with the standard k-space, the spatial axis k_z is defined as the area under the gradient $G_z(t)$, except that by convention the integration proceeds from right to left:

$$k_z = \frac{\gamma}{2\pi} \int\limits_{T_{\text{end}}}^{t} G_z(t') \, dt' \qquad (5.25)$$

It is often convenient to select T_{end} to be the end of the slice-rephasing gradient lobe to ensure that the center of each gradient plateau of the SPSP pulse corresponds to $k_z = 0$.

The spectral axis of the 2D SPSP k-space can be defined by analogy to the spatial dimension. Recall from Eq. (5.25) that the phase (in radians) accumulated from spatial displacement z is $\phi = 2\pi k_z z$, whereas the phase accumulated by magnetization with a frequency offset f during a time interval t is $\phi = 2\pi f t$.

By convention, we set $k_f(t = T_{\text{end}}) = 0$, so we define:

$$k_f = T_{\text{end}} - t \qquad (5.26)$$

Equation (5.26) implies that traversal along the spectral dimension of the SPSP k-space is accomplished simply by waiting. Therefore, separating the RF subpulses in time ensures that they are distributed along the k_f axis.

The Oscillating Gradient: True and Opposed Null Designs   Just as completion of a 2D image acquisition requires filling the standard k-space with signal data, the design of an SPSP pulse requires filling the 2D SPSP k-space with RF data. The process of designing an SPSP pulse begins with the selection of the oscillating gradient waveform, which in turn determines the k-space trajectory according to Eqs. (5.25) and (5.26) and as shown on Figure 5.15. Unless limited by physiological constraints such as peripheral nerve stimulation, we typically choose trapezoidal lobes with the maximal gradient amplitude $\pm h$ and use the minimal rise time r. These choices maximize the extent in k_z, which generates the thinnest slices, because $\Delta z \propto 1/k_{z,\text{max}}$. Naturally, to obtain thicker slices the gradient amplitude and slew rate (i.e., h/r) can be scaled down, but a more optimal result can be achieved by redesigning the SPSP pulse to make full use of the maximal gradient performance.

An important parameter of the oscillating gradient is its period T, which is determined by the type of SPSP design and the frequency separation of the excited and suppressed chemical species. As derived in Meyer et al. (1990) and illustrated in Figure 5.16, the magnetization response to the SPSP pulse has a main peak at $f = 0$ (i.e., on-resonance), as well as periodic replicates.

Assuming that spatial subpulses are played under both the positive and negative gradient lobes, the frequency separation between the replicates is

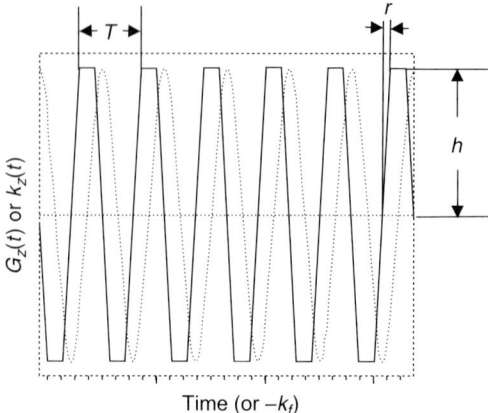

FIGURE 5.15 A spatial-spectral pulse is constructed by first generating an oscillating gradient (solid line) that has period T or lobe width $T/2$. Here the gradient is composed of trapezoidal lobes of amplitude h and rise time r. For the plot of the trapezoidal gradient, the horizontal axis represents time and the vertical axis represents gradient amplitude. The spatial-spectral k-space (dotted line) trajectory generated by this gradient waveform is superimposed. The horizontal axis for the k-space trajectory represents k_f and the vertical axis represents k_z. Note that the center of the each gradient plateau corresponds to $k_z = 0$. The slice-rephasing lobe, a negative-polarity trapezoid with one-half the area of each gradient lobe, is not shown.

given by $2/T$, so the main peaks appear at:

$$f_{\text{main}} = 0, \pm\frac{2}{T}, \pm\frac{4}{T}, \pm\frac{6}{T}, \cdots \tag{5.27}$$

Phase cycling techniques (Block et al. 1997; Schick 1998; Zur 2000) of the spatial RF subpulses can be used to shift these values and even to suppress the $f = 0$ peak (Zur 2000). Halfway between the main replicates are the secondary peaks (see Figure 5.16). The frequency offset of the secondary peaks is related to the period of the oscillating gradient by:

$$f_{\text{scnd}} = \pm\frac{1}{T}, \pm\frac{3}{T}, \pm\frac{5}{T}, \cdots \tag{5.28}$$

The secondary peaks are smaller in height than the main peaks. At each secondary-peak frequency location, there are two peaks with opposite polarities; that is, the polarity of the magnetization response approximately reverses sign when z is negated:

$$M_y(-z, f_{\text{scnd}}) \approx -M_y(z, f_{\text{scnd}}) \tag{5.29}$$

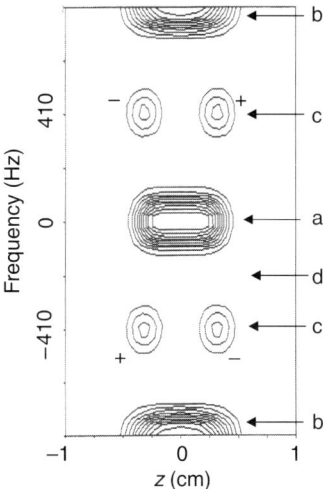

FIGURE 5.16 Contour plot of the magnetization response $|M_\perp|$ versus spatial and frequency coordinates obtained by numerically solving the Bloch equations for an SPSP pulse with a gradient oscillation period $T = 2.38$ ms. The main slice-selection peak (a) is located at $f = 0$ and has a slice thickness of approximately 7 mm. Replicates (b) of this main lobe are located at frequency $\pm 2/T = \pm 840$ Hz. Halfway between the main replicates at $f = \pm 1/T = \pm 420$ Hz are the asymmetric secondary peaks (c) The annotations $+$ and $-$ indicate the sign of the response of M_y. The frequency valley where lipids are placed for a true null SPSP pulse is indicated by (d) In this example, the valley occurs at $f = -210$ Hz, which is suitable for lipid suppression at 1.5 T.

(The relationship in Eq. 5.29 becomes an equality if the spectral envelope, the top graph in Figure 5.14, is symmetric about its center, as it is for a SINC or linear phase SLR pulse.) We also note another symmetry relationship that is always true as long as the B_1 field is applied in the x direction in the rotating frame and which is also apparent in Figure 5.16:

$$M_y(z, f) = M_y(-z, -f) \qquad (5.30)$$

Generally the period T is chosen so that if water is on-resonance the Larmor frequency of lipids falls in the valley halfway between $f = 0$ and the nearest secondary peak. This design is sometimes called a *true-null* SPSP pulse. As can be seen in Figure 5.16 (arrow d), the frequency separation f_{cs} is related to the period T by:

$$f_{cs} = \frac{1}{2T} \qquad \text{(true null)} \qquad (5.31)$$

Example 5.7 Water protons resonate at a frequency (in hertz) approximately $f_{cs} = 140 \times B_0$ (in teslas) higher than lipid protons. What is the period of the oscillating gradient to produce a true-null SPSP pulse at 3.0 T? What is the duration of each trapezoidal lobe (including ramps)?

Answer The chemical shift between fat and water at 3.0 T is approximately $f_{cs} \approx 420$ Hz. Using Eq. (5.31), we obtain:

$$T = \frac{1}{2 f_{cs}} = \frac{1}{2 \times 420 \, \text{Hz}} = 1.19 \, \text{ms}$$

Therefore, each trapezoidal lobe is approximately $T/2 = 595 \, \mu s$ in duration.

Sometimes the duration of the gradient lobe required by the true-null design is too short to provide the time-bandwidth product required for the spatial subpulses to yield the desired slice profile. In this case, an *opposed-null* design can be used. With the opposed-null design, the period of the oscillating gradient is selected so that the fat–water chemical shift corresponds to the closest secondary peak. From Eq. (5.28), the secondary peak is at a frequency:

$$f_{cs} = \frac{1}{T} \qquad \text{(opposed null)} \qquad (5.32)$$

The anti-symmetry of M_y with respect to z at the secondary peak (Eq. 5.29) means that a slice of lipid uniformly distributed in z gives no net signal because of cancellation within the slice.

Comparing Eqs. (5.31) and (5.32), the gradient oscillation period T can be doubled in the opposed-null design compared with the true-null design. Opposed-null SPSP pulses are useful for MR systems that operate with lower performance gradients, due to hardware or physiological constraints, or at higher field strength where the frequency separation f_{cs} is greater. The main drawback of opposed-null SPSP pulses is that they are prone to partial volume artifacts. Effective lipid suppression relies on the cancellation of the signal across the slice according to Eq. (5.29), and as illustrated in Figure 5.16. If lipids are not uniformly distributed across the entire slice thickness, then the cancellation can be incomplete. Finally, opposed-null designs also cannot be used as SPSP saturation pulses because, unlike the transverse magnetization, the longitudinal magnetization is an even function of z for both the main and secondary peaks. This is because the squaring of M_y in the relationship $M_z = \sqrt{M_0^2 - M_x^2 - M_y^2}$ means that the sign change described by Eq. (5.29) does not affect the longitudinal magnetization. More details about the symmetry properties of the magnetization response of SPSP pulses are given in Zur (2000).

The Spectral Envelope, Spatial Kernel, and Gradient Dwell Factor   The oscillating gradient determines the k-space trajectory, whereas the choices for the spectral RF envelope and spatial RF kernel complete the design of the SPSP pulse and determine the shape of the peaks. The product of four factors specifies the SPSP RF pulse $B_{1,\text{spsp}}(t)$ as a function of time:

$$B_{1,\text{spsp}}(t) = C(\theta) |G_z(t)| A_{\text{spec}}(t) A_{\text{spat}}(k_z(t)) \tag{5.33}$$

where $B_{1,\text{spsp}}(t)$ is in teslas (or microteslas). In this subsection, Eq. (5.33) and the factors that make up its right-hand side are described in more detail.

The constant normalization factor that gives the desired flip angle can be determined with integration, just as with any other real pulse:

$$C(\theta) = \frac{\theta}{\gamma \int_{\text{SPSPpulse}} A_{\text{spec}}(t) A_{\text{spat}}(t) |G_z(t)| \, dt} \tag{5.34}$$

where θ is the flip angle in radians. In the unusual situation where the SPSP pulse is complex (e.g., if the spatial kernel is itself complex), $C(\theta)$ can be determined by numerically solving the Bloch equations. Because A_{spec} and A_{spat} are in teslas (or microteslas), $C(\theta)$ is in distance per tesla^2.

The second factor in Eq. (5.33) is the absolute value of the slice-selection gradient $|G_z(t)|$, typically specified in milliteslas per meter. This factor is proportional to the absolute value of the time derivative of $k_z(t)$, and it compensates for the varying rate of the traversal of k-space. $|G_z(t)|$ is sometimes called the dwell-factor and is explained in more detail in Section 2.4 on variable rate pulses.

Typically the spectral modulation envelope $A_{\text{spec}}(t)$ is chosen to be a soft RF pulse, such as a SINC, or a linear or minimum-phase SLR pulse. Using an SLR pulse allows the designer to trade off stopband ripples against the spectral profile. Alternatively, the amplitude of the spatial subpulses can be determined by a set of discrete numbers rather than being derived from the continuous waveform $A_{\text{spec}}(t)$. For example, an FIR filter such as the binomial coefficients can be used, as described in Section 4.1 on composite pulses. The spectral selectivity of the RF envelope $A_{\text{spec}}(t)$ determines how rapidly the response of the main peak of the SPSP pulse (and its replicates) fall off versus the frequency. (The exact spectral response can be obtained by solving the Bloch equations with numerical methods.) Thus an efficient pulse such as a minimum-phase pulse SLR can provide good separation of the frequency islands while keeping the overall duration of the SPSP pulse to a minimum.

Figure 5.17 schematically illustrates the procedure for generating the SPSP pulse described by Eq. (5.33). Note how the spatial RF pulse kernel is evaluated at $k_z(t)$, which is periodic in t, so that the same kernel is repeatedly used

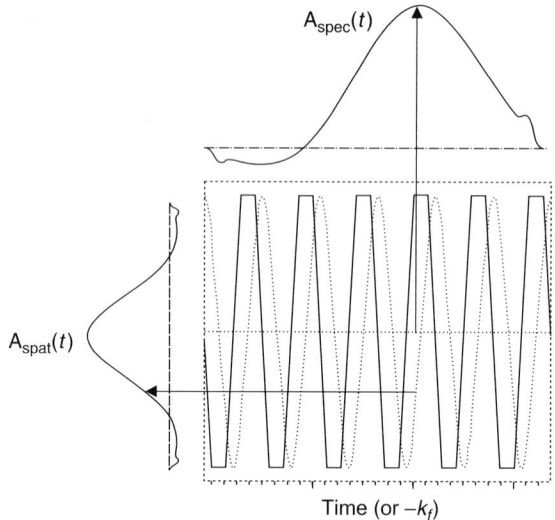

FIGURE 5.17 Generation of the spatial-spectral pulse. Along with the gradient and k-space depicted in Figure 5.15, a spectral RF envelope $A_{\text{spec}}(t)$ (top) and a spatial RF kernel $A_{\text{spat}}(t)$ (left) are plotted. At any time point, the value of the spatial-spectral pulse is generated according to Eq. (5.33). Note that A_{spat} is evaluated at $k_z(t)$. More design details can be found in Meyer et al. (1990).

to generate the spatial subpulses, in accordance with Eq. (5.33). The spatial kernel is often chosen to be a SINC or linear-phase SLR pulse. The spatial slice thickness can be calculated from the dimensionless time-bandwidth product of the spatial subpulse and the total extent in the spatial k-space:

$$\Delta z = \frac{T_{\text{spatial}} \Delta f_{\text{spatial}}}{k_{z,\text{max}}} \tag{5.35}$$

The SPSP pulse designer has two additional decisions concerning the spatial subpulses. First, should they be played during both the positive and the negative polarity gradient lobes? Playing the spatial subpulses during both ensures that the SPSP k-space will be densely packed, but requires excellent gradient fidelity. Playing the spatial subpulses only on the positive lobes sidesteps many of the gradient fidelity requirements, but doubles the data spacing in the RF k-space. In other words, the distance between the k_f samples doubles in the SPSP k-space, thereby halving the spectral field of view. This has the undesirable effect of cutting the frequency spacing in Eqs. (5.27) and (5.28) in half. To compensate for this problem, the period T can be halved, but then the minimum slice thickness is further increased.

Second, should the spatial subpulses be played during the gradient ramps? The advantage of playing RF during the gradient ramps is that the maximal gradient area is used, so the maximal extent in k_z-space is reached. Consistent with the RF k-space interpretation, this decreases the minimum slice thickness of the SPSP pulse.

Example 5.8 An SPSP pulse uses an oscillating gradient with a trapezoidal shape and a period of $T = 2.38$ ms. The gradient waveform has a maximal gradient amplitude $h = 20$ mT/m, and the duration of the ramp from 0 to h is $r = 100\,\mu$s. The spatial RF subpulse has a dimensionless time-bandwidth product of $T_{spatial}\Delta f_{spatial} = 4.0$. What is the slice thickness if the RF is played (a) only on the gradient plateau and (b) on both the plateau and the ramps?

Answer From Figure 5.15, each trapezoidal lobe has duration $T/2 = 1.19$ ms. Therefore, the duration of each gradient plateau is $1.19 - 2r = 0.99$ ms.

(a) From Eqs. (5.25) and (5.35), if RF is only played during the gradient plateau the slice thickness is:

$$\Delta z = \frac{4.0}{(\gamma/2\pi)(0.99\text{ ms})(20\text{ mT/m})} = 4.75\text{ mm}$$

(b) If RF is played during both the gradient ramps and the plateau, then maximal extent in k-space (i.e., the gradient area) is increased, so the slice thickness is correspondingly decreased:

$$\Delta z = \frac{4.0}{(\gamma/2\pi)(0.99\text{ ms} + 0.1\text{ ms})(20\text{ mT/m})} = 4.31\text{ mm}$$

Finally, we note the SPSP pulse given in Eq. (5.33) yields a slice centered at the gradient isocenter, $z = 0$. To offset the slice by a distance δz away from isocenter, according to the Fourier shift theorem, the pulse is modulated by:

$$B_{1,\text{spsp}}(t, \delta z) = e^{i2\pi k_z(t)\delta z} B_{1,\text{spsp}}(t, \delta z = 0) \tag{5.36}$$

where $k_z(t)$ is given by Eq. (5.25).

Note that the offset frequency in Eq. (5.36)

$$\frac{d}{dt}(2\pi k_z(t)\delta z) = \gamma G_z(t)\delta z \tag{5.37}$$

is directly proportional to the gradient amplitude, so it also varies with time. The exponential factor in Eq. (5.36) can be implemented either by phase or frequency modulation, depending on which methods are available or more convenient on a particular scanner.

5.4.2 PRACTICAL CONSIDERATIONS

A drawback of SPSP pulses is that the individual RF subpulses are not very spatially selective due to their short duration and consequently have small time-bandwidth products. Therefore the spatial profiles tend to have either broad transition regions, large minimum-slice thickness (e.g., 5–10 mm), or both. To partially address these deficiencies, SPSP pulses are typically played with a high RF duty cycle; that is, RF is played during as much of the pulse as possible. As mentioned earlier, spatial RF subpulses are typically played under both positive and negative gradient lobes. This, however, increases the sensitivity to system imperfections such as the B_0 and gradient eddy currents that perturb the B_0 and gradient fields. If gradient eddy currents are not accurately compensated, the actual k-space trajectory will deviate from theory and the SPSP pulse will not give the predicted performance.

To further increase the RF duty cycle, RF is usually played under the entire gradient lobe, including ramps, as implied in Eq. (5.33). Playing RF while the gradients are slewing not only requires excellent eddy-current compensation, but also requires that the RF and gradient waveforms be exactly synchronized. Playing RF during gradient ramps makes the offset SPSP pulses (Eq. 5.36) sensitive to extremely small (on the order of a few microseconds) mismatches between the group delays of the RF and gradient subsystems.

Any mismatch between the assumed waveform and the actual waveform (caused, for example, by eddy currents and gradient group delays) results in a lower water signal and higher lipid signal. As with eddy currents, the performance degradation from mismatches in group delay is most noticeable on offset slices, because the intended gradient waveform is used to calculate the time-dependent carrier frequency shift that offsets the slices (Eqs. 5.36 and 5.37). Calibration and correction methods have been developed (Block et al. 1997; Zur 2000) that increase the robustness of playing RF on both the positive and negative lobes. More details on this topic can be found in Section 10.3.

Another issue with playing RF during both positive and negative gradient lobes is that the first moment of the gradient cannot be nulled for both polarities. Moving spins therefore accumulate phase between the RF subpulses. The phase oscillates between positive and negative polarity lobes. In analogy with EPI, the result can be ghosting in the spectral direction that transfers energy from the central peak in Figure 5.16. Moving spins therefore have lower water signals than stationary spins. Playing the spatial subpulses during only one gradient polarity eliminates the problem at the cost of the drawbacks previously mentioned (Fredrickson et al. 1997).

Much of the recent work (Block et al. 1997; Schick 1998; Zur 2000) on SPSP pulses has dealt with adding phase cycles to suppress various peaks in the magnetization response. One method (Zur 2000) introduces a 0, 180°, 0, 180°, ... phase modulation onto the spatial subpulses. The alternating sign of the spatial RF subpulses suppresses the central main lobe of the magnetization response and the nearest asymmetric secondary peaks. With this method, the carrier frequency is adjusted so that fat is placed on-resonance and the water frequency corresponds to the next main peak.

Unlike the spectrally selective presaturation methods discussed in Section 4.3, a small resonance offset in either direction can cause a relatively large decrease in the water signal when SPSP pulses are employed. This is because of the relatively small width of the main spectral peak in Figure 5.16. The problem can be addressed by improving the spectral selectivity by increasing the time-bandwidth product of the spectral envelope or by allowing it to have higher stopband ripples in SLR pulse design. Increasing the time-bandwidth product usually requires more RF subpulses (and therefore a longer pulse). With suitable design trade-offs, SPSP pulses can sometimes offer improved tolerance to B_0 inhomogeneity compared to conventional fat-saturation pulses. The improvement, however, is not nearly as dramatic as for B_1 inhomogeneity. So, as with fat-saturation, good shimming is also required with SPSP pulses for effective lipid suppression.

As the main magnetic field decreases, using SPSP pulses for spectrally selective excitation becomes increasingly difficult. This is primarily because the reduced frequency separation results in an excessively long pulse width (Eqs. 5.31 and 5.32) and, accordingly, long TE values. For gradient systems with a slow slew rate (e.g., $<20\,\text{T}/\text{m}/\text{s}$), SPSP pulses may not be practical due to the extended pulse width required by the gradient waveform.

Finally, we mention that the SPSP excitation pulses can have two different isodelays. The minor isodelay is approximately equal to one-half the width of each spatial subpulse and is used to determine the slice-selection rephasing area. The major isodelay is approximately equal to the isodelay of the spectral envelope and is used to determine TE.

SELECTED REFERENCES

Block, W., Pauly, J., Kerr, A., and Nishimura, D. 1997. Consistent fat suppression with compensated spectral-spatial pulses. *Magn. Reson. Med.* 38: 198–206.

Fredrickson, J. O., Meyer, C., and Pelc, N. J. 1997. Flow effects in spectral spatial excitation. In *Proceedings of the 5th meeting of the ISMRM.* Vancouver, 1997, p. 113.

Meyer, C. H., Pauly, J. M., Makovski, A., and Nishimura, D. G. 1990. Simultaneous spatial and spectral selective excitation. *Magn. Res. Med.* 15: 287–304.

Schick, F. 1998. Simultaneous highly selective MR water and fat imaging using a simple new type of spectral-spatial excitation. *Magn. Reson. Med.* 40: 194–202.

Zur, Y. 2000. Design of improved spectral-spatial pulses for routine clinical use. *Magn. Reson. Med.* 43: 410–420.

RELATED SECTIONS

5.5 Tagging Pulses

RF tagging pulses are used to spatially label an image with a specified physical or physiological property. Most commonly, a tagging pulse places a series of parallel stripes or orthogonal grids on an image. These stripes or grids are known as *tags*. The deformation of the tags can be used to evaluate the properties of an imaged object, such as myocardial motion, fluid flow, and susceptibility variation. Tags on an image can also be used to evaluate the imaging system, such as measuring magnetic field inhomogeneity, gradient nonlinearity, B_1-field nonuniformity, or spatial resolution. In addition to placing tags on an image, a tagging pulse can also label the magnetization at a location distant from the imaged slice. The labeled magnetization then travels to the slice through the bloodstream and causes signal intensity changes. The differences in image intensity with and without a tagging pulse can be used to measure tissue perfusion parameters, such as cerebral blood flow, as described in Section 17.1.

Tags are typically applied as a magnetization preparation pulse prior to the actual imaging pulse sequence. Virtually any imaging pulse sequence can be combined with a tagging pulse or a train of tagging pulses. A gradient (known as a *tagging gradient*) is generally required to produce the desired spatial pattern. Depending on the tagging technique, the tagging gradient can be played out either concurrently or alternatively with the RF tagging pulses. After tagging, a time delay is often inserted prior to the start of the imaging pulse sequence. This delay time allows evolution of the spin system to sensitize the tags with motion, flow, relaxation, or other physiological and physical parameters.

Tagging pulses can take many forms. In this section, we focus on those tagging pulses that place stripes or grids on an image and discuss two tagging techniques: spatial modulation of magnetization (SPAMM) (Axel and Dougherty 1989a, 1989b) and delay alternating with nutation for tailored excitation (DANTE) (Morris and Freeman 1978; Mosher and Smith 1990). Composite pulses with a concurrent gradient can also be used to produce spatial tags. This can be readily inferred from Section 4.1, and thus it is not discussed in this section. Tagging pulses employed in phase contrast imaging and perfusion measurement are detailed in Sections 9.2 and 17.1, respectively.

5.5.1 SPAMM

Qualitative Description SPAMM, in its simplest form, consists of two nonselective RF pulses (e.g., rectangular pulses) with a gradient lobe sandwiched in-between (Figure 5.18). An optional spoiler gradient pulse (shown as dotted lines in Figure 5.18) is usually applied after the second RF pulse. Without loss of generality, let us assume that the two RF pulses in Figure 5.18 are both applied along the x axis in the rotating reference frame and have the same flip angle of 90°. The first RF pulse tips the magnetization to the transverse plane (Figure 5.19a). The tagging gradient then produces a phase dispersion in the excited transverse magnetization (Figure 5.19b); that is, the magnetization vector fans out to a degree that depends on its spatial location. The second RF pulse rotates the transverse plane by 90° about the x axis, moving the magnetization from the xy plane to the xz plane (Figure 5.19c). The magnetization vectors along the $\pm x$ axis are unaffected, whereas the transverse magnetization vectors along the $+y$ and $-y$ axes are rotated to the $-z$ and $+z$ axes, respectively. The transverse component of magnetization will continue to dephase through T_2 relaxation and eventually disappear. The dephasing process can be greatly accelerated by applying the optional spoiler gradient shown in Figure 5.18. At the end of the SPAMM sequence, the transverse magnetization is essentially destroyed and the longitudinal magnetization along the

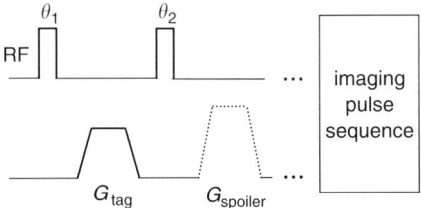

FIGURE 5.18 A SPAMM sequence with two RF pulses. The flip angles of the RF pulses are θ_1 and θ_2. A tagging gradient G_{tag} is placed between the RF pulses, and an optional spoiler gradient (dotted lines) $G_{spoiler}$ can be applied after the second RF pulse. Note that G_{tag} and $G_{spoiler}$ are not necessarily played out on the same gradient axis.

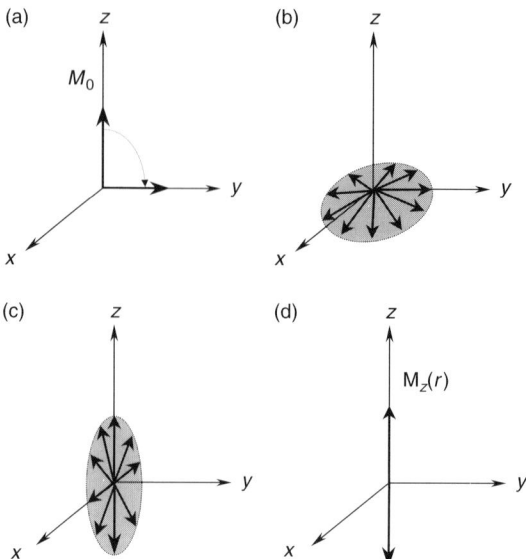

FIGURE 5.19 Evolution of the magnetization throughout the SPAMM sequence in Figure 5.18. The RF pulses are applied along the x axis with $90°$ flip angles. (a) The equilibrium magnetization M_0 is tipped to the transverse plane by the first RF pulse. (b) The tagging gradient produces a spatially dependent phase dispersion. Each arrow corresponds to a different spatial location. (c) The second RF pulse rotates the magnetization vectors from the xy plane to the xz plane. (d) After the transverse magnetization is dephased by a spoiler gradient, only the longitudinal magnetization remains. The amplitude of the longitudinal magnetization $M_z(r)$ is spatially modulated.

$\pm z$ axis is spatially modulated by the tagging gradient. The longitudinal magnetization then can be excited by an imaging pulse sequence, resulting in an image with periodic intensity modulations (i.e., peaks and troughs as illustrated in Figure 5.20).

Mathematical Description　After the first RF pulse in Figure 5.18 is applied, the three components of the magnetization in the rotating reference frame are given by:

$$\begin{bmatrix} M_x \\ M_y \\ M_z \end{bmatrix} = M_0 \begin{bmatrix} 0 \\ \sin \theta_1 \\ \cos \theta_1 \end{bmatrix} \tag{5.38}$$

where M_0 is the initial equilibrium magnetization, and θ_1 is the flip angle of the first RF pulse. The tagging gradient, G_{tag}, introduces a spatially dependent

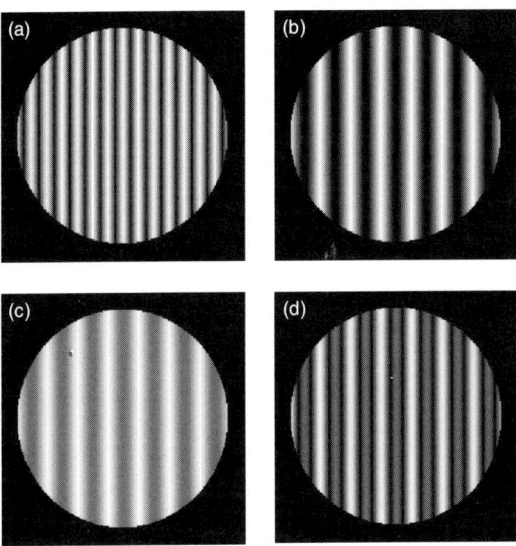

FIGURE 5.20 Simulated SPAMM images with tags produced under different conditions. (a) $\theta_2 = \theta_1 = 90°$. (b) $\theta_2 = \theta_1 = 45°$. (c) $\theta_2 = \theta_1 = 30°$. (d) $\theta_2 = \theta_1 = 60°$. The tagging gradient is applied along the horizontal direction.

phase into the transverse magnetization:

$$\phi(r) = \gamma r \int_0^T G_{\text{tag}} \, dt \qquad (5.39)$$

where r is the spatial variable along the gradient direction, and T is the duration of G_{tag}. After this phase dispersion, the transverse magnetization becomes:

$$\begin{bmatrix} M_x(r) \\ M_y(r) \\ M_z \end{bmatrix} = M_0 \begin{bmatrix} \sin\theta_1 \sin\phi(r) \\ \sin\theta_1 \cos\phi(r) \\ \cos\theta_1 \end{bmatrix} \qquad (5.40)$$

The second RF pulse rotates the magnetization vectors about the x axis (Section 1.2), yielding:

$$\begin{bmatrix} M_x(r) \\ M_y(r) \\ M_z(r) \end{bmatrix} = M_0 \begin{bmatrix} 1 & 0 & 0 \\ 0 & \cos\theta_2 & \sin\theta_2 \\ 0 & -\sin\theta_2 & \cos\theta_2 \end{bmatrix} \begin{bmatrix} \sin\theta_1 \sin\phi(r) \\ \sin\theta_1 \cos\phi(r) \\ \cos\theta_1 \end{bmatrix} \qquad (5.41)$$

Since the transverse magnetization is dephased by the subsequent spoiler gradient, we consider here only the longitudinal component:

$$M_z(r) = -M_0 \left[\sin\theta_1 \sin\theta_2 \cos\phi(r) - \cos\theta_1 \cos\theta_2 \right] \qquad (5.42)$$

which is spatially modulated by $\cos \phi(r)$. When an image is subsequently formed based on $M_z(r)$, periodic intensity variations occur in a direction parallel to the tagging gradient, as dictated by the cosine modulation of Eq. (5.42).

Equation (5.39) indicates that the period of the spatial modulation is given by:

$$\lambda = \frac{2\pi}{\gamma \int_0^T G_{\text{tag}} \, dt} \tag{5.43}$$

which is inversely proportional to the area of the tagging gradient pulse. For a magnitude image reconstruction, however, the spatial period of the tags does not always correspond to λ. For example, when $|\theta_1| = |\theta_2| = 90°$ (i.e., $|M_z(r)| = M_0|\cos \phi(r)|$), the spatial period of the tags becomes $\lambda/2$. The spins located at $r = n\lambda/2(n = 0, \pm1, \pm2, \ldots)$ give the bright (i.e., hyperintense) image signals, whereas spins at $r = (n/2 + 1/4)\lambda$ are saturated, producing dark (i.e., hypointense) tags. According to Eq. (5.42), the location of the tags, as well as the modulation pattern, also depends on the flip angle of the RF pulses. For example, if $\theta_1 = \theta_2 = 45°$, $M_z(r)$ becomes $\frac{M_0}{2}[1 - \cos \phi(r)]$. Therefore, the dark tags appear at $r = n\lambda$ (Figure 5.20b); that is, the period is doubled from the case of $|\theta_1| = |\theta_2| = 90°$ (Figure 5.20a). With certain combinations of θ_1 and θ_2 (e.g., $\theta_1 = 30°$ and $\theta_2 = 30°$), the tag intensity never reaches 0, resulting in gray instead of black tags in the image (Figure 5.20c). At other flip angle combinations (e.g., $\theta_1 = \theta_2 = 60°$), two interleaved sets of tags with different periods can occur (Figure 5.20d), as shown in the following example.

Example 5.9   A SPAMM sequence is implemented on a scanner with a maximum gradient amplitude $h = 22 \, \text{mT/m}$ and a slew rate $S_R = 120 \, \text{mT/m/ms}$. The flip angles of the two RF pulses in SPAMM are both 45°. If tags are desired at every 4 mm, (a) design a tagging gradient lobe that has the shortest pulse width. With this tagging gradient, what will happen if both the RF flip angles are (b) decreased to 30° and (c) increased to 60°?

Answer

(a) At 45° flip angles, the tags will occur at $r = n\lambda$. Substituting $\lambda = 4 \, \text{mm}$ into Eq. (5.43), the tagging gradient area S can be calculated as:

$$S = \int_0^T G_{\text{tag}} \, dt$$

$$= 2\pi/(\gamma \lambda) = \frac{2\pi}{2\pi \times 42.57 \, (\text{kHz/mT}) \times 0.004 \, (\text{m})} = 5.87 \, \text{mT} \cdot \text{ms/m}$$

Using the criteria given in Section 7.1, the most time-efficient gradient lobe is a trapezoid with amplitude, ramp time, and plateau duration given by:

$$G_{tag} = h = 22 \, \text{mT/m}$$

$$T_{ramp} = \frac{h}{S_R} = \frac{22}{120} = 0.183 \, \text{ms}$$

$$T_{plateau} = \frac{S}{h} - T_{ramp} = \frac{5.87}{22} - 0.183 \, \text{ms} = 0.084 \, \text{ms}$$

(b) When the flip angles are both reduced to $30°$, Eq. (5.42) becomes:

$$M_z(r) = \frac{M_0}{4} [3 - \cos \phi(r)] \qquad (5.44)$$

Therefore, the magnetization will be always positive, irrespective of spatial location. The cosine modulation produces troughs with nonzero intensities (Figure 5.20c). On a uniform phantom, the ratio between the maximal and minimal intensities is 2:1 and the spatial modulation frequency is the same as the in the case with $45°$ flip angles.

(c) When the flip angles are both increased to $60°$, Eq. (5.42) gives the following longitudinal magnetization:

$$M_z(r) = \frac{M_0}{4} [1 - 3 \cos \phi(r)] \qquad (5.45)$$

In this case, two sets of dark tags will appear, one at $\phi(r) = \cos^{-1}(1/3) = 70.5°$ and the other at $-70.5°$. The intensity between the tags in a magnitude image will oscillate among 0, $M_0/2$, and M_0 (Figure 5.20d).

Design Considerations

RF pulses. Although the simple two-pulse combination with $45°$ flip angles (Figure 5.18) is commonly used in SPAMM, those tags do not exhibit well-defined edges. This problem can be addressed by increasing the number of RF pulses to form a composite pulse, as discussed in Section 4.1. In fact, the two pulses in Figure 5.18 constitute the simplest (11) composite pulse (Axel and Dougherty 1989a). Figure 5.21 shows a SPAMM pulse train consisting of a (1331) composite pulse with tagging gradient lobes between the RF pulses. To produce simple tagging patterns with good tag-to-image contrast, the sum of the flip angle of all the composite pulses is typically chosen to be $90°$. Thus,

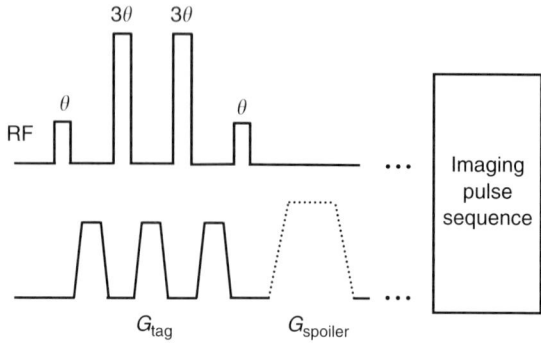

FIGURE 5.21 A SPAMM sequence with a (1331) composite RF pulse.

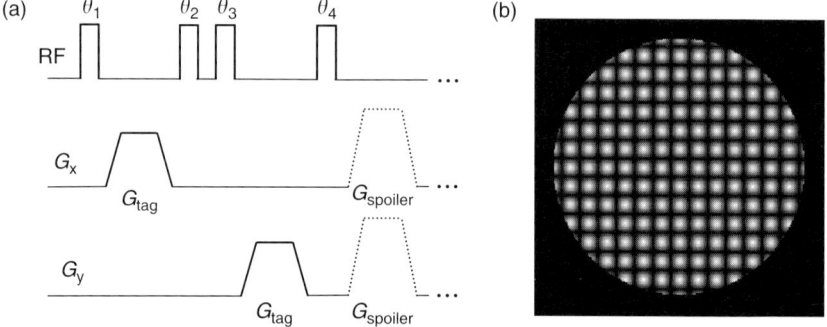

FIGURE 5.22 (a) A SPAMM pulse sequence that places two sets of orthogonal tags on an image. The phases of θ_3 and θ_4 can be shifted by 90° relative to the phases of θ_1 and θ_2 to avoid stimulated echoes (Axel and Dougherty 1989a). G_x and G_y are two orthogonal gradient axes. G_{tag} is the tagging gradient and $G_{spoiler}$ is an optional spoiling gradient (dotted lines). (b) A simulated image produced by the sequence in (a).

the flip angles for the four pulses in Figure 5.21 would be 11.25°, 33.75°, 33.75°, and 11.25°.

Tagging gradient. The tagging gradient can be applied in any direction. When the tag direction does not coincide with any of the physical (or logical) gradient axes, multiple physical (or logical) gradient axes can be simultaneously used to synthesize a vector pointing in the desired direction, as explained in Section 7.3 on oblique prescriptions. To minimize the adverse effects caused by flow, off-resonance, and relaxation, it is usually preferable to employ the most time-efficient gradient lobes. Multiple sets of tags can be placed along different directions on an image. For example, two orthogonal sets of tags (i.e., grids) can be produced using the sequence in Figure 5.22a. The area and axis of each gradient lobe are independent and are selected to acheive the desired grid pattern.

Spoiler gradient. An optional spoiler gradient accelerates the dephasing of the transverse magnetization after the last RF tagging pulse. The spoiler gradient area can be determined according to the principles outlined in Section 10.5. To minimize the chance of the phase dispersion from being accidentally unwound by a subsequent imaging gradient, the spoiler gradient can be applied along all three axes, provided gradient limitations such as heating and dB/dt are not problematic. Although the spoiler gradient is not mandatory, incomplete dephasing of the transverse magnetization can cause artifacts in the image. Thus, the spoiler gradient is highly recommended for SPAMM sequences.

Delay time. The delay time between SPAMM and the subsequent imaging pulse sequence is chosen based on specific applications. For example, in flow measurement, the time should be long enough to allow adequate deformation of the tags, yet not so long so that it causes aliasing, which occurs when flow causes the tags to move more than one spatial period. It is important to keep in mind that longitudinal relaxation does occur during this delay time. This can reduce the tag-to-image contrast or even change the patterns of the tags.

5.5.2 DANTE

Qualitative Description   DANTE consists of a series of short hard pulses (e.g., 16) separated by a constant interpulse delay time (Figure 5.23). The DANTE pulse train can be modulated by an envelope function, such as Gaussian, SINC, or RECT (rectangular function). Spins at periodic Larmor frequencies are excited, so when a constant gradient is played out

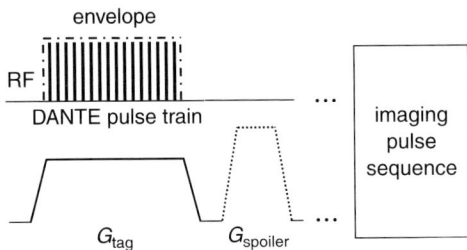

FIGURE 5.23 A DANTE sequence. The RF pulse train contains a series of equally spaced hard pulses under a shaped envelope (dotted-dashed line). The rectangular envelope shown here is one of many possible shapes. The tagging gradient is played out concurrently with the RF pulses, and an optional spoiler gradient (dotted line) can be applied after the RF pulse train.

concurrently with a DANTE pulse train, a series of parallel bands perpendicular to the gradient direction results. The excited signals (i.e., the transverse magnetization) can be destroyed (or dephased) with a spoiler gradient (Figure 5.23). The longitudinal magnetization has periodic spatial variation similar to that produced by the SPAMM sequence. A subsequent imaging pulse sequence produces an image that contains a series of dark tags at locations where the magnetization is saturated.

Mathematical Description   When the width of the DANTE pulses is very short (e.g., a few microseconds), the DANTE pulse train depicted in Figure 5.23 can be approximated by a series of delta functions multiplied by an envelope function $A(t)$:

$$B_1(t) = A(t, T) \sum_{n=-\infty}^{\infty} \delta(t - n\tau) \tag{5.46}$$

where τ is the interpulse delay (i.e., the time between the centers of two consecutive pulses in the DANTE pulse train), T is a measure of the width of the modulation function, and n is an integer. If $B_1(t)$ is used as an excitation pulse in the small flip angle approximation, its frequency response can be approximately obtained by a Fourier transform:

$$M(f) \propto \int_{-\infty}^{\infty} B_1(t)e^{-i2\pi ft} \, dt = W(f, F) \otimes \sum_{N=-\infty}^{\infty} \delta(f - N\Delta f) \tag{5.47}$$

where $W(f, F)$ is the Fourier transform of $A(t, T)$, F is a measure of the width of W, and Δf is the separation of the delta functions in the frequency domain (i.e., $\Delta f = 1/\tau$). According to Section 1.1, the convolution $\otimes$ on the right side of Eq. (5.47) gives a series of replicates of $W(f, F)$ separated by Δf. In the presence of a concurrent gradient G_{tag}, the frequency separation of these replicates is converted to different spatial locations along the gradient direction. Let r be the spatial location of the replicates, R be its width, and Δr be the gap between two neighboring tags. Then:

$$r = \frac{2\pi f}{\gamma G_{tag}}, \qquad R = \frac{2\pi F}{\gamma G_{tag}}, \qquad \Delta r = \frac{2\pi \Delta f}{\gamma G_{tag}} \tag{5.48}$$

Thus, the spatial locations corresponding to $W(r, R) \otimes \sum_{N=-\infty}^{\infty} \delta(r - N\Delta r)$ are excited, resulting in a series of stripes at $r = N\Delta r (N = 0, \pm 1, \pm 2, \ldots)$. After saturating these stripes with a spoiler gradient, only periodic longitudinal magnetization remains, and the final image will consist of a series of dark bands at the locations where the transverse magnetization has been saturated. These bands, which are perpendicular to the tagging gradient direction, constitute the tags.

Design Consideration

Tag locations. Because $\Delta f = 1/\tau$, the separation of the tagging bands is inversely related to the interpulse delay τ:

$$\Delta r = \frac{2\pi}{\gamma \tau G_{\text{tag}}} \tag{5.49}$$

A longer interpulse delay or stronger tagging gradient amplitude leads to an increase in tagging density within the image. Because prolonging τ exacerbates problems associated with motion, off-resonance, and relaxation, varying the gradient amplitude is more commonly used to control the density (or the spatial frequency) of the tags. Equation (5.49) assumes that all the pulses in a DANTE pulse train have the same phase. If the phase of every pulse is sequentially modulated with an increment $\Delta\phi$ (i.e., adding a phase ramp throughout the pulse train), then the tags will be shifted by $\delta_r = \Delta\phi/(\gamma \tau G_{\text{tag}})$. However, the gap between the tags does not change (Blondet et al. 1987). If the phase of every other pulse is modulated with an increment $\Delta\phi$ (i.e., adding a phase ramp only to the even pulses while leaving the odd pulses with a constant phase), then the gap between the tags will be decreased to:

$$\Delta r = \frac{\Delta\phi}{2\gamma \tau G_{\text{tag}}} \tag{5.50}$$

Note that the factor of 2 in the denominator is due to the fact that the spacing between even (or odd) echoes becomes 2τ. A DANTE pulse train with a phase ramp on every other pulse is called *double DANTE* (Geen et al. 1989). Double DANTE provides a convenient way to increase tagging density without changing G_{tag} or τ. A similar approach has also been adapted in spatial-spectral pulse design to alter the frequency response (Zur 2000).

Example 5.10   A DANTE pulse train with a constant phase is used for spatial tagging. Twenty tags are required on a field of view of 24 cm. (a) If an interpulse delay of 0.5 ms is used, what is the tagging gradient amplitude? (b) If all the pulses in the pulse train are phase modulated with a constant phase increment of 90°, how much will the tags be shifted? (c) If a second pulse train with an interpulse delay of 0.5 ms is interleaved with the original pulse train, what is the gap between the tags when the second pulse train is phase modulated with an increment of 90°?

Answer

(a) The desired gap between the tags is $\Delta r = 24/20 = 1.2$ cm. Substituting $\Delta r = 1.2$ cm and $\tau = 0.5$ ms into Eq. (5.49) and solving for G_{tag}, we obtain:

$$G_{tag} = \frac{2\pi}{\gamma \tau \Delta r} = \frac{2\pi}{2\pi \times 42.57\,\text{kHz/mT} \times 0.5\,\text{ms} \times 0.012\,\text{m}} = 3.92\,\text{mT/m}$$

(b) When the entire pulse train is phase modulated by $90°$, the spatial shift of the tags is $\delta_r = \Delta\phi/(\gamma\tau G_{tag}) = (\pi/2)\Delta r/(2\pi) = \Delta r/4 = 0.3$ cm.

(c) For the interleaved pulse train, the effective interpulse delay is $\tau = 0.25$ ms. Substituting $\tau = 0.25$ ms and $\Delta\phi = \pi/2$ into Eq. (5.50), we obtain $\Delta r = 0.3$ cm.

The width of the tags. The width of the tags is directly determined by $W(f, F)$, which is in turn related to $A(t, T)$. When an infinitely long DANTE train is used, $W(f, F)$ reduces to a delta function, leading to an infinitesimally thin tag width. In practical implementations, $A(t, T)$ must be truncated, which broadens $W(f, F)$. A narrower tag width can be achieved by a broader envelope function, which often requires a longer pulse train. The relationship between $A(t, T)$ and $W(f, F)$ for several common envelope functions is given in Table 5.2. For all functions shown in Table 5.2, the frequency domain width F is related to the time domain width T by $F \simeq 1/(2\pi T)$. With proper selection of the envelope function, DANTE generally gives sharper tag edges than SPAMM, especially when using SPAMM with only two RF pulses.

Tagging in multidimensions. DANTE pulses can be used to produce multiple sets of tags in different directions by concatenating two or more one-dimensional DANTE pulse trains in an analogous way to multidimensional SPAMM (Figure 5.22). The tags in each set behave independently, and

TABLE 5.2
Relationship Between $A(t, T)$ and $W(f, F)^a$

Function	$A(t, T)$	$W(f, F)$
Gaussian	$Ce^{-t^2/(2T^2)}$	$C'e^{-f^2/(2F^2)}$
RECT	$C\text{RECT}\left(\frac{t}{T}\right)$	$C'\text{SINC}\left(\frac{f}{F}\right)$
SINC	$C\text{SINC}\left(\frac{t}{T}\right)$	$C'\text{RECT}\left(\frac{f}{F}\right)$

^{a} C and C' are constants in microteslas.

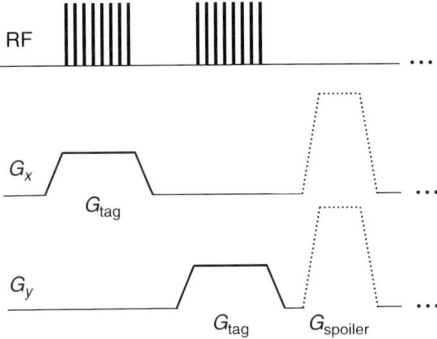

FIGURE 5.24 (a) A DANTE pulse sequence that places two sets of orthogonal tags on an image. G_x and G_y represent two orthogonal gradient axes. G_{tag} is the tagging gradient and $G_{spoiler}$ is an optional spoiling gradient. The imaging pulse sequence following the DANTE sequence is not explicitly shown.

the parameters for each set can be selected as if they were one-dimensional tags. Figure 5.24 shows a DANTE sequence that produces two sets of orthogonal tags.

Parameter selection. The individual RF pulses in the DANTE tagging train are usually kept very short (e.g., 1–$100\,\mu s$) in order to avoid edge blurring of the tags. The sum of all the flip angles in the pulse train is typically chosen as $90°$ to achieve a good tagging contrast. The interpulse delay, in conjunction with tagging gradient amplitude, is selected to yield the desired tag density. The choice of RF envelope function (Table 5.2) depends on the tolerance level of tag blurring. The tagging gradient amplitude is determined by the tag locations using Eq. (5.49) or (5.50). The spoiler gradient and the delay time are selected as outlined in Section 10.5 and subsection 5.5.1.

5.5.3 APPLICATIONS

SPAMM and DANTE have very similar applications. Both techniques can be used to evaluate myocardial motion, monitor flow, characterize gradient nonlinearity, and measure off-resonance effects caused by magnetic susceptibility variations, chemical shifts, and B_0-field inhomogeneity. All these applications are based on the deformity of the tags as a result of a physiological process (e.g., myocardial motion or fluid flow) or a system imperfection. In some applications (e.g., motion), the degree of tag deformity depends on the time delay between the tagging pulse train and the imaging pulse sequence. Because T_1 relaxation causes the tags to fade away over time, the time delay must be carefully chosen to maximize the measurement sensitivity without compromising the visibility of the tags. In other applications, such as the characterization of the gradient nonlinearity, the delay time does not affect the degree of tag deformity. Thus, a minimal time delay is preferred to maintain the best contrast between the image and the tags.

Tags produced by SPAMM are more sensitive to the RF flip angles than those generated by DANTE. As such, SPAMM can also be used to evaluate the B_1-field nonuniformity. On the other hand, the application of DANTE is not limited to spin tagging. For example, DANTE pulses are widely used in spectral editing (Blondet et al. 1987) and in ultra-fast imaging (Lowe and Wysong 1993).

SELECTED REFERENCES

Axel, L., and Dougherty, L. 1989a. Heart wall motion—improved method of spatial modulation of magnetization for MR imaging. *Radiology* 172: 349–350.

Axel, L., and Dougherty, L. 1989b. MR imaging of motion with spatial modulation of magnetization. *Radiology* 171: 841–845.

Blondet, P., Albrand, J. P., Vonkienlin, M., Decorps, M., and Lavanchy, N. 1987. Use of rotating-phase DANTE pulses for invivo proton nmr spectral editing with a single irradiation facility. *J. Magn. Reson.* 71: 342–346.

Geen, H., Wu, X. L., Xu, P., Friedrich, J., and Freeman, R. 1989. Selective excitation at 2 arbitrary frequencies—the double- DANTE sequence. *J. Magn. Reson.* 81: 646–652.

Lowe, I. J., and Wysong, R. E. 1993. DANTE ultra-fast imaging sequence (DUFIS). *J. Magn. Reson.* 101: 106–109.

Morris, G. A., and Freeman, R. 1978. Selective excitation in Fourier-transform nuclear magnetic resonance. *J. Magn. Reson.* 29: 433–462.

Mosher, T. J., and Smith, M. B. 1990. A DANTE tagging sequence for the evaluation of translational sample motion. *Magn. Reson. Med.* 15: 334–339.

Zur, Y. 2000. Design of improved spectral-spatial pulses for routine clinical use. *Magn. Reson. Med.* 43: 410–420.

RELATED SECTIONS

Section 1.1 Fourier Transforms
Section 4.1 Composite Pulses
Section 10.5 Spoiler Gradient
Section 17.1 Arterial Spin Tagging

6

ADIABATIC RADIOFREQUENCY PULSES

6.1 Adiabatic Excitation Pulses

In MRI, it is highly desirable to excite the magnetization uniformly over the imaged object. The excitation uniformity is primarily governed by the spatial homogeneity of the RF magnetic field (i.e., the B_1 field). In practice, a homogeneous B_1 field cannot be always achieved with RF coils. For example, when a surface coil is used to transmit a rectangular RF pulse into a uniform water phantom, the amplitude of the B_1 field can vary by several-fold across the imaged object. Even when a more homogeneous birdcage coil is used, the B_1 field variation is nonnegligible (e.g., $\sim$10% or more), especially when the imaged object occupies a large portion of the coil volume.

Conventionally, the flip angle (i.e., the angle in radians between the initial and final magnetization vectors) is given by:

$$\theta = \gamma \int\limits_{0}^{T} B_1(t)\, dt \qquad (6.1)$$

where T is the pulse width and γ is the gyromagnetic ratio. An inhomogeneous B_1 field therefore results in spatial variation of the flip angles. Because the amount of transverse magnetization excited is proportional to $\sin\theta$, the regions in which the flip angle is 90° produce a maximal MRI signal, whereas the regions with 0° or 180° flip angles generate no signal. This nonuniform excitation can lead to various problems, such as image shading, incomplete lipid suppression, and reduced signal-to-noise ratio (SNR). A natural question to ask is: Can RF pulses be designed to overcome these problems?

Adiabatic pulses are a special class of RF pulses that can excite, refocus, or invert magnetization vectors uniformly, even in the presence of a spatially nonuniform B_1 field. Unlike nonadiabatic RF pulses described in Sections 3.1, 3.2, and 3.3, adiabatic pulses do not obey the conventional relationship between the flip angle and the B_1 field amplitude described by Eq. (6.1). Instead, the flip angle of an adiabatic pulse depends on how the B_1 field varies its amplitude *and* modulation frequency (or the phase) during the pulse. By properly manipulating the modulation functions, spins that experience different B_1 fields can be excited with the same flip angle, as long as the amplitude of the B_1 modulation envelope exceeds a threshold. This property gives adiabatic pulses their excellent robustness to variation in B_1 field.

Similar to nonadiabatic pulses, adiabatic pulses can be divided into excitation, refocusing, and inversion pulses based on their effect on the magnetization. The waveforms of adiabatic excitation, refocusing, and inversion pulses generally differ from one another and may not be used interchangeably by simply stretching or scaling the pulse. For instance, halving the amplitude of an adiabatic 180° inversion pulse does not yield a 90° excitation pulse. In this section, we focus on *adiabatic excitation pulses*, the pulses that nutate the magnetization from the z axis (or the direction of B_0 field) into the transverse plane (Ugurbil et al. 1987, 1988; Bendall and Pegg 1986; Staewen et al. 1990; Garwood and Ke 1991). We also discuss several pulses that are capable of returning a transverse magnetization to the longitudinal axis, in addition to their function of exciting a longitudinal magnetization. These pulses are known as B_1-*independent rotation* (*BIR*) *pulses* (Ugurbil et al. 1987; Staewen et al. 1990; Garwood and Ke 1991). Because adiabatic excitation pulses are very sensitive to off-resonance effects, it has been challenging to design adiabatic excitation pulses for slice selection in which a large resonance offset is introduced by the slice-selection gradient (Johnson et al. 1989). Thus, we limit our discussion here to spatially nonselective adiabatic excitation pulses.

6.1.1 PRINCIPLES OF ADIABATIC EXCITATION

Effective Magnetic Field   The concept of effective magnetic field introduced in Section 1.2 is very helpful for understanding adiabatic pulses. Let us consider a transverse RF magnetic field with a time-dependent amplitude $A(t)$

and a carrier frequency $\omega_{rf}(t)$:

$$B_1(t) = A(t)e^{-i\omega_{rf}(t)t} \tag{6.2}$$

In a time-dependent rotating reference frame whose angular frequency equals $\omega_{rf}(t)$, the effective magnetic field can be decomposed into two orthogonal components. The component in the transverse plane is:

$$B_x(t) = A(t) \tag{6.3}$$

where, without loss of generality, we have assumed that the B_1 field is initially applied along the x axis. In general, the B_1 field can point in any direction in the transverse plane, depending on its initial phase. In the rotating reference frame, the component of the effective magnetic field along the z axis is:

$$B_z(t) = \frac{1}{\gamma}[\omega - \omega_{rf}(t)] = B_0 - \frac{\omega_{rf}(t)}{\gamma} \tag{6.4}$$

where ω is the Larmor frequency (i.e., $\omega = \gamma B_0$). Therefore, the effective magnetic field becomes:

$$\vec{B}_{eff}(t) = \vec{B}_x(t) + \vec{B}_z(t) = \hat{x}B_x(t) + \hat{z}B_z(t) \tag{6.5}$$

where $\hat{x}$ and $\hat{z}$ are the unit vectors along the x and z axes, respectively. The amplitude and the direction of the effective field are given by:

$$\left|\vec{B}_{eff}\right| = \sqrt{B_x^2(t) + B_z^2(t)} \tag{6.6}$$

$$\psi = \arctan\left(\frac{B_x(t)}{B_z(t)}\right) \tag{6.7}$$

respectively. Although the B_1 field is physically applied in the transverse plane, the direction of the effective field is not necessarily constrained to the transverse plane. In general, $\vec{B}_{eff}$ is tilted toward the z axis, except exactly at resonance (i.e., when $\omega_{rf} = \omega$) where the direction of $\vec{B}_{eff}$ coincides with that of the B_1 field.

As stated in Section 1.2, the magnetization vector precesses about $\vec{B}_{eff}$ in the rotating reference frame, just as the spins precess about the B_0 field in the absence of the B_1 field (Figure 6.1). This greatly simplifies the description of the interaction between the RF pulse of Eq. (6.2) and the magnetization.

Adiabatic Passage Principle and Adiabatic Condition   Adiabatic pulses operate under the *adiabatic passage principle*, which states that the magnetization vector of a spin system follows the direction of the effective magnetic

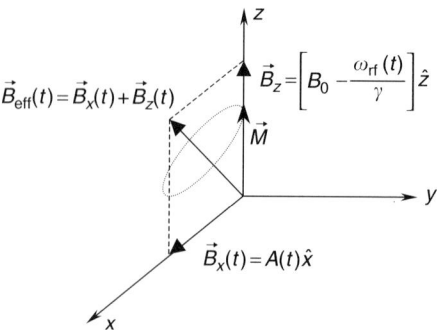

FIGURE 6.1 The relationship between the applied B_1 field with amplitude $A(t)$ and frequency $\omega_{rf}(t)$ modulations, the effective magnetic field $\vec{B}_{eff}$, and the magnetization $\vec{M}$ in the rotating reference frame. The magnetization vector precesses about the effective field and traces a cone, as indicated by the dotted path.

field (Figure 6.1), provided that the direction of the effective magnetic field does not change much during one period of precession of the magnetization about the effective field. Mathematically, this condition, also known as the *adiabatic condition*, is described by:

$$\left| \frac{d\psi}{dt} \right| \ll \gamma \left| \vec{B}_{eff} \right| \tag{6.8}$$

where ψ (in radians) is given by Eq. (6.7). In practice, it is often useful to define an adiabatic factor η:

$$\eta \equiv \frac{\gamma \left| \vec{B}_{eff} \right|}{\left| \dot{\psi} \right|} \tag{6.9}$$

where $\dot{\psi} = d\psi/dt$. To satisfy the adiabatic condition, η should be sufficiently larger than unity. When the adiabatic condition is satisfied, a magnetization that is initially collinear with $\vec{B}_{eff}$ will remain collinear with $\vec{B}_{eff}$, and a magnetization that is initially perpendicular to $\vec{B}_{eff}$ will precess about $\vec{B}_{eff}$ in a plane normal to $\vec{B}_{eff}$ during the course of the pulse. The second statement is particularly useful in analyzing adiabatic refocusing pulses (Section 6.3) and BIR pulses (subsection 6.1.4).

   Adiabatic Excitation   With the adiabatic passage principle in mind, let us consider the RF pulse given by Eq. (6.2), whose amplitude and carrier frequency are modulated by a sine and a cosine function, respectively:

$$A(t) = B_{x,0} \sin \xi t \tag{6.10}$$

$$\omega_{rf}(t) = \omega - \gamma B_{z,0} \cos \xi t \tag{6.11}$$

where ξ is the modulation frequency, and $B_{x,0}$ and $B_{z,0}$ are time-independent magnetic fields. Using Eqs. (6.3), (6.4), (6.6), and (6.7), it can be shown that the amplitude and direction of the effective field are:

$$\left| \vec{B}_{eff} \right| = \sqrt{(B_{x,0} \sin \xi t)^2 + (B_{z,0} \cos \xi t)^2} \tag{6.12}$$

$$\psi = \arctan \left(\frac{B_{x,0} \sin \xi t}{B_{z,0} \cos \xi t} \right), \tag{6.13}$$

respectively. At the beginning of the pulse, ψ is close to 0 and the effective field is aligned with the equilibrium magnetization along the z axis (Figure 6.2a). If the adiabatic condition is satisfied by choosing a sufficiently low modulation frequency ξ, a strong effective field, or both, the adiabatic passage principle dictates that the magnetization vector will track the direction of the effective field $\vec{B}_{eff}$ during the course of the RF pulse (Figure 6.2b). When $t = \pi/(2\xi)$, $\vec{B}_{eff}$ is rotated from the z axis to the x axis (Figure 6.2c) and so is the magnetization. If, at this point, the RF pulse is terminated, we have essentially achieved a 90° *adiabatic* excitation. For an adiabatic excitation pulse the flip angle (θ) at any moment during the pulse can be approximated by the instantaneous value of ψ.

Consider two locations that experience different B_1 field strengths as a result of a nonideal transmitting RF coil. One location receives $B_{1,a}$, and the other receives $B_{1,b}$. At the end of the RF pulse (i.e., $t = \pi/(2\xi)$ or $\psi = 90°$), the effective fields at both locations will be aligned along the x axis. Consequently, the magnetization vectors for the spins at these two locations are also parallel to the x axis, corresponding to a 90° excitation. This illustrates why adiabatic pulses can achieve uniform excitation even in the presence of B_1 field variation across the imaged object. Of course, both $B_{1,a}$ and $B_{1,b}$ must be sufficiently strong to satisfy the adiabatic condition (Eq. 6.8).

Comparison between Adiabatic and Nonadiabatic Excitations   Adiabatic excitation pulses differ from the conventional nonadiabatic excitation pulses (Section 3.1) in a number of ways. Some important differences are summarized here.

1. Adiabatic excitation requires both amplitude and frequency (or phase) modulation. Nonadiabatic excitation pulses typically do not require frequency modulation.

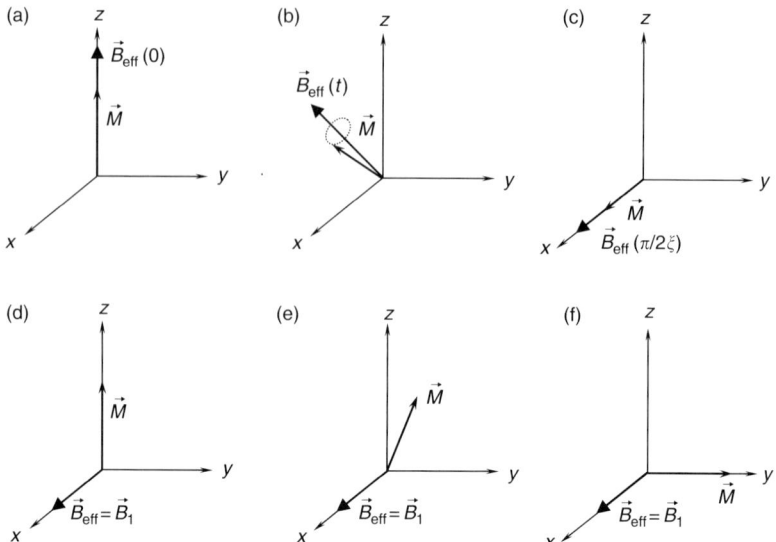

FIGURE 6.2 (a–c) The adiabatic excitation process and (d–f) the nonadiabatic excitation process. The figures in each row show the magnetization vector $\vec{M}$, the effective
magnetic field $\vec{B}_{eff}$, and the applied RF field $\vec{B}_1$ throughout the course of an excitation
pulse. (a) Beginning of an adiabatic pulse; (b) during the adiabatic pulse, showing the
magnetization precessing in a tight cone about the effective field; and (c) the end of
the adiabatic pulse. (d) Beginning of a nonadiabatic pulse, (e) during the nonadiabatic
pulse (assuming the spins are on-resonance), and (f) the end of the nonadiabatic pulse.

2. Adiabatic excitation pulses do not obey Eq. (6.1). As such, adiabatic
   pulses can achieve a uniform excitation even when the B_1 field is
   inhomogeneous.
3. At the end of an adiabatic excitation, the magnetization vector
   points in the same direction as the applied B_1 field (in the rotating
   frame), whereas in nonadiabatic excitation the final magnetization is
   perpendicular to the B_1 field (Figures 6.2d–f).
4. To satisfy the adiabatic condition, the adiabatic pulse amplitude (i.e.,
   $B_{x,0}$) is often considerably larger than that for nonadiabatic pulses. In
   addition, the pulse width can also be much longer, which increases the
   sensitivity to flow, off-resonance, and relaxation effects.

6.1.2 MODULATION FUNCTIONS

To achieve an adiabatic excitation, the B_1 amplitude modulation function
should start at 0, gradually increase during the pulse, and reach the maximal

value at the end of the pulse. In contrast, the frequency modulation function starts at the maximal value and then decreases to 0 (i.e., on-resonance) at the end of the pulse. Many functions can satisfy these criteria, including the sine and cosine functions shown in Eqs. (6.10) and (6.11) (Ugurbil et al. 1987) tan/sec pair, and tanh/sech pair (Ugurbil et al. 1987; Bendall and Pegg 1986). The quality of the modulation functions is evaluated based on how well they satisfy the adiabatic condition (Eq. 6.8) at a given B_1 amplitude and pulse width. Because $d\psi/dt$ changes throughout most modulation functions, the degree to which the adiabatic condition is satisfied varies during the pulse. To address this problem and improve the performance of adiabatic pulses, numerically optimized modulations (NOMs) have been developed. The details of NOMs can be found in Ugurbil et al. (1988).

6.1.3 DESIGN AND IMPLEMENTATION

To design an adiabatic excitation pulse, the initial step is to choose a pair of modulation functions, for example, a sine/cosine pair. Because not all the spins have the same resonance frequency, a tolerance level for the off-resonance effect κ is usually included in the frequency modulation function when analyzing the performance of an adiabatic excitation pulse with Bloch equations:

$$\Delta\omega_{\text{rf}}(t) = \omega - \omega_{\text{rf}}(t) = \gamma B_{z,0} \cos \xi t + \kappa \qquad (6.14)$$

The parameters that need to be determined include the B_1 field amplitude $B_{x,0}$, frequency modulation amplitude $\gamma B_{z,0}$, and the modulating frequency ξ. This can be done by first defining two dimensionless parameters, p and q:

$$p \equiv \frac{|B_{x,0}|}{|B_{z,0}|} \qquad (6.15)$$

$$q \equiv \frac{\gamma |B_{z,0}|}{\xi} \qquad (6.16)$$

and then solving the Bloch equations (Section 1.2) as a function of p and q. The efficiency of excitation (i.e., the amplitude of the transverse magnetization after the excitation as a percentage of the original longitudinal magnetization) can be plotted with respect to p and q. For a given efficiency (e.g., 95%) the range of p and q values can be determined from the 2D contour plot schematically shown in Figure 6.3. Generally, the allowed ranges for p and q depend on one another. To determine a value for q, we must consider the practical constraints, such as pulse width and SAR. The pulse width is determined by the modulation frequency $T = \pi/(2\xi)$, whereas the SAR is proportional to $B_{x,0}^2$. The latter is particularly important because an adiabatic excitation pulse typically requires

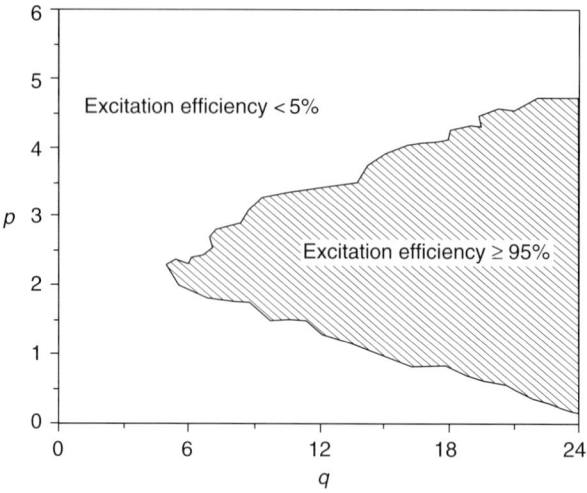

FIGURE 6.3 A schematic plot showing the 95% excitation efficiency contour as a function of p and q for an adiabatic excitation pulse. The excitation efficiency is defined as the amplitude of the transverse magnetization after the excitation as a percentage of the original longitudinal magnetization. (Adapted from Ugurbil et al. 1987.)

much higher RF power than its nonadiabatic counterpart. Once q is determined, the range of p gives the range of allowed B_1 field variation for the pulse. This design process can be integrated with NOMs, as discussed in Ugurbil et al. (1988).

   To implement adiabatic pulses on an MRI scanner, the frequency modulation (Eq. 6.14) is often replaced by phase modulation. This can be readily done by converting the frequency modulation to the corresponding phase modulation:

$$\Delta\phi_{\mathrm{rf}}(t) = \int_0^t \Delta\omega_{\mathrm{rf}}(t')\,dt' \qquad (6.17)$$

where time zero can be conveniently chosen as the beginning of the pulse. An example of an adiabatic excitation pulse, with all the modulation functions, is given in Figure 6.4.

6.1.4 B_1-INDEPENDENT ROTATION PULSES

   The adiabatic excitation pulses discussed thus far function well when the initial magnetization is collinear with the z axis (i.e., parallel or anti-parallel to the B_0 field). If the initial magnetization, or a component of the initial

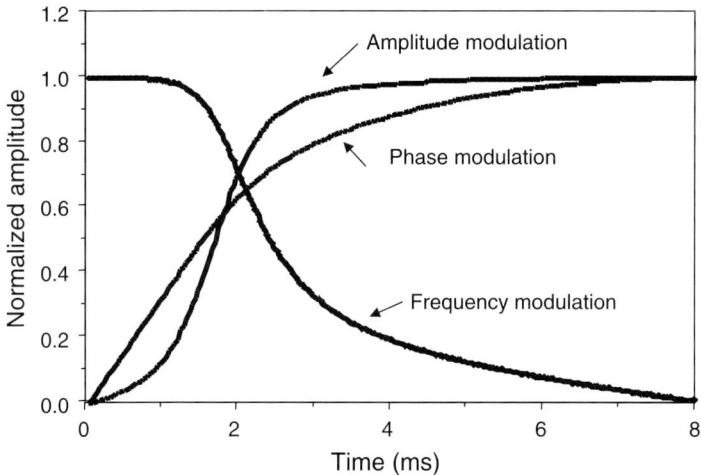

FIGURE 6.4 Modulation functions for a 90° adiabatic excitation pulse. The modulation functions are initially chosen as sine and cosine functions and subsequently optimized using the NOM algorithm.

magnetization, lies in the transverse plane, the transverse magnetization will fan out about the effective magnetic field during the adiabatic excitation pulse, dephasing the magnetization. If the pulse is played out with a reversed time course (i.e., $\vec{B}_{\text{eff}}$ starts from an axis in the transverse plane and ends along the z axis), then only the magnetization component that is initially parallel (or anti-parallel) to $\vec{B}_{\text{eff}}$ is returned to the z axis (or negative z axis), leaving all other components dephased. Thus, such a time-reversed adiabatic pulse cannot effectively restore the transverse magnetization to the longitudinal axis. Another limitation of the adiabatic excitation pulses discussed so far is that the flip angle is restricted to 90° (or multiples of 90°) in order to achieve insensitivity to B_1-field variations. For flip angles other than 90° (or multiples of 90°), the direction of $\vec{B}_{\text{eff}}$ will depend on the B_1-field amplitude as shown in Eqs. (6.7) and (6.13). Consequently, the flip angle is also B_1 dependent.

BIR pulses are a class of adiabatic pulses that can be used to both excite longitudinal magnetization to the transverse plane *and* to return transverse magnetization to the longitudinal axis (Ugurbil et al. 1987; Staewen et al. 1990; Garwood and Ke 1991). The BIR pulses are composed of multiple segments of the adiabatic excitation pulses described later. A phase discontinuity can be introduced at the juncture of the segments and adjusted to produce flip angles other than 90° without compromising the B_1-field insensitivity. Three examples of BIR pulses are given next. The BIR pulses operate very similarly to the 180° plane rotation pulses discussed in Section 6.3; the interested reader can analyze these pulses using the diagrams found there or consult Ugurbil et al. (1987).

BIR-1 Pulse   The BIR-1 pulse (Ugurbil et al. 1987) has two segments that can be described by:

Amplitude modulation:

$$\vec{A}(t) = \begin{cases} \hat{x} B_1 \cos \xi t & (0 \le t < T/2) \\ \hat{y} B_1 \cos \xi t & (T/2 < t \le T) \end{cases} \tag{6.18}$$

Frequency modulation:

$$\omega_{\text{rf}}(t) = \begin{cases} \omega - \gamma B_{z,0} \sin \xi t & (0 \le t < T/2) \\ \omega + \gamma B_{z,0} \sin \xi t & (T/2 < t \le T) \end{cases} \tag{6.19}$$

where B_1 is the peak amplitude of the B_1 field, the pulse width is $T = \pi/\xi$, and unit vectors $\hat{x}$ and $\hat{y}$ denote the axis along which the B_1 field is applied.

As indicated by Eq. (6.18), a 90° phase shift occurs at the mid-point of the pulse, resulting in a 90° flip angle. If this phase shift is adjusted, an arbitrary flip angle θ can be obtained (Garwood and Ke 1991).

BIR-2 Pulse   BIR-2 pulse (Ugurbil et al. 1987) has three segments with each segment based on a sinusoidal modulation function:

Amplitude modulation:

$$\vec{A}(t) = \begin{cases} \hat{x} |B_1 \cos \xi t| & (0 \le t < T/2) \\ \hat{y} |B_1 \cos \xi t| & (T/2 < t \le T) \\ -\hat{y} |B_1 \cos \xi t| & (T \le t < 2T) \end{cases} \tag{6.20}$$

Frequency modulation:

$$\omega_{\text{rf}}(t) = \omega - \gamma |B_{z,0} \sin \xi t| \quad (0 \le t \le 2T) \tag{6.21}$$

Compared to the BIR-1 pulse, the pulse width of the BIR-2 pulse is increased to $2T$ (note that the relation of $T = \pi/\xi$ still holds for the BIR-2 pulse). This pulse, however, provides better tolerance to off-resonance effects than the BIR-1 pulse.

Equation (6.20) indicates that there is a 90° phase shift at $t = T/2$, and a 180° phase shift at $t = T$. These phase shifts are required for a 90° rotation of the magnetization. The BIR-2 pulse can be generalized to produce an arbitrary flip angle θ if the phase shift at $t = T/2$ is adjusted (Garwood and Ke 1991).

BIR-4 Pulse The BIR-4 pulse is more frequently used than the other BIR pulses. Unlike the BIR-1 and BIR-2 pulses, the modulation functions for the BIR-4 pulse are symmetric with respect to the center of the pulse. It induces a plane rotation more accurately than other BIR pulses and typically requires less RF power. A BIR-4 pulse employing hyperbolic tangent (tanh) and tangent (tan) modulation functions (Staewen et al. 1990) is given next and schematically shown in Figure 6.5.

Amplitude modulation:

$$
A(t) = \begin{cases}
B_1 \tanh\left[\lambda(1 - 4t/T)\right] & (0 \le t < T/4) \\
B_1 \tanh\left[\lambda(4t/T - 1)\right] & (T/4 \le t < T/2) \\
B_1 \tanh\left[\lambda(3 - 4t/T)\right] & (T/2 \le t < 3T/4) \\
B_1 \tanh\left[\lambda(4t/T - 3)\right] & (3T/4 \le t \le T)
\end{cases}
\tag{6.22}
$$

Frequency modulation:

$$
\omega_{\text{rf}}(t) = \begin{cases}
\omega - \dfrac{\tan(4\beta t/T)}{\tan\beta} & (0 \le t < T/4) \\[2mm]
\omega - \dfrac{\tan[\beta(4t/T - 2)]}{\tan\beta} & (T/4 \le t < T/2) \\[2mm]
\omega - \dfrac{\tan[\beta(4t/T - 2)]}{\tan\beta} & (T/2 \le t < 3T/4) \\[2mm]
\omega - \dfrac{\tan[\beta(4t/T - 4)]}{\tan\beta} & (3T/4 \le t \le T)
\end{cases}
\tag{6.23}
$$

where β and λ are dimensionless constants that determine how well the pulse satisfies the adiabatic condition. For example, a pulse with $\lambda = 10$, $\tan\beta = 10$ and $T = 5$ ms can produce acceptable results when a surface coil is employed (Staewen et al. 1990).

The frequency modulation for BIR-4 pulses is often converted to a phase modulation to facilitate implementation:

$$
\phi(t) = \begin{cases}
\int\limits_0^t [\omega - \omega_{\text{rf}}(t')]dt' & (0 \le t < T/4) \\[2mm]
\int\limits_0^t [\omega - \omega_{\text{rf}}(t')]dt' + \Delta\phi_1 & (T/4 \le t \le 3T/4) \\[2mm]
\int\limits_0^t [\omega - \omega_{\text{rf}}(t')]dt' + \Delta\phi_2 & (3T/4 \le t \le T)
\end{cases}
\tag{6.24}
$$

where $\Delta\phi_1$ and $\Delta\phi_2$ are the phase offsets at $t = T/4$ and $t = 3T/4$, respectively (Figure 6.5c). Although not required, $\Delta\phi_1$ is typically set to $-\Delta\phi_2$

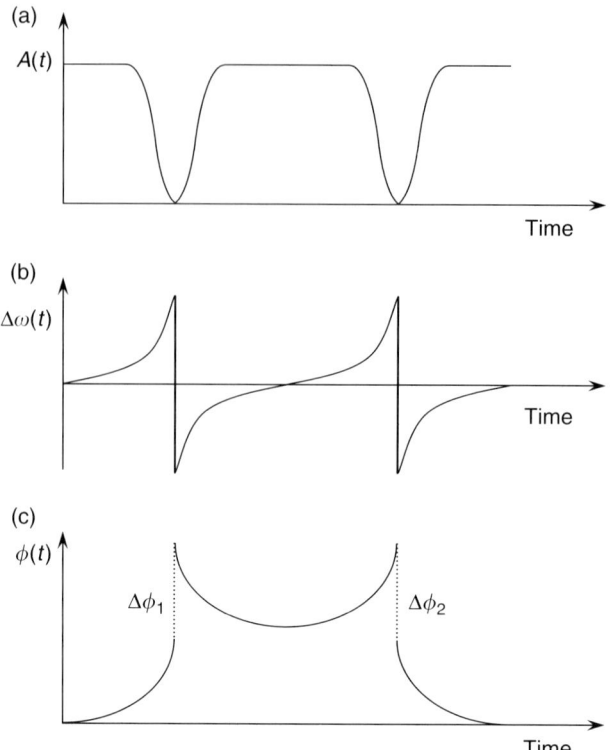

FIGURE 6.5 Schematic plots showing the (a) amplitude, (b) frequency, and (c) phase modulation functions for the BIR-4 pulse. The phase offsets $\Delta\phi_1$ and $\Delta\phi_2$ (denoted by the dotted lines) control the flip angle of the pulse.

in order to maintain pulse symmetry. The value of the phase offsets is quite important because it directly determines the flip angle of the BIR-4 pulse. To achieve a flip angle of θ, the phase offsets should be chosen as:

$$\begin{cases} \Delta\phi_1 = \pi + \dfrac{\theta}{2} \\ \Delta\phi_2 = -\pi - \dfrac{\theta}{2} \end{cases} \tag{6.25}$$

Alternative analytical expressions for BIR-4 pulses have also been reported (Garwood and Ke 1991). The shapes of the amplitude, frequency, and phase modulation functions are generally similar to those depicted in Figure 6.5.

6.1.5 APPLICATIONS

Adiabatic excitation pulses are often used when a surface coil is employed to transmit RF power to excite a desired volume. Although volume coils are more commonly used for RF excitation on modern clinical scanners, surface coil excitation is still occasionally employed for research applications. Even with volume coil transmitters (e.g., a birdcage coil), adiabatic excitation can reduce the sensitivity to B_1 field homogeneity in applications such as signal saturation. A drawback of adiabatic excitation is the substantially increased SAR as compared to nonadiabatic excitation. In addition, robust adiabatic excitation pulses for spatial selection are difficult to design due to the large off-resonance effect introduced by imaging gradients (Johnson et al. 1989). Thus, adiabatic excitation pulses are often limited to 3D volume imaging.

SELECTED REFERENCES

Bendall, M. R., and Pegg, D. T. 1986. Uniform sample excitation with surface coils for *in vivo* spectroscopy by adiabatic rapid half passage. *J. Magn. Reson.* 67: 376–381.

Garwood, M., and Ke, Y. 1991. Symmetric pulses to induce arbitrary flip angles with compensation for RF inhomogeneity and resonance offsets. *J. Magn. Reson.* 94: 511–525.

Johnson, A. J., Garwood, M., and Ugurbil, K. 1989. Slice selection with gradient-modulated adiabatic excitation despite the presence of large B_1-inhomogeneities. *J. Magn. Reson.* 81: 653–660.

Staewen, R. S., Johnson, A. J., Ross, B. D., Parrish, T., Merkle, H., and Garwood, M. 1990. 3-D flash imaging using a single surface coil and a new adiabatic pulse, BIR-4. *Invest. Radiol.* 25: 559–567.

Ugurbil, K., Garwood, M., and Bendall, R. 1987. Amplitude- and frequency-modulated pulses to achieve 90° plane rotation with inhomogeneous B_1 fields. *J. Magn. Reson.* 72: 177–185.

Ugurbil, K., Garwood, M., and Rath, A. R. 1988. Optimization of modulation functions to improve insensitivity of adiabatic pulses to variations in B_1 magnitude. *J. Magn. Reson.* 80: 448–469.

RELATED SECTIONS

6.2 Adiabatic Inversion Pulses

Adiabatic inversion pulses (Silver et al. 1984; Hardy et al. 1986; Rosenfeld and Zur 1996; Ordidge et al. 1996) are a special class of RF pulses that nutate the equilibrium magnetization vector from the $+z$ axis to the $-z$ axis (i.e., from along the B_0 direction to opposite to it). Unlike the conventional inversion pulses discussed in Section 3.2, adiabatic inversion pulses can *uniformly* invert the magnetization vector across an imaged object, even when the B_1 field is spatially nonuniform.

Adiabatic inversion pulses operate under the adiabatic passage principle. This principle, described in more detail in Section 6.1, states that a magnetization vector initially parallel to the effective magnetic field follows the direction of the effective magnetic field (see Section 1.2), provided that the effective field does not change its direction much during one rotational period of the magnetization about the effective field. In order to satisfy this condition, also known as the adiabatic condition, an adiabatic inversion pulse usually requires a relatively long pulse width and a rather high B_1 amplitude. As long as the B_1-field amplitude exceeds a minimum threshold, the resultant magnetization vector becomes immune to the B_1 field variations, leading to a spatially uniform inversion of the magnetization.

Adiabatic inversion is achieved by simultaneously modulating (i.e., varying) the amplitude and frequency of an RF pulse so that the orientation of the effective magnetic field changes from the $+z$ to the $-z$ axis in accordance with the adiabatic principle. As such, adiabatic pulses are sometimes called *frequency modulated* (FM) or *chirped pulses*. Depending on the choice of the modulation functions, adiabatic inversion pulses can take many different forms. In the rotating reference frame (Section 1.2), the frequency modulation function of an adiabatic inversion pulse always starts with a large positive value (i.e., above resonance), gradually decreases to 0 (i.e., on-resonance), and ends at a large negative value (i.e., below resonance). In contrast, the amplitude modulation function begins with a value of 0, increases to its maximum, and decreases to 0 at the end of the pulse.

The basic principles of adiabatic pulses are discussed in Section 6.1. In this section, we focus only on the issues specific to adiabatic inversion pulses. We first discuss the principles, then concentrate on the design issues, and finally provide an overview on the applications.

6.2.1 PRINCIPLES OF ADIABATIC INVERSION

Like all adiabatic pulses, the flip angle of an adiabatic inversion pulse does not obey the conventional relationship (see Section 3.1) between the flip angle (θ) and the B_1 field:

$$\theta \neq \gamma \int_0^T B_1(t)\,dt \tag{6.26}$$

where T is the pulse width, and γ is the gyromagnetic ratio. Instead, the flip angle of an adiabatic pulse depends on how the B_1 field varies its amplitude *and* modulation frequency (or phase) during the pulse. By properly manipulating the modulation functions, spins that experience different B_1 fields can be uniformly inverted with the same flip angle at the end of the pulse.

Consider an RF pulse, $B_1(t) = A(t)e^{-i\omega_{rf}(t)t}$, whose amplitude and frequency are modulated by a sine and a cosine function, respectively:

$$A(t) = B_x \sin \xi t \tag{6.27}$$

$$\omega_{rf}(t) = \omega - \gamma B_z \cos \xi t \tag{6.28}$$

where ξ is the modulation frequency, ω is the Larmor frequency, B_x is the time-independent magnetic field amplitude along the x axis (with no loss of generality, the transverse component is arbitrarily assigned to the x axis), and γB_z is the amplitude of the frequency modulation. Note that B_z is the equivalent magnetic field amplitude along the z axis arising from the off-resonance effect in the rotating reference frame. In that frame, which has an angular frequency $\omega_{rf}(t)$, the z component of the effective magnetic field is given by (see Eq. 1.79):

$$\frac{\Delta\omega}{\gamma} \equiv \frac{\omega - \omega_{rf}}{\gamma} = B_z \cos \xi t \tag{6.29}$$

If the transverse component of the effective field is along the x axis in the rotating frame, then:

$$B_{eff\perp} = B_x \sin \xi t \tag{6.30}$$

In light of Eqs. (6.29) and (6.30), the amplitude and direction of the effective magnetic field, $\vec{B}_{eff}$, are given by:

$$|\vec{B}_{eff}| = \sqrt{(B_x \sin \xi t)^2 + (B_z \cos \xi t)^2} \tag{6.31}$$

$$\psi = \arctan \left(\frac{B_x \sin \xi t}{B_z \cos \xi t} \right) \tag{6.32}$$

At the beginning of the pulse, ψ is 0. Therefore, the effective field is aligned with the equilibrium magnetization $\vec{M}$ along the z axis (Figure 6.6a). If the adiabatic condition (see Section 6.1) is satisfied by choosing a slow modulation frequency ξ, a strong effective field, or both, the adiabatic passage principle dictates that the magnetization vector $\vec{M}$ will track the direction of the effective field $\vec{B}_{eff}$ during the course of the RF pulse (actually, $\vec{M}$ precesses about $\vec{B}_{eff}$ along a very tight cone as shown in Figure 6.6b). When $t = \pi/(2\xi)$,

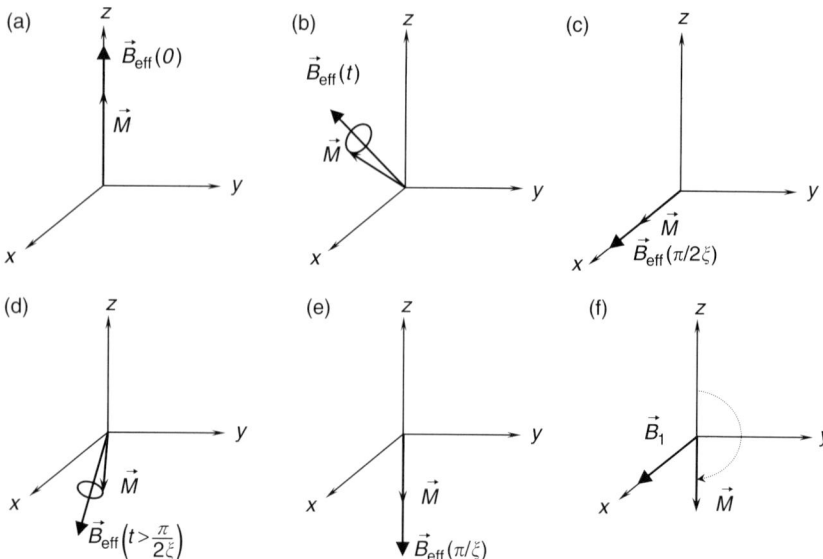

FIGURE 6.6 The inversion processes in (a–e) an adiabatic pulse and (f) a nonadiabatic pulse. (a) Beginning of the adiabatic inversion pulse; (b) during the first half of the adiabatic pulse, showing the magnetization precessing in a tight cone about the effective field (the size of the cone is exaggerated for better visualization); (c) at the mid-point of the adiabatic pulse; (d) during the second half of the adiabatic pulse; (e) at the end of the adiabatic pulse. (f) The trajectory of the magnetization $\vec{M}$ of a nonadiabatic pulse. Note that for adiabatic inversion, the magnetization vector $\vec{M}$ is approximately parallel to the effective field $\vec{B}_{\text{eff}}$ during the pulse, whereas for nonadiabatic inversion $\vec{M}$ is perpendicular to the applied B_1 field.

both $\vec{B}_{\text{eff}}$ and $\vec{M}$ point along the x axis (Figure 6.6c). As the RF pulse continues, $\vec{B}_{\text{eff}}$ rotates toward the negative z axis (Figure 6.6d) with ψ changing from 90° to 180°. At the end of the pulse ($t = \pi/\xi$), the effective magnetic field $\vec{B}_{\text{eff}}$ has experienced a 180° rotation. Because the magnetization vector tracks $\vec{B}_{\text{eff}}$, a 180° adiabatic inversion of the magnetization is achieved (Figure 6.6e). The trajectory of the magnetization vector during adiabatic inversion is quite different from that in nonadiabatic inversion (see Section 3.2), in which case $\vec{M}$ is always perpendicular to the B_1 field applied on resonance (Figure 6.6f).

To illustrate the immunity of adiabatic inversion pulses to spatial variation in the B_1 field, let us consider two locations that experience different B_1-field strengths. One location receives $B_{1,a}$, and the other receives $B_{1,b}$. At the end of the RF pulse (i.e., $t = \pi/\xi$ or $\psi = 180°$), the effective fields at both locations will be aligned along the negative z axis. Consequently, the magnetization vectors for the spins at these two locations are also parallel to the negative z axis, corresponding to a 180° inversion. This demonstrates why adiabatic pulses can achieve uniform inversion even in the presence of B_1-field variation across the imaged object. A condition is that both $B_{1,a}$ and $B_{1,b}$ must be sufficiently strong to satisfy the adiabatic condition.

6.2.2 DESIGN OF SPATIALLY NONSELECTIVE ADIABATIC INVERSION PULSE

Adiabatic inversion pulses can be either spatially selective or nonselective. The design procedure for spatially nonselective adiabatic inversion pulses is very similar to that discussed in Section 6.1 for nonselective adiabatic excitation pulses. The initial step is to choose a pair of modulation functions (e.g., a sine-cosine pair) for B_1-field amplitude and frequency. Because not all the spins have the same resonance frequency, a tolerance level for the off-resonance effect κ needs to be considered in the frequency modulation function:

$$\Delta\omega_{\mathrm{rf}}(t) = \omega - \omega_{\mathrm{rf}}(t) = \gamma B_z \cos \xi t + \kappa \qquad (6.33)$$

A simulation based on the Bloch equations with Eq. (6.33) as the off-resonant term can reveal the robustness of the adiabatic inversion pulse with respect to off-resonance. The other parameters, including the B_1-field amplitude B_x, frequency modulation amplitude γB_z, and modulating frequency ξ, can be determined using the method described in Section 6.1 on adiabatic excitation pulse design, except that the parameters p and q (defined by Eqs. 6.15 and (6.16), respectively) are chosen based on the inversion efficiency (i.e., the amplitude of the inverted magnetization as a percentage of the original longitudinal magnetization) instead of the excitation efficiency. To satisfy the adiabatic condition with minimal RF power, numerical optimization of the modulation functions can also be incorporated, as detailed in Ugurbil et al. (1988).

The design process of an adiabatic inversion pulse often can be simplified by first designing a 90° adiabatic excitation pulse and then concatenating this pulse with its mirror image. Although this simplified approach does not always give the same result as the conventional method, the performance of the pulse is acceptable for most applications.

Spatially nonselective adiabatic inversion pulses sometimes can also be designed using the modulation functions of an adiabatic refocusing pulse (Section 6.3). The reverse, however, is generally invalid—the modulation functions designed for an adiabatic inversion pulse generally cannot be used for adiabatic refocusing without modifications.

6.2.3 DESIGN OF SPATIALLY SELECTIVE ADIABATIC INVERSION PULSE

One of the most prevalent adiabatic pulses used in MRI is a spatially selective adiabatic inversion pulse, also known as a hyperbolic secant pulse or Silver-Joseph-Hoult pulse (Silver et al. 1984). We focus on this pulse in this subsection.

The Modulation Functions   A general hyperbolic secant pulse is given by:

$$B_1(t) = [A_0 \operatorname{sech}(\beta t)]^{1+i\mu} \tag{6.34}$$

where A_0 is the maximum B_1 field, β is an modulation angular frequency, μ is a dimensionless parameter, and the hyperbolic function sech is defined by $\operatorname{sech} x = 2/(e^x + e^{-x})$. Equation (6.34) can be recast to explicitly show the amplitude modulation $A(t)$ and the phase modulation $\phi(t)$:

$$B_1(t) = A(t)e^{i\phi(t)} \tag{6.35}$$

Comparing Eq. (6.35) with Eq. (6.34) and using the identity $b^z = e^{z \ln b}$, we obtain:

$$A(t) = A_0 \operatorname{sech}(\beta t) \tag{6.36}$$

$$\phi(t) = \mu \ln[\operatorname{sech}(\beta t)] + \mu \ln A_0 \tag{6.37}$$

The constant term $\mu \ln A_0$ in Eq. (6.37) drops out when the corresponding frequency modulation function is calculated by taking the time-derivative:

$$\Delta\omega(t) = \frac{d\phi}{dt} = -\mu\beta \tanh(\beta t) \tag{6.38}$$

where $\tanh x = (e^x - e^{-x})/(e^x + e^{-x})$. Thus, according to Eqs. (6.36) and (6.38), the hyperbolic secant pulse uses sech/tanh modulation functions. As the time variable t sweeps from $-\infty$ to $+\infty$, the amplitude modulation function goes from zero to the maximum (at $t = 0$) and then returns to zero. Meanwhile, the frequency modulation function decreases from its maximum value (i.e., $\mu\beta$) to zero, reverses its polarity, and finally reaches its minimum value (or negative maximum) $-\mu\beta$. These properties satisfy the requirement for adiabatic inversion pulses discussed previously.

To design an adiabatic inversion pulse based on hyperbolic secant modulations, we need to determine the three parameters A_0, β, and μ in a combination that meets the adiabatic condition as well as other practical constraints, such as the RF pulse bandwidth and RF power.

The Adiabatic Condition   According to Section 6.1, the adiabatic condition states:

$$\left| \frac{d\psi}{dt} \right| \ll \gamma \left| \vec{B}_{\text{eff}} \right|$$

Using $B_x = A_0$ and $B_z = -\mu\beta/\gamma$ and replacing the sin/cos modulation functions with sech/tanh in Eqs. (6.31) and (6.32) gives:

$$\left| \vec{B}_{\text{eff}} \right| = \sqrt{(A_0 \operatorname{sech} \beta t)^2 + \left(\frac{\mu\beta}{\gamma} \tanh \beta t \right)^2} \tag{6.39}$$

$$\psi = \arctan\left(-\frac{\gamma A_0 \operatorname{sech}\beta t}{\mu\beta \tanh \beta t} \right) = \arctan\left(-\frac{\gamma A_0}{\mu\beta \sinh\beta t} \right) \tag{6.40}$$

Combining Eqs. (6.38), (6.39) and (6.40), the adiabatic condition for the hyperbolic secant pulse can be derived (as shown in the appendix at the end of this section):

$$A_0 \gg \frac{\sqrt{\mu\beta}}{\gamma} \tag{6.41}$$

In practice, the performance of the adiabatic inversion pulse is acceptable as long as A_0 is greater than $\sqrt{\mu\beta}/\gamma$.

Parameter Selection   Similar to other spatially selective pulses, the dimensionless product of the pulse width and the RF bandwidth, $T\Delta f$, is a measure of the quality of the slice profile. An acceptable $T\Delta f$ can be found by numerically solving the Bloch equations using the B_1 field given by Eq. (6.34). The maximal pulse width is often fixed by other considerations, such as the minimal TR and TI requirements in the sequence, flow effects, and off-resonance perturbation. Once the pulse width and $T\Delta f$ are determined, the bandwidth can be readily calculated.

The RF bandwidth of a hyperbolic secant pulse, in conjunction with the amplitude of the slice-selection gradient, determines the slice thickness. Using Fourier or Bloch equation analysis of Eqs. (6.36) and (6.37), it can be shown that the RF bandwidth is related to the hyperbolic secant pulse parameters by the following equation:

$$\Delta f = \frac{\mu\beta}{\pi} \tag{6.42}$$

Combining Eqs. (6.41) and (6.42) yields:

$$A_0 \gg \frac{\pi \Delta f}{\gamma \sqrt{\mu}} \tag{6.43}$$

Equation (6.43) suggests that the largest μ value should be used to keep the RF amplitude and RF power minimal. This implies that β should take its smallest value, because the $\mu\beta$ product is constrained by the bandwidth requirement (Eq. 6.42). As β decreases, insufficient decay of the hyperbolic functions will result in discontinuity at the margins of the RF envelope due to truncation. In that case, the direction of the effective magnetic field will deviate from its required direction at the beginning and at the end of the pulse (see Eq. 6.39), causing signal loss in the inverted magnetization and poor slice profile.

In some cases, the conflicting requirements among the adiabatic condition, time-bandwidth product, off-resonance sensitivity, and the quality of slice profiles cannot be simultaneously satisfied. Alternative design methods can be used to help alleviate these problems (Rosenfeld and Zur 1996; Ordidge et al. 1996).

Figure 6.7 shows an example of a hyperbolic secant pulse with the following parameters: pulse width $= 8$ ms, $T\Delta f = 10$, $\beta = 800$ rad/s, $\mu = 4.9$, and $A_0 = 14\,\mu\text{T}$. This pulse works well for inverting the magnetization within a large imaging volume such as the whole human body.

Example 6.1 Determine whether the pulse in Figure 6.7 satisfies the adiabatic condition stated given by Eq. (6.43).

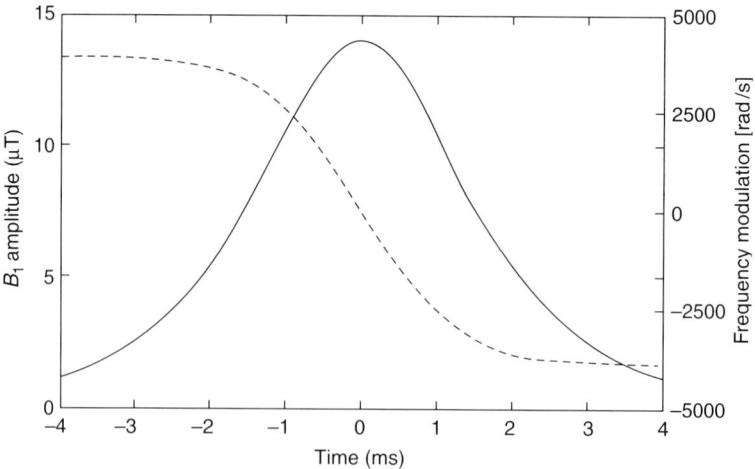

FIGURE 6.7 Modulation functions for a $180°$ hyperbolic secant adiabatic inversion pulse (pulse width $= 8$ ms, $T\Delta f = 10$, $\beta = 800$ rad/s, $\mu = 4.9$, and $A_0 = 14\,\mu\text{T}$). The amplitude modulation is shown as a solid line, and the frequency modulation is shown as a dashed line. Phase modulation can be obtained by integrating the frequency modulation function over time.

Answer The bandwidth of the pulse is:

$$\Delta f = \frac{T \Delta f}{T} = \frac{10}{8\,\text{ms}} = 1250\,\text{Hz}$$

Using the parameters of the pulse given in Figure 6.7, the right side of Eq. (6.43) is:

$$\frac{\pi \Delta f}{\gamma \sqrt{\mu}} = \frac{\pi (1250\,\text{Hz})}{(2\pi)(42.57\,\text{MHz/T})\sqrt{4.9}} = 6.6\,\mu\text{T}$$

which is smaller than A_0 by more than twofold. Thus, the adiabatic condition is met.

6.2.4 APPLICATIONS

Spatially nonselective adiabatic inversion pulses are often used when a surface coil is employed as an RF transmitter to invert magnetization within a desired volume. Because the B_1 field of a surface coil is highly nonuniform, adiabatic inversion pulses can produce considerably better inversion uniformity than their nonadiabatic counterpart. Sometimes, even with volume-coil transmitters (e.g., a transmit/receive birdcage body coil), adiabatic inversion pulses can exhibit improvement over nonadiabatic pulses in applications such as lipid suppression. The drawback of adiabatic pulses includes the longer pulse width, higher RF amplitude, and increased SAR. The issue with SAR can be addressed using variable rate design (Section 2.4) as illustrated by Conolly et al. (1988).

Spatially selective adiabatic inversion pulses are frequently employed in inversion recovery pulse sequences to null certain spin components with distinct T_1 values. For example, in a short TI inversion recovery (STIR) pulse sequence (Section 14.2), an adiabatic inversion pulse can be used to invert the signals from lipids. After a certain inversion time (e.g., ~150 ms at 1.5 T) when the longitudinal component of the lipid magnetization crosses zero during the recovery process, an imaging sequence is executed so that the acquired signal does not contain the contribution from the lipid. Because a large portion of the body lipid is located in the subcutaneous region where the B_1 field is often nonuniform, adiabatic pulses are especially useful to achieve good lipid suppression in that region. Figure 6.8 gives an example showing the improvement of lipid suppression afforded by an adiabatic inversion. Adiabatic inversion pulses can also be used in fluid-attenuated inversion recovery (FLAIR) pulse sequences (Section 14.2). In this case, spatially selective adiabatic inversion pulses are used to attenuate cerebrospinal fluid in the brain to improve the contrast between lesions and normal brain tissues.

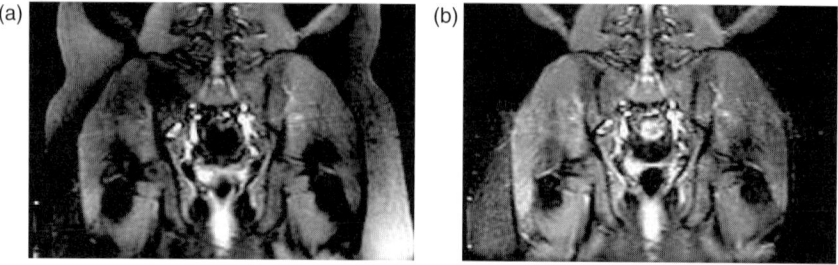

FIGURE 6.8 STIR images obtained with (a) a nonadiabatic inversion pulse and (b) an adiabatic inversion pulse. The imaging parameters are otherwise identical (TR = 2000 ms, TE = 25 ms, TI = 150 ms). The improved lipid suppression with an adiabatic inversion pulse is evident, even with the use of a whole-body birdcage RF transmit coil.

Adiabatic inversion pulses are also heavily used in pulsed arterial spin tagging (AST) experiments for tissue perfusion measurement. This application is detailed in Section 17.1.

6.2.5 APPENDIX

Taking a time derivative of Eq. (6.40) yields:

$$\left|\frac{d\psi}{dt}\right| = \frac{\gamma A_0}{\mu\beta}\cos^2\psi\left|\frac{d(\operatorname{csch}\beta t)}{dt}\right| \tag{6.44}$$

(Note that $\operatorname{csch}\beta t = 2/(e^{\beta t} - e^{-\beta t})$). Let:

$$\gamma A_0 = \lambda\mu\beta \tag{6.45}$$

where λ is a unitless parameter. Combining Eq. (6.44) with Eqs. (6.36) and (6.38), we obtain:

$$\left|\frac{d\psi}{dt}\right| = \left|\frac{\lambda\beta\,\operatorname{sech}(\beta t)}{1 + (\lambda^2 - 1)\operatorname{sech}^2(\beta t)}\right| \tag{6.46}$$

Using the relationship $\gamma A_0 = \lambda\mu\beta$, Eq. (6.39) becomes:

$$|\vec{B}_{\text{eff}}| = \frac{\mu\beta}{\gamma}[1 + (\lambda^2 - 1)\operatorname{sech}^2(\beta t)]^{1/2} \tag{6.47}$$

The adiabatic condition states that $|d\psi/dt| \cdot |\gamma\vec{B}_{\text{eff}}|^{-1} \ll 1$. Inserting Eqs. (6.46) and (6.47) into the adiabatic condition yields:

$$\left|\frac{\lambda\,\operatorname{sech}(\beta t)}{\mu[1 + (\lambda^2 - 1)\operatorname{sech}^2(\beta t)]^{3/2}}\right| \ll 1 \tag{6.48}$$

If we define a new variable:

$$\Gamma \equiv |\lambda| \mathrm{sech}(\beta t)[1 + (\lambda^2 - 1)\mathrm{sech}^2(\beta t)]^{-3/2} \qquad (6.49)$$

then the adiabatic condition reduces to $\Gamma \ll \mu$. Let us find the maximum Γ with respect to t by setting $\partial\Gamma/\partial t = 0$. This yields two conditions:

1. $\dfrac{d[\mathrm{sech}(\beta t)]}{dt} = 0$ \qquad\qquad (6.50)

2. $\dfrac{\partial\Gamma}{\partial[\mathrm{sech}(\beta t)]} = 0$ \qquad\qquad (6.51)

Condition 1 leads to $\mathrm{sech}(\beta t) = 1$ and $\Gamma = \lambda^{-2}$. Using Eq. (6.48) and the relationship $\gamma A_0 = \lambda\mu\beta$, we can readily derive the adiabatic condition in Eq. (6.41) (i.e., $A_0 \gg \sqrt{\mu}\beta/\gamma$). Condition 2 results in two scenarios:

2a. $\lambda \to 0$ \qquad if $\mathrm{sech}(\beta t) = 1$ \qquad\qquad (6.52)

2b. $\lambda = \sqrt{\dfrac{1 + 2\mathrm{sech}^2(\beta t)}{2\mathrm{sech}^2(\beta t)}}$ \qquad if $0 < \mathrm{sech}(\beta t) < 1$ \qquad (6.53)

Examining these two conditions reveals that Γ has a larger value under condition 2a. This leads to the same result (i.e., $A_0 \gg \sqrt{\mu}\,\beta/\gamma$) as condition 1.

SELECTED REFERENCES

Conolly, S., Nishimura, D., Macovski, A., and Glover, G. 1988. Variable-rate selective excitation. *J. Magn. Reson.* 78: 440–458.

Hardy, C. J., Edelstein, W. A., and Vatis, D. 1986. Efficient adiabatic fast passage for NMR population-inversion in the presence of radiofrequency field inhomogeneity and frequency offsets. *J. Magn. Reson.* 66: 470–482.

Ordidge, R. J., Wylezinska, M., Hugg, J. W., Butterworth, E., Franconi, F. 1996. Frequency offset corrected inversion (FOCI) pulses for use in localized spectroscopy. *Magn. Reson. Med.* 36: 562–566.

Rosenfeld, D., and Zur, Y. 1996. A new adiabatic inversion pulse. *Magn. Reson. Med.* 36: 124–136.

Silver, M. S., Joseph, R. I., and Hoult, D. I. 1984. Highly selective $\pi/2$ and π pulse generation. *J. Magn. Reson.* 59: 347–351.

Ugurbil, K., Garwood, M., and Rath, A. R. 1988. Optimization of modulation functions to improve insensitivity of adiabatic pulses to variations in B_1 magnitude. *J. Magn. Reson.* 80: 448–469.

RELATED SECTIONS

Section 1.2 Rotating Reference Frame
Section 3.2 Inversion Pulses
Section 6.1 Adiabatic Excitation Pulses
Section 6.3 Adiabatic Refocusing Pulses
Section 14.2 Inversion Recovery
Section 17.1 Arterial Spin Tagging

6.3 Adiabatic Refocusing Pulses

Adiabatic refocusing pulses are a special class of RF pulses that rotate the transverse (as well as longitudinal) magnetization vector by 180° about an axis in the transverse plane. Unlike the conventional refocusing pulses discussed in Section 3.3, adiabatic refocusing pulses can *uniformly* rotate the magnetization vector across an imaged object, even when the B_1 field is spatially nonuniform.

Similar to adiabatic excitation and inversion pulses (Sections 6.1 and 6.2), an adiabatic refocusing pulse operates under the *adiabatic passage principle*. This principle states that the magnetization vector follows the direction of the effective magnetic field, provided that the direction of the effective magnetic field does not change much during one precession cycle of the magnetization about the effective field. This condition, known as the adiabatic condition, is described in more detail in Section 6.1.

The adiabatic passage principle has three implications. First, if a magnetization vector is parallel to the effective field, then it will track the direction of the effective field. This property is exploited in designing adiabatic excitation and inversion pulses. Second, if a magnetization vector and the effective field are anti-parallel, then they will remain anti-parallel as the direction of the effective field varies. Third, if a magnetization vector is perpendicular to the effective field, then it will precess about and remain perpendicular to the effective field. Because any magnetization vector can be decomposed into components that are parallel (or anti-parallel) and perpendicular to the effective field, the behavior of magnetization during an adiabatic operation can be fully characterized.

To induce adiabatic refocusing of the transverse magnetization, the amplitude and frequency of an RF pulse must be modulated (i.e., varied) throughout the pulse in accordance with the adiabatic condition. Maintaining the adiabatic condition usually requires a relatively long pulse width and high B_1 amplitude. As long as the B_1 amplitude exceeds a threshold, the resultant magnetization vector is independent of B_1-field variations, leading to spatially uniform refocusing of the magnetization. Because of this property, adiabatic refocusing pulses are sometimes referred to as B_1-*i*ndependent *ref*ocusing (BIREF) pulses (Ugurbil, Garwood, Rath, and Bendall 1988).

For adiabatic excitation and inversion pulses, the initial direction of the magnetization coincides with that of the static magnetic field B_0 (or the z axis) (Figure 6.9a). The initial condition for an adiabatic refocusing pulse, however, is different. The magnetization already has been excited, fully or partially, to the transverse plane, and the transverse magnetization has dispersed (or dephased) into a set of isochromat vectors spanning a range of directions (Figure 6.9b). A challenge in designing adiabatic refocusing pulses

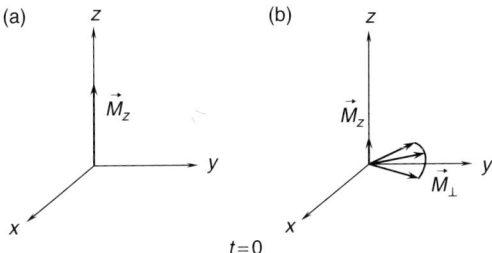

FIGURE 6.9 The initial conditions ($t = 0$) for (a) adiabatic excitation and inversion pulses and (b) adiabatic refocusing pulses. For both adiabatic excitation and adiabatic inversion pulses, the initial magnetization vector $\vec{M}_z$ is along the positive z axis. In adiabatic refocusing pulses, the initial transverse magnetization $\vec{M}_\perp$ consists of a set of isochromat vectors. In addition, a residual longitudinal magnetization $\vec{M}_z$ can remain along the z axis due to incomplete excitation.

is to induce a 180° rotation for all the transverse isochromat vectors so that they can be refocused at a later time. Such a rotation is known as *plane rotation* (Ugurbil, Garwood, Rath, and Bendall 1988). Although an adiabatic inversion pulse can also rotate the transverse plane, the transverse magnetization in the plane dephases during the pulse. Thus, adiabatic inversion pulses *cannot* be used for refocusing. Concurrent to plane rotation in adiabatic refocusing, the longitudinal magnetization vector along the z axis is inverted. Therefore, adiabatic refocusing pulses can be used for inversion. These relationships will become more apparent in the following discussion.

Although adiabatic refocusing pulses are amplitude modulated, their spatial or spectral selectivity is quite different from amplitude-modulated non-adiabatic refocusing pulses. Because off-resonance effects due to imaging gradients can greatly degrade the performance of adiabatic refocusing pulses (discussed in the next subsection), it has been challenging to design adiabatic refocusing pulses for slice selection. Spatially nonselective adiabatic refocusing pulses, however, can be employed for 3D imaging where slice selection is not necessary.

6.3.1 PRINCIPLES OF ADIABATIC REFOCUSING

An Example of an Adiabatic Refocusing Pulse   We can illustrate the principles of adiabatic refocusing by analyzing a specific pulse. Let us consider an RF pulse expressed in complex form, $B_1(t) = A(t)e^{-i\omega_{\mathrm{rf}}(t)t}$, whose amplitude and frequency are modulated by a sine and a cosine function, respectively

(Ugurbil, Garwood, Rath, and Bendall 1988):

$$A(t) = \begin{cases} B_x \sin \xi t & (0 \le \xi t < \pi/2) \\ -B_x \sin \xi t & (\pi/2 \le \xi t \le \pi) \end{cases} \tag{6.54}$$

$$\omega_{\mathrm{rf}}(t) = \omega - \gamma B_z |\cos \xi t| \quad (0 \le \xi t \le \pi) \tag{6.55}$$

where ξ is the modulation frequency that is related to the pulse width T by $\xi = \pi/T$, ω is the Larmor frequency of the spin system, B_x is the time-independent magnetic field amplitude along the x axis (with no loss of generality, the transverse component is arbitrarily assigned to the x axis), and B_z is the equivalent magnetic field amplitude along the z axis arising from the off-resonance effect in the rotating reference frame. This RF pulse is graphically shown in Figure 6.10. In the rotating reference frame with an angular frequency of $\omega_{\mathrm{rf}}(t)$, the z component of the effective magnetic field is given by (see Eq. 1.79):

$$\frac{\Delta\omega}{\gamma} \equiv \frac{\omega - \omega_{\mathrm{rf}}}{\gamma} = B_z |\cos \xi t| \tag{6.56}$$

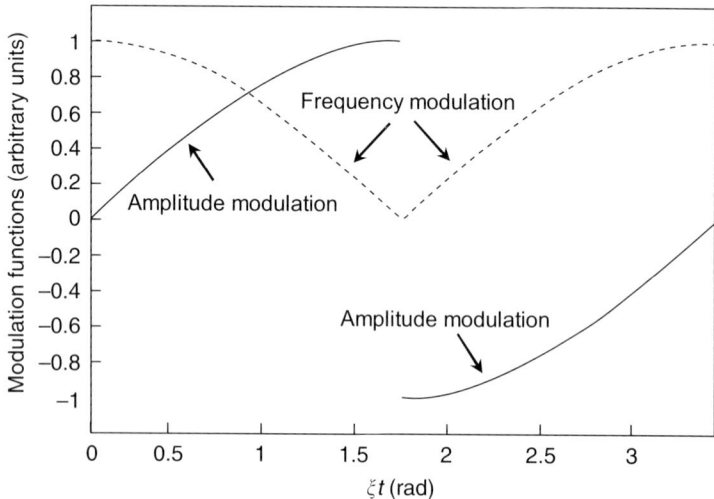

FIGURE 6.10 Modulation functions $A(t)$ and $\Delta\omega(t)$ for the adiabatic refocusing pulse shown in Eqs. (6.54) and (6.55). The solid lines show the amplitude modulation, and the dotted lines represent the frequency modulation. Both modulation functions are expressed in the rotating reference frame (i.e, the frequency modulation corresponds to $\omega - \omega_{\mathrm{rf}}$) and normalized between -1 and 1 with arbitrary units.

From Eq. (6.56), the amplitude and direction of the effective magnetic field can be expressed as:

$$|\vec{B}_{\text{eff}}| = \sqrt{(B_x \sin \xi t)^2 + (B_z \cos \xi t)^2} \tag{6.57}$$

$$\psi = (-1)^n \arctan\left(\frac{B_x \sin \xi t}{B_z |\cos \xi t|}\right) \qquad n = \begin{cases} 0 & (0 \le \xi t < \pi/2) \\ 1 & (\pi/2 \le \xi t \le \pi) \end{cases} \tag{6.58}$$

At the beginning of the pulse, ψ is zero. Therefore, the effective magnetic field is aligned along the z axis (Figure 6.11a). During the first half of the pulse (i.e., $0 \le \xi t < \pi/2$), $\vec{B}_{\text{eff}}$ rotates from the z axis to the x axis in the x, z plane (Figure 6.11b). Immediately after $\vec{B}_{\text{eff}}$ reaches the positive x axis (i.e., $\xi t = \pi/2$) (Figure 6.11c), the direction of $\vec{B}_{\text{eff}}$ is inverted to the negative x axis (Figure 6.11d). Finally, $\vec{B}_{\text{eff}}$ returns to the z axis through a 90° rotation in the $(-x, z)$ plane during the second half of the pulse (i.e., $\pi/2 \le \xi t \le \pi$) (Figure 6.11e and 6.11f).

Consider a spin system whose magnetization has been partially excited by an excitation pulse, producing a transverse magnetization component $M_\perp$ and a residual longitudinal component M_z (Figure 6.9b). After a certain time

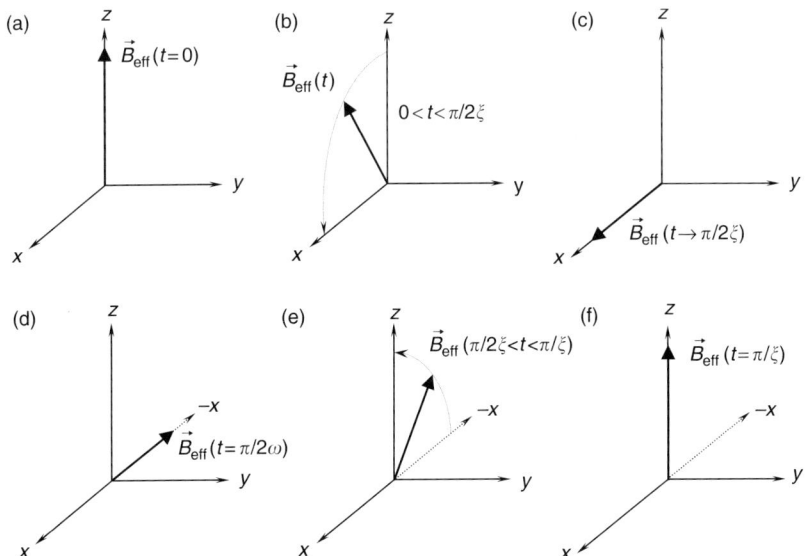

FIGURE 6.11 The trajectory of the effective magnetic field $\vec{B}_{\text{eff}}$ during the adiabatic refocusing pulse given by Figure 6.10 and Eqs. (6.54) and (6.55).

τ (i.e., TE/2) the transverse magnetization will be dispersed (or 'fanned out') into a set of isochomatic vectors spanning a certain angle as viewed in the rotating reference frame (Figure 6.9b). Our task is to demonstrate that the RF pulse shown in Figures 6.10 and 6.11 rotates *all* the vectors in the transverse plane by 180° so that the transverse magnetization can be refocused (or in phase) after another delay time τ, irrespective of the local B_1-field amplitude. In addition, we show that the pulse also adiabatically inverts the longitudinal magnetization M_z.

Interaction with the Longitudinal Magnetization At the beginning of the RF pulse (i.e., $t = 0$), $\vec{B}_{\text{eff}}$ and $\vec{M}_z$ are both along the z axis (Figure 6.12a). If we choose a sufficiently slow modulation frequency ξ and a strong effective field to satisfy the adiabatic condition, the adiabatic passage principle dictates that the magnetization vector $\vec{M}_z$ will track the direction of the effective field $\vec{B}_{\text{eff}}$ (within a very small cone) during the first half of the RF pulse (Figure 6.12b).

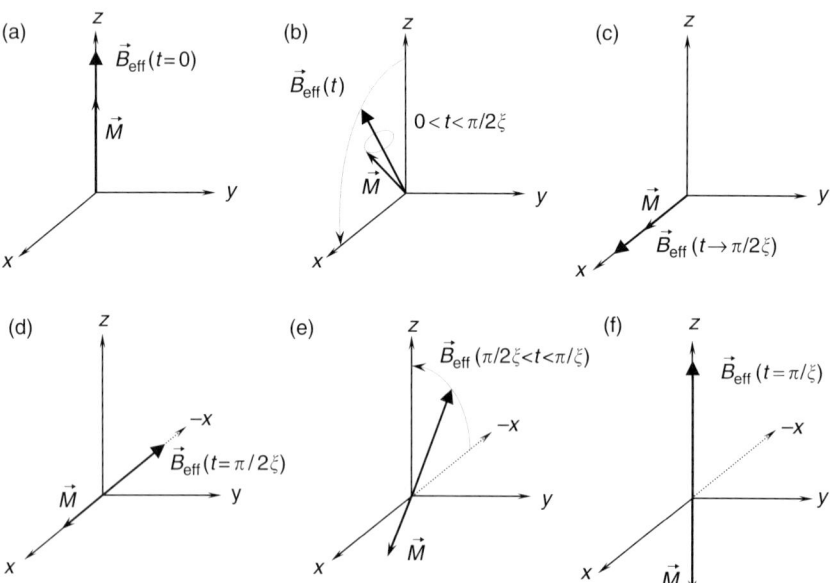

FIGURE 6.12 The trajectory of the longitudinal magnetization vector $\vec{M}_z$ during the adiabatic refocusing pulse described in Figure 6.10. All trajectories are described in the rotating reference frame. The magnetization $\vec{M}_z$ is parallel (or nearly parallel) to the effective field $\vec{B}_{\text{eff}}$ during the first half of the pulse (a–c), and anti-parallel (or nearly anti-parallel) during the second half of the pulse (d–f).

When $t = \pi/(2\xi)$, $\vec{M}_z$ follows $\vec{B}_{\text{eff}}$ onto the x axis (Figure 6.12c). At this point, $\vec{B}_{\text{eff}}$ instantaneously inverts its direction to the negative x axis, leaving $\vec{M}_z$ anti-parallel to $\vec{B}_{\text{eff}}$ (Figure 6.12d). According to the adiabatic passage principle discussed in the previous subsection, $\vec{M}_z$ remains anti-parallel to $\vec{B}_{\text{eff}}$ throughout the second half of the pulse (Figure 6.12e). When $\vec{B}_{\text{eff}}$ realigns with the positive z axis, $\vec{M}_z$ points to the negative z axis at the end of the RF pulse (Figure 6.12f). Therefore, the RF pulse in Figure 6.12 has performed an adiabatic inversion of the longitudinal magnetization.

Interaction with the Transverse Magnetization   Unlike the longitudinal magnetization, which can be represented by a single vector $\vec{M}_z$, the transverse magnetization can contain a set of isochromat vectors $\vec{M}_\perp(\varphi)$ because of different dephasing angles (φ). Let us focus on an arbitrary isochromat $\vec{m}_j$ within the $\vec{M}_\perp(\varphi)$ group and analyze its trajectory during the RF pulse given by Eqs. (6.54) and (6.55). At the beginning of the RF pulse, the magnetization $\vec{m}_j$ is perpendicular to the effective field $\vec{B}_{\text{eff}}$ and precesses about $\vec{B}_{\text{eff}}$ in the transverse plane. The initial position of $\vec{m}_j$ is shown as $\vec{m}_j(0)$ in each part of Figure 6.13 as a reference. If $\vec{B}_{\text{eff}}$ varies its direction while satisfying the adiabatic condition, the adiabatic passage principle indicates that $\vec{m}_j$ will remain perpendicular to $\vec{B}_{\text{eff}}$ and precess in a plane normal to $\vec{B}_{\text{eff}}$ (Figure 6.13b). At the end of the first half of the pulse (i.e., when $\vec{B}_{\text{eff}}$ points along the x axis), $\vec{m}_j$ precesses clockwise in the yz plane as viewed from the positive x axis (Figure 6.13c). Essentially, the transverse plane in which $\vec{m}_j$ initially precesses is rotated to the yz plane. If an observer follows the plane in which $\vec{m}_j$ precesses (i.e., the plane and $\vec{B}_{\text{eff}}$ appear static to the observer) and views the phase angle β_+ that $\vec{m}_j$ accumulates during the first half of the pulse, the phase angle is (Figure 6.13c):

$$\beta_+ = \gamma \int\limits_0^{\pi/2\xi} |\vec{B}_{\text{eff}}(t)|\, dt \qquad (6.59)$$

(Note that, although the phase angle is given by Eq. 6.59, the flip angle for adiabatic pulses does not obey the general relationship $\theta = \gamma \int B_1(t)\, dt$.) After $\vec{B}_{\text{eff}}$ abruptly changes its direction to the negative x axis, $\vec{m}_j$ remains perpendicular to $\vec{B}_{\text{eff}}$, but it begins to precess counter-clockwise in the zy plane as viewed from the positive x axis (Figure 6.13d). As $\vec{B}_{\text{eff}}$ returns to the positive z axis during the second half of the RF pulse, the precession plane of $\vec{m}_j$ is rotated accordingly (Figure 6.13e). At the end of the pulse, the precession plane coincides with the transverse plane again, but is flipped upside down with respect to the initial precession plane (Figure 6.13f). To distinguish the two sides of the plane in the diagram, one side is white and the other is shaded

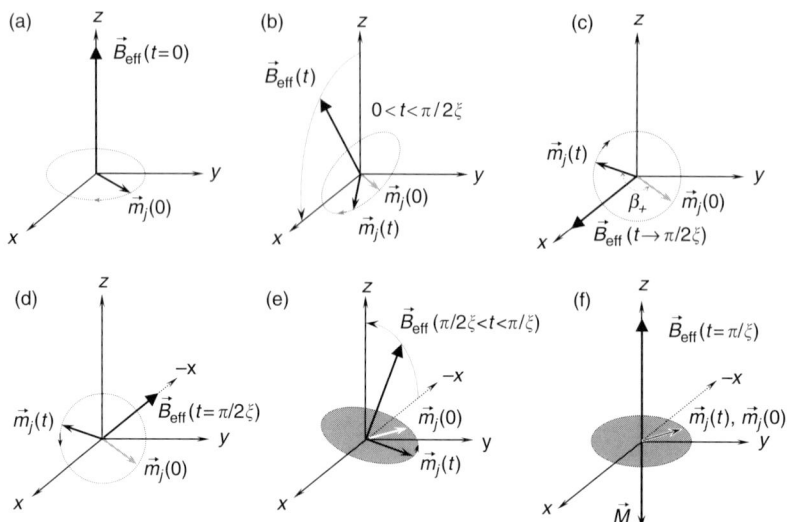

FIGURE 6.13 The trajectory of a transverse magnetization vector $\vec{m}_j$ during the adiabatic refocusing pulse given by Figure 6.10. All trajectories are described in the rotating reference frame. The magnetization $\vec{m}_j$ precesses clockwise about the effective field $\vec{B}_{\text{eff}}$ during the first half of the pulse (a–c). β_+ in (c) represents the phase accumulated by $\vec{m}_j$ halfway through the pulse (Eq. 6.59). The dotted circle denotes the precession plane of $\vec{m}_j$, which is always normal to $\vec{B}_{\text{eff}}$. The initial precession plane in (a) is rotated from the xy plane to the yz plane in (c) at the mid-point of the pulse. The abrupt change in $\vec{B}_{\text{eff}}$ direction at the middle of the pulse (c to d) causes $\vec{m}_j$ to precess counter-clockwise. (e) As $\vec{B}_{\text{eff}}$ returns to the z axis, the precession plane is turned upside down about the y axis. To distinguish the two sides of the precession plane, one side is shown as white (a–d) and the other as gray (e–f). (f) At the end of the pulse, the precession plane is completely flipped by 180° and the phase accumulated during the second half of the pulse cancels β_+. Effectively, $\vec{m}_j$ is flipped by 180° about the y axis. The initial position of $\vec{m}_j$, $\vec{m}_j(0)$, is shown as a reference in all figures. $\vec{m}_j(0)$ is static with respect to the precession plane (i.e., $\beta_+ = \beta_- = 0$ for $\vec{m}_j(0)$) and is rotated by 180° about the y axis when the precession plane is flipped like a pancake.

in Figure 6.13. If the observer who follows the precession plane calculates the phase angle β_- that $\vec{m}_j$ accumulates during the second half of the pulse, the result will be:

$$\beta_- = -\gamma \int_{\pi/2\xi}^{\pi/\xi} |\vec{B}_{\text{eff}}(t)|\, dt \qquad (6.60)$$

where the negative sign accounts for the counter-clockwise precession. Carrying out the integration in Eqs. (6.59) and (6.60) with the aid of Eq. (6.57), we can readily prove that the phase angle accumulated during the first half of the RF pulse is exactly cancelled by the second half of the pulse (i.e., $\beta_+ = -\beta_-$). Because there is no net phase accrual in the process of pancake flipping the precession plane, the net effect is that $\vec{m}_j$ is rotated by $180°$ about the y axis (Figure 6.13). In other words, the final position of $\vec{m}_j$ after the pancake flipping is the same as an isochromat vector that has not precessed in the precession plane (Figure 6.13f). Note that the positions of $\vec{m}_j(0)$ are different in Figures 6.13a and 6.13f due to the pancake flipping. Because the magnetization vector $\vec{m}_j$ is arbitrarily chosen, the effect of the RF pulse on $\vec{m}_j$ can be generalized to any transverse magnetization vectors. Therefore, at the end of the RF pulse, all the isochromat vectors in the transverse plane are flipped by $180°$ about the y axis. After a certain time τ, the flipped vectors will refocus and produce an echo signal. Because spins with different local B_1-field amplitudes experience the same change in the direction of the effective magnetic field, they will experience the same pancake flipping as $\vec{m}_j$, irrespective of their local B_1-field amplitude. The interested reader can perform a more detailed analysis using the approach given in Sections 6.1 and 6.2.

Off-Resonance Effects So far, we have only considered the on-resonance spins. For off-resonance spins, the actual frequency modulation function differs from Eq. (6.55) by an offset κ (in radians per second):

$$\omega_{\mathrm{rf}}(t) = \omega - \gamma B_z |\cos \xi t| - \kappa \qquad (0 \le \xi t \le \pi) \qquad (6.61)$$

The z component of the effective field (i.e., Eq. 6.56) is accordingly adjusted to:

$$\frac{\Delta \omega}{\gamma} \equiv \frac{\omega - \omega_{\mathrm{rf}}}{\gamma} = B_z |\cos \xi t| + \frac{\kappa}{\gamma} \qquad (6.62)$$

In the presence of off-resonance effects, it becomes increasingly challenging to satisfy the adiabatic condition. For example, if $\kappa < 0$, the z component of the effective field is reduced, assuming $B_z > 0$. When the x component of the effective field is also small (e.g., at the beginning of the pulse), the effective field amplitude decreases, leading to a possible violation of the adiabatic condition (see Eq. 6.8). This phenomenon does not occur when κ is positive. Thus, the adiabatic pulse discussed in this section has an asymmetric response to the off-resonance effect.

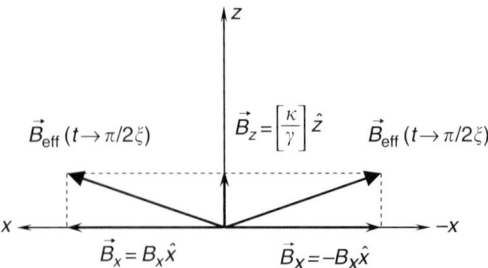

FIGURE 6.14 The off-resonance effect (κ) on the effective magnetic field $\vec{B}_{\text{eff}}$. Due to the off-resonance term, $\vec{B}_{\text{eff}}$ does not align with the x axis at the middle of the pulse. After the B_1 field ($\vec{B}_x$) is switched from the positive x axis to the negative x axis, $\vec{B}_{\text{eff}}$ is not flipped by 180°.

Off-resonance effects can also reduce the magnetization amplitude in adiabatic refocusing, resulting in a decreased echo amplitude. At the mid-point of the pulse, off-resonance effects prevent the effective field from being aligned along the x axis because of the nonvanishing term κ/γ (Figure 6.14). Therefore, the transverse magnetization cannot be completely rotated to the yz plane. Immediately after the B_1 field is inverted, the effective field will deviate from the negative x axis, also due to κ/γ (Figure 6.14). In that case, the effective field is no longer perpendicular to the spin precession plane, resulting in the diminishing intensity of the refocused magnetization and an additional longitudinal magnetization at the end of the pulse. Similarly, the longitudinal magnetization is not exactly anti-parallel to $\vec{B}_{\text{eff}}$ after the B_1-field polarity switch, leading to reduced intensity in the inverted signal, as well as an additional transverse magnetization. In MRI pulse sequences, this transverse magnetization can carry a different phase than the nominal transverse magnetization, causing signal dephasing and artifacts.

6.3.2 DESIGN PRINCIPLES OF ADIABATIC REFOCUSING PULSES

Adiabatic refocusing pulses can be designed in many different ways, depending on how the direction of the effective field is manipulated to achieve plane rotation. The pulse shown in Figure 6.10 illustrates one design strategy in which the effective field starts at the z axis, rotates to the x axis, inverts to the negative x axis, and ends at the z axis. This pulse is named BIREF-1 (Ugurbil, Garwood, Rath, and Bendall 1988).

The BIREF-2a pulse (Ugurbil, Garwood, Rath, and Bendall 1988), described by Eqs. (6.63) and (6.64), swaps the amplitude and frequency modulation functions of the BIREF-1 pulse. In this pulse, the effective magnetic field is initially along the x axis (in the rotating reference frame), rotates to the positive z axis between $t = 0$ and $t = \pi/(2\xi)$, then switches to the negative z axis, and finally returns to the x axis.

$$A(t) = B_x|\cos \xi t| \quad (0 \le \xi t \le \pi) \tag{6.63}$$

$$\omega_{\rm rf}(t) = \begin{cases} \omega - \gamma B_z \sin \xi t & (0 \le \xi t < \pi/2) \\ \omega + \gamma B_z \sin \xi t & (\pi/2 \le \xi t \le \pi) \end{cases} \tag{6.64}$$

Using similar analyses given in the previous subsection for the BIREF-1 pulse, it can be shown that the BIREF-2a pulse inverts the x magnetization and flips the yz plane by $180°$ about the y axis. Although the BIREF-2a pulse can achieve similar performance to the BIREF-1 pulse for on-resonance spins, its performance for off-resonance spins is much worse (Ugurbil, Garwood, Rath, and Bendall 1988). This is primarily because the x component of the initial transverse magnetization undergoes an inversion, whereas the y component experiences a plane rotation. In the presence of off-resonance effects, this difference leads to unequal phase angles between β_+ and $-\beta_-$ (see Eqs. 6.59 and 6.60). Consequently, the magnetization cannot be completely refocused. To address this problem, an additional pulse can be added immediately after the BIREF-2a pulse. Here is an example of such a concatenated pulse, referred to as BIREF-2b pulse (Ugurbil, Garwood, Rath, and Bendall 1988):

$$A(t) = \begin{cases} B_x|\cos \xi t| & (0 \le \xi t \le \pi) \\ -B_x \cos \xi t & (\pi \le \xi t \le 2\pi) \end{cases} \tag{6.65}$$

$$\omega_{\rm rf}(t) = \begin{cases} \omega - \gamma B_z \sin \xi t & (0 \le \xi t < \pi/2) \\ \omega + \gamma B_z \sin \xi t & (\pi/2 \le \xi t < 3\pi/2) \\ \omega - \gamma B_z \sin \xi t & (3\pi/2 \le \xi t \le 2\pi) \end{cases} \tag{6.66}$$

The second half of the BIREF-2b pulse ($\pi \le \xi t \le 2\pi$) helps to refocus the phase dispersion between β_+ and $-\beta_-$. Obviously, the width of the BIREF-2b pulse is twice that of BIREF-1 and BIREF-2a pulses.

The BIREF-3 pulse consists of two parts. The first part is a regular adiabatic inversion pulse (e.g., the hyperbolic pulse described in Section 6.2), and the second part is used to refocus the phase dispersion introduced by the inversion pulse among the transverse magnetization vectors. As the adiabatic inversion pulse inverts the longitudinal magnetization, the transverse plane is also flipped upside down at the end of the pulse. During this process, the phase accumulated by a transverse magnetization vector is:

$$\beta = \gamma \int_0^T |\vec{B}_{\text{eff}}(t)| \, dt \qquad (6.67)$$

where T is the pulse width of the adiabatic inversion pulse. Because the effective field $|\vec{B}_{\text{eff}}|$ is strong and the pulse width T is long (e.g., 10 ms), the phase β in Eq. (6.67) can be quite large. This phase dispersion among the transverse magnetization vectors can cause considerable signal loss. The second part of the BIREF-3 pulse essentially rewinds the phase to restore the transverse magnetization vectors to their proper positions so that they can be refocused to form an echo at a later time. Here is an example of the modulation functions that can be used in the second part of a BIREF-3 pulse (Ugurbil, Garwood, Rath, and Bendall 1988):

$$A(t) = B_x |\sin \xi t| \quad (\pi \le \xi t \le 2\pi) \qquad (6.68)$$

$$\omega_{\text{rf}}(t) = \omega - \gamma B_z |\cos \xi t| \quad (\pi \le \xi t \le 2\pi) \qquad (6.69)$$

Following an adiabatic inversion pulse (i.e., the first part of the BIREF-3 pulse when $0 \le \xi t < \pi$), the effective field $\vec{B}_{\text{eff}}$ is changed from the negative to the positive z axis. (Note that the z component of $\vec{B}_{\text{eff}}$ is defined as $(\omega - \omega_{\text{rf}})/\gamma$, as shown in Eq. 6.62.) The effective field then moves from the z axis to the x axis $(\pi < \xi t \le 3\pi/2)$ and returns to the z axis $(3\pi/2 < \xi t \le 2\pi)$. During the process, the inverted magnetization remains anti-parallel to $\vec{B}_{\text{eff}}$ and is returned to the negative z axis at the end of the pulse. Because of the polarity change of $\vec{B}_{\text{eff}}$ at $\xi t = \pi$, the transverse magnetization will accumulate a negative phase with respect to the phase in Eq. (6.67). If $|\vec{B}_{\text{eff}}|$ and (or) the pulse width is adjusted during the second half of the BIREF-3 pulse, the newly accumulated phase can cancel the phase accumulated during the first half of the BIREF-3 pulse.

In the presence of resonance offset κ, the performance of the adiabatic refocusing pulse can be analyzed by including κ in the frequency modulation function as shown in Eq. (6.61) or (6.62), followed by a simulation using Bloch equations to calculate the refocused magnetization as a function of κ. When $|\kappa|$ approaches the amplitude of frequency modulation (i.e., γB_z), the pulses typically can no longer refocus the magnetization. This analysis also is used to characterize the frequency selectivity of an adiabatic refocusing pulse.

In addition to the aforementioned pulses, other forms of adiabatic refocusing pulses are also possible. For example, a variation of the BIREF-1 pulse uses a constant amplitude modulation and a tangent frequency modulation

(Ugurbil, Garwood, Rath, and Bendall 1988). This pulse can alleviate certain problems with off-resonance effects.

6.3.3 PRACTICAL CONSIDERATIONS

Spatial Selectivity   Adiabatic refocusing pulses can be either spatially selective or nonselective. The spatial selectivity is largely determined by the off-resonance behavior of the adiabatic pulse in the presence of a slice-selection gradient. Of the adiabatic refocusing pulses discussed in the previous subsection, BIREF-2b is suitable for slice selection due to its symmetric response to spins above and below resonance (i.e., positive and negative κ in Eq. 6.62). In contrast, BIREF-3 is not appropriate for slice selection because of dephasing introduced by the off-resonance effect across the slice.

Modulation Functions   So far, we have employed simple analytical functions, such as sine and cosine, to illustrate the principles of adiabatic refocusing pulses. These modulation functions, however, are not optimal in terms of satisfying the adiabatic condition throughout the pulse. Various optimization techniques have been developed to numerically or analytically improve the modulation functions to best satisfy the adiabatic condition (Ugurbil, Garwood, and Rath 1988; Shen and Saunders 1992; Skinner and Robitaille 1992). The optimized modulation functions share the same boundary conditions (e.g., the effective field must be aligned with a certain axis at the beginning, mid-point, and end of a pulse) as their nonoptimized counterpart. They provide, however, a broader tolerance for B_1-field variation, decreased sensitivity to off-resonance effects, shorter pulse width, or less SAR. An in-depth discussion of the optimization techniques is beyond the scope of this section. The interested reader is referred to Ugurbil, Garwood, and Rath (1988); Shen and Saunders (1992); and Skinner and Robitaille (1992) for more details.

Parameter Selection   Once a type of adiabatic refocusing pulse has been selected and its modulation functions chosen, three parameters must be determined in order to implement the pulse. These parameters are the modulation frequency ξ, the minimum amplitude of the B_1-field modulation B_x, and the amplitude of the frequency modulation γB_z. The modulating frequency ξ is directly related to the total pulse width T. For BIREF-1 and BIREF-2a pulses $\xi = \pi/T$, whereas for BIREF-2b and BIREF-3 pulses $\xi = 2\pi/T$. A large ξ value is desirable in order to minimize the off-resonance, flow, and relaxation effects during the RF pulse. However, an excessively large ξ can violate the adiabatic condition. Thus, ξ is typically chosen as the maximum value that satisfies the adiabatic condition. The other two parameters, B_x and γB_z, can be determined using the method described in Section 6.1 on adiabatic excitation pulse design, except that the parameters p and q (defined by Eqs. 6.15 and 6.16) are selected based on the refocusing efficiency (i.e., the amplitude of the refocused magnetization as a percentage of the initial transverse magnetization) instead of the excitation efficiency. Once a pulse has been designed, its frequency selectivity and performance under off-resonant conditions can be evaluated using the Bloch equations with the inclusion of the frequency offset κ.

6.3.4 APPLICATIONS

Although adiabatic refocusing pulses can perform slice selection in conjunction with a gradient, they are rarely used for this purpose because of their sensitivity to off-resonance and very long pulse widths (e.g., >10 ms). Spatially nonselective adiabatic refocusing pulses can be used for applications in which a surface coil is employed as an RF transmitter. Examples include localized *in vivo* spectroscopy and imaging application with small coils. Adiabatic refocusing pulses are also useful in 3D volume imaging when there is considerable B_1-field nonuniformity in the transmitting RF coil. A drawback of adiabatic refocusing pulses is substantially increased SAR compared to their nonadiabatic counterparts. Because of this, adiabatic refocusing pulses are often limited to small local coils.

SELECTED REFERENCES

Shen, J. F., and Saunders, J. K. 1992. Analytical optimization of modulation functions for adiabatic pulses. *J. Magn. Reson.* 99: 258–267.

Skinner, T. E., and Robitaille, P.-M. L. 1992. General solutions for tailored modulation profiles in adiabatic excitation. *J. Magn. Reson.* 98: 14–23.

Ugurbil, K., Garwood, M., and Rath, A. R. 1988. Optimization of modulation functions to improve insensitivity of adiabatic pulses to variations in B_1 magnitude. *J. Magn. Reson.* 80: 448–469.

Ugurbil, K., Garwood, M., Rath, A. R., and Bendall, M. R. 1988. Amplitude- and frequency/phase-modulated refocusing pulses that induce plane rotations even in the presence of inhomogeneous B_1-fields. *J. Magn. Reson.* 78: 472–496.

RELATED SECTIONS

GRADIENTS

Introduction

Linear magnetic field gradients play a central role in MR imaging. Their primary function is to encode spatial information into NMR signals so that it later can be recovered during the reconstruction process to form an image. Magnetic field gradients are also used to sensitize the image contrast to coherent or incoherent motion. In addition, gradients can be employed to selectively choose or edit NMR signals and to minimize image artifacts.

Broadly interpreted, the term *linear magnetic field gradient* refers to any linear, spatial variation of the magnetic field. In MRI, however, we generally interpret the term more narrowly to mean only the spatial variation of the z component of the magnetic field, where the z direction corresponds to the main magnetic field B_0. We do this because B_0 is so large that magnetic field components perpendicular to it can usually be neglected. More discussion of and exceptions to this simplification are provided in Section 10.1.

The z component of the magnetic field (B_z) can vary in any of the three orthogonal directions. Mathematically, we can express a gradient vector $\vec{G}$ using:

$$\vec{G} = \frac{\partial B_z}{\partial x}\hat{x} + \frac{\partial B_z}{\partial y}\hat{y} + \frac{\partial B_z}{\partial z}\hat{z} \equiv G_x\hat{x} + G_y\hat{y} + G_z\hat{z}$$

where $\hat{x}$, $\hat{y}$, and $\hat{z}$ are the unit vectors of the Cartesian coordinate system and G_x, G_y, and G_z are the three orthogonal components of $\vec{G}$. Note that, regardless of the direction of the gradient, it produces a magnetic field in the z direction given by $\vec{B} = \left(B_0 + G_x x + G_y y + G_z z\right)\hat{z}$.

The three gradients G_x, G_y, and G_z are generated by three separate gradient coils. The coils are characterized by specific values of inductance and resistance. Each coil is driven by its own gradient amplifier, or driver. To an excellent approximation, the circuits of the three gradient drivers are independent of one another. When a gradient driver is producing its maximal current, its associated coil produces the maximal gradient strength, which we denote by h. Because the maximal current can be of either polarity, the available gradient amplitude ranges from $+h$ to $-h$. (Sometimes a small fraction of the gradient strength is held in reserve for eddy-current compensation; see Section 10.3.) Gradient amplitudes are typically measured in milliteslas per meter (mT/m), although sometimes the older unit gauss per centimeter (G/cm) is used. The conversion factor is 10 mT/m = 1 G/cm.

When a gradient driver produces its maximal voltage, the amplitude of the associated gradient field undergoes its largest rate of change. This rate of change is called the maximum gradient slew rate S_R and is measured in teslas per meter per second (T/m/s). Typical values for whole-body gradient systems are $h \sim 10$–50 mT/m, and $S_R \sim 10$–200 T/m/s. It is interesting to note that the product hS_R is proportional to the product of the gradient driver's peak voltage and current, or maximal power. That product therefore is a measure of the gradient system's performance.

Most gradient systems increase the gradient amplitude linearly with respect to time (i.e., linear slewing, which produces linear ramps), although other ramp shapes such as sinusoids have been used as well, particularly with resonant gradient systems. With linear ramps, the *rise time*, or duration of a ramp from zero amplitude to $+h$ (or $-h$), is given by $r = h/S_R$.

Sometimes the full performance of a gradient system cannot be used, due to physiological or hardware constraints. For example, in order to avoid possible peripheral nerve stimulation, pain, and other biological effects during gradient slewing, a limit on the maximal rate of change of the magnetic field (i.e., dB/dt) must be obeyed. This is because, according to Maxwell's equations, a time-varying magnetic field generates an electric field. Many regulatory agencies, such as the U.S. Food and Drug Administration, impose limits on the maximal amount of dB/dt that can be produced by clinical MRI scanners. An empirical model known as the Reilly curve (Reilly 1989) is sometimes used to predict whether peripheral nerve stimulation will result from a given pulse sequence. Note that because peripheral nerve stimulation and other biological effects are related to dB/dt (rather than dG/dt), a shorter gradient coil generally allows higher slew rates while still satisfying the regulatory limits.

A second constraint on gradient performance is known as the *gradient duty cycle*. The gradient duty cycle has been defined a variety of ways, but for simplicity we consider a square wave whose amplitude continually oscillates from $+h$ to $-h$ to have a duty cycle of 100% (i.e., it is maximally active all the time). Gradient amplifiers and gradient coils are subject to thermal heating, and generally each has its own duty cycle limit. Exceeding the duty cycle limit can temporarily shut down (or damage) the gradient amplifier, damage the gradient cables or coil, or cause unacceptable patient heating. With modern clinical MRI systems, however, gradient duty cycle limits have become much less severe (or have been eliminated) because many gradient coils and amplifiers are liquid-cooled and because of advances in amplifier technology.

We use the nomenclature *gradient lobe* to refer to a single gradient pulse shape that starts and ends with zero amplitude. Examples of lobes include a triangle, trapezoid, and half-sine. We use the nomenclature *gradient waveform* to refer to all (or at least multiple) gradient lobes on a single axis within a pulse sequence. For example, we refer to the slice-selection and slice-rephasing trapezoids as separate lobes, but we refer to all the lobes on the slice-selection axis collectively as the slice-selection gradient waveform. This nomenclature should be thought of as a general guideline rather than a rigorous definition. A spiral readout gradient, for example, does not fit easily into this classification.

Part III of the book contains four chapters. Chapter 7 describes several common strategies in the design of gradient lobes and waveforms. This chapter contains sections on simple gradient lobe shapes (Section 7.1) and on how multiple lobes can sometimes be combined on the same axis with a technique called bridging (Section 7.2). The bridged gradient lobes can perform the same gradient function, but in a more time-efficient fashion. The distribution of gradient waveforms among multiple axes to acquire oblique imaging planes is discussed in Section 7.3.

Chapter 8 includes the three basic functions that the gradients perform that achieve spatial localization: frequency encoding (Section 8.1), phase encoding (Section 8.2), and slice selection (Section 8.3). Each of these functions often requires more than one gradient lobe. For example, frequency encoding typically requires a prephasing (also known as a dephasing) lobe and a readout lobe. These three gradient functions are fundamental to MR imaging, and the results of these three sections are used throughout the book.

Chapter 9 discusses the gradients used to sensitize the image to motion. Diffusion-weighting gradients are discussed in Section 9.1. They are used to encode information about microscopic self-diffusion in tissues into the *magnitude* of the MR signal. Flow-encoding gradients (Section 9.2) are considered separately because they encode information about macroscopic flow and motion into the *phase* of the MR signal. These two gradient waveforms are used in the later sections on diffusion imaging (Section 17.2) and phase-contrast imaging (Section 15.2), respectively.

Chapter 10 covers a variety of gradient waveforms used to correct or prevent image artifacts. The correction gradients that compensate for concomitant magnetic field are described in Section 10.1. The concomitant field is unavoidable in MR imaging because it is a consequence of Maxwell's equations on electricity and magnetism. Eddy-current compensation (Section 10.3) addresses a very common cause of gradient waveform infidelity. Gradient moment nulling (Section 10.4), which is sometimes known as flow compensation, is used to reduce ghosting and signal loss in regions of flow and bulk motion. Crusher (Section 10.2), spoiler (Section 10.5), and twister gradients (Section 10.6) are also described. All three use gradient lobes to dephase unwanted signals. Sometimes the terms *crusher, spoiler*, and *killer* are used interchangeably in the literature; in this book we distinguish between crushers and spoilers (or killers). Crusher gradients are used to eliminate the FIDs that result from nonideal refocusing pulses or to select certain magnetization coherence pathways. Spoiler or killer gradients, on the other hand, are used to eliminate residual signal after a readout or after a spatial or chemical saturation pulse by making the average transverse magnetization over a voxel nearly zero. The correction gradients described in Chapter 10 are frequently employed in the pulse sequences discussed in Part V of the book.

SELECTED REFERENCE

Reilly, J. P. 1989. Peripheral nerve stimulation by induced electric currents: Exposure to time-varying magnetic fields. *Med. Biol. Eng. Comput.* 27: 101–110.

7

GRADIENT LOBE SHAPES

7.1 Simple Gradient Lobes

MR pulse sequences contain gradient waveforms such as frequency-encoding, phase-encoding, and slice-selection. Each waveform can be further decomposed into individual gradient pulses or lobes (Harvey and Mansfield 1994). This section describes three commonly used simple lobe shapes: trapezoidal, triangular, and sinusoidal.

7.1.1 TRAPEZOIDAL AND TRIANGULAR LOBES

The area A (in milliseconds-milliteslas per meter) of a gradient lobe when plotted versus time is typically determined by the prescribed imaging parameters (e.g., field of view, matrix size, and bandwidth). Often only the area, not the specific shape of the gradient lobe, is determined by imaging constraints. Under these conditions, the shortest duration gradient lobe is normally used in order to minimize timing parameters such as TE and TR. For the gradient systems that use linear ramps, the simple lobe shapes with the shortest duration will be triangular or trapezoidal (Figure 7.1), depending on the gradient area. If the area satisfies the condition:

$$0 < |A| < hr = \frac{h^2}{S_R} \tag{7.1}$$

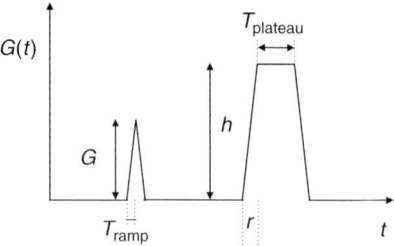

FIGURE 7.1 When the amplitude $G(t)$ is plotted versus time t, two common gradient lobe shapes are a triangle (left) and a trapezoid (right). The amplitude of the plateau of the trapezoid is h, which is equal to the maximal available gradient amplitude. The ramp time of the trapezoid is r, which is equal to h divided by the slew rate. The plateau duration $T_{plateau}$ can be calculated using Eq. (7.7). The triangle is the most time-efficient lobe when the desired gradient area is less than hr, otherwise the trapezoid is the preferred shape. Note that the slopes of the ramps of both the trapezoidal and triangular lobes are the same and have an absolute value equal to the slew rate S_R.

then the most time-efficient shape is a triangle, with ramp duration:

$$T_{ramp} = \sqrt{\frac{|A|r}{h}} = \sqrt{\frac{|A|}{S_R}} \tag{7.2}$$

and peak gradient amplitude:

$$G = \frac{A}{T_{ramp}} = \pm\sqrt{\frac{|A|h}{r}} = \pm\sqrt{|A|S_R} \tag{7.3}$$

(In principle the duration of the plateau or flat top of a triangular lobe is 0. Sometimes a duration of a few microseconds is used to reduce the discontinuity of the slope.)

If, instead, the gradient area exceeds the threshold:

$$|A| \geq hr = \frac{h^2}{S_R} \tag{7.4}$$

then the most time-efficient shape is a trapezoid. In that case, the gradient amplitude is maximized:

$$G = \pm h \tag{7.5}$$

and the ramp time (for both the ascending and descending ramps) is given by:

$$T_{ramp} = r = \frac{h}{S_R} \tag{7.6}$$

The duration of plateau of the trapezoidal lobe is given by:

$$T_{\text{plateau}} = \frac{|A|}{h} - r \qquad (7.7)$$

so the duration of the entire trapezoidal lobe is:

$$T = T_{\text{plateau}} + 2r = \frac{|A|}{h} + r \qquad (7.8)$$

Note that the ramps of the triangular and trapezoidal lobes both have the maximal slope. From Eqs. (7.2) and (7.3):

$$\frac{|G|}{T_{\text{ramp}}} = \frac{h}{r} = S_R \qquad (7.9)$$

We note that in the case of adjacent lobes of the same polarity, certain simple triangle and trapezoidal lobes can be combined, or *bridged*, together to further improve the time efficiency. A further discussion can be found in Section 7.2.

7.1.2 SINUSOIDAL LOBES

Occasionally, a sinusoidal gradient lobe shape is used. A *half-sine* lobe that starts at $t = t_0$ is given by:

$$G(t) = \begin{cases} G_0 \sin\left(\frac{\pi(t-t_0)}{T}\right) & t_0 \leq t \leq t_0 + T \\ 0 & \text{otherwise} \end{cases} \qquad (7.10)$$

where the peak amplitude is $G_0 \leq h$ and the duration is T (Figure 7.2). The sinusoidal lobe in Eq. (7.10) has an area given by the integral of Eq. (7.10):

$$A = \frac{2G_0 T}{\pi} \qquad (7.11)$$

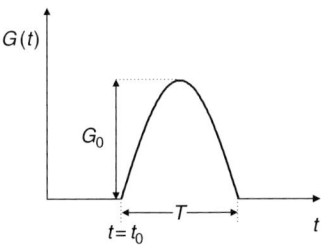

FIGURE 7.2 A sinusoidal gradient lobe.

Equation (7.11) states that for a fixed value of the gradient area A, a higher value of $|G_0|$ provides a shorter lobe duration T, as we would expect. Sometimes, however, we cannot simply set the value of G_0 in Eq. (7.11) equal to $\pm h$ because of slew-rate constraints. The maximal slew rate of the sinusoidal gradient lobe occurs at its beginning and end, and it is given by the derivative of Eq. (7.10):

$$\left| \frac{dG(t)}{dt} \right|_{\max} = \frac{\pi |G_0|}{T} \tag{7.12}$$

or equivalently:

$$\frac{\pi |G_0|}{T} \leq S_R \tag{7.13}$$

Combining Eqs. (7.11) and (7.13), we can conclude that the gradient amplitude for a sinusoidal lobe that satisfies both the gradient amplitude and slew-rate constraints is:

$$G_0 = \begin{cases} \pm h & |A| \geq \frac{2h^2}{S_R} \\ \pm \sqrt{\frac{S_R |A|}{2}} & |A| \leq \frac{2h^2}{S_R} \end{cases} \tag{7.14}$$

Substituting Eq. (7.14) into Eq. (7.11), we find the lobe duration:

$$T = \begin{cases} \frac{\pi |A|}{2h} & |A| \geq \frac{2h^2}{S_R} \\ \pi \sqrt{\frac{|A|}{2S_R}} & |A| \leq \frac{2h^2}{S_R} \end{cases} \tag{7.15}$$

Comparing Eqs. (7.8) and Eq. (7.15), and recalling that $\pi/2 \approx 1.57$, we can see why trapezoidal lobes carry more gradient area per unit time than sinusoidal lobes when both reach the maximal amplitude h while abiding by the slew-rate limit.

SELECTED REFERENCE

Harvey, P. R., and Mansfield, P. 1994. Resonant trapezoidal gradient generation for use in echo-planar imaging. *Magn. Reson. Imaging* 12: 93–100.

RELATED SECTION

Section 7.2 Bridged Gradient Lobes

7.2 Bridged Gradient Lobes

When a gradient hardware system generates linear ramps, triangles or trapezoids (Section 7.1) are typically the most time-efficient lobe shapes to generate a predetermined gradient area. An exception to this rule occurs when a gradient lobe with specified amplitude is adjacent to another lobe of the same polarity. This situation often arises for refocusing pulse slice-selection gradients and crusher gradient pairs (Section 10.2) and for readout gradients and end-of-sequence spoilers (Section 10.5). In this case, the most time-efficient shape is a compound lobe called a *bridged* gradient lobe. The important property is that not only the area but also the amplitude of at least one of the gradient lobes is determined by other imaging constraints such as slice thickness.

Figure 7.3 shows two adjacent trapezoidal lobes of the same polarity. Note that the descending ramp from the first lobe returns to 0 amplitude before the ascending ramp of the second lobe begins. Clearly, the duration of the bridge r_b depicted in Figure 7.4 offers a time savings over the duration of the two separate ramps, $r_1 + r_2$. The bridged lobe also may produce less acoustic

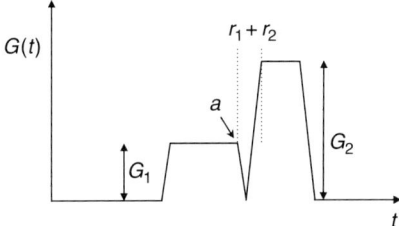

FIGURE 7.3 Two adjacent trapezoidal gradient lobes with the same polarity (unbridged). The amplitude G_1 of the first lobe is fixed by imaging constraints, such as slice thickness. The gradient area to the right of point a is normally preserved before and after bridging.

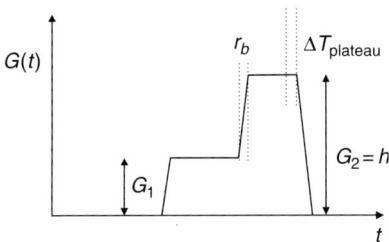

FIGURE 7.4 The two adjacent trapezoidal gradient lobes from Figure 7.3 are bridged to form a trapezoid-like bridged lobe. A bridge replaces the descending ramp of the first lobe and the ascending ramp of the second lobe in Figure 7.3. This results in a more compact gradient waveform, even if the plateau duration of the second lobe must be increased to preserve gradient area. Here the plateau length is increased by $\Delta T_{\text{plateau}}$. The bridged gradient waveform can be used for slice-selection gradients and crushers.

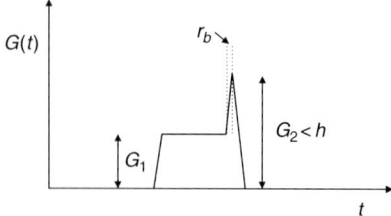

FIGURE 7.5 Under some circumstances, the area of the bridged lobe is insufficient for its amplitude to reach the maximal value h. In that case, a triangle-like bridged lobe results.

noise, reduced eddy currents, and less gradient heating than the two separate lobes.

In analogy to the simple gradient lobes described in Section 7.1, bridged lobes can be divided into trapezoid-like (Figure 7.4) and triangle-like cases. Figure 7.5 shows the case of a triangle-like bridged lobe. In this case, the area to the right of the plateau is insufficient for G_2 to reach the maximum gradient value h. We see next that there is also a third, intermediate case in which one of the unbridged gradient lobes (e.g., the second lobe) is triangular, but the bridged waveform becomes two trapezoid-like lobes as shown in Figure 7.4.

Naturally, bridged lobes are equally useful when occurring to the left or to the right (as depicted in Figures 7.4 and 7.5) of the plateau gradient. The mathematics presented next applies equally well to both cases.

7.2.1 MATHEMATICAL DESCRIPTION

Consider two adjacent gradient lobes of the same polarity, as shown in Figure 7.3. Without loss of generality assume that:

$$G_2 > G_1 > 0 \qquad (7.16)$$

If the slew rate is S_R, then the combined duration of the adjacent descending and ascending ramps is:

$$r_1 + r_2 = \frac{G_1 + G_2}{S_R} \qquad (7.17)$$

A single bridge, as shown in Figure 7.4, can replace these two ramps. The duration of the bridge is:

$$r_b = \frac{G_2 - G_1}{S_R} \qquad (7.18)$$

To calculate the amplitude of the bridged lobe and the net time savings gained by bridging, it is necessary to consider three separate cases. In all three cases, we assume that (1) the maximum slew rate is always used for the gradient ramps and (2) the gradient area to the right of the first plateau in Figure 7.3 (i.e., from point a to the end of the gradient waveform) is preserved before and after bridging.

Case 1: Rightmost Lobe Is Trapezoidal, Whether or Not It Is Bridged
If the total area A to the right of the first plateau in Figure 7.3 (from point a to the right) is sufficiently high, the rightmost lobe will be trapezoidal whether or not bridging is used. We can calculate the threshold for A by adding the area under a slew-rate-limited descending ramp from G_1 to 0 plus the area of a triangle whose base is $2r$ and whose height is h. (This triangle can be considered a trapezoid with zero plateau duration, i.e., the limiting case.) Recalling that $r = h/S_R$ is the ramp time from 0 to the maximal amplitude h, the threshold area for this case is:

$$A > hr \left(1 + \frac{G_1^2}{2h^2}\right) = \frac{h^2}{S_R}\left(1 + \frac{G_1^2}{2h^2}\right) \qquad (7.19)$$

For this case, the most efficient bridged lobe has its own plateau (Figure 7.4), so it is trapezoid-like. Also in this case, the amplitude of the second plateau is equal to the maximum gradient amplitude:

$$G_2 = h \qquad (7.20)$$

If there are no constraints other than the gradient amplitudes, the direct time savings by using the bridge (from Eqs. 7.17 and 7.18) is then:

$$\Delta T_{\text{ramp}} = r_1 + r_2 - r_b = \frac{2G_1}{S_R} \qquad (7.21)$$

Usually, the gradient lobe to the right of the plateau of the first lobe performs a function such as crushing and its area has a specified value. In that case, the plateau duration of the bridged lobe should be extended to compensate for the reduced gradient area of the bridged ramp. At the slew-rate limit, the total area of the two separate ramps is:

$$A_{R,\text{tot}} = \frac{1}{2S_R}(G_1^2 + G_2^2) \qquad (7.22)$$

whereas the area of the bridge is:

$$A_b = \left(\frac{G_1 + G_2}{2}\right)\left(\frac{G_2 - G_1}{S_R}\right) = \frac{1}{2S_R}(G_2^2 - G_1^2) \qquad (7.23)$$

Therefore, to maintain net area, the duration of the plateau of the second lobe should be increased by:

$$\Delta T_{\text{plateau}} = \frac{\frac{1}{2S_R}(G_1^2 + G_2^2) - \frac{1}{2S_R}(G_2^2 - G_1^2)}{G_2} = \frac{G_1^2}{S_R G_2} = \frac{G_1^2}{S_R h} \tag{7.24}$$

Combining Eqs. (7.21) and (7.24), the net time savings from using the bridge is:

$$\Delta T_{\text{net}} = \Delta T_{\text{ramp}} - \Delta T_{\text{plateau}} = \frac{G_1}{S_R}\left(2 - \frac{G_1}{h}\right) > 0 \qquad G_2 = h > G_1 > 0 \tag{7.25}$$

Case 2: Rightmost Lobe Is Triangular When Unbridged, but Becomes Trapezoidal When Bridged

The upper limit on the area A for this case is the same as the lower limit for case 1 (Eq. 7.19). The lower limit can be calculated by adding the area under a slew-rate-limited ramp from G_1 to h to the area under a descending ramp from h to 0. Thus, the second case arises when the area A to the right of the first plateau in Figure 7.3 (from point a to the right) is in the range:

$$\frac{h^2}{S_R}\left(1 - \frac{G_1^2}{2h^2}\right) \le A \le \frac{h^2}{S_R}\left(1 + \frac{G_1^2}{2h^2}\right) \tag{7.26}$$

Under this condition, the bridged lobe is trapezoid-like so, as in case 1:

$$G_2 = h \tag{7.27}$$

When unbridged, however, the rightmost lobe has an area less than $hr = h^2/S_R$, so according to Section 7.1 it is triangular. With some straightforward algebraic manipulation, it can be shown that the net time saved by bridging the two lobes, while keeping the area to the right of the plateau fixed, is given by:

$$\Delta T_{\text{net}} = \frac{2}{S_R}\sqrt{A S_R - \frac{G_1^2}{2} - \frac{A}{h} + \frac{2G_1}{S_R} - \frac{G_1^2}{2h S_R} - \frac{h}{S_R}} \tag{7.28}$$

Case 3: Rightmost Lobe Is Triangular, Whether or Not It Is Bridged

The upper limit on the area A for this case is the same as the lower limit in case 2. The lower limit for this case is the minimal possible area, that is, the area under a slew-rate-limited descending ramp from G_1 to 0. Thus, if the area to the right of the first plateau in Figure 7.3 (from point a to the right) is in the range:

$$\frac{G_1^2}{2S_R} < A < hr\left(1 - \frac{G_1^2}{2h^2}\right) = \frac{h^2}{S_R}\left(1 - \frac{G_1^2}{2h^2}\right) \tag{7.29}$$

then the bridged lobe will be triangle-like (Figure 7.5). In this case, the amplitude of the bridged lobe is related to the area to the right of the plateau by the relationship:

$$G_2 = \sqrt{AS_R + \frac{G_1^2}{2}} \qquad (7.30)$$

Following a procedure analogous to the derivation of Eq. (7.25), it can be shown that, if the area to the right of the plateau is maintained, the net time savings is given by:

$$\Delta T_{net} = \frac{2}{S_R}\left(\sqrt{G_2^2 - G_1^2} - (G_2 - G_1)\right) > 0 \qquad h > G_2 > G_1 > 0 \qquad (7.31)$$

Sometimes it is more convenient to recast Eq. (7.31) into the equivalent form:

$$\Delta T_{net} = \frac{2}{S_R}\left(\sqrt{AS_R - \frac{G_1^2}{2}} - \sqrt{AS_R + \frac{G_1^2}{2}} + G_1\right) \qquad (7.32)$$

Finally, we mention that there are cases when the overriding design consideration is not to make the most time-efficient waveform but rather some other factor such as the reduction of errors from the concomitant (i.e., Maxwell) field. In that case, a trapezoidal bridged lobe with a derated amplitude:

$$G_2 < h \qquad (7.33)$$

might be optimal. An example of this type of application is described in (Zhou et al. 1998).

Example 7.1 A gradient system has maximal slew rate of $S_R = 95\,\text{T/m/s}$ and a maximal amplitude of $h = 30\,\text{mT/m}$. A crusher with total gradient area of $A = 50\,\text{ms} \cdot \text{mT/m}$ is desired to the right of a slice-selection plateau, which has amplitude of $G_1 = 15.0\,\text{mT/m}$. If the lobes are bridged, what is the duration of the bridge ramp and how much time is saved compared to using two separate ramps?

Answer First we find that the desired area to the right of the plateau, 50 ms · mT/m, exceeds the lower limit for case 1 (Eq. 7.19) given by:

$$\frac{h^2}{S_R}\left(1 + \frac{G_1^2}{2h^2}\right) = 10.66\,\text{ms} \cdot \text{mT/m}$$

so this example falls under case 1. From Eq. (7.18), the duration of the bridge ramp is:

$$r_b = \frac{G_2 - G_1}{S_R} = \frac{(30.0 - 15.0)\,\text{mT/m}}{95\,\text{T/m/s}} = 0.158\,\text{ms} \qquad (7.34)$$

The net time savings is given by Eq. (7.25), so:

$$\Delta T_{\text{net}} = \frac{15\,\text{mT/m}}{95\,\text{T/m/s}} \left(2 - \frac{15}{30} \right) = 0.237\,\text{ms}$$

SELECTED REFERENCE

Zhou, X. J., Tan, S. G., and Bernstein, M. A. 1998. Artifacts induced by concomitant magnetic field in fast spin-echo imaging. *Magn. Reson. Med.* 40: 582–591.

RELATED SECTIONS

Section 7.1 Simple Gradient Lobes
Section 10.2 Crusher Gradients

7.3 Gradients for Oblique Acquisitions

Unlike computed tomography, MR can acquire images in any plane. In addition to the standard axial, sagittal, and coronal orthogonal planes, any arbitrary oblique imaging plane can be selected. Those acquisitions, and the images that result, are known as *obliques* (Edelman et al. 1986). The selection of the imaging plane is based on the operator's prescription and is implemented by digitally modifying the gradient waveforms that are sent to the gradient amplifiers. Because this modification is performed electronically, without the need for moving parts, the time required to switch acquisition planes in MRI is negligible. For example, it is even possible to collect views of data from different slice orientations in an interleaved fashion within a single TR period. This type of MRI scan is known as *multislice, multiangle* (MSMA) oblique acquisition. An example of an MSMA graphic prescription and two of the resulting images are shown in Figure 7.6.

7.3.1 QUALITATIVE DESCRIPTION

Most pulse sequences can be described in terms of their frequency-encoding, phase-encoding, and slice-selection gradient waveforms (Figure 7.7a). These pulse sequences are sometimes called Cartesian acquisitions

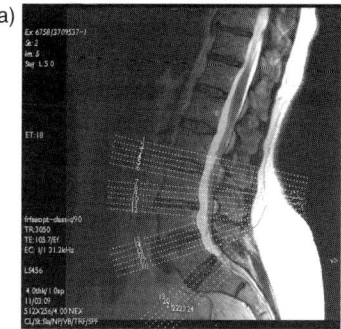

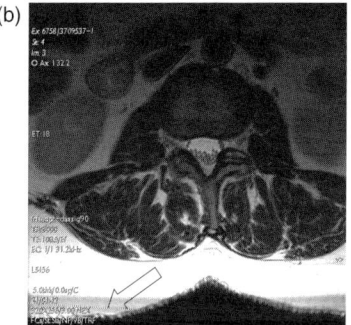
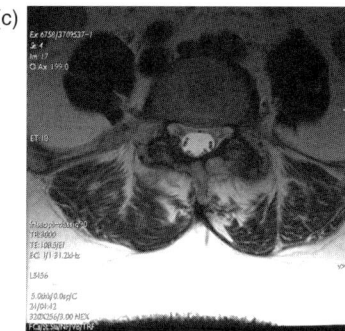

FIGURE 7.6 A multislice, multiangle prescription for a lumbar spine exam. (a) Four groups of oblique axial-coronal slices are deposited on a sagittal localizer exam so that the resulting images will show the disks in true cross section. (b–c) Two of the resulting oblique images. The annotated image numbers (e.g., Im: 17) correspond to the line labels on the localizer image. The dark band (hollow arrow) is the loss of signal due to saturation where two of the interleaved oblique slices intersected.

because their k-space trajectories are aligned with a Cartesian coordinate system (named after Rene Descartes, 1596–1650, the French philosopher and mathematician who introduced analytical geometry). That set of three gradient waveforms goes by a variety of names including *functional, imaging*, or *logical waveforms*, and the axes along which the waveforms are played out are often referred to as *functional, imaging*, or *logical axes*. We denote the logical axes by lowercase letters x, y, and z. Distinct from the three logical axes are the three *physical* axes, X, Y, and Z, which lie in another Cartesian coordinate system that is fixed to the magnet (Figure 7.8) and is usually rotated with respect to the logical axes. The (0,0,0) origin of the physical coordinate system is chosen to be the gradient isocenter, where the gradients produce zero magnetic field and which typically corresponds to the center of the magnet. By convention,

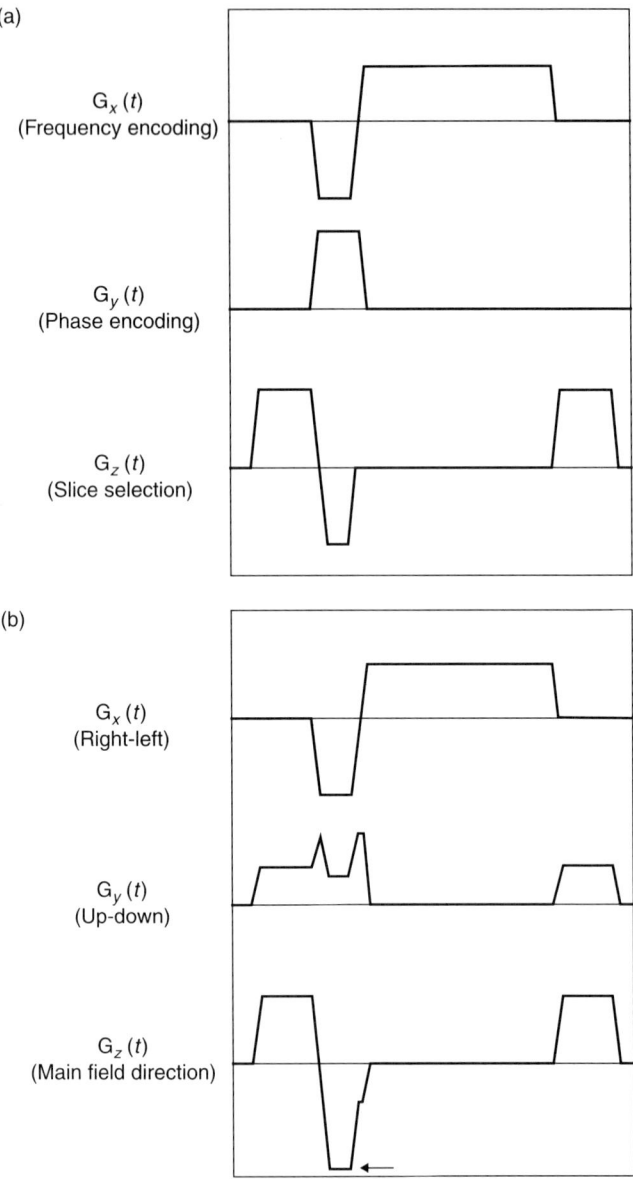

FIGURE 7.7 (a) 2D gradient echo pulse sequence diagram shown in the logical gradient coordinate system (frequency-encoding, phase-encoding, and slice-selection or x, y, and z, respectively). (b) The same pulse sequence after application of a 3×3 rotation matrix to transform it to the physical coordinate system. Note the increased gradient amplitude for one of the lobes on the physical Z axis (arrow).

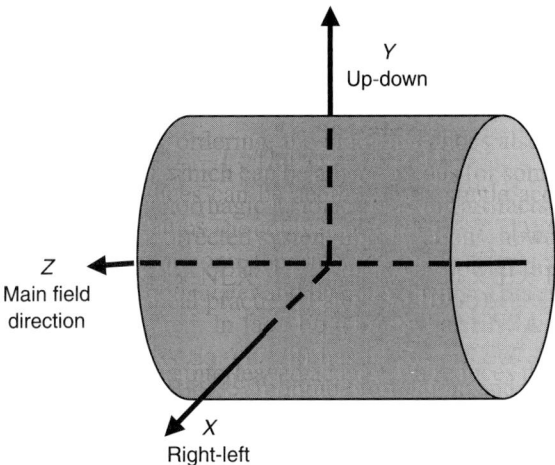

FIGURE 7.8 Physical X, Y, Z coordinate system that is fixed to the MRI magnet. By convention, the physical Z axis corresponds to the direction of the main magnetic field. The annotation in the figure assumes a horizontally placed, cylindrical magnet configuration.

the physical $+Z$ axis is chosen to be in the direction of the main magnetic field. Also by convention, the physical coordinates system is usually chosen to be right-handed. That means if we place our right hand on the system so that the fingers of the right hand curl from $+X$ to $+Y$, the right thumb points in the $+Z$ direction. Each of the three physical axes has its own associated gradient coil, which in turn is driven by its own dedicated gradient amplifier. Table 7.1 summarizes a few typical choices for the X, Y, and Z physical axes for horizontally oriented cylindrical magnets and for vertical-field open-sided MRI systems.

The physical X, Y, and Z magnet coordinate system does not necessarily correspond to the patient coordinate system. For example, if the magnet right-to-left also corresponds to a supine patient's right-to-left, it will be a prone patient's left-to-right. Similarly, the anterior-to-posterior (i.e., front-to-back) direction of the patient does not lie along the physical Y axis unless the patient is supine in a cylindrical magnet. These relationships are sometimes referred to as *patient geometries*. The associated bookkeeping required for proper image annotation (e.g., to indicate the patient's left) can get quite involved because of the large number of patient-positioning options available (e.g., head-first or feet-first, and prone, supine, right- or left-lateral decubitus). To standardize image viewing, MRI usually follows the same conventions for image orientation as do other medical images and illustrations (listed in Table 7.2).

TABLE 7.1

Typical Directions for the Physical Axes X, Y, and Z in Cylindrical and Vertical Field Magnets[a]

Magnet Type	Physical Axis		
	X	Y	Z
Horizontally oriented cylindrical magnet	Right-to-left or left-to-right	Up-to-down or down-to-up	Along B_0
Vertical-field open-sided magnet	Right-to-left or left-to-right	Head-to-foot or foot-to-head	Along B_0

[a] As viewed by a subject lying in the magnet (supine or prone). The choice between right-to-left or left-to-right, for example, is made so that the physical axes form a right-handed coordinate system.

TABLE 7.2

Conventional Image Orientations[a]

Image Plane	Apparent Location of the Viewer	Top of Image	Right Side of Image
Axial and axial-like oblique	Patient's feet	Patient's front	Patient's left
Sagittal and sagittal-like oblique	Patient's left	Patient's head	Patient's back
Coronal and coronal-like oblique	Patient's front	Patient's head	Patient's left

[a] These conventions are usually followed regardless of the patient positioning.

The three logical waveforms (Figure 7.7a) are digitally mixed in ratios determined by angulation of the prescribed imaging plane to yield the three physical waveforms along the X, Y, and Z axes (Figure 7.7b). The physical waveforms shown in Figure 7.7b are an example of a *single-angle* oblique prescription, in that only two of the waveforms (phase-encoding and slice-selection) are mixed, while the frequency-encoding waveform is not. Oblique prescriptions that mix all three logical waveforms are called *double-angle* or *compound-angle* obliques. (Note that either single- or double-angle oblique slices can make up the MSMA prescription described earlier in this section.) The mathematics of the mixing of the logical waveforms to yield the desired physical waveforms is described by a 3×3 orthogonal rotation matrix, which is discussed next.

Although Figure 7.7 and the preceding discussion focus on Fourier-encoded Cartesian acquisitions, obliques are also important for non-Cartesian acquisition strategies such as projection (i.e., radial) and spiral scans. Even for an axial radial projection acquisition, the necessary tilting of the frequency-encoding gradient in k-space required to generate the multiple spokes can be accomplished with the rotation matrix methods that are used for oblique imaging of Cartesian trajectories. More details are provided in Sections 17.5 and 17.6.

7.3.2 Mathematical Description

A 3×3 orthogonal rotation matrix $\Re$ describes the transformation from the logical gradient waveforms to the physical gradient waveforms:

$$\begin{bmatrix} G_X(t) \\ G_Y(t) \\ G_Z(t) \end{bmatrix} = \begin{bmatrix} a_{11} & a_{12} & a_{13} \\ a_{21} & a_{22} & a_{23} \\ a_{31} & a_{32} & a_{33} \end{bmatrix} \begin{bmatrix} G_x(t) \\ G_y(t) \\ G_z(t) \end{bmatrix}$$

or

$$\begin{bmatrix} G_X(t) \\ G_Y(t) \\ G_Z(t) \end{bmatrix} = \Re \begin{bmatrix} G_x(t) \\ G_y(t) \\ G_z(t) \end{bmatrix} \tag{7.35}$$

where the subscripts x, y, and z denote the coordinate system based on the image, or the logical coordinate system. For example, in a 2D Fourier-encoded pulse sequence, x, y, and z correspond to the frequency-encoded, phase-encoded, and slice-selection axes, respectively. The indices of the matrix elements should be interpreted from right to left—for example, the element a_{13} indicates the contribution from the third logical element to the first physical one, from z to X. Another way to express this property is to label the rows and the columns of the rotation matrix with *from* and *to*, as in Table 7.3.

Physically, the matrix $\Re$ describes a rotation in three-dimensional space. As the name suggests, the rotation matrix for a single-angle oblique can be parameterized by a single angle (one that is not equal to 0, ± 90, ± 180, ...) and has exactly one matrix element that is equal to ± 1. For a double-angle oblique, the rotation matrix has no elements that are equal to ± 1. The rotation matrix for an orthogonal prescription has three elements equal to ± 1, while the other six elements are always 0. (Because of the constraint described next, it is not possible for the rotation matrix to have exactly two elements equal to ± 1.)

All rotation matrices are *orthogonal* and *normal* (also called *orthonormal*); that is, the product of the matrix with its own transpose is equal to the identity

TABLE 7.3
Indices of Rotation Matrix Elements[a]

	From x	From y	From z
To X	a_{11}	a_{12}	a_{13}
To Y	a_{21}	a_{22}	a_{23}
To Z	a_{31}	a_{32}	a_{33}

[a] The indices of the rotation matrix elements should be interpreted from right to left. For example, the element a_{13} indicates the contribution from z to X, that is, from slice selection (the third logical axis) to X (the first physical axis).

matrix $\mathbb{I}$:

$$\Re\Re^{T} = \mathbb{I} = \begin{bmatrix} a_{11} & a_{12} & a_{13} \\ a_{21} & a_{22} & a_{23} \\ a_{31} & a_{32} & a_{33} \end{bmatrix} \begin{bmatrix} a_{11} & a_{21} & a_{31} \\ a_{12} & a_{22} & a_{32} \\ a_{13} & a_{23} & a_{33} \end{bmatrix} = \begin{bmatrix} 1 & 0 & 0 \\ 0 & 1 & 0 \\ 0 & 0 & 1 \end{bmatrix} \quad (7.36)$$

Similarly, $\Re^{T}\Re = \mathbb{I}$ as well. Equation (7.36) implies that the dot product of any two row (or column) vectors that make up $\Re$ is equal to 0, unless the row (or column) index is the same, in which case the dot product is equal to 1. This relation can be expressed compactly with the Kronecker delta form of the identity matrix (named after Leopold Kronecker, 1823–1891, a German mathematician):

$$\sum_{k=1}^{3} a_{ik} a_{jk} = \delta_{ij} = \begin{cases} 1 & i = j \\ 0 & i \neq j \end{cases} \quad (7.37)$$

An arbitrary 3D rotation has three degrees of freedom, which can be parameterized by the three Euler angles (named after Leonhard Euler, 1707–1783, a Swiss mathematician) (Goldstein 1980, chap. 4). Equation (7.37) represents a total of six independent constraints, which is consistent with the nine elements of the matrix because $9 - 6 = 3$ degrees of freedom. The product of any two orthogonal matrices is also an orthogonal matrix. Also, the determinant of any orthogonal matrix must have absolute value equal to 1:

$$\det(\Re) = \pm 1 \quad (7.38)$$

Next consider two examples of rotation matrices. For a cylindrical bore, horizontal magnet and a supine patient position, the rotation matrix for an axial acquisition with the frequency-encoding direction anterior to posterior is given by:

$$\begin{bmatrix} 0 & \pm1 & 0 \\ \pm1 & 0 & 0 \\ 0 & 0 & \pm1 \end{bmatrix} \tag{7.39}$$

where the signs are determined by specifics such as the direction of the main magnetic field and the direction of patient entry so that the image orientation conventions in Table 7.2 are followed. The example of gradient waveform mixing given in Figure 7.7 is an oblique axial-coronal, with the slice direction tilted 30° away from the Z axis. Its rotation matrix is:

$$\Re = \begin{bmatrix} 1 & 0 & 0 \\ 0 & \cos 30° & \sin 30° \\ 0 & -\sin 30° & \cos 30° \end{bmatrix} \approx \begin{bmatrix} 1 & 0 & 0 \\ 0 & 0.866 & 0.5 \\ 0 & -0.5 & 0.866 \end{bmatrix} \tag{7.40}$$

Example 7.2 Write a rotation matrix for a sagittal acquisition with the frequency encoding in the up-down direction (i.e., anterior-posterior for a supine patient in a cylindrical bore horizontal magnet).

Answer A sagittal acquisition has slice-selection gradient along the physical X axis, so from Table 7.3 the matrix element $a_{13} = \pm1$. The other elements of the rotation matrix are deduced similarly, yielding:

$$\Re = \begin{bmatrix} 0 & 0 & \pm1 \\ \pm1 & 0 & 0 \\ 0 & \pm1 & 0 \end{bmatrix} \tag{7.41}$$

The actual signs of the rotation matrix elements will be determined based on the magnet coordinate (e.g., the direction of the B_0 field) and patient geometry in accordance with the guidelines given in Tables 7.1 and 7.2.

Graphic Prescriptions Here we describe methods to generate the rotation matrix $\Re$ based on the operator's graphic prescription of a slice location. Consider unit vectors in the frequency-encoded, phase-encoded, and slice-selection directions:

$$\hat{u}_x = \begin{bmatrix} 1 \\ 0 \\ 0 \end{bmatrix} \qquad \hat{u}_y = \begin{bmatrix} 0 \\ 1 \\ 0 \end{bmatrix} \qquad \hat{u}_z = \begin{bmatrix} 0 \\ 0 \\ 1 \end{bmatrix} \tag{7.42}$$

When a slice is prescribed (usually graphically), it provides the unit vectors in the physical coordinate system:

$$\hat{u}_X = \mathfrak{R}\hat{u}_x = \begin{bmatrix} a_{11} \\ a_{21} \\ a_{31} \end{bmatrix} \qquad \hat{u}_Y = \mathfrak{R}\hat{u}_y = \begin{bmatrix} a_{12} \\ a_{22} \\ a_{32} \end{bmatrix} \qquad \hat{u}_Z = \mathfrak{R}\hat{u}_z = \begin{bmatrix} a_{13} \\ a_{23} \\ a_{33} \end{bmatrix}$$

$$(7.43)$$

The three physical axis vectors in Eq. (7.43) contain all the elements of the rotation matrix, so once they are determined $\mathfrak{R}$ is known.

Line Deposit Prescription   Perhaps the most common slice prescription procedure is to graphically deposit one or more lines on a reference image, as illustrated in Figure 7.6. (When this is the main purpose of the reference image, it often called a *scout, survey, basic,* or *localizer* image, especially if it is acquired in the first series of the exam.) Each deposited line represents the intersection between the prescribed slice and the localizer image. It is assumed that the physical coordinates are known for every location on the localizer image. Suppose $\hat{u}_{LOC}$ is a known unit vector normal (i.e., perpendicular) to the plane of the localizer image and $\hat{u}_{DEP}$ is a unit vector along the deposited line. (Both $\hat{u}_{LOC}$ and $\hat{u}_{DEP}$ are defined in the physical coordinate system.) The operator must also specify whether the deposited line represents the frequency-encoded or phase-encoded direction of the desired slice. If, for example, it represents the frequency-encoded direction, then the unit vectors in Eq. (7.43) are calculated with a vector cross product:

$$\hat{u}_X = \hat{u}_{DEP}$$
$$\hat{u}_Y = \hat{u}_{LOC} \qquad\qquad (7.44)$$
$$\hat{u}_Z = \hat{u}_{DEP} \times \hat{u}_{LOC}$$

Equation (7.44) completely specifies the rotation matrix for the prescribed slice. If the localizer image is orthogonal (i.e., it is axial, sagittal, or coronal), then the graphically prescribed slice will be either orthogonal as well or a single-angle oblique. If, however, the localizer is an oblique, then the prescribed slice can be either a single- or double-angle oblique.

Three-Point Prescription   Sometimes the operator desires a slice that includes landmarks that are only visible on more than one localizer image. One common procedure used to accomplish this is known as three-point localization or a *three-point prescription* (Busse et al. 1999). The operator graphically deposits three (non-collinear) points, which define a plane. The three points can be described by the vectors $\vec{r}_1$, $\vec{r}_2$, and $\vec{r}_3$ in the physical coordinate system. Because the vector difference of any pair lies within the desired imaging plane, the unit slice-selection vector is given by the vector cross product:

$$\hat{u}_Z = \pm \frac{(\vec{r}_1 - \vec{r}_2) \times (\vec{r}_3 - \vec{r}_2)}{\|(\vec{r}_1 - \vec{r}_2) \times (\vec{r}_3 - \vec{r}_2)\|} = \pm \frac{\vec{r}_1 \times \vec{r}_3 - \vec{r}_1 \times \vec{r}_2 - \vec{r}_2 \times \vec{r}_3}{\|(\vec{r}_1 - \vec{r}_2) \times (\vec{r}_3 - \vec{r}_2)\|} \quad (7.45)$$

There are an infinite number of choices for the frequency- and phase-encoding directions within the plane specified by $\vec{r}_1$, $\vec{r}_2$, and $\vec{r}_3$. For example, we can take:

$$\hat{u}_X = \frac{(\vec{r}_1 - \vec{r}_2)}{\|(\vec{r}_1 - \vec{r}_2)\|} \quad (7.46)$$
$$\hat{u}_Y = \hat{u}_Z \times \hat{u}_X$$

(Ideally, we would like to follow the image orientation conventions in Table 7.2, in which case appropriate linear combinations of the unit vectors in Eq. 7.46 can be used instead.)

The graphic prescription also contains information about the shortest distance δz from gradient isocenter to the prescribed slice plane (Figure 7.9). This information is also retained and is used to calculate RF frequency offset, as described in Section 8.3 on slice-selection gradients. For example, the slice

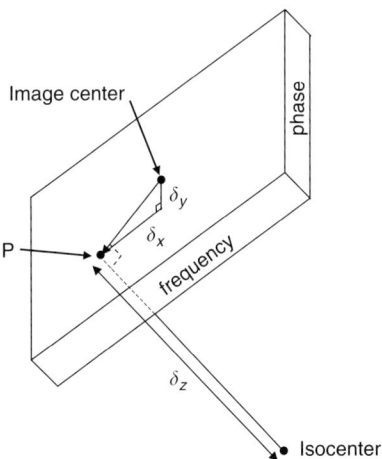

FIGURE 7.9 Given the prescription of a slice plane relative to isocenter, we can define offsets in the frequency-encoding, phase-encoding, and slice-selection directions. The slice offset δz is the nearest distance from gradient isocenter to the slice plane. The frequency and phase offsets δx and δy, respectively, are determined by decomposing a line from the image center to the intersection point (P).

offset can be calculated for a three-point prescription by finding the shortest distance from the prescribed plane to isocenter:

$$\pm\delta z = \vec{r}_1 \cdot \hat{u}_Z = \vec{r}_2 \cdot \hat{u}_Z = \vec{r}_3 \cdot \hat{u}_Z \tag{7.47}$$

which the interested reader can show with the aid of Eq. (7.45). Equation (7.47) is a special case of a general result from analytic geometric (Salas and Etgen 1998) that states that if a plane is defined by the vector equation:

$$\vec{r} \cdot \hat{u}_z = a \tag{7.48}$$

then the shortest distance between the origin (i.e., the isocenter) and the plane is given by:

$$\delta z = |a| \tag{7.49}$$

The off-center distances in the frequency- and phase-encoded directions (δx and δy, respectively) can also be obtained from the graphic prescription. These quantities are used to calculate frequency and phase modulation during image acquisition (Sections 11.1 and 11.5). They can be found by extending a line parallel to $\hat{u}_z$ from isocenter until it intersects the imaging plane at point (P), as shown on Figure 7.9. The lengths of the components in the frequency- and phase-encoded directions of a vector from the image center to P provide δx and δy, respectively.

Restrictions on the Logical Amplitudes and Distributed Loads   The rotation matrix mixes multiple logical waveforms to yield a single physical-axis gradient waveform. So for oblique prescriptions it is possible for the gradient amplitude on a physical-axis gradient waveform to exceed any of the logical-axis waveform amplitudes. An example is shown on the physical Z axis waveform in Figure 7.7b (arrow). There, the maximal absolute value of the amplitude is 1.366 times the largest gradient amplitude on any of the logical waveforms. Care must be exercised so that the maximal gradient amplitude of $\pm h$ is never exceeded on any of the three physical axes. The worst case situation occurs when all the logical gradient amplitudes are maximized and the prescribed slice orientation is such that all three of the matrix elements along a row of $\Re$ are equal. Then the logical amplitudes must be limited to $h/\sqrt{3} \approx 0.577h$.

Conversely, in some oblique prescriptions, the redistribution of the logical gradient waveforms can actually ease amplitude restrictions. For example, if only a single logical waveform is active at a certain time, then the rotation matrix can *distribute* that logical load onto multiple physical axes. Then the maximum logical amplitude can exceed h without problems. Again in the extreme case when the three matrix elements along a row of $\Re$ are all equal, that single logical gradient amplitude can be as high as $\sqrt{3}h \approx 1.73h$. The permissible range of logical gradient amplitudes therefore varies by a factor of 3 (i.e., from $h/\sqrt{3}$ to $\sqrt{3}h$). Because this is a very wide range and the hardware required to generate gradient performance is quite expensive, it is worthwhile to consider these limits in more detail.

The simplest method to ensure that the maximal gradient amplitude is never exceeded on each of the three physical axes is to restrict all the logical amplitudes so that they lie within the range $\left[-h/\sqrt{3}, +h/\sqrt{3}\right]$, regardless of which logical waveforms are active or dormant and the specific angulation of the prescription. Although simple to implement, this method is quite wasteful of gradient performance.

A more sophisticated algorithm that is still simple to implement is described in Bernstein and Licato (1994). This method calculates a target amplitude based on the *maximum absolute row sum* (MARS) for the rotation matrix. Suppose, for example, the middle column of the rotation matrix contains a 1, for example, $a_{12} = 1$. We can infer that this is a single-angle oblique in which the phase-encoding function is unmixed by the rotation. The rotation matrix can be expressed:

$$\mathfrak{R} = \begin{bmatrix} 0 & 1 & 0 \\ a_{21} & 0 & a_{23} \\ a_{31} & 0 & a_{33} \end{bmatrix} \tag{7.50}$$

The target amplitude for the phase-encoding function is simply the maximal gradient amplitude h:

$$-G_{y,\text{target}} \leq G_y(t) \leq G_{y,\text{target}} \qquad G_{y,\text{target}} = h \tag{7.51}$$

Suppose also that the pulse sequence contains a frequency-encoding lobe and a slice-selection lobe that (at least partially) overlap in time. Then, according to the MARS method in a feasible target amplitude for those two logical lobes can be calculated using:

$$G_{xz,\text{target}} = \frac{h}{\max\left(|a_{21}| + |a_{23}|, |a_{31}| + |a_{33}|\right)} \tag{7.52}$$

By substituting Eqs. (7.52) and (7.51) into Eq. (7.50), the reader can verify that all three physical gradient amplitudes are guaranteed to lie within the range $[-h, +h]$, as required. Although this discussion has focused on gradient amplitude restrictions, similar methods can be used to set limits for gradient slewing as well.

Example 7.3 Consider the oblique prescription depicted in Figure 7.7 and described by the rotation matrix in Eq. (7.40). What logical target amplitude should be used for gradient lobes on the phase-encoding and slice-selection axes if the two lobes temporally overlap? What logical target amplitude can be used on an isolated gradient lobe on the slice-selection axis?

Answer   Calculating the MARS on the second and third columns of the rotation matrix in Eq. (7.40) yields:

$$G_{yz,\ target} = \frac{h}{\max(|\cos 30°| + |\sin 30°|,\ |-\sin 30°| + |\cos 30°|)} = 0.732h \tag{7.53}$$

Note that because $0.732 \times 1.366 = 1$, the target amplitude in Eq. (7.53) prevents the physical Z axis gradient overrange depicted on Figure 7.7b.

The target amplitude for the isolated lobe on the slice-selection axis is:

$$G_{z,\ target} = \frac{h}{\max(|\cos 30°|,\ |\sin 30°|)} = 1.155h \tag{7.54}$$

Because of the distributed load, the maximal slice-selection amplitude in Eq. (7.54) can exceed the physical-axis limit h.

Although the MARS method offers a substantial improvement compared to the draconian restriction of setting all the logical target amplitudes to $h/\sqrt{3}$, it is not guaranteed to be optimal in all cases. Other powerful methods have been developed. For example, the *hardware optimized trapezoid* (HOT) method (Atalar and McVeigh 1994; Bolster and Atalar 1999) recognizes that in those time periods when both RF transmission and data acquisition are dormant, the net gradient area is the important factor rather than the exact shape of the gradient waveforms. The HOT method designs an optimal gradient subwaveform for each of these time periods, often providing a substantial time savings. A drawback to the HOT method is engineering complexity because, in general, the same optimized gradient designs cannot be reused for each phase-encoding step.

7.3.3 APPLICATIONS

Oblique prescriptions are widely used. A well-known application is lumbar, sacral, and thoracic spine imaging, in which oblique axial-coronal planes are graphically prescribed from a sagittal localizer so that the spine is imaged in true cross section (Figure 7.6). Another common application of oblique imaging is cardiac MR of the left ventricle (Figure 7.10). Often that prescription begins with a sagittal or coronal localizer, on which single-angle oblique images are graphically prescribed, providing long-axis views of the

(a)   (b)   (c)

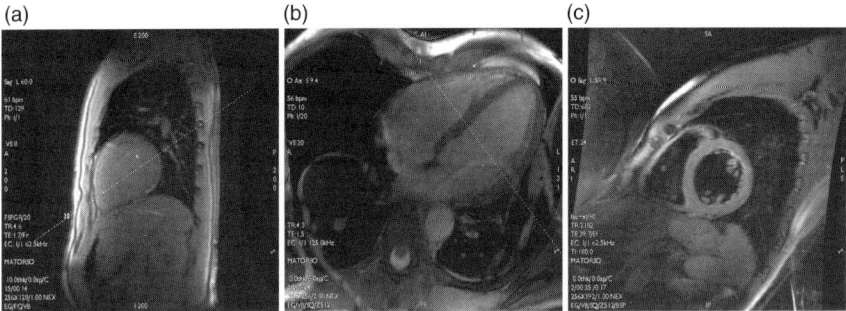

FIGURE 7.10 Example of a cardiac graphic prescription. (a) Sagittal localizer.
(b) Single-angle oblique long axis view. (c) Double-angle oblique short-axis view.
Note the progressively complicated patient-position labels on the edges of the images,
from S/I-A/P on the sagittal image to SA/IP- ARI/PLS on the double-angle oblique.
S, superior; I, inferior; A, anterior; P, posterior; L, left; R, right.

left ventricle. Then double-angle oblique short-axis view can be graphically
prescribed from a long-axis image. Oblique gradients are also quite useful in
diffusion-weighted imaging, in which two or three physical gradients can be
activated simultaneously to provide a much higher b-value than when using
a single-axis gradient alone. Even for brain examinations, axial prescriptions
are often given a slight coronal tilt to better align the corpus callossum with
the imaging plane.

With the advent of 3D volume imaging and the ability to reformat the
resulting contiguous slices into any arbitrary plane, it may seem somewhat
surprising that 2D oblique imaging continues to enjoy widespread popularity. It is sometimes stated that 3D volume acquisition has an SNR efficiency
advantage over 2D imaging equal to the square root of the number of slices.
As explained in Section 11.6, however, this is an oversimplification, and in
fact the signal-to-noise per unit time efficiency of the 3D and interleaved 2D
strategies is approximately equal for gradient echo acquisitions. Instead, it is
the linear relation between voxel volume and SNR that explains the peren-
nial popularity of 2D oblique acquisitions. Partial-volume artifacts are often
minimized when the slice is properly oriented; for example, the spinal cord
is imaged in cross section as in Figure 7.6. This reduction in partial-volume
artifact in turn allows oblique 2D imaging to use thicker slices and hence to
have increased SNR. 3D imaging, however, requires a smaller voxel volume to
provide the same quality views in multiple planes with retrospective reformat.
Moreover, retrospectively averaging voxels together in MR provides only a
square root, rather than a linear increase, in SNR. Thus 2D oblique imaging is
a particularly efficient acquisition mode for many applications.

Oblique 3D acquisitions have become increasingly popular as well. Oblique 3D acquisitions offer advantages in two separate regimes. First, as with 2D obliques, 3D oblique acquisitions can allow thicker slices (to increase the SNR) if the desired anatomy can be imaged in true cross section throughout the imaging volume. The second and more commonly exploited application advantage is that it allows full coverage of obliquely oriented anatomy with fewer or thinner slices, thereby saving acquisition time or increasing the spatial resolution. For example, in contrast-enhanced MRA the carotid-vertebral-basilar arterial circulation can often be covered with fewer or thinner oblique slices than with straight coronals.

SELECTED REFERENCES

Atalar, E., and McVeigh, E. R. 1994. Minimization of dead-periods in MRI pulse sequences for imaging oblique planes. *Magn. Reson. Med.* 32: 773–777.

Bernstein, M. A., and Licato, P. E. 1994. Angle-dependent utilization of gradient hardware for oblique MR imaging. *J. Magn. Reson. Imaging* 4: 105–108.

Bolster, B. D., Jr., and Atalar, E. 1999. Minimizing dead-periods in flow-encoded or -compensated pulse sequences while imaging in oblique planes. *J. Magn. Reson. Imaging* 10: 183–192.

Busse, R. F., Debbins, J. P., Kruger, D. G., Fain, S. B., and Riederer, S. J. 1999. Interactive three-point localization of double-oblique sections using MR fluoroscopy. *Magn. Reson. Med.* 41: 846–849.

Edelman, R. R., Stark, D. D., Saini, S., Ferrucci. J. T., Jr., Dinsmore, R. E., Ladd, W., and Brady, T. J. 1986. Oblique planes of section in MR imaging. *Radiology* 159: 807–810.

Goldstein, H. 1980. *Classical mechanics*. 2nd ed. Reading: Addison-Wesley.

Salas, L. S., and Etgen, G. J. 1998. *Calculus, one and several variables*. 8th ed. New York: John Wiley.

RELATED SECTIONS

8

IMAGING GRADIENTS

8.1 Frequency-Encoding Gradients

Frequency encoding is a common spatial encoding method employed by many MRI pulse sequences, including projection acquisition (Lauterbur 1973) and Fourier imaging (Kumar et al. 1975; Edelstein et al. 1980). Frequency encoding is accomplished by applying a *frequency-encoding gradient* to the imaged object. This gradient spatially encodes NMR signals by assigning a unique precession frequency (i.e., Larmor frequency) to each spin isochromat at a distinct spatial location along the gradient direction (a spin isochromat is a cluster of spins that precess with the same frequency). Under the influence of this gradient, time-domain NMR signals will consist of a range of frequencies, each corresponding to a different spatial location. An inverse Fourier transform of the time domain NMR signal reveals the frequency content. Each frequency is linearly related to the corresponding spatial location along the gradient direction.

A frequency-encoding gradient can be applied along any physical direction. In projection acquisitions, the direction of the gradient is varied during the course of imaging, as described in Section 17.5. In Fourier-encoded pulse sequences, the direction of the gradient is typically held fixed and repeats itself while the phase-encoding value is incremented. Even for the MSMA oblique prescriptions described in Section 7.3, the frequency-encoding gradient direction is held fixed during the data acquisition of any given slice. The polarity of the frequency-encoding gradient can be either positive or negative. When the polarity of a frequency-encoding gradient is reversed, the image simply flips in the frequency-encoded direction, which can be corrected for during image reconstruction.

8.1.1 QUALITATIVE DESCRIPTION OF FREQUENCY-ENCODING GRADIENTS

To qualitatively understand the effect of a frequency-encoding gradient on a spin system, let us consider two plates of water placed in a uniform magnetic field B_0 as shown in Figure 8.1a. In the absence of a frequency-encoding gradient, protons in both plates resonate with the same frequency (i.e., the Larmor frequency), producing a single-frequency NMR signal (Figure 8.1b). After a Fourier transform, this frequency is revealed in the spectrum (Figure 8.1c), which does not contain any spatial information regarding the two water plates. In the presence of a frequency-encoding gradient G applied along the

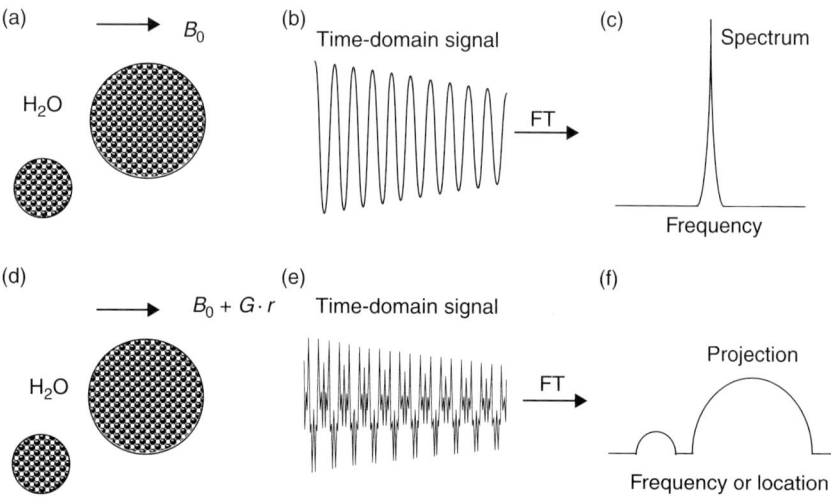

FIGURE 8.1 NMR signal characteristics for two plates of water in the absence (top row) and presence (bottom row) of a frequency-encoding gradient. B_0 denotes the main magnetic field, G the applied frequency-encoding gradient, r the spatial location along the gradient direction, and FT the Fourier transform. Without the gradient (a), only a single resonant frequency is contained in the time-domain signal (b) and its frequency-domain spectrum (c). With the gradient (d), a range of resonance frequencies is present in the time-domain signal (e) and its spectrum (f). Each frequency in the spectrum corresponds to a spatial location along the direction of the gradient. Thus, the spectrum gives a projection of the imaged object.

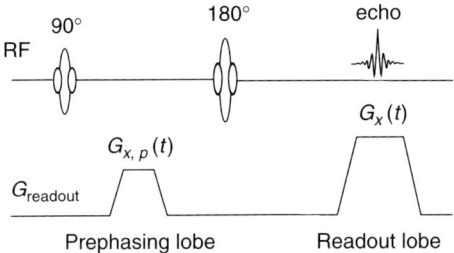

FIGURE 8.2 A frequency-encoding gradient waveform in a spin-echo pulse sequence. The waveform consists of two lobes; a prephasing gradient lobe $G_{x,p}(t)$ and a readout gradient lobe $G_x(t)$, both of which have the same polarity.

horizontal direction (Figure 8.1d), the resonant frequency of the spins becomes linearly related to their location along the direction of the gradient. Thus, the time-domain NMR signal consists of a range of frequencies (Figure 8.1e), each corresponding to spin isochromats at a specific location. A Fourier transform of the time-domain signal produces a spectrum that reveals the density of spins at these frequencies, thereby producing a projection of the objects (Figure 8.1f). Spatial information is encoded into the NMR signal by the frequency-encoding gradient, and decoded by a subsequent Fourier transform.

A frequency-encoding gradient waveform typically consists of two portions, a *prephasing gradient* lobe (also known as dephasing gradient lobe) and a *readout gradient* lobe. In an RF spin-echo pulse sequence, these two lobes are usually separated by an RF refocusing pulse with the prephasing gradient lobe before the pulse and the readout gradient lobe after it (Figure 8.2). This design is popular because it allows a shorter minimum TE (or echo spacing, in echo train pulse sequences), and the FID artifact from an imperfect 180° refocusing pulse can be more efficiently dephased. Because the RF refocusing pulse negates the accumulated phase from the prephasing lobe, both the prephasing and the readout gradient lobes have the same polarity. In a gradient-echo pulse sequence, the two gradient lobes can be combined into a single continuous waveform (Figure 8.3). The polarity of the prephasing gradient lobe is opposite to that of the readout gradient lobe. In pulse sequences with multiple spin echoes or gradient echoes, such as EPI, RARE, and GRASE, the second half of a readout gradient can also serve as a prephasing gradient for the subsequent readout. Thus, only a single separate prephasing gradient lobe is used at the beginning of the sequence, regardless of the length of the echo train (see Sections 16.1, 16.2, and 16.4).

The purpose of the prephasing gradient lobe is to prepare the transverse magnetization so that an echo signal can be created at a later time. This can

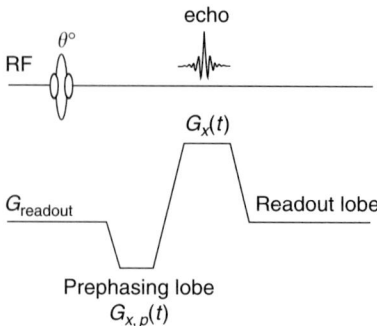

FIGURE 8.3 A frequency-encoding gradient waveform in a gradient-echo pulse sequence. The two gradient lobes, the prephasing lobe $G_{x,p}(t)$ and readout lobe $G_x(t)$, have the opposite polarity.

be intuitively understood by considering two spin isochromats, *I* and *II*, at different locations. When the prephasing gradient is applied, the two spin isochromats will begin to accumulate phase. The phase accumulation rate will be different if the isochromats are at locations that have different field strengths due to the prephasing gradient. Suppose isochromat *I* accumulates phase faster than isochromat *II* (Figure 8.4a). This scenario is analogous to two sprinters when one runs faster than the other, as depicted in Figure 8.5a. When the prephasing gradient is terminated, the spin isochromats will stop accumulating phase and remain, one at point *A* and the other at *B* (Figure 8.4a). In our analogy, this is equivalent to a situation in which sprinter *I* stops at point *A* and sprinter *II* stops at point *B* (Figure 8.5a).

In an RF spin-echo pulse sequence, the refocusing RF pulse negates the phase of the spin isochromats (Figure 8.4b); this is analogous to the two sprinters' swapping lanes (Figure 8.5b). When a readout gradient is applied, the two spin isochromats will continue to accumulate phase under the influence of the readout gradient or, equivalently, the two sprinters will continue to run (Figure 8.5b). When the two spin isochromats *I* and *II* meet (i.e., they are in phase), an echo is formed (Figure 8.4d); in our analogy, because sprinter *I* is still faster than sprinter *II*, sprinter *I* will catch up to sprinter *II* after a certain time (Figure 8.5b).

In a gradient-echo pulse sequence, the polarity change between the prephasing gradient lobe and the readout gradient lobe reverses the directions of phase accumulation of the spin isochromats (Figure 8.4c); in our analogy, this is equivalent to the two sprinters reversing their running directions (Figure 8.5c). The rapidly dephasing spin isochromat will meet the slowly dephasing spin isochromat (Figure 8.4d), producing an echo signal; similarly, with the reversal

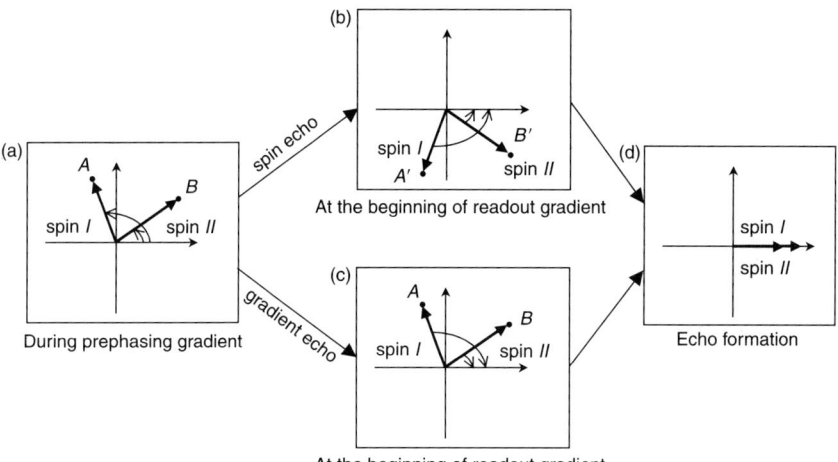

FIGURE 8.4 A diagram showing the effect of prephasing and readout gradients on a spin system consisting of two spin isochromats, *I* and *II*. (a) The prephasing gradient introduces a phase dispersion. In a spin-echo pulse sequence, the phase dispersion is reversed by the 180° RF pulse (b). When a readout gradient with the same polarity is applied, the spins *I* and *II* continue the phase accumulation in the same direction, producing an echo in (d). In a gradient-echo pulse sequence, the polarity of the readout gradient is the opposite to that of the prephasing gradient. The directions of phase accumulation of the spins are reversed (c), producing an echo as shown in (d).

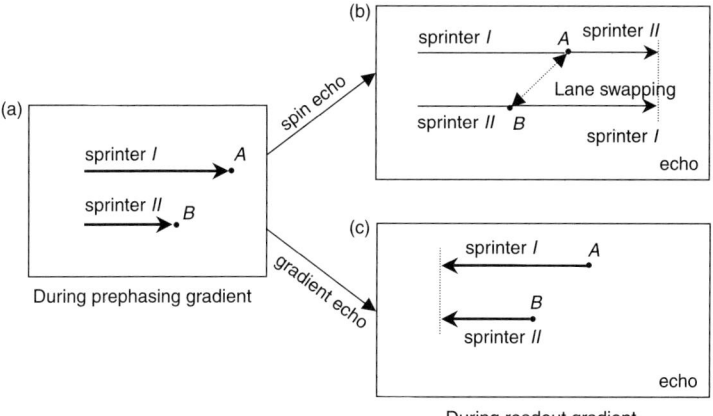

FIGURE 8.5 A diagram showing the effect of prephasing (a) and readout gradients (b and c) on spin systems using the analogy of two sprinters (two spin isochromats) and the action of 'running' (spin phase accumulation).

in direction the faster sprinter *I* will catch the slower sprinter *II* after a certain time (Figure 8.5c).

In both spin-echo and gradient-echo sequences, we can see that the prephasing gradient is a prerequisite for echo formation, while the readout gradient creates the echo. For the spin-echo case, the 180° RF pulse refocuses phase accumulation from chemical shift, B_0-field inhomogeneity, and susceptibility variations (collectively known as off-resonance effects). Because the gradient echoes do not employ a refocusing RF pulse, the off-resonance effects continue to cause phase accumulation throughout the frequency-encoding process. This difference between spin echo and gradient echo gives rise to different contrast mechanisms (e.g., T_2 vs. T_2^*) and artifacts in MR images (Sections 14.1 and 14.3).

Although a prephasing gradient is used in most pulse sequences to generate echo signals, some pulse sequences using FID signals do not require prephasing gradient lobes. An example can be found in some projection-acquisition pulse sequences (Section 17.5) in which FID signals, instead of echoes, are frequency-encoded (Lauterbur 1973; Boada et al. 1997). Such pulse sequences can achieve a very short TE time and are particularly useful for imaging tissues with short T_2 or T_2^* values, such as the lung.

The area under the prephasing gradient lobe determines the time at which the echo peak forms. The echo signal reaches its maximum when the area under the readout lobe is equal to the area of the prephasing lobe. Thus, increasing the area of the prephasing lobe delays the echo (or shifts the echo peak to the right). Conversely, decreasing the prephasing gradient area advances the echo (or shifts the echo peak to the left). It is worth noting that the position of the echo does not have to coincide with that of an RF spin echo in a spin-echo pulse sequence. When the echo produced by balancing the prephasing and readout gradients does match an RF spin echo, the off-resonance effects are minimized. Sometimes, a mismatch is intentionally introduced to make the pulse sequence more sensitive to chemical shift, magnetic susceptibility, or T_2^* effects.

The amplitude and duration of the readout gradient lobe are related to image resolution, receiver bandwidth, fields of view (FOVs), and gyromagnetic ratio. These relationships can be more clearly seen next, as well as in Section 11.1.

8.1.2 Quantitative Description of Frequency-Encoding Gradients

Consider a series of spin isochromats arranged in a one-dimensional array at locations $x_1, x_2, x_3, \ldots, x_n$ along the x axis with spin densities

$\rho_{x_1}, \rho_{x_2}, \rho_{x_3}, \ldots, \rho_{x_n}$. When the prephasing gradient $G_{x,p}(t)$ (Figure 8.2) is applied, each spin isochromat j will have a distinct precession frequency given by the Larmor equation:

$$\omega'_{x_j} = \gamma \left(B_0 + G_{x,p}(t)x_j \right) \tag{8.1}$$

where B_0 is the main magnetic field, and γ is the gyromagetic ratio in radians per second per tesla. In a reference frame rotating with frequency of $\omega = \gamma B_0$, the precession frequencies of the spin isochromats are simplified to:

$$\omega_{x_j} = \gamma G_{x,p}(t)x_j \tag{8.2}$$

The phase (measured in radians) accumulated by spin isochromat j due to the prephasing gradient is:

$$\phi_{x_j,p} = \int_0^T \omega_{x_j} dt = \gamma x_j \int_0^T G_{x,p}(t)dt = 2\pi x_j k_{x,p} \tag{8.3}$$

where T is the duration of the prephasing gradient, and $k_{x,p} \equiv (\gamma/2\pi)\int_0^T G_{x,p}(t)\, dt$ is the k-space offset, which is proportional to the prephasing gradient area. With the phase given by Eq. (8.3), the NMR signal $S_{x,p}$ in the transverse plane can be obtained by summing up all the isochromat vectors weighted by their spin densities: $\rho_{x_1}, \rho_{x_2}, \rho_{x_3}, \ldots, \rho_{x_n}$. Thus, we have:

$$S_{x,p} = \sum_{j=1}^n \rho_{x_j} e^{-i\phi_{x_j,p}} \approx \int_{-\infty}^{+\infty} \rho(x)e^{-i\phi_p(x)}dx \tag{8.4}$$

where $\rho(x)$ and $\phi_p(x)$ are the continuous representations of the spin density and the phase dispersion, respectively.

In a spin-echo pulse sequence, the 180° RF refocusing pulse negates the phase dispersion $\phi_p(x)$. After the 180° pulse, Eq. (8.4) becomes:

$$S'_{x,p} = \int_{-\infty}^{+\infty} \rho(x) e^{i\phi_p(x)}dx \tag{8.5}$$

At this point, when a readout gradient lobe $G_x(t)$ is applied, an additional phase dispersion is introduced to the spin isochromats:

$$\phi(x, t) = \gamma x \int_0^t G_x(t')dt' = 2\pi x k_x(t) \tag{8.6}$$

where the time origin is defined at the initial point of the readout gradient lobe (Figure 8.2). With this new phase, the NMR signal previously given by Eq. (8.5) becomes:

$$S(t) = \int_{-\infty}^{+\infty} \rho(x) e^{-i\left(\phi(x,t)-\phi_p(x)\right)} dx = \int_{-\infty}^{+\infty} \rho(x) e^{-i2\pi x\left(k_x(t)-k_{x,p}\right)} dx \quad (8.7)$$

At a specific time t_{echo} corresponding to $k_x(t_{echo}) = k_{x,p}$, the phase-dispersion term in Eq. (8.7) becomes 0, indicating that all spin isochromats are in phase and form an echo. Using the k-space expressions in Eqs. (8.3) and (8.6), we can readily see that at t_{echo}, the readout gradient area equals the prephasing gradient area:

$$\int_0^{t_{echo}} G_x(t) dt = \int_0^T G_{x,p}(t') dt' \quad (8.8)$$

t_{echo} defines the time point when the center of the k-space is sampled. If k-space is sampled symmetrically with respect to its center, then the readout gradient must be on for a time period $T_{acq}/2$, prior to t_{echo} (T_{acq} is the data acquisition time). This requires the readout gradient area to the left of t_{echo} be the same as the area of the entire pre-phasing gradient. During the time period $[t_{echo} - T_{acq}/2, t_{echo}]$, data points on the negative k_x axis are sampled (Figure 8.6). To sample the k-space points on the positive k_x axis, the readout gradient remains active for an additional time period $T_{acq}/2$ after t_{echo}. This produces a symmetric k-space line spanning $-k_{x,p}$ to $+k_{x,p}$ (Figure 8.6). If the pulse sequence is designed so that the peak of the 180° refocusing pulse occurs exactly midway between the peak of the 90° pulse and t_{echo}, then the off-resonance effect is minimized, which is highly desirable for many applications.

In a gradient-echo sequence, because the prephasing gradient and the readout gradient have opposite polarities, the magnetization during the readout gradient can also be described by Eq. (8.7). In this case, a gradient echo is produced when:

$$-\int_0^T G_{x,p}(t) dt = \int_0^{t_{echo}} G_x(t) dt \quad (8.9)$$

where the time point t_{echo} is defined similarly to that of the spin-echo pulse sequence. Although the readout gradient can be applied symmetrically with respect to t_{echo} in order to acquire the k-space data from $-k_{x,p}$ to $+k_{x,p}$

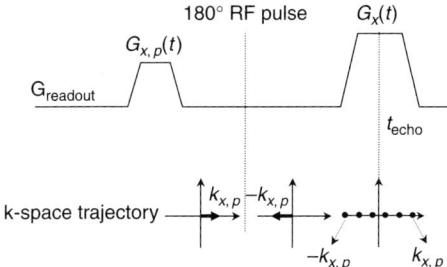

FIGURE 8.6 k-space sampling during the frequency-encoding gradients in a spin-echo pulse sequence. The k-space offset $k_{x,p}$ is determined by the prephasing gradient lobe $G_{x,p}(t)$ and negated by the 180° refocusing RF pulse. k-space sampling is accomplished during the readout gradient lobe, as denoted by the dots ranging from $-k_{x,p}$ to $k_{x,p}$.

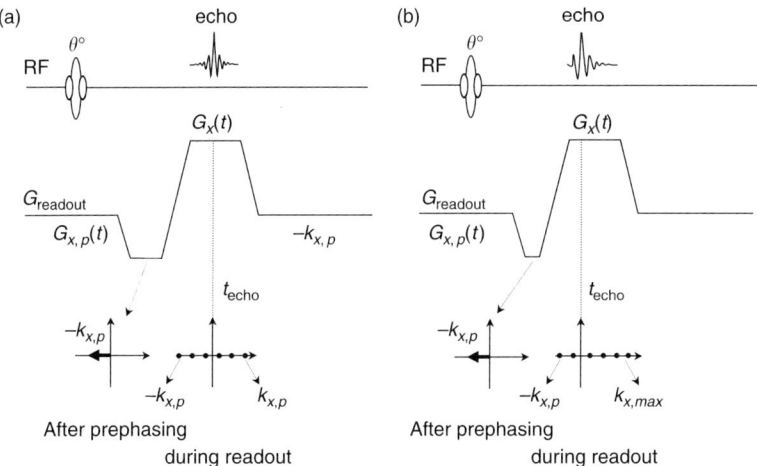

FIGURE 8.7 k-space sampling during the frequency-encoding gradients in a gradient-echo pulse sequence. (a) Full echo acquisition. (b) Partial echo acquisition. The k-space offset $k_{x,p}$ is determined by the prephasing gradient lobe $G_{x,p}(t)$, and k-space sampling is accomplished during the readout gradient lobe. The absolute value of the prephasing gradient area in (b) is smaller than in (a).

(Figure 8.7a), it can also be applied asymmetrically to acquire fewer data points before t_{echo} (Figure 8.7b). This acquisition technique, known as partial or fractional echo (Section 14.1), can considerably reduce the minimum echo time and the gradient moments. Thus, it is widely used for angiographic and cardiac applications.

8.1.3 IMPLEMENTATION

Readout Gradient Design   The duration of data acquisition T_{acq} is determined by the receiver bandwidth $\pm\Delta\nu$ and the number of k-space data points along the readout direction n_x:

$$T_{\text{acq}} = \frac{n_x}{2\Delta\nu} = \frac{1}{\Delta\nu_{\text{pp}}} \tag{8.10}$$

where $\Delta\nu_{\text{pp}}$ is the bandwidth per pixel. Given the FOV along the readout direction L_x, the amplitude of the readout gradient plateau can be readily derived from Eq. (1.30):

$$\Delta k_x = \frac{1}{n_x \Delta x} = \frac{1}{L_x} \tag{8.11}$$

and the k-space expression for a constant readout gradient is given by:

$$\Delta k_x = \frac{\gamma G_x \Delta t}{2\pi} = \frac{\gamma G T_{\text{acq}}}{2\pi n_x} \tag{8.12}$$

where Δt is the sampling time or dwell time (i.e., the time it takes to acquire one complex point of data), and $T_{\text{acq}} = \Delta t \cdot n_x$. Combining Eqs. (8.10), (8.11), and (8.12), we obtain:

$$G_x = \frac{4\pi \, \Delta\nu}{\gamma L_x} \tag{8.13}$$

Equation (8.13) can also be obtained by simply matching the spin precession bandwidth across the FOV (i.e., $(\gamma/2\pi)G_x L_x$) with the full receiver bandwidth (i.e., $2\Delta\nu$).

Equation (8.13) indicates that the higher the readout gradient amplitude, the smaller the FOV that can be achieved. Thus, when the receiver bandwidth is fixed, a strong readout gradient amplitude is crucial to imaging small subjects. Although a smaller FOV can also be achieved by reducing the receiver bandwidth, that approach leads to a longer data acquisition time (Eq. 8.10) and makes the image more susceptible to flow effects and off-resonance (e.g., chemical shift) artifacts.

The finite maximal slew rate of any practical gradient system does not allow the readout gradient to reach its target value instantaneously. Thus, a gradient ramp is required to increase the readout gradient from 0 to its plateau amplitude. Similarly, at the end of acquisition, another gradient ramp is needed to return the gradient to 0 amplitude. When linear gradient ramps are used, the minimal duration of the ramp (T_{ramp}) is limited by the maximal gradient slew rate S_R; $T_{\text{ramp}} \geq G_x/S_R$.

Pre-phasing Gradient Design   Once the readout gradient lobe has been determined, the prephasing gradient lobe can be calculated depending on whether a full echo or fractional echo is acquired. In a full-echo acquisition where $t_{echo} = T_{acq}/2$, the prephasing gradient area is calculated using Eqs. (8.8) and (8.9) for spin echo and gradient echo, respectively. In a partial-echo acquisition, if $n_{x,f}$ points are acquired prior to the center of the echo $(n_{x,f} \leq n_x/2)$, then t_{echo} can be calculated:

$$t_{echo} = T_{ramp} + \frac{n_{x,f}}{2\Delta\nu} \tag{8.14}$$

Once t_{echo} is known, the area of the prephasing gradient can be determined using Eq. (8.8) or Eq. (8.9). Theoretically, there is no requirement on the amplitude of the prephasing gradient as long as the area satisfies Eq. (8.8) or Eq. (8.9). This gives us some flexibility in choosing prephasing gradient lobes. For example, the maximal gradient amplitude can be used to minimize the echo time for applications such as angiography. Alternatively, a smaller gradient amplitude with a longer duration can be employed to reduce the effects of eddy currents and concomitant magnetic fields. The latter is particularly important in fast imaging at low magnetic field or with strong gradients (Section 10.1). An example on how to design readout gradient and prephasing gradient waveforms is given next.

Example 8.1   An MRI scanner has a maximal gradient amplitude of 22 mT/m and a slew rate of 120 T/m/s. An image reconstructed with 256^2 matrix is acquired from this scanner using a receiver bandwidth of $\Delta\nu = \pm62.5$ kHz on a FOV of 24 cm. Partial Fourier k-space data acquisition is employed to sample a k-space matrix of 224 (readout) by 256 (phase-encoding). Assume 96 points are acquired before the echo peak. If a gradient-echo pulse sequence is used, design (a) trapezoidal readout and (b) prephasing gradient waveforms that minimize the TE.

Answer

(a) Readout gradient. The readout gradient plateau amplitude can be readily calculated using Eq. (8.13):

$$G_x = \frac{4\pi\,\Delta\nu}{\gamma\,L_x} = \frac{4\times\pi\times62.5\times10^3}{2.675\times10^8\times0.24} = 1.223 \times 10^{-2}\,\text{T/m} = 12.23\,\text{mT/m} \tag{8.15}$$

This gradient strength is well below the maximum allowed (22 mT/m) on the scanner. The duration of the data acquisition can be obtained from Eq. (8.10):

$$T_{acq} = \frac{n_x}{2\Delta\nu} = \frac{224}{2\times62.5\times10^3} = 1.792\times10^{-3}\,\text{s} = 1.792\,\text{ms} \tag{8.16}$$

To minimize the TE, the maximal slew rate will be used. Thus, the trapezoidal gradient ramps (ascending and descending ramps) are:

$$T_{\text{ramp}} = \frac{G_x}{S_R} = \frac{1.223 \times 10^{-2}}{120} = 1.019 \times 10^{-4}\,\text{s} = 101.9\,\mu\text{s} \quad (8.17)$$

At this point, all the parameters for a trapezoidal readout waveform are determined.

(b) Prephasing gradient. To design the prephasing gradient, we first determine the center of echo t_{echo} using Eq. (8.14). Because we assume that 96 points are acquired prior to the echo center, $n_{x,f}$ in Eq. (8.14) equals 96. Accordingly, t_{echo} is:

$$t_{\text{echo}} = T_{\text{ramp}} + \frac{n_{x,f}}{2\Delta\nu} = 1.019 \times 10^{-4} + \frac{96}{2 \times 62.5 \times 10^3}$$

$$= 8.699 \times 10^{-4}\,\text{s} \quad (8.18)$$

The area (absolute value) of the prephasing lobe is equal to the area of the readout lobe to the left of the echo peak, and is given by:

$$A_p = G_x \left(\frac{T_{\text{ramp}}}{2} + \frac{n_{x,f}}{2\Delta\nu} \right) = 1.002 \times 10^{-5}\,\text{Ts/m} \quad (8.19)$$

Because:

$$A_p \geq hr = \frac{h^2}{S_R} = \frac{(0.022\,\text{T/m})^2}{120\,\text{T/m/s}} = 4.033 \times 10^{-6}\,\text{Ts/m} \quad (8.20)$$

Section 7.1 indicates that the most efficient shape for the prephasing lobe is a trapezoid with plateau amplitude:

$$G_{x,p} = -22\,\text{mT/m} \quad (8.21)$$

and ramp time:

$$T_{\text{ramp},p} = \frac{|G_{x,p}|}{S_R} = \frac{22 \times 10^{-3}}{120} = 1.833 \times 10^{-4}\,\text{s} \quad (8.22)$$

Finally, the plateau duration T_p of the prephasing gradient can be determined from:

$$T_p = \frac{A_p}{|G_p|} - T_{\text{ramp},p} = 2.720 \times 10^{-4}\,\text{s} = 272\,\mu\text{s} \quad (8.23)$$

Off-Center FOV In many applications, the region of interest (e.g., the shoulder) cannot be positioned at or near the gradient isocenter. To center the object in the FOV along the frequency-encoded direction, the frequency-encoding gradient waveform does not need to be redesigned. Instead, to offset the FOV by δx in the readout direction, the RF receiver frequency is offset by δv_{oc}:

$$\delta v_{oc} = \frac{\gamma}{2\pi} G_x \delta x \qquad (8.24)$$

This approach is analogous to adjusting the transmitter frequency for an off-center slice or modulating the receiver phase to achieve off-center FOV in the phase-encoded direction.

Time-Varying Readout Gradient Although the readout gradient is typically held constant during data acquisition, time-varying gradients can also be used during readout. Examples of time-varying readout gradient can be found in spiral scans (Section 17.6), echo planar imaging with sinusoidal gradients (Section 16.1), sampling during the gradient ramps (Section 16.1), twisted projection imaging (Boada et al. 1997), and concentric circular sampling (Zhou et al. 1998). With a time-varying readout gradient, the k-space sampling often becomes nonuniform. Data resampling is typically required prior to image reconstruction using fast Fourier transforms. Time-varying readout gradients and data resampling are discussed in more detail in Sections 16.1, 17.6, and 13.2.

SELECTED REFERENCES

Boada, F. E., Gillen, J. S., Shen, G. X., Chang, S. Y., and Thulborn, K. R. 1997. Fast three dimensional sodium imaging. *Magn. Reson. Med.* 37: 706–715.

Edelstein, W. A., Hutchison, J. M. S., Johnson, G., and Redpath, T. 1980. Spin warp nmr imaging and applications to human whole-body imaging. *Phys. Med. Biol.* 25: 751–756.

Kumar, A., Welti, D., and Ernst, R. 1975. NMR fourier zeugmatography. *J. Magn. Reson.* 18: 69–83.

Lauterbur, P. C. 1973. Image formation by induced local interactions—examples employing nuclear magnetic resonance. *Nature* 242: 190–191.

RELATED SECTIONS

8.2 Phase-Encoding Gradients

Spatial localization in MR usually employs both phase and frequency encoding. With frequency encoding, the precession frequency of the magnetization is spatially varied across the object in a linear relation with position by applying a gradient lobe during the data readout, as described in Section 8.1. The idea behind phase encoding is to also create a linear spatial variation of the phase of the magnetization, as shown in Figure 8.8. (The phase is the angle made by the transverse magnetization vector with respect to some fixed axis in the transverse plane). Phase encoding is implemented by applying a gradient lobe while the magnetization is in the transverse plane (Figure 8.9), but before the readout. By varying the area under the phase encoding gradient lobe, different amounts of the linear phase variation are introduced. The resultant signals can be reconstructed with Fourier transforms to recover spatial information about the object. Phase encoding is used with Cartesian k-space sampling (Section 11.2) and is typically used to spatially encode information orthogonal to the frequency-encoded direction.

Phase encoding is also sometimes called Fourier encoding. 3D volume acquisitions use phase or Fourier encoding in the slice direction, sometimes called *slice encoding* or *secondary phase encoding* to distinguish it from the primary phase-encoded direction. In principle, there is no difference between

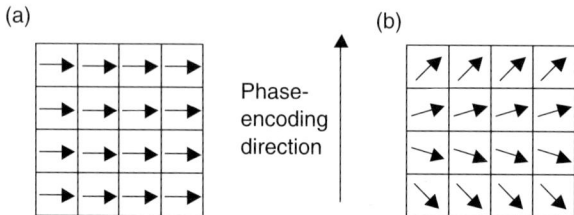

FIGURE 8.8 The object is divided into 16 pixels. The arrows represent transverse magnetization at the center of each pixel. (a) At the end of the RF excitation pulse, the transverse magnetization has the same phase (direction) in each pixel. (b) After a phase-encoding gradient is applied, the phase of the transverse magnetization varies at each location along the phase-encoded direction.

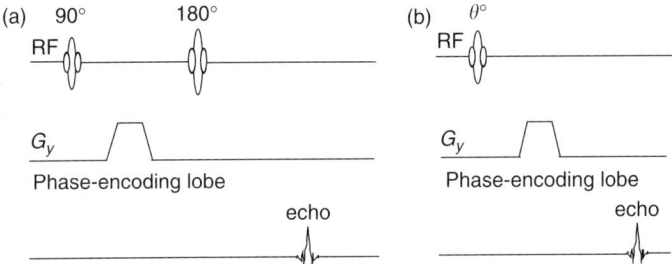

FIGURE 8.9 A phase-encoding gradient lobe in (a) a spin-echo pulse sequence and (b) a gradient-echo pulse sequence. For the spin-echo pulse sequence, the gradient lobe can occur either before or after the RF refocusing pulse.

the phase encoding applied in the two directions. In this section, phase encoding for 2D acquisitions is discussed. More information about the two-axis phase encoding used in 3D volume acquisitions is found in Section 11.6. In some applications, such as some spectroscopic imaging (or chemical-shift imaging) techniques (Brown, Kincaid, Ugurbil 1982), spatial localization is achieved without frequency encoding, and only phase encoding is used. Non-Cartesian k-space trajectories, such as spirals (Section 17.6), do not use phase encoding, except sometimes in the slice direction for 3D scans.

8.2.1 MATHEMATICAL DESCRIPTION

Despite the fact the phase and frequency encoding both introduce a spatially varying linear phase, they can be analyzed independently from one another. Therefore, in the following analysis we ignore the frequency-encoded direction and consider an object that varies only in one direction. For this analysis we use the convention that the object's effective magnetization includes the B_1 receive-field weighting, relaxation effects, and diffusion weighting. During the application of the phase-encoding gradient lobe, the nuclear spin precession frequency varies linearly in the direction of the gradient. For a y phase-encoding gradient G_y, the angular frequency of precession in the B_0 rotating reference frame (Section 1.2) is:

$$\omega = \gamma G_y y \tag{8.25}$$

The phase ϕ (in radians) of the transverse magnetization at the end of the phase-encoding pulse is:

$$\phi(y) = y\gamma \int_0^T G_y(t')dt' = 2\pi k_y y \tag{8.26}$$

where the G_y lobe has duration T, and k-space location k_y is defined as in Section 11.2. The signal detected is the vector sum of the magnetization of all the nuclear spins in the object. It is conventional to combine the two spatial components of the magnetization that are perpendicular to the static field into a complex number (see Section 1.2). The effective magnetization becomes $M_\perp = M_x + i M_y$. The signal is then the phase-sensitive or complex sum of the magnetization of all the spins. For a one-dimensional object, the k-space signal $S(k_y)$ is:

$$S(k_y) = \int M_\perp(y)\, e^{-i\phi(y)}\, dy \tag{8.27}$$

Approximating the integral in Eq. (8.27) as a discrete sum and using Eq. (8.26) gives:

$$S(k_y) = \sum_{n=0}^{N-1} M_\perp(n\Delta y)e^{-2\pi i (n\Delta y)k_y} \tag{8.28}$$

where $y = n\Delta y$, and Δy and N are the pixel size and number of pixels, respectively. Repeating the phase encoding N times for N different values of G_y produces N different sets of phase-encoding twists, or k_y values (Figure 8.10). This provides sufficient information for $M_\perp(n\Delta y)$ to be reconstructed.

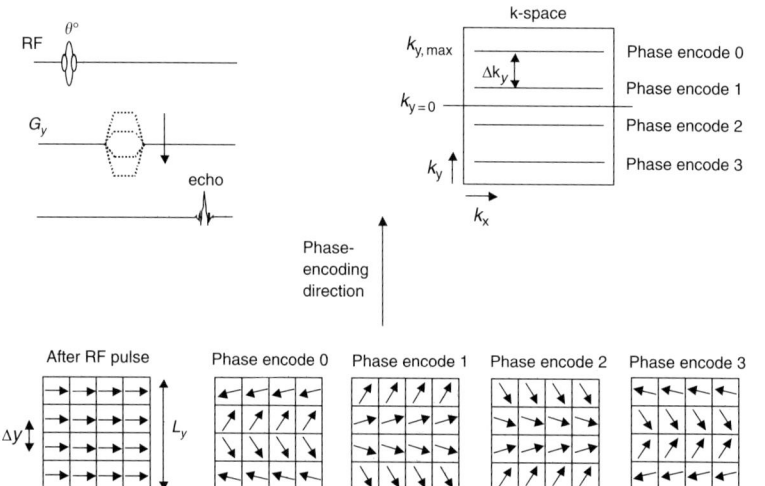

FIGURE 8.10 A gradient-echo pulse sequence with four phase-encoding steps. Each step corresponds to one of the four phase-encoding lobes (dotted lines), with the arrow indicating the view order for a sequential acquisition. Each phase-encoding step is associated with a separate k-space line and imparts a different twist in magnetization phase across the object in the y direction.

For N phase-encoding lines, the area covered in k-space is $(N-1)\Delta k_y$, where Δk_y is the k-space phase-encoding step size (Figure 8.10). Usually an even number of phase-encoding lines are used and the locations are usually chosen to straddle the $k_y = 0$ location. For N phase-encoding steps that are acquired sequentially starting at the top edge of k-space:

$$k_y(m) = k_{y,\max} - m\Delta k_y \qquad m = 0, 1, \ldots, N-1 \qquad (8.29)$$

where $k_{y,\max}$ is the starting (top edge) phase-encoding location (Figure 8.10) given by:

$$k_{y,\max} = \frac{1}{2}(N-1)\Delta k_y \qquad (8.30)$$

The resulting phase-encoding k-space locations are:

$$k_y(m) = \left(\frac{N-1}{2} - m\right)\Delta k_y \qquad (8.31)$$

The signal is:

$$S(m) = \sum_{n=0}^{N-1} M_\perp(n\Delta y)e^{-2\pi i(n\Delta y)((N-1)/2-m)\Delta k_y} \qquad m = 0, \ldots, N-1$$

$$(8.32)$$

To satisfy the Nyquist criterion, and as explained in Section 1.1, the phase-encoding step size Δk_y must be chosen so that:

$$\Delta k_y = \frac{1}{L_y} = \frac{1}{N\Delta y} \qquad (8.33)$$

where $L_y = N\Delta y$ is the y FOV. Equation (8.33) also implies that the maximum k-space sampling extent is related to image pixel size by:

$$N\Delta k_y = \frac{1}{\Delta y} \qquad (8.34)$$

Using Eq. (8.33), Eq. (8.32) becomes:

$$S(m) = \sum_{n=0}^{N-1} M_\perp(n\Delta y)e^{-\pi in(N-1)/N}e^{-2\pi imn/N} \qquad (8.35)$$

The factor $e^{-\pi in(N-1)/N}$ in Eq. (8.35) can be thought of as simply part of the phase of $M_\perp$ and can be ignored when a magnitude image is reconstructed.

(The factor must be accounted for when complex images are reconstructed.) An image representing the resulting effective magnetization can be recovered from the discrete inverse Fourier transform (Section 1.1) of the k-space phase-encoded data:

$$M_\perp(n\Delta y)e^{-\pi in(N-1)/N} = \frac{1}{N}\sum_{m=0}^{N-1} S(m)e^{2\pi imn/N} \qquad (8.36)$$

The factor $e^{-\pi in(N-1)/N}$ in Eq. (8.36) can be rewritten as $e^{-\pi in(N-1)/N} = (-1)^n e^{-\pi in/N}$. The factor $(-1)^n$ toggles the sign of every pixel. For the visualization of real, imaginary, or phase images, this factor is usually removed after the image is reconstructed. The remaining phase factor $e^{-\pi in/N}$ in Eq. (8.36) is usually ignored because it only puts a small phase slope across the image.

If the phase-encoding step size is chosen so that it is larger than in Eq. (8.33), aliasing will occur, in which replicates of the object overlap or wrap around in the phase-encoded direction of the image (Figure 8.11). Some aliasing is tolerable if anatomy of interest is not obscured. Note that aliasing is removed in the frequency-encoding direction using the anti-aliasing bandpass filter in the receiver (Section 11.1). This is not possible for phase encoding.

8.2.2 IMPLEMENTATION

The phase-encoding gradient may occur any time after the RF excitation pulse and before the readout. For spin-echo pulse sequences, it may be placed either before or after the refocusing pulse. The advantage of placing the phase-encoding gradient after the refocusing pulse is a decrease in oblique flow displacement artifacts (Section 10.4). The disadvantage is that the FID coming from the nonideal refocusing pulse (i.e., flip angle $\neq 180°$), as well as any stimulated echoes, are also phase-encoded. This may result in image artifacts that are more difficult to remove than if the FID and stimulated echoes were not phase-encoded. The phase-encoding gradient waveform can overlap other gradient lobes such as the slice-selection rephasing, crusher, and readout dephasing lobes. In contrast, the frequency-encoding gradient cannot overlap with any other gradient lobes during the readout. Many pulse sequences such as true FISP (Section 14.1) or RARE (Section 16.4) rewind the phase-encoding gradient after the readout (Figure 8.12) to rephase the transverse magnetization and make it more consistent between phase-encoding steps. In doing so, certain signal loss can be avoided and artifacts can be minimized.

For practical implementation, the phase-encoding gradient lobe usually has the same shape and time duration for each phase-encoding step and the amplitude is scaled to give the desired k_y. This method, called spin-warp

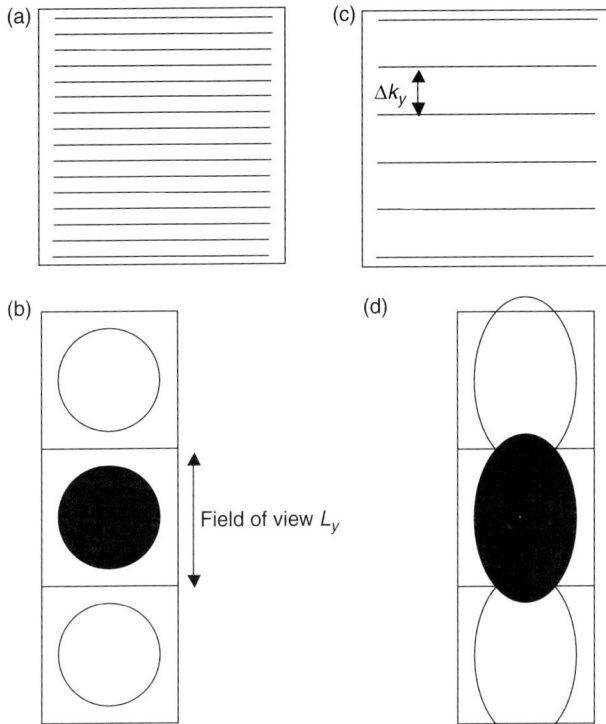

FIGURE 8.11 Discrete Fourier sampling causes the object to replicate in the phase-encoded direction. In (a) the phase-encoding steps are close enough that in the image (b) the replicates do not overlap and no aliasing occurs. In (c) the phase-encoding steps are further apart and in the image (d) the replicates do overlap and aliasing or wraparound artifacts result.

imaging (Edelstein et al. 1980) is different from earlier MRI pulse sequences (Kumar et al. 1975) that used constant amplitude but unequal time duration for the phase-encoding gradients in order to vary k_y. By keeping the phase-encoding lobe duration fixed, the spin-warp method keeps TE fixed for all phase-encoding steps, which has the advantage of providing the same T_2 decay and off-resonant phase accumulation. The lobe shape is typically chosen to be a trapezoid, although other choices such as one-half of a sine-wave cycle have also been used.

Pulse sequences that collect a single Cartesian line of k-space for each excitation typically collect the k_y lines starting at one edge of k-space and moving continuously to the other edge (sometimes called a *sequential* or

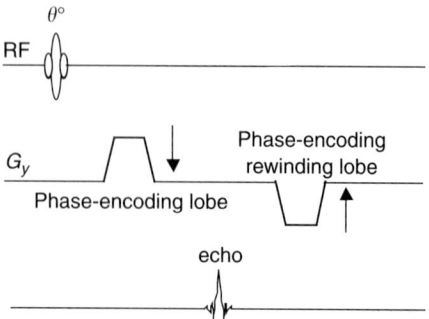

FIGURE 8.12 A gradient-echo pulse sequence that uses a phase-encode rewinding gradient. For each phase-encoding step, the rewinding gradient area is the negative of the phase-encoding gradient area. Therefore they are stepped in opposite directions (arrows).

top-down method). Echo train pulse sequences that collect multiple k_y lines for each excitation, such as echo planar imaging (EPI), (Section 16.1) or RARE (Section 16.4), may collect the lines in a different order. Phase-encoding orders that first acquire the central lines of k-space are called *centric* (Holsinger and Riederer 1990). Those view orders that start acquisition from the k-space edge and end at the central k-space lines are called *reverse-centric*. A more detailed discussion on phase-encoding orders for 2D imaging can be found in Section 11.5. In 3D acquisitions, the view orders for both phase-encoding axes are sometimes sorted to start at the center of the $k_y - k_z$ plane and then to move radially outward based on the distance to the center of k-space (the *elliptical centric* view order, Section 11.6).

The area under the largest phase-encoding lobe $A_{y,\max}$ can be calculated from:

$$\frac{\gamma}{2\pi} A_{y,\max} = k_{y,\max} \tag{8.37}$$

Using Eqs. (8.30), (8.33), and (8.37) gives:

$$A_{y,\max} = \frac{\pi (N - 1)}{\gamma L_y} \tag{8.38}$$

To minimize TR, the phase-encoding lobes are made as short as possible. The phase-encoding steps at the edges of k-space therefore use the maximum gradient amplitude and maximum slew rate.

In full Fourier encoding, lines are collected symmetrically around the $k_y = 0$ line (Figure 8.13). In partial Fourier encoding, one-half of k-space is fully filled and the other half is only partially filled. The missing data are

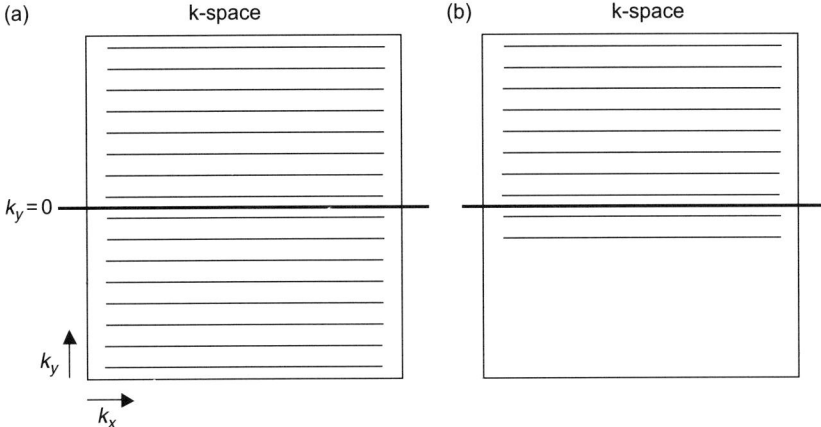

FIGURE 8.13 (a) Full Fourier encoding with 16 lines collected in k-space. (b) Partial Fourier encoding with 10 lines collected in k-space. Each line of k-space corresponds to a frequency-encoded readout.

either replaced with zeros or restored using an algorithm based on Hermitian conjugate symmetry or some other consistency criterion (Section 13.4). The number of phase-encoding steps does not have to be a power of two, but it is typically an even number. If a power of two is not used, the uncollected k-space lines can be symmetrically zero-filled on both sides of k-space so that the Fourier transform size is a power of two, enabling the use of FFTs (Section 13.1).

In 2D imaging, k-space is usually sampled so that the FOV is the same in both directions; that is, $\Delta k_x = \Delta k_y$. If the object extent is smaller in one direction (e.g., it has an oval shape), the total acquisition time can be reduced by selecting the phase-encoding direction along the smaller extent and increasing Δk_y to reduce the phase-encoding FOV. The frequency-encoding FOV and the spatial resolution determined by the maximal extent in k-space are also held fixed in both directions. This is sometimes called *rectangular* or *fractional field of view*. Because the image SNR is proportional to the voxel volume and the square root of the imaging time, fractional FOV carries an SNR penalty. For example, the SNR in a 3/4 FOV image is $\sqrt{0.75} = 86.6\%$ of the full FOV value.

In many applications, the region of interest (e.g., the shoulder) cannot be positioned at or near the gradient isocenter. In this case, an off-center FOV is required. According to the shift theorem for Fourier transforms (Section 1.1), to shift the image in the FOV along the phase-encoded direction, a linear phase ramp is applied to the data prior to the Fourier transform. The phase can be added at a variety of stages during the imaging processing, including the RF carrier during excitation or demodulation, or during the reconstruction prior to the Fourier transform in the phase-encoded direction. If the required FOV offset is δy in the phase-encoded direction, Eq. (8.36) is modified according to the shift theorem:

$$|M_\perp(\delta y + n\Delta y)| = \left| \frac{1}{N} \sum_{m=0}^{N-1} S(m)e^{2\pi i m(n + \delta y/\Delta y)/N} \right|$$

$$= \left| \frac{1}{N} \sum_{m=0}^{N-1} \left[S(m)e^{2\pi i m \delta y/L_y} \right] e^{2\pi i mn/N} \right| \qquad (8.39)$$

From Eq. (8.39), the applied phase increment to achieve an off-center FOV is $2\pi \delta y/L_y$ per phase-encoding step. Note that δy need not be an integer multiple of the pixel dimension.

Example 8.2 An MRI scanner has a maximal gradient amplitude of 22 mT/m and a slew rate of 120 T/m/s. A 256^2 image is acquired with a FOV of 24 cm and 256 phase-encoding steps. If a trapezoidal phase-encoding pulse is used, calculate the gradient waveform parameters (amplitudes and time durations) for each phase-encoding step, assuming a sequential phase-encoding order.

Answer To simplify the implementation, the same ramp and plateau widths will be used for each encoding step. From Eq. (8.38), $A_{y,\max} > hr$ (see Section 7.1), so for the maximal phase-encoding step, an amplitude of $\pm h = \pm 22$ mT/m will be used. The ramp time is therefore equal to r:

$$r = \frac{2.2 \times 10^{-2} \text{ T/m}}{120 \text{ T/m/s}} = 1.83 \times 10^{-4} \text{ s} = 183 \text{ } \mu\text{s} \qquad (8.40)$$

The k_y location for phase-encoding step n is:

$$k_y(n) = \frac{\gamma}{2\pi} \int_0^T G_y(n, t')dt' = \frac{\gamma}{2\pi} G_y(n) (r + T_{\text{plateau}}) \qquad (8.41)$$

where T_{plateau} is the plateau time for the phase-encoding lobe and $G_y(n)$ is the plateau amplitude for step n ($n = 0, \ldots, 255$). Also, according to Eq. (8.31):

$$k_y(n) = (127.5 - n)\Delta k_y \qquad (8.42)$$

where the phase-encoding step size is:

$$\Delta k_y = \frac{1}{L_y} = \frac{1}{0.24} \text{ m}^{-1} \qquad (8.43)$$

For the maximal phase-encoding step ($n = 0$), Eq. (8.42) gives:

$$k_y(0) = 127.5 \times \Delta k_y = \frac{127.5}{0.24} \, \text{m}^{-1} \tag{8.44}$$

Also for the maximal phase-encoding step, $G_y(0) = 22 \, \text{mT/m}$. The plateau time is then found using Eqs. (8.41) with Eq. (8.44):

$$\frac{127.5}{0.24} \, \text{m}^{-1} = (42.57 \, \text{MHz/T})(2.2 \times 10^{-2} \text{T/m})(1.83 \times 10^{-4} \, \text{s} + T_{\text{plateau}}) \tag{8.45}$$

$$T_{\text{plateau}} = 3.84 \times 10^{-4} = 384 \, \mu\text{s}.$$

The phase-encoding gradient step size is found from:

$$\Delta k_y = \frac{\gamma}{2\pi} \Delta G_y (r + T_{\text{plateau}}) \tag{8.46}$$

$$\Delta G_y = 1.73 \times 10^{-4} \, \text{T/m} = 0.173 \, \text{mT/m}$$

Alternatively ΔG_y can be found by using:

$$\Delta G_y = [G_y(0) - G_y(255)]/255$$

$$= [22 \, \text{mT/m} - (-22 \, \text{mT/m})] / 255 = 0.173 \, \text{mT/m}$$

SELECTED REFERENCES

Brown, T. R., Kincaid, B. M., and Ugurbil, K. 1992. NMR chemical shift imaging in three dimensions. *Proc. Natl. Acad. Sci. (USA).* 79: 3523–3526.

Edelstein, W. A., Hutchison, J. M., Johnson, G., and Redpath, T. 1980. Spin warp NMR imaging and applications to human whole-body imaging. *Phys. Med. Biol.* 25: 751–756.

Holsinger, A. E., and Riederer, S. J. 1990. The importance of phase-encoding order in ultra-short TR snapshot MR imaging. *Magn. Reson. Med.* 16: 481–488.

Kumar, A., Welti, D., and Ernst, R. R. 1975. NMR Fourier zeugmatography. *J. Magn. Reson.* 18: 69–83.

RELATED SECTIONS

Section 1.1 Fourier Transforms
Section 8.1 Frequency-Encoding Gradients
Section 11.2 k-Space
Section 11.5 Two-Dimensional Acquisition
Section 11.6 Three-Dimensional Acquisition
Section 13.1 Fourier Reconstruction
Section 13.4 Partial Fourier Reconstruction

8.3 Slice Selection Gradients

8.3.1 QUALITATIVE DESCRIPTION

Spatially selective RF pulses are used for many purposes in MR imaging, including excitation, refocusing, inversion, and spatial presaturation of magnetization. Each of these applications requires a *slice-selection gradient* (Wood and Wehrli 1999, 5–6; Lauterbur et al. 1975; Mansfield et al. 1976; Hoult 1977) to achieve the desired spatial localization. (In imaging, slices are perhaps more properly called sections, or partitions, but the term slice is in common use, especially in conjunction with the selection gradient.) The slice-selection gradient is typically a constant gradient that is played concurrently with the selective RF pulse (Figure 8.14). (An exception is the gradient for a variable-rate RF pulse, which is not constant and which is described in Section 2.4.) Typically the slice-selection gradient is straddled by ramps to form a slice-selection lobe. If the RF pulse performs excitation, then a *slice-rephasing* lobe usually follows the slice-selection gradient.

Modulating the RF envelope with a predetermined shape, such as the SINC waveform shown in Figure 8.14 generates a selective RF pulse. This process is described in more detail in Sections 2.2 and 3.1. The RF *bandwidth* Δf (expressed in hertz) is a measure of the range of frequencies contained in the RF pulse. The slice-selection gradient translates the band of frequencies into the desired band of locations, corresponding to the slice (see Figure 4.12). As

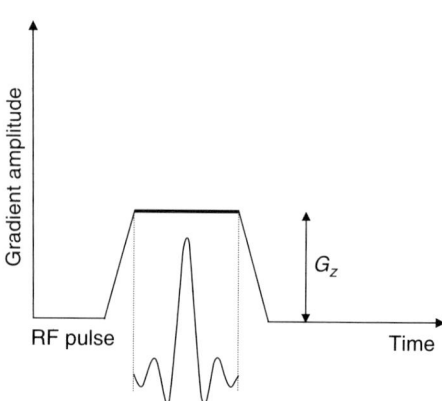

FIGURE 8.14 The slice-selection gradient (boldline) is a constant gradient played concurrently with a selective RF pulse. The amplitude of the slice-selection gradient, G_z, and RF pulse bandwidth determine the slice thickness.

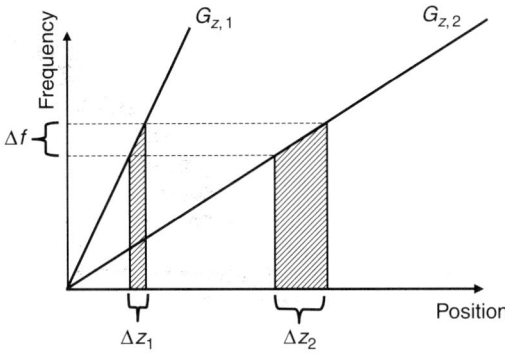

FIGURE 8.15 Plot of Larmor frequency versus position along the direction of the slice-selection gradient. The slope of each of the two lines represents the strength of a slice-selection gradient ($G_{z,1}$ and $G_{z,2}$). For any given bandwidth Δf of the RF pulse, the stronger gradient produces a thinner slice Δz_1.

shown on Figure 8.15 increasing the amplitude of the slice-selection gradient decreases the thickness of the slice for a fixed RF bandwidth.

Any of the three orthogonal gradients (or a vector combination of the gradients) can be used for slice selection. The gradient direction determines the *normal*, or line perpendicular to the plane of the slice. For example, in a horizontal cylindrical bore magnet, using the Z physical gradient for slice selection produces an axial slice. In order to produce a slice oriented in any arbitrary oblique direction, a linear combination of the three physical gradients is applied simultaneously.

Usually the desired slice plane does not pass through the point where all three gradient coils produce zero magnetic fields (i.e., the isocenter of the gradients), which typically is the same point as the isocenter of the magnet. In this case, the desired slice offset δz is obtained by shifting the carrier frequency of the RF by an amount δf, as shown in Figure 8.16. The required amount of frequency shift is proportional to the desired offset (e.g., in centimeters) and the amplitude of the slice-selection gradient.

8.3.2 MATHEMATICAL DESCRIPTION

The Larmor frequency of precession is related to the net magnetic field B by:

$$f = \frac{\gamma}{2\pi} B \tag{8.47}$$

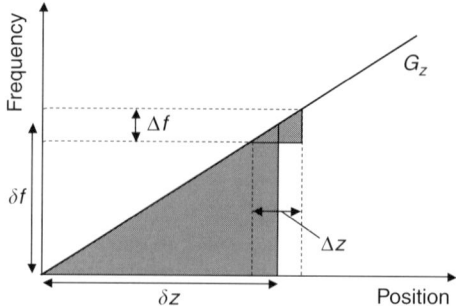

FIGURE 8.16 In order to offset the center of a slice by a distance δz from gradient isocenter, the RF carrier frequency is offset by an amount δf from the Larmor frequency. The two shaded triangles are similar, which is the origin of the proportionality relationship in Eq. (8.54).

Denoting the slice-selection gradient by the vector $\vec{G}_s$ the Larmor frequency can be expressed in terms of the vector dot product:

$$f = \frac{\gamma}{2\pi}\left(B_0 + \vec{G}_s \cdot \vec{r}\right) \qquad (8.48)$$

where B_0 is the main magnetic field, and $\vec{r}$ is a displacement vector from the gradient isocenter, that is, $\vec{r} = (0, 0, 0)$, to location (X, Y, Z) in a physical coordinate system (see Section 7.3). If the RF carrier frequency is set to the Larmor frequency at gradient isocenter, then the B_0 term in Eq. (8.48) vanishes in the rotating reference frame (Section 1.2):

$$f_{\text{ROT}} = f - \frac{\gamma B_0}{2\pi} = \frac{\gamma \vec{G}_s \cdot \vec{r}}{2\pi} \qquad (8.49)$$

The displacement vector can be decomposed into the two components that are parallel and perpendicular to the slice direction:

$$\vec{r} = \vec{r}_{\parallel} + \vec{r}_{\perp} \qquad (8.50)$$

Because $\vec{G}_s \cdot \vec{r}_{\perp} = 0$, Eq. (8.49) becomes:

$$f_{\text{ROT}} = f - \frac{\gamma B_0}{2\pi} = \frac{\gamma \vec{G}_s \cdot \vec{r}_{\parallel}}{2\pi}. \qquad (8.51)$$

If the RF pulse contains a bandwidth of frequencies Δf, then:

$$\Delta f_{\text{ROT}} = \Delta f = \frac{\gamma}{2\pi}\vec{G}_s \cdot \Delta \vec{r}_{\parallel} \qquad (8.52)$$

From Eq. (8.52), only displacement along the direction of the slice-selection gradient affects the resonant frequency. Therefore, the normal of the selected slice is parallel to the slice-selection gradient. Denoting the magnitude of the slice-selection gradient by G_z and the slice thickness by Δz, from Eq. (8.52), we can readily obtain:

$$\Delta z = \frac{2\pi \, \Delta f}{\gamma G_z} \tag{8.53}$$

(Recall that we use lowercase z to denote the slice direction, while uppercase Z denotes the physical Z axis. The two axes correspond only if an axial slice is prescribed, again assuming a horizontal cylindrical-bore magnet.) Equation (8.53) is a mathematical description of the situation depicted graphically in Figure 8.15: For a fixed RF bandwidth, thinner slices can be obtained by increasing the strength of the slice-selection gradient.

If the desired slice passes through the gradient isocenter, the RF carrier frequency is set to the nominal Larmor frequency of a set of spins (i.e., the precession frequency without any slice-selection gradient). For a more general slice that does not pass through the gradient isocenter, the RF carrier frequency must be changed. To determine the proper carrier frequency offset for those slices, we can set up a proportionality relationship between the sides of similar triangles shown in Figure 8.16, which yields:

$$\frac{\delta z}{\Delta z} = \frac{\delta f}{\Delta f} \tag{8.54}$$

From Eqs. (8.53) and (8.54), to offset the slice by a distance δz from the gradient isocenter the carrier frequency is adjusted by the amount:

$$\delta f = \frac{\gamma G_z \delta z}{2\pi} \tag{8.55}$$

or

$$\delta z = \frac{2\pi \, \delta f}{\gamma G_z} \tag{8.56}$$

Equation (8.56) has several interesting consequences. If the slice-selection gradient is not spatially uniform, the offset δz will also vary and the selected slice will not be planar. Instead, a potato-chip-shaped slice can result. This effect often occurs for large values of δz due to gradient nonlinearity and also whenever local gradient fields induced by magnetic-susceptibility variations perturb the slice-selection gradient. Also, if the system of spins contains multiple Larmor frequencies, selected slices for each component will be offset from one another. A common example is the chemical shift in the slice direction experienced by off-resonance spins in lipids (see Example 8.5.)

Example 8.3   Suppose the RF bandwidth is 1.0 kHz, and a 3-mm-thick slice is desired. What gradient amplitude should be used for the slice selection?

Answer   From Eq. (8.53):

$$G_z = \frac{2\pi \Delta f}{\gamma \Delta z} = \frac{1.0 \times 10^3 \text{ Hz}}{42.57 \times 10^6 \text{Hz/T} (0.003 \text{ m})} = 7.83 \text{ mT/m}$$

We note that gradient amplitude of -7.83 mT/m can be used as well, with the consequence that any nonzero carrier frequency offsets δf must also be negated, according to Eq. (8.55).

Example 8.4   The slice prescribed in Example 8.3 is oblique and includes the three points:

$$\vec{r}_1 = (11.1, 3.2, 4.7 \text{ cm})$$
$$\vec{r}_2 = (13.1, 2.0, 4.7 \text{ cm})$$
$$\vec{r}_3 = (9.1, 2.0, 6.2 \text{ cm})$$

What is the slice-selection gradient vector?

Answer   The direction of the slice-selection gradient vector is perpendicular to any vector that lies within the plane of the slice. Such in-plane vectors can be found by pairwise subtraction of the displacement vectors stated in the example. Therefore the desired slice-selection gradient vector can be calculated from the cross product:

$$\vec{G}_s = 7.83 \text{ mT/m} \frac{(\vec{r}_2 - \vec{r}_1) \times (\vec{r}_2 - \vec{r}_3)}{\|(\vec{r}_2 - \vec{r}_1) \times (\vec{r}_2 - \vec{r}_3)\|} = (2.373, 3.955, 6.328 \text{ mT/m})$$

$$(8.57)$$

The overall sign of the vector is determined by the choice of the sign of the offset frequency δf.

Example 8.5   At 1.5 T, water resonates approximately $f_{cs} = 210$ Hz higher than lipids (i.e., fat). If the amplitude of the slice-selection gradient is $+11$ mT/m, what is the slice-selection offset caused by chemical shift?

Answer   Setting $\delta f = f_{cs}$ in Eq. (8.56), the offset due to chemical shift is:

$$\delta z = \frac{2\pi f_{cs}}{\gamma G_z} = \frac{210 \text{ Hz}}{42.57 \times 10^6 \text{Hz/T} (11 \text{ mT/m})} = 0.45 \text{ mm}$$

If the slice-selection gradient takes a negative value instead (i.e., -11 mT/m), then the offset due to chemical shift will reverse its sign; that is, the shift will be in the opposite direction. Plots such as Figure 8.15 are very useful for determining the direction of the shift.

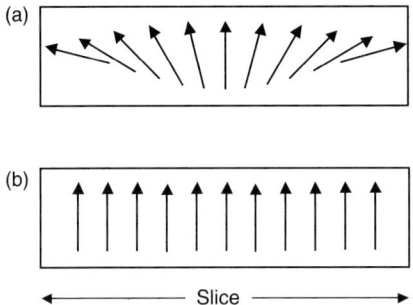

FIGURE 8.17 After the application of a spatially selective excitation pulse, there is phase dispersion of the transverse magnetization across the slice profile (a). This leads to signal loss. The slice-rephasing gradient lobe can restore the signal by re-aligning the phases of the transverse magnetization (b).

8.3.3 SLICE-REPHASING GRADIENT

The slice-selection gradient typically results in some phase dispersion of transverse magnetization across the slice (Figure 8.17). The exact nature of the dispersion is determined by the phase properties of its spatial response, which in turn depends on the shape of the RF excitation pulse. For example, when a linear phase RF excitation pulse is used in conjunction with a constant slice-selection gradient, the resultant slice is linearly phase modulated across the slice.

A *slice-refocusing or -rephasing* lobe is associated with the slice-selection gradient of an excitation pulse (Hutchinson et al. 1978). The slice-rephasing gradient lobe has opposite polarity compared to the slice-selection gradient and is used to compensate for the phase dispersion caused by the slice-selection gradient. Without the slice-rephasing gradient lobe, there is intravoxel phase dispersion across the slice and signal loss results, as if a spoiler gradient (Section 10.5) were present. In fact, the slice-selection gradient after the isodelay point of an excitation RF pulse functions as a spoiler gradient. The gradient area of the slice-rephasing lobe is calculated based on the isodelay Δt_I value of the excitation pulse, as described in more detail in Section 3.1 and illustrated in Figure 3.4.

Example 8.6 Estimate the phase dispersion across an excited slice in terms of the isodelay parameter and the RF bandwidth. Assume that the transverse magnetization is created at the isodelay point and undergoes dephasing until the end of the RF pulse.

Answer At a location z along the slice, the selection gradient introduces phase dispersion:

$$\phi(z) = \gamma \, G_z \, z \, \Delta t_\mathrm{I} \tag{8.58}$$

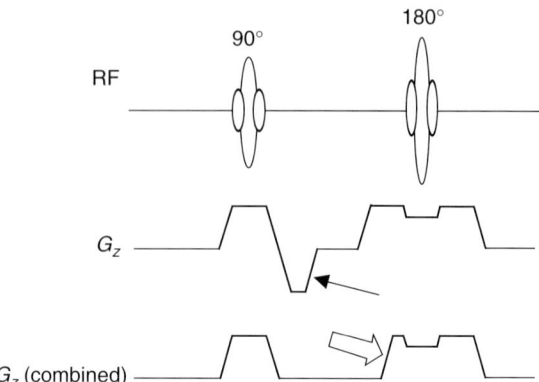

FIGURE 8.18 A slice-rephasing lobe (thin arrow) is used to compensate for the phase dispersion introduced by a slice-selection gradient. The gradient area of the lobe is calculated as described in Section 3.1. For some RF spin-echo pulse sequences, the slice-rephasing lobe can be combined with the left element of the crusher pair to form a combined lobe (hollow arrow).

The total phase dispersion across the slice is therefore proportional to the slice thickness:

$$\Delta\phi = \gamma\, G_z\, \Delta z\, \Delta t_1 \tag{8.59}$$

Eliminating the slice thickness from Eq. (8.59) with Eq. (8.53) produces:

$$\Delta\phi = 2\pi\, \Delta f\, \Delta t_1 \tag{8.60}$$

Equation (8.60) states that the phase dispersion (in cycles) across the slice is approximately given by the product of the RF bandwidth and the isodelay.

Spatially selective refocusing pulses (Section 3.3) generally do not require rephasing lobes. This is because the phase accumulated during the first half of the pulse is cancelled during the second half. This also explains why refocusing pulses are invariably symmetric, that is, why their isodelay point is located halfway through the pulse.

For RF spin-echo pulse sequences, sometimes the slice-rephasing gradient lobe for the excitation pulse is combined with the left element of the crusher pair (Figure 8.18) so that the net gradient area between the excitation and refocusing pulses is preserved. Combining the two lobes has several potential advantages including reduced minimum TE, acoustic noise, gradient heating, and eddy currents. The pulse programmer should be cognizant, however, that the combination can increase the net first-gradient moment of the entire waveform because of the moment arm between the slice-selection gradient and the right element of the crusher pair. The increased first moment can increase signal loss due to intravoxel dephasing for spins flowing perpendicular to the slice plane. Another problem with combined gradient waveforms is that the effect of concomitant magnetic field can be exacerbated because the uncombined crushers cancel their self-squared concomitant field, provided that the crushers are symmetrical about a refocusing pulse. This effect is described in more detail in Section 10.1.

SELECTED REFERENCES

Hoult, D. I. 1977. Zeugmatography—criticism of concept of a selective pulse in presence of a field gradient. *J. Magn. Reson.* 26(1): 165–167.

Hutchinson, J. M. S., Sutherland, R. J., and Mallard, J. R. 1978. NMR imaging: Image recovery under magnetic fields with large non-uniformities. *J. Phys. E* 11: 217–221.

Lauterbur, P. C., Kramer, D. M., House, W. V., and Chen, C.-N. 1975. Zeugmatographic high-resolution nuclear magnetic-resonance spectroscopy—images of chemical inhomogeneity within macroscopic objects. *J. Am. Chem. Soc.* 97: 6866–6868.

Mansfield, P., Maudsley, A. A., and Baines, T. 1976. Fast scan proton density imaging by NMR. *J. Phys. E* 9: 271–278.

Wood, M. L., and Wehrli, F. W. 1999. Principles of MRI. In *Magnetic resonance imaging*, Vol. 1, 3rd ed., edited by D. D. Stark and W. G. Bradley, pp. 5–6. St. Louis: Mosby.

RELATED SECTIONS

9

MOTION-SENSITIZING GRADIENTS

9.1 Diffusion-Weighting Gradients

Although magnetic field gradients are primarily used for spatial encoding, they can also be used for other purposes, such as the preparation of magnetization to produce MRI signals with specified contrast. One such application is diffusion imaging in which *a diffusion-weighting gradient* is incorporated into a pulse sequence to sensitize MRI signals to molecular diffusion within tissues.

A diffusion-weighting gradient typically consists of two lobes with equal area. In pulse sequences based on spin echoes, the two lobes have the same polarity and are placed at either side of a refocusing RF pulse (Figure 9.1a). In gradient-echo-based sequences, however, the two lobes must have opposite polarity and are often concatenated (Figure 9.1b). The diffusion-weighting gradient is sometimes referred to as a *bipolar gradient* (or Stejskal-Tanner gradient; Stejskal and Tanner 1965), even though it is unipolar in the spin-echo case, as shown in Figure 9.1a. Waveforms with more than two lobes can also be used as diffusion-weighting gradients, as long as they follow the guidelines given in this section. The amplitude of the diffusion-weighting gradient is typically the maximum allowed by the system, and its pulse width is considerably longer than that of most imaging gradients.

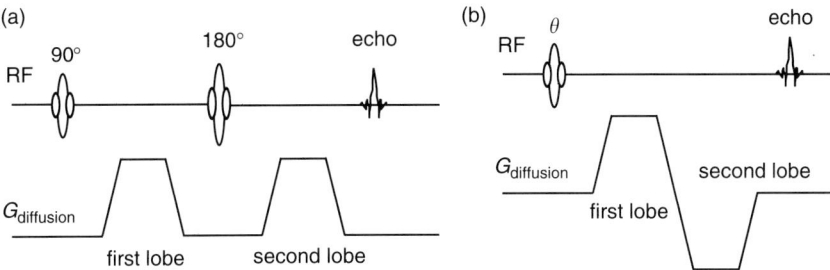

FIGURE 9.1 Examples of diffusion-weighting gradient waveforms used in a (a) spin-echo pulse sequence and (b) gradient-echo pulse sequence.

When a diffusion-weighting gradient is included in a pulse sequence, water diffusion (i.e., random or Brownian motion of water molecules) can cause an attenuation in proton MRI signals. The degree of attenuation depends on the dimensionless product of the diffusion coefficient D (in millimeters squared per second) and a quantity known as the *b-factor* or *b-value* (in seconds per millimeter squared). The b-factor is determined by the diffusion-weighting gradient waveform and can be adjusted in the pulse sequence. Increasing the diffusion gradient amplitude, the separation of its lobes, or the pulse width of each lobe results in a higher b-value. The b-value is analogous to TE in a T_2-weighted pulse sequence; the extent of diffusion-weighing increases with b just as the degree of T_2-weighting increases with TE.

9.1.1 QUANTITATIVE DESCRIPTION

Effects of Diffusion-Weighting Gradient on Spins   A gradient G can alter the Larmor resonant frequency of a spin isochromat in the transverse plane. A change in the resonant frequency $\Delta\omega$ accumulates a phase ϕ over time t:

$$\phi = \int_0^t \Delta\omega \, dt' = \gamma \int_0^t \vec{G}(t') \cdot \vec{r}(t') dt' \tag{9.1}$$

where γ is the gyromagnetic ratio, and $\vec{r}$ is the location of the spins. For coherent motion, the spatial displacement $\vec{r}(t)$ can be expanded with respect to t in a Taylor series, which yields terms that are linearly proportional to velocity, acceleration, and so on. This forms the basis of phase-contrast angiography (Section 15.2). If the spins within a voxel are moving randomly due to molecular diffusion, then the phases accumulated by different spins within the voxel will cause signal cancellation. The resultant MRI signal S is exponentially related to the variance of a Gaussian phase distribution, $<\phi^2>$, which is equal to the product bD:

$$S = S_0 e^{-<\phi^2>} = S_0 e^{-bD} \qquad (9.2)$$

where S_0 is the signal intensity in the absence of diffusion. Any imaging gradients contribute to the b-factor in Eq. (9.2) and hence to the diffusion-induced signal attenuation. The degree of attenuation from imaging gradients is usually small, however, except for acquisitions with very small FOV or thin slices. To increase the sensitivity to diffusion, a dedicated diffusion-weighting gradient must be applied.

Diffusion-Weighting Gradient Waveforms   Diffusion-weighting gradient waveforms can be designed according to the following guidelines:

1. In a spin-echo pulse sequence (e.g., conventional spin echo, spin-echo EPI, and RARE or fast spin echo), the net area of the diffusion-weighting gradient waveform before a refocusing RF pulse must be equal to the net area after the refocusing pulse.
2. In a gradient-echo pulse sequence (e.g., conventional gradient echo and gradient-echo EPI), the net area of the entire diffusion gradient waveform must be zero.

These rules are mathematically expressed as:

$$\int_{t_{ex}}^{t_{refocus}} G_d(t)dt = \int_{t_{refocus}}^{TE} G_d(t)dt \qquad (9.3)$$

for spin echo sequences, and

$$\int_{t_{ex}}^{TE} G_d(t)dt = 0 \qquad (9.4)$$

for gradient-echo sequences, where t_{ex}, $t_{refocus}$, and TE are the times at the center (or isodelay center) of the excitation pulse, refocusing pulse, and echo, respectively. Any gradient lobe shape (e.g., trapezoid, triangle, and half-sine) can be used to construct a diffusion-weighting gradient waveform, as long as the requirement in Eq. (9.3) or Eq. (9.4) is met. The trapezoidal shape is widely used due to its time efficiency. The diffusion-weighting gradient lobes can also be combined with other gradient waveforms, such as a crusher gradient, to reduce the minimum TE of the sequence.

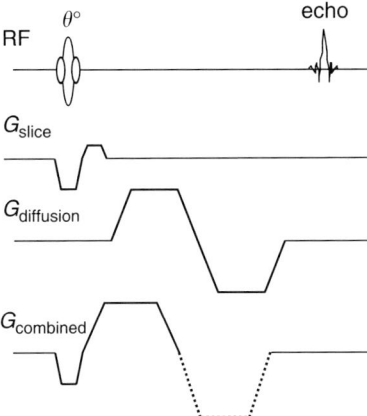

FIGURE 9.2 Gradient waveform for Example 9.1. The slice-selection gradient and the diffusion-weighting gradient are individually shown. The combined waveform is also illustrated. The gradient lobe to be calculated is indicated by dashed lines.

Example 9.1 A trapezoidal diffusion-weighting gradient lobe that will be placed on the slice-selection axis is combined with a slice-refocusing gradient lobe in a gradient-echo pulse sequence to minimize the echo time. The two lobes both have positive polarity (Figure 9.2). The refocusing gradient area is $10 \, \text{ms} \cdot \text{mT}/\text{m}$. The combined gradient lobe (Figure 9.2) has the following parameters: ramp width $= 2 \, \text{ms}$, plateau width $= 5 \, \text{ms}$, and amplitude $= 30 \, \text{mT}/\text{m}$. If the slew rate (S_R) of the system is $150 \, \text{T}/\text{m/s}$ and the maximal gradient amplitude (h) is $40 \, \text{mT}/\text{m}$, design the negative diffusion-gradient lobe (dashed lines in Figure 9.2) that has the shortest width.

Answer The area of the combined gradient lobe is $A_{\text{com}} = (2 + 5) \times 30 = 210 \, \text{ms} \cdot \text{mT}/\text{m}$. The area attributed to the positive diffusion lobe is $A_{\text{pos}} = 210 - 10 = 200 \, \text{ms} \cdot \text{mT}/\text{m}$. According to Eq. (9.4), the area of the negative lobe must be $A_{\text{neg}} = -200 \, \text{ms} \cdot \text{mT}/\text{m}$. Because the absolute value of the area is greater than $h^2/S_R = 40^2/150 \approx 10.7 \, \text{ms} \cdot \text{mT}/\text{m}$, the most time-efficient gradient lobe should be a trapezoid with gradient amplitude, ramp time, and plateau width given by (see Section 7.1):

$$G_d = -h = -40 \, \text{mT}/\text{m}$$
$$T_{\text{ramp}} = h/S_R = 40/150 = 0.267 \, \text{ms}$$
$$T_{\text{plateau}} = |A_{\text{neg}}| / h - T_{\text{ramp}} = 200/40 - 0.267 = 4.733 \, \text{ms}$$

b-Value   The *b*-value is related to an arbitrary gradient waveform $\vec{G}(t')$ by the following equations:

$$b = (2\pi)^2 \int_0^{TE} \vec{k}(t) \cdot \vec{k}(t)\,dt \tag{9.5}$$

$$\vec{k}(t) = \frac{\gamma}{2\pi} \int_0^t \vec{G}(t')\,dt' \tag{9.6}$$

When the gradient waveform is played along a single axis, Eqs. (9.5) and (9.6) can be simplified to:

$$b = \gamma^2 \int_0^{TE} \left[\int_0^t G(t')\,dt' \right]^2 dt \tag{9.7}$$

Equations (9.5), (9.6), and (9.7) are used to calculate the *b*-value for any gradient waveform in the pulse sequence. The details on how to carry out the integral can be found in Le Bihan (1995, chap. 5). The *b*-values for several common diffusion-weighting gradient waveforms are given in Figures 9.3 and 9.4.

Example 9.2   A pair of rectangular (i.e., trapezoidal lobes where the ramp time is negligible compared to the plateau duration) gradient lobes are used

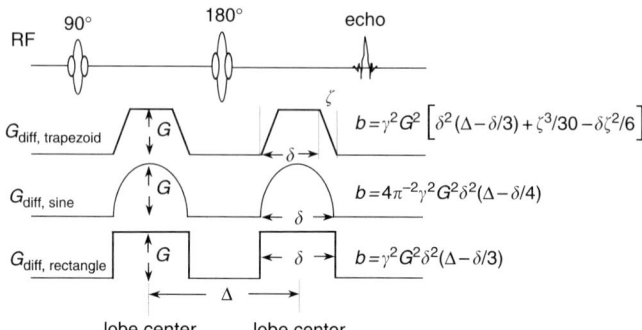

FIGURE 9.3 Commonly used diffusion-gradient waveforms in spin-echo pulse sequences and their corresponding *b*-values. Note that the expression for *b*-value from trapezoidal gradient lobes reduces to the value for the rectangular lobes if the ramp duration goes to 0. (The δ in the *b*-value expressions should be distinguished from chemical shift used in other sections of the book.)

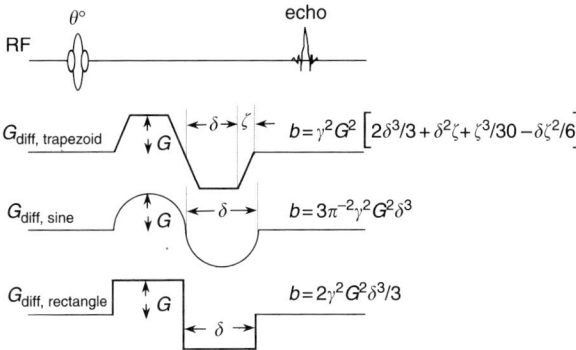

FIGURE 9.4 Commonly used diffusion-gradient waveforms in gradient-echo pulse sequences and their corresponding b-values. Note that the expression for the b-value from trapezoidal gradient lobes reduces to the value for the rectangular lobes if the ramp duration goes to 0.

as diffusion-weighting gradients in a spin-echo sequence. The lobes both have an amplitude of 25 mT/m and are separated by 50 ms. To achieve a b-value of 1000 s/mm^2, what is the width of each gradient lobe?

Answer According to Figure 9.3, the b-value for rectangular gradient lobes in a spin-echo pulse sequence is given by:

$$b = \gamma^2 G^2 \delta^2 (\Delta - \delta/3) \tag{9.8}$$

Substituting $b = 1000\,\text{s/mm}^2$, $\Delta = 50\,\text{ms}$, $\gamma/2\pi = 42.57\,\text{kHz/mT}$, and $G = 25\,\text{mT/m}$ into Eq. (9.8) and solving the cubic equation with respect to the gradient lobe width δ, we obtain a single physically meaningful solution, $\delta = 22.99\,\text{ms}$.

9.1.2 PRACTICAL CONSIDERATIONS

The b-value used in most diffusion imaging sequences is on the order of 1000 s/mm^2. To achieve this b-value, the diffusion-weighting gradient lobe is typically several tens of milliseconds in length (see Example 9.2), which inevitably leads to a rather long TE. This, in turn, reduces the SNR and introduces unwanted T_2 contrast in the diffusion-weighted image (the T_2 effect in diffusion-weighted imaging is also called T_2 *shine-through*). To minimize TE, the maximum gradient amplitude available on the MRI scanner is usually employed for diffusion imaging. Although using the maximum gradient slew rate can also reduce the TE value, the improvement is usually much less than employing the maximum gradient amplitude because the plateau duration typically greatly exceeds the ramp width. In addition, employing the maximum slew rate contributes to the overall dB/dt value, which may induce unwanted peripheral nerve stimulation or excessive eddy currents. For these reasons, maximum slew rate is often not used in diffusion-weighting gradients, especially for imaging human subjects.

The large diffusion-weighting gradient amplitude can induce substantial eddy currents even in a system with good eddy-current compensations. The eddy currents can lead to a number of image-quality problems in certain diffusion pulse sequences. For example, geometric distortion can be observed in diffusion-weighted EPI pulse sequences. An effective way to address this problem is to break the diffusion-weighting gradient waveform into multiple lobes so that eddy currents produced by different lobes can partially cancel one another using two refocusing pulses. This approach is further discussed in Section 17.2 and in Reese et al. (2003). Alternatively, the imaging gradient waveforms can be preadjusted to offset the eddy-current magnetic field (Zhou et al. 1997).

The diffusion-weighting gradient can also produce nonnegligible concomitant magnetic fields (Bernstein et al. 1998). If the diffusion gradient lobes before and after a refocusing pulse are identical, their phase accumulation from the concomitant field is completely canceled in spin-echo pulse sequences. In gradient-echo sequences, however, the phase accumulation from the concomitant field cannot be easily cancelled, which results in image artifacts, especially with a large b-value.

SELECTED REFERENCES

Bernstein, M. A., Zhou, X. J., Polzin, J. A., King, K. F., Ganin, A., Pelc, N. J., and Glover, G. H. 1998. Concomitant gradient terms in phase contrast MR: Analysis and correction. *Magn. Reson. Med.* 39: 300–308.

Le Bihan, D. 1995. *Diffusion and perfusion magnetic resonance imaging: Applications to functional MRI.* New York: Raven Press.

Reese, T. G., Heid, O., Weisskoff, R. M., and Wedeen, V. J. 2003. Reduction of eddy-current-induced distortion in diffusion MRI using a twice-refocused spin echo. *Magn. Reson. Med.* 49: 177–182.

Stejskal, E. O., and Tanner, J. E. 1965. Spin diffusion measurements: Spin echoes in the presence of a time-dependent field gradient. *J. Chem. Phys.* 42: 288–292.

Zhou, X., Maier, J. K., and Reynolds, H. G. 1997. Reduction of image misregistration in diffusion-weighted EPI. *Proc. Int'l. Soc. Magn. Reson. Med.* 3: 1724.

RELATED SECTIONS

9.2 Flow-Encoding Gradients

A *flow-encoding* (FE) or *flow-sensitizing gradient* is a waveform that encodes information about macroscopic flow or coherent motion into the phase of the MR signal. We consider this class of motion-sensitizing gradient waveforms separately from the diffusion-weighting gradient (Section 9.1), which encodes information about incoherent (or random) motion into the magnitude of the MR signal. With FE gradients, each of the three logical axes (readout, phase encoding, and slice selection) is treated independently. Therefore FE gradients can be added to a single axis, to any two, or to all three axes during a given pulse sequence.

FE gradients can encode information about velocity, acceleration, or higher derivatives of motion. The most common FE gradient is a *bipolar* velocity-encoding gradient (Figure 9.5a), which comprises two lobes of equal area and opposite polarity. Because the net area under the bipolar gradient is 0, it produces no net phase accumulation for stationary spins (Figure 9.5b). For spins moving along the direction of the gradient, however, the bipolar gradient produces a phase accumulation that is linearly proportional to their velocity. The bipolar velocity-encoding gradient is used in phase-contrast angiography (Section 15.2), in which both the speed and the direction of flow or motion along the gradient direction can be mapped. Sometimes the bipolar gradient is combined with other lobes in the waveform (Figure 9.6), in order to reduce the minimum TE of the pulse sequence.

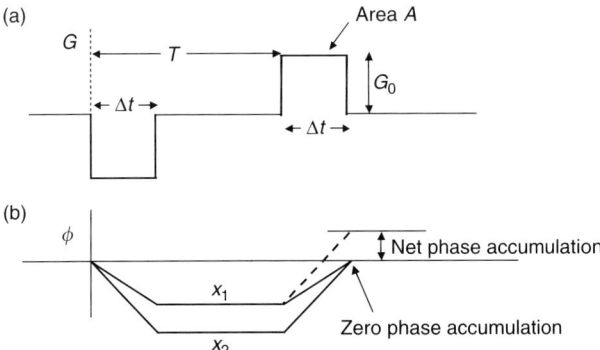

FIGURE 9.5 Bipolar velocity encoding gradient plotted versus time. (a) Two gradient lobes of equal area and opposite polarity form a bipolar velocity-encoding gradient. (b) Stationary spins acquire no net phase from the bipolar gradient, regardless of whether their location is x_1 or x_2. If, however, spins move from x_1 to x_2 during the bipolar gradient, a net phase is accumulated (dashed line).

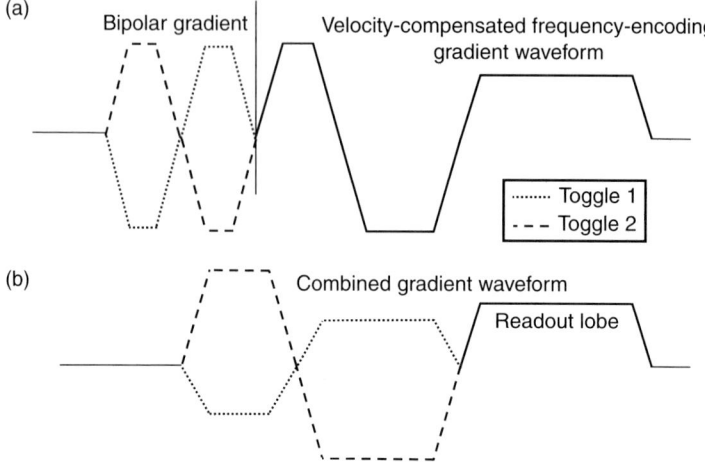

FIGURE 9.6 (a) Toggled bipolar gradient (dashed and dotted lines) is appended in front of a velocity-compensated frequency-encoding waveform (solid line). (b) The five-lobe waveform in (a) can be combined into three lobes, reducing the minimum TE. The readout lobe remains unchanged by the combination because it is determined by imaging parameters such as FOV, image matrix size, and receiver bandwidth.

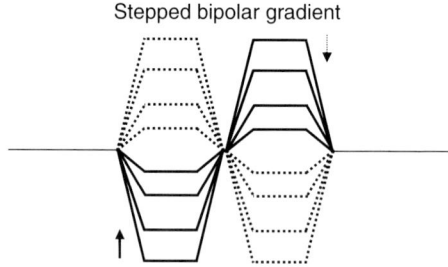

FIGURE 9.7 Fourier velocity-encoding waveform. The amplitude of a bipolar velocity-encoding waveform is stepped or incremented analogously to a phase-encoding waveform in standard imaging. The later increments are shown as dotted lines for clarity.

The amplitude of the bipolar gradient can be toggled as shown in Figure 9.6a, and described in Section 15.2 on phase-contrast angiography. Alternatively, in the Fourier velocity-encoding method (Moran 1982), the amplitude of the bipolar gradient is incremented (Figure 9.7), like the amplitude of the phase-encoding gradient in standard imaging. This concept enables many other options for imaging sequences that measure combinations of velocity and spatial information. For example, if a Fourier-velocity-encoding gradient replaces the standard phase-encoding gradient, then the resulting images will be spatially-encoded in the readout direction, whereas the phase-encoded direction will provide a velocity scale for motion along the applied velocity-encoding gradient direction. Another possibility is to obtain a 3D acquisition with two spatially encoded directions and one velocity-encoded direction. All these imaging sequences can be considered special cases of a general six-dimensional data acquisition, with three spatially encoded and three velocity-encoded directions, as described in Moran (1982).

As shown in Figure 9.8, a bipolar velocity-encoding waveform can be used as a preparation pulse (Guilfoyle et al. 1991; Korosec et al. 1993), much the

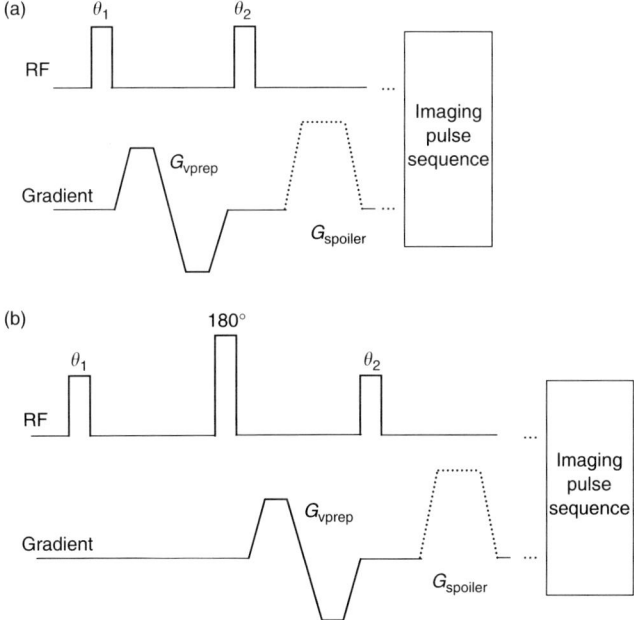

FIGURE 9.8 Velocity preparation. (a) A bipolar gradient after an RF excitation pulse θ_1 can be used to encode information about velocity into the longitudinal magnetization, much the same way a unipolar gradient is used for spatial tagging. The second RF pulse θ_2 stores the velocity-encoded magnetization along the axis. The subsequent spoiler gradient (dotted lines) dephases the residual transverse magnetization. Typical flip angles for θ_1 and θ_2 are 90°. A fast sequence such as echo planar or fast gradient echo follows this velocity preparation module. (b) Sometimes to minimize off-resonance effects, a 180° refocusing pulse is played halfway between θ_1 and θ_2.

same way a unipolar gradient pulse is used for spatial tagging (Section 5.5). In this method, the amplitude of the longitudinal magnetization is modulated by a function that depends on velocity. The first RF pulse θ_1 tips some of the longitudinal magnetization into the transverse plane. The bipolar gradient then encodes a phase into the transverse magnetization. (The velocity-induced phase change is described in more detail later in this section.) The second RF pulse θ_2 then tips some of this transverse magnetization back along the z axis, where it becomes velocity-modulated longitudinal magnetization. Any residual transverse magnetization is dephased by the spoiler gradient (dotted gradient lobe in Figure 9.8). A subsequent imaging sequence that uses this longitudinal magnetization will be intensity-modulated by a function of velocity.

Another type of FE gradient is called the *cyclic* or *synchronous motion-sensitizing* gradient waveform. This gradient waveform consists of a long train of small, concatenated bipolar elements. Although any single bipolar element in the train by itself produces only a miniscule phase accumulation, the net effect of the entire train is easily measurable. In MR elastography (Muthupillai et al. 1995), the train is synchronized (i.e., phase-locked with an adjustable delay) to the oscillation of a mechanical driver that produces shear waves in the object. In this way, wave motion with amplitudes on the order of hundreds of nanometers or less can be mapped, allowing noninvasive measurement of the shear modulus of the object.

FE gradients can also encode information about higher-order time derivatives of motion into the phase of the MR signal. For example, acceleration encoding can be accomplished with a three-lobed velocity-compensated gradient waveform with alternating polarity. The amplitude of the acceleration-encoding waveform can be either toggled (Figure 9.9) for acceleration phase-contrast imaging or incremented for Fourier acceleration imaging (Tsau et al.

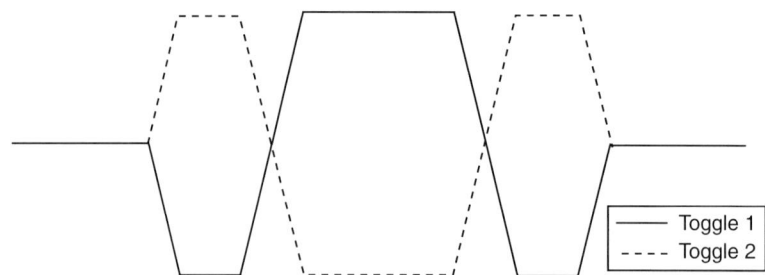

FIGURE 9.9 Toggled acceleration-encoding waveform. The gradient area and first moment of each waveform are zero, whereas the second moment m_2 changes sign when the waveform is toggled.

1997). In this section we primarily focus on velocity-encoding waveforms, because they are the most commonly used in pulse sequences.

9.2.1 QUALITATIVE DESCRIPTION

The phase behavior of moving spins in the presence of bipolar FE gradient can be understood by plotting the accumulated phase as a function of time for two locations, x_1 and x_2, where x_1 is closer to the gradient isocenter. As shown in Figure 9.5b, phase is accumulated at a linear rate whenever the rectangular gradient is active, that is, from $t = 0$ to Δt and from $t = T$ to $T + \Delta t$. The spins at x_2 accumulate phase at a faster rate because they are farther from the gradient isocenter. For stationary spins, the phase accumulated during the first lobe is exactly unwound during the second lobe, resulting in zero net phase accumulation. If, however, a spin moves from x_1 to x_2 during the time interval between the lobes, a net phase accumulation is produced (dashed line).

Next we show that the phase accumulation is linearly proportional to the gradient area under one of the lobes, the temporal separation of the lobes, and the velocity along the direction of the gradient.

9.2.2 QUANTITATIVE DESCRIPTION

Flow-Induced Phase and the Gradient First Moment   In this subsection we use the definitions and translation rules for the gradient moments presented in Section 10.4 to calculate the first moment of velocity-encoding waveforms. The moment expansion presented there states that the phase of a spin isochromat is given by:

$$\phi(t) = \gamma \int_0^t G(u)x(u)du$$

$$= \gamma \left(m_0 x_0 + m_1 v_0 + \cdots + \frac{1}{n!} m_n \left(\frac{d^n x}{dt^n} \right)_{t=0} + \cdots \right) \quad (9.9)$$

where m_n is the nth gradient moment, and x_0 and v_0 are the initial displacement and velocity of the spin isochromat respectively, along the direction of the gradient.

Typically the flow-encoding waveform is designed so that all the moments that are of lower order than the desired encoding are 0. For example, the bipolar velocity-encoding waveform has zero gradient area; that is, $m_0 = 0$. The first moment of the bipolar gradient waveform in Figure 9.5a can be calculated directly:

$$m_1 = \int_{t=0}^{\Delta t} -G_0 t \, dt + \int_{t=T}^{T+\Delta t} G_0 t \, dt$$

$$= \frac{G_0}{2} \left(-\Delta t^2 + (T+\Delta t)^2 - T^2 \right) = G_0 \Delta t T \qquad (9.10)$$

Because the total area under the bipolar waveform is 0, the value for the first moment in Eq. (9.10) is independent of the choice of temporal origin (Section 10.4). Recognizing that $G_0 \Delta t$ is equal to the area A of an individual gradient lobe, Eq. (9.10) becomes:

$$m_1 = AT \qquad (9.11)$$

By combining Eqs. (9.11) and (9.9), and selecting only the velocity term, the result for the phase shift depicted in Figure 9.5

$$\phi = \gamma A T \, v \qquad (9.12)$$

is readily obtained.

Although Eq. (9.11) was derived for rectangular lobe shapes starting at $t = 0$, it is a general result. This can be demonstrated by decomposing an arbitrary bipolar waveform into multiple pairs of rectangles with very thin width, as shown in Figure 9.10. The rectangles that make up any pair are also separated by the time T. The net first moment of the arbitrary bipolar waveform

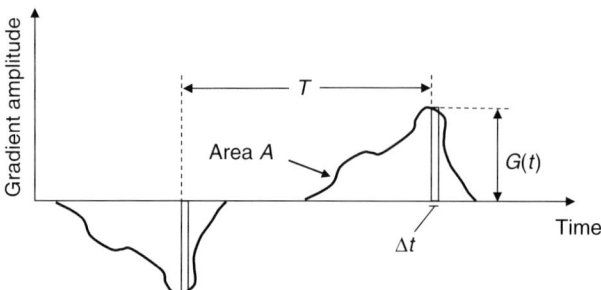

FIGURE 9.10 Bipolar velocity-encoding waveform composed of gradient lobes of arbitrary shape. Decomposing the waveform into multiple pairs of rectangles demonstrates that Eq. (9.11) is a general result that is valid regardless of the shape of the lobes that make up the bipolar waveform.

can be approximated by the sum of the first moments of all the pairs, which from Eq. (9.10) is:

$$m_1 \approx \sum_{n \text{ pairs}} m_{1,n} = \sum_{n \text{ pairs}} G_n \Delta t \, T = T \sum_{n \text{ pairs}} G_n \Delta t \qquad (9.13)$$

At the limit as $\Delta t \to 0$ the number of pairs goes to infinity, Eq. (9.13) becomes exact, and the sum approaches the integral for the gradient area under one lobe. This demonstrates that Eq. (9.11) is in fact a general result, independent of the shape of the lobes that make up the bipolar waveform. Because the total area under the arbitrary bipolar waveform is also 0, the value in Eq. (9.11) is independent of the choice of temporal origin. Also note that the sign of m_1 will always match the sign of the gradient lobe that is played last. Thus, when the bipolar waveform is toggled, as in phase-contrast angiography, the sign of the first moment is negated.

Aliasing Velocity VENC   A toggled bipolar velocity-encoding waveform is often characterized by its *aliasing velocity* parameter, sometimes denoted by VENC (for velocity encoding). By definition, when the velocity component along the gradient direction is equal to $\pm$VENC, the resulting phase difference is $\pm\pi$. The value $\pm\pi$ is used in the definition because it is the unaliased dynamic range of the phase difference reconstruction (Section 13.5). If the *change* in the first moment of the bipolar velocity gradient (when toggling the gradient waveform) is Δm_1, then:

$$\text{VENC} = \frac{\pi}{\gamma |\Delta m_1|} \qquad (9.14)$$

For quantitative flow analysis (i.e., measurement of flow in milliliters per minute), VENC is usually selected to be slightly higher (e.g., 30%) than the expected peak vessel velocity to avoid flow-related aliasing. This restriction can be relaxed if a postprocessing unwrapping algorithm is available. More details about selecting the value of VENC can be found in Section 15.2.

Example 9.3   Suppose the toggled bipolar gradient shown in Figure 9.6a is composed of gradient lobes, each of which has area $A = 6.0 \, \text{ms} \cdot \text{mT/m}$. The lobe width is 3 ms. What is the aliasing velocity in centimeters per second?

Answer   Because the lobes in Figure 9.6a are adjacent, the interlobe delay time T is equal to the lobe width, 3 ms. From Eq. (9.11), the first moment of the dotted bipolar waveform is:

$$m_1 = AT = 3 \, \text{ms} \times 6.0 \, \text{ms} \cdot \text{mT/m} = 1.8 \times 10^{-8} \, \text{s}^2 \text{T/m} \qquad (9.15)$$

The change in the first moment when the bipolar gradient is toggled is:

$$\Delta m_1 = m_1 - (-m_1) = 2AT \qquad (9.16)$$

which implies that:

$$\text{VENC} = \frac{\pi}{2\gamma AT}$$

$$= \frac{\pi}{2 \times (2\pi \times 42.57\,\text{MHz/T}) \times 1.8 \times 10^{-8}\,\text{s}^2\text{T/m}} = 32.6\,\text{cm/s}$$

Fourier Velocity Encoding   With the Fourier velocity-encoding method, parameters analogous to pixel size and FOV for standard imaging can be defined. Because the discrete Fourier transform is used to reconstruct velocity-encoded images, the basic relationship derived in Sections 1.1 and 8.2 between k-space step size Δk_v and pixel size Δv still applies:

$$\Delta k_v \Delta v = \frac{1}{N} \qquad (9.17)$$

where N is the number of total data points used in the discrete Fourier transform. (The values of the pixel size Δv and N are both taken before zero filling or other interpolation.) Because m_0 is equal to the gradient area in the moment expansion for the phase (Eq. 9.9), we can obtain spatially resolved velocity maps from Fourier-velocity-encoded acquisitions simply by replacing the phase-encoding lobe by the incremented bipolar gradient lobe of Figure 9.7. Moreover, quantities such as the velocity FOV and pixel size can be obtained by replacing the gradient area (zeroth moment) by the first moment in expressions derived in Section 8.2 on phase encoding (see Example 9.4). Similarly, spatial maps of acceleration can be obtained by using a stepped acceleration-encoding gradient based on a waveform such as the one in Figure 9.9. According to Eq. (9.9), the quantities of acceleration FOV and pixel size are obtained by replacing the phase-encoding area by $m_2/2! = m_2/2$.

Standard spatial encoding, velocity encoding, acceleration encoding, and higher-order flow encoding are not mutually exclusive within a single acquisition. The position and flow parameters can be encoded into the MRI signals by independently varying $m_0, m_1, m_2, \ldots, m_n$. In practice, however, the acquisition time for such a multidimensional data set quickly becomes prohibitive, unless a small number of encoding steps is used (Bittoun et al. 2000). Thus, Fourier flow-encoded acquisitions are often limited to specific spatial directions and to lower-order time derivatives of motion, such as velocity.

Example 9.4   A Fourier velocity acquisition with $N = 128$ increments is obtained. The first moment is incremented from $m_{1,\text{max}} = 5 \times 10^{-7}\,\text{s}^2\text{T/m}$

to $-m_{1,\max}$. What are the unaliased extent of sampled velocities (i.e., the velocity FOV) and the pixel size?

Answer In analogy to the methods in Section 8.2, (e.g., Eq. 8.38):

$$m_{1,\max} = \frac{\pi (N - 1)}{\gamma L_v} \tag{9.18}$$

So the velocity FOV is:

$$L_v = \frac{\pi (N - 1)}{\gamma m_{1,\max}} = \frac{\pi \times (128 - 1)}{(2\pi \times 42.57 \text{ MHz/T}) \times 5 \times 10^{-7} \text{ s}^2\text{T/m}} = 2.983 \text{ m/s}$$

Therefore each (uninterpolated) pixel represents a velocity bin of $L_v/N = 2.33 \text{ cm/s}$.

Velocity-Preparation Gradient Just as Fourier velocity-encoding parameters can be extracted from standard imaging relationships by analogy, the relationships for velocity-selective preparation (Figure 9.8) can be obtained by analogy to the relationships developed in Section 5.5 on tagging. In particular, the phase accumulation useful for analyzing spatial tags:

$$\phi(x) = \gamma x \int_0^T G_{\text{tag}} dt = \gamma x m_{0,\text{tag}} \tag{9.19}$$

can be adapted to phase for velocity preparation:

$$\phi(v) = \gamma v \int_0^T G_{\text{vprep}}(t) \, t \, dt = \gamma v m_{1,\text{vprep}} \tag{9.20}$$

In practice, using velocity-preparation pulses is similar to applying spatial tags. One difference is that a 180° pulse can be inserted in between the two velocity-tagging gradient lobes, in which case the gradient lobes must have the same polarity. The 180° pulse minimizes off-resonance effects and concomitant phase errors. However, to avoid artifacts introduced by B_1 inhomogeneity, sometimes both lobes of the bipolar gradient are placed on the same side (Korosec et al. 1993) of the 180°, as shown on Figure 9.8b.

A second deviation from spatial tagging is that two sets of velocity-tagged images are often acquired with slightly different values of the first moment and reconstructed with a phase difference (or complex difference) method, as in phase-contrast angiography. For a sufficiently small value of Δm_1, the phase difference corresponding to Eq. (9.20) will not alias and the range of velocities will be represented by the gray scale rather than by tagging bands. Images that are velocity prepared in this manner have the same appearance as standard phase-contrast images. Guilfoyle et al. (1991) and Korosec et al. (1993) provide more details about the use of velocity-preparation pulses.

9.2.3 COMBINED VELOCITY-ENCODING WAVEFORMS AND OTHER PRACTICAL CONSIDERATIONS

The most common application of FE is for velocity-encoding with gradient-echo pulse sequences. When the bipolar velocity-encoding gradient is appended to a velocity-compensated slice-selection or frequency-encoding waveform, the resulting five lobes can be combined into three lobes (Figure 9.6). This combination always reduces the minimum TE and often reduces higher-gradient moments as well. A drawback of combining the gradient lobes is that the phase error from the concomitant field (Section 10.1) is not necessarily equal for the two toggled settings of the FE gradient, as it is for the simple bipolar gradient waveform of Figure 9.6a. Therefore, the phase error does not automatically subtract out during the phase difference reconstruction. Luckily, phase errors from the concomitant field can be calculated exactly and then removed during the phase difference reconstruction (Section 13.5).

Design details for the combined waveform in Figure 9.6b are given in Bernstein et al. (1992). Given a desired amount of VENC and the corresponding Δm_1, there are three general design choices. They are called the *one-sided*, *two-sided*, and *minimum-TE* designs. The first moments of the combined waveform for the two toggles distinguishes these three designs. For example, in the two-sided design, the first moment (at the peak of the echo) symmetrically straddles zero (velocity compensation) for the two toggled waveforms. In the one-sided method, one of the two velocity encodings is velocity-compensated ($m_1 = 0$), while the other waveform produces the desired Δm_1. In the minimum-TE design, the most compact waveform is used, irrespective of where the individual first moments lie. Although all three designs can work well in phase-contrast angiography, the choice among them is often determined by how the accompanying magnitude images are reconstructed. If a magnitude image is reconstructed from a single data set, the one-sided method is desirable because a velocity-compensated data set will have the least severe flow artifacts. If, however, two data sets are averaged to produce the magnitude image, then the two-sided method is a good choice because the flow artifacts of the two sets will be comparable. The minimum-TE design should be used when minimizing the pulse sequence TE and TR is the overriding consideration. Another benefit of the minimum TE design is that higher-order gradient moments are often reduced.

Adding FE to the incremented phase-encoding waveform presents different design challenges compared to the frequency-encoding and slice-selection waveforms. The bipolar gradient is usually not combined with the stepped phase-encoding waveform. One popular method, however, is to place the phase-encoding gradient lobe in between the two FE lobes. This increases the moment arm T of the bipolar gradient, which, according to Eq. (9.11), allows a net reduction in gradient area A (with m_1 and VENC fixed) and hence a decrease in minimum TE.

SELECTED REFERENCES

Bernstein, M. A., Shimakawa, A., and Pelc, N. J. 1992. Minimizing TE in moment-nulled for flow-encoded two- and three-dimensional gradient echo imaging. *J. Magn. Reson. Imaging* 2: 583–588.

Bittoun, J., Jolivet, O., Herment, A., Itti, E., Durand, E., Mousseaux, E., and Tasu, J. P. 2000. Multidimensional MR mapping of multiple components of velocity and acceleration by Fourier phase encoding with a small number of encoding steps. *Magn. Reson. Med.* 44(5): 723–730.

Guilfoyle, D. N., Gibbs, P., Ordidge, R. J., and Mansfield, P. 1991. Real-time flow measurements using echo-planar imaging. *Magn. Reson. Med.* 18: 1–8.

Korosec, F. R., Grist, T. M., Polzin, J. A., Weber, D. M., and Mistretta, C. A. 1993. MR angiography using velocity-selective preparation pulses and segmented gradient-echo acquisition. *Magn. Reson. Med.* 30: 704–714.

Moran, P. R. 1982. A flow velocity zeugmatographic interlace for NMR imaging in humans. *Magn. Reson. Imaging* 1: 197–203.

Muthupillai, R., Lomas, D. J., Rossman, P. J., Greenleaf, J. F., Manduca, A., and Ehman, R. L. 1995. Magnetic resonance elastography by direct visualization of propagating acoustic strain waves. *Science* 269: 1854–1857.

Tasu, J. P., Jolivet, O., Mousseaux, E., Delouche, A., Diebold, B., and Bittoun, J. 1997. Acceleration mapping by Fourier acceleration-encoding: In vitro study and initial results in the great thoracic vessels. *Magn. Reson. Med.* 38: 110–116.

RELATED SECTIONS

Section 5.5 Tagging Pulses
Section 8.2 Phase-Encoding Gradient
Section 13.5 Phase Difference Reconstruction
Section 10.4 Gradient Moment Nulling
Section 15.2 Phase Contrast

10

CORRECTION GRADIENTS

10.1 Concomitant-Field Correction Gradients

Any magnetic field can be decomposed into its three orthogonal components B_x, B_y, and B_z. Each of these components can in turn exhibit spatial dependence along the three Cartesian axes, x, y, and z.[1] The linear gradients G_x, G_y, and G_z employed in MRI create spatial variations of B_z along the x, y, and z axes, respectively. When a linear gradient is applied (e.g., G_x, which creates variation of B_z with respect to x), other gradients (e.g., variation of B_x with respect to z) are unavoidably produced as a result of the Maxwell equations. (The equations are named after James Clerk Maxwell (1831–1879), a Scottish physicist and mathematician.) These other gradients are generated concurrently with the applied gradient and produce magnetic field components perpendicular to B_z, causing the net magnetic field vector to deviate from the direction of the applied B_0 field (i.e., along the z axis). They also cause the amplitude of the magnetic field to exhibit higher-order spatial dependence, such as x^2 and y^2. The magnetic field corresponding to the higher-order terms is known as a *concomitant magnetic field*, or simply *concomitant field*, and the higher-order spatial terms are referred to as *concomitant field-terms* or *Maxwell terms* (Norris and Hutchinson 1990; Wiesskoff et al. 1993; Bernstein et al. 1998).

The strength of the concomitant magnetic field is proportional to the square of the intentionally applied gradient and inversely proportional to the main magnetic field B_0. As such, the concomitant field can be negligible

---

[1] Note that in this section we denote the physical axis coordinates with lower case letters to make the symbols more easily readable.

at high field strength (e.g., 3.0 T) especially when a moderate gradient is used (e.g., 20 mT/m). At lower fields or with stronger gradients, however, the concomitant field can be substantial (e.g., ~10 ppm). The concomitant magnetic field represents a fundamental physics effect that is not related to imperfections in the hardware design and manufacture. Unlike eddy currents (discussed in Section 10.3), concomitant fields occur only when a gradient is active and disappear immediately when the gradient waveform returns to zero amplitude. Thus, there is no time constant associated with the concomitant fields. Also unlike eddy currents, the concomitant field at a specified spatial location can be exactly calculated for a given gradient waveform, without the need for measurement or calibration.

Because of the concomitant field, the transverse magnetization of a spin system accumulates an extra phase that is both spatially and temporally dependent. This is known as the *concomitant-field phase* or *Maxwell phase* (Bernstein et al. 1998). The concomitant-field phase, if not corrected, can cause a number of image artifacts, including geometric distortion, image shift, ghosting, intensity loss, blurring, and shading (Bernstein et al. 1998; Zhou, Du, et al. 1998; Zhou, Tan, et al. 1998; King et al. 1999; Du et al. 2002). Techniques to remove the concomitant-field phase include phase correction during image reconstruction (Bernstein et al. 1998; King et al. 1999; Du et al. 2002), hardware compensation (Classen-Vujcic et al. 1995), and alteration of the gradient waveforms in the pulse sequence. A discussion of a phase correction method during image reconstruction is given in Section 13.5. Approaches based on alteration of the pulse sequence are the focus of this section.

10.1.1 MATHEMATICAL DESCRIPTION OF CONCOMITANT MAGNETIC FIELD

According to the Maxwell equations, a magnetic field $\vec{B}$ must satisfy the following two conditions (Jackson 1975):

$$\vec{\nabla} \cdot \vec{B} = 0 \qquad \text{(div equation)} \qquad (10.1)$$

$$\frac{1}{\mu_0}\vec{\nabla} \times \vec{B} = \varepsilon_0 \frac{\partial \vec{E}}{\partial t} + \vec{J} \qquad \text{(curl equation)} \qquad (10.2)$$

where $\vec{\nabla}$ is the derivative operator (i.e., $\vec{\nabla} = \hat{x}\partial/\partial x + \hat{y}\partial/\partial y + \hat{z}\partial/\partial z$), $\vec{E}$ is the electric field, $\vec{J}$ is the current density, and μ_0 and ε_0 are the permeability and permittivity of free space, respectively. (Equation 10.2 assumes that the current source is embedded in a vacuum.) The first term on the right of Eq. (10.2) is usually called the displacement current density. If the displacement and real current densities are negligible, then Eq. (10.2) reduces to:

$$\vec{\nabla} \times \vec{B} = \vec{0} \tag{10.3}$$

Equations (10.1) and (10.3) can then be expanded into four scalar equations:

$$\frac{\partial B_x}{\partial x} + \frac{\partial B_y}{\partial y} + \frac{\partial B_z}{\partial z} = 0 \tag{10.4}$$

$$\frac{\partial B_x}{\partial y} = \frac{\partial B_y}{\partial x} \tag{10.5}$$

$$\frac{\partial B_y}{\partial z} = \frac{\partial B_z}{\partial y} \tag{10.6}$$

$$\frac{\partial B_z}{\partial x} = \frac{\partial B_x}{\partial z} \tag{10.7}$$

where B_x, B_y, and B_z are the components of $\vec{B}$ along the three orthogonal axes x, y, and z, respectively. Equations (10.4)–(10.7) contain a total of nine partial derivatives, among which only five are independent. Three of the independent partial derivatives are the intentionally applied linear gradients: $\frac{\partial B_z}{\partial x} \equiv G_x$, $\frac{\partial B_z}{\partial y} \equiv G_y$, and $\frac{\partial B_z}{\partial z} \equiv G_z$. The remaining two independent variables can be selected as a dimensionless parameter α:

$$\alpha \equiv -\frac{1}{G_z}\left(\frac{\partial B_x}{\partial x}\right) \quad \text{or} \quad 1 - \alpha = -\frac{1}{G_z}\left(\frac{\partial B_y}{\partial y}\right) \tag{10.8}$$

and a transverse gradient term:

$$G_\perp \equiv \frac{\partial B_x}{\partial y} = \frac{\partial B_y}{\partial x} \tag{10.9}$$

With these five independent variables, the partial derivatives in Eqs. (10.4)–(10.7) can be expressed as:

$$\begin{bmatrix} \dfrac{\partial B_x}{\partial x} & \dfrac{\partial B_x}{\partial y} & \dfrac{\partial B_x}{\partial z} \\[2mm] \dfrac{\partial B_y}{\partial x} & \dfrac{\partial B_y}{\partial y} & \dfrac{\partial B_y}{\partial z} \\[2mm] \dfrac{\partial B_z}{\partial x} & \dfrac{\partial B_z}{\partial y} & \dfrac{\partial B_z}{\partial z} \end{bmatrix} = \begin{bmatrix} -\alpha G_z & G_\perp & G_x \\ G_\perp & (\alpha - 1)G_z & G_y \\ G_x & G_y & G_z \end{bmatrix} \tag{10.10}$$

Consider a B_0 field applied along the z axis and three linear gradients G_x, G_y, and G_z. The net magnetic field vector is given by:

$$\vec{B} = \hat{x} B_x + \hat{y} B_y + \hat{z} B_z \tag{10.11}$$

If we neglect higher-order terms, the three magnetic field components B_x, B_y, and B_z are given by:

$$\begin{bmatrix} B_x \\ B_y \\ B_z - B_0 \end{bmatrix} = \begin{bmatrix} \dfrac{\partial B_x}{\partial x} & \dfrac{\partial B_x}{\partial y} & \dfrac{\partial B_x}{\partial z} \\ \dfrac{\partial B_y}{\partial x} & \dfrac{\partial B_y}{\partial y} & \dfrac{\partial B_y}{\partial z} \\ \dfrac{\partial B_z}{\partial x} & \dfrac{\partial B_z}{\partial y} & \dfrac{\partial B_z}{\partial z} \end{bmatrix} \begin{bmatrix} x \\ y \\ z \end{bmatrix}$$

$$= \begin{bmatrix} -\alpha G_z & G_\perp & G_x \\ G_\perp & (\alpha - 1)G_z & G_y \\ G_x & G_y & G_z \end{bmatrix} \begin{bmatrix} x \\ y \\ z \end{bmatrix} \tag{10.12}$$

Equation (10.12) has two important implications. First, because the transverse fields B_x and B_y are not necessarily 0, the net magnetic field is no longer aligned along the z axis, even when B_0, G_x, G_y, and G_z are all applied in the z-axis direction. Second, the amplitude of the overall magnetic field is not simply given by $B = B_0 + G_x x + G_y y + G_z z$. Instead, it must be calculated with:

$$B(x, y, z) = \sqrt{B_x^2 + B_y^2 + B_z^2} \tag{10.13}$$

If we perform a Taylor series expansion of Eq. (10.13), as detailed in Bernstein et al. (1998), we find that $B(x, y, z)$ not only has its nominal zeroth- and first-order spatial dependence, but also shows higher-order spatial components. The result of the Taylor expansion to the second order is given by:

$$B = B_0 + G_x x + G_y y + G_z z$$

$$+ \frac{1}{2B_0} \left[\left(\alpha^2 G_z^2 + G_\perp^2 \right) x^2 + \left((1 - \alpha)^2 G_z^2 + G_\perp^2 \right) y^2 + \left(G_x^2 + G_y^2 \right) z^2 \right]$$

$$+ \frac{1}{B_0} \left[-G_\perp G_z xy + \left(G_\perp G_x - (\alpha - 1)G_y G_z \right) yz \right.$$

$$\left. + \left(G_\perp G_y - \alpha G_x G_z \right) xz \right] \tag{10.14}$$

For cylindrical gradient coils used in MRI, $G_\perp \approx 0$ and $\alpha \approx 0.5$. Thus, Eq. (10.14) can be simplified to:

$$B = B_0 + G_x x + G_y y + G_z z$$

$$+ \frac{1}{2B_0} \left[\frac{G_z^2}{4} \left(x^2 + y^2 \right) + (G_x^2 + G_y^2)z^2 - G_x G_z xz - G_y G_z yz \right]$$

$$\text{(10.15)}$$

$$= B_0 + \vec{G} \cdot \vec{r} + B_c$$

where $\vec{G} = \hat{x}G_x + \hat{y}G_y + \hat{z}G_z$, $\vec{r} = \hat{x}x + \hat{y}y + \hat{z}z$, and B_c is the concomitant field that corresponds to the term in the bracket. Note that as long as B_0 is positive, the concomitant field B_c is a nonnegative quantity (i.e., it can be factored):

$$B_c = \frac{1}{2B_0} \left[\left(G_x z - \frac{G_z x}{2} \right)^2 + \left(G_y z - \frac{G_z y}{2} \right)^2 \right] \geq 0 \qquad \text{(10.16)}$$

It should be emphasized that the spatial variables x, y, and z in Eq. (10.15) are the physical, magnet coordinates. For example, z refers to the direction of the main magnetic field, which is not necessarily the same as the slice-selection axis. Thus, the concomitant field generated by the gradient waveforms in a pulse sequence depends not only on the choice of the slice, phase, and frequency directions, but also on the magnet geometry (i.e., standard horizontal cylindrical bore versus vertical-field open system).

The spatially quadratic and hyperbolic terms in Eqs. (10.14) and (10.15), as well as other higher-order terms not shown, are the concomitant-field terms. The concomitant field exhibiting x^2, y^2, or z^2 dependence has been called *on-axis* terms or *self-squared* terms, whereas the hyperbolic spatial terms (i.e., xz and yz) are called *cross terms* (Bernstein et al. 1998). Unlike self-squared terms, in order for a cross term to be nonzero, the waveforms of two applied gradients must be simultaneously active. As qualitatively described at the beginning of the section and mathematically shown in Eq. (10.14), all concomitant-field terms increase with gradient strength and spatial offset from the gradient isocenter and decrease with the static B_0 field. An example demonstrating these relationships is given next.

Example 10.1 At a distance of $z = 20$ cm from the gradient isocenter, calculate the z^2 concomitant-field term (in parts per million) produced by a G_x gradient of $40\,\text{mT/m}$ at $B_0 = 1.5$ T. Repeat the calculation for cases when (a) the gradient is reduced to 10 mT/m and (b) the main magnetic field is decreased to 0.7 T.

Answer With a G_x gradient of 40 mT/m, the z^2 concomitant-field term is calculated using Eq. (10.15):

$$\frac{G_x^2 z^2}{2B_0} = \frac{(40 \times 10^{-3} \times 0.2)^2}{2 \times 1.5} = 2.13 \times 10^{-5} \text{ T} = 14.2 \text{ ppm (at 1.5 T)}$$

(a) If the gradient is reduced to 10 mT/m, then:

$$\frac{G_x^2 z^2}{2B_0} = \frac{(10 \times 10^{-3} \times 0.2)^2}{2 \times 1.5} = 1.33 \times 10^{-6} \text{ T} = 0.889 \text{ ppm (at 1.5 T)}$$

(b) If the main magnetic field is decreased to 0.7 T, then:

$$\frac{G_x^2 z^2}{2B_0} = \frac{(40 \times 10^{-3} \times 0.2)^2}{2 \times 0.7} = 4.57 \times 10^{-5} \text{ T} = 65.3 \text{ ppm (at 0.7 T)}$$

Like all other perturbations in the magnetic field, concomitant field B_c causes transverse magnetization to accrue an additional phase over time. This phase (i.e., the *concomitant phase* or *Maxwell phase*) is given by:

$$\phi_c = \gamma \int_0^t B_c(G_x, G_y, G_z, x, y, z) \, dt' \tag{10.17}$$

Example 10.2 A trapezoidal gradient lobe $G_z(t)$ is applied to a spin system along the z direction at 1.5 T. The gradient amplitude is G_0, and the ramp time and plateau duration are δ and Δ, respectively. At the end of the gradient lobe, what is the concomitant phase for a point whose coordinates are (x, y, z) with respect to the gradient isocenter?

Answer The concomitant field produced by G_z is:

$$B_c = \frac{G_z^2(t)}{8B_0}(x^2 + y^2)$$

The corresponding concomitant phase can be calculated from Eq. (10.17):

$$\phi_c = \gamma \int_0^{2\delta + \Delta} \frac{G_z^2(t)}{8B_0}(x^2 + y^2) \, dt = \frac{\gamma G_0^2}{8B_0}\left(\Delta + \frac{2}{3}\delta\right)(x^2 + y^2)$$

When the concomitant phase ϕ_c is accounted for, the two-dimensional MR signal becomes:

$$S(k_x, k_y) = \iint_{x,y} \rho(x, y) e^{-i(k_x x + k_y y)} e^{-i\phi_c} \, dx \, dy \tag{10.18}$$

As implied by Eq. (10.17), ϕ_c depends on the amplitude of B_c, which is determined by the details of the pulse sequence. Unless the concomitant-field phase in Eq. (10.18) is negligible, it becomes a source of image artifacts, including intensity loss, shading, image shift, distortion, and ghosting.

10.1.2 CONCOMITANT-FIELD CORRECTION GRADIENT

To produce artifact-free images, the concomitant-field phase error must be eliminated or reduced to a negligible level. In this subsection, we present several strategies to cancel or substantially reduce the phase errors by altering existing gradient lobes or adding new gradient lobes to the gradient waveforms. The following discussion is largely based on Zhou, Tan, et al. (1998).

Waveform Symmetrization   If two identical gradient waveforms straddle a refocusing RF pulse (Figure 10.1), then the concomitant-field phases produced by the two waveforms are equal. Since a refocusing RF pulse negates the phase of an NMR signal, the net phase error after the second gradient waveform is zero. Thus, as long as the gradient waveforms are symmetrical before and after a refocusing RF pulse, the concomitant-field phase error is always nulled. This simple strategy has been referred to as *waveform symmetrization* (Zhou, Tan, et al. 1998). Examples of waveform symmetrization include diffusion-weighting gradients in a spin-echo pulse sequence, crusher gradients placed symmetrically around a refocusing pulse, and the slice-selection gradient that is played concurrently with a symmetric refocusing RF pulse.

Phase Subtraction   Related to the concept of waveform symmetrization is concomitant-field cancellation using *phase subtraction*. In phase difference imaging, often the gradient lobes that make up the waveforms used to acquire

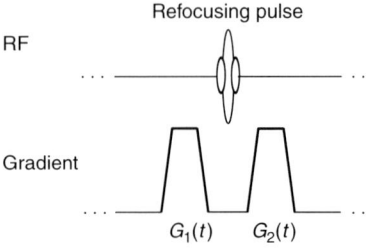

FIGURE 10.1 An example of waveform symmetrization. The gradient lobes $G_1(t)$ and $G_2(t)$ are identical and are placed on either side of a refocusing RF pulse.

the two sets of data are either identical or toggled (i.e., negated). The concomitant phase from any two identical lobes in a pair of pulse sequences will cancel during the phase difference reconstruction. The concomitant phase resulting from self-squared terms will also subtract out for lobes that are negated, but this is not necessarily true for a concomitant phase resulting from the cross terms. A more general procedure to correct phase-contrast images for the concomitant phase error is given in Bernstein et al. (1998).

Examples of two acquisitions employing identical gradient waveforms include phase-sensitive temperature imaging and B_0-field mapping sequences that use two different TEs (Figure 10.2). However, when the two data sets used for a phase difference calculation are acquired within a single excitation (e.g., sequences employing multiple RF spin echoes), the concomitant-field phase is generally *not* cancelled. This is partially why B_0-field mapping pulse sequences usually acquire two separated data sets rather than the more time-efficient method of using two echoes from a single acquisition. Examples of gradient waveforms with toggled gradient lobes can be found in pulse sequences used to measure eddy currents (Jehenson et al. 1990) and in phase-contrast angiography, provided that the bipolar flow-sensitizing gradient is not combined with any other imaging gradients.

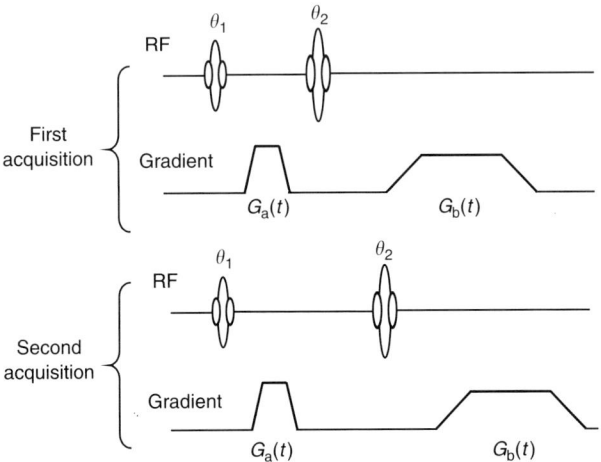

FIGURE 10.2 An example of phase subtraction employing two acquisitions with identical gradient lobes, differing only by a temporal shift. The TEs of the two acquisitions are different, but the concomitant phase arising from the gradient lobes $G_a(t)$ and $G_b(t)$ is cancelled during the phase difference calculation. $G_a(t)$ and $G_b(t)$ can be any gradient lobes in the pulse sequence.

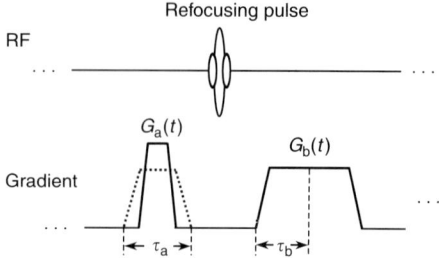

FIGURE 10.3 An example of waveform reshaping. The gradient lobe $G_a(t)$ can be adjusted or reshaped to cancel the concomitant phase introduced by $G_b(t)$. Similar to waveform symmetrization, the phase cancellation relies on the phase reversal effect of a refocusing RF pulse. The dotted lines indicate the gradient lobe after reshaping.

Waveform Reshaping   Unlike waveform symmetrization, which often occurs inherently in a pulse sequence without requiring conscious design, *waveform reshaping*, as the name implies, requires modification of the existing gradient lobes or waveforms to null the concomitant-field phases. This strategy is usually employed in conjunction with a refocusing RF pulse.

Consider the gradient waveform shown in Figure 10.3. If the lobe after the refocusing RF pulse represents a frequency-encoding gradient, then imaging considerations such as the prescribed FOV and receiver bandwidth determine the amplitude of the second gradient lobe G_b. With the amplitude of the second lobe fixed, waveform symmetrization may be impossible because of constraints such as the balancing of gradient area and minimization of TE. If the area of the gradient lobe G_a, for example, must be one-half of the total area of the lobe G_b, as in the case for a full echo readout prephasing gradient, then the shape of G_a can be adjusted to simultaneously satisfy the following two conditions:

$$\int_0^{\tau_a} G_a(t)\, dt = \int_0^{\tau_b} G_b(t')\, dt' \qquad (10.19)$$

$$\int_0^{\tau_a} G_a^2(t)\, dt = \int_0^{\tau_b} G_b^2(t')\, dt' \qquad (10.20)$$

where τ_a is the full duration of the lobe G_a and τ_b is the half duration of lobe G_b. Equation (10.20), together with the phase-reversal effect of the refocusing RF pulse, ensures that the self-squared concomitant phase is canceled at the center of G_b. Although we have used gradient area as a constraint to demonstrate the concept, other constraints can also be incorporated in the reshaping technique as long as enough freedom is present in the gradient waveform design so that Eq. (10.20) can be satisfied.

Waveform reshaping often involves solving quadratic or cubic equations. An example of solving a quadratic equation is given in Example 10.3; examples of solving cubic equations can be found in Zhou, Tan, et al. (1998).

Example 10.3 Assume that the gradient lobes G_a and G_b in Figure 10.3 all have the same ramp time δ. If the amplitude of G_b is fixed at G_0 and half the duration of the plateau is Δ, calculate the amplitude g and the plateau duration T of lobe G_a based on waveform reshaping criteria given by Eqs. (10.19) and (10.20).

Answer Substituting the gradient lobe parameters into Eqs. (10.19) and (10.20) and carrying out the integration, we obtain:

$$g(T + \delta) = G_0(\Delta + \delta/2)$$

$$g^2 \left(T + \frac{2}{3}\delta \right) = G_0^2 \left(\Delta + \frac{1}{3}\delta \right)$$

Combining these equations to eliminate the unknown T yields a quadratic equation with respect to g:

$$g^2 - 3G_0 \left(\frac{\Delta}{\delta} + \frac{1}{2} \right) g + G_0^2 \left(\frac{3\Delta}{\delta} + 1 \right) = 0$$

The solutions for the quadratic equation are:

$$g = \frac{3(2\Delta + \delta) \pm \sqrt{36\Delta^2 - 12\Delta\delta - 7\delta^2}}{4\delta} G_0$$

If both solutions are real and positive, then the sequence designer has the flexibility to choose either the smaller value of g to minimize the gradient heating, acoustic noise, and eddy currents or the larger value of g to reduce the sequence time. If only one solution makes physical sense, that solution is chosen as the reshaped gradient amplitude. If neither solution is real and positive, then the gradient lobe cannot be re-shaped to completely null the concomitant phase. However, some value of g always can be chosen that minimizes the phase, as discussed in Zhou, Tan et al. (1998). Once the value of g is specified, the plateau duration T can be calculated from:

$$T = \frac{G_0}{g} \left(\Delta + \frac{\delta}{2} \right) - \delta$$

Quadratic Nulling   When a gradient is applied on only one side of a refocusing RF pulse (G_c in Figure 10.4), such as a phase-encoding gradient, its self-squared phase can be canceled by introducing an additional gradient waveform G_d on the other side of the RF pulse, provided that the new waveform satisfies the following conditions:

$$\int_0^{\tau_d} G_d(t)\, dt = 0 \tag{10.21}$$

$$\int_0^{\tau_d} G_d^2(t')\, dt' = \int_0^{\tau_c} G_c^2(t)\, dt \tag{10.22}$$

where τ_c and τ_d are the waveform durations for G_c and G_d, respectively. This strategy has been referred to as *quadratic nulling* (Zhou, Tan, et al. 1998).

There are many waveforms that satisfy Eqs. (10.21) and (10.22). The simplest one is a bipolar gradient waveform shown in Figure 10.4a. Alternatively, a gradient waveform with three lobes whose area ratios are $1 : -2 : 1$ can also be used for quadratic nulling (Figure 10.4b). That waveform provides the additional benefit of velocity compensation as discussed in Section 9.2. It is worth noting that the quadratic nulling lobes can be applied on a different gradient axis. For example, a z^2 phase error caused by the x gradient can be canceled

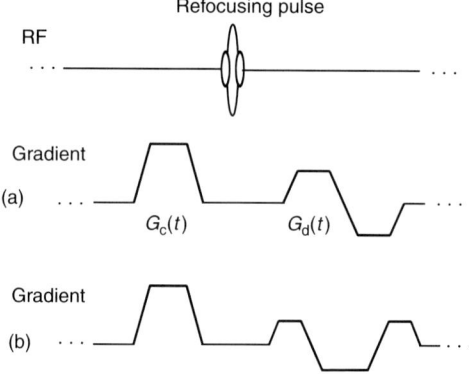

FIGURE 10.4 Two examples of quadratic nulling. To cancel the concomitant phase introduced by a gradient lobe $G_c(t)$ (e.g., the phase-encoding gradient), another gradient waveform $G_d(t)$ with zero net area can be introduced on the other side of a refocusing pulse. The waveform $G_d(t)$ in (a) is used to avoid net phase dispersion for static spins, whereas the waveform $G_d(t)$ in (b) has the additional advantage of rephasing spins moving with a constant velocity.

with a quadratic nulling gradient on the y gradient because both gradients contribute to the z^2 concomitant field. We refer to this approach as *cross-axis quadratic nulling*. When minimum sequence time, gradient duty cycle, or heating becomes a constraint, the cross-axis quadratic nulling approach can be employed to balance the gradient load among the coils and amplifiers.

Gradient Derating   In cases in which exact phase cancellation is difficult to achieve, an alternative approach to reduce the concomitant-field phase errors is to decrease the gradient amplitude, that is, *gradient derating*. As shown in Bernstein et al. (1998, app. B), the concomitant-field phase produced by a trapezoidal gradient lobe is approximately proportional to the maximum gradient amplitude when the gradient area is held constant. Because many applications require the gradient area to be held constant, decreasing the gradient amplitude often results in increased waveform duration. Thus, some limits must be imposed on the extent of gradient derating. Unlike the previously discussed strategies that are sometimes limited to self-squared terms, gradient derating can reduce both self-squared and cross-term phases.

Gradient derating does not always reduce the net concomitant phase in a pulse sequence. For example, if a strong gradient pulse is present before a refocusing RF pulse, derating the gradient amplitude after the refocusing pulse may increase the imbalance of the concomitant-field phase, leading to a larger net phase error. The details of the pulse sequence must be carefully examined before applying the gradient derating strategy.

Gradient Separation   Another effective way to reduce, or even eliminate, the cross-term phase errors is to minimize the temporal overlap of gradient lobes on different axes (Figure 10.5). Similar to the derating strategy, some practical limits must be imposed to prevent prolonging the interecho spacing,

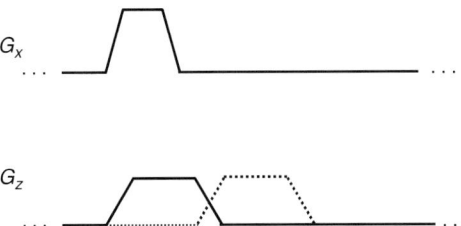

FIGURE 10.5 Waveform separation. The G_z gradient waveform is shifted (dotted lines) with respect to the G_x gradient to minimize the overlap. In doing so, concomitant phase due to the $G_x G_z$ cross term can be reduced or even eliminated.

or the minimum TE, of the sequence. It should be noted that the strategy with gradient separation cannot be used for oblique scan protocols because a gradient waveform on one logical (i.e, imaging, or functional) axis is produced by multiple physical gradient axes simultaneously.

Other Correction Techniques   Under special circumstances, concomitant-field phase errors are reduced from a spatially quadratic (or hyperbolic) term to a spatially linear term or even a constant term. For example, the z^2 term becomes spatially constant for a slice perpendicular to the z axis, and an xz term reduces to a linear phase error with respect to the x coordinate. Although the strategies already discussed still apply under these conditions, simpler phase correction techniques can be used to remove or reduce the linear and constant phase errors. For example, in an echo planar pulse sequence, the linear phase error can be corrected by using an additional gradient lobe or changing the existing gradient area, and the constant phase errors can be eliminated by adjusting the receiver phase or frequency as shown in Zhou, Du, et al. (1998).

Because the concomitant-field phase errors can be exactly calculated from the gradient waveforms in the pulse sequence, the errors can also be removed in the stage of image reconstruction, provided that the k-space signals do not contain multiple coherent pathways with varying concomitant-field phase errors (e.g., in RARE or fast-spin echo pulse sequences). Methods for phase correction during image reconstruction can be found in Bernstein et al. (1998), King et al. (1999), and Du et al. (2002).

SELECTED REFERENCES

Bernstein, M. A., Zhou, X. J., Polzin, J. A., King, K. F., Ganin, A., Pelc, N. J., and Glover, G. H. 1998. Concomitant gradient terms in phase contrast, MR: Analysis and correction. *Magn. Reson. Med.* 39: 300–308.

Claasen-Vujcic, T., Slotboom, J., and Mehlkopf, A. F. 1995. Reduction of concomitant field gradient effects by main magnetic field alternation. *Proc. Soc. Magn. Reson. Med.* 1: 315.

Du, Y. P., Zhou, X. J., and Bernstein, M. A. 2002. Correction of concomitant magnetic field induced image artifacts in non-axial echo planar imaging. *Magn. Reson. Med.* 48: 509–515.

Jackson, J. D. 1975. *Classical electrodynamics.* 2nd ed. New York: John Wiley & Sons.

Jehenson, P., Westphal, M., and Schuff, N. 1990. Analytical method for the compensation of eddy-current effects induced by pulsed magnetic field gradients in NMR systems. *J. Magn. Reson.* 90: 264–278.

King, K. F., Ganin, A., Zhou, X. J., and Bernstein, M. A. 1999. Concomitant gradient field effects in spiral scans. *Magn. Reson. Med.* 41: 103–112.

Norris, D. G., and Hutchison, J. M. S. 1990. Concomitant magnetic field gradients and their effects on imaging at low magnetic field strengths. *Magn. Reson. Imaging* 8: 33–37.

Weisskoff, R. M., Cohen, M. S., and Rzedzian, R. R. 1993. Nonaxial whole-body instant imaging. *Magn. Reson. Med.* 29: 796–803.

reference frame becomes:

$$\omega_L(r) = \gamma G_L r \tag{10.23}$$

where r is the spatial variable along the gradient direction (the time dependence of G_L is not explicitly expressed for simplicity). The spatially dependent
frequency $\omega_L(r)$ results in a phase dispersion of the transverse magnetization:

$$\phi_L(r) = \int_0^{t_L} \omega_L(r)\, dt = \gamma r \int_0^{t_L} G_L\, dt = \gamma A_L r \tag{10.24}$$

where t_L and A_L are the duration and the area of the left crusher lobe, respectively. Similarly, the phase dispersion created by the right crusher gradient lobe
is given by:

$$\phi_R(r) = \int_0^{t_R} \omega_R(r)\, dt = \gamma r \int_0^{t_R} G_R\, dt = \gamma A_R r \tag{10.25}$$

For a spin-echo signal, the magnetization is in the transverse plane before
and after the refocusing pulse. Thus, the phases in Eqs. (10.24) and (10.25)
both apply. Because the refocusing RF pulse negates the phase, the net phase
accumulation after the crusher pair is given by $\phi_R(r) - \phi_L(r)$. If the two crusher
lobes have equal area, the net phase is zero irrespective of r and the spin-echo
signal is formed as usual.

For the FID signal produced by the nonideal refocusing pulse, only $\phi_R(r)$
applies. If $\phi_R(r)$ is sufficiently large, the phase dispersion can completely
destroy the signal coherence when averaged over an image voxel, removing
the FID from the data-acquisition window.

Crusher Gradient for Multiple Refocusing Pulses   Consider the pulse
sequence with three RF pulses (an excitation pulse θ_1 followed by two nonideal
refocusing pulses θ_2 and θ_3) in Figure 10.9a. According to Section 16.4, the
three-pulse combination produces three primary spin echoes, one secondary
spin echo, one stimulated echo, and three FIDs. These signal pathways are
graphically shown in Figure 10.9b–e and summarized in Table 10.1 where
M_z and $M_\perp$ represent the longitudinal and the transverse magnetization,
respectively, and $\tilde{M}_\perp$ denotes the phase-negated transverse magnetization. For
example, the stimulated echo pathway is denoted by $M_z \to M_\perp$ (i.e., excited
by the first RF pulse), $M_\perp \to \tilde{M}_\perp \to M_z$ (i.e., phase-reversed and restored to
the longitudinal axis by the second pulse), and $M_z \to \tilde{M}_\perp$ (i.e., reexcited by
the third pulse).

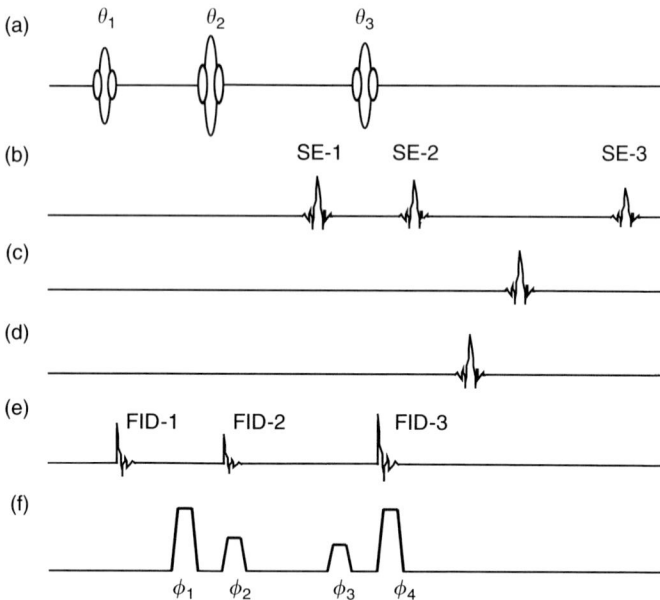

FIGURE 10.9 (a) A pulse sequence consisting of three RF pulses, one excitation pulse θ_1 followed by two refocusing pulses θ_2 and θ_3. The signal pathways—(b) primary spin echoes, (c) secondary spin echo, (d) stimulated echo, and (e) FIDs—produced by the sequence are summarized in Table 10.1. (f) The phase produced by each crusher gradient lobe surrounding the refocusing RF pulses is sequentially denoted by ϕ_1, ϕ_2, ϕ_3, and ϕ_4.

TABLE 10.1

Signal Pathways for a Sequence with Three RF Pulses[a]

Signal Pathways	θ_1	θ_2	θ_3
Primary SE-1	$M_z \rightarrow M_\perp$	$M_\perp \rightarrow \tilde{M}_\perp$	(no effect)
Primary SE-2	$M_z \rightarrow M_\perp$	$M_\perp \rightarrow \tilde{M}_\perp$	$\tilde{M}_\perp \rightarrow M_\perp$
Primary SE-3	$M_z \rightarrow M_\perp$	(no effect)	$M_\perp \rightarrow \tilde{M}_\perp$
Secondary SE	(no effect)	$M_z \rightarrow M_\perp$	$M_\perp \rightarrow \tilde{M}_\perp$
Stimulated echo	$M_z \rightarrow M_\perp$	$M_\perp \rightarrow \tilde{M}_\perp \rightarrow M_z$	$M_z \rightarrow \tilde{M}_\perp$
FID-1	$M_z \rightarrow M_\perp$	(no effect)	(no effect)
FID-2	(no effect)	$M_z \rightarrow M_\perp$	(no effect)
FID-3	(no effect)	(no effect)	$M_z \rightarrow M_\perp$

[a] The table shows the effect of each RF pulse on the magnetization. SE, spin echo; FID, free-induction decay.

With the aid of Table 10.1, we can illustrate how crusher gradients can be used to (1) eliminate the stimulated echo while preserving the first two primary spin echoes (SE-1 and SE-2), (2) eliminate the primary spin echoes while preserving the stimulated echo, or (3) preserve both the primary spin echoes and the stimulated echo. In all three cases, we dephase the signals from FID-2 and FID-3. In general, we show that each requirement leads to a set of linear equations for the crusher areas.

Case 1: Crushers to Select the Primary Echo Pathway

We denote the phases introduced by each crusher gradient lobe surrounding the refocusing pulses by ϕ_1, ϕ_2, ϕ_3, and ϕ_4, (Figure 10.9f). These phases can be calculated using Eq. (10.24) or (10.25). According to Table 10.1 and the guidelines listed in the previous subsection, the crusher phase experienced by the stimulated echo is:

$$\phi_{ste} = -\phi_1 + \phi_4 \qquad (10.26)$$

Equation (10.26) can be intuitively understood by recognizing that (1) the stimulated echo is excited by the first pulse and thus accumulates a phase ϕ_1 from the first crusher lobe, (2) the second RF pulse negates the phase ($\phi_1 \rightarrow -\phi_1$) and stores the magnetization on the longitudinal axis so that it is impervious to the second and third crusher lobes, and (3) the third RF pulse reexcites the magnetization that experiences the phase caused by the fourth crusher ϕ_4. To dephase the stimulated echo, ϕ_{ste} must be nonzero; that is:

$$\phi_1 \neq \phi_4 \qquad (10.27)$$

On the other hand, the phases experienced by the first two primary spin echoes are given by:

$$\phi_{pse1} = -\phi_1 + \phi_2 \qquad (10.28)$$
$$\phi_{pse2} = \phi_1 - \phi_2 - \phi_3 + \phi_4 \qquad (10.29)$$

To preserve the primary echoes, ϕ_{pse1} and ϕ_{pse2} must be both zero; that is:

$$\begin{cases} \phi_1 = \phi_2 \\ \phi_3 = \phi_4 \end{cases} \qquad (10.30)$$

In order to eliminate the FIDs following the refocusing pulses, we must have:

$$\begin{cases} \phi_2 \neq 0 \\ \phi_4 \neq 0 \end{cases} \qquad (10.31)$$

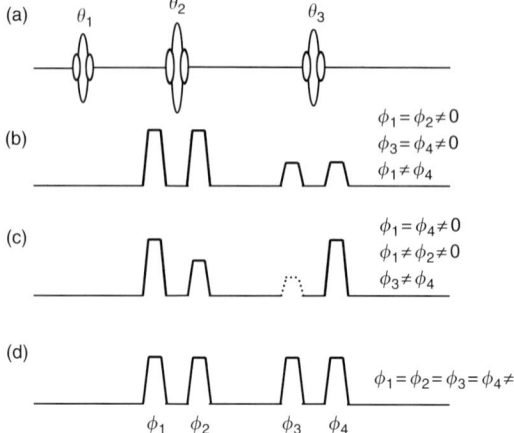

FIGURE 10.10 Examples of crusher gradient design based on the pulse sequence in Figure 10.9. (a) RF pulses. (b) Crushers to select only the primary spin echoes. (c) Crushers to select only the stimulated echo. The crusher gradient shown by the dashed line is optional. (d) Crushers to select both the primary spin echoes and the stimulated echo. In all three cases, the FIDs from the refocusing pulses are dephased.

Equations (10.27), (10.30), and (10.31) specify a set of design conditions for crusher gradients that selects the first two primary spin echoes while eliminating the stimulated echo and the FIDs. A set of crusher lobes that satisfies these conditions is graphically shown in Figure 10.10b.

Case 2: Crushers to Select the Stimulated Echo Pathway

In order to select the stimulated echo pathway while removing the primary spin echoes and the FIDs, the following conditions must be met: $\phi_{ste} = 0$, $\phi_{pse1} \neq 0$, $\phi_{pse2} \neq 0$, $\phi_{pse3} = -\phi_1 - \phi_2 - \phi_3 + \phi_4 \neq 0$, $\phi_2 \neq 0$, and $\phi_4 \neq 0$. Using Eqs. (10.26), (10.28) and (10.29), these conditions can be summarized as:

$$
\begin{cases}
\phi_1 = \phi_4 \\
\phi_1 \neq \phi_2 \\
\phi_3 \neq \phi_4 \\
\phi_2 \neq 0 \\
\phi_4 \neq 0
\end{cases}
\tag{10.32}
$$

A set of crusher lobes that satisfies Eq. (10.32) is graphically shown in Figure 10.10c. It is worth noting that the left crusher of the third RF pulse is optional (dashed line), as long as $\phi_3 \neq \phi_4$. When $\phi_3 = 0$, the third RF pulse has a one-sided crusher.

Case 3: Crushers to Select Both Primary and Stimulated Echo Pathways

To preserve both the primary and stimulated echoes while removing the FIDs, we must have $\phi_{ste} = 0$, $\phi_{pse1} = 0$, $\phi_{pse2} = 0$, $\phi_2 \neq 0$, and $\phi_4 \neq 0$. These conditions can be summarized by:

$$\phi_1 = \phi_2 = \phi_3 = \phi_4 \neq 0 \tag{10.33}$$

Crushers that satisfy Eq. (10.33) are illustrated in Figure 10.10d. They are widely used in pulse sequences employing multiple refocusing RF pulses, such as RARE or fast spin echo (Hennig 1988).

It is interesting to note that the condition in Eq. (10.33) does not preserve the third primary spin echo listed in Table 10.1 (i.e., $\phi_{pse3} = -\phi_1 - \phi_2 - \phi_3 + \phi_4 \neq 0$). In most multiecho pulse sequences, however, an additional RF pulse is applied prior to the formation of the third primary spin echo. If this RF pulse has the same crusher pair (denoted by their phase values ϕ_5 and ϕ_6) as the other two refocusing pulses (i.e., $\phi_5 = \phi_6 = \phi_1 = \phi_2 = \phi_3 = \phi_4$), the phase for the third primary spin echo becomes $\phi_{pse3} = -\phi_1 - \phi_2 - \phi_3 + \phi_4 + \phi_5 + \phi_6 = 0$. Therefore, this signal pathway is also preserved.

As the number of refocusing pulses increases in a pulse sequence, the number of signal pathways grows exponentially. For example, after applying n RF pulses, the maximum number of the signal pathways (M) following the nth pulse is:

$$M = \frac{3^{n-1} - 1}{2} \tag{10.34}$$

In spite of the large number of the signal pathways, the principles described here are equally applicable to designing crushers to select the desired coherence signal pathways.

10.2.3 DESIGN CONSIDERATIONS

Crusher gradients eliminate the unwanted signals by introducing intra-voxel dephasing. For a given crusher gradient area, the extent of signal dephasing is directly proportional to the voxel size along the crusher gradient direction, as implied by Eqs. (10.24) and (10.25). Although crusher gradients can be applied along any direction, in practice they are most commonly employed on the slice-selection axis, primarily because an imaging voxel typically has the largest dimension along this direction. To minimize the TE of a pulse sequence, the crusher lobes are often fused or bridged with the slice-selection gradient, as long as the area of the crusher lobe is not compromised. An example of bridging a crusher pair to a slice-selection gradient is given

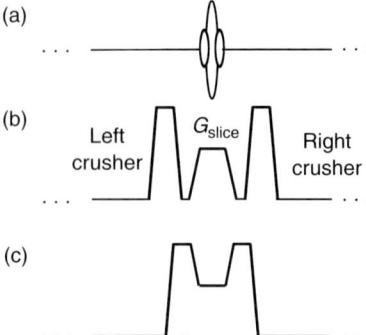

FIGURE 10.11 Crusher gradients before (b) and after (c) combination with the slice-selection gradient (G_{slice}) of a refocusing RF pulse (a).

in Figure 10.11. The quantitative details on how much pulse sequence time is saved by using a bridged gradient waveform can be found in Section 7.2.

The proper value of the crusher gradient area is commonly determined empirically. It has been suggested that the minimum phase dispersion within a voxel should be $\sim 4\pi$ (Hennig 1988). An example of how to use this guideline for crusher gradient design is given next.

Example 10.4 A subject is imaged on an MRI system with a maximum gradient amplitude $h = 22\,\text{mT/m}$ and a slew rate $S_R = 120\,\text{mT/m/ms}$. The desired image has a FOV of 24×24 cm, a matrix of 256×256, and a slice thickness of 0.5 cm. If a spin-echo pulse sequence is used, design an optimally time-efficient crusher gradient lobe (without bridging to the slice-selection gradient) to eliminate the FID signal arising from a nonideal refocusing pulse.

Answer The voxel size of the image is:

$$\Delta x = \Delta y = \frac{24\,\text{cm}}{256} = 0.094\,\text{cm}$$

$$\Delta z = 0.5\,\text{cm}$$

Because the slice-selection direction has the largest voxel dimension, the crusher gradient should be applied in that direction. To produce a 4π phase dispersion along the slice-selection direction, the crusher gradient area can be calculated from Eq. (10.25):

$$A_R = \frac{\Delta\phi_R}{\gamma\,\Delta z} = \frac{4\pi}{2\pi \times 42.57\,\text{kHz/mT} \times 0.005\,\text{m}} = 9.396\,\text{mT} \cdot \text{ms/m}$$

Because $A_R > h^2/S_R = 22^2/120 = 4.033\ \text{mT} \cdot \text{ms/m}$, according to Section 7.1, the most time-efficient crusher is a trapezoid with ramp time, plateau duration, and gradient amplitude given by:

$$T_{\text{ramp}} = h/S_R = 22/120 = 0.183\ \text{ms}$$
$$T_{\text{plateau}} = A_R/h - T_{\text{ramp}} = 9.396/22 - 0.183 = 0.243\ \text{ms}$$
$$G = h = 22\ \text{mT/m}$$

The left crusher should be identical to the right crusher.

As illustrated in Example 10.4, the crusher gradients can be quite large in many pulse sequences. As such, they can contribute to the diffusion-induced signal loss, eddy currents, and concomitant magnetic field. In a diffusion pulse sequence with crusher gradients, the contribution from the crusher pair to the b-value should be calculated and accounted for, if it is sufficiently large. Derating the crusher gradient amplitude and or the slew rate can reduce the eddy current problem. This approach sometimes leads to an increased minimum TE value or longer interecho spacing. Phase errors arising from concomitant magnetic fields (Section 10.1) of crusher gradients can be nonnegligible under certain imaging conditions, such as large FOV, low B_0 field, and high gradient strength. This problem can be addressed either by using identical crushers for each refocusing pulse or by reshaping the crusher lobes (Zhou et al. 1998).

10.2.4 APPLICATIONS

Crusher gradients are extensively used in pulse sequences containing RF refocusing pulses, such as spin-echo, multiple spin-echo (i.e., Carr-Purcell-Meiboom-Gill pulse train), RARE (or fast spin-echo), and GRASE sequences. In single-echo RF spin-echo pulse sequences, the primary function of the crusher gradient is to prevent the FID signal from intruding into the spin echo (Bottomley and Edelstein 1984). This can be done as shown in Example 10.4 and Figure 10.7. In multiple spin-echo pulse sequences, stimulated echoes are typically crushed out by varying the crusher gradient amplitude throughout the echo train (Poon and Henkelman 1992). In doing so, the acquired signals (i.e., the primary spin echoes) can exhibit pure T_2 exponential decay as a function of the TE, and the images at each echo can be used to calculate a T_2 map. In RARE, both stimulated echo and primary echo signals are commonly preserved in order to achieve the best SNR. This can be accomplished by using the same crusher amplitude throughout the echo train (Hennig 1988). Alternative crusher designs can also be used to select either primary (Zhou et al. 1993) or stimulated echoes (Norris et al. 1992) in fast spin echo sequences. These crusher designs are particularly useful in diffusion-weighted fast spin-echo pulse sequences (Beaulieu et al. 1993; Alsop 1997).

SELECTED REFERENCES

Alsop, D. C. 1997. Phase insensitive preparation of single-shot RARE: Application to diffusion imaging in humans. *Magn. Reson. Med.* 38: 527–533.

Beaulieu, C. F., Zhou, X., Cofer, G. P., and Johnson, G. A. 1993. Diffusion-weighted MR microscopy with fast-spin echo. *Magn. Reson. Med.* 30: 201–206.

Bottomley, P. A., and Edelstein, W. A. 1984. Methods of eliminating effects of spurious free induction decay NMR signal caused by imperfect 180 degree RF pulses. U.S. Patent 4,484,138.

Hennig, J. 1988. Multiecho sequences with low refocusing flip angles. *J. Magn. Reson.* 78: 397–407.

Norris, D. G., Bornert, P., Reese, T., and Leibfritz, D. 1992. On the application of ultra-fast RARE experiments. *Magn. Reson. Med.* 27: 142–164.

Poon, C. S., and Henkelman, R. M. 1992. Practical T_2 quantitation for clinical applications. *J. Magn. Reson. Imaging* 2: 541–553.

Zhou, X. J., Cofer, G. P., Suddarth, S. A., and Johnson, G. A. 1993. High-field MR microscopy using fast spin-echoes. *Magn. Reson. Med.* 30: 60–67.

Zhou, X. J., Tan, S. G., and Bernstein, M. A. 1998. Artifacts induced by concomitant magnetic field in fast spin-echo imaging. *Magn. Reson. Med.* 40: 582–591.

RELATED SECTIONS

10.3 Eddy-Current Compensation

10.3.1 EDDY CURRENTS

The time-varying magnetic fields from gradients in MRI pulse sequences induce currents in conducting structures within the magnet, gradient coils themselves, and RF coils. The induced currents are called *eddy currents* and create unwanted magnetic fields that are detrimental to image quality. With modern commercial scanners that use actively shielded gradients and gradient waveform preemphasis, eddy-current effects are minimal for most applications. Image-quality problems that have been caused by eddy currents include (but are not limited to) ghosting in EPI (Fischer and Ladebeck 1998), RARE and GRASE, slice-profile modulation with spatial-spectral RF pulses (Block et al. 1997; Zur 2000) geometric distortion in diffusion-weighted EPI (Haselgrove and Moore 1996), and quantitative velocity errors in phase-contrast imaging (Lingamneni et al. 1995).

Origin of Eddy Currents   The eddy currents are generated by the electric fields that result from changing magnetic flux (Faraday's law). They build up during the time-varying part of the gradient waveforms and decay during the constant portions. For a trapezoidal waveform, eddy currents are generated by the ramps and decay away at other times, as shown in Figure 10.12. The rate of eddy-current buildup is proportional to the gradient slew rate (i.e., the slope of the gradient ramp). The magnetic field produced by the eddy current always opposes the change in the field causing the eddy current (Lenz's law, named after Heinrich Friedrich Emil Lenz, 1804–1865, a Russian physicist).

Consider a trapezoidal pulse on the physical x gradient. (As in Section 10.1, we denote the physical axis coordinates with lowercase letters to make the equations more easily readable.) For the rising (i.e., ascending) ramp of the trapezoid shown in Figure 10.12, the field change is positive for $x > 0$, resulting in an eddy-current field that is negative. The opposite happens for the

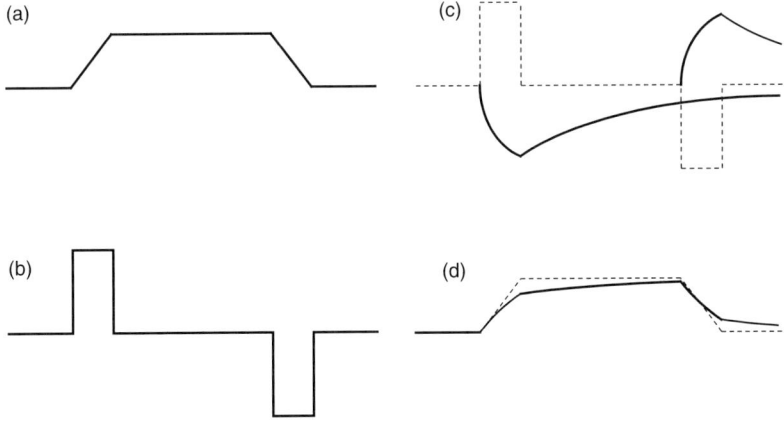

FIGURE 10.12 (a) A trapezoidal gradient waveform $G(t)$ plotted versus time. (b) The time derivative of the waveform dG/dt. (c) Eddy-current gradient (solid line) and exciting field dG/dt (dashed line). An independent eddy-current gradient is generated by each ramp. (d) Net gradient field (solid line) and ideal trapezoidal field (dashed line). The eddy-current field in (c) is added to the ideal field in (a). The amplitude of the eddy-current gradient in (c) and the degradation in the net field in (d) are exaggerated for clarity.

falling (i.e., descending) ramp. For a trapezoidal waveform, the net gradient field (ideal field plus eddy- current field) behaves as if it were passed through a low-pass filter, with the corners of the rising and falling ramps rounded off as shown in Figure 10.12. The eddy currents generated by the rising and falling ramps of any trapezoidal gradient lobe can be thought of as separate entities. Because the two eddy-current fields have opposite sign, they partially cancel after completion of the trapezoidal waveform. The degree of cancellation depends on the plateau length and the decay rate of the eddy current fields. This cancellation concept is used in some eddy-current reduction methods (Alexander et al. 1997; Koch and Norris 2000; Wider et al. 1994). An important point to note is that the eddy-current amplitude after completion of the trapezoid is proportional to the plateau amplitude and is therefore reduced by using lower-amplitude gradients.

It has been found that the time dependence of eddy currents is accurately modeled by an exponential function (Van Vaals and Bergman 1990; Jehenson et al, 1990). Using this model, eddy currents are characterized by a small number of *time constants* and coefficients that are called *amplitudes*. The time constant describes the rate of exponential buildup and decay after a gradient change. Eddy-current time constants on commercial scanners can range from a few microseconds to hundreds of seconds.

Eddy-current spatial dependence is mainly classified into B_0 eddy currents which are spatially constant over the imaging volume, and linear eddy currents, which have linear spatial variation, similar to the imaging gradient fields. Higher-order spatial dependence is possible but is not commonly measured or corrected.

Effect on Images   Because k-space location is related to the cumulative area under the gradient waveform, linear eddy currents can shift the actual k-space locations relative to the ideal locations. For example, when linear eddy currents are present in the readout direction, the center of k-space occurs later in the readout than expected. Also k-space readout intervals during the plateau of a trapezoid are compressed because the gradient amplitude is lower than ideal. Similar k-space shifts can also occur along the phase-encoding and slice-selection directions. B_0 eddy currents cause unwanted phase accumulation, but not k-space displacement like their linear counterparts.

For some applications, the eddy-current-induced k-space shift and phase accumulation are benign. For example, in conventional imaging with a rectilinear k-space raster, a uniform k-space shift in the frequency-encoded direction simply results in an additional phase slope in the frequency direction of the image that does not affect a magnitude image. However, for sequences such as EPI that traverse k-space in a back-and-forth raster, the k-space shift and phase accumulation cause ghosting. The eddy-current k-space shifts can also result in compression, shearing, or displacement in the image.

Although these effects are tolerable in many applications, if images with different distortions are combined during reconstruction or postprocessing, as in diffusion-weighted imaging (DWI) or diffusion tensor imaging (DTI), significant additional artifacts can result (see Section 17.2). Applications that require accurate phase images, such as phase-contrast imaging (Section 15.2) or B_0-field mapping, can also have artifacts from eddy currents.

10.3.2 REDUCING EDDY-CURRENT EFFECTS

Eddy currents increase with higher gradient amplitude and faster slew rate. Thus, they have become a bigger problem with the advent of higher-performance gradients. Without effective countermeasures, eddy currents would render many advanced pulse sequences unusable. Eddy currents are dealt with in four main ways: (a) shielded gradient coils, (b) gradient waveform preemphasis, (c) gradient waveform derating, and (d) application-specific calibrations and corrections during image acquisition or reconstruction.

Shielded Gradient Coils The idea behind shielded gradient coils (Mansfield and Chapman 1986) is to use two coils, a primary inner or main coil, and a secondary outer or shield coil (also sometimes called a bucking coil), which are connected in series. For horizontal-field (cylindrical) magnets, the two coils are arranged on concentric cylinders. For vertical field magnets, the two coils are arranged on coaxial disks. The same nomenclature for the coils is used for both types of systems. The shield coil produces a field that opposes the field from the main coil. The diameters, conductor wire patterns, and currents of the two coils are designed so that the net field outside the two coils (fringe field) is as close to zero as possible. Because eddy currents mainly flow in conducting structures outside the shield gradient coil, reducing the fringe field reduces eddy currents. The fields of the two coils also partially cancel one another within the imaging volume. More current is therefore required to produce the same field than for an unshielded gradient coil. This effect can be quantified by the gradient efficiency, which is sometimes defined as the product of peak gradient amplitude and slew rate. The loss in efficiency for a shielded configuration depends on the distance between the primary and secondary coils and the current ratio between the two coils. Increasing the distance increases the efficiency. For example, for cylindrical coils, the efficiency ratio between a shielded and unshielded configuration can be 1.5 or more. Shielded gradient coils typically reduce eddy current amplitudes by a factor of 10 to 100 relative to the amplitudes without shielding. Shielded gradient coils are used in almost all commercial scanners and provide the first line of defense against eddy currents.

Waveform Preemphasis   The idea underlying waveform preemphasis is to intentionally distort the current waveform that is input to the gradient coil, such that the preemphasis distortion cancels the subsequent eddy-current distortion. With an accurate characterization of eddy currents, waveform preemphasis can reduce eddy-current levels by one to two orders of magnitude. Accurate preemphasis requires a quantitative model of eddy currents. To simplify the model, spatial and temporal dependencies are usually separated.

Eddy-Current Spatial Dependence   If $B_e(\vec{x}, t)$ is the z component of the eddy-current magnetic field that results from pulsing the gradient coils, then a Taylor expansion gives:

$$B_e(\vec{x}, t) = b_0(t) + \vec{x} \cdot \vec{g}(t) + \cdots \tag{10.35}$$

The first term in Eq. (10.35) is usually called the B_0 *eddy current*. The second term is called the *linear eddy current*. The three components of $\vec{g}$, g_x, g_y, and g_z, represent the eddy-current gradient along the three physical gradient axes x, y, and z, respectively. Higher-order terms are not usually considered and do not have standard names. Most image-quality problems can usually be traced to one of the two terms in Eq. (10.35). The decomposition in terms of B_0 and linear eddy currents is useful because correction methods are sometimes different for the two components (see later discussion). Equation (10.35) can be equivalently thought of as a spherical harmonic expansion. That expansion differs from the Taylor series in how the second- and higher-order terms are grouped.

Eddy-Current Time Dependence   In a simple eddy-current model, the conducting structures that support the eddy currents are approximated as inductive-resistive (LR) circuits. Mutual inductance between the gradient coil and conducting structures allows current to be induced by the gradient coil. The resulting circuit model is shown in Figure 10.13. A straightforward analysis of this model (Van Vaals and Bergman 1990; Jehenson et al. 1990) shows that the field generated by the eddy currents is given by:

$$g(t) = -\frac{dG}{dt} \otimes e(t) \tag{10.36}$$

where G is the desired applied gradient waveform; $g(t)$ generically denotes one of the induced eddy-current terms in Eq. (10.35) with a specific spatial dependence; $\otimes$ denotes convolution (see Section 1.1); and $e(t)$ is the eddy-current impulse response, which is given by a sum of decaying exponentials:

$$e(t) = H(t) \sum_n \alpha_n e^{-t/\tau_n} \tag{10.37}$$

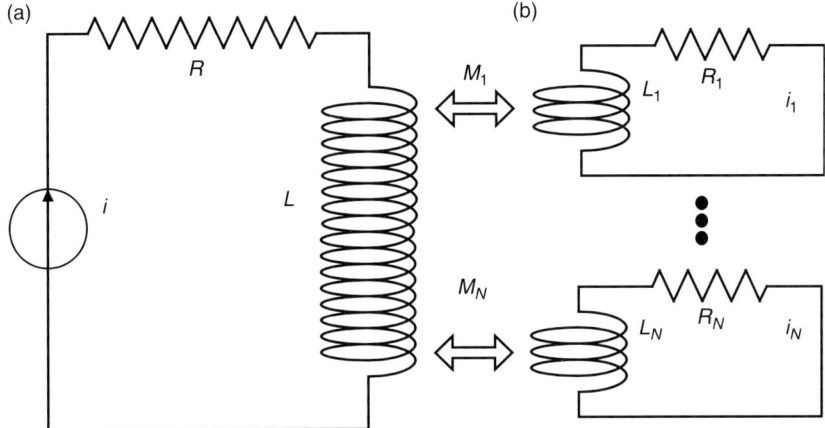

FIGURE 10.13 Lumped circuit model for eddy currents. The gradient coil (a) and each eddy-current conductor (b) are modeled as LR circuits. Eddy currents result from mutual inductance M_k between the gradient coil and each eddy-current conductor. The mutual inductance allows a current i in the gradient coil to induce currents i_k in the eddy-current conductors. Each conductor produces a magnetic field proportional to i_k. (Adapted from Van Vaals and Bergman 1990; Jehenson et al. 1990.)

where $H(t)$ is the unit step function given by:

$$H(t) = \begin{cases} 1 & t \geq 0 \\ 0 & t < 0 \end{cases} \tag{10.38}$$

A few terms in the summation in Eq. (10.37) (e.g., two to four) are sufficient to adequately characterize most eddy-current behavior.

In principle, the constants α_n and τ_n (called the amplitudes and time constants, respectively) could be calculated from the inductance and resistance of the equivalent circuits of Figure 10.13 if those parameters were known. In practice, amplitudes and time constants must be measured empirically. Eddy-current behavior can also be more complex than the decaying exponential description that results from the lumped LR circuit model. For example, oscillatory behavior has been observed (Ryner et al. 1996). Such behavior could arise either from capacitive coupling between conducting elements or from mechanical vibration.

All terms in Eq. (10.35) have a contribution of the form of Eq. (10.36) from eddy currents excited by each gradient coil. For example, the B_0 eddy current is:

$$b_0(t) = -\frac{dG_x}{dt} \otimes e_{0x}(t) - \frac{dG_y}{dt} \otimes e_{0y}(t) - \frac{dG_z}{dt} \otimes e_{0z}(t) \qquad (10.39)$$

whereas the x component of the linear eddy current g_x is:

$$g_x(t) = -\frac{dG_x}{dt} \otimes e_{xx}(t) - \frac{dG_y}{dt} \otimes e_{xy}(t) - \frac{dG_z}{dt} \otimes e_{xz}(t) \qquad (10.40)$$

with similar equations for the y and z linear components. Each of the impulse response functions $e_{ij}(t)$ is a sum of decaying exponentials as in Eq. (10.37), but each generally has a different set of α_n and τ_n. The first term in Eq. (10.40) is called the *direct linear term* because it represents an x eddy-current gradient caused by the applied x gradient. The second and third terms in Eq. (10.40) are called *cross-terms* and are typically much smaller than the direct terms. It should be noted that the B_0 eddy-current amplitude α_n can be either positive or negative. For unshielded gradient coils, the linear amplitudes are always positive due to Lenz's law, but for shielded gradient coils the linear amplitudes can be either positive or negative depending on whether the coil is slightly undershielded or overshielded (fringe field having the same or opposite sign as the imaging volume field). Equations (10.39) and (10.40) can also be generalized to include eddy-current fields created by pulsing coils other than the gradient coils (for example, resistive shim coils with nonlinear fields).

Eddy-current time dependence can be broadly described by long and short time constants. We exemplify the difference here using the linear eddy-current component. During the rising ramp of a trapezoid with amplitude G_0, the applied gradient is:

$$G_{\text{applied}}(t) = \frac{G_0 t}{r} \qquad 0 \le t \le r \qquad (10.41)$$

where r is the ramp duration and $t = 0$ corresponds to the beginning of the ramp. Using Eqs. (10.36) and (10.37) for a single eddy-current time constant, we obtain:

$$g(t) = -\frac{G_0}{r} \alpha \tau (1 - e^{-t/\tau}) \qquad 0 \le t \le r \qquad (10.42)$$

For $\tau \gg r$ (long time constants), the linear eddy current at the completion of the ramp is

$$g(t = r) \approx -G_0 \alpha \qquad (10.43)$$

where we have used $e^x \approx 1 + x$ for $x \ll 1$. In this case, the strength of the eddy-current magnetic field depends only on G_0 and α and is independent of the ramp time, slew rate, and time constant. The eddy currents (of all spatial orders: B_0, linear, etc.) created by the rising and falling ramps of a trapezoid always partially cancel as long as the plateau length is not much longer than τ. The shorter the plateau in comparison to τ, the better the cancellation.

For $\tau \ll r$ (short time constants) Eq. (10.42) gives:

$$g(t) \approx -\frac{G_0 \alpha \tau}{r} \tag{10.44}$$

Using Eqs. (10.41) and (10.44), the net gradient during the ascending ramp is:

$$G_{\text{net}}(t) = G_{\text{applied}}(t) + g(t) \approx \frac{G_0(t - \alpha\tau)}{r} = G_{\text{applied}}(t - \alpha\tau) \tag{10.45}$$

Therefore, to first order, a very short linear eddy current simply appears to delay the applied gradient waveform by an amount $\alpha\tau$.

It is almost impossible to distinguish linear eddy currents with very short τ from gradient amplifier impulse-response effects, such as group delays, feedback distortion, and waveform low-pass filtering due to the limited gradient amplifier bandwidth. Conversely, it is also very difficult to correct for very short linear eddy currents because the gradient amplifier bandwidth limits the correction. The first-order correction for very-short-time-constant linear eddy currents is to delay other waveforms such as RF pulses or the A/D converter window relative to the gradient waveforms. This is commonly done to center the echo within the A/D readout window and to avoid signal loss with spatial-spectral RF pulses that excite off-isocenter slices. The latter are sensitive to changes as small as a few microseconds in the relative RF-gradient subsystem group delays (Zur 2000). The relative group delay is usually empirically chosen rather than based on an eddy-current measurement. This is because the delay value compensates not only for eddy currents, but also for group delays in the gradient amplifier and in the transmit and receive electronics.

Eddy-Current Measurement The goal of eddy-current measurement techniques is to specify the α_n and τ_n that characterize each spatial component impulse response ($e_{0x}(t)$, $e_{xx}(t)$, etc). The most common technique uses one or more small samples placed at different locations in the imaging volume. A gradient coil is pulsed to generate eddy currents, followed by a nonselective (hard) RF pulse to excite the small samples. The phase of the resulting FID is:

$$\phi_1(t) = \gamma \int_0^t B_e(\vec{x}_s, t') \, dt' + \phi_0 \tag{10.46}$$

where $\vec{x}_s$ is the sample location, $t = 0$ occurs immediately after the RF pulse, and the term ϕ_0 accounts for the phase unrelated to eddy currents. To remove

ϕ_0, an additional FID signal can be acquired by negating the polarity of the testing gradient that produces the eddy currents. The phase of this FID is:

$$\phi_2(t) = -\gamma \int_0^t B_e(\vec{x}_s, t') \, dt' + \phi_0 \tag{10.47}$$

The phases of the two FID signals are subtracted, resulting in a phase that is purely related to eddy currents

$$\phi(t) = \frac{\phi_1(t) - \phi_2(t)}{2} = \gamma \int_0^t B_e(\vec{x}_s, t') \, dt' \tag{10.48}$$

The time derivative of the phase of the FID therefore gives a measurement of the decaying eddy currents during the FID. Typically, many consecutive FIDs are required to characterize the complete temporal variation of the eddy-current field. By either moving the samples or by using multiple samples simultaneously, the various spatial components of the eddy current can be measured and the respective amplitudes can be calculated for a series of time constants.

Preemphasis Compensation
  Linear component. Once the α_n and τ_n are measured, the linear spatial component of eddy-current fields can be compensated by adding a high-pass filter to the gradient amplifier input (Van Vaals and Bergman 1990; Jehenson et al. 1990) or by modifying the digital waveform input to the gradient amplifier. In either case, the compensation requires adding the negative of Eq. (10.36) to the original waveform. A subtlety is that we must use a slightly modified set of α_n and τ_n in the correction. (The reason that the measured and correction α_n and τ_n differ is that the eddy-current compensation itself generates an additional eddy current.) The correction α_n and τ_n can be obtained from the measured α_n and τ_n analytically using the method described in Jehenson et al. (1990). Alternatively, a simple iterative method can be used to obtain the set of α_n and τ_n. After a few iterations, α_n and τ_n will converge to the correct values. The convergence is fairly rapid (two to four iterations, typically) because the eddy currents are small compared to the desired gradient. The resulting preemphasized waveform looks like a high-pass-filtered version of the original gradient waveform (Figure 10.14).
  B_0 *component.* The B_0 component can be corrected by either using a B_0 coil with current control that can be varied in real time or shifting the exciter/receiver frequency (Crozier et al. 1992) in real time. The coil current

(a)   (b)

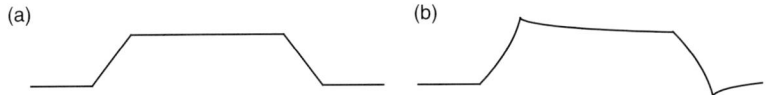

FIGURE 10.14 (a) Ideal gradient waveform. (b) Preemphasized (high-pass-filtered) waveform. The horizontal and vertical axes represent time and gradient, respectively. Preemphasis is exaggerated for clarity.

or frequency shift are both calculated using the same method as the linear compensation, using Eq. (10.36) with appropriate α_n and τ_n.

Other spatial orders. Correction for higher spatial orders such as the quadratic term is rarely done because it would require adding a dedicated coil with real-time current control that produces a field with the desired spatial dependence. Some commercial scanners have resistive shim coils that produce higher-order spatial fields, but there is seldom a control mechanism to vary the current for these coils in real time. Care must be taken in attempting to correct for higher-order eddy currents (as described for example in Section 10.5) because in imaging pulse sequences, their effects can be easily confused with the effects of concomitant fields (Section 10.1).

Gradient Waveform De-rating For gradient waveforms that require a fixed area instead of fixed amplitude, such as crushers (Section 10.2), one method for reducing eddy currents is to reduce the gradient amplitude (Figure 10.15). The rate of eddy current buildup is proportional to the slew rate. Decreasing the amplitude of the trapezoid while holding the slew rate fixed maintains the same buildup rate, but reduces the buildup time. This results in a lower eddy current after the ramp.

Reducing the slew rate but not the amplitude is usually not as effective as reducing the amplitude because the buildup rate is lower but the eddy current has more time to build up due to the resulting longer ramp to reach the desired gradient amplitude. In fact, for time constants much longer than the trapezoid ramp time, the eddy current increases almost linearly with time. Therefore, the eddy current after a ramp is approximately independent of the slew rate because a lower slew rate is compensated by a longer buildup time for the same gradient amplitude (see Eq. 10.43).

Example 10.5 A trapezoidal waveform has a plateau amplitude $G_0 = 50\,\mathrm{mT/m}$. The ramps use a slew rate $S_R = 200\,\mathrm{T/m/s}$. A linear eddy current with $\tau = 100\,\mathrm{ms}$ and $\alpha = 0.001$ is excited by the ramps. (a) Calculate the eddy-current gradient amplitude at the end of the rising ramp. (b) Repeat the calculation using the same amplitude but a lower slew rate of $S_R = 100\,\mathrm{T/m/s}$.

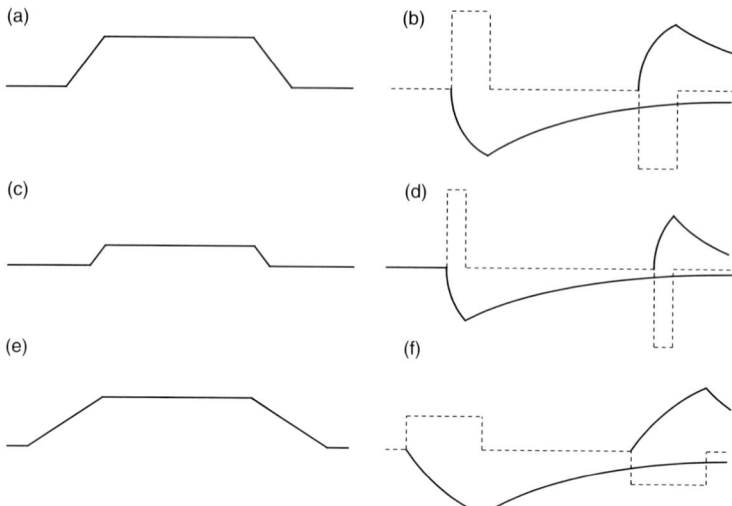

FIGURE 10.15 Schematic plots showing gradient derating methods to reduce eddy currents. (a) Original gradient waveform and (b) resulting eddy-current gradient. (c) Reduced amplitude waveform and (d) resulting eddy-current gradient. (e) Reduced slew-rate waveform and (f) resulting eddy-current gradient. The dashed lines in (b), (d), and (f) represent dG/dt for the gradient waveforms in (a), (c), and (e), respectively. The horizontal axis represents time.

(c) Repeat the calculation using a lower amplitude of $G_0 = 25$ mT/m and maintaining the slew rate of $S_R = 200$ T/m/s.

Answer

(a) For the first case, the ramp time is:

$$r = \frac{50 \text{ mT/m}}{200 \text{ T/m/s}} = 0.25 \text{ ms}$$

Because $\tau \gg r$, we can use Eq. (10.43). The eddy-current gradient amplitude at the end of the ramp is:

$$g \approx -(50 \text{ mT/m})(0.001) = -0.05 \text{ mT/m}$$

(b) For the second case, the ramp time doubles ($r = 0.5$ ms), but we still have $\tau \gg r$ so Eq. (10.43) still applies. Therefore $g \approx -0.05$ mT/m for this case as well.

(c) For the third case, from Eq. (10.43):

$$g \approx -(25 \text{ mT/m})(0.001) = -0.025 \text{ mT/m}.$$

Application-Specific Calibrations and Corrections   The combination of shielded gradient coils and eddy current preemphasis results in good image quality with almost all applications. A few applications are so sensitive to eddy currents that additional corrections are needed. A full discussion of application-specific corrections is beyond the scope of this book; we review here several key techniques.

Application Dependence of Eddy-Current Artifacts   Different applications are generally sensitive to eddy currents with different time constants. Whereas artifacts always increase with the eddy-current amplitude α, the dependence on time constant τ is more complicated. For any application, there is a range of time constants that results in maximal artifacts. Time constants outside this range cause lower artifact levels. Zhou (1996) shows an example of this time-constant sensitivity for EPI.

Phase Contrast Velocity Correction   In phase-contrast imaging, bipolar flow-encoding gradients create a velocity-dependent phase (see Section 15.2). A velocity map is calculated from the difference of the phase maps acquired with two different velocity-encoding waveforms. Because the eddy currents resulting from different velocity-encoding waveforms are usually different, the phase accrued by the eddy-current gradient does not subtract completely in the phase-difference image. For example, toggling the sign of the velocity-encoding gradient also toggles the sign of the associated eddy-current gradients, making the eddy-current error additive in the phase-difference image. The result is that the velocity map has an error due to eddy currents. In general the eddy-current error is spatially dependent, but the spatial dependence is determined by the direction of the velocity-encoding gradient.

It has been found that the eddy-current error has slow spatial dependence that can be modeled by constant, linear, and quadratic variation within the imaging plane (Lingamneni et al. 1995). Because of the slow variation, the error is usually not a significant problem unless quantitative velocity calculations are needed. Ideally the concomitant phase error is first removed in the phase-difference reconstruction, as described in Section 13.5. Then a low-order polynomial fit of a region of interest in the phase-difference image covering stationary tissue is calculated. In the absence of eddy currents, the fitted phase should be zero. The value of the phase is then extrapolated to the location of the vessel of interest and subtracted to provide more accurate velocity estimates.

Reference Scans for Echo Train Pulse Sequences   Eddy currents are one of the leading causes of ghosting and intensity loss in many sequences employing echo trains, such as EPI, RARE, and GRASE. In EPI, the readout gradient waveform alternates polarity and the data must be time-reversed on every other echo prior to the Fourier transform in the phase-encoded direction. Therefore, after time-reversal, the echo peak is alternately late (shifted toward $+k_x$) and early (shifted toward $-k_x$). The alternate shifting causes ghosting, as discussed in Section 16.1. In RARE, although there is no need to reverse k-space data for every other echo, the phase-reversal effect of RF refocusing pulses alternates the signal phase throughout the echo train. Under ideal conditions in which the phase is perfectly rewound to zero prior to applying a refocusing pulse (Section 16.4), the phase-reversal effect is not problematic. When eddy currents are present, however, a nonzero net phase is produced and its sign is alternated by the refocusing pulses. This gives rise to ghosting in RARE. In GRASE (Section 16.2), a combination of the phase problems of EPI and RARE are present, leading to ghosting as well. Furthermore, B_0 eddy currents cause a phase accumulation that varies among the various echoes of most echo train pulse sequences. The resulting phase inconsistency also causes ghosting.

Reference scans are commonly used to address the eddy-current problems for pulse sequences employing echo trains (Bruder et al. 1992; Zhou et al. 1993; Hinks et al. 1995). The reference scan usually consists of a complete scan, a single echo train, or a portion of an echo train acquired without phase-encoding gradients. Turning off the phase-encoding gradient waveforms makes each echo identical in principle (except for amplitude change due to T_2 or T_2^* relaxation) and allows calibration of the differences in location and phase between echoes. The phase-encoding gradient waveforms usually make a smaller contribution to the eddy currents than other waveforms because the maximal signal occurs when they have zero amplitude. Therefore, the reference scan calibration captures most eddy-current differences between echoes in the echo train. Alternatively, instead of a separate reference scan acquisition, two or more reference scan echoes can be included in the normal scan for calibration purposes (Jesmanowicz et al. 1993). For example, in EPI, one of the lines at or adjacent to $k_y = 0$ can be collected twice on consecutive echoes by appropriately modifying the phase-encoding lobes. More discussion on this topic can be found in Section 16.1.

The resulting data can be processed in several ways to estimate the k-space shift and phase shift for each echo that results from the linear and B_0 eddy currents, respectively. A 1D Fourier transform of each echo results in a projection of the object along the readout gradient direction. According to the Fourier shift theorem, the phase slope of the projection is proportional to the k-space shift. In addition, the intercept of the phase of the projection gives the approximate phase shift caused by B_0 eddy currents.

For RARE, the linear eddy-current k-space shift can be corrected by adjusting the readout prephasing area. The B_0 eddy-current phase shift can be corrected by adjusting the phase of the 180° refocusing pulses.

For EPI, the errors can be corrected during reconstruction by multiplying the data after the frequency Fourier transform in the (x, k_y) domain, by appropriate phase factors determined from the calibration scan. The simplest correction uses one phase slope and intercept for all even echoes and a different set for all odd echoes. This usually removes most of the ghosting due to eddy currents. More elaborate corrections can also be derived from the reference scan data including echo-specific phase slope and intercept or nonlinear phase corrections (Bruder et al. 1992). More elaborate methods run the risk of introducing additional artifacts and should be used with caution.

DWI Distortion Correction   The standard Stejskal-Tanner diffusion imaging pulse sequence uses two identical gradient lobes separated by a 180° RF refocusing pulse for diffusion sensitization (see Sections 9.1 and 17.2). The preparation period is followed by an imaging sequence, usually using single-shot EPI to minimize the sensitivity to bulk motion. To get the desired *b* value in the shortest TE, the diffusion lobes are played at the maximum gradient amplitude, resulting in large eddy currents. Each ramp of each diffusion lobe results in an eddy current. The net eddy current that persists during the EPI readout gives rise to geometric distortion, as further described in Section 17.2.

In general, the eddy currents and resulting geometric distortion depend both on the diffusion gradient direction and amplitude. In diffusion tensor imaging, the components of the diffusion tensor are measured by repeating the diffusion scan using at least two different diffusion gradient amplitudes and at least six directions. When eddy currents are present, the individual diffusion images are therefore misregistered. When these images are combined, the resulting diffusion trace or diffusion anisotropy maps can have artifacts, including increased apparent anisotropy and blurring, especially in the periphery of the image.

Several techniques for reducing DW-EPI eddy-current geometric distortion have been developed. These include image postprocessing, optimizing the waveform preemphasis for the diffusion pulse sequence, modifying the pulse sequence waveforms, k-space data corrections using reference scans, and replacing the unipolar diffusion lobes with bipolar lobes to obtain partial cancellation of eddy currents.

Spatial-Spectral RF Pulses   Spatial-spectral (SPSP) RF pulses use a bipolar slice-selection gradient similar to the EPI readout gradient (see Section 5.4). The eddy-current sensitivity of SPSP RF pulses is therefore very similar to EPI (Block et al. 1997; Zur 2000). In the case of SPSP excitation, eddy currents cause Nyquist ghosting in the temporal frequency domain, giving poor fat-saturation and water signal modulation with off-center slice location. The water signal modulation occurs because offsetting the slice away from the gradient isocenter requires that the instantaneous transmit frequency be shifted by an amount proportional to the slice-selection gradient amplitude. Any difference between the ideal and actual gradient amplitude causes artifacts in the form of excited signal modulation, that is, reduced signal at some slice locations. In fact, SPSP RF pulses can be used to develop a short eddy-current and group-delay calibration because of their extreme sensitivity (King and Ganin 2001).

Linear eddy-current effects can be eliminated by careful adjustment of the relative group delay between the SPSP gradient and RF waveforms. B_0 eddy-current effects can be eliminated by appropriately modulating the transmitted RF waveform (Block et al. 1997). The eddy-current sensitivity can also be eliminated by only playing RF pulses during one polarity of the slice-selection gradient (Zur 2000). This, however, degrades the efficiency of the SPSP pulse, as discussed in Section 5.4.

SELECTED REFERENCES

Alexander, A. L., Tsuruda, J. S., and Parker, D. L. 1997. Elimination of eddy current artifacts in diffusion-weighted echo-planar images: The use of bipolar gradients. *Magn. Reson. Med.* 38: 1016–1021.

Block, W., Pauly, J., Kerr, A., and Nishimura, D. 1997. Consistent fat suppression with compensated spectral-spatial pulses. *Magn. Reson. Med.* 38: 198–206.

Bruder, H., Fischer, H., Reinfelder, H-E, and Schmitt, F. 1992. Image reconstruction for echo planar imaging with nonequidistant k-space sampling. *Magn. Reson. Med.* 23: 311–323.

Crozier, S., Eccles, C. D., Beckey, F. A., Field, J., and Doddrell, D. M. 1992. Correction of eddy-current-induced B_0 shifts in receiver reference-phase modulation. *J. Magn. Reson.* 97: 661–665.

Fischer, H., and Ladebeck, R. 1998. Echo-planar imaging image artifacts. In *Echo-planar imaging*, edited by F. Schmitt, M. K. Stehling, and R. Turner, pp. 179–200. Berlin: Springer-Verlag.

Haselgrove, J. C., and Moore, J. R. 1996. Correction for distortion of echo-planar images used to calculate the apparent diffusion coefficient. *Magn. Reson. Med.* 39: 960–964.

Hinks, R. S., Kohli, J., and Washburn, S. 1995. Fast spin echo pescan for artifact reduction. *Proc. 3rd SMR*, p. 634.

Jehenson, P., Westphal, M., and Schiff, N. 1990. Analytical method for the compensation of eddy-current effects induced by pulsed magnetic field gradient in NMR systems. *J. Magn. Reson.* 90: 264–278.

Jesmanowicz, A., Wong, E. C., and Hyde, J. S. 1993. Phase correction for EPI using internal reference lines. *Proc. 12th SMRM*, p. 1239.

King, K. F., and Ganin, A. 2001. Method and apparatus for calibration of RF and gradient field time delays. U.S. Patent 6,288,545.

Koch, M., and Norris, D. G. 2000. An assessment of eddy current sensitivity and correction in single-shot diffusion-weighted imaging. *Phys. Med. Biol.* 45: 3821–3832.

Lingamneni, A., Hardy, P. A., Powell, K. A., Pelc, N. J., and White, R. D. 1995. Validation of cine phase-contrast MR imaging for motion analysis. *J. Magn. Reson. Imaging* 5: 331–338.

Mansfield, P., and Chapman, B. 1986. Active magnetic screening of coils for static and time-dependent magnetic field generation in NMR imaging. *J. Phys. E.* 19: 540–545.

Ryner, L. N., Stroman, P., Wessel, T., Hoult, D. I., and Saunders, J. K. 1996. Effect of oscillatory eddy currents on MR sprectroscopy. *Proc. 4th ISMRM*, p. 1486.

Van Vaals, J. J., and Bergman, A. H. 1990. Optimization of eddy-current compensation. *J. Magn. Reson.* 90: 52–70.

Wider, G., Doetsch, V., and Wuethrich, K. 1994. Self-compensating pulsed magnetic-field gradients for short recovery times. *J. Magn. Reson A* 108: 255–258.

Zhou, X. 1996. Quantitative analysis of eddy current effects on echo planar images. *Proc. 4th ISMRM*, p. 1486.

Zhou, X., Cofer, G. P., Hinks, R. S., MacFall, J. R., and Johnson, G. A. 1993. On phase artifacts of high-field fast spin-echo images. *Proc. 12th SMRM*, p. 1248.

Zur, Y. 2000. Design of improved spectral-spatial pulses for routine clinical use. *Magn. Reson. Med.* 43: 410–420.

RELATED SECTIONS

10.4 Gradient Moment Nulling

Gradient moment nulling (GMN) or *gradient motion rephasing* is the process of modifying a gradient waveform in order to make a pulse sequence more immune to image artifacts arising from motion (e.g., blood flow) (Pattany et al. 1987; Haacke and Lenz 1987; Wendt 1991). The modifications can include changing the amplitude, duration, shape, or number of gradient lobes that make up the waveform. With GMN, each of the three logical axes (readout, phase encoding, and slice selection) is treated independently. Therefore, GMN can be performed on a single axis, any two, or all three axes at once.

GMN can reduce signal loss and ghosting image artifacts that occur when there is pulsatile flow or periodic motion (Wood and Henkelman 1999). GMN is also useful for reducing artifacts that arise from non-periodic motion, which can introduce a phase shift that varies in k-space. Figure 10.16 shows a sagittal cervical spine image comparison, in which image with GMN (Figure 10.16b) displays brighter cerebral spinal fluid (CSF) and hence better cord-CSF contrast. GMN can be used alone or in conjunction with physiological monitoring techniques such as ECG triggering (Section 12.1) to further reduce pulsatile artifacts. GMN can also reduce or eliminate intravoxel phase dispersion that occurs when there is a range of flow velocities within a single voxel (Wood and Henkelman 1999). Finally, when a phase-encoding waveform is moment nulled, the flow displacement artifact can be eliminated (Nishimura et al. 1991).

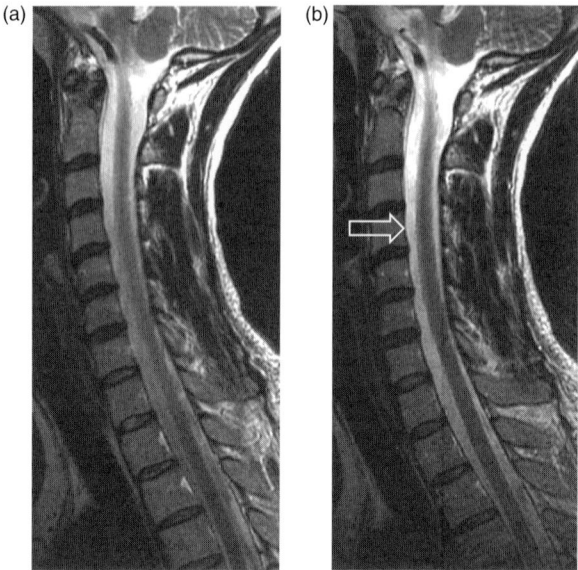

FIGURE 10.16 Sagittal T_2 weighted cervical spine images using a RARE (fast spin echo) technique. (a) Without GMN. (b) First-order gradient moment nulling (velocity compensation) on the readout axis (anterior-posterior). The CSF produces a more intense signal (arrow) when GMN is used.

A gradient waveform can be described by its *gradient moments*, which are a series of values calculated from the gradient waveform expressed as a function of time. The zeroth moment is equal to the gradient area, the first moment is the gradient area weighted linearly with time t, the second moment is the gradient area weighted by t^2, and so on. The concept of moments may also be familiar from its use in statistics and mechanics. For example, the location of the center of gravity for a physical object can be calculated by forming the ratio of its first to its zeroth mechanical moments.

Gradient waveforms can be moment-nulled to various degrees or orders. Zeroth-order GMN ensures that static spins are properly rephased after the application of a gradient. It is used in virtually all pulse sequence designs. First-order GMN compensates for motion or flow with constant velocity and is sometimes called *velocity compensation* or simply *flow compensation*. Second-order GMN compensates both for velocity and constant acceleration and is sometimes called *acceleration compensation*. Higher-order GMN is defined analogously. In this section, we primarily focus on GMN of the first order.

GMN beyond first order has not been commonly implemented because it has the drawback of increasing the minimum TE and also increasing any higher moments (e.g., the third and fourth) that are not deliberately nulled.

For example, a velocity-compensated frequency-encoding waveform can be constructed from a minimum of three gradient lobes, whereas acceleration-compensating that same waveform requires a minimum of four lobes. Because of the increase in the number of lobes, GMN beyond a certain order will invariably become counterproductive. The optimal order to which a waveform should be nulled depends on the specifics of the application and on the performance of the gradient hardware. In some applications it may not be necessary or desirable to null any moments (beyond the zeroth) at all. An example is contrast-enhanced MR angiography, in which gradient echo acquisitions with the shortest TR and TE are used.

10.4.1 QUALITATIVE DESCRIPTION AND BINOMIAL WAVEFORMS

A qualitative understanding of many common moment-nulled waveforms can be gained by studying the idealized example of a series of rectangular gradient lobes with equal widths and with areas arranged in the binomial patterns (Figure 10.17). Figure 10.17a shows a binomial pattern that has two equal and opposite lobes. Its gradient area (i.e., zeroth moment) is nulled. This pair of lobes is sometimes labeled $1\bar{1}$, where the 1s denote the area ratio of the two lobes and the bar above indicates that the second lobe is negative. In Figure 10.17a, the zeroth, first, and second moments are graphed versus time, with $t = 0$ chosen to be the beginning of the waveform. The curves representing the moments are normalized so that the maximal absolute values are equal, and the moments are labeled m_0, m_1, and m_2, respectively. At the end of the $1\bar{1}$ waveform, the zeroth moment is nulled, but the first and second moments both have residual nonzero values. Also note that near the beginning

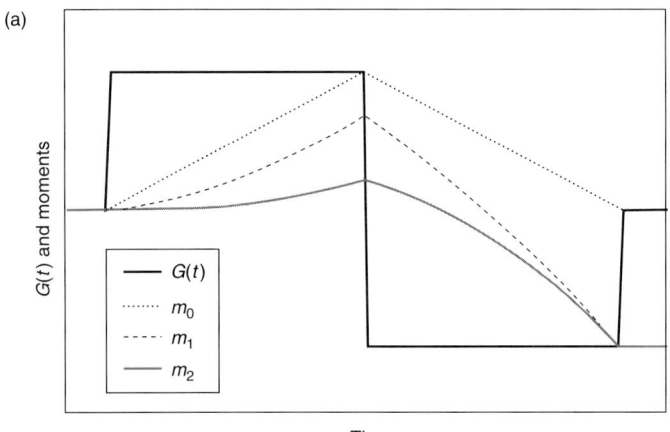

(a)

$G(t)$ and moments

Time

 — $G(t)$
 .... m_0
 - - - - m_1
 — m_2

FIGURE 10.17 Continued

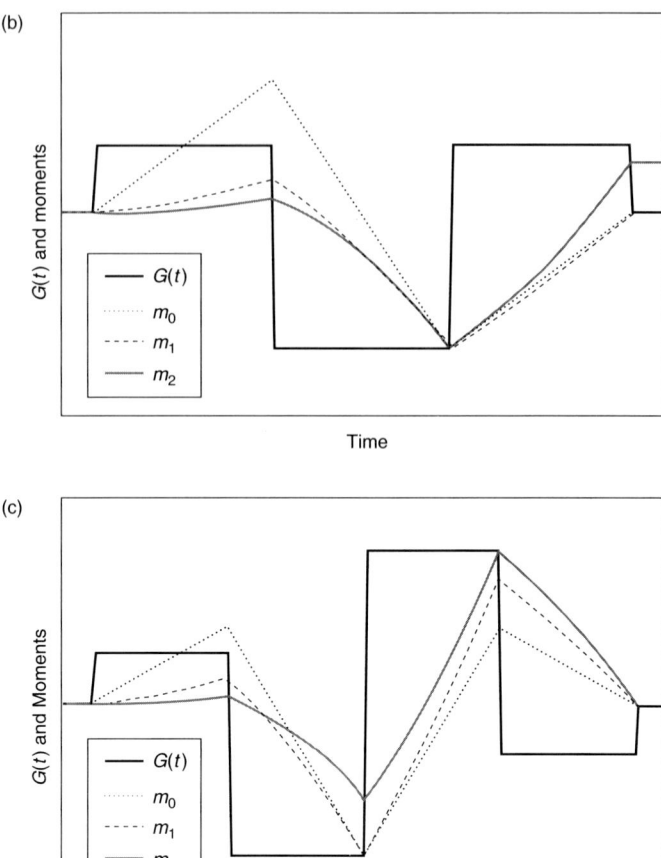

FIGURE 10.17 Continued. Binomial waveforms demonstrate various orders of GMN. (a) The $1\bar{1}$ waveform has zero net area (i.e. $m_0 = 0$ at the end of the waveform), but its first and second moment are not nulled. (b) The $1\bar{2}1$ waveform demonstrates velocity compensation; that is, its first moment is nulled at the end of the waveform. (c) The $1\bar{3}3\bar{1}$ waveform demonstrates acceleration compensation, because both its first and second moments are nulled.

of the gradient waveform, m_1 and m_2 do not deviate much from zero, but that as time progresses they take on larger and larger values during the first (positive) lobe and then decrease during the second (negative) lobe. The values of m_1 and m_2 at the end of the waveform are both negative because the later times are more heavily weighted.

Figure 10.17b shows the $1\bar{2}1$ binomial waveform. By adding a third lobe in this specific pattern, the waveform not only has zero net area, but also is velocity-compensated; that is, at the end of the waveform its zeroth and first moments are both nulled. The end of the rightmost lobe could correspond to the location in the data readout where the echo signal peaks. This example illustrates that a moment cannot be nulled for the entire readout, but only at a specific time point, which is typically chosen to be the peak of the echo (i.e., where the MR signal is strongest). The $1\bar{2}1$ waveform could also be used for slice-selection. In that case, its beginning would correspond to the isodelay point of the RF pulse, which usually corresponds to the peak amplitude of the pulse. (Because, to first order, the transverse magnetization is created at the RF isodelay point, the slice-selection gradient prior to the isodelay point does not contribute to the first moment and can be ignored.) In other words, the plateau width of leftmost lobe corresponds to the isodelay of the RF pulse. Again, the first moment cannot be nulled during the entire slice-selection gradient, but only for a specified point in time.

The binomial waveform shown in Figure 10.17c is known as $1\bar{3}3\bar{1}$. The zeroth, first, and second gradient moments of this waveform are all nulled at the end of the waveform. Therefore, it is both velocity- and acceleration-compensated.

The binomial waveforms serve as prototypical examples of GMN to various orders. For example, it is generally true that for a gradient echo pulse sequence a frequency-encoding waveform with GMN to order N requires a minimum of $N + 2$ gradient lobes with alternating polarity, just as in the binomial examples. This relation holds true even if the waveform is composed of more realistic lobe shapes such as trapezoids or triangles rather than the idealized rectangular lobes shown in Figure 10.17. (Waveforms for RF spin echo pulse sequences are discussed later.) Also, remnants of an underlying $1\bar{2}1$ pattern are apparent in many other velocity-compensated gradient waveforms. For example, Figure 10.18 shows a waveform that is closely related to the $1\bar{2}1$ waveform. It has a positive middle lobe that is twice as wide as either outer lobe. This waveform has practical importance for multiple-echo readouts in RF spin echo pulse sequences (Section 14.3). The first moment at the peak of

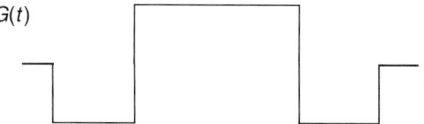

FIGURE 10.18 A FEER waveform characterized by a central lobe of twice the width of either end lobe. Like the binomial $1\bar{2}1$ waveform of Figure 10.17b, it is velocity-compensated. This waveform is of practical interest for multiple-echo RF spin echo.

the even-numbered echoes is much lower than at the peak of the odd-numbered echoes. Sometimes this effect is called field even-echo refocusing (FEER), and the waveform in Figure 10.18 is sometimes called the FEER waveform. Like the $1\bar{2}1$ waveform, the zeroth- and first-order moments of the FEER waveform are nulled. More information about the FEER waveform can be found in Simonetti et al. (1991).

10.4.2 QUANTITATIVE DESCRIPTION

Consider the one-dimensional motion of a small object under the influence of a gradient. Suppose the object moves along the x axis, and its displacement relative to the gradient isocenter is given by $x(t)$. If we know its initial position x_0, velocity v_0, and acceleration a_0 at an initial time $t = 0$, then its location at later times can be extrapolated with the Taylor series expansion:

$$x(t) = x_0 + v_0 t + \frac{1}{2} a_0 t^2 + \cdots \tag{10.49}$$

If a gradient along the x direction $G(t)$ is applied when $t > 0$, then the accumulated phase at time t is given by:

$$\phi(t) = \gamma \int_0^t G(u) x(u) \, du \tag{10.50}$$

where u is an integration variable denoting time. Substituting Eq. (10.49) into Eq. (10.50) yields:

$$\phi(t) = \gamma \int_0^t G(u) \left(x_0 + v_0 u + \frac{1}{2} a_0 u^2 + \cdots \right) du \tag{10.51}$$

Equation (10.51) can be decomposed into a *moment expansion*:

$$\phi(t) = \gamma m_0(t) x_0 + \gamma m_1(t) v_0 + \frac{\gamma}{2} m_2(t) a_0 + \cdots \tag{10.52}$$

where the nth gradient moment is:

$$m_n(t) = \int_0^t G(u) u^n \, du \tag{10.53}$$

(Some authors define the nth moment with an additional factor of $n!$ The definition we use in Eq. 10.53, without the factorial, is commonly used in statistics for the moments of a probability distribution.) Very often we are only interested in the value of the gradient moments at a single instant in time, such as at the center of the echo or at the end of a waveform, in which case the explicit time dependence in Eq. (10.53) is sometimes dropped. In that case, we simply write m_n and understand that the moments are calculated for the single time point of interest.

Equations (10.51) and (10.53) are conveniently generalized to three dimensions using vector notation. For example, for three-dimensional motion, Eq. (10.52) becomes:

$$\phi(t) = \gamma \left(\vec{m}_0 \cdot \vec{r}_0 + \vec{m}_1 \cdot \vec{v}_0 + \frac{1}{2}\vec{m}_2 \cdot \vec{a}_0 + \cdots \right) \tag{10.54}$$

where $\vec{r}_0 = (x_0, y_0, z_0)$, $\vec{v}_0 = (v_{0x}, v_{0y}, v_{0z})$, and $\vec{a}_0 = (a_{0x}, a_{0y}, a_{0z})$ are the initial vector displacement, velocity, and acceleration of the small object, respectively, and:

$$\vec{m}_n(t) = \int_0^t \vec{G}(u)u^n \, du \tag{10.55}$$

Translation Rules for Moments   Figure 10.19 shows an arbitrary gradient waveform $G_0(t)$, defined for $0 < t < T_L$. Assume that the moments of $G_0(t)$ are $m_0, m_1, m_2, \ldots$:

$$m_1 = \int_0^{T_L} G_0(u)u \, du \tag{10.56}$$

If this original waveform $G_0(t)$ is translated to the right by Δt, then the translated waveform can be described by the function $\tilde{G}(t) = G_0(t - \Delta t)$.

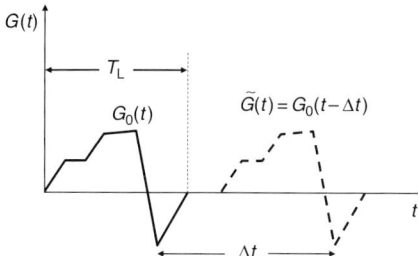

FIGURE 10.19 An arbitrary gradient waveform $G_0(t)$ is defined for $0 \leq t \leq T$. A duplicate of the waveform $\tilde{G}(t)$ is translated to the right by Δt.

As expected, the gradient area remains unchanged by the translation:

$$\tilde{m}_0 = \int_{\Delta t}^{\Delta t + T_L} \tilde{G}(u)\, du = \int_{\Delta t}^{\Delta t + T_L} G_0(u - \Delta t)\, du = \int_0^{T_L} G_0(w)\, dw = m_0$$

(10.57)

where $w = u - \Delta t$. The first moment of the translated waveform, however, is given by:

$$\tilde{m}_1 = \int_{\Delta t}^{\Delta t + T_L} \tilde{G}(u) u\, du = \int_{\Delta t}^{\Delta t + T_L} G_0(u - \Delta t) u\, du$$

$$= \int_0^{T_L} G_0(w)(w + \Delta t)\, dw = m_0 \Delta t + m_1$$

(10.58)

Similarly:

$$\tilde{m}_2 = \int_{\Delta t}^{\Delta t + T_L} \tilde{G}(u) u^2\, du$$

$$= \int_0^{T_L} G_0(w)(w + \Delta t)^2\, dw = m_0 \Delta t^2 + 2m_1 \Delta t + m_2$$

(10.59)

Note the appearance of the binomial coefficients in Eqs. (10.58) and (10.59).

Example 10.6 Based on the binomial pattern in Eqs. (10.58) and (10.59), write an expression for $\tilde{m}_4$ without performing the integration explicitly.

Answer Because the appropriate row in Pascal's triangle is 1-4-6-4-1 (i.e., the coefficients of the binomial expansion of $(x + y)^4$ are 1, 4, 6, 4, and 1):

$$\tilde{m}_4 = m_0 \Delta t^4 + 4m_1 \Delta t^3 + 6m_2 \Delta t^2 + 4m_3 \Delta t^3 + m_4$$

The expressions for the moments of a translated waveform have some important consequences (Simonetti et al. 1991). First, according to Eq. (10.58), the value of the first moment is invariant under translation ($\tilde{m}_1 = m_1$) if (and only if) the waveform has zero net area, that is, $m_0 = 0$. Another way to state this result is the value of the first moment is independent of the choice of the origin $t = 0$ when the waveform area is zero.

A second important consequence deals specifically with symmetric lobes, such as trapezoids or triangles whose ascending and descending ramps are equal in duration. If a lobe is symmetric with respect to the origin $t = 0$, then all its odd moments are zero because the contribution to the integral from positive and negative times exactly cancel. Applying Eq. (10.58) yields a simple expression for the first moment of a symmetric lobe centered at $t = \Delta t$:

$$\tilde{m}_1 = m_0 \Delta t, \qquad \text{(symmetric lobe)} \qquad (10.60)$$

As far as the first moment is concerned, all the area under a symmetric lobe can be treated as if it were concentrated at the single time point $t = \Delta t$, that is, at the centroid of the lobe (Bernstein et al. 1992). This rule can greatly simplify the design of velocity-compensated waveforms (see later discussion).

The translation rules can also be used to elegantly verify the moments of the binomial waveforms stated previously. Consider the $1\bar{1}$ waveform in Figure 10.17a, and an inverted copy of it, which we call $\bar{1}1$. The first moments of these two waveforms have the same magnitude, but opposite sign. Therefore, the sum of the first moments of the $1\bar{1}$ and $\bar{1}1$ waveforms is zero. Because they each have zero net gradient area, their first moments are also independent of translation, and any combination of these two waveforms has zero first moment. By arranging the two waveforms so that their negative lobes exactly overlap, the $1\bar{2}1$ waveform of Figure 10.17b is obtained, so the first moment of that waveform is indeed zero. (A similar argument can be used to show that the FEER waveform shown in Figure 10.18 has zero first moment by arranging the lobes of $\bar{1}1$ and $1\bar{1}$ waveforms so that their positive lobes touch but do not overlap.) This process can be continued in an iterative manner; that is, $1\bar{2}1$ and $\bar{1}2\bar{1}$ waveforms can be overlapped to form the $1\bar{3}3\bar{1}$ waveform in Figure 10.17c, demonstrating that the second moment of that waveform is zero. Alternatively, these same results can be obtained by direct calculation.

Finally, we note an analogy can be made between the moments of translated gradient lobes and the mechanical concepts of force, torque, and moment arm. In the analogy, the gradient area corresponds to a force acting at the centroid of a lobe, the translation time Δt corresponds to moment arm of the force, and the gradient first moment is analogous to the torque. Thus a three-lobe, velocity-compensated waveform ($m_0 = 0$ and $m_1 = 0$), such as the $1\bar{2}1$ waveform, is analogous to a set of three force vectors that produce zero net force and also produce no net torque about any point.

Calculation of Moments for Ramps, Plateaus, and Bridges   The basic gradient lobe shapes of triangles, trapezoids, and bridged lobes are described in Sections 7.1 and 7.2. Each of these basic shapes can be built from the components of ascending ramps, descending ramps, plateaus, and bridges (i.e., ramps between two plateaus of nonzero amplitude). A generic expression that covers all of these lobe components is:

$$G(t) = G_1 + \frac{(G_2 - G_1)t}{\tau} \qquad 0 \geq t \geq \tau \qquad (10.61)$$

where τ is the duration of the lobe component. From Eq. (10.61) $G(t)|_{t=0} = G_1$ and $G(t)|_{t=\tau} = G_2$. Thus, a positive ascending ramp is obtained by setting $G_2 > G_1 = 0$, a positive gradient plateau is obtained by setting $G_1 = G_2 > 0$ in Eq. (10.61), and a descending negative bridge is obtained when $0 > G_1 > G_2$.

The moments for the lobe components are obtained by substituting Eq. (10.61) into Eq. (10.53) and performing the integration from 0 to τ. The result is:

$$m_n = \frac{\tau^{n+1}}{n+2} \left(\frac{G_1}{n+1} + G_2 \right) \qquad (10.62)$$

The expression in Eq. (10.62) can be evaluated for the special cases of ramps, bridges, and plateaus. Table 10.2 gives several results that are commonly used. These results can be used in conjunction with the translation rules of Eqs. (10.57)–(10.59) to calculate the moments of segments that begin at times other than $t = 0$. A more extensive table, which includes sinusoidal lobes, is provided in Wendt (1991).

Example 10.7 (a) Use Table 10.2 and Eq. (10.58) to find the first moment of a positive trapezoid with amplitude h and ascending and descending ramp durations r. The plateau duration is T, and the trapezoid begins at $t = 0$.

TABLE 10.2
Gradient Moments for Commonly Used Lobe Segments

Shape	$G(t=0)$	$G(t=\tau)$	m_0	m_1	m_2
Ascending ramp	0	G	$\dfrac{G\tau}{2}$	$\dfrac{G\tau^2}{3}$	$\dfrac{G\tau^3}{4}$
Descending ramp	G	0	$\dfrac{G\tau}{2}$	$\dfrac{G\tau^2}{6}$	$\dfrac{G\tau^3}{12}$
Plateau	G	G	$G\tau$	$\dfrac{G\tau^2}{2}$	$\dfrac{G\tau^3}{3}$
Bridge	G_1	G_2	$\tau\left(\dfrac{G_1+G_2}{2}\right)$	$\tau^2\left(\dfrac{G_1}{6}+\dfrac{G_2}{3}\right)$	$\tau^3\left(\dfrac{G_1}{12}+\dfrac{G_2}{4}\right)$

(b) Then exploit the fact that this trapezoid is a symmetric lobe to find the same result using Eq. (10.60).

Answer

(a) We can add together the first moments of each of the components of the trapezoid to find the net first moment. The first moment of the ascending ramp starting at $t = 0$ is found from Table 10.2:

$$m_1 = \frac{hr^2}{3} \qquad \text{(ascending ramp)} \qquad (10.63)$$

The plateau starts at $t = r$, so it has first moment:

$$\tilde{m}_1 = m_0 r + m_1 = rhT + \frac{hT^2}{2} \qquad \text{(plateau)} \qquad (10.64)$$

Finally, the descending ramp, which starts at $t = r + T$, has first moment:

$$\tilde{m}_1 = m_0(r + T) + m_1 = \frac{hr}{2}(r + T) + \frac{hr^2}{6} \qquad \text{(descending ramp)}$$
$$(10.65)$$

Gathering terms in Eqs. (10.63), (10.64), and (10.65), the net first moment is:

$$m_{1,\text{trapezoid}} = h\left(r^2 + \frac{3rT}{2} + \frac{T^2}{2}\right) \qquad (10.66)$$

(b) The result in Eq. (10.66) can be obtained more simply by recognizing that the trapezoid is a symmetric lobe with area $h(T + r)$ centered at $\Delta t = r + T/2$. Applying Eq. (10.60):

$$m_{1,\text{trapezoid}} = m_0 \Delta t = [h(r+T)]\left(r + \frac{T}{2}\right) = h\left(r^2 + \frac{3rT}{2} + \frac{T^2}{2}\right)$$
$$(10.67)$$

10.4.3 METHODS FOR CALCULATING VELOCITY-COMPENSATED WAVEFORMS

This section gives representative examples illustrating techniques used to calculate velocity-compensated (i.e., first-order moment nulled) waveforms. We primarily use symmetric trapezoidal waveforms and exploit Eq. (10.60) to reduce the algebraic complexity. Waveforms using other symmetric lobe shapes (e.g., sinusoidal) can be obtained analogously.

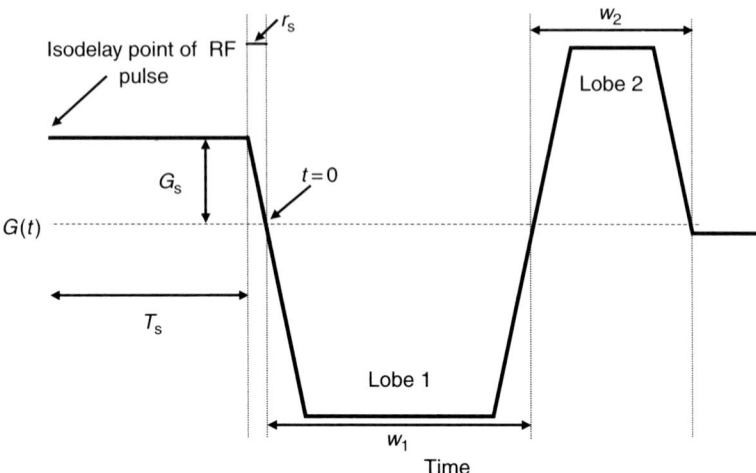

FIGURE 10.20 Definition of quantities used to calculate a velocity-compensated slice-selection waveform for a gradient-echo pulse sequence. By flipping the waveform from right to left, it can also serve as a velocity-compensated frequency-encoding waveform.

Slice-Selection Waveform Figure 10.20 shows a velocity-compensated slice-selection waveform, commonly used with gradient-echo pulse sequences. The amplitude G_s and duration T_s of the slice-selection lobe are determined by imaging considerations such as the isodelay of the RF excitation pulse, slice thickness, and RF bandwidth. The goal is to calculate the widths, amplitude, and shape of the two unknown lobes, labeled lobe 1 and lobe 2. Because proper rephasing requires that the net area of the waveform be zero, the first moment of the waveform is independent of the time origin. For convenience we choose $t = 0$ to be at the junction of the slice-selection lobe and lobe 1. If we denote the *absolute value* of the area under each lobe by A, then balancing the zeroth moment requires:

$$A_1 = A_2 + A_s \qquad (10.68)$$

where A_s is the gradient area from the RF isodelay point to the end of the slice-selection lobe and is given by $A_s = G_s (T_s + r_s/2)$. By recognizing that lobes 1 and 2 are symmetric trapezoids, we express their first moments by $-A_1 w_1/2$ and $A_2(w_1 + w_2/2)$, respectively, according to Eq. (10.60) where w_1 and w_2 are the widths of lobes 1 and 2, respectively, including both ramps. To balance the first moment, we have:

$$-m_s - \frac{A_1 w_1}{2} + A_2 \left(w_1 + \frac{w_2}{2} \right) = 0 \qquad (10.69)$$

where m_s is the absolute value of the first moment of the slice-select lobe from the RF isodelay point to the end of the slice-selection gradient lobe. (The minus sign in front of m_s in Eq. (10.69) accounts for the fact that the slice-selection lobe occurs at $t < 0$.) From Table 10.2 and Eq. (10.60) m_s is:

$$m_s = G_s \left(\frac{r_s^2}{3} + r_s T_s + \frac{T_s^2}{2} \right) \tag{10.70}$$

Often the most compact waveform is obtained when lobes 1 and 2 are trapezoidal with the maximal gradient amplitude and slew-rate-limited ramps. According to Section 7.1, the total width of such a trapezoidal lobe is related to the absolute value of its area by

$$w_i = \frac{A_i}{h} + r = \frac{A_i}{h} + \frac{h}{S_R} \qquad i = 1, 2 \tag{10.71}$$

where h is the maximal gradient amplitude, r is the minimal rise time from 0 to h, and S_R is the corresponding maximal slew rate.

Substituting Eqs. (10.71) and (10.68) into Eq. (10.69) yields a quadratic equation for the unknown lobe area:

$$A_2^2 + A_2 hr - \left(hm_s + \frac{hr A_s}{2} + \frac{A_s^2}{2} \right) = 0 \tag{10.72}$$

The physically significant root of Eq. (10.72) is:

$$A_2 = \frac{-hr + \sqrt{(hr)^2 + 2(hr A_s + A_s^2 + 2hm_s)}}{2} \tag{10.73}$$

The remaining unknowns, such as the area of lobe 1 and the width of the two lobes, can be obtained by substituting Eq. (10.73) into Eqs. (10.68) and (10.71). Figure 10.21 shows a resulting slice-selection waveform calculated with this method. For the purposes of the plot, $t = 0$ was selected to be the beginning of the waveform, but the first moments would be properly nulled at the end of the waveform regardless of where the time origin was selected because the net gradient area (i.e., the zeroth moment) is zero (Simonetti et al. 1991).

For very small slice-selection lobes that satisfy:

$$hr A_s + A_s^2 + 2hm_s < 4hr \tag{10.74}$$

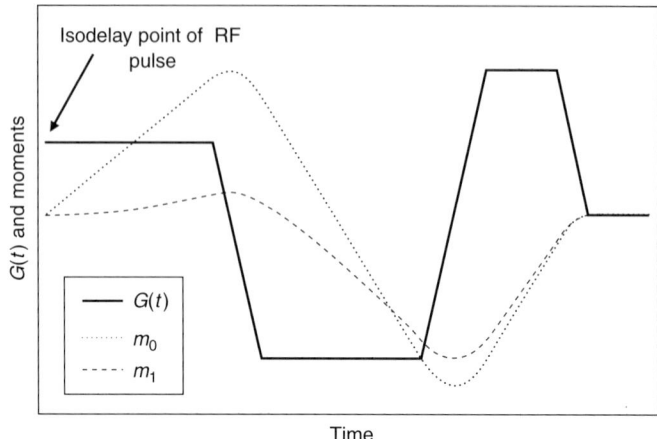

FIGURE 10.21 Velocity-compensated slice-selection waveform. The first moment m_1 is plotted assuming the $t = 0$ corresponds to the isodelay point of the RF pulse, which usually corresponds to its peak. Note that the $t = 0$ location is different from that in Figure 10.20. Because the net area under the waveform is zero, the first moment will be nulled at the end of the waveform, regardless of the choice of the temporal origin.

the optimal shape for lobe 2 will be a triangle rather than a trapezoid because $A_2 < hr$. In that case, Eq. (10.71) is replaced by:

$$w_2 = 2\sqrt{\frac{A_2 r}{h}} = 2\sqrt{\frac{A_2}{S_R}} \tag{10.75}$$

Substitution of Eq. (10.75) into (10.69) yields a quartic (fourth-order) expression. As long as $A_1 > hr$ (i.e., lobe 1 remains a trapezoid), then the closed-form expression (Bernstein et al. 1992) for A_2 is:

$$A_2 = \frac{hr + 2\sqrt{hr A_s + A_s^2 + 2hm_s} - \sqrt{(hr)^2 + 4hr\sqrt{hr A_s + A_s^2 + 2hm_s}}}{2} \tag{10.76}$$

(If $A_1 < hr$, there is still a closed-form solution to the resulting quartic equation, but several mathematical cases must be considered.)

The methods presented here also can be used to calculate a velocity-compensated, frequency-encoding waveform for gradient-echo pulse sequences. That waveform is essentially the time-reversed version of the slice-selection waveform, with imaging considerations such as FOV and receiver bandwidth determining the fixed portion. More details can be found in Bernstein et al. (1992).

Velocity-Compensated Phase-Encoding Waveform Although the algebra for a velocity-compensated phase-encoding waveform is somewhat more complex, the example is instructive because it illustrates how to deal with amplitude-stepped waveforms and also waveforms that do not have zero net gradient area. The maximal k-space signal occurs when the phase-encoding amplitude is at (or near) zero. Therefore, the phase-encoding waveform is approximately nulled to all orders at the center of k-space. It is still sometimes useful to velocity-compensate the phase-encoding waveform, however, to avoid the flow displacement artifact. This artifact occurs when there is flow in an oblique direction that has a component along the phase-encoding direction (Nishimura et al. 1991). For example, for oblique flow in the readout phase-encoded plane, the magnitude of the displacement artifact is given by:

$$\Delta D = v \Delta t \sin \delta \cos \delta \qquad (10.77)$$

where v is the flow velocity, Δt is the time between the centroid of the phase-encoding lobe and the echo peak, and δ is the angle between the flow vector and the phase-encoding axis. The maximum displacement artifact $v\Delta t/2$ occurs when $\delta = 45°$. When all three axes are first-moment nulled, the pulse sequence is sometimes said to have *tridirectional* flow compensation.

Figure 10.22 shows a velocity-compensated phase-encoding waveform. The goal is to determine the unknown lobe I and lobe II that null the first moment at the echo peak, which occurs at a time Δ after the end of lobe II. Lobe I is further from the nulling point, so it has a longer moment arm and will be smaller. This is helpful because the net area of the waveform must not be zero but rather equal to the phase-encoding area, A_j for step j. Many

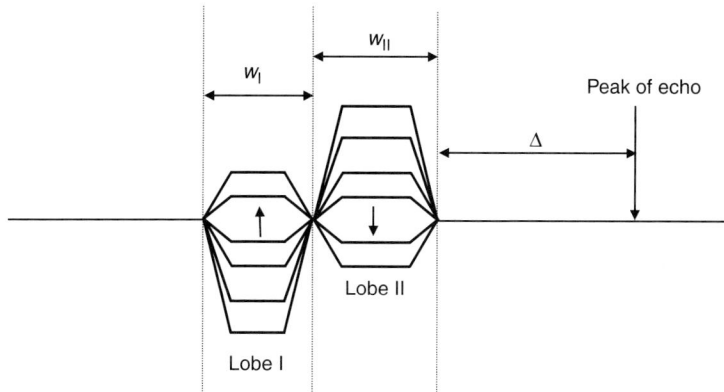

FIGURE 10.22 Velocity-compensated phase-encoding waveform. The arrows depict the direction of the stepping of the two lobes.

alternative sign conventions can be adopted; they all give the same final answer if applied consistently. We adopt the sign convention that the first step of each gradient lobe is described by a positive area and then account for bipolar nature of the waveform with the signs that appear in the equations. Balancing gradient areas gives:

$$-A_{\mathrm{I},j} + A_{\mathrm{II},j} = A_j = A_{\max}\left(1 - \frac{2j}{N-1}\right) \qquad j = 0, \ldots, N-1 \quad (10.78)$$

where the maximum gradient area is derived in terms of the phase-encoding FOV L_y (see Eq. 8.38 in Section 8.2):

$$A_{\max} = \frac{\pi(N-1)}{\gamma L_y} \tag{10.79}$$

Thus, the encoding area A_j ranges from $+A_{\max}$ to $-A_{\max}$ as j is stepped from 0 to $N-1$. We choose the temporal origin $t = 0$ to be at the echo peak. Nulling the first moment at the echo peak requires:

$$A_{\mathrm{I},j}\left(\frac{w_{\mathrm{I}}}{2} + w_{\mathrm{II}} + \Delta\right) - A_{\mathrm{II},j}\left(\frac{w_{\mathrm{II}}}{2} + \Delta\right) = 0 \tag{10.80}$$

where we are using the fact that both lobes I and II are symmetrical. Velocity compensation on the phase-encoding axis normally requires the maximal gradient amplitude, so for nearly all clinical applications the most time-efficient lobes will be trapezoidal rather than triangular.

Substituting Eq. (10.78) into Eq. (10.80) yields the gradient amplitudes for the jth step of lobes I and II:

$$A_{\mathrm{I},j} = A_j \frac{w_{\mathrm{II}} + 2\Delta}{w_{\mathrm{I}} + w_{\mathrm{II}}}$$
$$A_{\mathrm{II},j} = A_j \frac{w_{\mathrm{I}} + 2w_{\mathrm{II}} + 2\Delta}{w_{\mathrm{I}} + w_{\mathrm{II}}} \tag{10.81}$$

The unknown widths in Eq. (10.81) are obtained by solving for the largest absolute value of the areas of lobes I and II, which we call $A_{\mathrm{I,max}}$ and $A_{\mathrm{II,max}}$, respectively. For simplicity, the same ramp duration can be used for all the phase-encoding steps, as shown in Figure 10.22.

$$w_{\mathrm{I}} = \frac{A_{\mathrm{I,max}}}{h} + r$$
$$w_{\mathrm{II}} = \frac{A_{\mathrm{II,max}}}{h} + r \tag{10.82}$$

The maximum values for the area in Eq. (10.82) correspond to setting $j = 0$ in Eq. (10.78). The resulting expression for the maximum area for lobe II can then be obtained after some algebraic manipulation:

$$A_{\mathrm{II,max}} = \frac{-hr + 2A_{\max} + \sqrt{(hr - 2A_{\max})^2 + 4A_{\max}\left(h\Delta + \dfrac{3hr}{2} - \dfrac{A_{\max}}{2}\right)}}{2}$$

(10.83)

The value of $A_{\mathrm{I},max}$ can then be obtained from Eq. (10.78), and both widths can be obtained from Eq. (10.82).

Figure 10.23 shows a plot of a single phase-encoding step of a velocity-compensated waveform generated by this method, with $t = 0$ selected to be the echo peak. This is a convenient choice because the first moment must be nulled there. Note that from Eq. (10.53), as soon as $G(t)$ goes to zero, the values all of gradient moments can no longer change; this property is reflected in Figure 10.23.

GMN Waveforms for RF Spin Echo Sequences The calculation methods just illustrated can be readily extended to RF spin echo pulse sequences. It is important to remember, however, that each refocusing pulse negates the phase

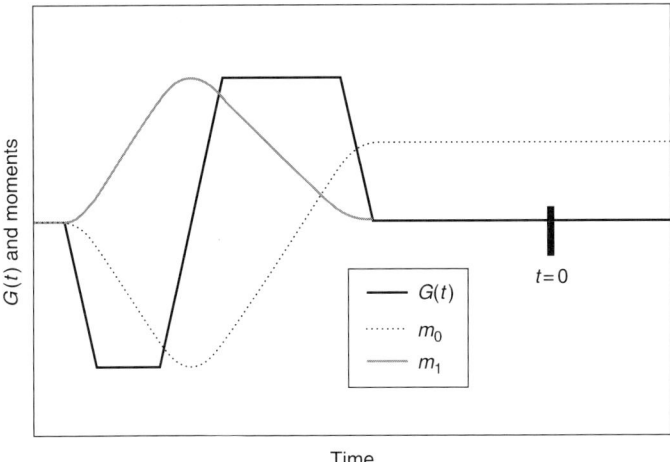

FIGURE 10.23 Example of a velocity-compensated phase-encoding step. The net area under the waveform is nonzero, but the first moment is nulled at the end of the waveform relative to the echo peak. Also, the graph of the first moment has the opposite sign as the first gradient lobe because that lobe is played when $t < 0$.

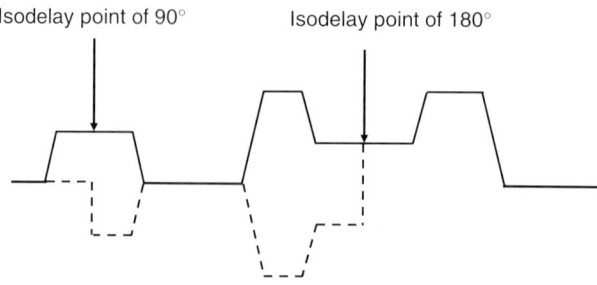

Isodelay point of 90°   Isodelay point of 180°

FIGURE 10.24 Slice-selection waveform for an RF spin echo pulse sequence. Because the refocusing pulse negates the phase accumulation from preceding gradient lobes, the waveform depicted by the dashed line is used to calculate moments for times after the peak of 180° Note also that the portion of the slice-selection gradient before the isodelay point of the 90° excitation pulse is not used in moment calculations.

accumulation from all the gradient lobes that precede it, all the way to the isodelay point of the RF excitation pulse, which is usually well approximated by the peak of the pulse. So, when calculating moments with Eq. (10.53), remember to invert any gradient lobe that is followed by an *odd* number of refocusing pulses up to time t. Figure 10.24 shows an example of a typical slice-selection waveform for a single-echo RF spin echo pulse sequence. The waveform consists of slice-selection gradients and a crusher pair. The dashed waveform accounts for the phase negation and is used to calculate the gradient moments for times to the right of the peak of 180° refocusing pulse.

10.4.4 PRACTICAL CONSIDERATIONS

Although GMN reduces the adverse effects caused by flow and motion, its use can result in other problems. First, the minimum TE and TR times of the sequence can be lengthened, especially in gradient-echo pulse sequences. This can limit its use in certain applications, such as breath-held cardiac imaging and contrast-enhanced angiography. Second, the increased number of gradient lobes required by GMN can exacerbate the eddy currents if the MR scanner is not well compensated. Third, the additional gradient lobes in GMN can contribute to the phase errors arising from concomitant magnetic fields (Section 10.1). Often these phase errors cannot be easily cancelled, particularly in pulse sequences without RF refocusing pulses, leading to image artifacts. These potential drawbacks should be considered before incorporating GMN into a pulse sequence. Finally, note that flow artifacts can often be reduced to an acceptable level by designing the gradient waveforms with reduced values of specific gradient moments, even if it is not practical to precisely null them.

SELECTED REFERENCES

Bernstein, M. A., Shimakawa, A., and Pelc, N. J. 1992. Minimizing TE in moment-nulled for flow-encoded two- and three-dimensional gradient echo imaging. *J. Magn. Reson. Imaging* 2: 583–588.

Haacke, E. M., and Lenz, G. W. 1987. Improving MR image quality in the presence of motion by using rephasing gradients. *Am. J. Roentgenol.* 148: 1251–1258.

Nishimura, D. G., Jackson, J. I., Pauly, J. M. 1991. On the nature and reduction of the displacement artifact in flow images. *Magn. Reson. Med.* 22: 481–492.

Pattany, P. M., Phillips, J. J., Chiu, L. C., Lipcamon, J. D., Duerk, J. L., McNally, J. M., and Mohapatra, S. N. 1987. Motion artifact suppression technique (MAST) for MR imaging. *J. Comput. Assisted Tomogr.* 11: 369–377.

Simonetti, O. P., Wendt, III R. E., and Duerk, J. L. 1991. Significance of the point of expansion in interpretation of gradient moments and motion sensitivity. *J. Magn. Reson. Imaging* 1: 569–577.

Wendt, R. E., III. 1991. Interactive design of motion-compensated gradient waveforms with a personal computer spreadsheet. *J. Magn. Reson. Imaging* 1: 87–92.

Wood, M. L., and Henkelman, M. R. 1999. Artifacts. In *Magnetic resonance imaging*, Vol. 1, edited by D. D. Stark and W. G. Bradley, chap. 10. St. Louis: Mosby.

RELATED SECTIONS

10.5 Spoiler Gradients

At the end of a pulse sequence or a preparatory RF pulse, residual transverse magnetization can remain. The residual transverse magnetization, if not eliminated, can produce a spurious signal that interferes with the desired signal in subsequent data acquisition, causing image artifacts (Figure 10.25a) (Haase et al. 1986; Haacke et al. 1991). A *spoiler gradient*, as the name implies, spoils or kills the unwanted MR signals that would otherwise produce artifacts in the image. Spoiler gradients are also known as *homospoil* and *killer* gradients.

Spoiler gradients are typically applied at the end of a pulse sequence (Figure 10.26a) or at the end of a preparatory RF pulse within a pulse sequence (Figure 10.26b). Examples of preparatory RF pulses include tagging pulses, inversion pulses, spatial saturation pulses, and spectral (or chemical) saturation pulses. Under the influence of a spoiler gradient, the transverse magnetization dephases along the direction of the gradient, leading to signal cancellation within a voxel. Meanwhile, the longitudinal magnetization experiences no effect from the spoiler gradient and thus is preserved to give rise to a signal in subsequent data acquisition.

The area of a spoiler gradient is usually very large so that it can adequately dephase the residual transverse magnetization. As such, a spoiler gradient often invokes the maximal available gradient amplitude or has a long pulse width. Trapezoidal, triangular, and half-sinusoidal waveforms can all be employed as spoiler gradients, although trapezoidal is most common because it yields the required gradient area in the shortest time (Section 7.1). Spoiler gradients are unipolar and can have either positive or negative polarity on a given gradient axis. The polarity is determined based on the other gradient waveforms within the pulse sequence (see later discussion). Although a spoiler gradient can be

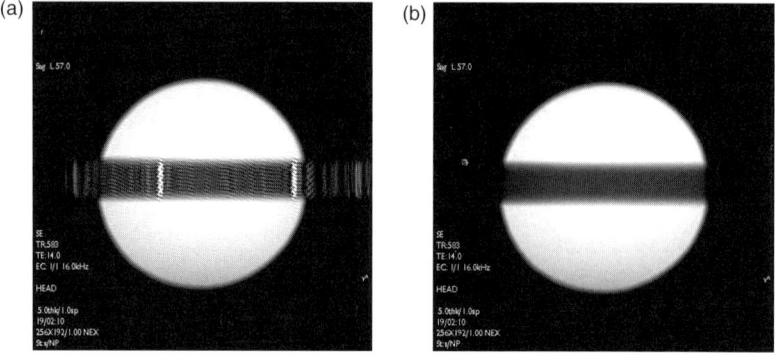

FIGURE 10.25 Two images of a phantom with a spatial saturation band visible as a horizontal stripe in the middle (a) without and (b) with a spoiler gradient following the spatial saturation RF pulse. The spoiler gradient eliminates the artifacts within the saturation band.

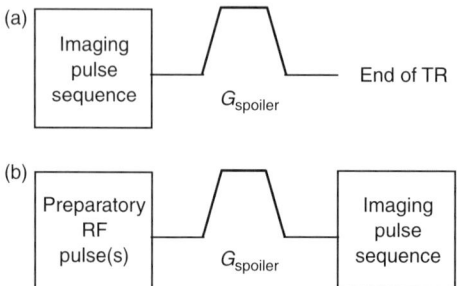

FIGURE 10.26 Two examples of spoiler gradients. (a) A spoiler gradient that is applied at the end of a pulse sequence. (b) A spoiler gradient that is applied after a preparatory RF pulse (or pulses) but prior to an imaging pulse sequence.

applied to any one, any two, or all three logical (i.e., readout, phase-encoding, and slice-selection axes) or physical gradient axes, it is often sufficient to employ a spoiler gradient along a single axis. When spoiler gradients are required on more than one axis, they are typically applied simultaneously to minimize the length of the pulse sequence.

In many aspects, spoiler gradients resemble the crusher gradients discussed in Section 10.2. Both types of gradients are used to eliminate unwanted magnetization in order to reduce or remove image artifacts. Thus, they are not always distinguished in the literature. In this book, we distinguish spoiler gradients from crusher gradients based on the following differences:

1. Spoiler gradients always dephase transverse magnetization, whereas crusher gradients can either dephase or rephase.
2. Spoiler gradients are used to nonselectively eliminate all unwanted transverse magnetization. Crusher gradients, on the other hand, are employed to select or filter a specific signal pathway.
3. Spoiler gradients can be employed in virtually any pulse sequence, but crusher gradients are specifically used in pulse sequences with at least one refocusing RF pulse.
4. Spoiler gradients are applied *at the end* of a pulse sequence or a preparatory RF pulse, prior to subsequent excitation. Crusher gradients, however, are played *during* a pulse sequence.

10.5.1 QUALITATIVE DESCRIPTION

Consider an arbitrary voxel in an image and assume there exists residual transverse magnetization $\vec{M}_\perp$ at the end of a data acquisition (i.e., a readout). This magnetization needs to be eliminated to avoid a spurious signal in subsequent readouts that can cause image artifacts. Within the voxel, the transverse magnetization consists of contributions from many spin isochromats, each represented by an arrow (i.e., a vector) in Figure 10.27a. The vector sum gives rise to $\vec{M}_\perp$ and contributes to the artifact intensity. If a spoiler gradient pulse is applied, the spin isochromats within the voxel will dephase (i.e., fan out) according to their location along the gradient direction (Figure 10.27b). Spin isochromats at one end of the voxel will accumulate more phase (e.g., $\vec{M}_1$ in Figure 10.27), while spin isochromats at the other end will accrue less (e.g., $\vec{M}_n$ in Figure 10.27). The overall phase dispersion across the voxel is determined by the product of the gradient area and the voxel dimension along the gradient direction. If the gradient area or the voxel dimension is sufficiently large, the phase dispersion will result in a greatly reduced net vector sum and consequently a decreased or nulled $\vec{M}_\perp$ (Figure 10.27c). In other words, the

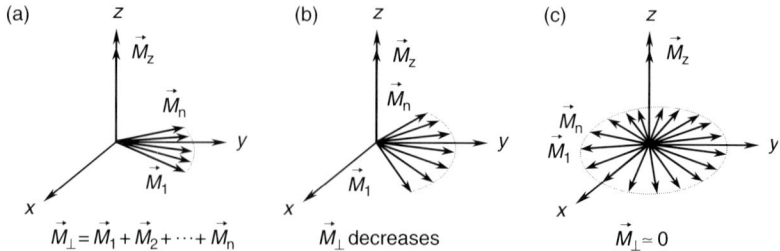

(a) $\vec{M}_\perp = \vec{M}_1 + \vec{M}_2 + \cdots + \vec{M}_n$ (b) $\vec{M}_\perp$ decreases   (c) $\vec{M}_\perp \approx 0$

FIGURE 10.27 Transverse ($\vec{M}_\perp$) and longitudinal ($\vec{M}_z$) magnetization within a voxel before (a), during (b), and after (c) the application of a spoiler gradient pulse. The net transverse magnetization $\vec{M}_\perp$ is equal to the vector summation of the individual magnetizations of the spin isochromats represented by arrows in the transverse plane.

transverse magnetization is spoiled or killed. This becomes more evident in the mathematical description given in the following subsection.

As outlined in Section 10.2, a gradient has no effect on the longitudinal (i.e., the z axis) component of the magnetization $\vec{M}_z$. During the dephasing process of the transverse magnetization, the longitudinal magnetization $\vec{M}_z$ remains unchanged (except for T1 relaxation if the longitudinal magnetization is not in equilibrium) (Figure 10.27). The longitudinal magnetization can be excited to produce signals for subsequent data acquisitions.

10.5.2 MATHEMATICAL DESCRIPTION

Let $\vec{M}_\perp(\vec{r})$ be residual, spatially dependent magnetization that remains in the transverse plane at the end of a pulse sequence or after a preparatory RF pulse. We show here how $\vec{M}_\perp(\vec{r})$ summed over an arbitrary image voxel can be greatly attenuated under the influence of a spoiler gradient $\vec{G}_{sp}$ applied along direction $\vec{r}$.

Within the arbitrary voxel, the total transverse magnetization $\vec{M}_\perp$ can be expressed as:

$$|\vec{M}_\perp| = \left| \sum_{n=1}^{N} \vec{M}_{\perp,n}(\vec{r}_n) \right| \approx \frac{\int\limits_{voxel} M_\perp e^{-i(\phi_0 + \phi)} dr}{\int\limits_{voxel} dr} \tag{10.84}$$

where index n represents different spin isochromats in the voxel (Figure 10.27), $M_\perp$ is the amplitude of $\vec{M}_{\perp,n}(\vec{r}_n)$, ϕ_0 is the phase before $\vec{G}_{sp}$ is applied, ϕ is the additional phase introduced by $\vec{G}_{sp}$, and dr is a linear differential along the direction of the gradient $\vec{G}_{sp}$. The integrals in Eq. (10.84) are performed over the voxel (assuming that the integrals over the other directions orthogonal to $\vec{r}$ have already been done), and $M_\perp$, ϕ_0, and ϕ are all dependent on the spatial location r. Prior to the application of the spoiler gradient, $\phi = 0$, and the range of ϕ_0 is generally not large enough to cause sufficient phase dispersion within the voxel (Figure 10.27a). Thus, $|\vec{M}_\perp|$ is nonzero and gives rise to signals that can cause image artifacts. After the spoiler gradient, ϕ becomes:

$$\phi(r) = \gamma \int_t \vec{G}_{sp}(t) \cdot \vec{r}\, dt = \gamma \int_t G_{sp}(t) r\, dt = \gamma r A_{sp} \qquad (10.85)$$

where γ is the gyromagnetic ratio, and A_{sp} is the spoiler gradient area. The phase dispersion ($\Delta\phi$) across a voxel is:

$$\Delta\phi(r) = \gamma A_{sp}\Delta r \qquad (10.86)$$

where Δr is the voxel dimension along the direction of $\vec{G}_{sp}$. Combining Eqs. (10.84), (10.85), and (10.86), ignoring ϕ_0, and assuming $M_\perp$ is uniform within the voxel, we obtain:

$$|\vec{M}_\perp| \approx M_\perp \left| \frac{\int_{r_0-\Delta r/2}^{r_0+\Delta r/2} e^{-i\gamma A_{sp} r}\, dr}{\int_{r_0-\Delta r/2}^{r_0+\Delta r/2} dr} \right| = M_\perp \left| \mathrm{SINC}(\gamma A_{sp}\Delta r/2) \right|$$

$$= M_\perp \left| \mathrm{SINC}(\Delta\phi/2) \right| \qquad (10.87)$$

where r_0 is the location of the voxel center. Equation (10.87) is virtually the same as Eq. (10.90) in Section 10.6, except that the slice thickness Δz is replaced by the voxel size Δr.

Equations (10.85) and (10.86) indicate that the phase introduced by $\vec{G}_{sp}$ is proportional to the area of the spoiler gradient. If A_{sp} is sufficiently large, the phase dispersion $\Delta\phi$ can cause considerable attenuation of the transverse magnetization, as indicated by the SINC function in Eq. (10.87). For example, when $\Delta\phi = 5\pi$, the transverse magnetization is attenuated by more than 87%. A further increase in A_{sp} results in a negligible $|\vec{M}_\perp|$. Thus, the residual magnetization is effectively dephased or spoiled.

It is interesting to note that, when $\Delta\phi = \pm 2m\pi$ ($m = 1, 2, \ldots$), $|\vec{M}_\perp|$ becomes zero, provided that the magnetization is uniform across the voxel. Equation (10.87) also indicates that either positive or negative spoiler gradients can be used to dephase the magnetization because the SINC is an even function.

10.5.3 DESIGN CONSIDERATIONS

Area of Spoiler Gradient   The minimal phase dispersion required to spoil the unwanted transverse magnetization is typically determined by experiments. To obtain a proper phase value, the spoiler gradient can be incremented in amplitude or pulse width until the observed image artifacts are sufficiently reduced or eliminated. For most applications, the minimal phase dispersion must be greater than 2π across an image voxel.

Equation (10.86) indicates that the required spoiler gradient area A_{sp} is inversely related to the voxel size. When the image matrix is held constant, the voxel size is directly proportional to the FOV. In that case, scans with a smaller FOV require a larger spoiler gradient area than scans with a larger FOV.

Example 10.8   It has been empirically found that a spoiler gradient with an area of 0.14 mT $\cdot$ s/m can effectively eliminate artifacts due to residual transverse magnetization remaining from previous excitations. If the FOV is reduced by 25% while keeping the same image matrix, what is the expected area of the spoiler gradient that is required for the reduced FOV?

Answer   With the new FOV, the voxel size Δr is reduced to 75% of its original value. To maintain the same phase dispersion given by Eq. (10.86), the new spoiler gradient area should be:

$$A'_{sp} = A_{sp}/75\% = 0.14/0.75 = 0.187\text{mT} \cdot \text{s/m}$$

Under the specific conditions given in this example, the calculated gradient area provides a good initial estimation in spoiler gradient design. The optimal spoiler gradient area can be determined empirically based on this initial guess.

Polarity of the Spoiler Gradient   Since either positive or negative spoiler gradients can dephase the transverse magnetization, a pulse sequence designer has the flexibility to choose the spoiler gradient polarity so as to avoid counteracting the phase dispersion (i.e., ϕ_0 in Eq. 10.84) already introduced by the proceeding gradients. This allows ϕ_0 and ϕ to add constructively, leading to a smaller spoiler gradient area A_{sp} to achieve a desired total phase dispersion. For example, if a spoiler gradient is applied along the readout axis in a pulse sequence, the spoiler gradient should have the same polarity as that of the readout gradient (Figure 10.28a). For the same reason, the spoiler gradient at the end of an echo planar imaging (EPI) pulse sequence should always match the polarity of the last readout gradient lobe (Figure 10.28b–c).

Axis Selection for the Spoiler Gradient   The axis of a spoiler gradient can be selected based on the following guidelines.

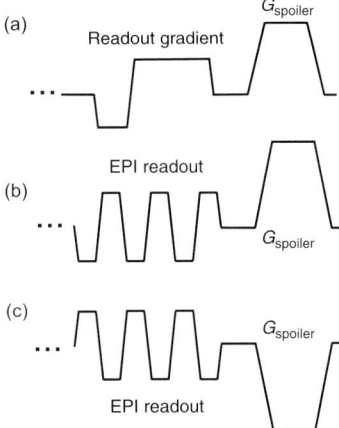

FIGURE 10.28 Spoiler gradients along the readout gradient axis at the end of (a) a gradient echo sequence and (b–c) EPI sequences. To maximize dephasing efficiency, the polarity of spoiler gradients should match the polarity of the last readout gradient lobe. As such, the polarity of the spoiler gradient changes from (b) to (c). This often occurs when the echo train length in EPI is changed from an odd number to an even number. In each case, the spoiler gradient lobe could be bridged with the adjacent readout gradient lobe.

1. The spoiler gradient direction is preferably applied along a direction that gives the largest phase dispersion.
2. If gradient coil or gradient amplifier heating is a concern, then the spoiler gradient is preferably played on the axis that has the lowest duty cycle.

Guideline (1) is demonstrated in Example 10.9.

Example 10.9 In an image, the voxel dimensions along the readout, phase-encoding, and slice-selection directions are $\Delta x = 0.5$ mm, $\Delta y = 0.5$ mm, and $\Delta z = 2.0$ mm, respectively. If a phase dispersion of 4π across the voxel is required to eliminate residual transverse magnetization, calculate the area of a spoiler gradient when it is applied along (a) the phase-encoding direction, (b) the slice-selection direction, and (c) the longest diagonal direction of the voxel.

Answer When a spoiler gradient is applied along the phase-encoding, slice-selection, and diagonal directions, Δr will have the following values, respectively:

(a) $\Delta r = \Delta y = 0.5$ mm
(b) $\Delta r = \Delta z = 2.0$ mm
(c) $\Delta r = \sqrt{(\Delta x)^2 + (\Delta y)^2 + (\Delta z)^2} = 2.12$ mm

The required gradient area to give a 4π phase dispersion can be obtained using Eq. (10.86):

(a) $A_{sp} = \dfrac{\Delta\phi}{\gamma\,\Delta r} = \dfrac{4\pi}{2\pi \times 42570 \text{ Hz/mT} \times 0.5 \times 10^{-3} \text{ m}}$
$= 0.0940 \text{ mT} \cdot \text{s/m}$

(b) $A_{sp} = \dfrac{\Delta\phi}{\gamma\,\Delta r} = \dfrac{4\pi}{2\pi \times 42570 \text{ Hz/mT} \times 2.0 \times 10^{-3} \text{ m}}$
$= 0.0235 \text{ mT} \cdot \text{s/m}$

(c) $A_{sp} = \dfrac{\Delta\phi}{\gamma\,\Delta r} = \dfrac{4\pi}{2\pi \times 42570 \text{ Hz/mT} \times 2.12 \times 10^{-3} \text{ m}}$
$= 0.0222 \text{ mT} \cdot \text{s/m}$

Example 10.9 shows that, by applying the spoiler gradient along a larger voxel dimension, a smaller gradient area can be used to achieve the same degree of signal dephasing. In practice, however, the spin distribution in a voxel can be nonuniform. Thus, the largest voxel dimension does not always correspond to the direction of most efficient dephasing. Even for a uniform spin density within the voxel, the signal intensity can be modulated by a SINC function along the readout and phase-encoding directions and by a non-rectangular slice profile along the slice direction, leading to deviations from that predicted by Eq. (10.86). All those deviations have been neglected in Example 10.9.

Guideline 2 is intended to better balance the gradient load among the gradient axes. Because the phase-encoding gradient axis usually has the lowest duty cycle, spoiler gradients along the phase-encoding direction are very popular. Based on the same guideline, spoiler gradients along the readout direction are rare, especially in pulse sequences with long readout echo trains. For imaging in oblique planes, balancing the load among the logical gradient axes, however, becomes less important.

Other Effects of a Spoiler Gradient   Similar to many gradient pulses with high amplitude, spoiler gradients can produce considerable eddy currents, concomitant magnetic fields, and gradient-induced vibration. Eddy currents produced by a spoiler gradient are generally detrimental because they can counteract the spoiler gradient and thus reduce the dephasing efficiency. (Ironically, eddy-current gradient fields along a direction other than that of the applied spoiler gradient may help accelerate the dephasing process. This effect is, however, very small.) In addition, eddy currents that have not fully decayed during the subsequent data acquisitions can perturb the desired magnetization, leading to image artifacts. These adverse effects, as well as gradient-induced vibration, can be mitigated by derating the spoiler-gradient amplitude at the expense of a prolonged pulse width. Unlike eddy currents, the concomitant magnetic fields can help spin dephasing because the spatial dependency of concomitant magnetic fields is orthogonal to that of the applied spoiler gradient, provided that the spoiler gradient is applied along a single physical axis.

SELECTED REFERENCES

Haacke, E. M., Weilopolski, P. A., and Tkach, J. A. 1991. A comprehensive technical review of short TR, fast magnetic resonance imaging techniques. *Rev. Magn. Reson. Med.* 3: 53–170.
Haase, A., Frahm, J., Matthaei, D., Hänicke, W., and Merboldt, K. D. 1986. FLASH imaging: Rapid NMR imaging using low flip angle pulses. *J. Magn. Reson.* 67: 258–266.

RELATED SECTIONS

10.6 Twister (Projection Dephaser) Gradients

A *projection dephaser* or *twister gradient* (Dixon et al. 1986) acts to attenuate signals from larger structures while leaving smaller structures relatively unaffected. Thus, the twister gradient functions as a spatial high-pass filter. Although twister gradients can be applied along any gradient axis, they are usually applied in the slice-selection direction and used in conjunction with thick 2D slices that are sometimes called *projections* or *slabs*. This is because a twister gradient is effective only when the dimension of the voxel in the gradient direction is greater than the size of the structure (e.g., a blood vessel) whose conspicuity we are trying to enhance. Figure 10.29 shows an example of a pair of coronal 2D phase-contrast angiograms and their corresponding magnitude images. They show the head and neck of a healthy volunteer, acquired with a slice thickness of 100 mm, with and without a twister gradient applied in the slice direction. The twister gradient increases the contrast of the vessels relative to the surrounding stationary tissue. In addition to increasing the

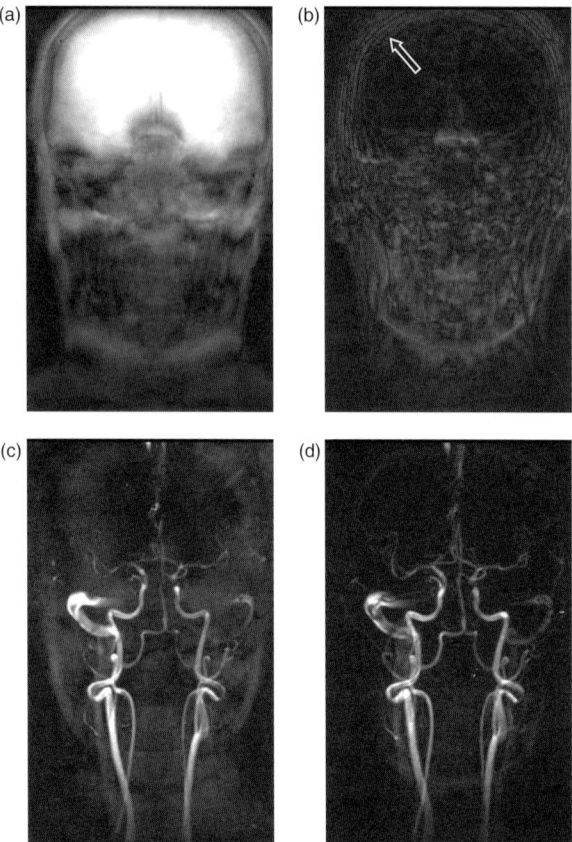

FIGURE 10.29 (c–d) 2D phase-contrast angiograms and (a–b) their corresponding magnitude images, without (left column) and with (right column) an applied twister gradient. The slice thickness is 100 mm, and the twister gradient applied in the slice direction produces a 2π phase shift over 15 mm. Note how the twister gradient suppresses the stationary tissue background to increase the conspicuity of the vessels. Also note the oscillating intensity (hollow arrow) in the magnitude image with the twister gradient, which is predicted by Eq. (10.90) and shown in Figure 10.31.

conspicuity of small structures, the twister gradient also reduces the dynamic range of the raw k-space signal, which can be advantageous if the number of bits in the digitizer is a limiting factor.

10.6.1 QUALITATIVE DESCRIPTION

As its name implies, the twister gradient produces a phase twist of the MR signal along the gradient direction. This phase twist produces à spatially

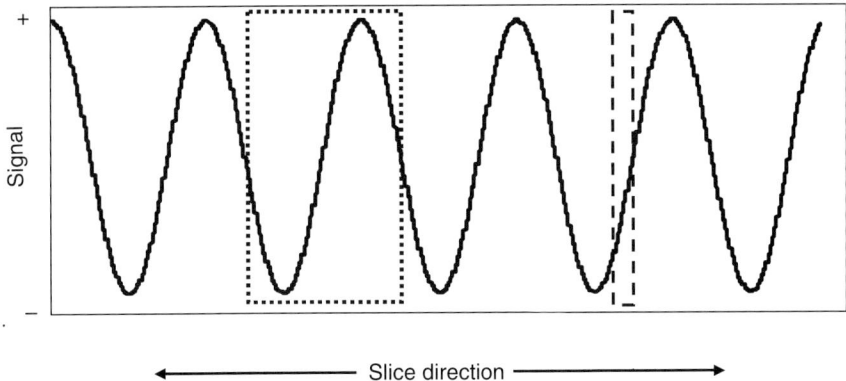

FIGURE 10.30 A twister gradient sets up a sinusoidal variation in the real or imaginary part of the MR signal. The signal intensity from a thicker structure (dotted line) is attenuated because the positive and negative contributions cancel. A thinner structure (dashed line), however, largely maintains its phase coherence. Thus, its signal is relatively unaffected.

dependent sinusoidal variation in each component of the complex MR signal. Figure 10.30 schematically illustrates this sinusoidal variation. A uniform thick structure, depicted by the dotted-line box, experiences both the positive and negative influence of the sinusoidal variation, causing signal cancellation, or *destructive interference*. A thin structure such as a small blood vessel, depicted by the dashed-line box, experiences either the positive or the negative influence of the sinusoidal variation, depending on its location. Therefore, the MR signal largely maintains phase coherence and suffers little signal loss.

10.6.2 MATHEMATICAL DESCRIPTION

The effect of the twister gradient can be modeled by calculating the dimensionless attenuation ratio:

$$r(\Delta z) = \frac{\left| \int\limits_{0}^{\Delta z} e^{i\phi} dz \right|}{\int\limits_{0}^{\Delta z} dz} \tag{10.88}$$

where Δz is the *smaller* of the voxel dimension in the direction of the twister gradient or the dimension of the structure of interest within the voxel. The denominator of Eq. (10.88) represents the linear growth of the signal with

Δz when there is no twister gradient present. The numerator is the magnitude of the phase-sensitive sum that accounts for the phase dispersion due to the twister gradient. Although Eq. (10.88) is a somewhat simplified model, because it does not account for nonuniformity of the structure or variation in the slice profile, it does capture the main effect of the twister gradient.

According to the Larmor equation, the phase angle in Eq. (10.88) (for stationary spins) is given by:

$$\phi = \gamma A z \tag{10.89}$$

where γ is the gyromagnetic ratio, A is the gradient area (in milliteslas-milliseconds per meter) under the twister gradient, and z is the displacement from isocenter in the direction of the gradient. Substituting Eq. (10.89) into Eq. (10.88), with $dz = d\phi/(\gamma A)$, the integrals can be readily evaluated. Using the identity $\sin \theta = (e^{i\theta} - e^{-i\theta})/(2i)$, we obtain:

$$r(\Delta z) = \left| \frac{2 \sin \left(\frac{\gamma A \Delta z}{2} \right)}{\gamma A \Delta z} \right| = \left| \mathrm{SINC} \left(\frac{\gamma A \Delta z}{2} \right) \right| \tag{10.90}$$

Figure 10.31 shows a plot of $r(\Delta z)$ when $\gamma A = 8.4$ rad/cm. The maximal value of $r = 1$ occurs when $\Delta z = 0$, that is, when the structure is infinitesimally thin. At this maximum, the twister gradient does not attenuate the signal at all. As the structure becomes thicker (i.e., as Δz increases), signal attenuation tends to increase, as shown in Figure 10.31. The effect, however, is not monotonic because the attenuation ratio oscillates, that is, $r(\Delta z)$ has periodic zeros at $\Delta z = 2\pi n/\gamma A$, where n is a positive integer. The signal attenuation is very similar to that caused by a spoiler gradient (Section 10.5).

10.6.3 PRACTICAL CONSIDERATIONS AND APPLICATIONS

The gradient area A of a twister gradient is an adjustable parameter that must be tailored to the specific imaging application. Typically γA is set so that it produces a 2π phase wrap over a distance approximately twice as long as the dimension of the (thin) structure to be enhanced. For example, if vessels with cross-sectional diameter less than or equal to $\Delta z = 10$ mm are to be imaged, we might initially set the area:

$$A \approx \frac{2\pi}{\gamma(2\Delta z)} = \frac{2\pi}{2\pi \times 42.57 \text{ MHz/T} \times 2 \times 0.01\text{m}} = 1.17 \times 10^{-3} \text{ s} \cdot \text{mT/m} \tag{10.91}$$

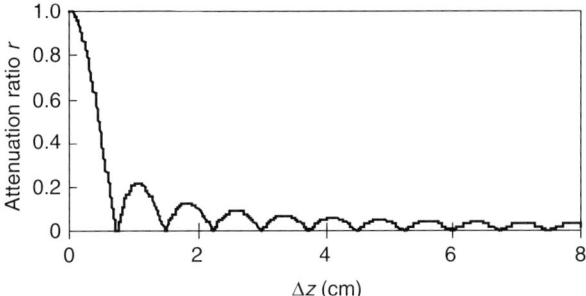

FIGURE 10.31 Plot of the attenuation ratio $r(\Delta z)$ calculated in Eq. (10.90) for $\gamma A = 8.4\,\mathrm{rad/cm}$.

Equation (10.91) provides a reasonable starting point in practical implementation; the optimal area can then be empirically determined by adjusting A to enhance the desired structures in the image. Often the twister gradient can be implemented simply by reducing the gradient area of the slice-rephasing lobe by an amount A.

Twister gradients have found application mainly in MR angiography (Dumoulin and Hart 1987) because blood vessels are usually much smaller than the stationary tissue structures surrounding them. Thick-slab 2D phase-contrast angiography (Figure 10.29) is a common application of twister gradients. Twister gradients are also useful in fluoroscopic triggering of 3D contrast-enhanced exams. Employing a thick 2D slice in the real-time fluoroscopic mode (Section 11.4) virtually ensures that the vessels of interest will be included in the imaging volume. The twister gradient increases the conspicuity of those vessels, making it easier to determine exactly when the contrast material arrives in the arteries and when the 3D acquisition should be initiated. Other applications of twister gradients arise in catheter tracking (Unal et al. 1998) because, like a vessel, a catheter is usually much thinner than the tissue structures that surround it.

SELECTED REFERENCES

Dixon, W. T., Du, L. N., Faul, D. D., Gado, M., and Rossnick, S. 1986. Projection angiograms of blood labeled by adiabatic fast passage. *Magn. Reson. Med.* 3: 454–462.

Dumoulin, C. L., and Hart, H. R. 1987. Rapid scan magnetic resonance angiography. *Magn. Reson. Med.* 5: 238–245.

Unal, O., Korosec, F. R., Frayne, R., Strother, C. M., and Mistretta, C. A. 1998. A rapid 2D time-resolved variable-rate k-space sampling MR technique for passive catheter tracking during endovascular procedures. *Magn. Reson. Med.* 40: 356–362.

RELATED SECTIONS

PART
IV

DATA ACQUISITION, K-SPACE SAMPLING, AND IMAGE RECONSTRUCTION

Introduction

Part IV describes pulse sequence features other than RF and gradient pulses, including data acquisition sampling strategies and data acquisition controls. Part IV also discusses processes that work in close conjunction with pulse sequences, such as physiological monitoring, motion suppression, and image reconstruction.

Chapter 11 describes data acquisition modes and k-space sampling. Bandwidth and sampling related to signal reception are described in Section 11.1. The concept of k-space is explored in Section 11.2; this concept is used throughout the book because it conveniently describes a variety of data acquisition strategies. Partial k-space updating strategies (e.g., keyhole) in a time-course study are presented in Section 11.3. Real-time imaging and fluoroscopic triggering are covered in Section 11.4. The properties of 2D and 3D data acquisition modes are described in Sections 11.5 and 11.6, respectively. Many of the properties described in these two sections are general and apply regardless of the specifics of the pulse sequence used, for example, whether it is gradient echo or RF spin echo.

Chapter 12 covers the basics of physiological gating, triggering, and monitoring. These methods are used to reduce motion-related artifacts, as well as to image moving organs such as the heart. Although the terms *gating* and *triggering* are often used interchangeably, we make a distinction between them in this book. We use the term *triggering* when an event (e.g., the detection of the R-wave) initiates pulse-sequence activity of predetermined duration, as in electrocardiogram (ECG) triggering (Section 12.1). We use the term *gating* when pulse-sequence activity of an indeterminate duration is allowed only when a physiological parameter lies within predetermined limits, as in respiratory gating (Section 12.3). Respiratory compensation by view reordering and motion suppression by breath-holding are also described in Section 12.3. Navigator echoes, which use MR data (rather than external devices) to detect and correct motion, are the subject of Section 12.2.

Chapter 13 provides an introduction to the commonly used image reconstruction methods. MR image reconstruction is the mathematical process that transforms the raw k-space data into the desired image data. Fourier reconstruction (Section 13.1) is a commonly used reconstruction method that can be efficiently applied when k-space data are acquired in a rectilinear fashion (e.g., with phase- and frequency-encoded acquisitions). The reconstruction of data from other k-space trajectories (e.g., spirals and radial projection acquisition) typically uses gridding, as described in Section 13.2. That method maps the non-Cartesian k-space data back onto a rectilinear grid, followed by Fourier reconstruction to yield an image. Phase difference reconstruction

(Section 13.5) is used to reconstruct phase maps that accentuate a desired quantity (e.g., flow, B_0 shim, or temperature change) encoded in the phase of the signal while suppressing the unwanted phase variation that is unavoidable in MR images.

A variety of reconstruction methods have been developed for data acquired in an accelerated manner, and these are also described in Chapter 13. Parallel-imaging reconstruction (Section 13.3) is used to reconstruct images acquired with sensitivity encoding (SENSE), simultaneous acquisition of spatial harmonics (SMASH), and related methods. Partial Fourier reconstruction (Section 13.4) can be used with either partial-echo acquisition, which reduces TE, or partial k_y acquisition, which reduces scan time. The latter is also called a partial NEX acquisition, where NEX denotes the number of excitations, i.e., the number of signal averages. View-sharing reconstruction is described in Section 13.6. That method increases the number of reconstructed phases in a cardiac study or the frame rate in a real-time study. It should be noted that Chapter 13 is intended to be an introduction to reconstruction techniques most likely to be encountered by the pulse-sequence designers and users. Thus, we have chosen to focus on reconstruction techniques that are either commonly used or are becoming prevalent.

SIGNAL ACQUISITION AND K-SPACE SAMPLING

11.1 Bandwidth and Sampling

The readout bandwidth is the range of spin precession frequencies across the FOV in the readout (i.e., the frequency-encoded) direction. This precession frequency range depends on the FOV and the amplitude of the frequency-encoding gradient (see Section 8.1). The readout bandwidth is specified as either the full bandwidth or the half-bandwidth. We use the latter convention here, denoting the half-bandwidth by $\Delta \upsilon$. The full bandwidth is then $2\Delta \upsilon$, and the bandwidth of the scan prescription is $\pm \Delta \upsilon$. In discussing MRI data acquisition, we frequently treat the data as if they were continuously acquired during the readout, but in reality the signal is discretely sampled with an analog-to-digital (A/D) converter. The resulting sampling time per complex point Δt (also known as the *dwell time*) is the inverse of the full readout bandwidth.

11.1.1 MATHEMATICAL DESCRIPTION

The Nyquist theorem states that the spectrum of a discretely sampled signal is replicated in the Fourier conjugate domain (see subsection 1.1.8). For example, Figure 11.1 shows a time-domain signal and its Fourier transform.

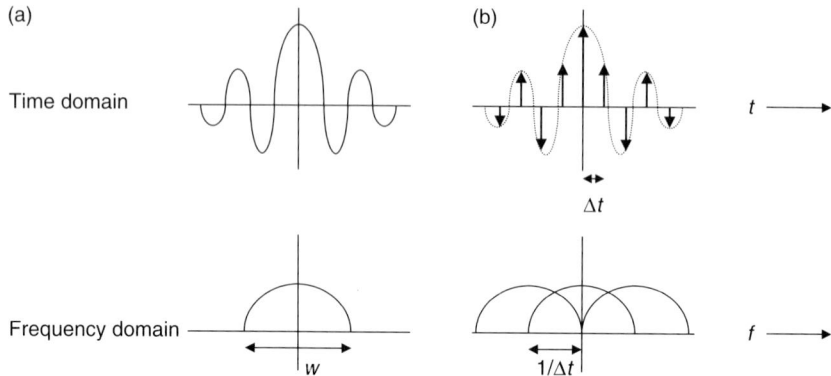

FIGURE 11.1 A time-domain signal and its Fourier transform (a) before discrete sampling and (b) after sampling. The frequency-domain replication interval is the inverse of the sampling time Δt. Because the width of the frequency-domain spectrum w is greater than $1/\Delta t$, the replicates overlap and aliasing results.

If the signal is sampled at intervals Δt, the Fourier transform of the sampled signal is replicated at intervals $1/\Delta t$. If the frequency bandwidth of the spectrum w (its area of compact support) is greater than $1/\Delta t$, the replicates overlap (i.e., aliasing results). This overlap can be prevented by windowing the spectrum before sampling so that the bandwidth w is less than or equal to the replication distance $1/\Delta t$ (Figure 11.2). This result can be directly applied to the readout process in MRI by calculating the bandwidth of the signal resulting from spin precession in the presence of the readout gradient, as shown in Section 8.1.

    In frequency encoding, the precession frequency is varied linearly in one direction, say x, by applying a readout gradient G_x in that direction. The full range of precession frequencies, or bandwidth, across the object in the x direction is $(\gamma/2\pi)G_x D$, where D is the object length (Figure 11.3). In the frequency-encoding process, precession frequency is used to recover the spin location. If an FOV L_x smaller than D is desired, the signal bandwidth must be reduced. This bandwidth reduction is an essential feature of an MRI receiver and requires the receiver to apply a bandlimiting filter (sometimes also called an analog *anti-alias* or hardware filter) prior to the sampling step. (In contrast, with phase encoding, the object signal coming from outside the FOV cannot be eliminated by a filter and the aliased replicates overlap in the image, causing wrap-around artifacts as discussed in Section 8.2.) After applying the anti-alias filter, the signal bandwidth is:

$$\Delta \upsilon = \frac{1}{2}\frac{\gamma}{2\pi}G_x L_x \tag{11.1}$$

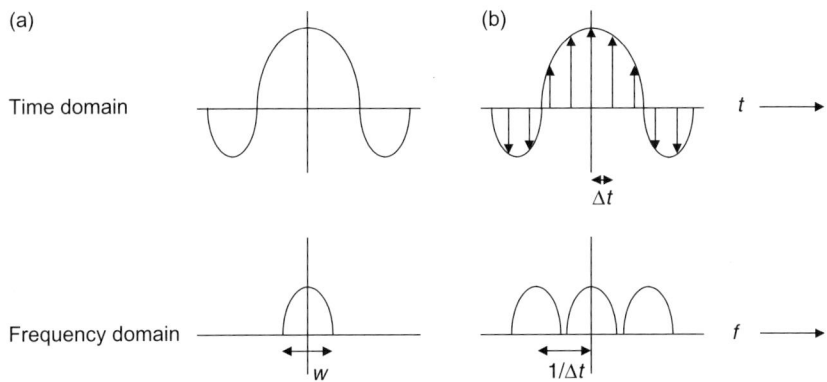

FIGURE 11.2 A time-domain signal and its Fourier transform (a) before sampling and (b) after sampling. The width of the frequency domain spectrum w is less than $1/\Delta t$, preventing aliasing.

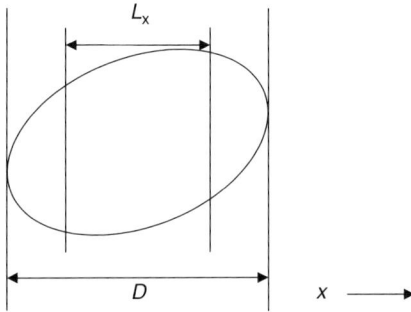

FIGURE 11.3 The object (ellipse) has length D in the frequency-encoded direction. The frequency-encoded FOV L_x is less than D. In this case, applying a bandlimiting filter prevents aliasing.

The A/D converter then samples the signal at intervals:

$$\Delta t = \frac{1}{2\Delta \upsilon} \tag{11.2}$$

as dictated by the Nyquist theorem.

The sampling requirements of the Nyquist theorem apply both to the k-space and spatial domains. For example, the temporal Nyquist sampling requirement is related to the k-space sampling Nyquist requirement as follows. Assuming a constant readout gradient, the interval between readout points in k-space Δk_x is:

$$\Delta k_x = \frac{\gamma}{2\pi} G_x \Delta t \tag{11.3}$$

Combining Eq. (11.3) with Eqs. (11.1) and (11.2), we obtain the k-space Nyquist requirement:

$$\Delta k_x = \frac{1}{L_x} \tag{11.4}$$

If we acquire N_x readout points, the maximum extent of the acquired k-space is:

$$N_x \Delta k_x = \frac{N_x}{L_x} = \frac{1}{\Delta x} \tag{11.5}$$

where Δx is the image resolution in the readout direction, that is, the pixel size after the Fourier transform without zero filling. Equations (11.4) and (11.5) state that the k-space (or image space) sampling interval is the inverse of the length of compact support in image space (or k-space). Equations (11.4) and (11.5) can be compared to Eq. (1.30), Eq. (8.11), and Eqs. (8.33) and (8.34).

11.1.2 RECEIVER DESIGN

An MRI receiver removes the Larmor precession frequency of the transverse magnetization. This has the same effect as if the received data were acquired in the rotating frame (Section 1.2) and is called *demodulation*. The receiver converts the real signal induced in the receive coil into a complex signal suitable for Fourier transformation to reconstruct the MR image. This process is called *quadrature detection*. Finally, the receiver performs data sampling and bandlimiting to prevent aliasing.

Many different receiver designs are possible; only one design, illustrating many of these concepts, is discussed here. To allow flexibility in the choice for bandwidth, the bandlimiting is always done in several steps and partly using digital hardware. In all designs, prior to A/D sampling, the signal is bandlimited with the analog anti-alias filter (hardware filter) to the maximum bandwidth allowed by the A/D converter sample time. The purpose of the anti-alias filter is to prevent wide-band noise such as white noise and spurious signals from aliasing into the imaging FOV. The A/D sample bandwidth is denoted here $\pm \Delta \upsilon_{ad}$ and the corresponding sample time is denoted Δt_{ad}. The maximum bandwidth allowed by the system $\pm \Delta \upsilon_{max}$ can be less than $\pm \Delta \upsilon_{ad}$. If the operator has prescribed a bandwidth less than $\Delta \upsilon_{max}$, the signal is then digitally filtered and sampled to the final bandwidth.

MR Signal   To understand how the receiver performs these functions, it is helpful to consider the MR signal generation process. A complete discussion can be found in Haacke et al. (1999). As shown there, ignoring relaxation effects, the signal $S(t)$ induced in the coil by the precessing magnetization is given by:

$$S(t) \propto \omega \int \left| \vec{M}_T(\vec{r}) \right| \left| \vec{B}_T(\vec{r}) \right| \sin(\phi_M(\vec{r}, t) - \phi_B(\vec{r})) \, d^3r \qquad (11.6)$$

In Eq. (11.6), $\omega = \gamma B_0$ is the Larmor frequency in radians per second; $\vec{M}_T(\vec{r}) = M_x \hat{x} + M_y \hat{y}$ is the transverse component of magnetization in the laboratory frame at time $t = 0$; $\vec{B}_T(\vec{r})$ is the transverse component of the receive coil B_1 field; $\phi_M(\vec{r}, t)$ is the phase of $\vec{M}_T(\vec{r})$, that is, its angle with respect to the x axis in the laboratory frame; and $\phi_B(\vec{r})$ is the phase of $\vec{B}_T(\vec{r})$ in the laboratory frame. The integration is performed over the entire volume of the sample (patient). Ignoring resonance offsets from susceptibility variation and chemical shift, the precession frequency of $\vec{M}_T(\vec{r})$ is the Larmor frequency plus a frequency offset due to imaging gradients $\vec{G}(t)$. The resulting phase is:

$$\phi_M(\vec{r}, t) = \phi_0(\vec{r}) + \omega t + \gamma \int_0^t \vec{G}(t') \cdot \vec{r} \, dt' \qquad (11.7)$$

where $\phi_0(\vec{r})$ is the transverse magnetization phase at $t = 0$. Equation (11.6) then becomes:

$$S(t) \propto \omega \int \left| \vec{M}_T(\vec{r}) \right| \left| \vec{B}_T(\vec{r}) \right| \sin \left[\omega t + \gamma \int \vec{G}(t') \cdot \vec{r} \, dt' \right.$$
$$\left. + \phi_0(\vec{r}) - \phi_B(\vec{r}) \right] d^3r \qquad (11.8)$$

Demodulation and Quadrature Detection   The ωt term in the sine function in Eq. (11.8), represents Larmor precession and is removed by multiplying the signal by (i.e., mixing it with) a sine or cosine oscillating at or near ω (called a local oscillator or LO signal), followed by low-pass filtering. Consider multiplying the function $\sin(\omega + \Delta\omega)t$ by $\sin \omega t$. Using the trigonometric identity:

$$\sin A \sin B = \frac{\cos(A - B) - \cos(A + B)}{2} \qquad (11.9)$$

yields:

$$\sin(\omega + \Delta\omega)t \times \sin \omega t = \frac{\cos \Delta\omega t - \cos(2\omega + \Delta\omega)t}{2} \qquad (11.10)$$

The second term on the right-hand side of Eq. (11.10) is a sideband at offset frequency 2ω and can be eliminated by a low-pass filter with the appropriate bandwidth. Even if $\Delta\omega$ is time-dependent, the second term can still be eliminated with a low-pass filter provided $\omega \gg \Delta\omega$. Similarly, multiplying by $\cos \omega t$ results in:

$$\sin(\omega + \Delta\omega)t \times \cos \omega t = \frac{\sin \Delta\omega t + \sin(2\omega + \Delta\omega)t}{2} \tag{11.11}$$

The second term in (11.11) can also be eliminated by using a low-pass filter. The resulting low-pass-filtered signal oscillates at $\Delta\omega$; that is, the frequency offset ω has been removed.

Demodulating the signal in Eq. (11.6) by multiplying by $\sin \omega t$ and $\cos \omega t$ followed by low-pass filtering results in two separate signals S_R and S_I given by

$$S_R(t) \propto \omega \int \left|\vec{M}_T(\vec{r})\right|\left|\vec{B}_T(\vec{r})\right| \cos\left[\gamma \int \vec{G}(t') \cdot \vec{r} \, dt' + \phi_0(\vec{r}) - \phi_B(\vec{r})\right] d^3r \tag{11.12}$$

and

$$S_I(t) \propto \omega \int \left|\vec{M}_T(\vec{r})\right|\left|\vec{B}_T(\vec{r})\right| \sin\left[\gamma \int \vec{G}(t') \cdot \vec{r} \, dt' + \phi_0(\vec{r}) - \phi_B(\vec{r})\right] d^3r \tag{11.13}$$

The two signals can be combined to give a complex demodulated signal given by:

$$S_\perp(t) = S_R - i S_I \propto \omega \int \left|\vec{M}_T(\vec{r})\right|\left|\vec{B}_T(\vec{r})\right| e^{-i\left[\gamma \int \vec{G}(t') \cdot \vec{r} \, dt' + \phi_0(\vec{r}) - \phi_B(\vec{r})\right]} d^3r \tag{11.14}$$

(Defining $S_\perp = S_R - i S_I$ instead of $S_\perp = S_R + i S_I$ is equivalent to adding an arbitrary $180°$ phase shift to S_I. We use the former definition for notational consistency with the rest of the book.) Using complex notation, the demodulated signal can be written:

$$S_\perp(t) \propto \omega \int M_\perp(\vec{r}) B_\perp(\vec{r}) e^{-i\gamma \int \vec{G}(t') \cdot \vec{r} \, dt'} d^3r \tag{11.15}$$

where $M_\perp(\vec{r}) = |\vec{M}_T(\vec{r})| e^{-i\phi_0(\vec{r})}$ and $\vec{B}_\perp(\vec{r}) = |\vec{B}_T(\vec{r})| e^{i\phi_B(\vec{r})}$ are complex numbers whose real and imaginary parts are equal to the x and y components of the vectors $\vec{M}_T(\vec{r})$ and $\vec{B}_T(\vec{r})$, respectively. Identifying the k-space vector (Section 11.2):

$$\vec{k}(t) = \frac{\gamma}{2\pi} \int_0^t \vec{G}(t') \, dt' \tag{11.16}$$

as a spatial frequency directly leads to the interpretation that the complex demodulated signal is the Fourier transform of the transverse magnetization, weighted by the receive coil B_1 field.

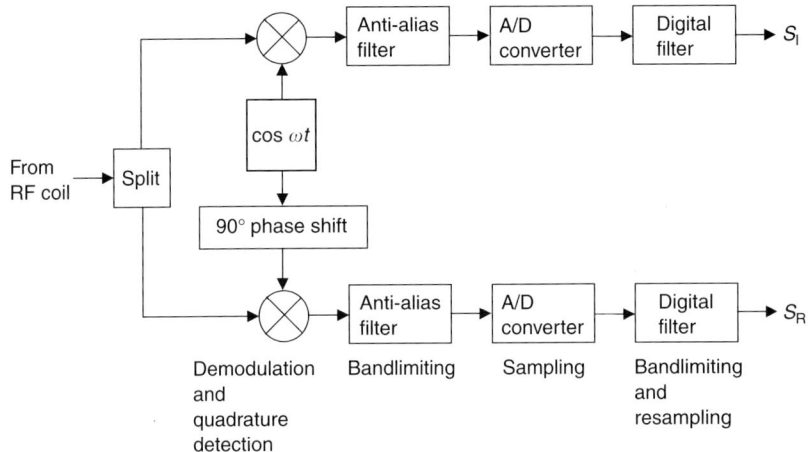

FIGURE 11.4 Direct-conversion analog receiver. The signal from the RF coil oscillating at the Larmor frequency ω is split and then mixed with sine and cosine reference signals oscillating at frequency ω to remove the Larmor frequency oscillation. Separate anti-alias filters then bandlimit each signal to $\pm\Delta\upsilon_{ad}$ prior to A/D sampling in order to eliminate demodulation sidebands and avoid aliasing. The sampled signals are digitally filtered to further bandlimit and resample the data if $\Delta\upsilon_{max} < \Delta\upsilon_{ad}$ or if the operator has selected a bandwidth less than $\Delta\upsilon_{max}$.

Direct-Conversion Analog Receiver In this design, S_R and S_I are computed with separate analog demodulation and digitization hardware (Figure 11.4). Demodulation to remove the Larmor frequency is done by multiplying the signal by $\sin \omega t$ and $\cos \omega t$. Both S_R and S_I are separately bandlimited to $\pm\Delta\upsilon_{ad}$ to remove the unwanted sidebands in Eqs. (11.10) and (11.11) and to prevent aliasing prior to digitization. The resulting signals, now centered at zero frequency (also known as baseband or DC), are digitized by the A/D converters at intervals Δt_{ad}. Further bandlimiting and resampling use digital processing as shown in Figure 11.4 if $\Delta\upsilon_{max} < \Delta\upsilon_{ad}$, or if the operator has selected a bandwidth less than $\Delta\upsilon_{max}$.

A drawback to this design is that the two analog paths can have different gains (in-phase/quadrature, or I/Q mismatch) resulting in an amplitude difference between S_R and S_I. The phase shift between the local oscillator signals for the two paths may not be exactly 90°. These problems cause an artifact called a quadrature ghost. The artifact consists of a very-low-amplitude copy of the object, reflected in both readout and phase-encoded directions and superimposed on the image (Henkelman and Bronskill 1987).

Another drawback to this design is that A/D converters usually have a DC offset (i.e., a nonzero output voltage even with zero input voltage) that can drift due to thermal changes. The effect of DC offset is a spurious super-imposed signal at zero frequency. This results in an artifact that consists of a dot at the center of the image if the DC offset is constant throughout the scan. Alternatively, the artifact can be a slight spreading of the dot in the phase-encoded direction if the DC offset drifts slowly during the scan. Frequent recalibration of the offset voltage between scans can minimize, but often does not eliminate, the problem. The artifact can be removed or reduced by phase cycling or chopping the RF pulse (see Section 11.5). A DC offset can also result from leakage of the LO signal into the MR signal (input to the preamp) or from leakage of the MR signal into the LO (input to the mixer) because the leaked signal is demodulated to baseband at the output of the mixer.

Alternative Receiver Designs   To avoid these problems, the receiver on most modern MRI scanners does not use the design in Figure 11.4. Many receivers use an intermediate frequency (IF) to partially demodulate the signal to a baseband value that is on the order of 100 kHz. An A/D converter digitizes the signal, followed by further bandlimiting and demodulation that uses digital processing. DC offset is eliminated because the output of analog-mixing hardware, as well as the input to the A/D converter, is centered at an intermediate frequency rather than at DC. Because quadrature is created using digital processing, I/Q mismatch is also eliminated. Another receiver design (direct digital receiver) does not use any analog demodulation but bandlimits and digitizes the data centered at the Larmor frequency. Demodulation to baseband and creation of quadrature data are accomplished using digital processing. A complete discussion of these designs is outside the scope of this book, but more information can be found in Hoult (1978), Holland and MacFall (1992), Michal et al. (2002), and Morris et al. (2002).

Design Trade-Offs   In most MR scanners, $\Delta\upsilon_{max}$ is somewhat larger than required for most applications. The cost of the A/D converter depends on the number of bits and minimum sampling time per complex point. On many systems, the minimum sampling time per complex point is 1 μs or longer and the number of bits is 16 or fewer. The requirements for the number of bits and minimum sampling time are interdependent and are determined by the maximum SNR as well as typical readout bandwidths. A full discussion is beyond the scope of this book; however, the A/D sampling time is usually limited by a cost trade-off made by the manufacturer.

11.1.3 OPERATOR PARAMETER SELECTION

Choosing any two of the three parameters—bandwidth $\Delta\upsilon$, gradient amplitude G_x, and FOV L_x—in Eq. (11.1) fixes the third parameter. Usually only certain values of Δv and L_x are allowed on most scanners. For example, L_x can usually be changed in increments of 1 cm or finer. Typical allowed values of $\pm\Delta v$ for a 1.5-T scanner might be ±16 kHz, ±32 kHz, ±64 kHz, and so forth. Some commercial MRI scanners allow the operator to choose any combination of allowed parameter values consistent with Eq. (11.1). Other scanners allow only fixed combinations of the parameters. For most pulse sequences, it is customary to let the operator choose Δv and L_x and fix G_x accordingly. Note that we must limit the choices of Δv and L_x so that G_x does not exceed the maximum gradient amplitude h that the system can produce. Similarly, the choice of G_x and L_x are also limited by the maximum receiver bandwidth that the MR system can provide. L_x is typically chosen based on the size of the object, the spatial resolution requirements, and SNR (Section 11.2).

The bandwidth Δv is typically chosen based on requirements for chemical shift artifact, as well as SNR and minimum echo time. The chemical shift artifact is the displacement of off-resonant spins that occurs when frequency encoding is used for spatial localization and spatial selection (slice or slab selection). Similar displacement can also occur when there is a spatial magnetic susceptibility variation or B_0 inhomogeneity. Chemical shift artifacts occur in the readout direction and in the slice-selection (Section 8.3) or slice-encoded (Section 11.6) direction in most pulse sequences. It can also appear along the phase-encoded direction in some echo-train pulse sequences, such as EPI. The cause of chemical shift in the readout direction is schematically shown in Figure 11.5. The frequency-encoding gradient creates a linearly varying precession frequency across the FOV. A spin at location x_1 precesses with

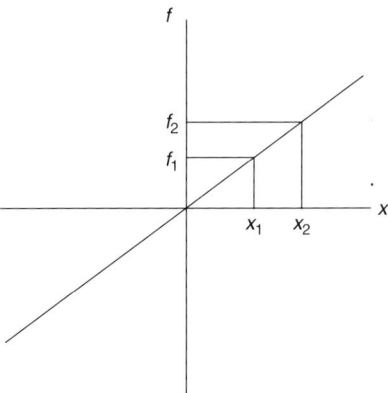

FIGURE 11.5 Frequency-encoding gradient gives a precession frequency that varies linearly across the FOV. A spin at location x_1 precesses with frequency f_1 if the spin is on-resonance. If the spin is off-resonance and precesses instead with frequency f_2, it will appear in the image at location x_2.

frequency f_1 if it is on-resonance. If the spin is off-resonance and instead precesses with frequency f_2, it will be mapped to location x_2 in the image. The shift distance $\delta x = x_2 - x_1$ is given by:

$$\delta x = \frac{2\pi \delta f}{\gamma G_x} \tag{11.17}$$

where $\delta f = f_2 - f_1$. Using Eq. (11.1), the shift in units of the FOV is the dimensionless quantity:

$$\delta x_{\text{FOV}} = \frac{\delta x}{L_x} = \frac{\delta f}{2\Delta \upsilon} \tag{11.18}$$

Alternatively, because N_x pixels cover the FOV, the shift in pixels is:

$$\delta x_{\text{pixel}} = \frac{N_x \delta x}{L_x} = \frac{N_x \delta f}{2\Delta \upsilon} \tag{11.19}$$

The shift distance can be reduced by increasing the bandwidth at the expense of lower SNR.

The selection of the receiver bandwidth also depends on the B_0-field strength. At low fields (e.g., 0.2 T), chemical shift artifacts and magnetic susceptibility artifacts are less pronounced, allowing a lower receiver bandwidth to be selected (e.g., ± 2 kHz). The narrow bandwidth also helps to increase the SNR, which is particularly needed at low fields. Conversely, at high fields (e.g., 1.5 T or 3 T), a wider receiver bandwidth (e.g., 16 kHz) is required to reduce chemical shift and magnetic susceptibility artifacts. The higher SNR at high magnetic fields facilitates the choice of a wider receiver bandwidth. To keep the chemical shift (in pixels) constant for a particular FOV and matrix size, a receiver bandwidth that is linearly proportional to field strength is selected.

For pulse sequences that use a train of gradient echoes, such as EPI, chemical shift occurs primarily in the phase-encoded direction. This is because off-resonant spins continue to accrue phase during the train of gradient echoes. The resulting additional phase twist accrued by the spins at any phase encoding is the same as would be accrued by an on-resonant spin displaced in the phase-encoded direction. The chemical shift displacement is calculated using Eq. (11.18), except that the bandwidth $\Delta \upsilon$ corresponds to the inverse of twice the echo spacing. Although chemical shift in the readout direction also occurs, the readout bandwidth is usually much higher than the effective bandwidth along the phase-encoded direction. For example, for a 0.5 ms echo spacing, the effective phase-encoding bandwidth is $\pm 1/(2 \times 0.5\,\text{ms}) = \pm 1$ kHz, whereas the readout bandwidth is typically ± 100 kHz or more. Chemical shift in the readout direction is therefore usually negligible for such pulse sequences. (More discussion can be found in Section 16.1.)

For some pulse sequences, such as EPI or spiral, that are extremely sensitive to off-resonance effects, it may be preferable to set the readout gradient equal to the system maximum h and allow the operator to choose either the bandwidth or FOV. The remaining parameter is then fixed. This is because the readout gradient determines the traversal speed of k-space trajectory. From Eq. (11.16), the readout gradient is:

$$G_x(t) = \frac{2\pi}{\gamma} \frac{dk_x}{dt} \tag{11.20}$$

For EPI or spiral, the use of the maximum k-space speed, and therefore the maximum gradient, is desirable to minimize the accumulation of phase from off-resonant spins. For EPI this means setting $G_x = h$, whereas for a 2D spiral it means setting $\sqrt{G_x^2 + G_y^2} = h$ (see Section 17.6). Note that sometimes the limit of $\sqrt{G_x^2 + G_y^2} = h$ can be exceeded for an oblique prescription (Section 7.3).

Example 11.1   A scanner has a maximum gradient amplitude of $h = 40\,\text{mT/m}$ and a maximum bandwidth of $\Delta\upsilon_{max} = \pm 125\,\text{kHz}$. The operator has selected $\Delta\upsilon = \pm 125\,\text{kHz}$ and $L_x = 18\,\text{cm}$. What readout gradient will be used?

Answer   Using Eq. (11.1),

$$G_x = \frac{125000\,\text{Hz}}{(0.5)(42.57 \times 10^6\,\text{Hz/T})(0.18\,\text{m})} = 0.0326\,\text{T/m} = 32.6\,\text{mT/m}$$

Example 11.2   A scanner has a maximum gradient amplitude of $h = 30\,\text{mT/m}$. The operator has selected an EPI scan with $L_x = 24\,\text{cm}$. If the scanner automatically uses the maximum gradient amplitude for the EPI readout, what bandwidth will be used for the readout?

Answer   Using Eq. (11.1),

$$\Delta\upsilon = \pm(0.5)(42.57 \times 10^6\,\text{Hz/T})(30 \times 10^{-3}\,\text{T/m})(0.24\,\text{m}) = \pm 153\,\text{kHz}.$$

SELECTED REFERENCES

Haacke, E. M., Brown, R. W., Thompson, M. R., and Venkatesan, R., 1999. *Magnetic resonance imaging physical principles and sequence design*. New York: Wiley-Liss.
Henkelman, R. M., and Bronskill, M. J. 1987. Artifacts in magnetic resonance imaging. *Rev. Magn. Reson. Imaging* 2: 1–126.

Holland, G. N., and MacFall, J. R. 1992. An overview of digital spectrometers for MR imaging. *J. Magn. Reson. Imaging* 2: 241–246.

Hoult, D. I. 1978. The NMR receiver: A description and analysis of design. *Prog. Nucl. Magn. Reson. Spectrosc.* 12: 41–77.

Michal, C. A., Broughton, K., and Hansen, E. 2002. A high performance digital receiver for home-built nuclear magnetic resonance spectrometers. *Rev. Sci. Instr.* 73: 453–458.

Morris, H. D., Derbyshire, J. A., Kellman, P., Chesnick, A. S., Guttman, M. A., and McVeigh, E. R. 2002. A wide-bandwidth multi-channel digital receiver and real-time reconstruction engine for use with a clinical MR scanner. In *Proceedings of the 10th ISMRM*, p. 61.

RELATED SECTIONS

11.2 k-Space

Early in the development of MRI it was recognized that the time-varying signals detected from precessing magnetization could be analyzed by following trajectories that evolve in a 2D or 3D space. That space corresponds to a domain that is Fourier conjugate to the standard spatial domain that contains the object magnetization (Likes 1981; Ljunggren 1983). The Fourier transform variables were given the symbol k, and the domain was called *k-space*. The k-space concept greatly simplifies the understanding of many pulse sequences such as echo planar imaging (EPI) or spiral, which are very cumbersome to analyze without it. The requirements for sampling and the effects of partial sampling (e.g., partial Fourier acquisition or parallel imaging) are relatively straightforward when viewed from the k-space perspective.

Later it was shown that selective excitation with small flip angles also can be described using a k-space formalism (Pauly et al. 1989). The k-space concept is especially beneficial for designing and understanding variable-rate (Section 2.4), multidimensional (Section 5.1), and spatial-spectral (Section 5.4) RF pulses. In this section, we discuss k-space as it applies to MRI signal reception for 2D acquisition. The extension of this to 3D acquisition is straightforward and is discussed in Section 11.6.

11.2.1 MATHEMATICAL DESCRIPTION

After demodulation to remove the rapid signal oscillation caused by the B_0 field (see Section 11.1), the time-domain signal created by transverse magnetization is:

$$S(t) = \int M_\perp(\vec{r}) B_\perp(\vec{r}) e^{-i\phi(\vec{r},t)} d^3r \qquad (11.21)$$

where $M_\perp(\vec{r})$ is the transverse magnetization, $B_\perp(\vec{r})$ is the component of the receive coil B_1 field that lies in the transverse plane, and the accumulated phase (in radians) is:

$$\phi(\vec{r}, t) = \gamma \int_0^t \vec{r} \cdot \vec{G}(t') \, dt' \qquad (11.22)$$

In Eq. (11.21), $M_\perp$ and $B_\perp$ are complex quantities, $\vec{r}$ is a spatial variable; and d^3r is a shorthand notation for the product of spatial differentials, for example, in three dimensions, $d^3r = dx\,dy\,dz$. We have neglected relaxation and diffusion effects, and the integral is taken over the entire excited portion of the sample. Defining:

$$\vec{k}(t) = \frac{\gamma}{2\pi} \int_0^t \vec{G}(t') \, dt' \qquad (11.23)$$

the space that $\vec{k}(t)$ resides in is known as k-space. (Some authors omit the factor of 2π in the denominator from the definition of k-space and absorb it into the definition of γ or else use the angular frequency representation of the Fourier transform, see Section 1.1.) Note that k-space has units of inverse distance, typically inverse centimeters (cm^{-1}). Also keep in mind that in Eq. (11.23) timekeeping begins anew whenever transverse magnetization is created by an excitation pulse. (Typically we take $t = 0$ to be the isodelay point of the RF excitation pulse.) With the definition of k-space, Eq. (11.21) becomes:

$$S(t) = \int M_\perp(\vec{r}) B_\perp(\vec{r}) e^{-i2\pi \vec{k}(t) \cdot \vec{r}} d^3r \qquad (11.24)$$

The signal $S(t)$ is the Fourier transform (Section 1.1) of the weighted transverse magnetization $M_\perp(\vec{r}) B_\perp(\vec{r})$. The function $\vec{k}(t)$ in Eq. (11.24) is the Fourier conjugate variable to the spatial variable $\vec{r}$. As time evolves, $S(t)$ traces a path $\vec{k}(t)$ in k-space. For nuclei with a positive γ, the direction of motion in k-space is the same as the gradient direction. The speed of k-space traversal is determined by the gradient amplitude $\|\vec{G}(t)\|$ as well as by γ because, from Eq. (11.23), $\|d\vec{k}/dt\| = \|\gamma \vec{G}\|/(2\pi)$. Equation (11.23) also shows that the total distance in k-space covered during any time interval is determined by the area under the gradient waveform $\vec{G}(t)$ during that time interval. Note that k-space can be interpreted as the spatial rate of change of the phase (when it is measured in cycles) that stationary spins accumulate as a result of the gradients. Specifically, if $\vec{r}$ does not depend on time and we neglect gradient nonuniformity, then from Eqs. (11.22) and (11.23):

$$\vec{k}(t) = \frac{1}{2\pi}\vec{\nabla}\phi(\vec{r}, t) \tag{11.25}$$

Note that, because ϕ is linearly proportional to $\|\vec{r}\|$, $\vec{\nabla}\phi$ is independent of $\|\vec{r}\|$ but it does depend on time. The direction of the k-space vector is therefore the same as the direction of the spatial variation of the phase at time t. The case of phase accumulation for spins moving in a gradient field is discussed in Sections 9.2 and 10.4.

11.2.2 K-SPACE TRAJECTORY

The k-space trajectory is the path traced out by $\vec{k}(t)$. This path illustrates the acquisition strategy, influences which types of artifacts can result, and determines the image reconstruction algorithm to be employed. k-Space is filled along the path only when MR data are actively being sampled, but it is traversed even when the data sampling is dormant. The most popular k-space trajectory is a Cartesian raster in which each line of k-space (Figure 11.6a) corresponds to the frequency-encoding readout at each value of the phase-encoding gradient, with signal averaging (if any). All lines in the raster are parallel and separated by equal distance in k-space. The image can be reconstructed using FFTs if the lines of the raster and samples along each line are equally spaced (see Section 13.1 for a general description of FFT-based reconstruction methods). A typical Cartesian raster uses between 128 and 512 phase-encoded views. The Cartesian trajectory is popular because (unless echo-train spin refocusing is used, e.g., EPI, RARE, or GRASE) its artifacts are less objectionable than those from other trajectories in the presence of resonance offset, eddy currents, and other imperfections. One drawback of the Cartesian raster is relatively long scan times unless echo train spin refocusing is used because each line requires a separate RF excitation pulse (or multiple pulses, if signal averaging is used). The use of echo trains greatly increases the sensitivity to several artifacts.

If a spatially selective RF pulse is used for excitation, then immediately after the RF pulse the transverse magnetization is dephased by the portion of the slice-selection gradient after the isodelay point, effectively displacing the k-space trajectory away from the origin in the k_z direction. In 2D pulse sequences, a slice-rephasing lobe (Section 8.3) is usually applied to bring the trajectory back to $k_z = 0$. 2D pulse sequences therefore sample the $k_z = 0$ plane of a 3D k-space, so the k_z dependence can be ignored.

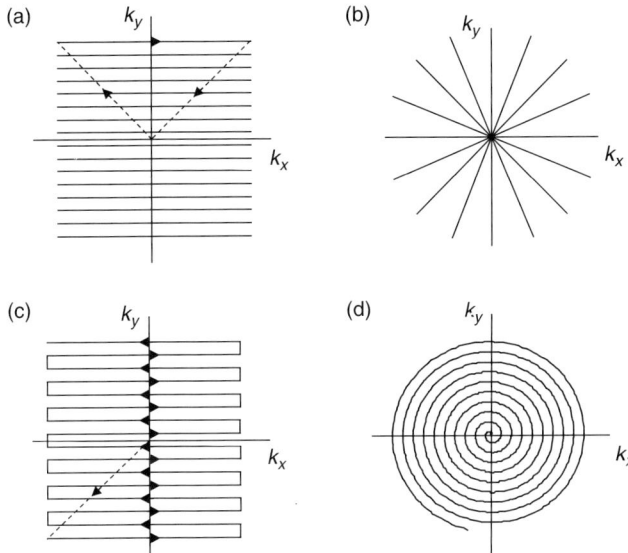

FIGURE 11.6 k-Space trajectories for some commonly used 2D pulse sequences. (a) Cartesian raster using non-echo-train pulse sequences, (b) radial projection acquisition, (c) echo planar imaging, and (d) spiral. The dashed lines show prephasing or rephasing trajectories. The arrows indicate the direction of k-space traversal.

If a Cartesian raster is used, a frequency-axis prephaser (also called a dephaser) gradient lobe (Section 8.1) and a phase-encoding lobe (Section 8.2) are applied to bring the k-space trajectory to the start of the raster line being sampled, as shown by the left dashed line in Figure 11.6a. After traversing the raster line, some pulse sequences such as RARE or steady-state free precession (SSFP) return the k-space trajectory to the origin using gradient rephasing lobes, as shown by the right dashed line in Figure 11.6a. More detailed discussion is provided in the sections on these pulse sequences.

Another k-space trajectory example is projection acquisition (PA) (Section 17.5), consisting of spokes that radiate out from the origin (Fig. 11.6b). PA was the first k-space trajectory used for MRI (Lauterbur 1973). Because of the nonuniform sampling density (the spokes are closer together near the origin than at the edge of k-space), PA is somewhat less efficient than a Cartesian raster, resulting in longer scans if the Nyquist criterion is satisfied at the edge of k-space. Artifacts from undersampling in the azimuthal direction are streaks instead of the replication or wraps that result from undersampling a Cartesian raster. If the streaks are not objectionable, this can result in shorter scans without sacrificing spatial resolution compared to a Cartesian raster. Because of the high vessel intensity relative to the stationary tissue background, contrast-enhanced MRA is an application where angularly undersampled PA can be used for scan-time reduction because the resulting streaks are usually of low intensity and are mostly hidden by the use of maximum intensity projections. Different methods for traversing the radial spokes are discussed in Section 17.5.

The EPI trajectory (Section 16.1) was developed to decrease scan time by speeding up the raster so that k-space is covered with a single (or few) RF excitation pulse(s). The number of excitation pulses required to cover k-space is called the number of *shots*. This trajectory uses a series of gradient echoes to cover a large number of raster lines with one RF excitation, reversing the direction of travel on each line (Figure 11.6c). The main drawback of EPI is geometric distortion caused by off-resonant spins and Nyquist ghosts due to alternating k-space trajectory reversal. Additional discussion can be found in Section 16.1.

The spiral trajectory (Section 17.6) was developed to decrease scan time and covers k-space somewhat more efficiently than the Cartesian trajectory. The number of shots in a spiral scan is also called the number of *interleaves*. Most of the efficiency comes from the fact that a relatively small number of interleaves (usually about 16) is sufficient. The trajectory usually starts at the origin of k-space and spirals outward. Some of the efficiency improvement is sacrificed because the limited-gradient slew rate results in points sampled closer than the Nyquist limit near the center of k-space. Spiral trajectories give blurring (resolution loss) when the spins are off-resonance rather than the geometric shifts and distortion that result with a Cartesian raster. Spiral use has been limited to applications with small FOVs that are near the center of the magnet (cardiac imaging and fMRI, for example) where blurring is minimal.

In addition to those just discussed, many other k-space trajectories have been developed, such as PROPELLER (Pipe 1999), rosette (Noll 1997), and circular (Zhou et al. 1998). Some of these trajectories are discussed in Part V of this book. New trajectories have continued to emerged—a trend that will probably continue.

11.2.3 K-SPACE SAMPLING AND COVERAGE

Although k-space trajectories traverse a continuous path, the signal is sampled only at discrete intervals along the path. Elements of the path, whether straight or curved, are also spaced at discrete distances. The requirement for sampling distance is governed by the Nyquist criterion, discussed in more detail in Sections 1.1, 8.1, 8.2, and 11.1. Generally, sample distances in k-space should be equal to (or smaller than) the inverse of the desired FOV. k-Space is sometimes undersampled to reduce scan time. If multiple receive coils are used, parallel-imaging reconstruction techniques (Section 13.3) can be used to remove the resulting aliasing.

If k-space is covered symmetrically in both the k_x and k_y directions for 2D pulse sequences, the acquisition is called full Fourier. Asymmetric sampling, covering a smaller area in either direction is called partial Fourier and is frequently used to reduce echo time or scan time. Special reconstruction methods are usually used with partial Fourier acquisition (Section 13.4).

SELECTED REFERENCES

Lauterbur, P. C. 1973. Image formation by induced local interactions: Examples employing nuclear magnetic resonance. *Nature* 242: 190–191.

Likes, R. S. 1981. Moving gradient zeugmatography, U.S. patent 4307343.

Ljunggren, S. 1983. A simple graphical representation of Fourier-based imaging methods. *J. Magn. Reson.* 54: 338–343.

Noll, D. C. 1997. Multishot rosette trajectories for spectrally selective MR imaging. *IEEE Trans. Med. Imaging* 16: 372–377.

Pauly, J., Nishimura, D., and Macovski, A. 1989. A k-space analysis of small-tip-angle excitation. *J. Magn. Reson.* 81: 43–56.

Pipe, J. G. 1999. Motion correction with PROPELLER MRI: Application to head motion and free-breathing cardiac imaging. *Magn. Reson. Med.* 42: 963–969.

Zhou, X., Liang, Z. -P., Gewalt, S. L., Cofer, G. P., Lauterbur, P. C., and Johnson, G. A. 1998. A fast spin echo technique with circular sampling. *Magn. Reson. Med.* 39: 23–27.

RELATED SECTIONS

Section 1.1 Fourier Transforms
Section 5.1 Multidimensional Pulses
Section 8.1 Frequency-Encoding Gradients
Section 8.2 Phase-Encoding Gradients
Section 11.1 Bandwidth and Sampling

11.3 Keyhole, BRISK, and TRICKS

It is often desirable to acquire a time-resolved study to image dynamic or time-varying processes such as cardiac motion, fMRI task activation, contrast enhancement after a bolus injection, joint motion, or catheter tracking. High spatial resolution or large coverage is also frequently desirable in such studies, but both decrease the maximal achievable temporal resolution. Therefore, imaging dynamic processes usually involves a compromise among temporal resolution, spatial resolution, and spatial coverage.

One way of achieving the compromise is through the use of *partial k-space updating* methods. These methods are frequently accompanied by reconstruction processing that attempts to recover some of the sacrificed spatial resolution or coverage based on reasonable assumptions or *a priori* knowledge. The methods that compromise spatial resolution are called *keyhole* methods (Jones et al. 1993; Van Vaals et al. 1993), of which the blocked regional interpolation scheme for k-space (BRISK) and time-resolved imaging of contrast kinetics (TRICKS) are extensions. The methods that compromise spatial coverage are called *reduced field of view* (rFOV) methods (Hu and Parrish 1994). Keyhole acquisition is based on the assumption that dynamic information is bandlimited in k-space (i.e., image changes have low spatial resolution), whereas rFOV acquisition is based on the assumption that dynamic information is bandlimited in image space (image changes occur only within a limited FOV). Keyhole and rFOV acquisition can also be combined (Parrish and Hu 2000). Although a detailed discussion of rFOV methods is beyond the scope of this book, the interested reader is encouraged to consult other references because keyhole and rFOV methods give different artifacts and each is better suited to particular applications. For example, rFOV may be more appropriate for cardiac imaging because the heart is often small compared to the FOV.

The keyhole methods repeatedly update data in the center of k-space more frequently than in other parts of k-space. The various keyhole methods are differentiated by their k-space updating schemes and reconstruction methods. In comparison to parallel imaging (Section 13.3), partial k-space updating methods can be used with a single receiver channel, but they generally sacrifice some information as a result.

11.3.1 KEYHOLE ACQUISITION

Data Acquisition   In the original keyhole method (Jones et al. 1993; Van Vaals et al. 1993), a small number of views, called the *keyhole* views, are repeatedly collected to monitor the dynamic process. The keyhole views are symmetrically located about the center of k-space. By themselves, the keyhole views provide a time-series of images with reduced spatial resolution (Figure 11.7). A *reference* data set with the full number of views (providing full spatial resolution) is also collected, usually before (but in some cases during or after) the collection of the keyhole data. The number of keyhole views is usually approximately 25% of the full number of views. The high spatial frequencies of the reference data are combined with each set of keyhole data to generate a complete set of k-space data that is used to reconstruct sets of images. The combination can be simple substitution or more complicated methods, discussed later.

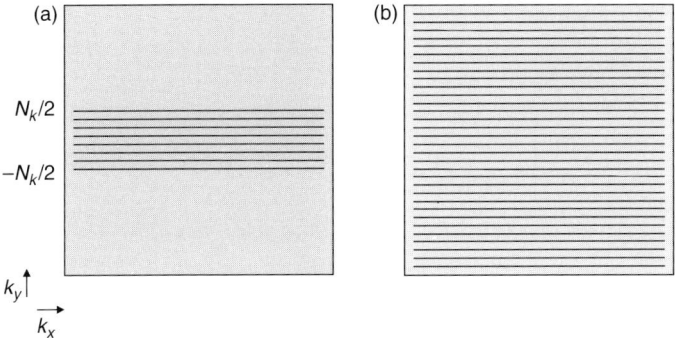

FIGURE 11.7 Example keyhole acquisition with (a) 8 keyhole views, and (b) 32 reference views (full resolution).

Keyhole acquisition was initially introduced to improve the temporal resolution of contrast-enhanced imaging, based on the assumption that most of the information about the contrast bolus is contained in the low spatial frequencies and that information in the high spatial frequencies is relatively static. Although the reconstructed images have the appearance of full spatial resolution, the dynamically changing data are actually reconstructed with the reduced spatial resolution of the keyhole acquisition (Hu 1994). The high-frequency information can serve as an anatomic reference, but does not convey any dynamic information.

Ideally, the extent of the keyhole is determined by the size of the smallest dynamic object to be resolved. For a given keyhole size, the smaller the object, the greater the error in the reconstructed image (underestimation of the image intensity) (Spraggins 1994). For 3D acquisitions, keyhole methods can be used in the phase-encoded, the slice-encoded direction, or both. Because spatial resolution in the slice-encoded direction is usually lower than in the phase direction, the keyhole fraction in the slice-encoded direction is usually larger, typically approximately 50%.

Although the keyhole data are usually centered in k-space, this constraint is not necessary and can be a disadvantage for following the dynamic changes of small objects such as biopsy needles (Duerk et al. 1996). Partial-Fourier-type acquisitions can be used for the keyhole data, as well as for acquisition of k-space segments that are completely displaced from the center of k-space. For simplicity in the following discussion, we assume all keyhole data are centered.

Reconstruction   Three main reconstruction methods that have been applied to keyhole data (Bishop et al. 1997) are substitution, weighted substitution, and generalized series. A more sophisticated algorithm that requires iteration can be found in Oesterle and Hennig (1998). In *substitution*, the reference k-space data are substituted for the missing high spatial frequencies of the keyhole data set to create composite k-space data $\hat{S}$:

$$\hat{S}(k_m) = \begin{cases} S_{\text{keyhole}}(k_m) & -N_k/2 \leq m < N_k/2 \\ S_{\text{reference}}(k_m) & \text{otherwise} \end{cases} \qquad (11.26)$$

where S_{keyhole} and $S_{\text{reference}}$ are keyhole and reference raw data, respectively; m is the index of the phase encode line number k_m; and N_k is the number of key-hole views (assumed to be even). For contrast-enhanced scans, the intensity of S_{keyhole} changes relative to the reference as the contrast bolus enters the imaging plane. This results in a discontinuity of $\hat{S}$ that can cause ringing artifacts.

In *weighted substitution*, the discontinuity between S_{keyhole} and $S_{\text{reference}}$ is reduced by using a weighted combination of pre- and postcontrast references S_{pre} and S_{post}:

$$\hat{S}(k_m) = \begin{cases} S_{\text{keyhole}}(k_m) & -N_k/2 \leq m < N_k/2 \\ w_{\text{pre}} S_{\text{pre}}(k_m) + w_{\text{post}} S_{\text{post}}(k_m) & \text{otherwise} \end{cases} \qquad (11.27)$$

The weighting coefficients w_{pre} and w_{post} are obtained by least-squares fitting of the following equation for each acquisition of S_{keyhole}:

$$S_{\text{keyhole}}(k_m) = w_{\text{pre}} S_{\text{pre}}(k_m) + w_{\text{post}} S_{\text{post}}(k_m) \qquad -N_k/2 \leq m < N_k/2 \qquad (11.28)$$

In general, the fit results in a different set of w_{pre} and w_{post} for each point in the time series. Near the beginning of the time series w_{pre} is close to 1, and near the end w_{post} is close to 1. A constraint such as $w_{\text{pre}} + w_{\text{post}} = 1$ can be included if desired.

In the *generalized series* method (reduced-encoding imaging by generalized-series reconstruction or RIGR) (Liang and Lauterbur 1994; Webb et al. 1993), the discontinuity is reduced by reconstructing the image from basis functions that incorporate *a priori* information from the reference image. The reconstructed image I_{GS} is given by:

$$I_{\text{GS}}(y) = \sum_{m=-N_k/2}^{N_k/2-1} c_m \phi_m(y) \qquad (11.29)$$

where the basis functions ϕ_m are:

$$\phi_m(y) = |I_{\text{ref}}(y)| e^{i 2\pi k_m y} \qquad (11.30)$$

and I_{ref} is the reference image. The coefficients c_m are determined by requiring that the measured data within the keyhole $S_{\text{keyhole}}(k_m)$ equal the resulting k-space data found from Fourier transforming I_{GS}. It is straightforward to show that this constraint results in the relation:

$$S_{\text{keyhole}}(k_m) = \sum_{n=-N_k/2}^{N_k/2-1} c_n S_{\text{ref}}(k_{|m-n|}) \qquad -N_k/2 \leq k < N_k/2 \quad (11.31)$$

Equation (11.31) can be efficiently solved for c_n by using standard numerical methods. The high spatial frequency data resulting with I_{GS} are forced to be continuous with the keyhole data to order $N_k/2$, which reduces artifacts compared to the substitution method.

Although outside the scope of this discussion, non-Fourier encoding methods such as singular value decomposition (SVD) (Hanson et al. 1977) or wavelet encoding (Shimizu et al. 1999) can also be modified to use a reduced set of encodings, or keyhole-type acquisition, for improved temporal resolution in dynamic imaging.

Applications   Although keyhole acquisition has been applied to fMRI (Xiong et al. 1999) and cardiac imaging (Suga et al. 1999); the most common application is contrast-enhanced imaging. Studies suggest that keyhole acquisition should be applied cautiously for quantitative assessment of contrast kinetics. One study showed that keyhole acquisition introduces substantial errors into the calculation of contrast kinetic model parameters, even though the reconstructed images appear relatively artifact-free (Bishop et al. 1997). In that study, weighted substitution and generalized series modeling did not improve the accuracy of the fitted model parameters, even though the reconstructed images had fewer artifacts than with simple substitution. Increasing the keyhole size to match the spatial extent of the enhancing lesion improved model parameter accuracy. Caution is also warranted when applying keyhole methods to contrast-enhanced angiography because the k-space representations of small structures such as aneurysms and tight stenoses contain high spatial frequencies.

In the most common situation, k-space data are assumed to be centered within the keyhole window. When this assumption is violated, for example, due to poor shim or susceptibility gradients in scans with long echo times, severe distortion in the contrast uptake curve can result (Oesterle et al. 2000).

11.3.2 BRISK

Block regional interpolation scheme for k-space (BRISK) is an extension of the fundamental keyhole idea that the edges of k-space need less frequent updating than the center when tracking most dynamic processes. BRISK was originally developed to shorten acquisition times with 2D multiphase cardiac scans that do not use segmented k-space acquisition (Doyle et al. 1995). In the conventional nonsegmented scan, one view of k-space is acquired N_{cp} times per heartbeat for each slice, where N_{cp} is the number of cardiac phases. The number of heartbeats required to acquire a full k-space data set for each slice is therefore equal to the number of k-space lines (see Section 11.5 and Figure 11.23a later in this chapter). For a typical heartbeat of 80 beats per minute (bpm) and 256 phase-encoding lines, the number of heartbeats is $256 \times 60/80 = 192$ s or slightly over 3 min per slice.

Figure 11.8 shows the k-space sampling schedule for BRISK. k-space is divided into 16 segments in this example. The cardiac cycle is divided into 20 phases. Views in the shaded blocks are sampled; those in the unshaded blocks are filled in by interpolation. Views near the center of k-space (blocks 8 and 9) are sampled on each cardiac phase. Views further from the center of k-space are sampled less frequently. In this example, views near the edge of k-space (blocks 1–4 and 12–16) are sampled only once per cardiac cycle. The sampling frequency is increased to five and ten per cardiac cycle for

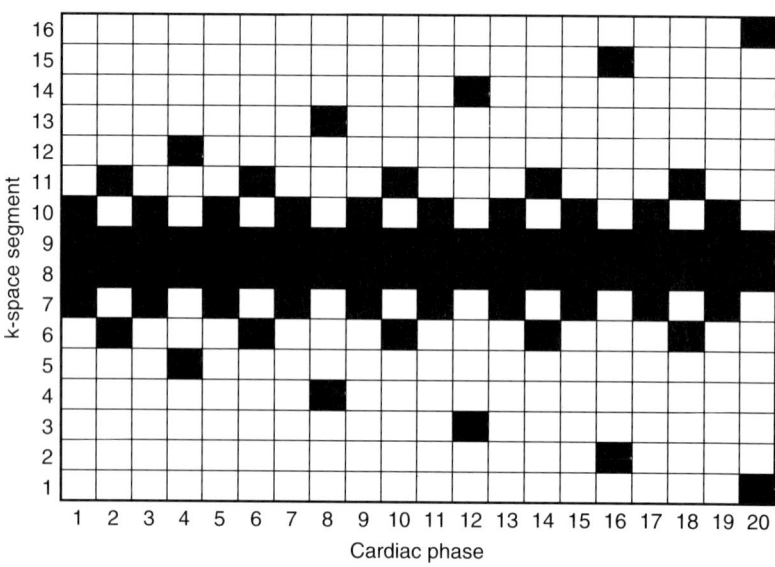

FIGURE 11.8 BRISK k-space sampling schedule. In this example, k-space is divided into 16 segments. The cardiac cycle is divided into 20 phases. Dark blocks indicate k-space segments that are sampled. Views in the segments near the middle of k-space are sampled on each cardiac phase (segments 8 and 9). Other views are sampled less frequently. Views in the segments near the edge of k-space (segments 1–5 and 12–16) are sampled only once per cardiac cycle. (Adapted from Doyle et al. 1995.)

blocks 6 and 11 and blocks 7 and 10, respectively. In doing so, the scan time per slice is one-fourth the conventional scan time (i.e., the number of the shaded blocks is one-fourth the total number of blocks in Figure 11.8). The original implementation of BRISK used Fourier interpolation to fill in the missing views at each cardiac phase. Later, linear interpolation was also used to increase reconstruction speed, but it was found to slightly degrade image quality (Doyle et al. 1997).

BRISK can also be combined with segmented k-space acquisition (turbo-BRISK). One way to achieve this is to simply vary the number of views per segment depending on which block of k-space is collected (Doyle et al. 1997). Views near the center of k-space use the fewest number of views per segment, whereas views near the edge use the most. Missing data at each phase are filled in by interpolation, as usual. In addition to cardiac imaging, turbo-BRISK has been used for quantitative phase-contrast (velocity-encoded) imaging of aortic flow (Polzin et al. 1995; Doyle et al. 1999).

BRISK has not been widely used for cardiac imaging even though, in principle, it allows dramatic improvements in temporal resolution. One reason may be that the basic assumption of keyhole techniques (that high-frequency information is relatively static) might be less valid for cardiac imaging than for contrast-enhanced imaging.

11.3.3 TRICKS

Time-resolved imaging of contrast kinetics or TRICKS (Korosec et al. 1996) is another variation of the general ideas of keyhole acquisition and BRISK. TRICKS is usually applied to improve the time resolution of 3D contrast-enhanced scans. The $k_y - k_z$ plane is divided into equal areas that are cyclically sampled in time (here k_y and k_z denote the primary and secondary phase-encoded directions, respectively, in 3D rectilinearly sampled k-space). Similar to BRISK, the center area of k-space is acquired with the highest temporal frequency. In the original implementation, the $k_y - k_z$ plane was divided only in the k_y direction (Figure 11.9a), but more recent work uses an elliptical-centric division (Section 11.6) as shown in Figure 11.9b. Usually four divisions are used, labeled A, B, C, and D, where section A corresponds to the center of k-space. Prior to the contrast injection, k-space is fully sampled (i.e., all views in all four sections are acquired). The resulting image can be used as a mask for subtraction. Subsequently, the four sections are acquired in the order $ABACADABACAD\ldots$ until the scan terminates.

For example, if the time to acquire all four segments is $4T$, then segment A is acquired at intervals $2T$, whereas segments B, C, and D are acquired at intervals $6T$ (Figure 11.10a). A sliding window reconstruction (Section 13.6)

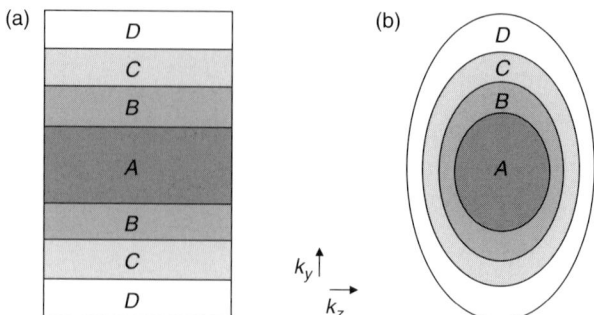

FIGURE 11.9 Segmentation of k-space into four sections labeled A, B, C, and D for TRICKS acquisition. (a) Segmentation along a single dimension (e.g., the first phase-encoded axis k_y), and (b) elliptical-centric segmentation. (Adapted from Korosec et al. 1996.)

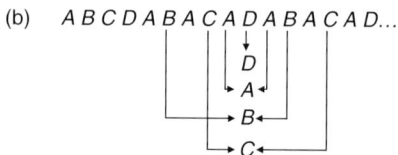

FIGURE 11.10 (a) Temporal resolution of TRICKS k-space segments. The time to acquire a full k-space set is $4T$. The center section of k-space A is acquired at intervals $2T$. Other sections are acquired at intervals $6T$. (b) Interpolation to reconstruct images at each temporal frame uses views from the two nearest acquired frames, indicated by arrows for each k-space segment. Note that segment D has an interpolation weight of unity because it is acquired during the frame being reconstructed.

is used to calculate images at time intervals T by linearly interpolating between data for each k-space segment at the two nearest acquired frames, as shown in Figure 11.10b. Therefore segment A is used in the reconstruction with temporal resolution $2T$, whereas segments B, C, and D are used with temporal resolution $6T$. The temporal resolution of the center of k-space (low-spatial-frequency information) is therefore increased from $4T$ to $2T$, relative to a conventional scan, in exchange for degraded temporal resolution of the higher spatial frequencies. In the example in Figure 11.10b, segments A, B, and C are interpolated from the two nearest acquired segments, indicated by arrows.

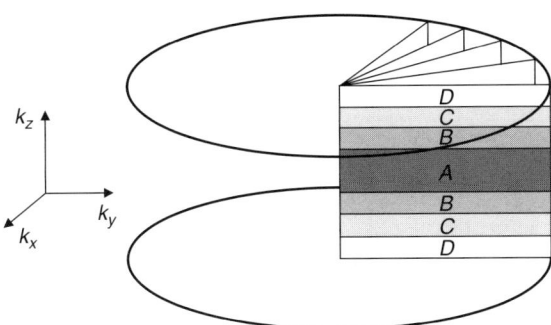

FIGURE 11.11 Segmentation of k-space for TRICKS with stacked projection acquisition. Spokes are collected in the $k_x - k_y$ plane, with segmentation in the k_z direction. The first five spokes are shown. (Adapted from Vigen et al. 2000.)

In this case, segment D does not require interpolation (or equivalently it has an interpolation weight of 1) because it is acquired in the temporal frame being reconstructed.

Another variation, called 3D PR-TRICKS, uses stacked projection acquisition (Section 17.5), that is, projection acquisition within the $k_x - k_y$ plane along with Fourier encoding in the slice-encoded direction k_z. In this case, TRICKS is applied to the k_z direction, which is divided into equal segments as shown in Figure 11.11. This method can also be combined with angular undersampling to further increase temporal resolution (Vigen et al. 2000).

TRICKS has found application in the bilateral imaging of the vessels of the lower legs, where temporal resolution is very useful due to the different filling rates in each leg. With the relatively slow flow in the legs, the temporal resolution allowed by TRICKS (as high as 8 s for typical spatial resolution) is sufficiently good that a timing bolus is usually not needed. Figure 11.12 shows six consecutive frames from a TRICKS acquisition. Each image is a maximum intensity projection of a stack of coronal slices. The interval between frames is $T = 13.2$ s, giving a true temporal resolution of $2T = 26.4$ s for the center of k-space (segment A). In this example, very fast flow results in a venous enhancement only a few frames after arterial enhancement (arrows in frame Figure 11.12f). Without TRICKS, the temporal resolution would be $4T = 52.8$ s and would be insufficient to reliably capture the peak arterial phase.

On the other hand, TRICKS is more difficult to apply to scans requiring breath-holding, such as imaging aorta and renal arteries. The breath-holding must be timed to coincide with the scan and bolus arrival and therefore requires either a timing bolus or other synchronization method. For contrast-enhanced imaging of the carotid, vertebral, and basilar arteries, the temporal resolution

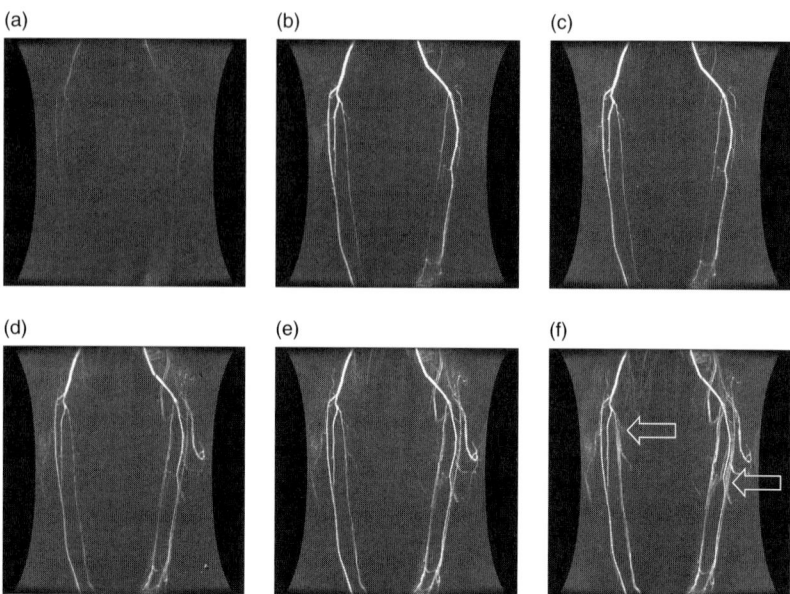

FIGURE 11.12 Six consecutive frames of a TRICKS acquisition at intervals $T = 13.2$ s. Each image is a maximum intensity projection of the stack of 40 coronal slices. Spatial resolution is $1.14 \times 0.85 \times 2.2$ mm. Fast flow results in a venous enhancement (arrows in f) only a few frames after arterial enhancement. (Images courtesy of J. Kevin DeMarco, M. D. Laurie Imaging Center.)

of conventional TRICKS is sometimes insufficient because of the fast (e.g., 5 to 9-s) venous return that causes jugular enhancement. In order to guarantee that a single phase is free of venous contamination and also catches the peak enhancement of the arterial bolus, faster methods such as PR-TRICKS with angular undersampling can be used.

SELECTED REFERENCES

Bishop, J. E., Santyr, G. E., Kelcz, F., and Plewes, D. B. 1997. Limitations of the keyhole technique for quantitative dynamic contrast-enhanced breast MRI. *J. Magn. Reson. Imaging* 7: 716–723.

Doyle, M., Kortright, E., Anayiotos, A. S., Elmahdi, A. M., Walsh, E. G., Fuisz, A. R., and Pohost, G. M. 1999. Rapid velocity-encoded cine imaging with turbo-BRISK. *J. Cardiovasc. Magn. Reson.* 1: 223–232.

Doyle, M., Walsh, E. G., Blackwell, G. G., and Pohost, G. M. 1995. Block regional interpolation scheme for *k*-space (BRISK): A rapid cardiac imaging technique. *Magn. Reson. Med.* 33: 163–170.

Doyle, M., Walsh, E. G., Foster, R. E., and Pohost, G. M. 1995. Rapid cardiac imaging with turbo BRISK. *Magn. Reson. Med.* 37: 410–417.

Duerk, J. L., Lewin, J. S., and Wu, D. H. 1996. Application of keyhole imaging to interventional MRI: A simulation study to predict sequence requirements. *J. Magn. Reson. Imaging* 6: 918–924.

Hanson, J. M., Liang, Z.-P., Magin, R. L., Duerk, J. L., and Lauterbur, P. C. 1997. A comparison of RIGR and SVD dynamic imaging methods. *Magn. Reson. Med.* 38: 161–167.

Hu, X. 1994. On the "keyhole" technique. *J. Magn. Reson. Imaging* 4: 231.

Hu, X., and Parrish, T. 1994. Reduction of field of view for dynamic imaging. *Magn. Reson. Med.* 31: 691–694.

Jones, R. A., Haraldseth, O., Mueller, T. B., Rinck, P. A., and Oksendal, A. N. 1993. k-space substitution: A novel dynamic imaging technique. *Magn. Reson. Med.* 29: 830–834.

Korosec, F. R., Frayne, R., Grist, T. M., and Mistretta, C. A. 1996. Time-resolved contrast-enhanced 3D MR angiography. *Magn. Reson. Med.* 36: 345–351.

Liang, Z.-P., and Lauterbur, P. C. 1994. An efficient method for dynamic magnetic resonance imaging. *IEEE Trans. Med. Imaging* 13: 677–686.

Oesterle, C., and Hennig, J. 1998. Improvement of spatial resolution of keyhole effect images. *Magn. Reson. Med.* 39: 244–250.

Oesterle, C., Strohschein, R., Koehler, M., Schnell, M., and Hennig, J. 2000. Benefits and pitfalls of keyhole imaging, especially in first-pass perfusion studies. *J. Magn. Reson. Imaging* 11: 312–323.

Parrish, T. G., and Hu, X. 2000. Hybrid technique for dynamic imaging. *Magn. Reson. Med.* 44: 51–55.

Polzin, J. A., Frayne, F., Grist, T. M., and Mistretta, C. A. 1995. Phase-contrast flow measurements with variable rate k-space sampling. In *Proceedings of the 3rd Meeting of the SMR*, p. 593.

Shimizu, K., Panych, L. P., Mulkern, R. V., Yoo, S.-S., Schwartz, R. B., Kikinis, R., and Jolesz, F. A. 1999. Partial wavelet encoding: A new approach for accelerating temporal resolution in contrast-enhanced MR imaging. *J. Magn. Reson. Imaging* 9: 717–724.

Spraggins, T. A. 1994. Simulation of spatial and contrast distortions in keyhole imaging. *Magn. Reson. Med.* 31: 320–322.

Suga, M., Matsuda, T., Komori, M., Minato, K., and Takahashi, T. 1999. Keyhole method for high-speed human cardiac cine MR imaging. *J. Magn. Reson. Imaging* 10: 778–783.

Van Vaals, J. J., Brummer, M. E., Dixon, W. T., Tuithof, J. J., Engels, J., Nelson, R. C., Gerety, B. M., Chezmar, J. L., and den Boer, J. A. 1993. "Keyhole" method for accelerating imaging of contrast agent uptake. *J. Magn. Reson. Imaging* 3: 671–675.

Vigen, K. K., Peters, D. C., Grist, T. M., Block, W. F., and Mistretta, C. A. 2000. Undersampled projection-reconstruction imaging for time-resolved contrast-enhanced imaging. *Magn. Reson. Med.* 43: 170–176.

Webb, A. G., Liang, Z.-P., Magin, R. L., and Lauterbur, P. C. 1993. Applications of reduced-encoding MR imaging with generalized-series reconstruction (RIGR). *J. Magn. Reson. Imaging* 3: 925–928.

Xiong, J., Fox, P. T., and Gao, J.-H. 1999. The effects of k-space data undersampling and discontinuities in keyhole functional MRI. *Magn. Reson. Imaging* 17: 109–119.

RELATED SECTIONS

11.4 Real-Time Imaging

Imaging modalities such as ultrasound and x-ray fluoroscopy provide the operator with real-time feedback to tailor the examination to the specific needs of the patient. These real-time imaging modalities can be used to monitor dynamic processes, guide interventional procedures, or interactively select a specific imaging plane. A *real-time MRI* acquisition (Riederer 1997) has the ability to (1) continually acquire data, (2) rapidly reconstruct and display the resulting images, and (3) provide the operator control to interactively alter the image acquisition based on the displayed images (i.e., a feedback loop). Thus, real-time imaging is not a particular pulse sequence but rather an acquisition strategy that can replace the standard paradigm of prescribing, acquiring, and displaying images one series at a time. One use of real-time imaging is to improve the efficiency of the entire examination. Several other applications of real-time MRI are outlined later in this section.

Although early prototype real-time systems developed at academic institutions (Riederer 1997; Kerr 1997; Gmitro 1996) required customized hardware and software, many MR manufacturers have integrated real-time functionality into their standard commercial products. In addition to a rapid reconstruction engine and data buses, real-time MR systems must also include a pathway for operator-prescribed parameter changes to take effect while the acquisition is in progress. Figure 11.13 shows an example of a real-time control screen for a commercially available MRI system. The operator can interactively adjust the scan plane, acquisition parameters including the field of view and slice thickness, and others that affect the image contrast.

In order to achieve a high temporal resolution, most real-time MRI is acquired in 2D sequential mode—that is, data from only one slice location are collected during a TR interval, as discussed in Section 11.5. Although other real-time acquisition modes are certainly possible (e.g., interleaved 2D or 3D), they are not in common use and are not discussed here.

11.4.1 REAL-TIME TERMINOLOGY

There are several terms used to discuss real-time systems. The *true temporal resolution* is the number of times that a complete set of k-space views is acquired per unit time. Temporal resolution is measured in frames per second (fps) or in hertz, with 1 fps = 1 Hz. For a 2D phase-encoded acquisition the true temporal resolution is given by the expression:

$$R = \frac{1}{N_{\text{shot}}\,\text{TR}\,\text{NEX}} \tag{11.32}$$

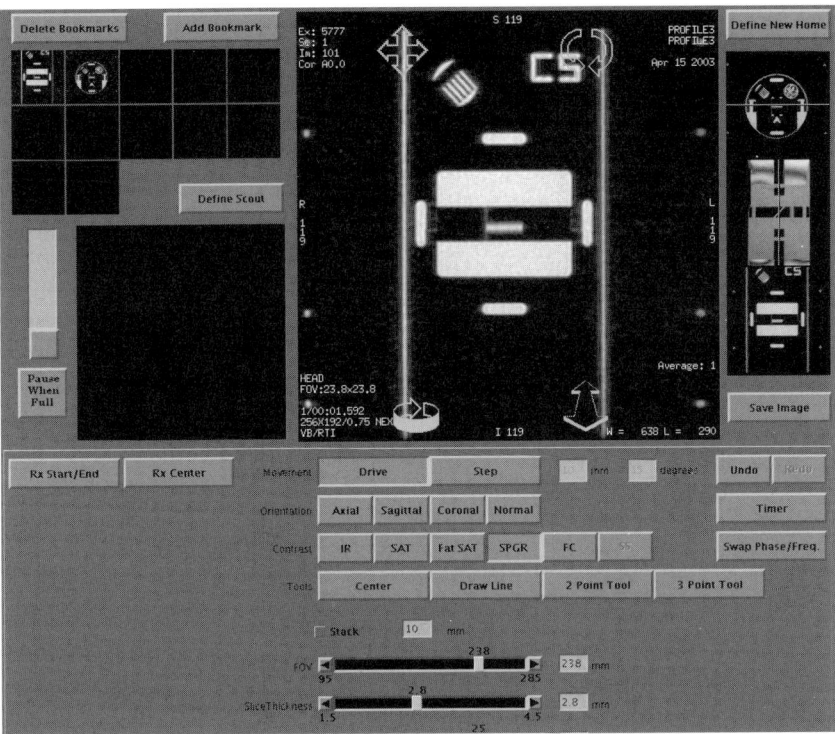

FIGURE 11.13 Example of a user interface for interactive control of a real-time acquisition. The hollow arrows on the image display window allow various rotation and translations of the image plane. (Courtesy of GE Healthcare.)

where N_{shot} is the number of RF excitations (i.e., TR intervals) per complete k-space traversal, and NEX is the number of signal averages. Note that for a standard 2D Fourier acquisition (i.e., echo train length $= 1$), the number of shots is simply equal to the number of phase-encoding lines, $N_{shot} = N_{phase}$. By using N_{shot}, however, Eq. (11.32) is generalized to include EPI, spiral, RARE, and radial acquisitions.

The use of rectangular FOV, parallel imaging, and partial Fourier acquisition all can increase the true temporal resolution because each reduces N_{shot}. Parallel imaging reconstruction (Section 13.3) and partial Fourier reconstruction (Section 13.4), however, both increase computational complexity, so the temporal resolution improvement is only useful if the reconstruction engine can keep pace.

Real-time acquisitions are also characterized by their *frame rate*, which is the number of images reconstructed and displayed per second, also measured in frames per second or hertz. Sometimes the frame rate is called the *apparent*, or *effective*, temporal resolution. The frame rate can be greater than the true temporal resolution if a *partial k-space updating* technique (e.g., keyhole, see Section 11.3, or sliding window reconstruction, see Section 13.6) is used. The number of phase-encoded views that are updated for each reconstructed frame is called the *glimpse* size.

Example 11.3   Consider a 2D gradient-echo real-time acquisition with 1 signal average, 128 phase-encoding steps, and TR = 10 ms. (a) What is the true temporal resolution? (b) If the glimpse size is 64, what is the apparent temporal resolution? Assume that the reconstruction and display hardware can keep pace, so they are not the limiting factor.

Answer

(a) From Eq. (11.32), the true temporal resolution is:

$$R = \frac{1}{(128)(10 \times 10^{-3} \text{ s})(1.0)} = 0.78 \text{ fps}$$

(b) If an image is reconstructed after every 64 views are acquired, the apparent temporal resolution is twice as great, or 1.56 fps.

Frame rates in the 1–10 fps range are commonly achieved with real-time MRI. It continues to strive for the 30-fps frame rate that is typical in x-ray fluoroscopy, which can depict the beating heart without motion artifacts. Real-time MR with higher frame rates is sometimes called MR *fluoroscopy*, in analogy to x-ray fluoroscopy. Although the name *real-time* seems to imply a very rapid frame rate (e.g., 10 fps or higher), slower acquisitions can be classified as such provided they meet all three criteria listed earlier. An example is the MRI-guided breast biopsy shown in Figure 11.14. Despite the very slow frame rate (~0.02 fps), the spin echo series can be considered real-time because the images served as an interactive guide for needle placement.

Lag or *latency* also characterizes a real-time system. Latency is defined as the time interval between when an event occurs and when an operator viewing the real-time images can first detect it. If the latency is too long (e.g., ~0.5 s or longer), the operator often makes a second parameter adjustment before the first one has worked its way through the system. This unwanted effect is familiar to anyone who has ever tried to adjust the temperature of the water while taking a shower.

The total latency has several contributions, which are schematically depicted in the time line shown in Figure 11.15. If the event is an operator-initiated command to change a parameter (e.g., to increase the FOV), then the command takes some finite amount of time L_P to be recognized and played by the pulse-sequence hardware that controls the gradients and RF.

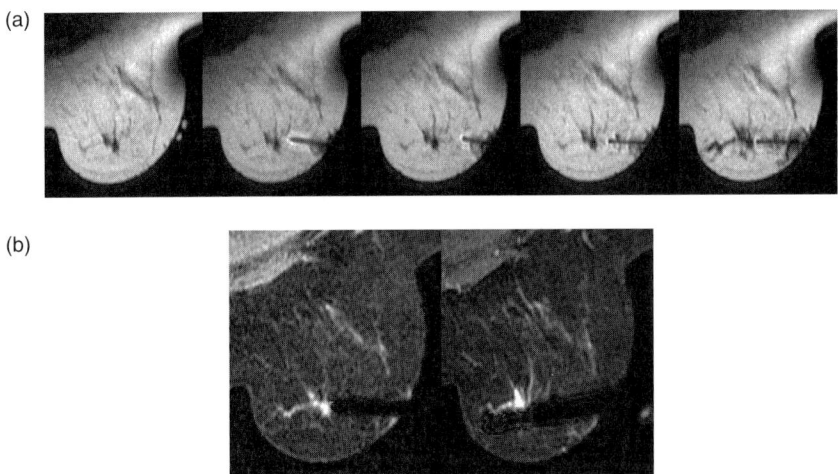

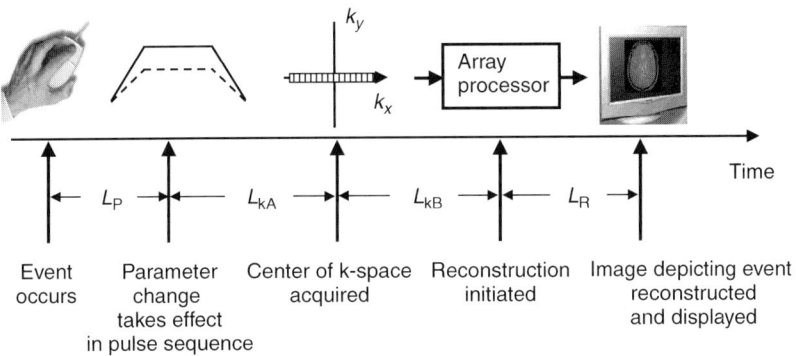

FIGURE 11.14 Breast biopsy needle placement under MRI guidance. (a) An initial sequence of RF spin echo images used to place the needle. (b) Three-point Dixon water-specific images (Section 17.3) that confirm the contrast-enhancing lesion was indeed what was being biopsied. The 14-gauge core biopsy revealed infiltrating adenocarcinoma. (Courtesy of Bruce Daniel, M.D., Karl Vigen, Ph.D., Claudia Cooper, Kim Butts, Ph.D., and the Stanford Interventional MRI team.)

FIGURE 11.15 Time line depicting various contributions to the latency of a real-time MRI acquisition. In this example, the event is a pulse-sequence parameter change initiated by an operator's mouse click. If, instead, the event is initiated within the magnet bore (e.g., patient motion), then the parameter latency L_P should be set equal to 0.

Usually the parameter latency L_P is simply the time interval between the event and the next time that the affected gradient lobe(s) or RF pulse(s) are played. An exception occurs if *waveform buffering* is used. To keep pace with waveform updates (such as incrementing the phase-encoding gradient's amplitude), some MRI systems with limited computational power store ahead, or buffer, two or three copies of gradient and RF waveforms into memory. (Streaming audio broadcast over the World Wide Web similarly uses buffering to prevent interruptions during periods of heavy network traffic.) On MR systems that buffer waveforms, the parameter latency L_P can be increased by several seconds. Also note that if the event is not a parameter change but rather is initiated from within the bore of the magnet (e.g., a change in patient position or an advancing biopsy needle), then L_P does not contribute at all to total latency for that acquisition.

The k-space order also affects the total latency (Busse et al. 1999). The gross features of an image are determined by the central k-space data. In phase-encoded Fourier imaging, the gross image features are controlled by the roughly 10% of the central k-space lines acquired with phase-encoding amplitude closest to zero. The k-space latency has two contributions to this type of acquisition: the waiting period L_{kA} until the center of k-space is acquired again and the interval L_{kB} between that acquisition of the center of k-space and the initiation of the reconstruction. The value of the first component L_{kA} depends on when the event occurs, so it is a randomly distributed variable. The second component L_{kB}, however, is determined solely by the view order. For example, a real-time image acquired with a reverse-centric view order (i.e., the center of k-space acquired last; see Section 11.5 and Figure 11.25 later in this chapter) will have a smaller value of L_{kB} than one acquired with a centric or sequential view order. Note that L_{kA} is zero if the event fortuitously occurs during the acquisition of the center of k-space, giving the minimal possible k-space latency (equal to L_{kB}). Any of these relationships between view order and latency can be modified if a sliding window reconstruction (Section 13.6) is used because in that case a reconstruction process can be initiated at any time during the acquisition.

The amount of time L_R that it takes to reconstruct and display an image is the last contribution to the total latency of the real-time acquisition. Depending on the computer architecture, L_R also might include data transfer times if the functions are performed by dedicated hardware components, for example, if the reconstruction is on an array processor. Although faster reconstruction engines and data buses are continually becoming available, the advent of larger imaging matrices (512 and 1024), parallel imaging techniques, and increased number of receiver channels (e.g., 8 or 16) all place heavy demands on the reconstruction processors. Consequently we should not assume that L_R is necessarily negligible, even with modern hardware. To summarize, the total latency L_T of a real-time acquisition is the sum of the terms:

$$L_T = L_P + L_{kA} + L_{kB} + L_R. \tag{11.33}$$

Although the central k-space views predominantly determine the gross structure and contrast, all of the acquired phase-encoded views contribute to the image. Because they are acquired at different times, *dispersion* artifacts can result, especially when imaging moving structures. If the real-time display of a uniformly moving (or changing) object appears to move (or change) uniformly, the acquisition is said to be *consistent*. Specific view orders can be designed that minimize dispersion and maximize consistency (Busse et al. 1999).

Even when partial k-space updating is used, the center of k-space typically is acquired exactly once per reconstructed frame. More frequent acquisition of the center of k-space is wasteful because important information is acquired but never displayed; less frequent acquisition of the center of k-space unnecessarily increases the latency.

11.4.2 ACQUISITION AND RECONSTRUCTION STRATEGIES

Almost any MR pulse sequence can be used for real-time acquisition, although the temporal resolution can vary widely. This subsection describes several that are more commonly used.

2D Gradient Echo   Its simplicity, robustness, and speed make 2D gradient echo (Section 14.1) a popular pulse sequence for real-time acquisitions. Because TR values in the range of 2–5 ms are readily obtainable with modern gradient hardware, temporal resolution of 5 fps or more can be achieved with 2D gradient echo, even with full k-space acquisition (i.e., NEX = 1). Another advantage of a 2D gradient-recalled echo is that the Cartesian k-space raster simplifies reconstruction because no gridding (Section 13.2) or sophisticated phase correction (Section 16.1) is required.

Real-time 2D gradient echo images are usually obtained with spoiled gradient echo acquisitions (Section 14.1), yielding moderately T_1-weighted contrast. 2D gradient echo real-time images with other contrast mechanisms have also been demonstrated. Steady-state free precession (SSFP) pulse sequences such as true FISP (also described in Section 14.1) set up a steady state not only for the longitudinal but also for the transverse magnetization. This class of pulse sequences has the advantage of producing a more intense signal and the option of obtaining a bright fluid signal. One issue is that the steady state can take longer to establish than in the spoiled pulse sequences, which can be problematic for some dynamic imaging. True FISP has generally proved to be robust for cardiac imaging, however (Lee et al. 2002;

Schaeffter et al. 2001). RF power deposition is another issue at field strengths of 1.5 T and higher. Because true FISP acquisitions are ideally acquired with the minimum TR, sometimes SAR restrictions require the flip angle to be reduced below the range of 70–90° that typically maximizes fluid signal.

HASTE   In some applications gradient echo acquisitions are suboptimal because contrast weighting obtained only with RF spin echoes is desired, susceptibility artifacts cannot be tolerated, or both. For standard RF spin echo, however, the temporal resolution given by Eq. (11.32) is too slow for the majority of real-time applications, so echo train methods are used instead. In order to increase the frame rate to the range of 1–2 fps, half-Fourier acquired single turbo spin echo (HASTE, also known as single-shot fast spin echo with half-Fourier acquisition; see Section 16.4) can be used.

The string of refocusing pulses required for HASTE carries considerable RF energy, especially at field strengths of 1.5 T or higher. Even in non-real-time HASTE applications, the flip angle of the refocusing pulses is usually reduced from 180° to a value in the range of 120–160°. To further minimize patient heating, several additional strategies can be employed in real-time applications. These include varying the flip angle of the refocusing pulses as a function of position in the echo train and only acquiring an updated image when the operator makes a parameter change (Busse et al. 2000).

Other k-*Space Trajectories*   Fast imaging methods such as EPI, (Section 16.1), spirals (Section 17.6), and radial projection acquisition (Section 17.5) all can be used for real-time acquisitions. As described in each of their sections, these methods require additional reconstruction processing (e.g., row-flipping and phase correction for EPI and gridding for spirals). With single-shot EPI, k-space can be completely traversed in 50 ms or less, allowing a frame rate of 20 fps or more, provided the reconstruction is not the limiting factor. The SNR, however, of these acquisitions is generally low due to the high receiver bandwidth. Also its long readout train makes single-shot EPI very prone to geometrical distortion from susceptibility variation and imperfect shim. The use of multishot EPI can reduce these drawbacks, with a corresponding reduction in the true temporal resolution by the number of shots. (Also, parallel imaging can help alleviate geometrical distortion in single-shot EPI.) Multishot spirals and the related trajectory of circular EPI have been used for real-time coronary imaging (Nayak et al. 2001). True temporal resolution in the range of 5–10 fps is achieved with spatial resolution in the range of 1 mm, which is sufficient to visualize the coronary arteries.

Radial projection acquisition is becoming a more popular real-time acquisition method (Schaeffter et al. 2001; Shankaranarayanan et al. 2001).

As described in Section 17.5, radial acquisitions can be accelerated with the use of angular undersampling. The less dense the angular sampling, the closer streak artifacts appear to the source that generates them. With moderate angular undersampling, the streak artifacts are usually tolerable and true temporal resolution in the range of 10–20 fps is readily obtainable. The method is compatible with a variety of gradient-echo contrast types, including true FISP contrast, and has been applied to real-time cardiac imaging.

Parallel-Imaging Reconstruction   Parallel-imaging methods that reduce the number of phase-encoding steps can be used to increase the true temporal resolution. In standard, non-real-time applications, SENSE (Section 13.3) is one of the most widely used parallel-imaging techniques. Its use for real-time imaging is more challenging because the reconstruction time is prolonged, because of not only the high number of receiver channels (e.g., 16) but also the complexity of the SENSE reconstruction itself. Thus, the available temporal resolution can be limited by the reconstruction. Unaliasing by Fourier encoding the overlaps using the temporal dimension (UNFOLD) (Section 13.3) is a parallel-imaging technique that is specifically designed to operate on time-series of images and does not require multiple receiver channels. A low-latency real-time system using UNFOLD is described in (Kellman et al. 2000).

M-Mode Imaging   In motion-mode (M-mode) ultrasound, the vertical axis of the gray-scale display is a spatial dimension and the horizontal axis represents time. Because only one spatial dimension is acquired, very high temporal resolution (on the order of 1 kHz) can be obtained. Real-time MRI has an analogous M-mode acquisition (Hardy et al. 1993). The MR M-mode imaging acquisition usually employs a two-dimensional RF spiral excitation pulse (Section 5.1) that excites a pencil-beam-shaped volume. A gradient-echo readout then provides spatial encoding along the long axis of the beam. No phase encoding is applied, so the resulting image is a line scan that has only one spatial dimension. Because $N_{shot} = 1$ and TR is short (10 ms or less), Eq. (11.32) implies that very high true temporal resolution can be achieved, even with signal averaging. The resulting image lines are displayed analogously to M-mode ultrasound.

11.4.3 EXAMPLE APPLICATIONS OF REAL-TIME MRI

This subsection outlines two examples of widely used applications of real-time imaging. Many other applications have been described in review articles such as Riederer (1997). A detailed description of these methods is beyond the scope of this book. In particular, interventional MR (Schwartz et al. 1999; Debatin and Adams 1998), real-time navigator echoes (Section 12.2) for f MRI studies (Ward et al. 2000), and real-time tracking of kinematic imaging of joint motion (Shellock et al. 1993) are very active areas.

Interactive Scan Plan Prescription   Real-time MRI allows interactive control of imaging parameters including the scan plane. The details of the control mechanisms depend on the specific interface, but the operator always has some ability to interactively adjust the oblique angle as well as the FOV and slice offsets. The operator might also have the ability to jump at any time to the standard axial, coronal, and sagittal planes or to other previously bookmarked planes. New scan planes can be conveniently defined by depositing points, for example, the three-point prescription described in Section 7.3.

Interactive scan plane control has applications to a variety of imaging situations. Because the orientation of the heart is quite patient-dependent, cardiac imaging has been a natural application. Fetal imaging (Figure 11.16) is another application well suited to use of real-time imaging because the coordinate system that produces the anatomical axial, sagittal, and coronal planes varies as the fetus moves. Moreover, if the fetus moves frequently, a series-based scan plane selection is impractical.

How widely real-time interactive scan plane control will eventually supplant series-based scan plane selection remains to be seen. Although it is less efficient, series-based scan plane selection is nearly operator-independent, which can be both an advantage and disadvantage.

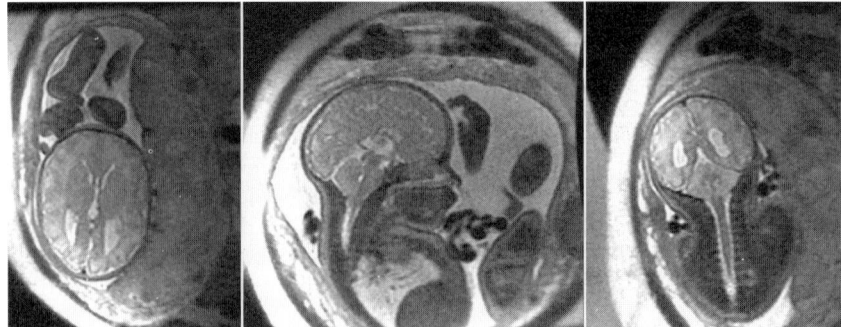

FIGURE 11.16 Single-shot fast spin-echo images of a fetus shown in three planes. The fetus has agenesis of the corpus callosum (seen in the axial and sagittal planes) and nodular irregularities of the lateral ventricles (seen in the coronal plane), consistent with heterotopia. A three-point graphic prescription was used to obtain the three standard imaging planes in the reference frame of the fetus. (Courtesy of Reed Busse, Ph.D., GE Healthcare, and Orit Glenn, M.D., University of California San Francisco.)

Fluoroscopically Triggered MR Angiography   Fluoroscopically trigger-ing contrast-enhanced 3D MR angiography is another commonly used applica-tion of real-time imaging. In this method, a series of real-time 2D gradient echo images of the artery of interest are acquired. A bolus of contrast agent is injected (e.g., 20 mL of a gadolinium chelate). When the arrival of the bolus is detected by increased signal intensity in the artery, the operator issues a single command that stops the 2D acquisition and starts a 3D acquisition. Usually the elliptical centric view order (Section 11.6) is used because this will provide a high degree of venous suppression (Wilman et al. 1998). Minimizing the latency of the real-time acquisition is important, especially for imaging the carotid arteries, where the jugular veins can enhance in as little as 5 s after the carotids enhance.

The 2D real-time acquisition can be performed with a thin slice to image the arteries of interest in cross section. If an axial slice is used (e.g., to monitor the bolus arrival in the carotid arteries), spatial saturation pulses (Section 5.3) should be applied both superior and inferior to the slice in order to min-imize spurious arterial and venous signals before the arrival of the bolus. Alternatively, the thin slice can be replaced by a thick slice that covers the entire anatomy, typically in the coronal plane. In this case, a twister gradient (Section 10.6) is used as a high-pass spatial filter to accentuate the vessel. Figure 11.17 shows examples of both types of 2D real-time acquisitions and the resulting 3D MR angiogram.

(a)   (b)

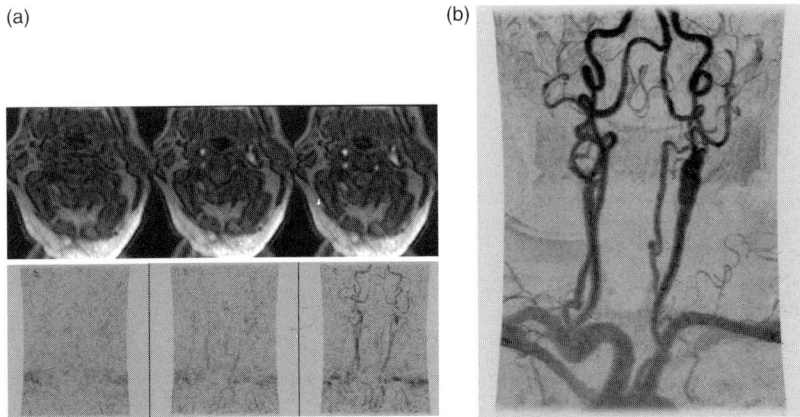

FIGURE 11.17 Fluoscopically triggered MR angiography of the carotids. (a) The arrival of the contrast bolus is tracked either with a real-time set of axial images (top row) or a coronal projection with a twister gradient (bottom row). When the bolus is detected, the 2D real-time acquisition terminates and a 3D elliptical centric acquisition immediately begins. (b) A coronal maximum intensity projection from the resulting 3D acquisition. Because of the accurate fluoroscopic timing of the bolus, there is little venous contamination, even though the 3D acquisition time was 50 s. (Courtesy of John Huston, III, M.D., Mayo Clinic College of Medicine.)

Fluoroscopic triggering replaces the method of test bolus timing. In test bolus timing, a small test dose (e.g., 2 mL of a gadolinium chelate) is injected simultaneously with the start of a series of time-stamped 2D images. The 2D images are retrospectively examined, and the circulation time of the contrast agent is determined. Then the main bolus is injected, and the 3D acquisition is started after waiting the measured circulation time. Fluoroscopic triggering has the advantage over test bolus timing that only one injection is required, so the overall exam time is reduced. Also, the 2- mL test dose sometimes can cause an unwanted increase in background signal (e.g., in the bladder). On the other hand, test bolus timing has the advantage over fluoroscopic triggering in that the time interval between arterial and venous enhancement can be considered when the optimal circulation time is selected.

SELECTED REFERENCES

Busse, R. F., Kruger, D. G., Debbins, J. P., Fain, S. B., and Riederer, S. J. 1999. A flexible view ordering technique for high-quality real-time 2DFT MR fluoroscopy. *Magn. Reson. Med.* 42: 69–81.

Busse, R. F., Riederer, S. J., Fletcher, J. G., Bharucha, A. E., and Brandt, K. R. 2000. Interactive fast-spin echo imaging. *Magn. Reson. Med.* 44: 339–348.

Debatin, J. F., and Adam, G., eds. 1998. *Interventional magnetic resonance imaging.* Heidelburg: Springer-Verlag.

Gmitro, A. F., Ehsani, A. R., Berchem, T. A., and Snell, R. J. 1996. A real-time reconstruction system for magnetic resonance imaging. *Magn. Reson. Med.* 35: 734–740.

Hardy, C. J., Darrow, R. D., Nieters, E. J., Roemer, P. B., Watkins, R. D., Adams, W. J., Hattes, N. R., and Maier, J. K. 1993. Real-time acquisition, display, and interactive graphic control of NMR cardiac profiles and images. *Magn. Reson. Med.* 29: 667–673.

Kellman, P., Sorger, J. M., Epstein, F. H., and McVeigh, E. R. 2000. Low latency temporal filter design for real-time MRI using UNFOLD. *Magn. Reson. Med.* 44: 933–939.

Kerr, A. B., Pauly, J. M., Hu, B. S., Li, K. C., Hardy, C. J., Meyer, C. H., Macovski, A., and Nishimura, D. G. 1997. Real-time interactive MRI on a conventional scanner. *Magn. Reson. Med.* 38: 355–367.

Lee, V. S., Resnick, D., Bundy, J. M., Simonetti, O. P., Lee, P., and Weinreb, J. C. 2002. Cardiac function: MR evaluation in one breath hold with real-time true fast imaging with steady-state precession. *Radiology* 222: 835–842.

Nayak, K. S., Pauly, J. M., Yang, P. C., Hu, B. S., Meyer, C. H., and Nishimura, D. G. 2001. Real-time interactive coronary MRA. *Magn. Reson. Med.* 46: 430–435.

Riederer, S. J. 1997. Real-time MR imaging. In *The RSNA categorical course in physics: The basic physics of MR imaging.* Reiderer, S. J., and Wood, M. L., Eds., Oak Brook, IL: RSNA Publications. pp. 175–186.

Schaeffter, T., Weiss, S., Eggers, H., and Rasche, V. 2001. Projection reconstruction balanced fast field echo for interactive real-time cardiac imaging. *Magn. Reson. Med.* 46: 1238–1241.

Schwartz, R. B., Hsu, L., Wong, T. Z., Kacher, D. F., Zamani, A. A., Black, P. M., Alexander, E., III, Stieg, P. E., Moriarty, T. M., Martin, C. A., Kikinis, R., and Jolesz, F. A. 1999. Intraoperative MR imaging guidance for intracranial neurosurgery: Experience with the first 200 cases. *Radiology*.211: 477–488.

Shankaranarayanan, A., Simonetti, O. P., Laub, G., Lewin, J. S., and Duerk, J. L. 2001. Segmented k-space and real-time cardiac cine MR imaging with radial trajectories. *Radiology* 221: 827–836.

Shellock, F. G., Mink, J. H., Deutsch, A. L., Foo, T. K., and Sullenberger, P. 1993. Patellofemoral joint: Identification of abnormalities with active-movement, "unloaded" versus "loaded" kinematic MR imaging techniques. *Radiology* 188: 575–578.

Ward, H. A., Riederer, S. J., Grimm, R. C., Ehman, R. L., Felmlee, J. P., and Jack, C. R., Jr. 2000. Prospective multiaxial motion correction for fMRI. *Magn. Reson. Med.* 43: 459–469.

Wilman, A. H., Riederer, S. J., Huston, J., III, Wald, J. T., and Debbins, J. P. 1998. Arterial phase carotid and vertebral artery imaging in 3D contrast-enhanced MR angiography by combining fluoroscopic triggering with an elliptical centric acquisition order. *Magn. Reson. Med.* 40: 24–35.

RELATED SECTIONS

11.5 Two-Dimensional Acquisition

MRI is a very versatile imaging modality, capable of acquiring images in one, two, or three spatial dimensions. Despite its historical importance, 1D MR imaging (also known as *line scan*) is rarely used today except for a few applications such as signal tracking (Foo et al. 1997) and line-scan diffusion imaging (Maier et al. 1998). The vast majority of present MR applications employ 2D and 3D acquisitions (Section 11.6).

2D imaging, also known as planar or slice imaging, involves two main steps: slice selection and spatial encoding within the selected slice. Slice selection is typically accomplished by a gradient played concurrently with a selective RF pulse, as detailed in Section 8.3. Occasionally, slice selection is also accomplished by spatially saturating or canceling signals outside the slice of interest (Johnson et al. 1989). The former approach can be used for single- or multislice imaging, whereas the latter method is limited to a single slice, unless TR is much longer than T_1 to allow the longitudinal magnetization to substantially recover to its equilibrium value. For example, in order for inverted magnetization to recover to 99% of its equilibrium value, TR must be $\sim 5 \times T_1$. For saturated magnetization, the required TR is reduced to $\sim 4 \times T_1$ for the same level of recovery. Following slice selection, any of several 2D spatial-encoding strategies (e.g., RF spin echo, gradient echo, EPI, projection acquisition, or spiral) can be used to sample k-space. A 2D image is then produced with an inverse 2D Fourier transform, gridding, or filtered back-projection of the k-space data, as described in Chapter 13 and Herman (1980).

11.5.1 SEQUENTIAL VERSUS INTERLEAVED ACQUISITION

To cover an imaging volume with a 2D acquisition, multiple sections or slices must be acquired. The spatial information for each slice location is individually encoded into its own k-space data matrix. Multislice 2D imaging can be performed one slice at a time by acquiring all required k-space *lines* (also called k-space *views*) for a given slice before moving to the next slice. This approach is often referred to as *sequential acquisition* (Figure 11.18a). If signal averaging is desired, it is typically performed before moving on to the next k-space line. Therefore, the looping order for sequential acquisition from innermost to outermost is (1) signal averaging, (2) k-space lines, and (3) slice location, as shown in Figure 11.18a.

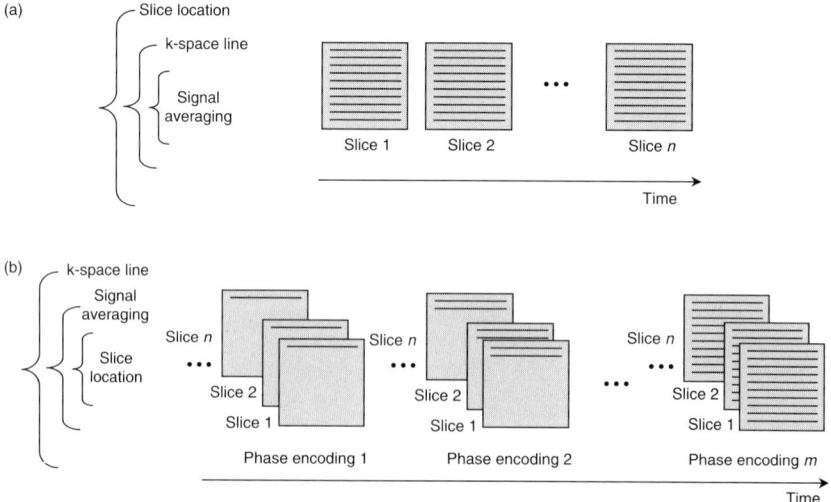

FIGURE 11.18 (a) Sequential acquisition and (b) interleaved acquisition in 2D imaging. Each box represents a slice, and each line within the box denotes a k-space line (also called a k-space view; each k-space line includes signal averaging, if any). The time axes in (a) and (b) are not to the same scale. The looping orders for each of these acquisitions are summarized on the left.

Alternatively, the acquisition can be performed by obtaining a specific k-space line for multiple slice locations and then repeating the acquisition for the next k-space line during the next TR interval. This is known as an *interleaved acquisition* (Figure 11.18b). As in sequential acquisitions, signal averaging (if desired) is usually performed before moving to the next k-space line. Its looping order is shown on Figure 11.18b.

In sequential acquisition, the magnetization within a slice is repeatedly excited once every TR. When TR is longer than the actual length of the pulse sequence waveforms (T_{seq}), the scanner becomes inactive for a period of ($TR - T_{seq}$), which is often called *idle time* (or *dead time*) (Figure 11.19). If we define data acquisition efficiency as the scanner-active time divided by the total scan time, then the longer TR is relative to T_{seq}, the smaller the efficiency becomes for sequential acquisition (see Example 11.4). If, however, TR is approximately equal to T_{seq}, the idle time diminishes and high data acquisition efficiency can be achieved. Therefore, in practice, sequential acquisition is used only when $TR \simeq T_{seq}$.

Example 11.4 A gradient-echo pulse sequence with a sequence length of $T_{seq} = 5$ ms is employed to acquire a total of 28 slice locations from the abdomen. The acquisition matrix is 256^2 for each slice. (a) If sequential acquisition is used with a TR of 150 ms and number of signal averages NEX $= 1$, what is the idle time as a percentage of the total acquisition time and what is the data acquisition efficiency? (b) Repeat the calculation for $TR = 6$ ms.

Answer

(a) The acquisition of each slice takes 256 sequences to complete. Thus, the total acquisition time is $256 \times 28 \times TR = 7168 \times TR$. As can be seen from Figure 11.19, the idle time is:

$$256 \times 28 \times (TR - 5\,ms) = 7168 \times (TR - 5\,ms)$$

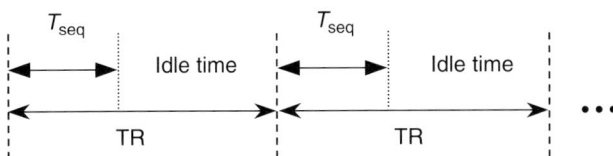

FIGURE 11.19 Relationship among sequence length (T_{seq}), TR, and idle time in sequential acquisition. Only two TR periods are shown in the figure.

If TR $= 150$ ms, the total data acquisition time and the idle time are:

$$T_{scan} = 7168 \times 150\,ms = 1075.2\,s = 17.92\,min$$
$$T_{idle} = 7168 \times (150 - 5)\,ms = 1039.4\,s = 17.32\,min$$
$$= 96.7\%\,of\,T_{scan}$$

Accordingly, the data acquisition efficiency is $1 - 96.7\% = 3.3\%$. Thus, the high percentage of the idle time prolongs the acquisition time ($\sim$18 min.), resulting in a low acquisition efficiency.

(b) When TR is reduced to 6 ms:

$$T_{scan} = 7168 \times 6\,ms = 43.0\,s$$

$$T_{idle} = 7168 \times 1\,ms = 7.2\,s$$

Or $T_{idle} = 16.7\%$ of T_{scan}, improving the data acquisition efficiency to 83.3%.

Unless a single-shot pulse sequence is used (e.g., single-shot EPI, Section 16.1), a very short TR is needed to achieve high data-acquisition efficiency with sequential acquisitions, as illustrated in Example 11.4. Sequential acquisition is most commonly used with gradient-echo pulse sequences, in which the desired image contrast can be obtained when TR $\simeq T_{seq}$. In sequential acquisition, all k-space data for a given slice are acquired within a time given by TR $\times N_{phase} \times$ NEX, where N_{phase} is the number of phase-encoding gradient steps, and NEX is the number of signal averages. (Note that we have assumed each pulse sequence accomplishes only one phase-encoding step as in conventional spin-echo or gradient-echo sequences. For echo train pulse sequences, the time is reduced to TR $\times N_{phase} \times$ NEX/N_{etl}, where N_{etl} is the echo train length.) Sequential 2D acquisitions are preferred for some applications such as 2D time-of-flight angiography (Section 15.3). Sequential acquisition also can suppress motion artifacts if the motion is slow relative to the imaging time for a slice (i.e., TR $\times N_{phase} \times$ NEX).

In many pulse sequences, a TR time considerably longer than T_{seq} must be used to achieve the desired image contrast and signal-to-noise ratio. For example, TR in RF spin-echo pulse sequences typically ranges from 400 to 600 ms for good T_1 contrast in human tissues. In comparison, the minimum sequence length T_{seq} of a single-echo RF spin-echo sequence is only approximately 15–30 ms. Under these circumstances, sequential acquisition is prohibitively slow and interleaved acquisition becomes the method of choice.

In interleaved acquisition mode, data from multiple slice locations can be acquired within each TR (Crooks et al. 1983). Each sequence produces a k-space line (or lines) at a *different* slice location (Figure 11.18b). In other word, the 'idle time' of a sequential acquisition is now used to acquire k-space data at other slice locations. As described in Section 7.3, the slice locations and orientations can be flexible—the slice planes need not be evenly spaced or parallel. The maximum number of slices $N_{\text{slice,acq}}$ that can be acquired within a TR can be obtained from:

$$N_{\text{slice,acq}} = \text{int}\left(\frac{TR}{T_{\text{seq}}}\right) \qquad (11.34)$$

where int stands for 'the integer part' of its argument. If the number of the prescribed slices N_{slice} is less than or equal to $N_{\text{slice,acq}}$, all the prescribed slices can be acquired within the scan time given by:

$$T_{\text{scan}} = TR \times N_{\text{phase}} \times \text{NEX} \qquad (11.35)$$

(Note that we have assumed that each sequence acquires one k-space line. Further acceleration can be achieved with echo train pulse sequences such as EPI and RARE.) If $N_{\text{slice}} > N_{\text{slice,acq}}$, additional time is required to collect data for the remaining slices. In this case, the total scan time becomes:

$$T_{\text{scan}} = TR \times N_{\text{phase}} \times \text{NEX} \times N_{\text{acq}} \qquad (11.36)$$

where N_{acq} is the total number of acquisitions required to obtain all of the prescribed slices. N_{acq} is also called the number of *passes* or *packs*.

Depending on the pulse sequence, the transmitting RF coil, the main magnetic field strength, and the patient weight, Eq. (11.34) is sometimes overridden by SAR limitations. If the SAR exceeds a regulatory limit for a desired value of $N_{\text{slice,acq}}$ given by Eq. (11.34), then the maximum number of slices per TR must be reduced or TR must be increased. Either solution increases the total scan time, provided that the total number of slices is held constant. Sometimes a slight increase in TR can actually reduce the total scan time because more slices can be incorporated into each pass and fewer passes are required to accommodate all the slices.

Example 11.5 A 2D gradient-echo pulse sequence is used to acquire 24 slices from the liver with the following parameters: TR $= 150\,$ms, TE $= 2.0\,$ms, NEX $= 1$, $N_{\text{phase}} = 160$, and $T_{\text{seq}} = 6\,$ms. (a) Assuming SAR is not the limiting factor, what is the total scan time for interleaved acquisition? (b) If SAR limits the maximum number of slices per acquisition to 13, what is the total scan time?

Answer

(a) According to Eq. (11.34):

$$N_{\text{slice,acq}} = \text{int}\left(\frac{\text{TR}}{T_{\text{seq}}}\right) = \text{int}\left(\frac{150}{6}\right) = 25$$

Because the prescribed number of slices is less than $N_{\text{slice,acq}}$, the total scan time can be calculated from Eq. (11.35):

$$T_{\text{scan}} = 150\,\text{ms} \times 160 \times 1 = 24\,\text{s}$$

With this scan time, sometimes all slices can be acquired within a single breath-hold of the patient.

(b) With the SAR limit, two acquisitions ($N_{\text{acq}} = 2$) are required to complete the prescribed 24 slices. Thus, the total scan time, calculated from Eq. (11.36), is 48 s.

11.5.2 CROSS-TALK AND SLICE ORDERING

As discussed in Part II of this book, no selective RF pulse used in practice provides a perfectly rectangular slice profile. When an RF pulse is applied to a desired slice location, the regions adjacent to the slice are inevitably affected (Figure 11.20). Magnetization in the neighboring regions (B and B′ in Figure 11.20) can be partially excited or even inverted. Unless a very long TR time (e.g., TR $\geq$ 4–5 $\times$ T_1) is used, the perturbed magnetization will not fully return to its equilibrium value. When those locations are imaged in subsequent acquisitions, decreased image intensity and altered contrast result, as shown in Figure 11.21a. This effect is called *slice cross-talk*, or simply *cross-talk*.

One way to reduce cross-talk is to place a spatial gap between adjacent slices. The gaps serve as a buffer against cross-talk and are not imaged during that acquisition (i.e., pass). Slice gaps in 2D imaging can be filled in with slices from a subsequent acquisition, but then, according to Eq. (11.36), the number of acquisitions N_{acq} is increased, prolonging the total scan time. With gaps present, the multiple sections become discontinuous along the slice-selection direction, causing poor image quality when the slices are reformatted to other viewing planes. (This problem is avoided in 3D acquisitions, discussed in Section 11.6.) When a SINC pulse is used for slice selection, cross-talk can be rather severe due to the suboptimal slice profile (Figure 11.21a). Gaps as much as 50% of the slice thickness are often needed to compensate for cross-talk (Figure 11.21b). With the use of SLR (Section 2.3) or other tailored

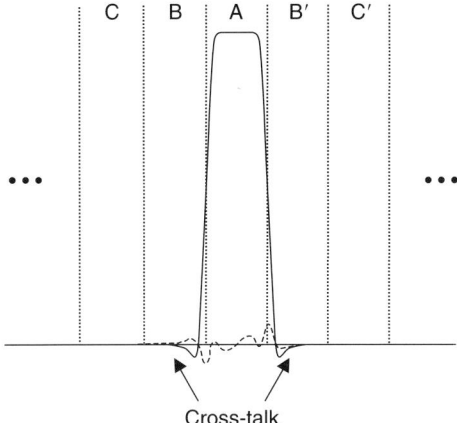

FIGURE 11.20 Cross-talk due to out-of-slice contamination in 2D imaging. When slice location A is imaged, magnetization of its two neighboring slices (B and B′) are also affected. This out-of-slice interference progressively decreases as the slices move away from slice A (e.g., C and C′). The slice profile at slice A is shown with a solid line and a dashed line denoting real and imaginary magnetization components, respectively.

pulses, however, the slice profile is considerably improved. A much smaller gap (e.g., 10% of the slice thickness) is usually adequate to produce images free from cross-talk (Figure 11.21c).

Another approach to reducing cross-talk is to modify the *slice acquisition order*. After acquiring k-space data for a given slice location using either sequential or interleaved acquisition, we can choose which slice to image next. If we choose an immediately adjacent slice (i.e., region B or B′ in Figure 11.20), the magnetization at this location is perturbed the most, resulting in severe cross-talk. If, however, we skip the immediately adjacent slice and start acquiring the next adjacent slice (i.e., region C or C′ in Figure 11.20), cross-talk can be substantially reduced because the out-of-slice excitation usually decays rapidly along the slice-selection direction. After acquiring every other slice (e.g., all slices indexed with odd numbers) in a stack of prescribed slices (Figure 11.22), the cross-talk effect in the remaining slices (e.g., all slices indexed with even numbers) can be substantially reduced by the T_1-relaxation process. At this point, we can return to the previously omitted slices (e.g., all slices indexed with even numbers, as shown in Figure 11.22) and acquire them to complete the scan. This technique is often referred to as *odd/even slice acquisition order* (also called *interleaved slice acquisition order*; this should not be confused with interleaved acquisition).

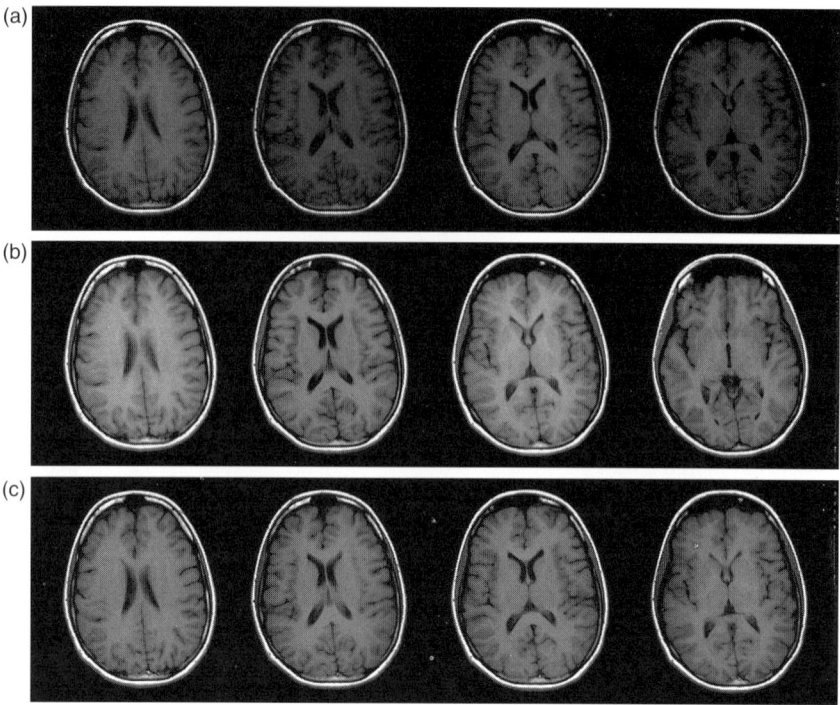

FIGURE 11.21 Three groups of four consecutive slices (5 mm each) acquired with a spin-echo pulse sequence (TR/TE = 400 ms/9 ms at 1.5 T) using (a) SINC pulses with 0.5-mm gaps, (b) SINC pulses with 2.5-mm gaps, and (c) SLR pulses with 0.5-mm gaps. (a) When SINC pulses with 0.5-mm gaps are used, cross-talk causes image-intensity loss and fluctuation as well as image-contrast degradation. (b) These image artifacts are reduced when the gaps are increased to 2.5 mm. (c) In comparison, SLR pulses produce virtually no cross-talk with 0.5-mm gaps. All images are displayed at the same window and level.

Odd/even slice acquisition order relies on both the rapid *spatial* decay of out-of-slice interference and efficient *temporal* recovery of the perturbed magnetization through T_1-relaxation. If the slices are acquired without skipping, then the perturbed magnetization outside the slice has a short time, on the order of T_{seq}, for T_1 relaxation. This is true for either sequential or interleaved acquisition (assuming TR is not limited by other factors such as SAR). With odd/even slice ordering, however, the magnetization recovery time is increased to:

$$\sim \frac{N_{slice} N_{phase} \text{NEX}}{2} \text{TR}$$

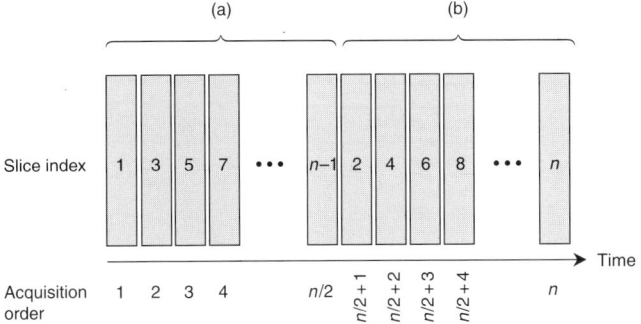

FIGURE 11.22 Relationship between slice index and data acquisition order in odd/even slice ordering. The slice index represents the sequential slice location in an imaging volume. Slices with odd numbers are acquired first (a), followed by slices with even numbers (b). In interleaved acquisition, if all slices cannot be accommodated in a single TR, they are divided into multiple groups to fit each group into a TR duration. Although the diagram assumes the total number of the slices is even, the same principle is also applicable to an odd number of slices.

in sequential acquisition and $\sim$ TR/2 in interleaved acquisition with $N_{\text{acq}} = 1$. For $N_{\text{acq}} > 1$, the recovery time can be considerably longer than TR/2.

Example 11.6 Ten image slices are acquired from a phantom using a gradient-echo sequence with the following parameters: NEX $= 1$, $N_{\text{phase}} = 128$, and $T_{\text{seq}} = 5$ ms. The RF pulse excites 20% of the longitudinal magnetization in regions immediately adjacent to the slice. The T_1 of the phantom material is 300 ms. (a) If sequential acquisition is used with TR $= 5$ ms, calculate the percentage of signal saturation with and without odd/even slice ordering. (b) Repeat the calculation for interleaved acquisition assuming all slices can be accommodated within a TR of 300 ms. (c) Tabulate the start of the acquisition time for each slice in interleaved acquisition with odd/even slice ordering.

Answer

(a) The longitudinal magnetization in the region immediately adjacent to the imaging slice is:

$$M_z(t) = M_0 - (M_0 - M_z(0)) \, e^{-t/T_1} \qquad (11.37)$$

where M_0 is the equilibrium magnetization and t is the recovery time. Using $M_z(0) = 0.8M_0$ gives:

$$M_z = M_0 \left(1 - 0.2e^{-t/T_1}\right) \qquad (11.38)$$

TABLE 11.1

Aquisition Start Times for the Slices in Example 11.6

Slice 1	Slice 2	Slice 3	Slice 4	Slice 5	Slice 6	Slice 7	Slice 8	Slice 9	Slice 10
0 TR	0.5 TR	0.1 TR	0.6 TR	0.2 TR	0.7 TR	0.3 TR	0.8 TR	0.4 TR	0.9 TR

Without odd/even slice ordering, the recovery time $t \simeq T_{seq} = 5$ ms. Using $T_1 = 300$ ms, Eq. (11.38) gives $M_z = 0.8 M_0$, indicating 20% of the signal is still saturated. With odd/even slice ordering, the recovery time becomes:

$$ t \simeq \frac{N_{slice} N_{phase} \text{NEX}}{2} \text{TR} = \frac{1}{2} \times 10 \times 128 \times 1 \times 5 \text{ ms} = 3.2 \text{ s} $$

Substituting $T_1 = 300$ ms and $t = 3.2$ s into Eq. (11.38), we obtain $M_z \simeq M_0$. Thus, the perturbed magnetization is fully recovered.

(b) Without odd/even slice ordering, the result for interleaved acquisition is the same as that for sequential acquisition. With odd/even slice ordering, the recovery time is $t \simeq \text{TR}/2 = 150$ ms. The corresponding longitudinal magnetization is $\sim 0.88 M_0$, which is improved from the case without odd/even slice ordering.

(c) The start of acquisition time for each slice is given in Table 11.1.

Although odd/even slice ordering is the most popular, methods that skip more than one slice can also be used. For example, two slices can be skipped within a single pass, resulting in an acquisition order of (1, 4, 7, 10, 2, 5, 8, 11, 3, 6, 9, 12) for a total of 12 slices.

In interleaved acquisitions with $N_{acq} > 1$, the slices imaged within each acquisition (or pass) can be grouped analogously to odd/even slice ordering. For example, when $N_{acq} = 2$, the first pass includes all odd slices and the second pass contains all even slices. Similarly, when $N_{acq} = 3$, the first, second and third passes may include slices with indices (1, 4, 7, 10, ...), (2, 5, 8, 11, ...), and (3, 6, 9, 12, ...), respectively. This allows more time for the magnetization perturbed by out-of-slice excitation to undergo longitudinal relaxation.

Within each acquisition, cross-talk can be further reduced by carefully distributing or *scrambling* the slice order. For example, suppose slice locations (1, 4, 7, 10, 13) are to be acquired in a pass. To reduce cross-talk, slice locations can be acquired in temporal order (1, 10, 4, 13, 7) or (1, 7, 13, 4, 10). The former is a variation of odd/even slice ordering, and the latter is very similar to the odd/even slice ordering described in Figure 11.22.

11.5.3 Acquisition with Cardiac Triggering

In cardiac-triggered 2D pulse sequences, either sequential or interleaved acquisition modes can be used. The data acquisition schemes, however, are somewhat different from those discussed in the previous subsection due to the need to synchronize each image to a specific cardiac phase. (Note that the term *cardiac phase* as used here is analogous to a phase of the moon and should not be confused with the phase of a complex signal.)

Sequential Acquisition with Cardiac Triggering   In sequential acquisition, an ECG signal (see Section 12.1) triggers a pulse sequence. The sequence excites a specific slice and acquires a specific k-space line or view for that slice. Identical pulse sequences (i.e., excitation of the same slice and acquisition of the same k-space line) are repeated until the next trigger signal is received (Figure 11.23). With the new trigger signal, a different k-space line is acquired, but the slice location remains the same. This process is repeated until all k-space lines are acquired for the slice location. Thus, for an image with N_{phase} k-space lines, a total of N_{phase} trigger signals are required to complete one slice. After the completion of the slice, acquisition will advance to the next slice and the same process continues until all slices are acquired, as illustrated by the looping structures in Figure 11.23.

The number of times that data from a specific image location are acquired between two consecutive cardiac triggers is sometimes called the *number of cardiac phases* N_{cp}. As depicted in Figure 11.23, a total of N_{cp} k-space data sets (denoted by the cardiac phase index in Figure 11.23) are acquired, each consisting of a group of k-space lines corresponding to approximately the same temporal point in the cardiac cycle. At each slice location, images reconstructed from the N_{cp} k-space data sets can be viewed as a CINE loop to reveal the dynamics during an averaged cardiac cycle. If there is arrhythmia, interpolation using temporal information from the ECG prior to image reconstruction can help to align all k-space lines of a data set to the same time point. This technique is referred to as *CINE imaging* (Waterton et al. 1985; Bohning et al. 1990).

In order to reduce the total imaging time of CINE, the acquisition can be *segmented*; that is, more than one k-space line can be acquired at each cardiac phase, as shown in Figure 11.23b (Atkinson and Edelman 1991; Hernandez et al. 1993). This shortens the total scan time at the expense of reduced temporal resolution and increased image blurring. Segmented cardiac acquisitions are sometimes called *FASTCARD* (Foo et al. 1995). The number of k-space lines acquired at each cardiac phase is called the *views per segment*. To increase the effective temporal resolution or shorten the scan time, view sharing (Section 13.6) is often employed in the reconstruction of segmented cardiac acquisitions.

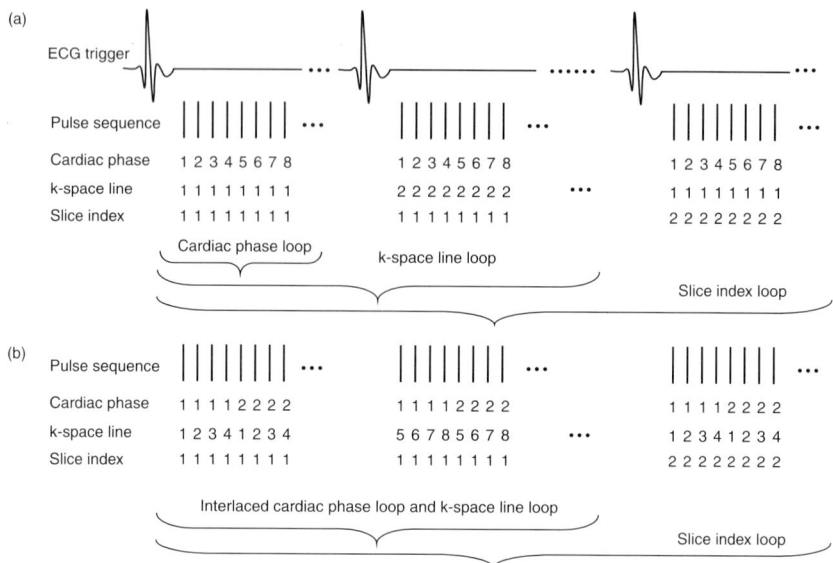

FIGURE 11.23 Sequential acquisition with cardiac trigging for (a) CINE and (b) segmented k-space. Four views per segment are used in (b). The looping structure is schematically shown at the bottom of each figure.

Example 11.7 A pulse sequence with $T_{seq} = 20$ ms is used to sequentially acquire 2D images with cardiac triggering. The R-R interval (T_{RR}) is 1 s, and triggering starts 40 ms (T_{delay}) after a QRS complex is detected. Assume that the heart rate is constant (i.e., no arrhythmia) and neglect the trigger window (discussed in Section 12.1). (a) What is the maximal number of cardiac phases and what is the maximal temporal resolution? (b) If the k-space data set consists of 128 lines, what is the CINE data acquisition time for a single slice and for eight slices? (c) If the acquisition is segmented with four views per segment, recalculate the data acquisition times in (b). (d) What is the temporal resolution in (c)?

Answer

(a) The maximal number of cardiac phases is:

$$N_{cp,max} = \frac{T_{RR} - T_{delay}}{T_{seq}} = \frac{1000 - 40}{20} = 48$$

The maximal temporal resolution is determined by T_{seq}, i.e., 20 ms.

(b) For a single slice, the total imaging time is $T_{scan} = 128 \times T_{RR} = 128\,\text{s}$. For eight slices in sequential acquisition, the total imaging time becomes $T_{scan} = 8 \times 128 \times T_{RR} = 1024\,\text{s}$.

(c) With four views per segment, the imaging times in (b) are both reduced by a factor of 4:

$$T_{scan} = 128 \times T_{RR}/4 = 32\,\text{s} \qquad \text{for single slice}$$

and

$$T_{scan} = 8 \times 128 \times T_{RR}/4 = 256\,\text{s} \qquad \text{for eight slices}$$

(d) With four views per segment, the true temporal resolution is reduced by a factor of 4 from that calculated in **(a)**:

$$20\,\text{ms} \times 4 = 80\,\text{ms}$$

In segmented k-space acquisition, pulse-sequence designers usually try to put the views corresponding to the center of k-space within the same segment. For example, if there are two views per segment and a total of eight views, the segments might be arranged as (2, 3), (4, 5), (6, 7), and (1, 8). Placing the center of k-space (views 4 and 5 in this case) within the same segment can reduce image artifacts if there is cardiac arrhythmia or bulk motion.

Interleaved Acquisition with Cardiac Triggering   Interleaved acquisitions are typically faster than sequential acquisitions because multiple slices can be acquired between triggers. Two interleaved acquisition schemes with cardiac triggering are illustrated in Figure 11.24. For CINE, several slices (two slices are shown in Figure 11.24a) are grouped together and acquired at each cardiac phase. The same group of slices is repeated for the subsequent cardiac phases after each trigger (Figure 11.24a). A new k-space line is acquired each time a trigger signal is received. As can be seen in Figure 11.24a, multislice interleaved acquisition is achieved at the expense of decreased temporal resolution (i.e., reduced N_{cp}). In addition, the slices in the group are acquired at different time points, although they are assigned to the same cardiac phase. Increasing the number of slices in the group exacerbates these problems. Thus, a small number of slices (e.g., 2–4) are typically included in the group. The remaining slices can be acquired in the next pass (as discussed later in this section). For segmented acquisitions, multislice interleaved acquisition can be accomplished analogously. For the acquisition scheme shown in Figure 11.24b, each slice in the group is again acquired at a different time point, although they are treated as the same cardiac phase. The total number of slices per pass is limited by the time available for imaging after each trigger, as well as by number of

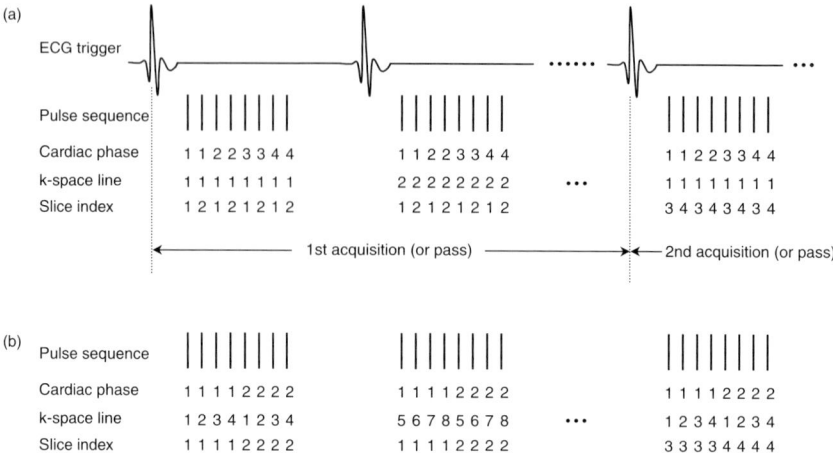

FIGURE 11.24 Interleaved acquisition schemes with cardiac trigging for (a) CINE and (b) segmented k-space. Four views per segment are used in (b). Two slices per pass are assumed, although more slices can be employed in some applications.

views per segment for each slice. For a large number of slices, multiple passes are required and the scan time is prolonged. To reduce the cross-talk, the same strategies as discussed previously can be employed.

Cross R-R Acquisition   For noncardiac applications such as neuroimaging, sometimes cardiac triggering is also required to reduce image artifacts from pulsatile flow but the specific time within the R-R does not matter. Moreover, for T_2-weighted imaging, the desired TR should be longer than a single R-R interval. Under these conditions, a method called *cross R-R cardiac trigger* can be used.

The first step in cross R-R triggering is to select the number of R-R intervals based on the desired TR and the patient's heart rate. For example, if the heart rate is 80 beats per minute (bpm), and a TR of 2000 ms is desired, then the best choice of TR is three R-R intervals. The actual TR is $3 \times (60/80) = 2.25$ s, which is the closest value to the desired TR. The second step is to distribute the slices within the R-R intervals. This is analogous to dealing cards in a game of poker. For example, if 11 slices are desired in the three R-R intervals, then view 1 for slices (1, 4, 7, 10) is played in the first R-R interval, view 1 for slices (2, 5, 8, 11) is played in the second, and view 1 for slices (3, 6, 9) is played in the third. The fourth to sixth R-R intervals contain view 2 for slices (1, 4, 7, 10), (2, 5, 8, 11), and (3, 6, 9), and so on. As described previously, the slices within any R-R interval can be scrambled to further reduce slice cross-talk; that is, within the first R-R interval we can play the slices in the order (1, 7, 10, 4).

11.5.4 K-Space View Order

In 2D imaging, there are many different ways to sample 2D k-space. Commonly used trajectories include a raster of parallel lines in Cartesian coordinates, and non-Cartesian rasters such as zigzag lines, spirals, and radial spokes, to name a few. The details of these trajectories can be found in the corresponding pulse sequence sections in Part V of this book. For each k-space pattern, there are multiple ways to arrange the order of the trajectories. This is often referred to as the *k-space order, view order*, or *phase order*. In the popular rectilinear k-space trajectory of a raster of parallel lines, there are three commonly used k-space orders: *sequential order* (from the maximum to minimum phase-encoding values, or vice versa; Figure 11.25a), *centric order* (from the center of the k-space alternatively propagating to the two edges; Figure 11.25b), and *reverse centric order* (from the two edges of k-space going in toward the center; Figure 11.25c). Some of the advantages and drawbacks

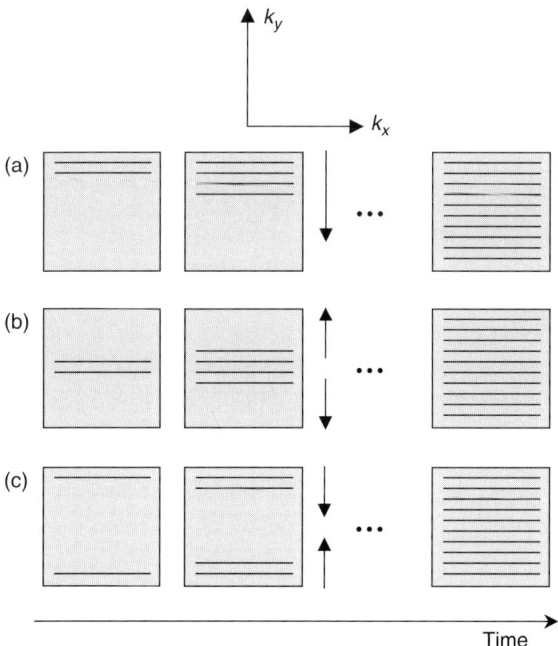

FIGURE 11.25 Three schemes to cover a 2D rectilinear k-space. (a) Top-to-bottom sequential. (b) Centric ordering (also known as center-out ordering). (c) Reverse centric ordering. Each box represents a 2D k-space raster. The arrows indicate the order of the k-space lines to be scanned as time progresses. k_x and k_y are the frequency and phase-encoding axes, respectively.

of these view orders are discussed further in Holsinger and Riederer (1990). Additional discussion of k-space ordering can also be found in Sections 12.3, 16.2, and 16.4.

Phase Cycling   Unless a single-shot pulse sequence is used, 2D imaging requires more than one RF excitation to sample k-space. Repeated RF excitations might also be needed to average the signals in order to increase the SNR. Although identical RF pulses can be used, it is often beneficial to alter the phase of the RF pulse in successive excitations. Changing the phase of the RF pulses within a sequence or between sequences is known as *phase cycling*, a technique that has been extensively used in NMR spectroscopy. A comprehensive discussion on phase cycling is beyond the scope of this book. Instead, we present here several simple examples to illustrate how phase cycling can be employed to eliminate image artifacts.

Phase of the RF Pulse and Its Notation   In the rotating reference frame, when an RF pulse with a flip angle θ is applied along the x axis, the phase of the RF pulse is defined as zero by convention and denoted by θ_x or $\theta(0°)$. Similarly, RF pulses along the $+y$, $-x$, and $-y$ axes have phase angles of 90°, 180°, and 270° and are denoted by θ_y, $\theta_{\bar{x}}$, and $\theta_{\bar{y}}$, respectively. RF excitation pulses with different phases produce transverse magnetization with different orientation in the rotating reference frame. The relationship between the phase of an excitation RF pulse and the direction of its resultant magnetization vector is summarized in Table 11.2.

Phase Cycling to Remove DC Artifacts   In 2D Fourier imaging with rectilinear sampling, any constant (i.e., DC) signal in the receiver can produce a bright spot in the center of the image (Figure 11.26a), which often interferes

TABLE 11.2

Radiofrequency Phase and the Direction of
Transverse Magnetization[a]

Phase of RF excitation pulse	x	y	$\bar{x}$	$\bar{y}$
Transverse magnetization		y	$\bar{x}$	$\bar{y}$	x

[a] In this table, we assume that the gyromagnetic ratio γ is positive. For spins with negative γ, the direction of the transverse magnetization in the table is reversed.

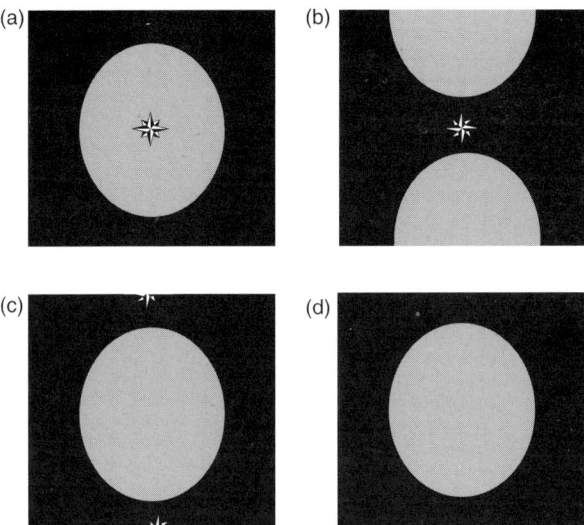

FIGURE 11.26 DC artifact removal by phase cycling. (a) A 2D image with a DC artifact (the star) in the center of the FOV. (b) With phase cycling, the image is shifted by one-half of the FOV along the phase-encoding direction (the vertical direction), but the DC artifact remains at the center. (c) After shifting the image by one-half of the FOV, the image is restored to its nominal position and the artifact is relocated to the edges. (d) The artifact is removed by discarding a few lines at the edges.

with image interpretation. The artifact can also appear as a central line or *zipper* parallel to the frequency-encoded direction when the spurious signal does not vary as a function of phase-encoded view but varies within each readout window. The spot or zipper artifacts can also be broadened slightly along the phase-encoding direction due to slight view-to-view modulations. Examples of signals that produce such artifacts are receiver baseline offsets and FID or stimulated echo signals that are not phase-encoded (Henkelman and Bronskill 1987). Proper phase cycling can push these artifacts to the edge of the FOV, where they can be cropped off by discarding a few lines at the image edge. For example, the phase of the RF excitation pulse can be alternated between x and $\bar{x}$ (or any other two opposite directions in the transverse plane) for adjacent phase-encoded k-space lines. This causes the 2D k-space signal to be modulated by an alternating positive and negative sign (see Table 11.2) along the phase-encoded direction, which is equivalent to a linear phase modulation $e^{-i\pi k_y}$ (where k_y is the phase-encoding index, 0, 1, 2, ...). According to the shift theorem for Fourier transforms (Section 1.1), the linear phase shifts the reconstructed image by one-half of the FOV, resulting in the image in Figure 11.26b. Because the DC offset does not experience the linear phase modulation, it remains at the center of the FOV, as shown in Figure 11.26b. If we shift the image in Figure 11.26b by one-half of the FOV, the image is restored to its nominal position and the DC offset is placed at the edges of the FOV (Figure 11.26c). Because the edge of the FOV typically does not contain important information, a few lines (e.g., 2–4) can be discarded. This produces an image free of DC artifacts (Figure 11.26d). Similarly, FID artifacts produced by incomplete crushing (Section 10.2) can be removed if the excitation pulse is phase cycled but the refocusing pulse is not.

If an even number of signal averages is employed in the data acquisition, the DC artifact can also be removed by using a different method, which is sometimes called RF *chopping*. For example, if NEX = 2, the phases of the RF excitation pulses for each signal average can be offset by 180° (e.g., x and $\bar{x}$), resulting in a positive and negative signal, each with a DC offset s_0:

$$s_x = s + s_0 \tag{11.39}$$

$$s_{\bar{x}} = -s + s_0 \tag{11.40}$$

Subtracting Eq. (11.40) from Eq. (11.39) eliminates the DC offset and yields a signal twice as strong. Thus, this phase-cycling technique removes the DC artifacts while providing the same SNR benefit as two RF excitations with the same phase. Note that this phase-cycling approach does not require any image lines to be cropped.

Phase Cycling within a Pulse Sequence   Phase cycling can also be applied to multiple RF pulses played out within a single pulse sequence. An example is a multi-spin-echo pulse sequence where the phases of the excitation and refocusing pulses are offset by 90° with respect to one another. This phase-cycling approach is denoted by:

$$(\theta_{\text{excitation},x}) - (\theta_{\text{refocus},y}) - (\theta_{\text{refocus},y}) \cdots (\theta_{\text{refocus},y})$$

and is known as a CPMG (Carr-Purcell-Meiboom–Gill) sequence (Meiboom and Purcell 1958). It compensates for imperfections in refocusing pulse flip angles and suppresses the corresponding image artifacts. Imperfections in refocusing pulses can also be compensated for with an alternative phase-cycling approach:

$$(\theta_{\text{excitation},x}) - (\theta_{\text{refocus},x}) - (\theta_{\text{refocus},\bar{x}}) - (\theta_{\text{refocus},x}) - (\theta_{\text{refocus},\bar{x}}) \cdots$$

which is known as a CP (Carr-Purcell) sequence (Carr and Purcell 1954).

Intrasequence phase cycling is often combined with intersequence phase cycling discussed previously to remove image artifacts arising from stimulated echoes. An example can be found in Zur and Stokar (1987).

SELECTED REFERENCES

Atkinson, D. J., and Edelman, R. R. 1991. Cineangiography of the heart in a single breath hold with a segmented turboflash sequence. *Radiology* 178: 357–360.

Bohning, D. E., Carter, B., Liu, S. S., and Pohost, G. M. 1990. PC-based system for retrospective cardiac and respiratory gating of NMR data. *Magn. Reson. Med.* 16: 303–316.

Carr, H. Y., and Purcell, E. M. 1954. Effects of diffusion on free precession in nuclear magnetic resonance experiments. *Phys. Rev.* 94: 630.

Crooks, L. E., Ortendahl, D. A., Kaufman, L., Hoenninger, J., Arakawa, M., Watts, J., Cannon, C. R., Brantzawadzki, M., Davis, P. L., and Margulis, A. R. 1983. Clinical efficiency of nuclear magnetic resonance imaging. *Radiology* 146: 123–128.

Foo, T. K. F., Bernstein, M. A., Aisen, A. M., Hernandez, R. J., Collick, B. D., and Bernstein, T. 1995. Improved ejection fraction and flow velocity estimates with use of view sharing and uniform repetition time excitation with fast cardiac techniques. *Radiology* 195: 471–478.

Foo, T. K. F., Saranathan, M., Prince, M. R., and Chenevert, T. L. 1997. Automated detection of bolus arrival and initiation of data acquisition in fast, three-dimensional, gadolinium-enhanced MR angiography. *Radiology* 203: 275–280.

Henkelman, R. M., and Bronskill, M. J. 1987. Artifacts in magnetic resonance imaging. *Rev. Magn. Reson. Med.* 2: 1–126.

Herman, G. T. 1980. *Image reconstruction from projections: The fundamentals of computerized tomography.* New York: Academic Press.

Hernandez, R. J., Aisen, A. M., Foo, T. K. F., and Beekman, R. H. 1993. Thoracic cardiovascular anomalies in children—evaluation with a fast gradient-recalled-echo sequence with cardiac-triggered segmented acquisition. *Radiology* 188: 775–780.

Holsinger, A. E., and Riederer, S. J. 1990. The importance of phase-encoding order in ultra-short TR snapshot MR imaging. *Magn. Reson. Med.* 16: 481–488.

Johnson, A. J., Garwood, M., and Ugurbil, K. 1989. Slice selection with gradient-modulated adiabatic excitation despite the presence of large B1-inhomogeneities. *J. Magn. Reson.* 81: 653–660.

Maier, S. E., Gudbjartsson, H., Patz, S., Hsu, L., Lovblad, K. O., Edelman, R. R., Warach, S., and Jolesz, F. A. 1998. Line scan diffusion imaging: Characterization in healthy subjects and stroke patients. *Am. J. Radiol.* 171: 85–93.

Meiboom, S., and Purcell, E. M. 1958. Modified spin-echo method for measuring nuclear relaxation times. *Rev. Sci. Instrum.* 29: 688–691.

Waterton, J. C., Jenkins, J. P. R., Zhu, X. P., Love, H. G., Isherwood, I., and Rowlands, D. J. 1985. Magnetic-resonance (MR) cine imaging of the human-heart. *Br J Radiol* 58: 711–716.

Zur, Y., and Stokar, S. 1987. A phase-cycling technique for canceling spurious echoes in NMR imaging. *J. Magn. Reson.* 71: 212–228.

RELATED SECTIONS

11.6 Three-Dimensional Acquisition

A 3D or 3D volume MR acquisition simultaneously excites an entire set of contiguous slices each TR interval. The set of slices is called a *chunk* or a *slab*, and an individual element within the slab is called a *partition, section*, or simply a *slice*. The most common acquisition strategy for 3D MR imaging is to use rectilinear sampling (den Boef et al. 1984). In that case, the 3D volume is spatially encoded with phase encoding along two perpendicular spatial directions and with frequency encoding along the third. The *secondary phase encoding* is also called *phase encoding 2*, or *slice encoding*, to distinguish it from the primary phase encoding (i.e., the in-plane phase-encoding). The resulting raw data fills a 3D k-space matrix, which is reconstructed by a 3D Fourier transform (Figure 11.27). Even though the slices in the 3D slab are acquired and reconstructed quite differently than 2D acquisitions, they both can be displayed as individual slices.

3D volume acquisition can also be accomplished using a variety of non-rectilinear sampling methods. One method is to apply phase encoding along the slice direction while sampling the in-plane direction with radial projections or spirals. This method is sometimes called a *stack* of projections or spirals. Alternatively, phase encoding can be abandoned completely by using a 3D-projection acquisition, in which the frequency-encoding direction varies in three dimensions by incrementally changing the azimuthal and

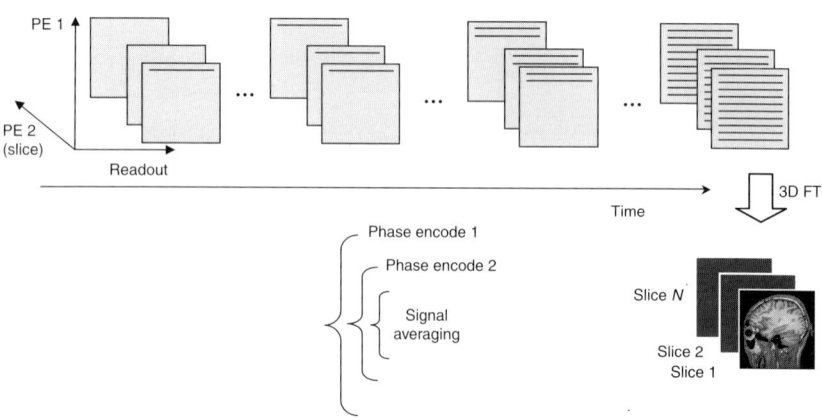

FIGURE 11.27 Schematic depiction of the filling of a 3D k-space with nested looping of the in-plane and slice-direction phase encodings. On the top row, each line represents a frequency-encoded readout. When the entire 3D k-space is filled with data, a set of 3D images can be obtained with a 3D discrete Fourier transform.

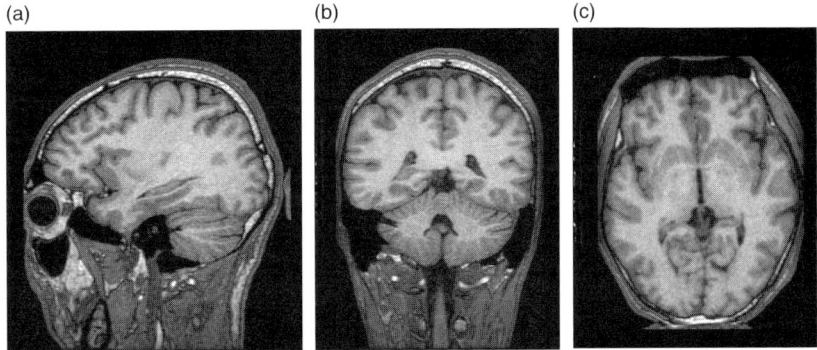

FIGURE 11.28 A slab of 128 1.2-mm-thick 3D images is acquired in the sagittal plane at 1.5 T in 6 min. The images can be displayed in the original (a) sagittal plane or reformatted into the (b) coronal, (c) axial, or any oblique plane. In this acquisition, frequency encoding is superior-inferior, in-plane phase encoding is anterior-posterior, and the second phase encoding (i.e., the slice encoding) is right-left. (Courtesy of Chen Lin, Ph.D., Mayo Clinic College of Medicine.)

polar angles (Lai and Lauterbur 1981; Barger et al. 2002). Each gradient orientation produces a k-space line in the polar coordinate. Thus, 3D k-space is sampled by a set of radial lines. The corresponding 3D image can be reconstructed using methods such as filtered back-projection or gridding (Section 13.2) followed by a 3D Fourier transform. In this section, we focus primarily on rectilinear k-space trajectories because they are more commonly used.

3D volume acquisitions share many features with their 2D counterparts. Consequently this section uses the concepts phase encoding (Section 8.2) and slice-selection gradients (Section 8.3). The main advantage of 3D acquisitions is their ability to acquire thin contiguous slices that are ideal for volume rendering, multiplanar reformatting (Figure 11.28), or maximum intensity projection (MIP). The best viewing plane for a reformatted image and the best viewing angle for a MIP can be chosen retrospectively, after the acquisition. 3D reconstruction also allows zero-filled interpolation that provides overcontiguous (i.e., overlapping) slices and can further improve the quality of postprocessed images such as MIPs. Finally, 3D acquisition carries SNR implications, which are explored later in this section.

11.6.1 COMPARISON BETWEEN 2D AND 3D ACQUISITION

Acquisition Time   Because phase encoding is performed along two spatial directions, the acquisition time for 3D scans is prolonged. Suppose that the number of phase-encoding steps in the in-plane and slice directions are N_{phase1} and N_{phase2}, respectively. Then the total time needed to acquire the data for the 3D slab is:

$$T_{scan} = N_{phase1} \times N_{phase2} \times NEX \times TR \qquad (11.41)$$

Equation (11.41) is similar to the expression for 2D acquisitions (Section 11.5), except for the additional factor N_{phase2}, which arises because the two phase-encoding gradients are incremented independently. That is, for each value of the in-plane phase encoding, the slice encoding must be incremented through all of its values. As described later in this section, a variety of view orders can be used. In order to generalize Eq. (11.41) to cases such as a slice-encoded stack of spirals, N_{phase1} is replaced by the number of interleaves (i.e., shots). This also accounts for the reduction of imaging time when echo train methods are used.

Most 3D pulse sequences use gradient echoes because their short minimum TR allows the acquisition to be completed in several minutes or less. 3D RF spin-echo acquisitions are also obtained in a reasonable scan time when echo train methods (e.g., RARE) are used (Oshio et al. 1991).

Minimum Slice Thickness   Thin slices can be desirable because they reduce partial volume averaging and reduce intravoxel phase dispersion resulting from susceptibility variations (i.e., T_2^*) or complex flow. In 2D imaging, the RF bandwidth Δf and the gradient amplitude G determine the slice thickness Δz_{2D} (see Section 8.1):

$$\Delta z_{2D} = \frac{2\pi \, \Delta f}{\gamma G} \qquad (11.42)$$

Thus, thin 2D slices are obtained by using a large gradient amplitude or a narrow RF bandwidth. The gradient amplitude cannot be arbitrarily increased because it is a property of the gradient hardware. The maximal amplitude is typically 10–50 mT/m for whole-body gradient coils. The RF bandwidth also cannot be arbitrarily reduced because the slice profile suffers (e.g., see Eq. 2.36 from Section 2.3) and the chemical shift artifact in the slice direction increases.

As derived in Section 8.2 on phase-encoding gradients, the slice or partition thickness for a 3D acquisition is inversely proportional to the area under the largest phase-encoding lobe. Applying Eq. (1.30) to the slice encoding process yields:

$$\Delta z_{3D} = \frac{1}{N_{phase2} \, \Delta k_z} \qquad (11.43)$$

where Δk_z is the step size in k-space from each slice encoding. The conversion from step size in k-space to step size in gradient area is:

$$\Delta A = \frac{2\pi \,\Delta k}{\gamma} \qquad (11.44)$$

If the slice-encoding area ranges from $+A_{max}$ to $-A_{max}$ in N_{phase2} steps, then the gradient area of each step is:

$$\Delta A = \frac{2\,A_{max}}{N_{phase2} - 1} \qquad (11.45)$$

Combining Eqs. (11.43), (11.44), and (11.45) yields:

$$\Delta z_{3D} = \frac{(N_{phase2} - 1)\pi}{\gamma\, N_{phase2}\, A_{max}} \qquad (11.46)$$

Example 11.8 illustrates why 3D acquisition is often used when very thin slices are desired.

Example 11.8 Suppose the maximal gradient amplitude and slew rate are $h = 25$ mT/m and $S_R = 100$ T/m/s, respectively, so that the ramp time is $r = h/S_R = 250\,\mu$s. (a) Assuming the maximal gradient amplitude is used for slice selection, what RF bandwidth is required to obtain a 0.5-mm-thick slice with a 2D acquisition? (b) If a dimensionless time-bandwidth product of 3.0 is required to produce an acceptable slice profile, what is the RF pulse duration? (c) What fraction of the slice thickness is the fat-water chemical shift in the slice direction at 3.0 T? (d) If the 0.5-mm slice is instead obtained with a 64-slice 3D acquisition, what is the total duration of a trapezoidal slice-encoding gradient lobe?

Answer

(a) Substituting the maximum gradient amplitude into Eq. (11.42), yields:

$$\Delta f = (42.57\,\text{MHz/T})(0.5 \times 10^{-3}\,\text{m})(25 \times 10^{-3}\,\text{T/m}) = 532\,\text{Hz}$$

(b) The pulse duration in this case is:

$$T = \frac{T\Delta f}{\Delta f} = \frac{3.0}{532\,\text{Hz}} = 5.6\,\text{ms}$$

(c) The fat-water chemical shift at 3.0 T is approximately 420 Hz. Therefore, the chemical shift artifact in the slice direction for the RF pulse bandwidth calculated in (a) is 420/532, or approximately 79% of the slice thickness. Often this creates an artifact level that is higher than is clinically acceptable.

(d) From Eq. (11.46), the area under the largest phase-encoding step is:

$$A = \frac{(N_{\text{phase2}} - 1)\pi}{\gamma \, \Delta z \, N_{\text{phase2}}}$$

From Eq. (7.8) (Section 7.1 on simple gradient lobes), its duration is:

$$T_{\text{lobe}} = \frac{|A|}{h} + r = \frac{\pi(63/64)}{\gamma \, \Delta z \, h} + r$$

$$= \frac{(63/64)}{2(42.57\,\text{MHz/T})(0.5 \times 10^{-3}\,\text{m})(25 \times 10^{-3}\,\text{T/m})} + 250\,\mu s$$

$$= 1.175\,\text{ms}$$

Note that duration of the slice-encoding lobe calculated in Example 11.8 is almost five times shorter than the duration of the 2D RF excitation pulse. This illustrates that for sufficiently thin slices, 3D imaging provides a shorter minimum TE. (The value of the slice thickness for which 3D shows a substantial TE advantage depends on the details of the gradient hardware and the pulse sequence. For example, the duration of the RF pulse in a 3D gradient-echo pulse sequence can vary widely, e.g., from 0.5 to 5 ms.) Also (as explained later), the chemical shift artifact in the slice direction is less problematic for 3D. One limitation on the minimum slice thickness for 3D acquisitions is anatomical coverage because the slices are contiguous and scan time is proportional to the number of slices. Another limitation on minimum slice thickness is the SNR, which is discussed next.

SNR Efficiency   The SNR of MR acquisitions obeys the scaling relationship (Edelstein et al. 1986):

$$\text{SNR} \propto \Delta x \, \Delta y \, \Delta z \, \sqrt{T_{\text{acq,total}}} \tag{11.47}$$

where the product of the three pixel dimensions (without zero-filled interpolation) $\Delta x \, \Delta y \, \Delta z$ is the voxel volume, and $T_{\text{acq,total}}$ is the total amount of time that the data acquisition window is open to sample data. (To calculate $T_{\text{acq,total}}$ we consider all the data that are later reconstructed with a single Fourier transform, regardless of the dimension of that transform.) The scaling relationship in Eq. (11.47) does not contain any information about the RF coil, the main magnetic field, or the physical properties of the object (e.g., relaxation times), so it cannot provide an absolute SNR value.

Because the entire 3D slab of slices is reconstructed with a single 3D Fourier transform, the total acquisition time includes the number of slice-encoding steps. Thus, for 3D acquisitions:

$$\text{SNR}_{3D} \propto \Delta x \, \Delta y \, \Delta z \, \sqrt{N_{\text{phase1}} \, N_{\text{phase2}} \, \text{NEX} \, T_{\text{acq}}} \qquad (11.48)$$

where T_{acq} is the time that the data acquisition window is open during each readout, that is, the number of frequency-encoded points divided by the full receiver bandwidth. For comparison, for 2D acquisitions:

$$\text{SNR}_{2D} \propto \Delta x \, \Delta y \, \Delta z \, \sqrt{N_{\text{phase1}} \, \text{NEX} \, T_{\text{acq}}} \qquad (11.49)$$

Dividing Eq (11.48) by (11.49) yields:

$$\frac{\text{SNR}_{3D}}{\text{SNR}_{2D}} = \sqrt{N_{\text{phase2}}} \qquad (11.50)$$

Because N_{phase2} is typically 16–128, its square root represents a very large increase in SNR (e.g., 400–1100%), especially because many observers can detect SNR differences of as little as 10%. This SNR efficiency advantage is illustrated by the following example: A 3D slab of 32 slices can be acquired with NEX = 1 in the same time (and with the same SNR) as a single 2D slice acquired with NEX = 32 signal averages, provided that the TR time is the same for both acquisitions.

If 3D has such a great SNR efficiency advantage, then why is it not used more frequently? The answer is that the comparison in Eq. (11.50) is naive because multiple 2D slices can be interleaved (Section 11.5), which allows more time for T_1 relaxation, and 2D regains much (if not all) of the SNR deficit. Recall that during 3D volume acquisitions the entire volume is excited each TR. If the 3D pulse sequence contains no dead time, then the sequence time T_{seq} and the repetition time TR are equal. As discussed in Section 11.5 for 2D interleaved acquisitions, however, TR can be much longer than T_{seq} without adding pulse sequence dead time. If we neglect slice cross-talk for the 2D interleaved acquisition, then TR $= N T_{\text{seq}}$, where N is the number of 2D slices. Therefore, for pulse sequences with long TR, multislice interleaved 2D acquisition can be more time efficient than 3D acquisition.

To account for interleaving and to obtain a less naive comparison of the SNR for 2D and 3D acquisitions requires knowledge of the T_1 of the object and the specifics of the pulse sequence. Here we assume a single value of T_1 and a spoiled gradient-echo pulse sequence (Section 14.1). Spoiled gradient echoes are commonly used for 2D and 3D acquisitions and have a simple analytical expression (Section 14.1) for the signal, which facilitates the calculation:

$$S(\text{TR}, T_1, \theta) \propto M_0 \frac{\sin\theta(1 - e^{-\text{TR}/T_1})e^{-\text{TE}/T_2^*}}{1 - \cos\theta \, e^{-\text{TR}/T_1}} \qquad (11.51)$$

The flip angle θ that maximizes Eq. (11.51) is called the Ernst angle and is given by:

$$\theta_E = \arccos(e^{-TR/T_1}) \tag{11.52}$$

Accounting for the increase in TR due to interleaving, the Ernst angle for the interleaved 2D is higher than for the 3D acquisition:

$$\theta_{2D} = \arccos(e^{-NT_{seq}/T_1}) \tag{11.53}$$

$$\theta_{3D} = \arccos(e^{-T_{seq}/T_1}) \tag{11.54}$$

Substituting Eq. (11.52) into Eq. (11.51) and using $\sin\theta = \sqrt{1 - \cos^2\theta}$, the maximum signal is:

$$S(TR, T_1, \theta_E) \propto M_0 \frac{(1 - e^{-TR/T_1})e^{-TE/T_2^*}}{\sqrt{1 - e^{-2TR/T_1}}} \tag{11.55}$$

Assuming that the 2D and 3D acquisitions have roughly the same TE, the T_2^* dependence in Eq. (11.55) does not affect the relative SNR. Then, the result is to replace Eq. (11.50) by:

$$\frac{SNR_{3D}}{SNR_{2D}} = \sqrt{N_{phase2}} \sqrt{\frac{1 - e^{-2NT_{seq}/T_1}}{1 - e^{-2T_{seq}/T_1}} \frac{(1 - e^{-T_{seq}/T_1})}{(1 - e^{-NT_{seq}/T_1})}} \tag{11.56}$$

To complete the comparison, we set the number of 2D and 3D slices equal to one another. The values of the relative SNRs calculated from Eq. (11.56) with $N_{phase2} = N$ are provided in Table 11.3. Note that in many typical combinations of T_{seq}/T_1 and the number of slices, the SNRs of 3D and interleaved 2D

TABLE 11.3
The Relative SNRs of Spoiled Gradient
Echo 3D and 2D Interleaved
Acquisitions[a]

	T_{seq}/T_1			
N	0.001	0.01	0.1	1.0
16	1.00	1.00	1.10	2.72
32	1.00	1.00	1.32	3.85
64	1.00	1.02	1.79	5.44
128	1.00	1.06	2.53	7.69

[a]Calculated with Eq. (11.56) with $N_{phase2} = N$.

are equal to within a few percent. Situations in which 2D oblique acquisition is preferable to 3D acquisition are discussed in Section 7.3.

If $T_1 \ll T_{seq}$ all the exponential factors in Eq. (11.56) are negligible compared to 1. Then, the 3D pulse acquisition truly has a $\sqrt{N_{phase2}}$ SNR advantage compared to 2D. This is one of the reasons that 3D acquisitions are the method of choice for nuclei with very short T_1, such as sodium-23 (Perman et al. 1986). If T_1 is much longer than the sequence time T_{seq}, then 3D acquisitions have no SNR advantage. We can see from Table 11.3 that 3D acquisitions also become more favorable as the number of slices increases.

Truncation Artifacts and Fourier Leakage in the Slice-Encoded Direction Because 3D images are Fourier-encoded in all three dimensions, they can suffer truncation artifacts (i.e., Gibbs ringing, Section 13.1) in all three dimensions. Truncation artifacts arise when the spatial resolution is insufficient to depict rapidly varying structures, such as edges, in the object.

Whereas in-plane truncation artifacts act the same for 3D and 2D acquisitions, truncation artifacts in the slice direction are unique to 3D. Truncation artifacts in the slice-encoded direction in 3D can be difficult to recognize when the images are viewed as standard slices because the ringing propagates from slice to slice. Often the truncation artifact can be more easily recognized on reformatted images (Figure 11.29).

The best countermeasure against truncation artifact is to reduce the slice thickness (or to use a 2D acquisition). Thus for slice thickness greater than approximately 3 mm, 2D acquisitions are usually preferred. Also, as explained in Section 13.1, windowing the raw data prior to the Fourier transform in the slice-encoded direction can reduce truncation artifacts, but at the expense of spatial resolution. Note that zero-filled interpolation does not reduce truncation artifacts because it provides overlapping slices of the original slice thickness. In fact, the reduced partial-volume averaging of the zero-filled reconstruction can make the ringing artifacts more conspicuous on reformatted images.

Whereas Gibbs ringing places a practical upper limit on the slice thickness, Fourier leakage artifacts place a practical lower limit on the number of encoded slices. Rarely are 3D acquisitions with fewer than eight phase-encoded slices per slab used. Bracewell (1978) discusses Fourier leakage effects in more detail. When fewer than approximately eight slices per slab are desired, alternative methods to 3D Fourier encoding such as Hadamard encoding (Souza et al. 1988) and phase offset multiplanar (POMP, as described in Glover 1991) should be considered.

Receiver Dynamic Range Requirements Because 3D acquisitions excite an entire volume, the peak signal at the center of k-space is approximately

(a)   (b)

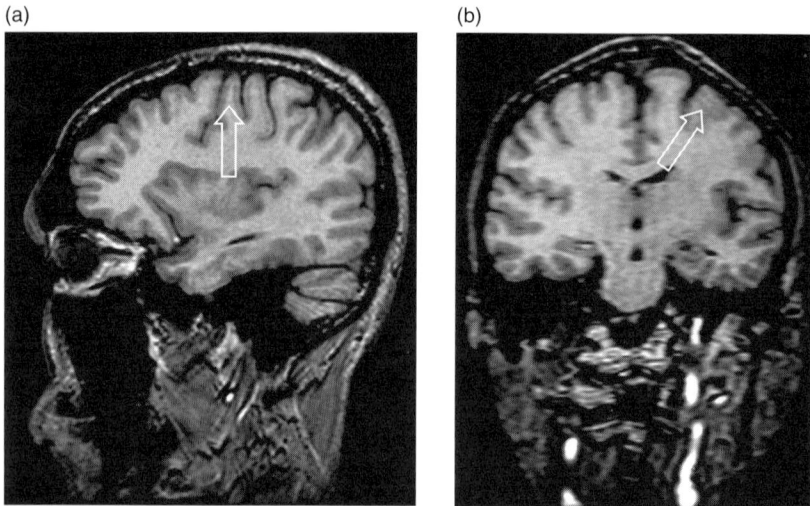

FIGURE 11.29 (a) One slice from a set of 60 3-mm-thick 3D sagittal slices. A ripple artifact (arrow) appears as if it is caused by patient motion. (b) Reformatted coronal image shows the true cause of the artifact—Gibbs ringing (arrow) due to the relatively large slice thickness. The reformatted coronal image appears blurred due to anisotropic spatial resolution.

N_{phase2} times stronger than for the corresponding 2D acquisition, assuming equal slice thickness. This places special requirements on the dynamic range of the A/D converter of the receiver (Mugler et al. 2000; Oh et al. 1992).

Many MR systems have 16-bit A/D converters, meaning digitized signals are represented as an integer between $-2^{15} + 1$ and 2^{15}. Therefore the smallest positive signal that they can represent is $2^0 = 1$ and the largest is $2^{15} = 32,768$, or 32k. This dynamic range is sufficient for most 2D acquisitions, but it is often insufficient for 3D imaging. To prevent overranging, the peak 3D signal must be scaled down to below 32k, which causes useful information that falls within the range of 0 to 1 to be represented as 0 and therefore lost. This increases quantization noise, which degrades the SNR.

Several strategies can be used to avoid quantization noise in 3D acquisitions. One method is simply to use an A/D converter with more dynamic range (e.g., 20 bits or deeper). Such A/D converters are available, but tend to be more expensive and can have slower digitization rates, which limits the maximal receiver bandwidth. A different method is to dynamically adjust the receiver gain throughout the acquisition (Mugler et al. 2000). For example, a lower receiver gain is used to acquire the center of k-space than the periphery.

This nonconstant receiver gain must be corrected during the reconstruction. If the receiver gain adjustment introduces a phase shift, it must be measured and also corrected for during reconstruction because the MR data are phase-sensitive.

A third strategy to reduce quantization noise in 3D is to use an RF excitation pulse with a nonlinear phase response (Oh et al. 1992), such as a minimum or quadratic phase pulse (Section 2.3). This strategy relies on the phase dispersion across the slab to reduce the peak signal. This can be an effective method, but is more difficult to implement for some applications such as 3D RARE (Oshio et al. 1991) for which it is important to maintain specific phase relationships between the excitation and refocusing RF pulses.

11.6.2 3D ACQUISITION STRATEGIES

Selective and Nonselective 3D   Most 3D pulse sequences use selective RF excitation in order to limit aliasing (i.e., wrap-around) artifacts in the slice-encoded direction (Figure 11.30). This is called a *selective 3D* acquisition.

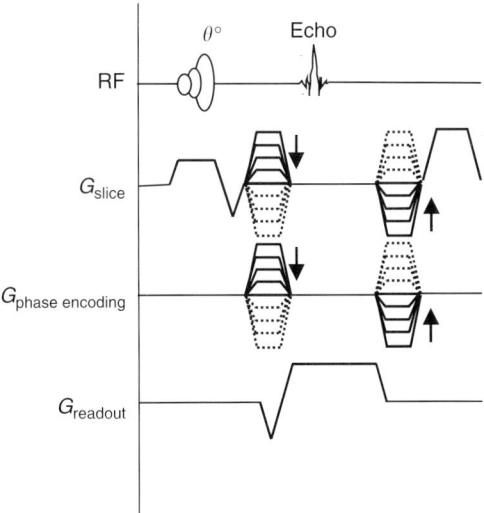

FIGURE 11.30 Pulse sequence diagram for a selective 3D gradient-echo acquisition. The frequency-encoded readout and in-plane phase-encoding waveforms are the same as a 2D pulse sequence. The slice axis has both a slab selection and a phase encoding gradient. In order to minimize TE, the slice-encoding gradient can be combined with the slice-rephasing lobe; to minimize TR, the slice-rewinding lobe can be combined with the end of sequence spoiler.

(a)   (b)

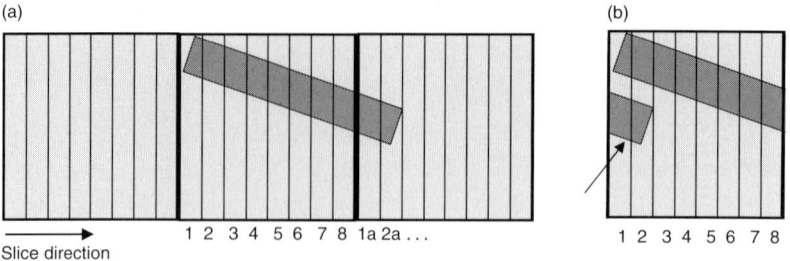

Slice direction   1 2 3 4 5 6 7 8 1a 2a ...   1 2 3 4 5 6 7 8

FIGURE 11.31 In nonselective 3D imaging, wrap-around or aliasing artifacts in the slice-encoded direction can result if the object extends beyond the FOV. (a) Each vertical rectangle schematically represents one slice. In this example, there are eight slices. The object extends into the adjacent replicate (i.e., slices 1a and 2a). (b) As a result, image numbers 1 and 2 have aliasing artifacts.

Alternatively, *nonselective 3D* uses a hard pulse (Section 2.1) or a spectrally-selective pulse (Harms et al. 1993) for excitation. To limit aliasing, the user of nonselective 3D must either (1) select a field of view in both phase-encoding directions that is larger than the object, sometimes called *oversampling the object*, or (2) use an RF coil with a sensitive region that is smaller than the FOV, sometimes called *oversampling the coil*. Figure 11.31 schematically illustrates the result of aliasing in nonselective 3D. The main advantage of nonselective 3D is its very short minimum TE because the duration of a hard pulse is typically on the order of 100 ms. This section, however, focuses on selective 3D because it is more commonly used.

The gradient for selective 3D excitation (sometimes called the *slab-selection gradient*) is applied along the same gradient axis as slice encoding and limits aliasing, as depicted in Figure 11.32. The amplitude of the slab-selection gradient is chosen so the slab thickness approximately matches the FOV in the slice-encoded direction $N_{\text{phase2}} \times \Delta z$:

$$G_{\text{slab}} = \frac{2\pi \, \Delta f}{\gamma \, (N_{\text{phase2}} \Delta z)} \qquad (11.57)$$

where Δz is the thickness of one slice.

No practical RF pulse has a perfect profile. Instead, every profile has a nonzero transition width between the stopband and the passband, and sometimes ripples and side lobes as well. These imperfections can cause aliasing in 3D imaging, especially on the end slices of the slab. Also, the flip angle applied to the slices that lie in the transition band of the RF profile is lower than in the passband, which changes the image contrast. To hide these artifacts, a few (i.e., 1–4) slices are typically dropped from each end of the slab, like discarding the end crusts from a loaf of bread. For example, if 32 slices

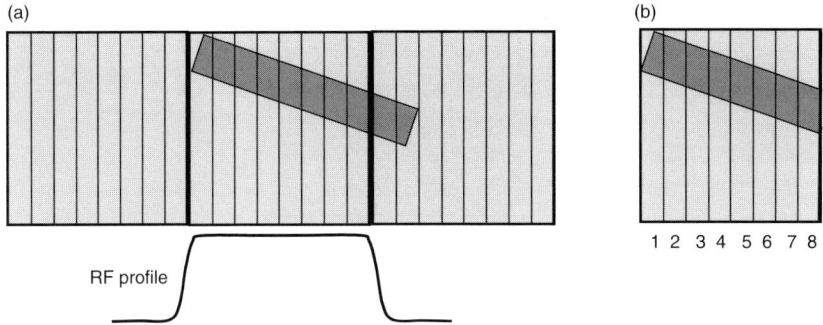

FIGURE 11.32 In selective 3D imaging, the RF profile of the slab-selection pulse reduces aliasing artifacts. If the RF profile is ideal, aliasing can be avoided completely. Here the RF profile covers the desired eight slices, so (unlike in Figure 11.31) the signal from the outside replicates does not wrap back in.

are Fourier-encoded and reconstructed, we may choose only to display the central 28 slices. Sometimes the gradient amplitude calculated in Eq. (11.57) is increased slightly to account for the discarded slices. Because the end slices will be dropped anyway, it is convenient to phase cycle the DC artifact described in Section 11.5 to the end slices (i.e., the edge of the FOV in the slice-encoded direction) instead of the edge of the in-plane FOV.

Example 11.9 Consider an excitation pulse whose slice profile has a side lobe, as schematically illustrated in Figure 11.33a. Suppose that the side lobe's amplitude and width are 10 and 5% of the passband, respectively. (a) Estimate how much signal in a 2D image is coming from outside the desired slice because of the side lobe. (b) If the flip angle of the excitation pulse is 90°, estimate how much the side lobe would disturb the longitudinal magnetization of a neighboring 2D slice. (c) If the 3D slab comprises 64 slices, how many slices will the side lobe affect? (d) Estimate the strength of the image artifact that the side lobe produces on those 3D slices.

Answer

(a) The partial volume contribution from the side lobe can be estimated by calculating the ratio of its area to the total area under the passband. This ratio is approximately 10% of 5%, or 0.5%, which is usually negligible.

(b) The flip angle produced by the side lobe is 10% of 90° $= 9°$. The remaining longitudinal magnetization in neighboring slices after experiencing the side lobe will be approximately $\cos(9°) = 0.988$ of its original value.

(c) Based on the width of the side lobe, the number of slices that are affected is 5% of N_{phase2}, or about 3 slices out of a slab of 64.

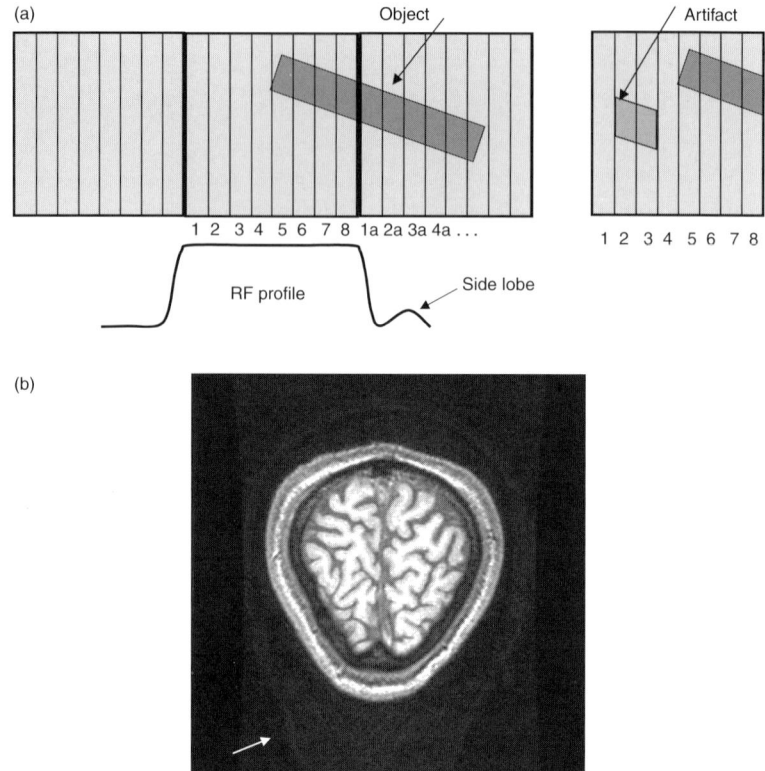

FIGURE 11.33 In selective 3D imaging, imperfect RF profiles of the slab-selection pulse cause aliasing artifacts to reappear, but at a lower intensity than nonselective 3D. (a) A side lobe causes aliasing artifacts on image numbers 2 and 3. Similar artifacts can also be caused by a broad transition region of the slice profile. (b) A coronal slice from the posterior part of the brain is contaminated with wraparound artifact from more anterior slices. A faint ghost image including the neck is seen (arrow).

(d) Each affected slice will suffer an admixture of the true signal and an artifact with intensity on the order of $\sin(9°) = 16\%$ wrapped in from outside the slab, which is usually strong enough to be seen in the image as a faint ghost, as shown in Figure 11.33b.

For the reasons illustrated in Example 11.9, a 3D RF excitation pulse should be designed with special attention to its profile. High values of the dimensionless time-bandwidth products ($T \Delta f = 5$–20) are used unless overriding requirements for short TE and TR demand a lower $T \Delta f$. As described in Section 2.3, minimum phase SLR pulses make excellent 3D excitation pulses because they can produce good slice profiles with short pulse duration, due to a small value of D_∞. Because the isodelay of a minimum phase pulse is less than one-half of its pulse width, the minimum TE is reduced. Although the phase dispersion across the slab is nonlinear and cannot be completely refocused by a linear gradient, this is rarely a problem for 3D acquisitions. Intravoxel dephasing in 3D is calculated by integrating the phase over a single slice rather than the whole slab, so it is usually negligible. Over any one slice, the phase dispersion can be approximated as a linear function of z, in which case the mathematical methods used in Section 10.6 on twister gradients can be used to quantify the signal loss due to intravoxel phase dispersion. As previously discussed, the nonlinear phase of the excitation profile paradoxically can improve the SNR if a dynamic range-limited digitizer introduces quanitization noise.

Although the slab profile determines the amount of aliasing in the slice-encoded direction, it has no effect on the individual slice profile. Instead, that is determined by the Fourier encoding and reconstruction (Section 13.1). For example, if no windowing is used, each slice profile will be SINC shaped. The idealized rectangular representation shown in Figure 11.31 is schematic and cannot be obtained in practice, even if windowing is applied prior to Fourier transform along the slice-encoded direction.

Chemical Shift in the Slice-Encoded Direction   Chemical shift in the slice-encoded direction displaces the profile of the selective excitation pulse, but does not offset the slice-encoded replicates. As illustrated by Figure 11.34, this mismatch results in chemical shift artifacts on the end slices of the 3D slab.

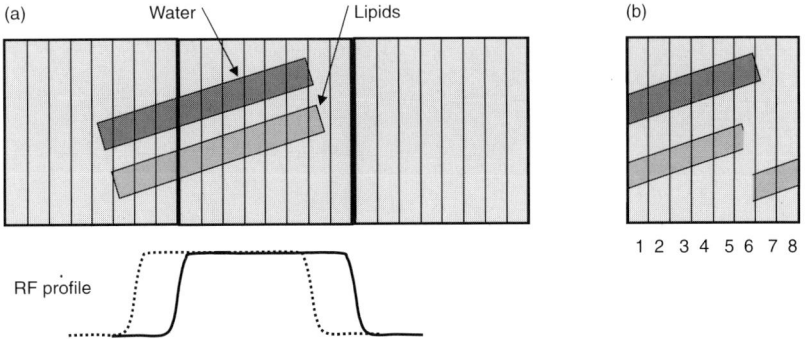

FIGURE 11.34 Chemical shift artifact in selective 3D. (a) The RF profile that lipids experience (dotted line) is offset to the left due to chemical shift. (b) This causes a chemical shift artifact on image numbers 6, 7, and 8. The amount of chemical shift is exaggerated for illustration purposes.

The central slices in the slab are not affected, although naturally they are also prone to the standard chemical shift artifact in the frequency-encoded direction (and the blip direction in the case of 3D echo planar imaging). Effective ways to counteract chemical shift in the slice direction in 3D include increasing the RF bandwidth of the slab-selection pulse and discarding the end slices, as discussed previously.

Example 11.10   A 3D slab-selection pulse has a bandwidth of $\Delta f = 2700\,\text{Hz}$. If 64 slices are Fourier-encoded, how many slices on each end will have an inaccurate depiction of lipid structures at 1.5 T? 3.0 T? Neglect the transition region of the RF profile and assume no end slices are discarded.

Answer
The fat-water chemical shift is approximately 140 Hz/T. So at 1.5 T, the number of affected slices is:

$$\frac{140\,\text{Hz/T} \times 1.5\,\text{T}}{2700\,\text{Hz}} \times 64\,\text{slices} = 5\,\text{slices}$$

At 3.0 T the chemical shift frequency is doubled, so 10 slices on each end are affected.

Offset Slabs   Sometimes we need to offset a 3D slab to cover anatomy that does not lie at the isocenter of the gradients. Offsets in the frequency-encoded and in-plane phase-encoded directions can be accomplished as described in Sections 8.1 and 8.2, respectively. The theory and practice of those two offsets are the same for 2D and 3D imaging.

As shown on Figure 11.35, however, two steps carried out in concert are required to offset in the slab direction for 3D. First, all RF pulses must be offset as described in Section 8.3 by adjusting their carrier frequencies. Second, a linear phase ramp is applied as a function of the slice encode index, just as off-center FOV can be achieved in the in-plane phase-encoded direction. (See Eq. 8.39 in Section 8.2 and replace y by z, e.g., the offset δy becomes δz.) The applied phase modulation shifts the encoded slices within the replicates, so one set of slices properly aligns with the offset profile of the RF pulse (Figure 11.35a). The phase shifts can be applied during reconstruction, demodulation, or even excitation. If the receiver has a DC baseline artifact, however, it is best to apply the phase shift after the A/D conversion (e.g., during reconstruction), so that the baseline artifact is not offset onto the retained central slices. Note that both the RF slab profile and the phase-encoded slices can be offset by an arbitrary amount—the offset is not restricted to an integer multiple of the slice thickness. The linear phase ramp is often used to correct for the half-pixel offset described in Section 1.1. That correction is particularly

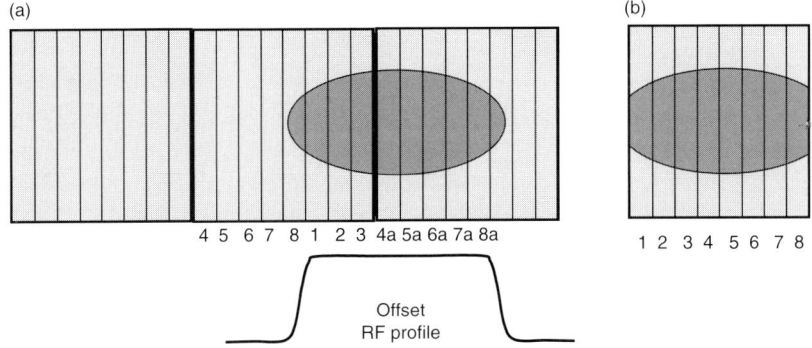

FIGURE 11.35 Slab offset in 3D. To image a set of slices that are not centered at gradient isocenter, the RF profile is offset by adjusting the carrier frequency and the encoded slices are shifted by applying a linear phase ramp to the k-space data. Note that images 4–8 are obtained from an adjacent replicate (i.e., image 4 on the right is obtained from 4a, etc.).

important when there are a small number of slices per slab (e.g., eight) because the error is a relatively high fraction of the slab thickness.

11.6.3 OTHER TECHNICAL CONSIDERATIONS FOR THREE-DIMENSIONAL IMAGING

View orders   With 2D Cartesian acquisitions (Section 11.5), the lines of k-space can be collected in a variety of different view orders including sequential, centric, and reverse centric. In 3D imaging, the view order has even more flexibility. One class of 3D view orders is implemented by stepping though each of the values on one phase-encoding axis before incrementing the value on the other phase-encoding axis. This is called *nesting* the phase-encoding loops. There are many possible view orders that use nested loops (Wilman et al. 2001). For example, either the in-plane phase encoding or the slice encoding can be the inner (i.e., most frequently incremented) loop. Also, the view order on each axis can be sequential, centric, reverse centric, and so forth. One strategy is to choose the slice-encoding loop to be the inner one and to begin the reconstruction concurrently with the acquisition by performing the 1D FTs along the slice-encoded direction. This method has the advantage that at the completion of the acquisition, the raw data can be processed as if it were a set of multiple 2D slices.

The *elliptical centric* view order (Wilman et al. 1997) and related view orders such as contrast enhanced timing robust angiography (CENTRA) (Willinek et al. 2002) replace the two nested loops with a single loop. In

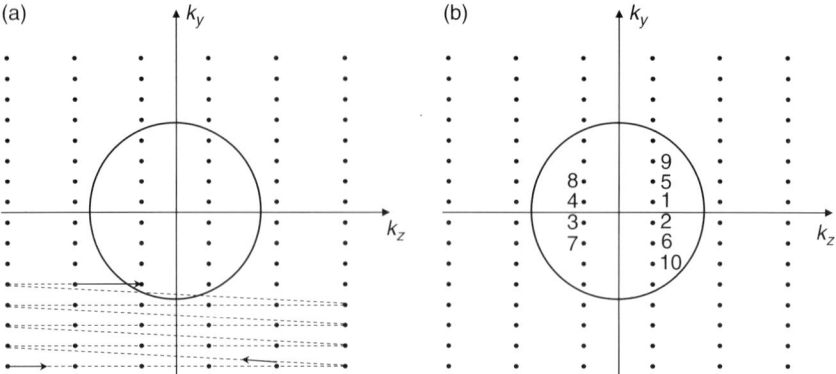

FIGURE 11.36 (a) With sequential view order and nested loops (slice-encoding is the innermost loop), the center of k-space (circle) is acquired approximately halfway through the scan. (b) With the elliptical centric view order, the center of k-space is acquired at the beginning of the scan by design. Each dot represents a frequency-encoded k-space line perpendicular to the plane. The k-space variables k_y and k_z correspond to the in-plane and slice phase-encoded directions, respectively.

the elliptical centric view order, its distance to the origin in the k_y-k_z plane (Figure 11.36) determines the order that a particular view is played. Thus, elliptical centric is a true centric k-space ordering for 3D. Figure 11.36 illustrates the difference between standard nested loops and the elliptical centric view order. It is convenient to plot each frequency-encoded readout as a point, that is, to view the k-space lines shown in Figure 11.27 head-on. Then unequal FOVs for the in-plane and slice-encoded directions can be represented because each FOV is equal to the inverse of its k-space step size $1/\Delta k$. In the *reverse elliptical centric* view order, the view order is reversed so that the acquisition starts at the periphery of k-space and ends at the center. Elliptical centric has found applications in contrast-enhanced MR angiography because the center of k-space can be acquired after arterial but before venous enhancement, providing a high degree of venous suppression.

Multislab 3D Acquisition Sometimes it is convenient to acquire more than one 3D volume during a single scan. This is called *multiple-chunk* or *multiple-slab (multislab)* acquisition. Analogous to 2D multislice acquisitions (Section 11.5), 3D multislab acquisitions can be acquired in sequential or interleaved mode. The most well-known example of sequential multislab 3D is MOTSA (multiple overlapping thin slab acquisition), which is used for MR angiography and is described in Section 15.3. Interleaved multislab 3D is convenient to use when a long TR is required. A commonly used example of interleaved 3D multislab acquisition is 3D RARE (Oshio et al. 1991).

For sequential multislab 3D and interleaved 3D requiring multiple passes, Eq. (11.41) is modified to:

$$T_{scan} = N_{phase1} \times N_{phase2} \times NEX \times TR \times N_{acqs} \qquad (11.58)$$

where N_{acqs} is the number of passes, in analogy to Eq. (11.36) in Section 11.5. The number of passes in a sequential 3D acquisition is equal to the number of slabs.

Parallel Imaging Parallel-imaging techniques such as SENSE (Section 13.3) are often combined with 3D acquisitions. One reason of this is that SENSE does not add value when signal averaging is used (NEX ≥ 2) because the same scan time versus SNR trade-off can be made more simply by eliminating the averaging. 3D acquisitions rarely use signal averaging because according to Eq. (11.48), the same SNR advantage can be obtained by encoding more slices. Also, 3D acquisitions have two phase-encoded directions, and SENSE can be applied on either one or both, which adds flexibility. If SENSE is applied along a single direction, then that direction is typically chosen to be the one with the greatest separation of the coil elements. Often this is the in-plane phase-encoded direction because its FOV is usually longer. An exception occurs in the case of sagittal bilateral breast imaging, in which SENSE is better applied along the slice-encoded direction because the coil separation is larger.

SELECTED REFERENCES

Barger, A. V., Block, W. F., Toropov, Y., Grist, T. M., and Mistretta, C. A. 2002. Time-resolved contrast-enhanced imaging with isotropic resolution and broad coverage using an undersampled 3D projection trajectory. *Magn. Reson. Med.* 48: 297–305.

Bracewell, R. N. 1978. The Fourier transform and its applications. New York. McGraw-Hill.

den Boef, J. H., van Uijen, C. M., and Holzscherer, C. D. 1984. Multiple-slice NMR imaging by three-dimensional Fourier zeugmatography. *Phys. Med. Biol.* 29: 857–867.

Edelstein, W. A., Glover, G. H., Hardy, C. J., and Redington, R. W. 1986. The intrinsic signal-to-noise ratio in NMR imaging. *Magn. Reson. Med.* 3: 604–618.

Glover, G. H. 1991. Phase-offset multiplanar (POMP) volume imaging: A new technique. *J. Magn. Reson. Imaging* 1: 457–461.

Harms, S. E., Flamig, D. P., Hesley, K. L., Meiches, M. D., Jensen, R. A., Evans, W. P., Savino, D. A., Wells, R. V. 1993. MR Imaging of the breast with rotating delivery of excitation off resonance: clinical experience with pathologic correlation. *Radiology* 187: 493–501.

Lai, C. M., and Lauterbur, P. C. 1981. True three-dimensional image reconstruction by nuclear magnetic resonance zeugmatography. *Phys. Med. Biol.* 26: 851–856.

Mugler, J. P., III, Bao, S., Mulkern, R. V., Guttmann, C. R., Robertson, R. L., Jolesz, F. A., and Brookeman, J. R. 2000. Optimized single-slab three-dimensional spin-echo MR imaging of the brain. *Radiology* 216: 891–899.

Oh, C. H., Hilal, S. K., Wu, E. X., and Cho, Z. H. 1992. Phase-scrambled RF excitation for 3D volume-selective multislice NMR imaging. *Magn. Reson. Med.* 28: 290–299.

Oshio, K., Jolesz, F. A., Melki, P. S., and Mulkern, R. V. 1991. T2-weighted thin-section imaging with the multislab three-dimensional RARE technique. *J. Magn. Reson. Imaging* 1: 695–700.

Perman, W. H., Turski, P. A., Houston, L. W., Glover, G. H., and Hayes, C. E. 1986. Methodology of in vivo human sodium MR imaging at 1.5 T. *Radiology* 160: 811–820.

Souza, S. P., Szumowski, J., Dumoulin, C. L., Plewes, D. P., and Glover, G. H. 1988. SIMA: Simultaneous multislice acquisition of MR images by Hadamard encoded excitation. *J. Comput. Assist. Tomogr.* 12: 1026–1030.

Willinek, W. A., Gieseke, J., Conrad, R., Strunk, H., Hoogeveen, R., von Falkenhausen, M., Keller, E., Urbach, H., Kuhl, C. K., and Schild, H. H. 2002. Randomly segmented central k-space ordering in high-spatial-resolution contrast-enhanced MR angiography of the supraaortic arteries: Initial experience. *Radiology* 225: 583–588.

Wilman, A. H., Riederer, S. J., King, B. F., Debbins, J. P., Rossman, P. J., and Ehman, R. L. 1997. Fluoroscopically triggered contrast-enhanced three-dimensional MR angiography with elliptical centric view order: Application to the renal arteries. *Radiology* 205: 137–146.

Wilman, A. H., Yep, T. C., and Al-Kwifi, O. 2001. Quantitative evaluation of nonrepetitive phase-encoding orders for first-pass, 3D contrast-enhanced MR angiography. *Magn. Reson. Med.* 46: 541–547.

RELATED SECTIONS

CHAPTER

12

BASICS OF PHYSIOLOGIC GATING, TRIGGERING, AND MONITORING

12.1 Cardiac Triggering

Cardiac triggering (also known as *cardiac gating*) synchronizes a pulse sequence to the cardiac cycle of the patient (Lanzer et al. 1985; Shellock and Kanal 1996; Gatehouse and Firmin 2000). The devices most commonly used for cardiac triggering are the electrocardiograph and peripheral monitors. Cardiac triggering is used to minimize motion artifacts arising from cardiac motion and from pulsatile flow of arterial blood or cerebrospinal fluid. Cardiac triggering is also used to study cardiac motion by forming images at various cardiac phases. The goal of cardiac triggering is to acquire an entire set of k-space data at approximately the same portion of the cardiac cycle, even though the duration of the entire acquisition is longer than a single R-R interval. As discussed in Section 11.5, there are many methods to distribute the acquisition of the required k-space data over the multiple R-R intervals.

When cardiac triggering is successful, we obtain a *consistent* set of k-space data, which yields images free of motion artifacts (Figure 12.1). That is, the entire set of k-space raw data is acquired when the object (e.g., the heart)

443

(a)   (b)

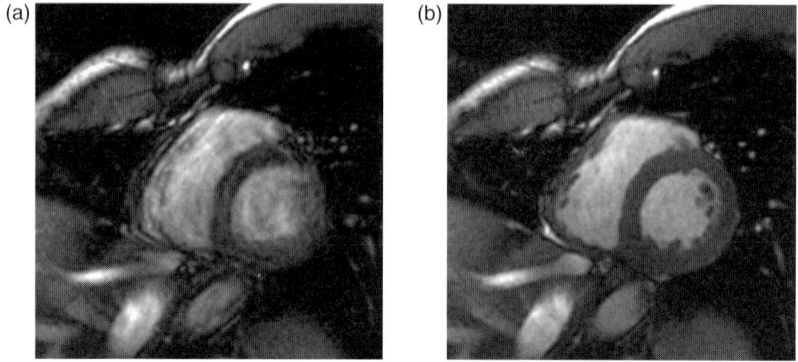

FIGURE 12.1 Cardiac triggering can improve image quality by providing raw data in which the interview motion is consistent. Short-axis view of the heart (a) without ECG triggering and (b) with successful ECG triggering. (Courtesy of Kiaran McGee, Ph.D., Mayo Clinic College of Medicine.)

is approximately in the same location and moving with the same velocity, acceleration, jerk, and so on. Even if the motion introduces a nonzero phase shift, as long as it is consistent throughout the entire k-space it will not cause any artifacts on magnitude images.

Cardiac triggering is sometimes used in conjunction with motion compensation methods such as gradient moment nulling, respiratory gating, and navigators. Gradient moment nulling (Section 10.4) can further suppress motion artifacts because in practice it is difficult to obtain a perfectly consistent set of k-space data due to the beat-to-beat deviation from the normal rhythm of the heart known as arrhythmia. Even if the heart rate is perfectly regular, methods such as segmented k-space cardiac acquisition (Sections 11.5 and 13.6) preclude obtaining perfect consistency because the data are acquired over an extended time. Gradient moment nulling is complementary to cardiac triggering because it can reduce intravoxel phase dispersion that occurs when there is rapid spatial variation of motion-induced phase. Because the heart moves during the respiratory cycle, cardiac triggering is also used in conjunction with respiratory gating or compensation (e.g., see Yuan et al. 2000) or with navigator echoes (Section 12.2) to image the heart.

12.1.1 TRIGGERING METHODS

ECG Triggering   An electrocardiogram (EKG or ECG) is a plot of voltage versus time indicating the electrical activity of the heart muscle, as

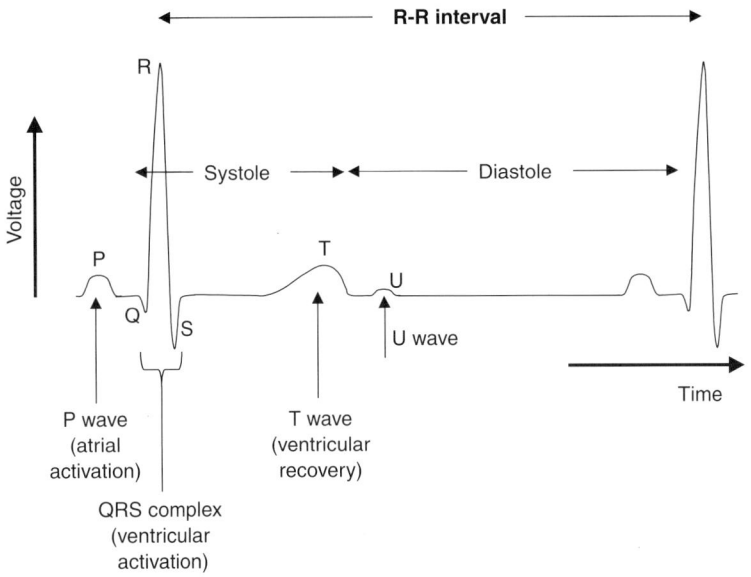

FIGURE 12.2 Schematic depiction of the ECG waveform over an R-R interval.

measured at the surface of the body (Malmivuo and Plonsey 1995) with an electrocardiograph. Figure 12.2 shows a schematic diagram of a normal ECG. The time scale of the ECG can be calculated from the patient's heart rate, or vice versa, because the duration of the R-R interval is:

$$\text{R-R interval [ms]} = \frac{60{,}000}{\text{Heartrate [bpm]}} \qquad (12.1)$$

For example, a heartrate of 80 bpm corresponds to an R-R interval of 750 ms. The peak amplitude of an ECG depends on the specifics of the patient and measurement technique, but values on the order of 1–2 mV are typical. This voltage is often amplified prior to being displayed on a monitor or recorded on paper.

The waves labeled in Figure 12.2 have physiological interpretations (Malmivuo and Plonsey 1995). The P wave indicates the activation of the atria, corresponding to their contraction. Activation (also called excitation or *depolarization*) is associated with the flow of positively charged sodium ions into cells, making the electrical potential outside negative. The QRS complex indicates the activation of the ventricles and is normally the strongest peak of the ECG waveform. Both the P wave and the QRS complex are known as depolarization waves. During the cardiac cycle, the heart muscle also recovers or repolarizes. *Repolarization* is caused by the flow of positively charged potassium ions out of cells and indicates the start of muscle relaxation. Repolarization of the atria occurs during ventricular activation, so the relatively weak ECG signal is entirely hidden by the QRS complex. Repolarization of the ventricles, however, can be detected as the T wave, which is known as a repolarization wave. At this time, the physiological origin of the U wave is still an area of scientific investigation (Di Bernardo and Murray 2002).

The cardiac cycle can be divided into two parts, called systole and diastole. *Systole* corresponds to contraction of the heart muscle, whereas *diastole* corresponds to its dilatation. Electrically, ventricular systole covers the period from the onset of the QRS complex to the end of the T wave (Figure 12.2).

Usually the pulse sequence is triggered when the amplitude of the R wave reaches its maximum voltage. To simplify the processing, sometimes triggering occurs when the ECG waveform exceeds a predetermined voltage threshold, which is called *threshold detection*. The QRS complex usually corresponds to the greatest slope of the ECG waveform, so, alternatively, triggering can occur when the time derivative of the voltage waveform reaches a maximum or exceeds a predetermined threshold. This is called *peak-slope* detection. Noise filtering of the ECG waveform prior to differentiation is especially important for peak-slope detection to avoid false triggers.

The effect of the complex electrical activity of the heart at the surface of the body can be modeled to a reasonably good approximation by an electric dipole vector (Malmivuo and Plonsey 1995), indicated by the hollow arrow in Figure 12.3a. The strength and direction of the electric dipole vector varies throughout the R-R interval. For example, during the QRS complex the depolarization front travels from the right ventricle to the left ventricle, and the electric dipole vector points toward the left and reaches its maximal amplitude.

The electric dipole produces an electric field, which creates a potential difference that is measured at the surface of the body by attaching multiple electrodes to the skin. Figure 12.3a shows an idealized placement of the electrodes on the right arm (RA), the left arm (LA), and the left leg (LL). This forms the *Einthoven triangle* (named for Willem Einthoven, 1860–1927, a Dutch physiologist and pioneer of the ECG). In practice, cardiac triggering in MRI is accomplished with three electrodes placed on the patient's chest (or back), separated from one another by about 10 cm (e.g., see Figure 12.3b). The labels RA, LA, and LL, however, are used for the upper right, upper left, and lower left electrodes, respectively. To add redundancy, some systems use four electrodes. In that case, the fourth electrode is sometimes placed a few centimeters to the (patient's) right of the LL electrode.

From the three electrodes we can obtain voltage (i.e., potential difference) measurements called *leads*, as shown in Figure 12.3a. With the RA, LA, and

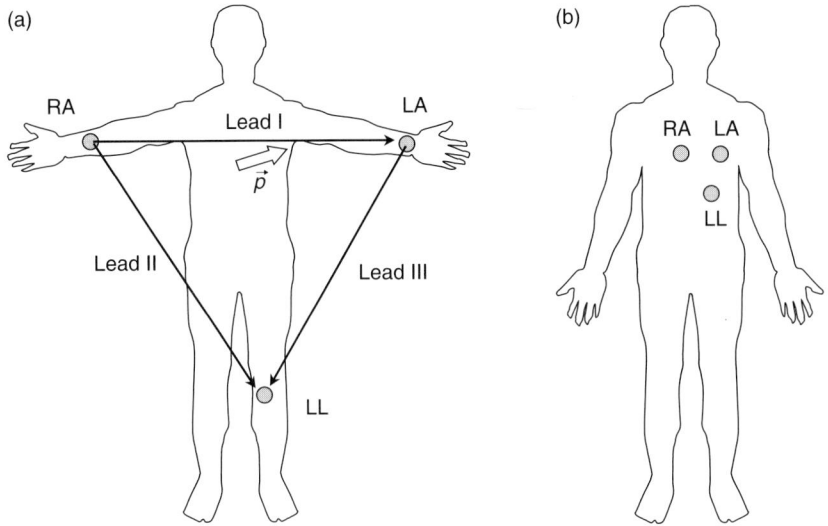

FIGURE 12.3 (a) Einthoven triangle shown on an anterior view with electrodes attached to the right arm (RA), left arm (LA), and left leg (LL). Measuring potential differences between these electrodes provides the three leads (see Eq. 12.2). The electric dipole vector $\vec{p}$ (hollow arrow) is used to approximate the electrical activity of the heart. (b) Three-electrode placement. For ECG-triggering in MRI, the electrodes are often placed approximately 10 cm apart from one another on the patient's chest. Some systems use four electrodes instead.

LL electrodes, we can measure:

$$
\begin{aligned}
V_{\mathrm{I}} &= V_{\mathrm{RA}} - V_{\mathrm{LA}} && \text{(lead I)} \\
V_{\mathrm{II}} &= V_{\mathrm{RA}} - V_{\mathrm{LL}} && \text{(lead II)} \\
V_{\mathrm{III}} &= V_{\mathrm{LA}} - V_{\mathrm{LL}} && \text{(lead III)}
\end{aligned}
\tag{12.2}
$$

The following mnemonic device might be useful: The total number of subscript Ls in Eq. (12.2) matches the Roman numeral of the lead. Note that only two of the three leads in Eq. (12.2) are independent because the sum of the voltage drops around any closed loop is zero. For example, from Eq. (12.2), we can readily verify that:

$$
V_{\mathrm{II}} = V_{\mathrm{I}} + V_{\mathrm{III}}
\tag{12.3}
$$

In ECG triggering, we often have the option of selecting lead I, II, or III to obtain the best waveform. Physically, each lead corresponds to a projection of the electric dipole vector onto a side of the Einthoven triangle. Alternatively, we can use information from two leads simultaneously to extract the magnitude and direction of the electric dipole vector. This is called a vectorcardiogram (VCG) and has proved useful in rejecting false triggers from arrhythmia (Chia et al. 2000).

Peripheral Triggering   The setup time to attach electrodes to the patient for ECG-triggering can be appreciable. As an alternative, cardiac triggers can be detected with a peripheral monitor. As its name suggests, this device is attached to the periphery of the body, for example, to a finger, toe, or earlobe. Peripheral monitors do not measure electrical activity but rather the optical properties of the blood (Shellock and Kanal 1996).

There are two main types of peripheral monitors. The most commonly used is the *cutaneous blood flow meter*, which measures blood flow through the capillary bed by detecting the Doppler frequency shift of reflected light. The other class, known as *pulse oximeters*, is widely used in anesthesiology, but can be used as triggering devices as well. Pulse oximeters measure the attenuation of transmitted laser light. The use of two different wavelengths of light (e.g., 650 and 805 nm) and proper calibration allows the determination of the percent oxygenation of the blood.

Due to delays in pressure wave propagation, the systolic pulse at the finger or toe is not simultaneous with the contraction of the left ventricle. Consequently the triggers detected with peripheral monitors are usually not synchronized with the ECG waveform and can have substantially different delays depending on where the probe is attached. Also the width of the peak of the waveform detected with peripheral monitors is much broader than that detected with ECG-waveforms, leading to imprecision in the triggering time. Still, the convenience of peripheral monitors makes them popular, particularly for neurological applications requiring triggering, such as, the cross R-R cardiac triggering described in Section 11.5.

12.1.2 PULSE SEQUENCE CONSIDERATIONS

When a valid trigger is detected, real-time information is provided to the pulse sequence controller. Usually the trigger can be considered an external event—whether it was detected from an ECG waveform or peripheral pulse is not important. How the trigger is used, however, depends on whether the pulse sequence is *prospectively triggered* or *retrospectively gated*. For example, segmented k-space cardiac acquisition (discussed in Section 11.5) uses prospective triggering, whereas the CINE acquisition is retrospectively gated.

Prospectively triggered ECG pulse sequences divide the R-R interval into several subintervals (Figure 12.4). The time when the pulse sequence is waiting for and will accept a valid trigger is called the *trigger window* (TW). The trigger

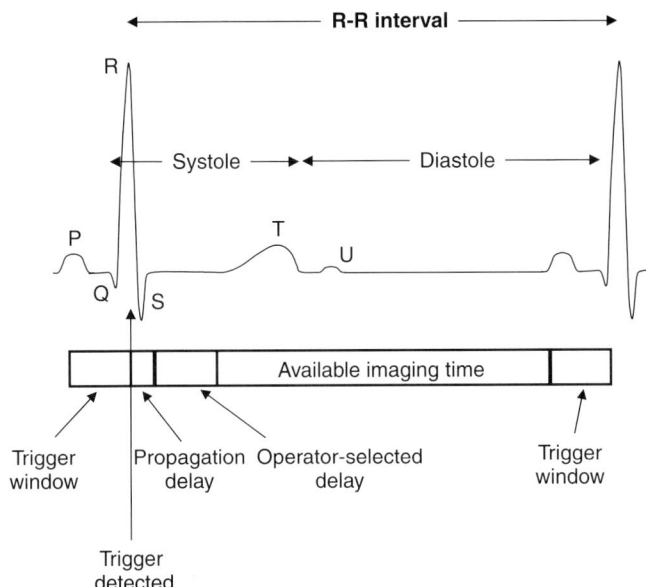

FIGURE 12.4 In a prospectively triggered ECG pulse sequence, the R-R interval is divided into several subintervals. The pulse sequences are played during the available imaging time.

window closes when a valid trigger is detected. The time between the triggering event and the confirmation that a valid trigger has been detected is called the *hardware delay* or the *propagation delay* (PD). The propagation delay can include delays from digital signal processing, including noise filtering and other processing such as calculating the VCG from multiple leads. The smaller the PD the better. Typically the amount of calculation is restricted to keep the PD under 10 ms.

The *operator-selected delay* (OSD) is the next subinterval in the R-R. If the goal is to maximize acquisition efficiency, then zero is selected for the OSD. A nonzero value of the OSD is often chosen to restrict the acquisition to diastole, when the heart muscle is more quiescent.

The remainder of the R-R interval for a prospectively triggered pulse sequence is the *available imaging time* (AIT). This is the interval when the triggered ECG pulse sequences can play out gradient and RF waveforms and acquire MR data. The longer the AIT the better. From Figure 12.4 and the preceding discussion:

$$\text{AIT} = \text{RR} - \text{PD} - \text{OSD} - \text{TW} \tag{12.4}$$

where RR is the duration of the R-R interval calculated in Eq. (12.1). After the AIT, the trigger window opens again, and the cycle repeats until the end of the scan.

Typically the trigger window is selected by the operator to be 5–20% of the duration of average R-R interval. According to Eq. (12.4), a longer trigger window reduces AIT. If, however, the heart rate increases during the scan and the trigger window is too short, then the next QRS complex will occur during the AIT before the trigger window is open, resulting in a *missed beat*, as well as possible motion contamination in the acquired data. The trigger window will remain open throughout that next R-R interval and trigger off the following QRS complex. To a listener, a missed beat sounds like a long gap in the rhythm of the gradient's acoustic noise. (With some ECG systems, the trigger signal is converted to audible tone, so a missed trigger can be easily heard that way as well.) The acquisition is prolonged by the product of the number of missed beats and the duration of an R-R interval. If a scan contains many missed beats, it indicates that the trigger window is too narrow.

Occasionally the pulse sequence is too long to fit into the AIT given by Eq. (12.4). In that case, we can increase the AIT by intentionally triggering less frequently than every heart beat. If we trigger off every nth QRS complex ($n = 2, 3, \ldots$) then the available imaging time becomes:

$$\text{AIT} = n\,\text{RR} - \text{PD} - \text{OSD} - \text{TW} \qquad (12.5)$$

Although this procedure increases the available imaging time, it usually prolongs the total scan time compared to triggering every heartbeat. Also, triggering less frequently than every heartbeat increases the chance of image artifacts, especially in the presence of arrhythmia.

An alternative approach to triggering less frequently than every QRS complex is to prospectively estimate when the next trigger(s) would occur based on the current heart rate. For example, when the heart rate is ∼80 bpm, the QRS complex is predicted to occur 750 ms, 1500 ms, 2250 ms, and so on after a trigger is detected. Based on this prediction, acquisition will proceed immediately after the trigger, as well as at delays of 750 ms, 1500 ms, and 2250 ms. If the pulse sequence fits within a single R-R interval, this method can be used to acquire data from multiple views or slice locations. This triggering method can reduce variability in TR, which can be advantageous for quantitative imaging, such as T_1 mapping. Its primary drawback is that the QRS complex and data acquisition can easily get out of synch with a large number (e.g., three or more) of skipped triggers, especially in the presence of arrhythmia.

In retrospective gating (also called retrospective triggering), pulse sequences are continually played while the time stamps of the ECG triggers are stored along with the raw data. Consequently the trigger window remains open throughout the entire scan. The ECG triggers are used to accept, reject, or interpolate data, for example as used in the CINE phase contrast method (Pelc et al. 1991).

An algorithm called *arrhythmia rejection* is frequently used with retrospective gating. For example if two detected triggers are separated in time by much less than the nominal R-R interval given by Eq. (12.1), the algorithm can assume that either a false trigger (e.g., from gradient noise) was detected or that the patient experienced an arrhythmia. In either case, the raw data associated with that time interval can be discarded and reacquired.

12.1.3 PRACTICAL CONSIDERATIONS

Reliable ECG triggering is difficult to obtain on some patients. Often elderly patients or patients with cardiovascular disorders produce low-amplitude ECG waveforms from which reliable triggers are difficult to extract. In this sense, ECG triggering is the opposite of gradient moment nulling, which is often least effective on young healthy patients who generally have the strongest pulsatile flow. When using the ECG hardware, it is important to follow the manufacturer's recommendations, which often include details about electrode pad placement and patient's skin condition. Normally the skin should be dry and shaved if necessary. It also may be helpful to prepare the patient's skin with a mildly abrasive cleanser. If the electrodes contain an electrolyte gel to aid electrical conductivity, they should be inspected prior to placement to ensure that they have not dried out.

On some patients reliable ECG triggers can be obtained outside the MRI scanner, but are more difficult to obtain during the acquisition. Figure 12.5a shows the ECG trace of a healthy volunteer outside the magnet. When the volunteer is brought inside the field (a cylindrical-bore 1.5-T magnet in this case), the ECG waveform is distorted (Figure 12.5b). This distortion is due to surface potentials arising from Lorentz force (named after Hendrik Antoon Lorentz, 1853–1928, a Dutch physicist) $\vec{F}$ on ions in the flowing blood in the magnetic field $\vec{B}_0$:

$$\vec{F} = q\,\vec{v} \times \vec{B}_0 \qquad (12.6)$$

where $\vec{v}$ is the velocity of the blood. Ions of opposite charge q are deflected in opposite directions, which sets up an electric field. (This is analogous to the Hall effect in metals, which is explained in most college-level general physics texts. The effect is named after Edwin Herbert Hall, 1855–1938, an American physicist.) The net result of this electric field is to create a surface potential that distorts the ECG waveform. Because the T wave is usually the most severely distorted, this effect is sometimes called the *elevated T wave*. As can be seen from the vector cross product in Eq. (12.6), the amount of ECG distortion increases with the strength of the main magnetic field B_0.

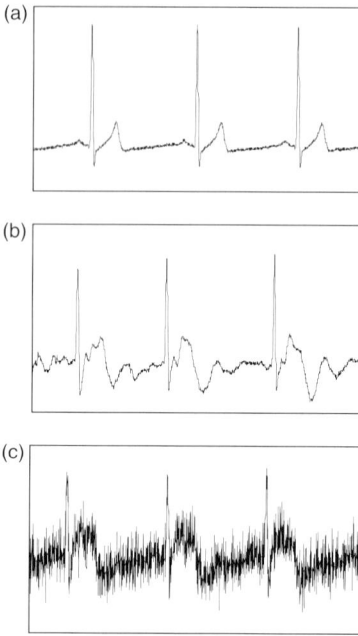

FIGURE 12.5 ECG waveforms from lead II of a healthy volunteer with heart rate of 50 bpm. (a) The volunteer is outside the main magnetic field, and a good ECG waveform is obtained. (b) The volunteer is inside the 1.5-T B_0 field, leading to an elevated T wave and other distortion. (c) During application of the imaging gradients the ECG waveform is further distorted. (Courtesy of Kiaran McGee, Ph.D., Mayo Clinic College of Medicine.)

The ECG waveform is further distorted when the imaging pulse sequence begins and gradient waveforms are activated (Figure 12.5c). This is because the changing magnetic field associated with gradient slewing induces spurious voltage in conducting wires that carry the ECG voltage signal from the electrodes to the processing hardware outside the magnet. The use of fiber optic (Amoore and Ridgeway 1989) or wireless links can minimize the length of the conducting cables and greatly reduce this distortion.

Many filtering methods have been applied to the ECG waveform to improve the extraction of reliable triggers (Rokey et al. 1988; Kreger and Giordano 1995). *Adaptive filtering* is a digital signal-processing method that is also used to reduce the gradient noise on the ECG waveform (Rokey et al. 1988). The concept behind adaptive filtering is that the pulse sequence controls the gradients, so it has detailed knowledge about the shape and timing of those waveforms. The inputs to each of three physical gradient waveforms are sent to hardware that processes the ECG signal, where they are used as a noise reference to help provide a cleaner ECG waveform. In the method described in Kreger and Giordano (1995), the gradient signals are individually differentiated and low-pass filtered. The resulting signal is then input to a digital filter that has adjustable coefficients. The output of the filter is subtracted from the ECG signal.

Because of the distortions caused by the B_0 and gradient magnetic fields, the ECG trace generally should not be used for diagnostic purposes or for physiological monitoring (other than triggering). It should be assumed that the waveform distortion masks subtleties that are apparent on a diagnostic ECG waveform, such as Q waves and the QRS duration.

The RF field can cause heating of conducting wires. In addition to picking up spurious voltage signals from gradient slewing, conducting wires used to carry ECG signals have also caused patient burns (Dempsey and Condon 2001) during MRI exams. Burns have also been reported with the use of pulse oximeters that have conducting cables. The use of fiber optic links or high-impedance carbon fiber cables can reduce the likelihood of burns. (The fiber optic cable itself does not conduct electricity, so it does not heat up at all.) Again, it is important to follow the manufacturer's recommendations, which often include not looping any conducting cables and also keeping them away from the bore wall where the RF electric field tends to be highest when the RF body coil is used for transmission.

Peripheral pulse monitoring tends to be less challenging for the operator than ECG triggering. The patient setup time is much shorter, and most patients produce a usable signal. A common exception occurs when the patient wears opaque nail polish that blocks the light, but that can usually be removed easily. Because the triggers obtained with peripheral pulse monitoring are delayed relative to the electrical activity of the heart, it is not the primary choice for cardiac imaging. Often peripheral triggering serves as a backup when a good ECG signal cannot be obtained. As long as the heart rate is constant, any delays in the peripheral triggers relative to the ECG are not especially problematic. If, however, the patient experiences arrhythmia, cardiac images usually contain artifacts when peripheral triggering is used. This is because the delayed peripheral trigger is not truly a real-time monitor but rather provides information about a previous heartbeat.

SELECTED REFERENCES

Amoore, J. N., and Ridgeway, J. P. 1989. A system for cardiac and respiratory gating of a magnetic resonance imager. *Clin. Phys. Physiol. Meas.* 10: 283–286.

Chia, J. M., Fischer, S. E., Wickline, S. A., and Lorenz, C. H. 2000. Performance of QRS detection for cardiac MRI with a novel vectorcardiographic triggering method. *J. Magn. Reson.* 12: 678–688.

Dempsey, M. F., and Condon, B. 2001. Thermal injuries associated with MRI. *Clin. Radiol.* 56: 457–465.

Di Bernardo, D., and Murray, A. 2002. Origin on the ECG of U-waves and abnormal U-wave inversion. *Cardiovasc. Res.* 53: 202–208.

Gatehouse, P. D., and Firmin, D. N. 2000. The cardiovascular MR machine: Hardware and software requirements. *Herz* 25: 317–330.

Kreger, K. S., and Giordano, C. R. 1995. Bio-potential signal processor for MRI. U.S. patent 5,436,564.

Lanzer, P., Barta, C., Botvinick, E. H., Wiesendanger, H. U., Modin, G., and Higgins, C. B. 1985. ECG-synchronized cardiac MRI: Method and evaluation. *Radiology* 155: 681–686.

Malmivuo, J., and Plonsey, R. 1995. *Bioelectromagnetism: Principles and applications of bioelectric and biomagnetic fields.* New York: Oxford University Press.

Pelc, N. J., Herfkens, R. J., Shimakawa, A., and Enzmann, D. R. 1991. Phase contrast cine magnetic resonance imaging. *Magn. Reson. Q.* 7: 229–254.

Rokey, R., Wendt, R. E., and Johnston, D. L. 1988. Monitoring of acutely ill patients during nuclear MRI: Use of a time-varying filter ECG gating device to reduce gradient artifacts. *Magn. Reson. Med.* 6: 240–245.

Shellock, F. G., and Kanal, E. 1996. *MR bioeffects, safety, and patient management,* 2nd ed. Philadelphia: Lippincott-Raven.

Yuan, Q., Axel, L., Hernandez, E. H., Dougherty, L., Pilla, J. J., Scott, C. H., Ferrari, V. A., and Blom, A. S. 2000. Cardiac-respiratory gating method for magnetic resonance imaging of the heart. *Magn. Reson. Med.* 43: 314–318.

12.2 Navigators

Patient motion is a common source of MRI artifacts, including ghosting, blurring and image misregistration. Examples of patient motion include large-scale motion (sometimes called bulk motion), cardiac motion, respiration, gastrointestinal peristalsis, blood flow, CSF flow, and brain motion due to CSF pulsations. Bulk motion artifacts can sometimes be reduced by using patient restraints (common in fMRI studies). Fiducial markers can be used for dynamic scan plane tracking and retrospective bulk motion correction (Korin et al. 1995; Derbyshire et al. 1998), but the technique has never become widely used in clinical practice. Blood flow effects can be reduced by use of pulse sequences with gradient moment nulling (Section 10.4) (i.e., flow compensation). Blood flow, cardiac motion, and CSF pulsation artifacts can be reduced or eliminated using cardiac triggering (Section 12.1). Respiration artifacts can be reduced using ultrafast imaging, breath-holding, respiratory gating, or respiratory phase encode reordering (Section 12.3). However, uncooperative patients may induce large bulk motion artifacts and make breath-holding problematic. Even with cooperative patients and careful breath-holding, small amounts of residual motion can create substantial artifacts.

There are several different types of motion that corrupt MR images. For most pulse sequences, *interview motion* (motion between views) is a bigger problem than *intraview motion* (motion within a view). For multishot diffusion-weighted imaging (DWI), the large diffusion-weighting gradients at each shot create substantial phase errors if motion occurs during their application. This is called *intrashot motion*. Variation in the phase errors among shots creates image artifacts. For multishot DWI, intrashot motion is usually the dominant source of motion artifacts.

Navigators (or *navigator echoes*) are a method to monitor and correct motion artifacts (Ehman and Felmlee 1989). A navigator acquires a partial set of k-space data that is processed to track one or more effects of patient motion, for example, head translation and rotation or diaphragm position. The navigator echoes are interleaved within the normal acquisition of the image data. A key assumption in the use of navigators is that negligible motion takes place between the navigator and the acquired view(s) to be corrected.

The navigator data are used either prospectively or retrospectively. In *prospective* correction, the navigator data are used to modify the subsequent imaging acquisition to prevent artifacts. *Retrospective* navigator data are used to correct the image or raw data after the scan is completed. Prospective correction requires sufficient real-time processing capability to complete any required computations, so that the acquisition of subsequent views can be modified in time. This can limit the complexity of the algorithm or impose a minimum time between the navigator and subsequent imaging acquisition.

The choice of navigator and the processing method both depend on the specific application. In the following discussion, we consider general methods for navigator acquisition and processing and the methods to correct motion using the navigator results. Additional details for the use of navigators in cardiac imaging (Firmin and Keegan 2001), fMRI (Ward et al. 2000), and diffusion-weighted imaging (Norris 2001) are then given. Although these are the most common applications, navigators have also been used for motion correction in spectroscopy (Thiel et al. 2002), microscopy (Song and Wehrli 1999), and arterial spin tagging (Spuentrup et al. 2002); for real-time shim adjustment (Ward et al. 2002); and for B_0-shift correction (Hinks et al. 2001). Navigators are also used to monitor signals in dynamic studies and bolus arrival in contrast-enhanced angiography. The discussion of navigators in this section is limited to motion monitoring and correction.

12.2.1 Rigid Body Motion

Before discussing navigator pulse sequences and processing, let us briefly review the effects of motion on MRI data. In some applications, especially for head imaging, both interview and intraview patient motion can be modeled as rigid body motion, consisting of a translation plus a rotation. According to the Fourier shift theorem, a displacement of the object by vector distance $\vec{T}$ results in motion-corrupted raw data $S_m(\vec{k})$ given by:

$$S_m(\vec{k}) = S_s(\vec{k})e^{i2\pi\vec{k}\cdot\vec{T}}$$
(12.7)

where $S_s(\vec{k})$ is the data for a stationary object. Interview translation therefore results in k-space data that has a linear phase shift that is proportional to the object translation distance.

Consider a rotation whose axis passes through the center of the imaging volume. Interview rotation of the object rotates the k-space data about the same rotation axis and by the same rotation angle as the object. In a 2D acquisition, the rotation- and translation- corrupted k-space data $S_m(k, \theta)$ are given in polar coordinates (k, θ) by (Ward et al. 2000):

$$S_m(k, \theta) = S_s(k, \theta - \alpha)e^{i2\pi k(x_0 \cos\theta + y_0 \sin\theta)}$$
(12.8)

where α is the rotation angle and (x_0, y_0) are the coordinates of any translation that might have occurred. The magnitude of the k-space data is thus affected only by rotation, whereas the phase is affected by both rotation and translation. Rotations whose axes do not pass through the center of the imaging volume can be expressed as a three-step process: translation to register the rotation axis with the image center, rotation, and translation back. The net effect of the two additional translations will modify, but can be absorbed into, parameters (x_0, y_0) in Eq. (12.8) (Lee et al. 1998).

The effects of rigid body motion in multishot DWI are dominated by intrashot motion due to the large diffusion-weighting gradients and typically have a negligible contribution from the imaging gradients. These effects are somewhat different than the ones already discussed. For intrashot motion with DWI, the corrupted raw data $S_m(\vec{k})$ are given by (Anderson and Gore 1994):

$$S_m(\vec{k}) = S_s(\vec{k} + \Delta\vec{k})e^{i\phi}$$
(12.9)

The phase ϕ (in radians) and k-space shift $\Delta\vec{k}$ are given by:

$$\phi = \gamma \int \left(\vec{G}_d \cdot \vec{T}\right) dt$$
(12.10)

and, for small-angle rotations:

$$\Delta \vec{k} = \frac{\gamma}{2\pi} \int \left(\vec{G}_d \times \vec{\Theta} \right) dt \qquad (12.11)$$

where $\vec{G}_d(t)$ is the diffusion-sensitizing gradient (negated in sign by an odd number of subsequent refocusing RF pulses). $\vec{T}(t)$ is the object translation vector, and $\vec{\Theta}(t)$ is a vector that points in the direction of the rotation axis and whose magnitude equals the rotation angle (in radians).

12.2.2 Navigator Data Acquisition and Processing

Navigators can use 1D, 2D, or 3D k-space trajectories. The simplest navigator is a 1D or *linear* navigator (Ehman and Felmlee 1989), which acquires one line of data passing through the origin of k-space (Figure 12.6a), usually along the k_x, k_y, or k_z axis. The RF excitation pulse for a linear navigator can excite a column, a slice, or a thick slab of spins. Note that linear navigators are the same as the 1D projections that are sometimes used as reference acquisitions for echo train pulse sequences (see Section 10.3). The Fourier

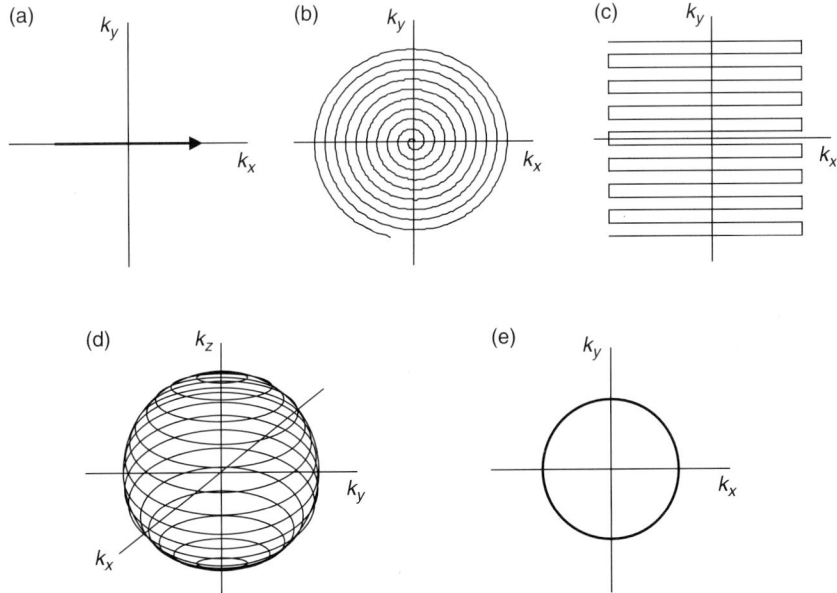

FIGURE 12.6 k-space trajectories for (a) linear, (b) 2D spiral, (c) 2D EPI, (d) 3D spherical, and (e) 2D orbital navigators.

transformation of the navigator data is a projection orthogonal to the navigator readout gradient direction. A linear navigator allows object translation in the navigator readout direction to be monitored during the scan.

The linear navigator data can be processed in several ways to determine the object translation. The most common methods are correlation and least-squares fitting. In the correlation method, the estimated object translation distance d maximizes:

$$c(d) = \sum_j \left| P_n(x_j - d) \right| \left| P_r(x_j) \right| \tag{12.12}$$

where $P_n(x_j)$ is the complex navigator projection (Fourier transform of the navigator raw data) for the current view and $P_r(x_j)$ is the projection of a reference navigator, usually acquired at the beginning of the scan. The sum in Eq. (12.12) is usually taken over a subset of the projection containing the highest signal or desired edges (e.g., the diaphragm).

In the least-squares method the estimated object displacement d minimizes:

$$l(d) = \sum_j \left(\left| P_n(x_j - d) \right| - \left| P_r(x_j) \right| \right)^2 \tag{12.13}$$

where, again, the sum is usually taken over an appropriate subset of the projection. Least-squares fitting can be preferable if the navigator SNR is low (Wang et al. 1996), for example, because of a short TR.

Depending on the available computer hardware, the calculations in Eqs. (12.12) and (12.13) used for prospective navigators can lead to delays of the subsequent data acquisition. This has led to the development of faster alternative algorithms (Foo and King 1999; Thanh et al. 2001).

2D navigators (Figure 12.6b–c) acquire data over a small region near the center of k-space. They are sometimes used in DWI studies (Butts et al. 1997; Atkinson et al. 2000) to monitor shifts of the origin of k-space, as well as the average phase of the data (see Eq. 12.9). The shift can be computed by calculating the centroid of the k-space data.

Although consecutive linear navigators in three directions can track any general translation, they cannot efficiently track rotation. Complete tracking of rotation and translation in three directions can be achieved using a *spherical navigator*. The k-space trajectory traces all or part of the surface of a sphere (Figure 12.6d). Interview rotations of the object result in rotations of the data on the navigator sphere, whereas translations of the object shift the phase of the navigator data (without rotating it). One implementation uses a helical trajectory that covers the sphere in two interleaves, with each covering a hemisphere starting at the equator (Welch et al. 2002).

An alternative to a spherical navigator is a set of *orbital navigators* (Figure 12.6e), each using a circular k-space trajectory (Fu et al. 1995). An orbital navigator can track translations and rotations in two dimensions (i.e., in a plane). By applying three orbital navigators in different planes, translation and rotation in all three dimensions can be monitored (Ward et al. 2000). The slice thickness of the multiple orbital navigators should be wide enough to encompass the entire object, otherwise saturation bands from the initial navigator can corrupt the signal from subsequent navigators, making motion detection difficult.

One disadvantage of orbital navigators compared to spherical navigators is that translation and rotation out of the plane formed by the two navigator gradient directions are difficult to track. Such motion corrupts the navigator data, giving slightly inaccurate in-plane motion estimates. When a prospective correction is used, this drawback can be overcome by rotating and translating the navigator scan plane as predicted by one set of navigators and then repeating the navigators a second time, giving a total of six navigators prior to the imaging acquisition (Ward et al. 2000). This reduces the through-plane motion for the second set of navigators and gives an improved estimate of the object position, which is then used to translate and rotate the plane a second time prior to the imaging acquisition.

For either spherical or orbital navigators, the optimal radius of the sphere or circle represents a compromise between sensitivity and SNR. The larger the radius, the larger the distance a k-space location moves for a given rotation angle and hence the greater its sensitivity to motion. However, because k-space signal intensity typically decreases away from the center of k-space, the larger the radius, the lower the k-space SNR. Typically the k-space radius of orbital or spherical navigators is on the order of $10 \, \Delta k$, where $\Delta k = 1/L$ is the distance between k-space samples for a FOV L. The optimal value has been found to depend on the scan plane and the object (Ward et al. 2000).

For orbital navigators, the rotation angle can be determined from the navigator magnitude using either correlation or least-squares fitting. For example, with least-squares fitting the estimated rotation angle α minimizes:

$$l(\alpha) = \sum_j \left(\left| S_n(k_\rho, \theta_j - \alpha) \right| - \left| S_r(k_\rho, \theta_j) \right| \right)^2 \qquad (12.14)$$

where $S_n(k_\rho, \theta_j)$ and $S_r(k_\rho, \theta_j)$ now represent k-space data acquired over a circle of radius k_ρ for the orbital navigator and reference navigator, respectively. The summation in Eq. (12.14) is taken over the circle of data in the k-space trajectory. Once α is determined, the translation components x_0 and y_0 are determined from the difference between the navigator and reference phases. The reference navigator is first rotated by α to line up with the current navigator; otherwise the phase difference would also contain a contribution due to rotation. Let $\psi_n(k_\rho, \theta)$ and $\psi_r(k_\rho, \theta - \alpha)$ be the phase of the current navigator and rotated reference navigators, respectively. From Eq. (12.8), the phase difference is:

$$\Delta\psi_j = \psi_n(k_\rho, \theta_j) - \psi_r(k_\rho, \theta_j - \alpha)$$
$$= 2\pi k_\rho \left[x_0 \cos(\theta_j - \alpha) + y_0 \sin(\theta_j - \alpha) \right] \tag{12.15}$$

The sine and cosine terms in Eq. (12.15) are orthogonal, and can be determined from:

$$x_0 = \frac{1}{k_\rho} \frac{2}{N_\rho} \sum_j \Delta\psi_j \cos(\theta_j - \alpha) \tag{12.16}$$

and

$$y_0 = \frac{1}{k_\rho} \frac{2}{N_\rho} \sum_j \Delta\psi_j \sin(\theta_j - \alpha) \tag{12.17}$$

where N_ρ is the number of points used in the summation.

Navigator RF excitation is usually spatially selective and can be read out using either a gradient or spin echo (Figure 12.7). However, in many cases the navigator does not require a separate RF excitation but can simply use the transverse magnetization excited by the imaging RF pulse, either before or after the imaging echo is acquired. In Figure 12.8, the transverse magnetization used for the imaging spin echo is rephased by a refocusing pulse and used as the subsequent navigator.

Navigators can be acquired multiple times for each k-space line or segment of k-space. For example, linear navigators in several directions or orbital navigators in several planes can be acquired for each k_y line of the imaging scan. To reduce the total repetition time of the navigator plus imaging acquisition, multiple navigators are sometimes acquired *cyclically*. For example, a linear navigator might be alternated between the k_x and k_y axes. This has the drawback of somewhat reducing the temporal resolution of both navigators.

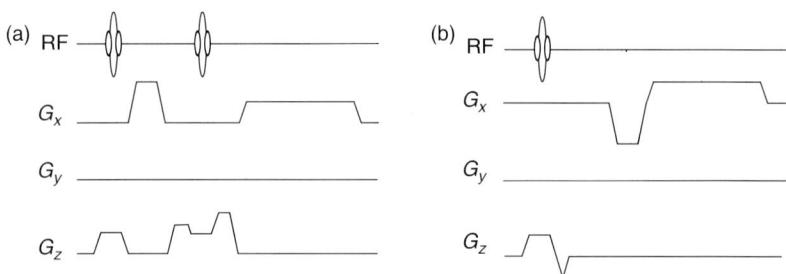

FIGURE 12.7   Linear navigators that excite a plane using (a) spin echo and (b) gradient pulse sequences.

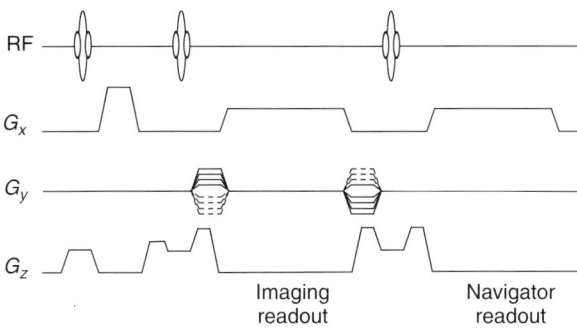

FIGURE 12.8 Spin-echo pulse sequence with a subsequent linear navigator. The transverse magnetization used for imaging is refocused and re-used for the navigator.

12.2.3 MOTION CORRECTION

Prospective Correction Navigator information can be used in numerous ways. *Prospective gating* leaves the scan volume fixed with respect to the magnet and gates the acquisition to achieve consistent anatomical location with respect to the scan volume. This method is used in cardiac imaging and works only with smooth periodic motion such as respiration, for which it can be assumed that the anatomy repeatedly moves through the scan volume.

Slice following (also called slice tracking) is used with either periodic or nonperiodic motion and moves the scan volume to lie at approximately the same location with respect to the patient anatomy on each acquisition. (Although the name implies 2D acquisition, slice following can also be used with 3D acquisition.) This method is used in cardiac imaging and fMRI.

Phase reordering methods (also known as view reordering, discussed in Section 12.3) modify the data acquisition order (k_y or, in 3D scans, k_z lines) in real time based on navigator data to yield a k-space data set that is more consistent with respect to the respiratory phase. The same phase reordering algorithms that are used with respiratory bellows can be used with navigators (see Section 12.3). For some phase reordering methods, all or part of k-space is sampled multiple times. For these methods, data acquisition is stopped, either after a fixed amount of time or when the data are sufficiently consistent according to the particular criterion employed. (The application of cardiac imaging is discussed later.)

Retrospective Correction Several general retrospective methods can be used. In the first method, each k_y or k_z line is acquired a fixed number of times (e.g., five) and is also interleaved with navigator acquisitions. After the scan completes, the navigator data are used to sort the acquisitions. Only the data from the most consistent anatomical positions are retained and used in image reconstruction.

In a second retrospective method, the navigator information is used to correct the data during reconstruction. Translation can be corrected retrospectively by multiplying the k-space data by a phase factor (see Eqs. 12.7 and 12.9). For the case of interview motion without diffusion weighting, the factor is $e^{-i2\pi \vec{k} \cdot \vec{T}}$, where $\vec{T}$ is the translation distance. For the case of DWI, the k-space data are multiplied by $e^{-i\phi}$, where ϕ is given by Eq. (12.10).

Retrospective correction for interview rotation requires remapping the k-space data using gridding or some other interpolation method. For the case of interview rotation without diffusion weighting, the remapping is a rotation of the k-space data. Depending on the acquisition technique used and the rotation axis, remapping of k-space according to the navigator data may result in regions of k-space devoid of data. With multishot DWI, the remapping is a shift by $\Delta \vec{k}$ for each shot, where $\Delta \vec{k}$ is given by Eq. (12.11). Although the shift by $\Delta \vec{k}$ could be done with a linear phase ramp in image space, this would require the reconstruction of separate images for each shot and is less convenient than performing the shift in k-space using gridding. Rotational motion correction is therefore best done prospectively. Another disadvantage of retrospective correction is that rotation or translation orthogonal to the scan plane is not possible with 2D data sets.

In dynamic imaging by model estimation (DIME) the temporally varying object $I(\vec{r}, t)$ is represented by a generalized harmonic model (Liang et al. 1997) as:

$$I(\vec{r}, t) = \sum_{m=1}^{M} a_m(\vec{r})\, e^{i2\pi f_m t} \qquad (12.18)$$

where $\{f_m\}$ is the set of all possible motion frequencies present over the entire object $(m = 1, 2, \ldots, M)$ and $a_m(\vec{r})$ incorporates the spatial dependence of each frequency. If the motion is periodic, only discrete frequencies are present given by $f_m = m f_0$. If the motion is nonperiodic, the f_m are arbitrary real numbers. In DIME, motion artifacts are thought of as arising from undersampling in a hybrid $(\vec{k}, t)$ space (Figure 12.9). The raw data $S(\vec{k}, t)$ are given by:

$$S(\vec{k}, t) = \int I(\vec{r}, t)\, e^{-i2\pi \vec{k} \cdot \vec{r}}\, d\vec{r} \qquad (12.19)$$

Inserting Eq. (12.18) into Eq. (12.19) gives:

$$S(\vec{k}, t) = \sum_{m=1}^{M} \hat{a}_m(\vec{k})\, e^{i2\pi f_m t} \qquad (12.20)$$

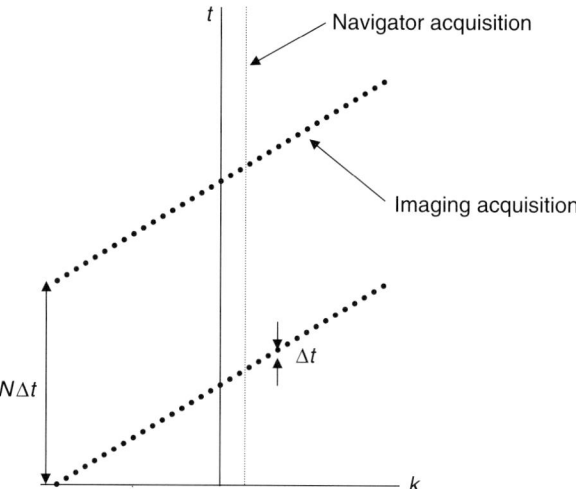

FIGURE 12.9 Simplified (k, t) space with one k-space dimension used for dynamic imaging by model estimation. The imaging scan acquires N points Δt apart to cover the full extent of k-space needed to reconstruct an image. Motion artifacts result from undersampling in the (k, t) space. The navigator acquires points at a single k value with time resolution Δt sufficient to freeze motion. (Adapted from Liang et al. 1997.)

where

$$\hat{a}_m(\vec{k}) = \int a_m(\vec{r}) \, e^{-i2\pi \vec{k} \cdot \vec{r}} d\vec{r} \tag{12.21}$$

Equation (12.20) indicates that $S(\vec{k}, t)$ is also represented by a generalized harmonic model. In DIME, f_m and $\hat{a}_m(\vec{k})$ are estimated and used to construct $S(\vec{k}, t)$ for abitrary time t using Eq. (12.20). The resulting image reconstructed by the Fourier transformation of $S(\vec{k}, t)$ has reduced artifacts.

The f_m can be estimated from ECG or respiration waveforms or from Nyquist-sampled $(\vec{k}, t)$ data that are collected with a navigator. The simplified 1D example in Figure 12.9 shows navigator data collected at a single point k, but with temporal sampling Δt that is much higher than the complete k-space temporal sampling interval $N \Delta t$ (where N is the number of imaging k-space points acquired).

Once the f_m are known, $\hat{a}_m(\vec{k})$ can be estimated using undersampled imaging measurements $S(\vec{k}, t)$. The estimation fits $S(\vec{k}, t)$ values measured with an imaging pulse sequence by writing Eq. (12.20) in matrix form and inverting to obtain $\hat{a}_m(\vec{k})$ (Liang et al. 1997).

12.2.4 CARDIAC IMAGING

Although ECG triggering removes the effects of cardiac motion, respiration also substantially changes the heart position. The acquisition is usually short enough with 2D scans that breath-holding can be used to eliminate artifacts due to respiration. However, 3D acquisition is sometimes preferable, particularly for coronary artery imaging. The coronary arteries are tortuous and move throughout the cardiac cycle, making them difficult to capture in a single imaging plane. 3D scans allow higher resolution and SNR, and make it easier to image the entire coronary artery tree. Unfortunately 3D scans may be too long (>20 s) to use breath-holding with many patients. Multiple breath-holds typically have as much as 8 mm in variation in diaphragm position (Liu et al. 1993), resulting in poor image quality with 3D scans because of the resulting inconsistency in cardiac position (Wang, Riederer, et al. 1995).

Even with 2D breath-held acquisitions, multiple breath-holds may be required to cover the entire coronary tree. Although each 2D scan is self-consistent, variation in breath-holding can result in slightly different coronary artery positions on each scan. This can lead to gaps in the coverage of the coronary artery tree. Navigators can give more consistent positioning of the arteries and reduce gaps.

Navigator tracking of the diaphragm position has been used to create a respiration feedback monitor (Liu et al. 1993; Wang, Grimm, et al. 1995). In this method, the diaphragm position calculated in real time from navigator data on each heartbeat is displayed visually to the patient, allowing the patient to give more consistent breath-holds during the scan. Unfortunately, respiration feedback only works with cooperative patients and therefore has not been used extensively.

Navigators are often used to gate data acquisition to a quiescent part of the respiratory cycle, thus allowing free breathing during the scan. Most commonly, a linear navigator acquires data along a column in the superior-inferior (SI) direction through the diaphragm. Diaphragm position along the SI direction is quantified and used to determine the respiratory phase. Acquisition during the same respiratory phase over multiple respiratory cycles provides consistent heart positioning.

Pulse Sequence and Processing   A linear navigator excites a 1 to 2-cm-wide column of spins in the SI direction, which is then read out along the column. Spatial resolution along the column is approximately 1 mm. One method for the 2D excitation uses a spin echo with the two slice selection gradients chosen so that their respective slices intersect (Figure 12.10a and Section 5.1), resulting in a rectangular column of refocused spins in the intersecting area (also called a line scan pulse sequence). The spin-echo method

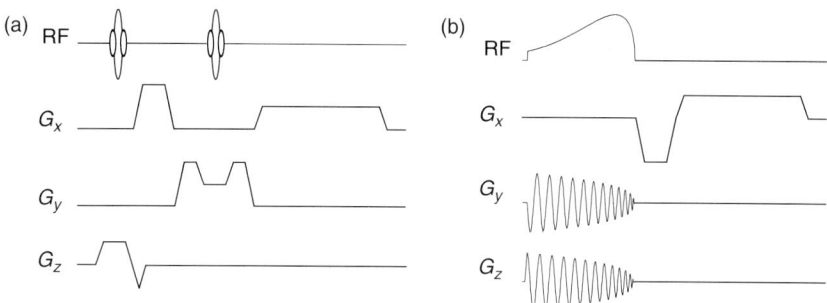

FIGURE 12.10 Linear navigators that excite a column using (a) a spin echo with orthogonal planes for the excitation and refocusing pulses and (b) a spiral k-space trajectory.

can result in saturated bands in the image if one of the navigator planes crosses the imaging plane.

A more common method excites a circular column of spins or 2D pencil beam (see Section 5.1) using a spiral excitation k-space trajectory (Figure 12.10b). The spiral pencil beam creates less extensive saturation artifacts and, if used with a small flip angle, can be repeated with shorter TR than the spin echo. A disadvantage of the spiral pencil beam is flaring of the circular cross section from resonance offsets. The processing methods described previously are used to extract the diaphragm displacement. The sums in Eqs. (12.12) and (12.13) are usually taken over a subset of the projection containing the diaphragm edge.

For prospective use, the navigator is played prior to data acquisition within the same the cardiac cycle. For imaging multiple cardiac phases or acquiring multiple slices per cardiac phase, using more than one navigator within the cardiac cycle can be beneficial (Figure 12.11).

Prospective Gating   Diaphragm location data can be used prospectively in several ways. The simplest is to acquire data only when the respiratory phase is within a predefined acceptance window (accept/reject algorithm). A window location near the end-expiration phase is usually chosen because it is held longer and is found to be somewhat more consistent over time than other phases. The acceptance window width (typically 2–5 mm) and window location are determined from navigator data acquired over a period of free breathing prior to the gated scan. An acceptance window that is too wide results in poor image quality. Conversely, a smaller acceptance window gives better image quality but results in longer scan time to acquire a complete set of data (reduced efficiency). A key assumption in the use of navigators is that the

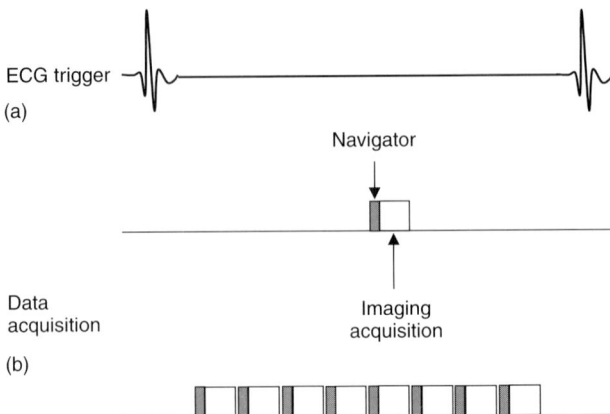

FIGURE 12.11 Navigator placement for cardiac imaging. Shaded boxes represent the navigator pulse sequence. Unshaded boxes represent the imaging pulse sequence that acquires multiple phase encoding steps (k_y or k_z). (a) One navigator and acquisition per cardiac cycle. (b) Eight acquisitions per cardiac cycle (either eight phases or eight slices), each with its own navigator.

respiration pattern is constant throughout the scan. Unfortunately, even with cooperative patients this is sometimes not the case. Inconsistency or drift in the respiratory pattern that moves the acceptance window location over the course of the scan is a significant problem.

Slice Following   Slice following moves the data acquisition volume to follow the anatomy of interest and can be used with 2D or 3D scans that use either free breathing or breath-holding. Combining slice following with prospective respiratory gating allows the gating window width to be increased without loss of image quality, resulting in reduced scan time (Danias et al. 1997).

The coronary arteries move in the SI and anterior-posterior AP directions by roughly 60 and 20% of the diaphragm displacement, respectively (Wang, Riederer, et al. 1995). Left-right (LR) displacement is usually negligible. The scan volume is prospectively moved in the SI and AP directions by a fraction (called a *correction factor*) of the diaphragm SI displacement relative to the center of the window (McConnell et al. 1997). Although generic correction factors can be used, better results are obtained when the correction factors are measured on each patient (Taylor et al. 1999).

Phase Reordering   One method for phase reordering maps the respiratory phase to the k_y line (Section 12.3). The type of mapping determines the type of residual artifact. The mapping can take into account the frequency of each respiratory phase for more efficient scanning. (See Jhooti et al. 1999 for an example.)

A variation of the accept/reject algorithm uses multiple acceptance window widths for different areas of k-space (weighted gating). Narrower windows are used near the center of k-space where consistency is more critical to good image quality. When weighted gating is used, the phase-encoding order can be prospectively chosen to improve the scan efficiency. This forms the basis of motion-adapted gating (MAG), which reduces the scan time by as much as 60% relative to an accept/reject algorithm using a single acceptance window (Weiger et al. 1997). MAG is only applicable to Cartesian k-space trajectories where different RF excitations sample different areas of k-space. Trajectories such as spiral or projection acquisition, which sample low and high spatial frequencies on each excitation, must use a different method. MAG has also been enhanced to incorporate real-time evaluation of the respiratory pattern during the scan. This allows the automatic moving of the acceptance window location or termination of the scan if the respiration pattern changes sufficiently (Sinkus and Boernert 1999).

Another prospective algorithm that attempts to overcome the problem of respiration drift is the diminishing variance algorithm (DVA) (Sachs et al. 1995). In this method, there is a predefined window acceptance width, but no predefined window location. A complete set of k-space data is acquired once without respiratory gating, along with corresponding navigator data. A histogram determines the most frequent diaphragm position (i.e., the mode of the distribution). k-space data along with navigator data are then reacquired beginning with the data farthest from the mode, and the histogram is updated. As time progresses, the range of diaphragm positions becomes narrower. The acquisition progresses for a fixed time or until all the views fall within the same window width. Unfortunately, significant respiratory drift results in very long scans if all data are to lie within the acceptance window. DVA can be used with any k-space trajectory.

Retrospective Respiratory Gating   For retrospective use, navigator placement either before or after the acquisition is possible. k-space is fully sampled several times (e.g., five) without respiratory gating. The corresponding navigator data are acquired along with the imaging data and used to retrospectively determine diaphragm position. The imaging data are sorted based on diaphragm position. In one method (Li et al. 1996), a histogram of diaphragm positions is used to determine the most frequent position. All acquisitions of each k-space location (k_y and k_z) collected within a certain diaphragm window (e.g. ± 1 mm) of this position are used (with averaging if multiple acquisitions are available). If no data are within the window, the closest acquisition is used. Retrospective gating has been found to give inferior image quality compared to prospective gating (Du et al. 2001).

Navigator Placement   Although the entire diaphragm moves in the same direction with respiratory motion, it is not a rigid body. Therefore the motion measured by the navigator strongly depends on where it is placed. In most work, the navigator is placed at the dome of the liver (right hemidiaphragm) because the diaphragm is most perpendicular to the SI direction there.

The navigator may also be placed over the heart itself. The proximity of the navigator and coronary arteries for this placement eliminates the need for slice-following correction factors. A disadvantage is the possibility of greater saturation of the cardiac structures being imaged. Studies of the effect of navigator placement with free-breathing 3D acquisition and slice following show little difference in scan time or image quality scores for placement in the right hemidiaphragm versus the left ventricle (Stuber et al. 1999).

Because respiration causes the heart to move in both the SI and AP directions, multiple linear navigators have been placed over the heart to monitor three directions of motion (Sachs et al. 1998). Multiple navigators result in longer scans, increasing the possibility of drift in the respiratory pattern.

12.2.5 FUNCTIONAL MRI (FMRI)

With fMRI, small head movements can either give a spurious activation or mask real activation. Although single-shot EPI freezes motion within a scan, motion causes the misregistration of images within a time series that results in activation errors. Even though head restraints are typically used, involuntary head motion can still take place even with cooperative patients. In addition to head motion, fMRI is also degraded by apparent activation that correlates with respiratory and cardiac motion.

In one approach to navigated fMRI, the effects of all types of motion (rigid-body head motion, respiration, and cardiac motion) are modeled as general phase and frequency shifts. The shifts are found to be slowly varying over the brain (Noll et al. 1998) and are usually modeled as spatially constant. Early work of this type (Hu and Kim 1994) with a gradient-echo pulse sequence used a single data point from the refocused FID immediately after the excitation to track the phase of the subsequent echo (Figure 12.12). Because activation based on blood oxygen level dependence (BOLD) can change the magnitude of the FID over the course of time, only the phase of the navigator point is used to correct fMRI data. The phase is also measured during a reference navigator acquisition and differences between any other navigator phase and

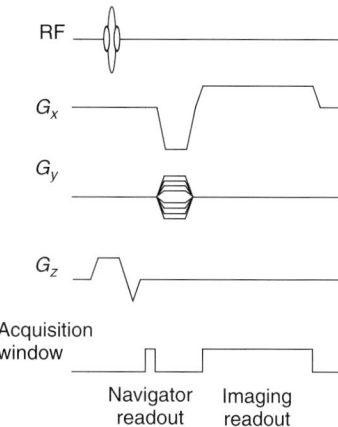

FIGURE 12.12 Gradient-echo pulse sequence using a single refocused FID navigator point (or group of points). The transverse magnetization is subsequently spatially encoded for imaging.

the reference phase are subtracted from the corresponding fMRI data phase. When used with Cartesian k-space trajectories, a separate reference is used for each k_y line.

When used with an interleaved spiral k-space trajectory, the navigator point is simply the first sample point in the spiral readout (Glover and Lai 1998). In this case, no extra data collection is needed and the pulse sequence is effectively self-navigated. A single reference is obtained by averaging the complex signals from each spiral interleaf of the reference time frame. Differences between the navigator phase of each spiral interleaf and the reference phase are removed from the imaging data. Dynamic off-resonance in k-space (DORK) extends this idea, using two navigator measurements per fMRI acquisition (e.g., one immediately after the RF pulse and one at the center of k-space), which allows frequency shifts as well as baseline phase shifts to be corrected (Pfeuffer et al. 2002). Comparison to a reference acquisition allows additional phase shifts due to eddy currents to be removed. This navigation method has been used for both EPI and spiral imaging.

In a somewhat different approach, navigators have been used to track head motion. Head motion is usually modeled as rigid body motion, consisting of a translation plus a rotation. Early work used linear navigators to measure head translation (Lee et al. 1996), but recent work uses orbital or spherical navigators to measure both rotation and translation. A prospective correction is preferable and requires rotating and shifting the imaging plane before the subsequent fMRI acquisition (Ward et al. 2000).

12.2.6 Diffusion-Weighted Imaging

DWI frequently uses single-shot EPI to minimize the effects of patient motion. Single-shot EPI suffers from low spatial resolution, geometric distortion, and low SNR, however. Although multishot (usually interleaved) EPI has much less distortion, patient motion results in severe image artifacts. The artifacts are a result of intrashot motion effects described previously (a phase error and shift in the center of k-space) that are inconsistent between shots. (Intrashot motion is also present in single-shot DW-EPI, but the resulting phase error and k-space shift are constant and thus do not cause artifacts.)

Navigators are sometimes used with multishot DWI methods (including both EPI and FSE) to minimize motion artifacts. As with f MRI, head motion is modeled as rigid body motion. Brain motion from pulsatile CSF flow caused by the beating of the heart is not rigid body motion. Although this motion is usually negligible for anatomical brain imaging, the extreme motion sensitivity introduced by the diffusion-weighting gradients causes it to be a substantial problem from 100 to 300 ms after systole (Norris 2001). (Although CSF itself does not always create a signal in DWI, CSF pulsation causes brain motion that creates artifacts affecting other brain tissues.) DWI navigator methods therefore work best if ECG triggering is also used to reduce nonrigid body motion associated with cardiac pulsatility. Even with navigators and ECG triggering, acceptable image quality may be difficult to achieve until shortly after end-systole.

Any navigator that measures the data phase for each view can provide the information to correct the phase ϕ in Eq. (12.10). In the early application of navigators to DWI (Ordidge et al. 1994), a linear navigator was used to measure ϕ in Eq. (12.10), followed by a correction for translational motion by removing ϕ from the diffusion acquisition data. Because a linear navigator only measures the component $\Delta \vec{k}$ that is along the navigator readout axis, according to Eq. (12.11) a linear navigator is insensitive to rotation ($\Delta \vec{k} = 0$) when the navigator readout axis is along either $\vec{\Theta}$ or $\vec{G}_d$. Even multiple linear navigators along different axes (Butts et al. 1996) have problems measuring $\Delta \vec{k}$ accurately. This is because eddy currents and patient motion can create a sufficiently large $\Delta \vec{k}$ that linear navigators along multiple axes (e.g. along k_x, k_y, and k_z) can completely miss the true (shifted) origin of k-space (Butts et al. 1997), with a resulting low sensitivity. A 2D navigator is therefore preferable for measuring both $\Delta \vec{k}$ and ϕ.

Both a single-shot spiral navigator (Butts et al. 1997) and a single-shot EPI navigator (Atkinson et al. 2000) have been successfully used to sample data within a small area near the origin of 2D k-space. A retrospective correction for the two in-plane components of $\Delta \vec{k}$ is obtained by shifting the data in k-space using gridding or direct data resampling using matrix inversion (described in Atkinson et al. 2000). The through-plane component of $\Delta \vec{k}$ gives a linear phase across the slice that results in signal loss and cannot be corrected. Discarding views for which the navigator signal falls below some threshold can minimize the effect of this motion component. One problem with this approach is that phase-encoding lines are not evenly spaced (uneven Δk_y) due to random motion and discarding views and may not obey the Nyquist criterion. This can be somewhat alleviated by sampling at smaller Δk_y than required for the final image FOV and by sampling each phase-encoding step multiple times.

SELECTED REFERENCES

Anderson, A. W., and Gore, J. C. 1994. Analysis and correction of motion artifacts in diffusion weighted imaging. *Magn. Reson. Med.* 32: 379–387.

Atkinson, D., Porter, D. A., Hill, D. L. G., Calamante, F., and Connelly, A. 2000. Sampling and reconstruction effects due to motion in diffusion-weighted interleaved echo planar imaging. *Magn. Reson. Med.* 44: 101–109.

Butts, K., Crespigny, A., Pauly, J. M., and Moseley, M. 1996. Diffusion-weighted interleaved echo-planar imaging with a pair of orthogonal navigator echoes. *Magn. Reson. Med.* 35: 763–770.

Butts, K., Pauly, J., Crespigny, A., and Moseley, M. 1997. Isotropic diffusion-weighted and spiral-navigated interleaved EPI for routine imaging of acute stroke. *Magn. Reson. Med.* 38: 741–749.

Danias, P. G., McConnell, M. V., Khasgiwala, V. C., Chuang, M. L., Edelman, R. R., and Manning, W. J. 1997. Prospective navigator correction of image position for coronary MR angiography. *Radiology* 203: 733–736.

Derbyshire, J. A., Wright, G. A., Henkelman, R. M., and Hinks, R. S. 1998. Dynamic scan-plane tracking using MR position monitoring. *J. Magn. Reson. Imaging* 8: 924–932.

Du, Y. P., McVeigh, E. R., Bluemke, D. A., Silber, H. A., and Foo, T. K. F. 2001. A comparison of prospective and retrospective respiratory navigator gating in 3D coronary angiography. *Inte. J. Cardiovasc. Imaging* 17: 287–294.

Ehman, R. L., and Felmlee, J. P. 1989. Adaptive technique for high-definition MR imaging of moving structures. *Radiology* 173: 255–263.

Firmin, D., and Keegan, J. 2001. Navigator echoes in cardiac magnetic resonance. *J. Cardiovasc. Magn. Reson.* 3: 183–193.

Foo, T. K. F., and King, K. F. 1999. A computationally efficient method for tracking reference position displacements for motion compensation in magnetic resonance imaging. *Magn. Reson. Med.* 42: 548–553.

Fu, Z. W., Wang, Y., Grimm, R. C., Rossman, P. J., Felmlee, J. P., Riederer, S. J., and Ehman, R. L. 1995. Orbital navigator echoes for motion measurements in magnetic resonance imaging. *Magn. Reson. Med.* 34: 746–753.

Glover, G. H., and Lai, S. 1998. Self-navigated spiral fMRI: interleaved versus single-shot. *Magn. Reson. Med.* 39: 361–368.

Hinks, R. S., Kraft, R. A., and Kurucay, S. 2001. Compensation of variations in polarizing magnetic field during magnetic resonance imaging. U.S. patent 6,294,913.

Hu, X., and Kim, S-G. 1994. Reduction of signal fluctuation in functional MRI using navigator echoes. *Magn. Reson. Med.* 31: 495–503.

Jhooti, P., Keegan, J., Gatehouse, P. D., Collins, S., Rowe A., Taylor, A. M., and Firmin, D. N. 1999. 3D coronary artery imaging with phase reordering for improved scan efficiency. *Magn. Reson. Med.* 41: 555–562.

Korin, H. W., Felmlee, J. P., Riederer, S. J., and Ehman, R. L. 1995. Spatial-frequency-tuned markers and adaptive correction for rotational motion. *Magn. Reson. Med.* 33: 663–669.

Lee, C. C., Grimm, R. C., Manduca, A., Felmlee, J. P., Ehman, R. L., Riederer, S. J., and Jack, C. R. 1998. A prospective approach to correct for inter-image head rotation in FMRI. *Magn. Reson. Med.* 39: 234–243.

Lee, C. C., Jack, C. R., Grimm, R. C., Rossman, Felmlee, F. P., Ehman, R. L., and Riederer, S. J. 1996. Real-time adaptive motion correction in functional MRI. *Magn. Reson. Med.* 36: 436–444.

Li, D., Kaushikkar, S., Haacke, E. M., Woodard, P. K., Dhawale, P. J., Kroeker, R. M., Laub, G., Kuginuki, Y., and Gutierrez, F. R. 1996. Coronary arteries: Three-dimensional MR imaging with retrospective respiratory gating. *Radiology* 201: 857–863.

Liang, Z-P., Jiang, H., Hess, C. P., and Lauterbur, P. C. 1997. Dynamic imaging by model estimation. *Intl. J. Imaging Syst. Technol.* 8: 551–557.

Liu, Y. L., Riederer, S. J., Rossman, P. J., Grimm, R. C., Debbins, J. P., and Ehman, R. L. 1993. A monitoring, feedback and triggering system for reproducible breath-hold MR imaging. *Magn. Reson. Med.* 30: 507–511.

McConnell, M. V., Khasgiwala, V. C., Savord, B. J., Chen, M. H., Chuang, M. L., and Edelman, R. R., and Manning, W. J. 1997. Prospective adaptive navigator correction for breath-hold MR coronary angiography. *Magn. Reson. Med.* 37: 148–152.

Noll, D. C., Genovese, C. R., Vazquez, A. L., O'Brien, J. L., and Eddy, W. F. 1998. Evaluation of respiratory artifact correction techniques in multishot spiral functional MRI using receiver operator characteristic analysis. *Magn. Reson. Med.* 40: 633–639.

Norris, D. G. 2001. Implications of bulk motion for diffusion-weighted imaging experiments: Effects, mechanisms, and solutions. *J. Magn. Reson. Imaging* 13: 483–495.

Ordidge, R. J., Helpern, J. A., Qing, Z. X., Knight, R. A., and Nagesh, V. 1994. Correction of motional artifacts in diffusion-weighted MR images using navigator echoes. *Magn. Reson. Imaging* 12: 455–460.

Pfeuffer, J., Van de Moortele, P-F., Ugurbil, K., Hu, X., and Glover, G. 2002. Correction of physiologically induced global off-resonance effects in dynamic echo-planar and spiral functional imaging. *Magn. Reeson. Med.* 47: 344–353.

Sachs, T. S., Meyer, C. H., Irarrazabal, P., Hu, B. S., Nishimura, D. G., and Macovski, A. 1995. The diminishing variance algorithm for real-time reduction of motion artifacts in MRI. *Magn. Reson. Med.* 34: 412–422.

Sachs, T. S., Meyer, C. H., Pauly, J. M., Nishimura, D. G., and Macovski, A. 1998. Coronary angiography using the real-time interactive 3D DVA. In *Proceedings of the 6th ISMRM*, p. 20.

Sinkus, R., and Boernert, P. 1999. Motion pattern adapted real-time respiratory gating. *Magn. Reson. Med.* 41: 148–155.

Song, H. K., and Wehrli, F. W. 1999. In vivo micro-imaging using alternating navigator echoes with application to cancellous bone structural analysis. *Magn. Reson. Med.* 41: 947–953.

Spuentrup, E., Manning, W., Boernert, P., Kissinger, K. V., Botnar, R. M., and Stuber, M. 2002. Renal arteries: Navigator-gated balanced fast field-echo projection MR angiography with aortic spin labeling, initial experience. *Radiology* 225: 589–596.

Stuber, M., Botnar, R. M., Danias, P. G., Kissinger, K. V., and Manning, W. J. 1999. Sub-millimeter three-dimensional coronary MR angiography with real-time navigator correction: Comparison of navigator locations. *Radiology* 212: 579–587.

Taylor, A. M., Keegan, J., Jhooti, P., Firmin, D. N., and Pennell, D. J. 1999. Calculation of a subject-specific adaptive motion-correction factor for improved real-time navigator echo-gated magnetic resonance coronary angiography. *J. Cardiovasc. Magn. Reson.* 1: 131–138.

Thanh, D. N., Wang, Y., Watts, R., and Mitchell, I. 2001. *k*-space weighted least-squares algorithm for accurate and fast motion extraction from magnetic resonance navigator echoes. *Magn. Reson. Med.* 46: 1037–1040.

Thiel, T., Czisch, M., Elbel, G. K., and Hennig, J. 2002. Phase coherent averaging in magnetic resonance spectroscopy using interleaved navigator scans: Compensation of motion artifacts and magnetic field instabilities. *Magn. Reson. Med.* 47: 1077–1082.

Wang, Y., Grimm, R. C., Felmlee, J. P., Riederer, S. J., and Ehman, R. L. 1996. Algorithms for extracting motion information from navigator echoes. *Magn. Reson. Med.* 36: 117–123.

Wang, Y., Grimm, R. C., Rossman, P. J., Debbins, J. P., Riederer, S. J., and Ehman, R. L. 1995. 3D coronary MR angiography in multiple breath-holds using a respiratory feedback monitor. *Magn. Reson. Med.* 34: 11–16.

Wang, Y., Riederer, S. J., and Ehman, R. L. 1995. Respiratory motion of the heart: Kinematics and the implications for the spatial resolution in coronary artery imaging. *Magn. Reson. Med.* 33: 713–719.

Ward, H. A., Riederer, S. J., Grimm, R. C., Ehman, R. L., Felmlee, J. P., and Jack, C. R. 2000. Prospective multiaxial motion correction for fMRI. *Magn. Reson. Med.* 43: 459–469.

Ward, H. A., Riederer, S. J., and Jack, C. R. 2002. Real-time autoshimming for echo planar timecourse imaging. *Magn. Reson. Med.* 48: 771–780.

Weiger, M., Boernert, P., Proksa, R., Schaeffter, T., and Haase, A. 1997. Motion-adapted gating based on k-space weighting for reduction of respiratory motion artifacts. *Magn. Reson. Med.* 38: 322–333.

Welch, E. B., Manduca, A., Grimm, R. C., Ward, H. A., and Jack, C. R. 2002. Spherical navigator echoes for full 3D rigid body motion measurement in MRI. *Magn. Reson. Med.* 47: 32–41.

RELATED SECTIONS

12.3 Respiratory Gating and Compensation

Respiratory motion is a major source of artifacts in thoracic and abdominal MR imaging. If not compensated for or corrected, respiratory motion can produce image blurring, ghosting, intensity loss, and misregistration. These image artifacts can obscure important anatomic structures, making diagnosis difficult or impossible.

The problems caused by respiratory motion can be addressed in a number of ways. A straightforward strategy is to employ fast imaging. Because the typical breathing cycle for adult human subjects lasts 4–5 s, respiratory motion is essentially frozen if the *entire* k-space data can be acquired much faster than that. This can be accomplished with ultrafast pulse sequences, such as EPI and RARE with long echo trains (see Sections 16.1 and 16.4

for details). Although ultrafast imaging pulse sequences can effectively freeze respiratory motion, the resolution of the resultant image is usually poor (e.g., 128×128 with single-shot EPI) and artifacts inherent to fast imaging often become problematic. Another strategy to address respiratory motion is to retrospectively perform motion correction. In this strategy, the acquisition is modified to obtain some extra data beyond that required to reconstruct an image. The motion-contaminated k-space data are then corrected during image reconstruction using the information contained in the extra data. Examples of this approach include retrospective navigator echo correction (Section 12.2) and ghost phase cancellation (Xiang and Henkelman 1991; Xiang et al. 1993). A related technique in this category is to acquire data in two orthogonal k-space grids (Welch et al. 2002). Although it does not necessarily increase the total amount of data, the k-space data are arranged differently to facilitate motion correction. Alternatively, motion artifacts can also be corrected based solely on the nominal k-space data, without the extra data acquisition. Two examples of this strategy are motion corrections using projection data consistency (Glover and Pauly 1992) and autocorrelation (Manduca et al. 2000). If multiple receive coils are used, parallel imaging methods can also be used to correct motion by providing constraints that force data consistency (Bydder et al. 2003).

In this section, we focus on four techniques that suppress or compensate for respiratory motion artifacts during data acquisition: Breath-holding, respiratory gating, respiratory triggering, and k-space view reordering (also known as phase reordering and discussed in Section 12.2). In the context of this book, we collectively refer to the first three techniques as respiratory synchronization methods and to the last technique as respiratory compensation. Unlike motion correction, respiratory synchronization and compensation require little or no change in the image reconstruction algorithm. They do, however, require either patient cooperation or substantial modification of the data acquisition.

12.3.1 BASICS OF RESPIRATION

Lung expansion and contraction is accompanied by (1) SI movement of the diaphragm to change the vertical dimension of the chest cavity and (2) AP elevation and deflation of the ribs to increase and decrease the diameter of the chest cavity. The diaphragm motion is exploited for respiratory monitoring with navigators (Section 12.2), whereas changes in chest cavity diameter provide the basis for respiratory monitoring techniques employing pressure transducers such as pneumatic bellows.

Similar to cardiac motion, pulmonary ventilation also contains multiple phases, as shown in Figure 12.13 (Note that the term *phase* as used here is analogous to a phase of the moon and should note be confused with the phase

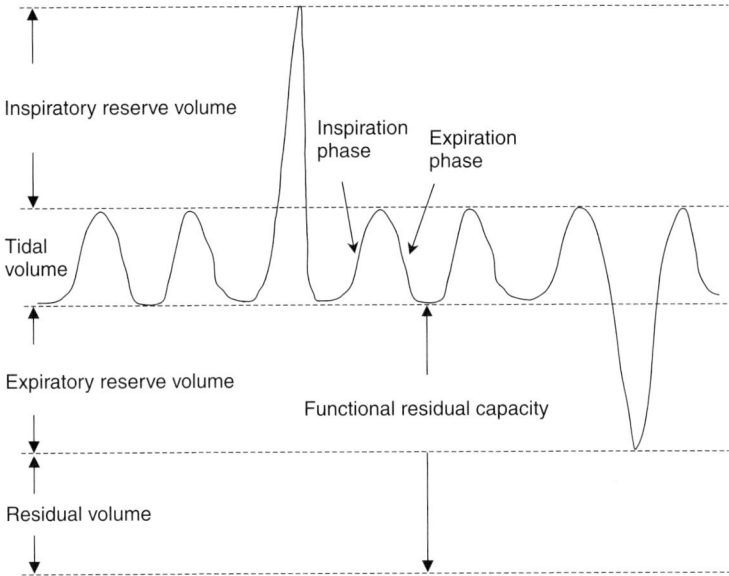

FIGURE 12.13 A schematic plot of a respiratory waveform showing the respiratory phases, various lung volumes, and functional residual capacity. The vertical and horizontal axes represent lung volume and time, respectively.

of a complex signal.) The inspiration (also known as inhalation) phase is characterized by a negative alveolar pressure (i.e., the pressure in the alveoli is approximately 2 mmHg less than the atmospheric pressure) and typically lasts ~2 s for a healthy adult human subject. The expiration (or exhalation) phase occurs, driven by a positive alveolar pressure, immediately following inspiration. Expiration takes approximately the same amount of time as inspiration. After the expiration, there is a brief pause (typically less than 1 s) before the next cycle begins. These phases are illustrated in Figure 12.13.

During a respiratory cycle, the lung volume changes with the respiratory phases (Figure 12.13). The *tidal volume* (~0.5 liter) is the volume of air inhaled or exhaled with each normal breath. The additional amount of air that can be forcefully inhaled beyond a tidal inspiration is called *inspiratory reserve volume* (~3.1 liters). Similarly, the extra amount of air that can be maximally exhaled after a tidal expiration is called *expiratory reserve volume* (~1.2 liters). Even after the maximal expiration, residual air remains in the lung. This air volume is known as *residual volume* (also ~1.2 liters). The combination of the expiratory reserve volume and residual volume is referred to as the *functional residual capacity* (FRC; ~2.4 liters). Note that even though the residual volume is not accessed, it constitutes part of FRC. As described later, respiratory gating typically occurs when the lung volume corresponds to FRC. The duration when the lung volume is at FRC also plays a very important role in centric k-space view reordering.

12.3.2 RESPIRATORY MOTION MONITORING

Respiratory gating and triggering and view reordering all rely on real-time monitoring of the respiratory cycles. Although not required, the real-time respiratory waveform can also guide operators to monitor a patient's response during breath-holding acquisitions. Two monitoring methods, pneumatic bellows and navigators, are commonly employed in MRI data acquisition.

A pneumatic bellows consists of an elastic belt that is secured around the patient's abdomen at a position caudal from the anterior costal margin. The belt is attached to a pressure transducer that produces an analog voltage related to lung expansion and contraction. The voltage signal is amplified, low-pass filtered (e.g., with a cut-off frequency of 60 Hz), and digitized. In some designs, optical coupling is used to convert the voltage to light, transmit the light signal through a fiber optic cable, and convert the signal back to voltage prior to digitization. The optical transmission minimizes spurious signals that can be picked up in electrically conducting cables when the gradients are pulsed. The digitized signal is processed to linearly relate the signal amplitude with the circumferential changes (or displacement) of the body wall associated with breathing. The processed signal is displayed on a monitor at or near the scanner console for real-time respiratory monitoring. A schematic plot of the body wall displacement as a function of time is shown in Figure 12.14, in which the peaks and the valleys correspond to the end of inspiration and the FRC, respectively. The sampling rate of the respiratory waveform in Figure 12.14 is typically a few tens of kilohertz (e.g, ~20 kHz) and the display window covers a few tens of seconds (e.g., 20 s).

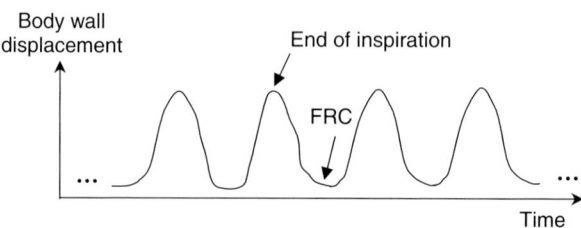

FIGURE 12.14 A schematic plot of the body wall displacement as a function of time, as monitored by a pneumatic bellows. FRC stands for functional residual capacity.

Navigator echoes monitor respiratory motion by repeatedly acquiring MR signals from an area that moves during respiration, such as the diaphragm. The navigator signals are processed to produce a spatial profile of the monitored region and may be displayed as a function of time for monitoring. The update rate of the navigator profiles depends on the pulse sequence length and processing time. It is typically much lower than that of a pneumatic bellows. The details of navigator acquisition and processing are described in Section 12.2.

12.3.3 BREATH-HOLDING

Unlike cardiac motion, respiratory motion can be voluntarily suspended or suppressed for a limited amount of time. Typically, an adult human subject can hold his or her breath for approximately 20–30 s, although this duration is challenging for some patients. If all k-space data can be acquired during this time window, respiratory motion artifacts can be eliminated from the image. An example of lower abdomen images without and with breath-holding is shown in Figure 12.15. Depending on applications, breath-holding can occur at the end of either the inspiration or expiration phase. Because most people can breath-hold longer at the inspiratory reserve volume (Figure 12.13) than any other point of the respiratory cycle, patients are often instructed to take a deep breath in and hold it before the operator starts the scans. Hyperventilation prior to breath-holding is also helpful to lengthen the breath-holding time and is often practiced in breath-hold data acquisitions. Although not necessary,

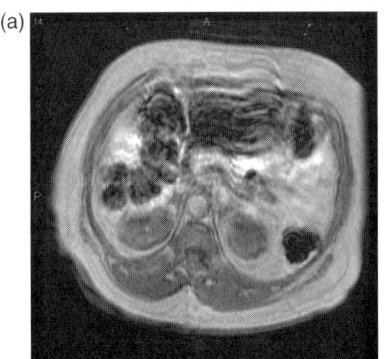 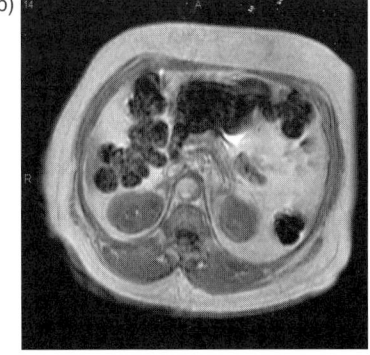

FIGURE 12.15 Two gradient-echo images of the lower abdomen (a) without and (b) with breath-holding. The imaging parameters are $TR/TE = 110/4.2$ ms (i.e., fat-water in-phase at 1.5 T), flip angle $= 80°$, matrix $= 256 \times 128$, NEX $= 1$, and $T_{scan} = 15$ s. Reduction of ghosting artifacts and image blurring is evident in (b).

monitoring the patient's breathing pattern before and during breath-holding is very helpful to ensure good motion suppression.

Because only an approximately 20 to 30-s window is available for breath-hold scans, fast pulse sequences are essential. Fast gradient-echo pulse sequences (Section 14.1) are commonly used in breath-hold scans to acquire multiple 2D slices or even a 3D volume to cover the desired imaging region, such as the liver. Parallel imaging (Section 13.3) can further accelerate data acquisition. The time saved by parallel imaging can be used to increase the number of slices, improve in-plane resolution, or shorten the breath-holding duration.

Example 12.1   A 2D fast gradient pulse sequence with a TR of 10 ms is used to acquire images with 128 phase-encoding steps in a single breath-hold of 26 s (assuming NEX $= 1$). (a) How many slices can be acquired? (b) If SENSE is used with an acceleration factor of 2, recalculate the number of slices that can be acquired.

Answer

(a) According to Section 11.5, the time required for a single slice is:

$$10 \text{ ms} \times 128 \times 1 = 1.28 \text{ s}$$

Within a breath hold of 26 s, a total of $26/1.28 = 20$ slices can be acquired.

(b) With an acceleration factor of 2, the time required for a single slice is halved and the total number of slices is doubled to 40. If fewer than 40 slices are needed, the required duration of the breath-hold can be reduced accordingly.

Even with fast pulse sequences and parallel imaging, sometimes conflicting requirements such as the desired number of slices, spatial resolution, and SNR cannot all be satisfied within a single breath-hold. In that case, the data acquisition is divided into multiple groups (or passes), each consisting of fewer slices that can be acquired in one breath-hold. Multiple breath-holds are used to obtain all desired slices. In multiple breath-hold acquisitions, it is important to instruct the patient to hold his or her breath at a consistent position in the respiratory cycle, especially when the 2D slices are reformatted into different viewing planes.

To reduce scan time, breath-hold acquisition is often limited to a relatively small number of phase-encoding steps (e.g., 128). Thus, the resolution can be rather poor along the phase-encoded direction. Breath-holding also relies on how well the patient can cooperate. For applications demanding higher resolution or for uncooperative patients (e.g., patients with compromised pulmonary function), alternative techniques such as respiratory gating, respiratory triggering, and view reordering can be used instead.

12.3.4 RESPIRATORY GATING

Respiratory gating acquires or retains data *only* within a predefined window during which the respiratory motion is minimal or the subject is at a consistent position. The window is often chosen in the vicinity of the FRC, between the downhill of an expiration and the uphill of the next inspiration (Figure 12.16). Compared to the other segments of a respiratory cycle, this window provides the greatest reduction of artifacts (Ehman et al. 1984).

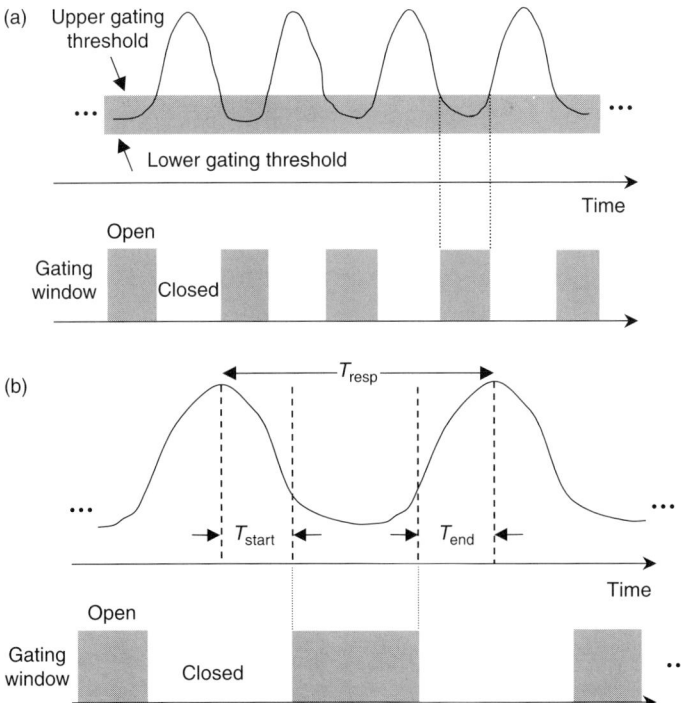

FIGURE 12.16 Schematic diagrams showing the selection of gating open/close points. (a) Selecting an upper and a lower threshold determines the gating window. The pair of vertical dotted lines illustrates the relationship between the thresholds and the gating window. (b) The gating window is selected by defining two time intervals T_{start} and T_{end} as a percentage of the average respiratory period T_{resp}.

Two time points must be specified to define the gating window—one opens the window and the other closes it. Two approaches can be used to determine these time points. In the first approach, upper and lower thresholds are selected based on the amplitude of the tidal respiration waveform (Figure 12.16a). For example, the upper and lower thresholds can be selected at 20% of the tidal volume above and below FRC (or the baseline), respectively. When the respiration waveform is within this range, the gating window is open; otherwise, the window is closed. Although the lower limit is rarely exceeded, it serves as a safeguard in case expiration activates the expiratory reserve volume. In the second approach, the average period of the respiratory cycle (T_{resp}) is first evaluated after monitoring the tidal respiration waveform for an extended period of time (e.g., 30 s). Then a gate-open point (T_{start}) is specified as a percentage of the average period (T_{resp}). After the scanner detects the end of an inspiration (or the beginning of expiration) by searching for the maximum in the tidal respiration waveform, the acquisition window will open following a delay of T_{start} (Figure 12.16b). Because the average period is already known, the scanner can predict when the next maximum occurs in the tidal respiration waveform. The scanner closes the gating window at a time T_{end} before the next predicted tidal maximum, where T_{end} is also defined as a percentage of the average period (T_{resp}) (Figure 12.16b). These timing relationships are further explained in Example 12.2.

Example 12.2 Over a period of 30 s, a tidal respiratory waveform showed six full cycles with period of 4.8, 4.7, 4.8, 4.9, 4.5, and 4.6 s. If T_{start} and T_{end} are selected as 30 and 35% of the averaged period, respectively, what is the duration of the respiratory gating window?

Answer The average period of the respiratory cycle is:

$$T_{resp} = (4.8 + 4.7 + 4.8 + 4.9 + 4.5 + 4.6)/6 = 4.72\,s$$

The gating window opens at:

$$T_{start} = 0.30\,T_{resp} = 1.42\,s$$

after the end of an inspiration, and closes at

$$T_{end} = 0.35\,T_{resp} = 1.65\,s$$

before the end of the next predicted inspiration. Because the predicted inspiration occurs at 4.72 s after the preceding inspiration, the duration of the gating window is

$$T_{resp} - T_{start} - T_{end} = 1.65\,s$$

When T_{start} or T_{end} is too short, considerable expiration or inspiration can intrude into the acquisition window, causing motion contamination of the acquired data. If, however, T_{start} or T_{end} is too long, data can only be acquired in a very narrow window, leading to a low acquisition efficiency. T_{end} is essentially the time allocated to the scanner to search for the next maximum in the tidal respiratory waveform. If the respiratory cycle shortens, data can be acquired when the next tidal maximum occurs and the next tidal signal can be missed. To balance these factors, T_{start} and T_{end} are typically chosen at $\sim 30\%$ of T_{resp}, as shown in Example 12.2. (Note that T_{start} and T_{end} do not have to be the same.)

Within the gating window, data can be acquired with 2D sequential, 2D interleaved, or 3D mode. When 2D interleaved acquisition is used, the effective TR time is governed by the period of the respiratory cycle. Because this period is typically ~ 4–5 s, respiratory gating corresponds nicely with the TR requirements of T_2-weighted pulse sequences such as spin echo or RARE. However, the maximum number of slices per acquisition (or per pass) can be greatly reduced due to the dead time taken by T_{start} and T_{end}. In sequential acquisitions, respiratory gating can be made compatible with a short TR pulse sequence, such as gradient echo. To maintain the image contrast and the steady state of the magnetization, RF pulses are continuously played out even when the gating window is closed and no data are acquired or retained. This approach has been referred to as *spin-conditioned respiratory gating* (Ehman et al. 1984).

A primary drawback of respiratory gating is the prolonged scan time because the acquisition window is open only for a fraction of the respiratory cycle. It is quite typical for a respiratory-gated acquisition to take approximately three times longer than its ungated counterpart because only approximately one-third of the respiratory cycle is used for data acquisition, as shown in Example 12.2. Because of this, respiratory gating is most commonly used with fast pulse sequences, such as RARE and fast gradient echo. Another approach used to increase the data acquisition efficiency is to instruct the patient to lengthen the time between expiration and the next inspiration; doing this can widen the data acquisition window. This approach, however, requires patient cooperation.

12.3.5 RESPIRATORY TRIGGERING

Similar to respiratory gating, respiratory triggering (Lewis et al. 1986) starts data acquisition after a predetermined event is detected. Unlike respiratory gating, however, respiratory triggering does not terminate data acquisition by detecting a second event. Instead, a predetermined number of pulse sequences are played, after which data acquisition terminates automatically.

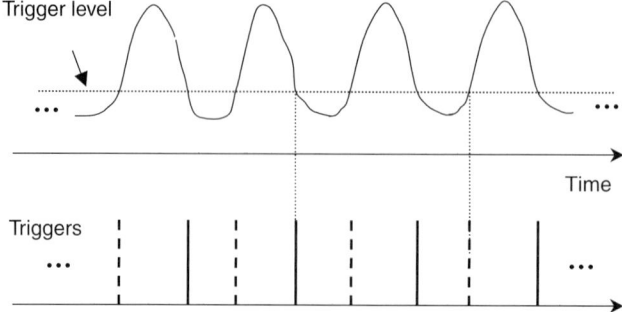

FIGURE 12.17 Respiratory triggering. The horizontal line shows the operator-selected trigger level. The solid and dashed vertical lines indicate trigger points on expiration and inspiration phases, respectively. The two dotted vertical lines illustrate the relationship between the trigger level and the trigger points.

The number of pulse sequences played out depends on the pulse sequence length, duration of the respiratory cycle, desired data acquisition efficiency, and applications. Following acquisition, the scanner reopens the trigger window and wait for the next trigger signal. Because respiration has no specific trigger event analogous to the R wave of the ECG, the operator must set the trigger point. The trigger level can be selected at any specified fraction of the tidal volume above the FRC. The dotted horizontal line in Figure 12.17 shows a trigger level at $\sim$25% of the tidal volume. Respiratory triggering can occur at the inspiration slope (dashed vertical lines in Figure 12.17), the expiration slope (solid vertical lines in Figure 12.17), or both. If data acquisition is preferred when the lung volume corresponds to the FRC, only the expiration slope is used for respiratory triggering. When both inspiration and expiration slopes are used for triggering, however, the data acquisition efficiency can be increased.

With respiratory triggering, the TR of the pulse sequence is limited by the trigger interval (i.e., $\sim T_{resp}$ if either inspiration or expiration slope is used or $\sim T_{resp}/2$ if both slopes are used). The long scan time, as well as a small number of slices that can be acquired (with an interleaved mode) after each trigger, considerably limits the acquisition efficiency when respiratory triggering is used.

12.3.6 VIEW REORDERING

Ghosting due to Periodic Motion   With standard Cartesian k-space trajectories, periodic (or nearly periodic) motion, such as respiration, causes ghosting in the phase-encoded direction (Figure 12.15a) (Wood and Henkelman 1985). The ghosts do not necessarily correspond to motion along the phase-encoded direction; they can be caused by motion along any direction. Theoretically, each motion frequency can produce a pair of ghosts symmetrically displaced about the imaged object. In practice, multiple motion frequencies coexist and the ghosts from each frequency can add up constructively or destructively, producing a complicated ghosting pattern. The separation of the ghosts depends on the period (or frequency) of the motion, as well as imaging parameters. The relationship between ghost separation (Δy_g) and several imaging parameters is given by (Wood et al. 1988):

$$\Delta y_g = \frac{L_y \text{ NEX TR}}{T_{m,a}} \tag{12.22}$$

where L_y is the FOV along the phase-encoded direction, NEX is the number of signal averages for each k-space line (or view), TR is the repetition time, and $T_{m,a}$ is the *apparent* motion period as perceived by the k-space data along the phase-encoded direction. For example, if the k-space is sampled in a sequential order (see Section 11.5 and Figure 11.25a), $T_{m,a}$ is the same as the period of the actual motion (T_m), provided that NEX $\times$ TR is substantially shorter than T_m. In a respiratory gated or triggered acquisition, $T_{m,a}$ approaches infinity (i.e., the periodic respiratory modulation is not seen by the k-space data), which causes zero ghost separation. In this case, the "ghosts" overlap with the image, and no ghosts will be observed. Using the relationship in Eq. (11.35), Eq. (12.22) can be equivalently expressed as:

$$\Delta y_g = \frac{L_y T_{\text{scan}}}{T_{m,a} N_{\text{phase}}} = \frac{L_y T_{\text{scan}} f_{m,a}}{N_{\text{phase}}} \tag{12.23}$$

where T_{scan} is the scan time, N_{phase} is the total number of phase-encoded k-space lines (or views) for an image, and $f_{m,a}$ is the apparent motion frequency in k-space.

Principles of View Reordering   The concept behind view reordering is to change $T_{m,a}$ (or $f_{m,a}$) by modifying the acquisition order of the k-space lines so that the separation of motion ghosts (Δy_g) is either minimized or maximized in the image (Bailes et al. 1985; Haacke and Patrick 1986; Pelc and Glover 1987; MacGowan and Wood 1996; Jhooti et al, 1998). The method that minimizes Δy_g is known as *low-frequency* (or *low-sort*) view reordering, whereas the method that maximizes Δy_g is called *high-frequency* (or *high-sort*) view reordering.

In low-frequency view reordering (i.e., low $f_{m,a}$ or long $T_{m,a}$), the ghosts are placed closer to the moving part of the imaged subject. The views are acquired in an order so that it appears that the patient took only one-half or

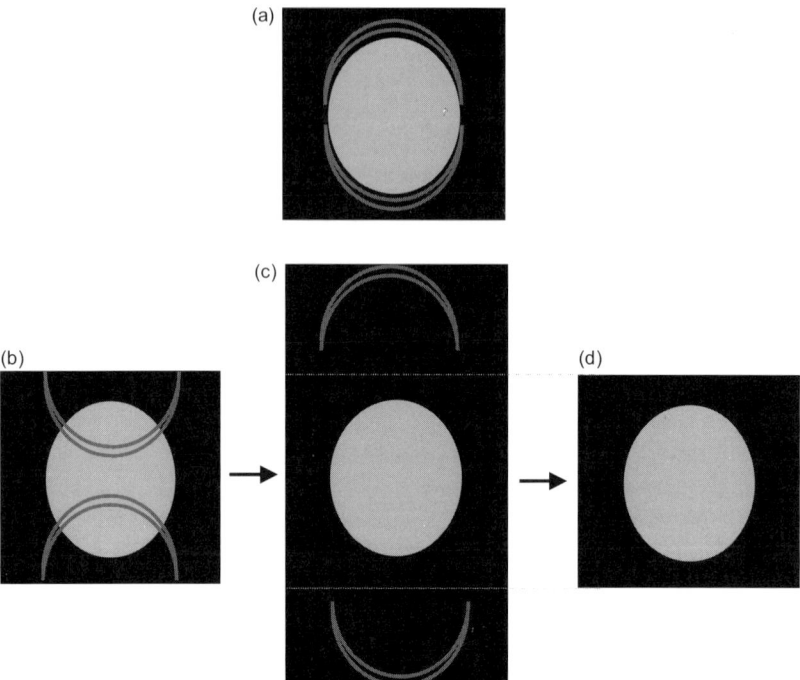

FIGURE 12.18 Respiratory motion ghosts in (a) low-frequency view reordering and (b–d) high-frequency view reordering. With low-frequency reordering, the ghosts are placed close to the source of motion to minimize its disturbance on other parts of the image. With high frequency-ordering, the ghosts are pushed far away from the image, but can alias back to obscure the image (b). If the FOV is increased, the ghosts can be separated from the image (c). Cropping the central part of image (c) results in a ghost-free image (d).

one breath over the entire acquisition. Thus, the ghosts will minimally perturb regions distant from the moving source (Figure 12.18a). Respiratory gating or triggering under ideal conditions can be treated as an extreme case of low-frequency view ordering where $f_{m,a}$ approaches zero and the ghosts coincide with the image.

In high-frequency view ordering (i.e., high $f_{m,a}$ or short $T_{m,a}$), the ghosts are placed far away from the desired image along the phase-encoded direction. The views are acquired in an order so that it appears that the patient breathes very rapidly, completing an entire respiratory cycle each $2 \times$ NEX $\times$ TR. Because these ghosts can alias back onto the desired image (Figure 12.18b), the FOV in the phase-encoded direction must be increased in order to separate

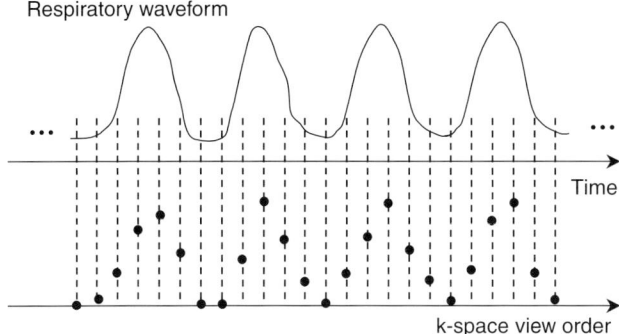

FIGURE 12.19 Conventional k-space view ordering in relation to the respiratory waveform.

the ghosts from the image (Figure 12.18c). The ghosts are then cropped from the image (Figure 12.18d).

Low-Frequency View Reordering   Consider the respiratory waveform with a frequency f_m as shown in Figure 12.19. If the k-space lines are acquired in a sequential order (see Section 11.5), then the k-space data are modulated by a similar function as the respiratory waveform (Figure 12.19). In this case, the apparent motion frequency $f_{m,a}$ is the same as f_m. If, however, the k-space lines are not acquired in sequential order, $f_{m,a}$ can be quite different from f_m. When the neighboring k-space lines are acquired at similar points of the respiratory cycles as shown in Figure 12.20a, the apparent motion frequency $f_{m,a}$ becomes much less than f_m. Therefore, the ghost separation Δy_g is reduced. For example, if $f_{m,a}$ corresponds to a full cycle of respiration during the scan (i.e., $T_{m,a} = T_{scan}$), then, as suggested by Eq. (12.23), Δy_g is only approximately one pixel in the image. In the view reordering scheme depicted in Figure 12.20a, the entire set of the k-space lines appears to be acquired within one half of a respiratory cycle, although the actual data acquisition spans many respiratory cycles. The most negative k-space views are acquired when the respiratory displacement is minimal (i.e., the end of expiration phase), while the most positive k-space views are obtained when the respiratory displacement is maximal (i.e., the end of inspiration phase). The intermediate k-space views are progressively acquired between the minimal and the maximal displacements, resulting in a monotonic k-space modulation function. This view-order scheme has been called *respiratory ordered phase encoding* (ROPE) (Bailes et al. 1985). Alternatively, the central region of k-space can be acquired when the respiratory

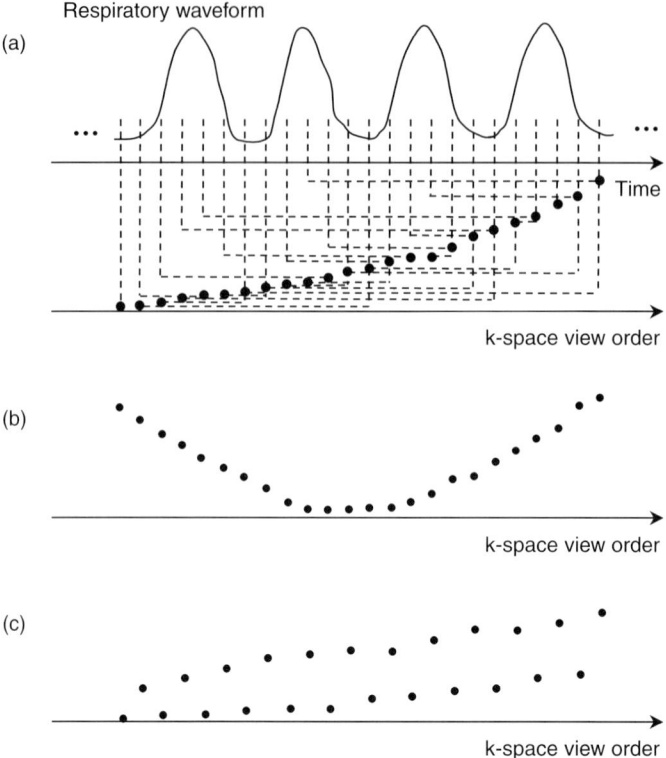

FIGURE 12.20 Low-frequency k-space (a–b) view reordering and (c) high-frequency reordering in relation to the respiratory waveform. The reordering schemes used in ROPE and COPE are shown in (a) and (b), respectively. The dashed lines in (a) indicate how data acquired at different respiratory phase are mapped to specific k-space views. For simplicity, this relationship is not shown in (b) and (c).

displacement is minimal and the edges of k-space acquired at the maximal respiratory displacement (Figure 12.20b). Thus, the entire k-space views appear to be sampled in a single respiratory cycle. This view-ordering scheme is known as *centric ordered phase encoding* (COPE) (Haacke and Patrick 1986). Because the end of the expiration lasts slightly longer than the end of inspiration and has minimal displacement, COPE acquires a large portion of central k-space views during this best window of the respiratory cycle. Since the image quality and contrast is largely determined by the central k-space data, COPE can provide better ghost reduction than ROPE, even though its apparent motion frequency $f_{m,a}$ is twice as high. Moreover, COPE keeps the best k-space data (i.e., those acquired during the best respiratory window) from being attenuated if k-space windowing is applied during image reconstruction (Section 13.1).

Unlike ROPE, COPE does not use a real-time displacement probability function (see later discussion) to guide view selection. Instead, it assumes a predefined probability in determining the k-space views. As such, mismatching between the respiratory displacement and k-space view often occurs, even when breathing is stable. This results in some high-frequency components contaminating the low-frequency k-space modulation function. To solve this problem, *hybrid ordered phase encoding* (HOPE), was introduced. It uses displacement probability profiling to minimize the high-frequency modulations in COPE. The details of the algorithm can be found in Jhooti et al. (1998).

High-Frequency View Reordering   In high-frequency view reordering, neighboring k-space lines are acquired at a different respiratory displacement so that motion appears to be at the highest possible frequency (i.e., maximizing $f_{m,a}$). For example, if a k-space line is acquired at the end of the expiration phase, then its neighboring k-space line can be acquired halfway between the end of expiration and the end of inspiration (i.e., the two k-space lines are separated by one quarter of the respiratory cycle). This view-ordering scheme (Figure 12.20c) results in an apparent motion frequency of $f_{m,a} = N_{phase}/(2T_{scan})$ (i.e., there are $N_{phase}/2$ cycles during the entire scan time). According to Eq. (12.23), the ghosts will be shifted by one-half of the FOV along the phase-encoded direction. If the FOV is approximately the same as the dimension of the imaged subject, the ghosts alias onto the desired structure, obscuring it in the image. If, however, the FOV is doubled in the phase-encoded direction, cropping can separate the desired image from the ghosts (Figure 12.18).

Doubling the FOV without increasing N_{phase} reduces the spatial resolution. This problem, however, can be solved when signal averaging is used. When NEX = 2, for example, an additional set of k-space lines with an offset of 1/(2FOV) can be obtained, instead of repeating the same k-space line twice. This doubles the FOV in the phase-encoded direction, while maintaining the image resolution and SNR gain. Thus, high-frequency view reordering is most conveniently used when NEX > 1. For acquisitions with NEX > 1, high-frequency ordering is usually preferred to low-frequency ordering because it places the ghosts one-half of the FOV away (and then crops the ghosts off) instead of one pixel away. A pair of abdominal images before and after applying high-frequency view ordering is shown in Figure 12.21.

Note that the high-frequency ordered k-space data also contain low-frequency components, as shown by the slowly increasing baseline in Figure 12.20c. This effect can cause image blurring. A method to reduce this effect is discussed in Pelc and Glover (1987).

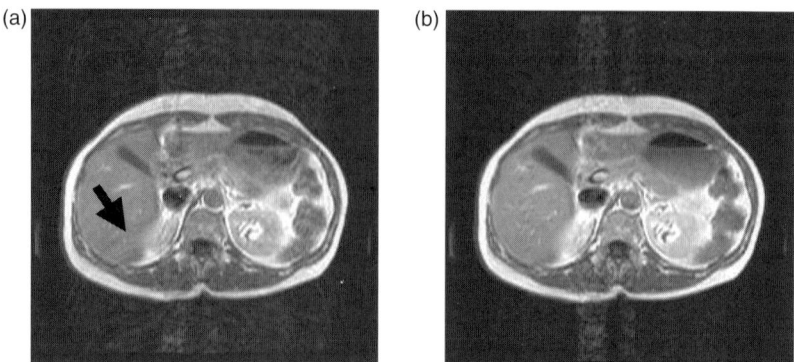

FIGURE 12.21 Two liver images (a) without and (b) with a high-frequency view reordering scheme. Note the reduced ghosting artifacts in the region indicated by the arrow.

Practical Considerations   View reordering algorithms monitor the respiratory waveform before the start of the scan as well as throughout the scan. By acquiring respiratory signals over several cycles just prior to the start of the scan, a histogram that relates the respiratory displacement to the frequency of occurrence can be constructed. This histogram is updated during the data acquisition to account for the changes in breathing patterns. Based on the histogram, a mapping function or a lookup table that relates respiratory displacement to a range of desired k-space views is generated. This can be done using a probability distribution function $p(r)$, which is defined as the number of occurrences at displacement r over the total number of measurements:

$$N_k(r) = p(r) N_{\text{phase}} \qquad (12.24)$$

where $N_k(r)$ is the number of k-space views that can be acquired when the respiratory cycle is at displacement r. The probability function $p(r)$ can be readily derived from the histogram.

During data acquisition, a reading from the respiratory waveform is obtained prior to playing out the first phase-encoding gradient pulse. The mapping function (or the lookup table) based on $p(r)$ guides the sequence to play out the phase-encoding gradient amplitude that corresponds to one of the views given by Eq. (12.24). Alternatively, the algorithm can determine the most appropriate k-space view at a specific displacement r without using the probability distribution function. If that view has already been acquired, the algorithm proceeds to find the next most appropriate view. This process is repeated until all the views are acquired. For signal averaging (i.e., low-frequency reordering with NEX > 1 and high-frequency reordering with

NEX > 2), the same k-space view is repeated at the closest possible respiratory displacement r.

View reordering does not require patient cooperation and does not necessarily lengthen the total scan time. These advantages result in frequent use of viewing reordering in many applications. For patients with irregular respiration, timely updating of the histogram of respiration is essential to obtain optimal artifact reduction. Note that although view reordering reduces ghosting artifacts, it does not in general reduce image blurring caused by subject motion.

Selected References

Bailes, D. R., Gilderdale, D. J., Bydder, G. M., Collins, A. G., and Firmin, D. N. 1985. Respiratory ordered phase encoding (ROPE)—a method for reducing respiratory motion artifacts in MR imaging. *J. Comput. Assist. Tomogr.* 9: 835–838.

Bydder, M., Atkinson, D., Larkman, D. J., Hill, D. L. G., and Hajnal, J. V. 2003. SMASH navigators. *Magn. Reson. Med.* 49: 493–500.

Ehman, R. L., McNamara, M. T., Pallack, M., Hricak, H., and Higgins, C. B. 1984. Magnetic-resonance imaging with respiratory gating—techniques and advantages. *Am. J. Radiol.* 143: 1175–1182.

Glover, G. H., and Pauly, J. M. 1992. Projection reconstruction techniques for suppression of motion artifacts. *Magn. Reson. Med.* 28: 275–289.

Haacke, E. M., and Patrick, J. L. 1986. Reducing motion artifacts in two-dimensional Fourier transform imaging. *Magn. Reson. Imaging* 4: 359–376.

Jhooti, P., Wiesmann, F., Taylor, A. M., Gatehouse, P. D., Yang, G. Z., Keegan, J., Pennell, D. J., and Firmin, D. N. 1998. Hybrid ordered phase encoding (HOPE): An improved approach for respiratory artifact reduction. *J. Magn. Reson. Imaging* 8: 968–980.

Lewis, C. E., Prato, F. S., Drost, D. J., and Nicholson, R. L. 1986. Comparison of respiratory triggering and gating techniques for the removal of respiratory artifacts in MR imaging. *Radiology* 160: 803–810.

MacGowan, C. K., and Wood, M. L. 1996. Phase-encode reordering to minimize errors caused by motion. *Magn. Reson. Med.* 35: 391–398.

Manduca, A., McGee, K. P., Welch, E. B., Felmlee, J. P., Grimm, R. C., and Ehman, R. L. 2000. Autocorrection in MR imaging: Adaptive motion correction without navigator echoes. *Radiology* 215: 904–909.

Pelc, N. J., and Glover, G. H. 1987. Method for reducing image artifacts due to periodic signal variations in NMR imaging. U.S. patent 4,663,591.

Welch, E. B., Felmlee, J. P., Ehman, R. L., and Manduca, A. 2002. Motion correction using the k-space phase difference of orthogonal acquisitions. *Magn. Reson. Med.* 48: 147–156.

Wood, M. L., and Henkelman, R. M. 1985. NMR image artifacts from periodic motion. *Med. Phys.* 12: 143–151.

Wood, M. L., Runge, V. M., and Henkelman, R. M. 1988. Overcoming motion in abdominal MR imaging. *Am. J. Radiol.* 150: 513–522.

Xiang, Q. S., Bronskill, M. J., and Henkelman, R. M. 1993. Two-point interference method for suppression of ghost artifacts due to motion. *J. Magn. Reson. Imaging* 3: 900–906.

Xiang, Q. S., and Henkelman, R. M. 1991. Motion artifact reduction with 3-point ghost phase cancellation. *J. Magn. Reson. Imaging* 1: 633–642.

RELATED SECTIONS

Section 8.2 Phase-Encoding Gradients
Section 11.5 Two-Dimensional Acquisition
Section 11.6 Three-Dimensional Acquisition
Section 12.1 Cardiac Triggering
Section 12.2 Navigators
Section 13.1 Fourier Reconstruction

COMMON IMAGE RECONSTRUCTION TECHNIQUES

13.1 Fourier Reconstruction

In MR imaging, the time domain signal corresponds to the Fourier transform (FT) of the transverse magnetization (suitably defined to include factors such as relaxation effects, flow effects, and diffusion weighting). As a consequence, MR image reconstruction simply requires a 2D- or 3D-IFT. If the Fourier transform space (k-space) is sampled along a rectilinear trajectory, the 2D- or 3D-IFT can be done with a series of FFTs. If k-space is sampled with a nonrectilinear trajectory such as a spiral or projection acquisition, the data are typically resampled to a rectilinear grid to enable the use of FFTs. This operation is known as gridding (Section 13.2). Projection acquisition data can also be reconstructed by filtered back-projection, which is commonly used in computed tomography (CT).

In this section, we discuss image reconstruction for rectilinear sampling using FFTs. Most of the material in this section applies either to data acquired with a rectilinear k-space trajectory or to rectilinear k-space samples estimated with gridding. We consider only the case of full Fourier acquisition, in which data are sampled symmetrically over both positive and negative spatial frequencies. Reconstruction for the partial Fourier case, in which the acquisition is not symmetric, is handled in Section 13.4.

13.1.1 ZERO FILLING

The 2D- or 3D-IFT is usually done with FFTs. Because FFTs typically require the input data length to be a power of 2, the acquired data are appended with zeros in any direction(s) necessary to fulfill this condition. This step is also called *zero padding* or *zero filling*. It is customary to center the data in the 2D or 3D array that is input to the FFT; that is, the data are zero-filled symmetrically.

Sometimes additional zeros are appended to extend the data length to a yet higher power of 2 for image-quality considerations. Because the object is of finite extent (i.e., it has compact support), its FT has infinite extent, so the measured k-space signal is invariably truncated. Truncation is equivalent to multiplication of the k-space data by a rectangle function (i.e., a boxcar), which is equivalent to convolution in image space with a SINC function (the FT of the RECT function). Therefore, zero filling results in upsampling of the image by SINC interpolation and provides additional SINC-interpolated pixels in the display matrix. Although it does not add any information content to the raw data, zero filling can improve the apparent spatial resolution (i.e., measured in line pairs per millimeter) by giving the image a smoother or less blocky appearance due to reduced partial volume artifacts (Du et al. 1994). Zero filling has no effect on the SNR, although because it is an interpolation method it can correlate the noise. Zero filling is commonly used to increase the image matrix size in the phase-encoded direction (e.g., from 256 to 512) or in the slice-encoded direction for 3D scans (e.g., from 32 to 64). The apparent gains in spatial resolution are greatest for the first doubling of the FT length. Increasing the FT length beyond a factor of 4 provides magnification of the image, but does not provide any further gains in apparent spatial resolution. This is sometimes called 'empty' magnification.

A drawback to zero filling is the increase in reconstruction time due to the increased FT length. Also, images with large matrices, for example, 1024×1024 or 2048×2048, can bog down system functions such as display and archive. Finally, zero filling can increase the conspicuity of truncation artifacts (i.e., Gibbs ringing) in MR images (discussed later in this section). Despite these minor drawbacks, zero filling is widely employed in modern MR reconstruction algorithms because of its computational convenience and its image-quality advantages.

13.1.2 PHASE SHIFTING

As discussed in Section 1.1 on FTs, when a sequence of numbers $S_0, S_1, \ldots, S_{N-1}$ is input to an FFT, the algorithm assumes that the DC point (the zero frequency or zero time point) is the initial point S_0. The zero and positive spatial frequency (or positive time) values are assumed to be $S_0, S_1, \ldots, S_{N/2-1}$; the negative spatial frequency (or negative time) values are assumed to be (going from most negative to least negative) $S_{N/2}, S_{N/2+1}, \ldots, S_{N-1}$. Discrete sampling in one domain causes replication in the Fourier conjugate domain. Note that because the output of the FFT is discretely sampled, the input sequence is replicated, as shown in Figure 13.1.

MRI data are not generally acquired or stored in the input order expected by an FFT. For example, the data measured in a single readout of a full echo are ordered from negative to positive k_x (or vice versa depending on the readout gradient polarity), with the $k_x = 0$ point (DC point) falling in the middle for a full echo acquisition. When applying FFTs to k-space data, the data array could be reordered to fit the FFT locations. It is more common, however, to store the data with the DC point in the middle in the k_x, k_y, and k_z directions (assuming full k-space sampling) and to apply phase corrections after the FFT that compensate for the shift by $N/2$.

According to the Fourier shift theorem (Section 1.1), for 1D data a displacement by m data points gives a phase shift of $e^{i2\pi nm/N}$ for the nth data point in the Fourier conjugate domain. Therefore a displacement of $N/2$ pixels

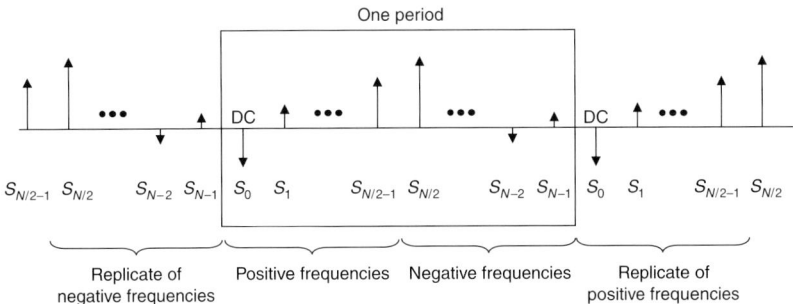

FIGURE 13.1 Raw k-space data sequence used as input for an FFT (indicated by the rectangular frame). The sequence values are $S_0, S_1, \ldots, S_{N-1}$. The DC value is S_0. Positive spatial frequencies (or times) are represented by $S_0, S_1, \ldots, S_{N/2-1}$. Negative spatial frequencies (or times) are represented by $S_{N/2}, S_{N/2+1}, \ldots, S_{N-1}$. The sequence can be thought of as a periodic array of replicates with the input to the FFT shifted by $N/2$ points relative to the conventional MR acquisition where DC is at the center of the array.

gives a phase shift of $e^{i2\pi n(N/2)/N} = e^{i\pi n} = (-1)^n$. This corresponds to a sign alternation of every other point. Therefore, it is not necessary to shift the array of input data to the FFT algorithm so long as the output of the FFT is sign alternated.

Similarly, the FFT algorithm creates an output sequence with the DC value as the initial point, not the center point. The output could be reordered to translate the DC point back the to the center. It is simpler, however, to apply a phase shift prior to the FFT that makes this happen automatically. The phase shift is just a sign alternation of every other k-space sample. For a 2D FFT, the resulting sign alternation for the entire 2D array is the combination for both directions, resulting in the checkerboard pattern illustrated in Figure 13.2. Similar extension applies to the third FFT direction. Note that if the half-pixel offset described in Section 1.1 cannot be neglected, it can be corrected for at this stage with appropriate phase shifts.

In summary, the FFT algorithm assumes that both input and output data are shifted by $N/2$ relative to the conventional ordering. The shifts are accomplished by sign alternation in the Fourier conjugate domain. Sign alternating the input gives the output shift; sign alternating the output gives the input shift. Note that for a magnitude reconstruction, the sign alternation step after the FT can be skipped, but the sign alternation before the FT must be performed.

13.1.3 WINDOWING

When measured data contain only a low-frequency subset of the complete set of magnetization Fourier components, the reconstructed image contains

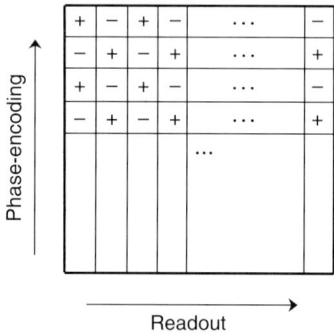

FIGURE 13.2 Sign alternation for 2D Fourier reconstruction. The matrix multiplies k-space data prior to the FFT to shift the DC point to the center of the image. The matrix multiplies the image after the FFT to compensate for the DC point of the k-space array being shifted to the center.

overshoot and ringing artifacts, particularly near sharp edges. The maximum overshoot (or undershoot) is approximately 9% of the intensity difference, irrespective of the number of data points used in the FFT. This artifact is also called *truncation artifact* or *Gibbs ringing* (after the American mathematician and physicist Josiah Willard Gibbs, 1839–1903, who first explained the phenomenon) (Oppenheim and Schafer 1989; Smith 1999). The truncation is equivalent to multiplying the k-space data by a rectangle function as previously discussed, and results in the convolution of the image with a SINC function. For small matrix sizes, which imply large pixel sizes, the rectangle has a relatively low cutoff frequency, giving a SINC that produces ringing with wide lobes. A useful rule of thumb is that truncation artifacts become substantial only when the edge transition width in the object is on the order of or smaller than the pixel size (without zero filling).

The ringing can be reduced by multiplying the k-space data by a filter or *window* function that smoothly attenuates the high spatial frequencies. This process is called *apodization* (literally translated as "cutting off the feet"). The signal from the spin density in the image is convolved with the FT of the window, which is known as the point-spread function. Because the window function smoothly rolls off toward zero, instead of abruptly truncating like the rectangle, the amplitude of the point-spread-function side lobes are smaller than those of a SINC function, which reduces the ringing. The trade-off is that the point-spread-function main lobe is wider than for the original SINC, thereby reducing the spatial resolution. The window is typically characterized by a cutoff distance k_c and a rolloff width w. These parameters are adjusted to trade spatial resolution for reduced ringing artifacts. A comprehensive list of useful window functions and their FTs can be found in Harris (1978). Windowing is usually applied in the k_x and k_y directions for 2D scans and in addition in the k_z direction for 3D scans. Note that the sign alternation matrix that places DC at the center of the output image can be conveniently built into the 2D or 3D window function.

An example of a window function from Harris (1978) suitable for use with MRI k-space data is the cosine taper or Tukey window. In one dimension, the Tukey window $W(k)$ is given by:

$$W(k) = \begin{cases} 1 & |k| < k_c \\ \cos^2\left(\dfrac{\pi(|k| - k_c)}{2w}\right) & k_c \le |k| < k_c + w \\ 0 & k_c + w \le |k| \end{cases} \qquad (13.1)$$

where k_c is the maximum unattenuated spatial frequency (cutoff), and w is the roll-off distance. The window transitions smoothly from 1 to 0 over the distance w (Figure 13.3). Applying the 1D window to 2D k-space data can be

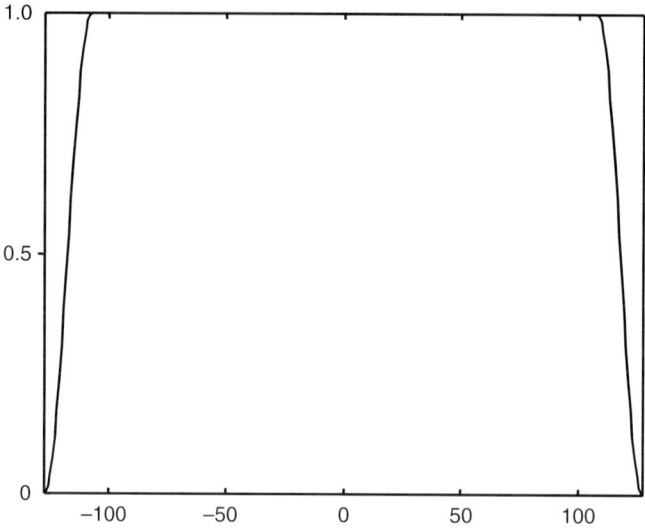

FIGURE 13.3 Plot of the 1D Tukey window in Eq. (13.1) with parameters $k_c = 108$ and $w = 20$. The window goes to 0 at $k = \pm 128$.

done in several ways. One way is to use a 2D window function $W_{2D}(k_x, k_y)$ that is a product of two 1D window functions (also called a *separable* window function):

$$W_{2D}(k_x, k_y) = W(k_x)W(k_y) \tag{13.2}$$

The window in Eq. (13.2) gives a point-spread function with a spatial resolution that is anisotropic (varies with direction in the image). Figure 13.4 shows an example of a 256×256 2D window function that corresponds to the point-spread function created using Eqs. (13.1) and (13.2) with the parameters $k_c = 108$ and $w = 20$. (In this section, k-space locations are given as indices in the k-space array, for example a 256×256 k-space array has k_x and k_y in the range $[-127, 128]$). As Figure 13.4 shows, the maximal cutoff extends further out along the diagonals of k-space. Correspondingly the lobes of the point-spread function are smaller, resulting in better spatial resolution along the diagonals than along the x and y axes.

A common choice is to use a window function with the same cutoff regardless of azimuthal angle to give isotropic spatial resolution. This is sometimes called a *radial* or *nonseparable* window. Because the noise power is relatively uniform over k-space and the signal power is concentrated near the center, the uniform cutoff also gives better SNR than a separable window with the same cutoff.

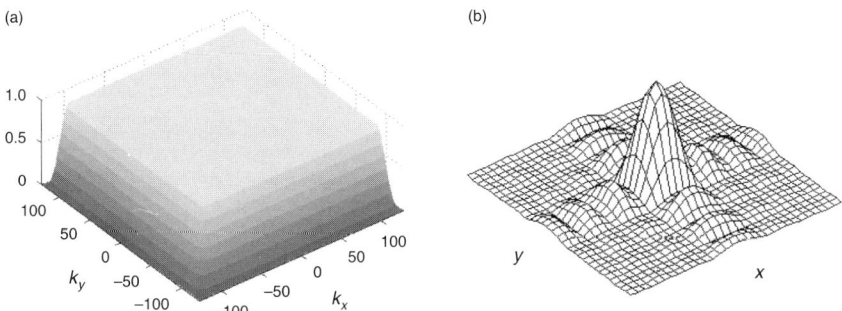

FIGURE 13.4 (a) 2D separable Tukey window function (256 × 256 k-space matrix) and (b) corresponding point-spread function (8 × 8 pixel display zoomed at the center with interpolation). The spatial resolution is anisotropic (varies with direction) because of inclusion of the corner areas of k-space. The window parameters are $k_c = 108$ and $w = 20$ for both k_x and k_y directions.

Note that using a uniform cutoff discards the corners of k-space. In fact, it can be shown that using the k-space corner data is not beneficial unless an interpolation method such as zero filling is used to increase the image matrix size (Bernstein et al. 2001). Interpolation by zero filling gives sufficient image sampling to use the data from the corners of k-space and results in higher diagonal resolution, provided those data are acquired and not discarded by windowing.

Even when zero filling is used, however, it is common practice to discard the corners of k-space with radial windowing to obtain isotropic resolution and improve SNR. This is one reason that some nonrectilinear k-space trajectories, such as spirals, are slightly more efficient than rectilinear trajectories when isotropic resolution is desired. Spirals do not waste time acquiring data in the corners of k-space. With rectilinear trajectories, if the corner data are discarded, the time spent acquiring these data is wasted because it does not contribute to improving the SNR. Efficiency can be improved for rectilinear trajectories by limiting the acquisition to a circular k-space area, for example with circular EPI (Section 16.1).

The radial window can be implemented using the 1D window function in Eq. (13.1) by setting:

$$|k| = \sqrt{k_x^2 + k_y^2} \tag{13.3}$$

where k_x and k_y are the usual Cartesian k-space coordinates. Figure 13.5 shows an example of using Eqs. (13.1) and (13.3) with a 256 × 256 k-space matrix, $k_c = 108$, and $w = 20$.

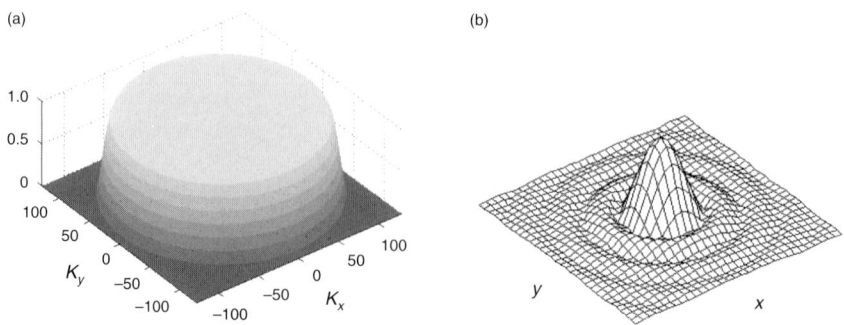

FIGURE 13.5 (a) 2D nonseparable (i.e., radial) Tukey window function and (b) corresponding point-spread function. The spatial resolution is isotropic because the window is circularly symmetric in k_x and k_y. The window parameters are $k_c = 108$ and $w = 20$.

So far we assumed that data were acquired over a square k-space matrix. To save scan time it is common to reduce the spatial resolution in the phase-encoded direction. To accommodate such scans with anisotropic resolution, the cutoff k_c varies with the k-space azimuthal angle θ. As before, a separable 2D window that retains the corners of k-space could be used:

$$W_{2D}(k_x, k_y) = W_1(k_x)W_2(k_y) \tag{13.4}$$

where W_1 and W_2 have different cutoffs k_c, corresponding to the different resolution limits (i.e., k-space extents) in the two directions. Alternatively, an elliptical cut-off variation that discards the k-space corners is described by:

$$\frac{k_{cx}^2}{k_1^2} + \frac{k_{cy}^2}{k_2^2} = 1 \tag{13.5}$$

where k_{cx} and k_{cy} are the k_x and k_y components of $k_c(\theta)$ and k_1 and k_2 are the ellipse radii (i.e. semimajor and semiminor axes) in the k_x and k_y directions, respectively. After some algebra, Eq. (13.5) can be rearranged to give:

$$k_c = k_1 \sqrt{\frac{k_x^2 + k_y^2}{k_x^2 + k_y^2/\varepsilon}} \tag{13.6}$$

where $\varepsilon = k_1/k_2$ is the resolution anisotropy. When $\varepsilon = 1$, we get $k_c = k_1$. Figure 13.6 shows an example of using Eqs. (13.1), (13.3), and (13.6) with $\varepsilon = 2$, $k_1 = 108$, and $w = 20$.

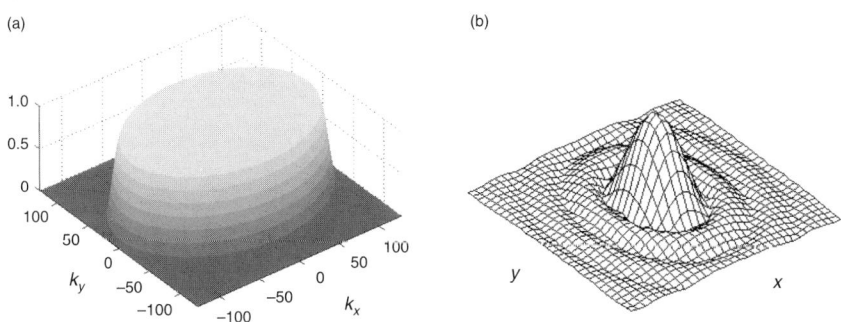

FIGURE 13.6 (a) 2D nonseparable Tukey window function and (b) corresponding point-spread function with anisotropic spatial resolution. The resolution is lower in the phase-encoded direction (k_y direction) by a factor of 2. The window has an elliptically varying cutoff that is correspondingly lower in k_y by a factor of 2. The window parameters are $\varepsilon = 2$, $k_1 = 108$, and $w = 20$.

13.1.4 RECTANGULAR FIELD OF VIEW

Many anatomical cross sections are better approximated by ellipses than by circles. A technique that exploits this fact to reduce scan time by decreasing the FOV in the phase-encoded direction is called *rectangular field of view*. If the FOV in the phase-encoded direction is reduced too much, rectangular FOV will result in aliasing or wrap-around artifacts. The technique is still useful if the wrapping artifacts are not superimposed on anatomy of interest. Rectangular FOV is mainly used for rectilinear k-space trajectories, but has been extended to some non-Cartesian trajectories (King 1998; Scheffler and Hennig 1998).

In the phase-encoded direction, the FOV is inversely proportional to the distance between measured k-space lines. For a fixed spatial resolution (fixed maximum k_y value $k_{y,max}$), the number of phase-encoding steps N is directly proportional to the FOV L_y:

$$N = 2L_y k_{y,\max} \tag{13.7}$$

Therefore scan time, which is proportional to N, can be shortened by reducing the phase-encoded FOV relative to the frequency-encoded FOV. This gives rise to an alternative name for rectangular FOV, *fractional FOV*.

It is straightforward to modify the pulse sequence to implement rectangular FOV by reducing N and increasing the step size between the phase-encoding gradient lobes to maintain the same $k_{y,\max}$ (i.e., the spatial resolution). The reconstruction changes are more substantial. If the reduced number of phase-encoded lines happens to be a power of two, an FFT can still be used in the phase-encoded direction. This will not usually be the case, however. In general there are three ways to perform the Fourier transform: (1) by discrete Fourier transform (DFT), (2) by k-space interpolation to give a power of 2 for the phase-encoded data dimension followed by an FFT, and (3) by zero filling to give a power of 2 for the phase-encoded data dimension, followed by an FFT and image space interpolation to restore the correct aspect ratio.

The first method is exact, but very time consuming because the DFT is much slower than the FFT. The second method is also time consuming because of the interpolation step. Because the object is compactly supported, SINC interpolation is the ideal choice. However, SINC interpolation is time consuming and a faster method such as gridding is the logical alternative. Some loss of image quality due to aliasing from the k-space resampling step typically results from gridding.

The third method may be the most practical with the computing hardware typically available on commercial scanners. As an example, if 256 phase-encoding steps are used with full FOV, selecting 3/4 FOV means that 192 phase-encoding steps are actually acquired. Let L_x and L_y be the frequency- and phase-encoded FOVs, respectively, and let Δx and Δy be the corresponding pixel sizes. Because 192 is not a power of 2, zero filling is required for the FFT. Zero filling and performing a 256-point FFT results in an image with $L_y = (3/4)L_x$. Because both frequency and phase FFTs have 256 points, the pixel sizes are related by:

$$\Delta y = L_y/256 = (3/4)L_x/256 = (3/4)\Delta x$$

The image is therefore magnified in the phase-encoded direction at this stage. The desired phase-encoded pixel size $\Delta y = \Delta x$ can be restored by interpolation (i.e., minification) in the y direction. For the special case of FOV fractions 1/2, 1/4, 1/8, and so on, reconstructed x and y matrix sizes (i.e., FFT lengths) are different, no stretching occurs, and no interpolation is needed. For example, selecting 1/2 FOV gives 128 phase-encoding steps and $L_y = (1/2)L_x$. Using a phase-encoding FFT with 128 points gives:

$$\Delta y = L_y/128 = (1/2)L_x/128 = L_x/256 = \Delta x$$

After the FFT and interpolation, the image will have unequal matrix sizes in x and y and must be zero-filled in the phase-encoding direction for display as a square matrix. Although the interpolation step is time consuming, depending on the algorithm chosen, the complete reconstruction may take less time than if a DFT were used. Because the interpolation takes place on the final image rather than in k-space, the artifacts from interpolation errors are less objectionable. A cubic spline interpolation is one possible choice (Parker et al. 1983). If an image-warping correction is used to compensate for gradient nonlinearity (see later discussion), the interpolation step can be conveniently included within it.

13.1.5 MULTIPLE-COIL RECONSTRUCTION

When multiple receivers are used, complex images from each coil-receiver pair are individually reconstructed as previously described. The final magnitude image is usually reconstructed using a square root of the sum of the squares algorithm (Roemer et al. 1990). If the image from each of the coils is $I_j(x, y)$, where j refers to the coil number, the final 2D image is:

$$I(x, y) = \sqrt{\sum_j \left(\frac{|I_j(x, y)|^2}{\sigma_j^2} \right)} \qquad (13.8)$$

where the sum runs over all the coils in the array, and σ_j^2 is the noise variance from coil j. The value of σ_j^2 depends on coil loading and therefore depends on the coil proximity to the patient anatomy. Therefore σ_j^2 is usually measured *in vivo* using:

$$\sigma_j^2 = E(x_j^* x_j) - E(x_j^*)E(x_j) \qquad (13.9)$$

where x_j is a complex random variable denoting noise from coil j, star (∗) denotes the complex conjugate, and E is the expectation operator (i.e., E operating on a random variable gives the mean of that variable). The measurement of σ_j^2 takes place during the calibration that is normally done for each patient scan to calibrate the RF power and transmit-receive frequency. The x_j are data collected without gradient or RF pulses at the readout bandwidth of the patient scan.

An image with slightly better SNR can be reconstructed if the receive coil B_1 fields $B_{1,j}(x, y)$ are known. The image is given by (Roemer et al. 1990):

$$I(x, y) = \frac{\sum_{j,k} B_{1,j}^*(x, y) \psi_{jk}^{-1} I_k(x, y)}{\sum_{j,k} B_{1,j}^*(x, y) \psi_{jk}^{-1} B_{1,k}(x, y)} \qquad (13.10)$$

where ψ_{jk} is the coil noise correlation matrix given by:

$$\psi_{jk} = E(x_j^* x_k) - E(x_j^*)E(x_k) \qquad (13.11)$$

Note that $\psi_{jj} = \sigma_j^2$. The reconstruction in Eq. (13.10) removes the receive coil B_1 weighting from the image. Therefore the final image $I(x, y)$ has different units than the individual images $I_k(x, y)$. The receive coil B_1 field $B_{1j}(x, y)$ can also be normalized so that the final image is weighted by the receive coil B_1 fields. Additional discussion of sensitivity measurement can be found in Section 13.3 on parallel imaging.

Due to the inconvenience of estimating $B_{1j}(x, y)$, the sum of squares approximation in Eq. (13.8) is more commonly used today. Roemer et al.

(1990) show that the SNR loss from using the sum of squares approximation is usually only a few percent. Eq. (13.10) reduces to Eq. (13.8) by approximating the receive fields using:

$$B_{1j} \approx \frac{I_j}{\sqrt{\sum_j \left(|I_j|^2 / \sigma_j^2 \right)}} \qquad (13.12)$$

by ignoring the coil noise cross-correlations, which are usually small, and by setting:

$$\psi_{jk} = \begin{cases} \sigma_j^2 & j = k \\ 0 & j \neq k \end{cases} \qquad (13.13)$$

The multiple-coil reconstruction in Eq. (13.10) is also the same as the reconstruction for SENSE when an acceleration factor of 1 is used.

Note that Eq. (13.10) gives a complex image, whereas Eq. (13.8) gives only a magnitude image, making its use problematic with methods that require phase images (e.g., phase contrast, temperature mapping, or shimming). Methods for estimating multiple-receive-coil phase difference images for such applications are described in Section 13.5.

13.1.6 IMAGE WARPING

MR imaging is based on the assumption that the z component of the total B field created by the gradient coils varies linearly with x, y, or z over the FOV. Linearity is high near the gradient coil isocenter, but degrades with off-center distance. The linearity fall off with distance depends on the gradient coil design. Substantially higher gradient amplitude and slew rate can be achieved by compromising a gradient coil's spatial linearity, effectively reducing the imaging volume over which a given linearity is achieved (Harvey 1999). Such a trade-off is attractive for applications that do not require a large FOV (e.g., for brain imaging).

With cylindrical magnets, the gradient field diminishes with off-center distance in z and increases with off-center distance in x and y due to proximity to the conductors. The effect is to increase the FOV or slice width with off-center distance in z and to decrease it with off-center radial distance. The image appears distorted both in size and intensity as a result. For example, in the z direction, the object in a sagittal image appears minified and brighter near the edge of the FOV in the superior-inferior (SI) direction (Figure 13.7). With 2D slice selection, the slice location is also shifted and is not planar (also called the potato chip effect). Depending on the coil design, gradient nonlinearity effects may be substantial enough to require correction.

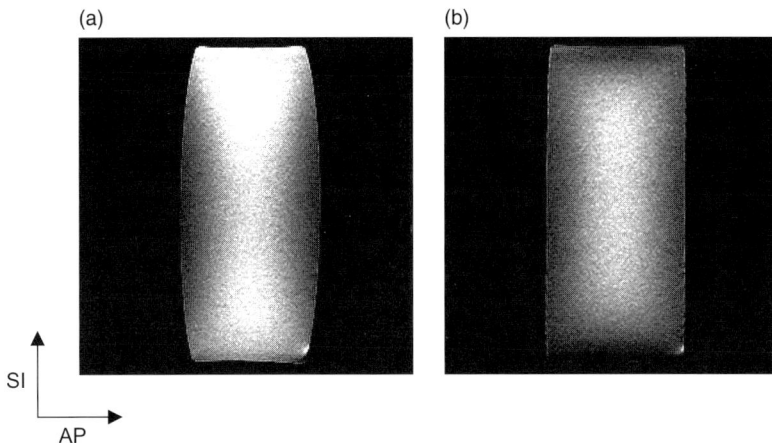

SI

AP

FIGURE 13.7 Sagittal image of a cylindrical phantom with a 48-cm FOV. The image was obtained from a horizontally oriented cylindrical magnet. Images are (a) without and (b) with a gradient warping correction. In (a) the object appears compressed in the anterior-posterior (AP) direction as well as brighter near the edges of the FOV in superior-inferior (SI) direction.

Image warping that is not directly related to the gradient coil can also occur in the phase-encoded direction with pulse sequences that use a train of gradient echoes (e.g., EPI) along with a rectilinear k-space trajectory. The warping can occur because of B_0 inhomogeneity, concomitant gradient fields, or eddy currents generated by large-amplitude gradient waveforms such as diffusion-sensitizing gradients.

Additional geometric distortion occurs in the readout direction with rectilinear k-space trajectories due to local resonant frequency variations arising from susceptibility differences within the object and chemical shifts.

For most clinical applications, only the warping due to gradient nonlinearity is routinely corrected. For some applications, such as DWI or stereotactic localization, other distortions must be corrected as well. Extensive work has been done on the measurement and correction of the various distortions. Hajnal et al. (2001) give a survey and list of references. Langlois et al. (1991) provide a correction algorithm for nonlinear gradient fields.

13.1.7 SCALING

MR acquisitions obey a well-known scaling relationship that states that the image SNR is proportional to the product of the voxel volume and the square root of the total time the data are sampled. (More discussion and an example of the use of this scaling relationship are provided in Section 11.6.) Separate scaling relationships can also be derived for the signal and for the noise. The MR signal intensity in a real, imaginary, or magnitude image is proportional to the receiver gain, the voxel volume, and the total acquisition time (which is proportional to the number of acquired k-space points in k_x, k_y, and k_z times the number of averages of each point). This scaling relationship for the signal is useful for image normalization in order to avoid the need for excessive window and level adjustment among various images, which simplifies image filming and display.

The image is also usually scaled to fit the dynamic range of the data storage and image display. (Note that image scaling here should be distinguished from the receiver-gain adjustment of the raw k-space signal, discussed in Section 11.6.) Images are typically stored in integer format (e.g., 2 or 4 bytes) and must be scaled so neither the greatest positive nor negative integer value is exceeded. Conversely, the scaling should not be too low, otherwise small-intensity fluctuations will map to less than one gray level change and the image will have a blocky appearance. The scaling factor used in image reconstruction is typically predetermined empirically based on receiver coil sensitivity, the allowable data dynamic range in the computer, and a representative imaging protocol.

13.1.8 BASELINE CORRECTION

With some receiver hardware, a DC offset (baseline) can be present in the measured k-space data. Although the baseline can be eliminated by phase cycling (Section 11.5), it is also sometimes measured either at the beginning or end of data acquisition and then subtracted from the raw data prior to all processing steps. This baseline is measured by collecting data without gradient or RF waveforms. The data collection time is chosen to give a baseline estimate with negligible noise. The baseline offset can also be estimated without acquiring additional data by taking the average of the last few points in a k-space line (FID or echo signals). A key assumption is that the magnetization has already decayed or dephased at the end of a k-space line and the remaining signal corresponds to the DC offset.

13.1.9 SUMMARY

The steps in the Fourier reconstruction of rectilinear k-space data are (Figure 13.8)

1. Subtract a baseline, if needed.
2. Zero-fill to the next power of 2 (or to an even higher power of 2 if image interpolation is desired).

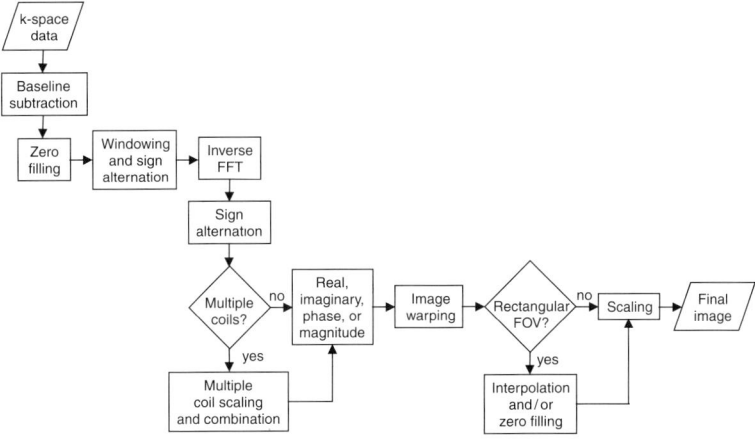

FIGURE 13.8 A flowchart summarizing the Fourier reconstruction steps.

3. Multiply by the window function to reduce Gibbs ringing. Sign alternation to translate DC to the center of the output array can be built into the window.
4. Apply a 2D or 3D inverse FFT to translate k-space data into an image.
5. Apply sign alternation of the output image if real or imaginary images are desired.
6. Combine multiple coil data, if appropriate.
7. Calculate the final image (real, imaginary, magnitude, or phase), including multiplication in the image domain by a sign alternation checkerboard, unless magnitude was chosen.
8. Apply image warping to correct for gradient nonlinearity, if needed.
9. Apply interpolation to restore the correct pixel-aspect ratio, if needed for rectangular FOV. This can be incorporated into the image-warping correction.
10. Apply scaling.

SELECTED REFERENCES

Bernstein, M. A., Fain, S. B., and Riederer, S. J. 2001. Effect of windowing and zero-filled reconstruction of MRI data on spatial resolution and acquisition strategy. *J. Magn. Reson. Imaging* 14: 270–280.

Du, Y. P., Parker, D. L., Davis, W. L., and Cao, G. 1994. Reduction of partial-volume artifacts with zero-filled interpolation in three-dimensional MR angiography. *J. Magn. Reson. Imaging* 4: 733–741.

Hajnal, J. V., Hill, D. L. G., and Hawkes, D. J. 2001. *Medical image registration*. New York: CRC Press.

Harris, F. J. 1978. On the use of windows for harmonic analysis with the discrete fourier transform. *Proc. IEEE* 66: 51–83.

Harvey, P. R. 1999. The modular (twin) gradient coil—high resolution, high contrast, diffusion weighted EPI at 1.0 tesla. *MAGMA* 8: 43–47.

King, K. F. 1998. Spiral scanning with anisotropic field of view. *Magn. Reson. Med.* 39: 448–456.

Langlois, S., Desvignes, M., Constans, J. M., and Revenu, M. 1991. MRI geometric distortion: A simple approach to correcting the effect of non-linear gradient fields. *J. Magn. Reson. Imaging* 9: 821–831.

Oppenheim, A. V., and Schafer, R. W. 1989. *Discrete-time signal processing*. Englewood Cliffs: Prentice-Hall.

Parker, J. A., Kenyon, R. V., and Troxel, D. E. 1983. Comparison of interpolating methods for image resampling. *IEEE Trans. Med. Imaging* 2: 31–39.

Roemer, P. B., Edelstein, W. A., Hayes, C. E., Souza, S. P., and Mueller, O. M. 1990. The NMR phased array. *Magn. Reson. Med.* 16: 192–225.

Scheffler, K., and Hennig, J. 1998. Reduced circular field of view imaging. *Magn. Reson. Med.* 40: 474–480.

Smith, S. W. 1999. *The scientist and engineer's guide to digital signal processing*. 2nd ed. San Diego: California Technical Publishing.

RELATED SECTIONS

13.2 Gridding Reconstruction

When the entire MR data set is acquired along a uniformly sampled rectilinear k-space trajectory, the image can be reconstructed using FFTs. If any part of the k-space trajectory is nonuniformly sampled, the reconstruction algorithm is more complicated. Examples of such trajectories are spiral, radial projection acquisition, and EPI with ramp sampling, sinusoidal readout gradient, or zig-zag k-space trajectory. Nonrectilinear or nonuniformly sampled k-space data could be reconstructed directly with a straightforward extension of the DFT, sometimes called a conjugate phase reconstruction (Maeda et al. 1988). However, this is usually far too slow to be practical. It is much faster to resample the data onto a uniform rectilinear grid to enable FFT reconstruction. The most common interpolation method is to resample the data after convolving them with a smooth function. The entire reconstruction process, including the FFT step, is frequently referred to as *gridding*.

Gridding is usually the method of choice for reconstructing data from nonrectilinear k-space trajectories. Radial projection MR data can also be reconstructed using filtered back-projection, but that method is currently less popular. In the following discussion we assume that k-space has been acquired using nonuniform sampling. The goal is to compute samples on a rectilinear k-space grid.

The problem of resampling a set of discrete data has been extensively studied and many methods have been developed (Matej and Bajla 1990; Rosenfeld 1998; Van de Walle et al. 2000; Sarty et al. 2001). Straightforward interpolation methods result in high artifact levels, although the artifacts can be reduced by using more sophisticated interpolation. A convolution-based method such as gridding is commonly used in MR imaging because it is relatively fast compared to other methods and gives adequate image quality. This technique uses a convolution in k-space to convert the input data to a uniform rectilinear data set. The choice of convolution function involves a trade-off between processing time and interpolation accuracy. Because the spin density itself is compactly supported (i.e., it is zero outside some finite region), the sampling theorem states that the k-space value at any location can be calculated exactly by SINC interpolation of the measured values (i.e., by convolving measured k-space values with a SINC function) as long as the measured values are sampled at or greater than the Nyquist frequency. The original nonuniform k-space sampling results in aliasing, which has an infinite extent in the image domain. If the original k-space data are sampled at the Nyquist limit, the aliasing lies outside the representation of the object (Figure 13.9a). Convolution of the measured k-space data with a SINC multiplies the image with a rectangle function, removing the aliasing that would result in the image domain (Figure 13.9b). Subsequent uniform rectilinear k-space resampling causes replication in the image domain after the 2D-FFT (Figure 13.9c). Because the aliasing has been removed, no overlap with the object occurs.

The disadvantage of SINC interpolation is that the SINC function is not compactly supported (i.e., it has infinite extent). Computing the k-space data at every new k-space location therefore requires multiplication of the SINC function by all measured k-space values, resulting in relatively long computation time.

In gridding, the SINC function is replaced by a compactly supported function (the gridding *kernel*) in order to reduce convolution time. Convolving the k-space data with the gridding kernel is equivalent to multiplying the image by the FT of the kernel, which is not compactly supported. Aliasing from the original sampling is therefore attenuated but not eliminated, as it is with a SINC convolution. The attenuated aliasing is replicated in the image domain (along with the object) after the FFT of the resampled rectilinear k-space data and therefore overlays the object.

Gridding therefore results in some loss of image quality compared to SINC convolution because resampling the convolved k-space results in an image with aliasing (discussed more extensively later in this section). The aliasing is usually reduced to an acceptable level by k-space oversampling to increase

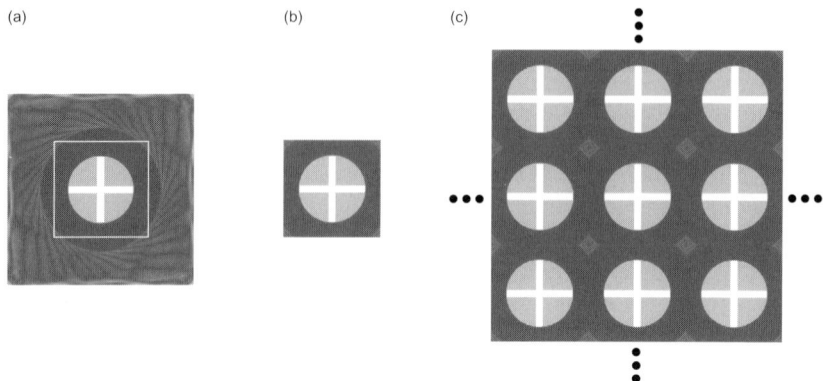

FIGURE 13.9 (a) Simulated spiral scan image showing aliasing artifacts (swirls). The aliasing extends to infinity even though only a finite section is shown. The box shows the FOV prescribed in the scan. (b) Image resulting from SINC interpolation of the k-space data used for image (a) without rectilinear resampling (i.e., continuous k-space data). (c) Image resulting from SINC interpolation plus rectilinear resampling. Image (b) is replicated at intervals determined by the k-space rectilinear resampling distance. If the k-space data corresponding to image (a) are convolved with a compactly supported function instead of a SINC, the aliasing artifacts will not be truncated as they are in (b). (c) Uniform rectilinear resampling results in the overlap of the object from one replicate and aliasing from other replicates.

the FOV (pushing rectilinear aliased replicates farther apart in the image) and then discarding the excess FOV after the FT. Because convolution results in multiplication of the image by the FT of the gridding kernel, usually resulting in substantial shading, the shading is removed by dividing the image by the FT of the kernel.

13.2.1   BASICS OF GRIDDING

Let us start with the 1D version of the algorithm; generalization to higher dimensions is straightforward. Let $g(k)$ be the gridding kernel and let $G(x)$ be its IFT. (Note that $G(x)$ should not be confused with the gradient notation used elsewhere in this book.). To begin with, consider the limiting case of continuous (not discretely sampled) data $S(k)$. Convolution with $g(k)$ gives:

$$S^{(c)}(k) = \int S(k')g(k - k')dk' \qquad (13.14)$$

where the superscript (c) is introduced to represent convolved data. Of course, if we really had continuous data instead of sampled data, the data could be sampled at uniform rectilinear locations without the convolution step. Now let the sampled k-space data be $S(k_j)$, where the locations k_j need not be uniformly spaced. Convolution of $S(k_j)$ with $g(k)$ can be approximated by converting Eq. (13.14) to a sum. Resampling the convolution at uniform locations $m\Delta k$, where m is an integer, gives:

$$S^{(c)}(m\Delta k) = \sum_j S(k_j)g(m\Delta k - k_j)\Delta k_j^{(s)} \qquad (13.15)$$

where the superscript (s) denotes the sampled data. If $g(k)$ has a compact support distance of w, the sum in Eq. (13.15) is taken over all the samples k_j that are located within a distance w of each output point $m\Delta k$. In other words, gridding is a local process that only needs to be performed near the original sample.

The factor $\Delta k_j^{(s)}$ is called the density compensation and corresponds to the discrete representation of the differential length element dk in Eq. (13.14). The density compensation is required because, otherwise, the convolution would give higher values in areas where the samples were denser and lower values in areas where they were sparser, even when the sampled k-space data S were constant. The density compensation is usually estimated from differences between adjacent sample locations, for example, in one dimension $\Delta k_j^{(s)} \approx |k_j - k_{j-1}|$. The factor $\Delta k_j^{(s)}$ is similar to the Jacobian dwell factor required for variable rate RF pulses (discussed in Section 2.4).

After evaluating the convolution in Eq. (13.15) at the desired uniform sampling points, a standard reconstruction is done (here a 1D-IFT is applied). To reduce aliasing, the uniform sampling distance Δk is usually chosen to be one-half the value needed for the final desired FOV L, $\Delta k = 1/(2L)$, resulting in $I(x)$ with twice the desired FOV. The excess FOV at the edges is discarded, and the central region with reduced aliasing is retained. The resulting image is the IFT of $S^{(c)}$ times the IFT of g, $G(x)$. Dividing by $G(x)$ gives the final image:

$$I(x) = FT^{-1}[S^{(c)}](x)/G(x) \qquad (13.16)$$

When gridding is extended to two or more dimensions, it is common to use a gridding kernel g_{2D} that is separable, that is, can be factored into a product of 1D kernels g_{1D}. For example, in two dimensions:

$$g_{2D}(k_x, k_y) = g_{1D}(k_x)g_{1D}(k_y) \qquad (13.17)$$

A nonseparable kernel can give slightly faster computation in some situations (Boada et al. 1999). In the following discussion we assume a separable kernel is used because it has the advantage of a slightly simpler implementation. The compact support length of the kernel can be different in different directions. For simplicity, we assume equal compact support lengths in all directions. The 2D resampled data are given by:

$$S^{(c)}(m\Delta k_x, n\Delta k_y)$$

$$= \sum_j S(k_{xj}, k_{yj})g_{1D}(m\Delta k_x - k_{xj})g_{1D}(n\Delta k_y - k_{yj})\Delta k_j^{(s)} \qquad (13.18)$$

The factor $\Delta k_j^{(s)}$ now represents the area around each of the nonuniformly sampled points. Details on how to obtain $\Delta k_j^{(s)}$ are given later in this section. The final image is obtained by performing a 2D inverse FFT of $S^{(c)}$, discarding the excess FOV as described before for the 1D case, and dividing by the inverse Fourier transform of g_{2D}. If the separable version of g_{2D} is used, its IFT is equal to the product of the IFTs of g_{1D}.

To reduce computation time, the gridding kernel value is usually not recalculated for each output point. Instead the kernel values are calculated for a relatively small number of points, say 256, and stored in a lookup table. Evaluation of $g_{1D}(k)$ in Eq. (13.18) is done by using the nearest value in the lookup table. Alternatively, if the same k-space trajectory is used for repeated reconstructions and sufficient memory is available, reconstruction time for all images after the first one can be reduced by storing the gridding kernel value appropriate for each input data sample and for each rectilinear location to which that sample is distributed.

In summary, the steps nrequired for gridding are the following (also see Figure 13.10 and Section 13.1 for a discussion of FT reconstruction steps).

1. Calculate the k-space locations and density compensation for each input data point.
2. Calculate the gridding kernel and its inverse Fourier transform. Either store the gridding kernel as a lookup table or store the values for each input and output data sample.
3. Subtract a baseline from the input data if needed.
4. Zero the output k-space matrix. For each input data sample, find all the uniform rectilinear output locations within the compact support distance of the input point. Distribute the product of the input data, the density compensation, and the appropriate gridding kernel weight to each of the output locations in a running sum as indicated by Eq. (13.18).
5. Apply a k-space window and sign alternation to the resampled rectilinear k-space data.
6. Inverse Fourier transform the uniform rectilinear samples to obtain an intermediate image.
7. If k-space oversampling is used to reduce aliasing, extract the center portion of the image corresponding to the desired final FOV.

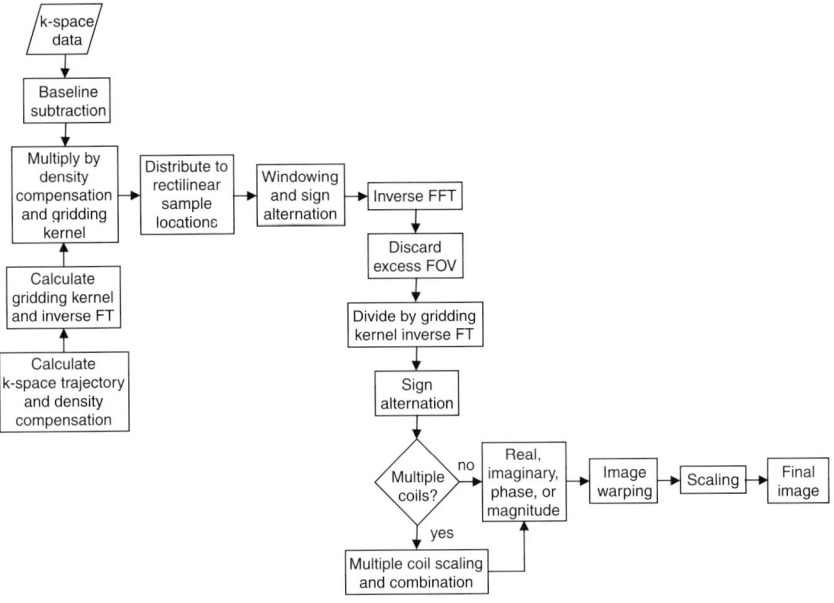

FIGURE 13.10 Flowchart of steps in gridding, including the subsequent image reconstruction using FFTs.

8. Divide the intermediate image by the Fourier transform of the gridding kernel.
9. Apply sign alternation if a real or imaginary image is needed.
10. Combine multiple coil data, if appropriate.
11. Calculate the final image (e.g., real, imaginary, magnitude, or phase, if appropriate).
12. Apply image warping if needed.
13. Apply image scaling.

13.2.2 RECONSTRUCTION TIME

The gridding reconstruction can be divided into three steps: convolution, FFT, and division by the IFT of the kernel. As an example, for the 2D case, the convolution in Eq. (13.18) is most conveniently done by taking each raw data sample, $S(k_{xj}, k_{yj})$, multiplying by the factor $g_{1D}(m\Delta k_x - k_{xj})g_{1D}(n\Delta k_y - k_{yj})\Delta k_j^{(s)}$ needed for k-space location $(m\Delta k_x, n\Delta k_y)$, and adding the product to a running sum over the raw data samples for that k-space location. This process is repeated for each uniform rectilinear sample location $(m\Delta k_x, n\Delta k_y)$

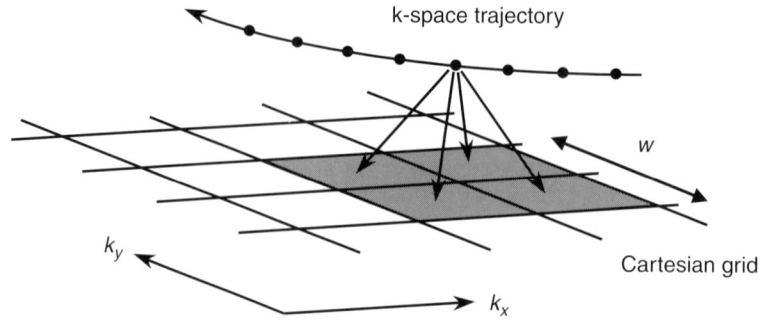

FIGURE 13.11 Diagram of gridding. Each input point is distributed to the uniform rectilinear output points that lie within the gridding kernel compact support distance w (shaded region). In this example, a separable kernel is used with $w = 2$ k-space sample points.

located within the compact support distance w of $S(k_{xj}, k_{yj})$ (Figure 13.11). The number of multiplications in the convolution step is therefore the number of input data samples N_s times the number of uniform rectilinear k-space locations located within a distance w of each input sample. If w is given in units of rectilinear k-space samples, the number of multiplications is $w N_s$ for 1D gridding, $w^2 N_s$ for 2D gridding, and so forth. Note that if sufficient memory is available, the factor $g_{1D}(m \Delta k_x - k_{xj}) g_{1D}(n \Delta k_y - k_{yj}) \Delta k_j^{(s)}$ can be computed in advance for each k-space sample. The factor does not need to be recomputed until a different k-space trajectory is used, and therefore we ignore its computation time. The FFT time for the 2D case is proportional to $\xi^2 N_x N_y \log_2(\xi^2 N_x N_y)$, where ξ is the k-space oversampling factor ($\xi \geq 1$), and N_x and N_y are the final matrix sizes in x and y. The division by the FT of the gridding kernel requires $N_x N_y$ divisions. The number of operations for the three steps is summarized in Table 13.1. The convolution step is usually the most time-consuming step. Improving image quality by increasing either w or ξ results in increased reconstruction time.

13.2.3 GRIDDING KERNEL

Extensive work has been done to determine the optimal 1D gridding kernel $g(k)$ (Jackson et al. 1991). The consensus is that a Kaiser-Bessel function gives nearly optimal results in the sense that the final image is closest to the ideal image (obtained with conjugate phase reconstruction or SINC interpolation, for example) using some suitably defined metric such as a least-squares difference.

TABLE 13.1
Approximate Number of Multiplications for Each of the Three Major
Steps in 2D Gridding

Step	Convolution	Fast Fourier Transform	Intensity Correction
Number of multiplications	$w^2 N_s$	$\xi^2 N_x N_y \log_2(\xi^2 N_x N_y)$	$N_x N_y$

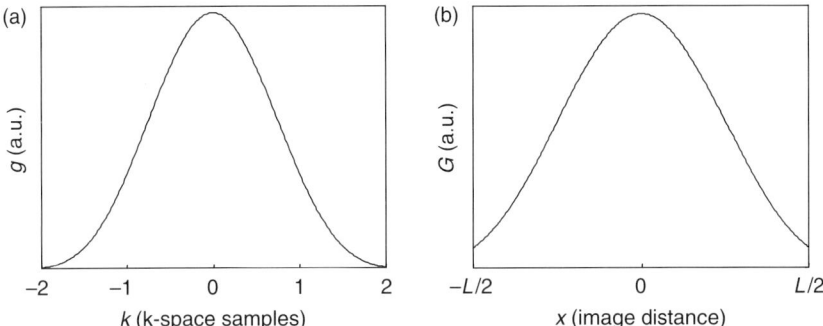

FIGURE 13.12 (a) Kaiser-Bessel function (in arbitrary units, a.u.) plotted as a function of k-space distance (in units of k-space samples). (b) Inverse Fourier transform of the Kaiser-Bessel function (in arbitrary units, a.u.) plotted as a function of image distance for FOV L. Kaiser-Bessel parameters are $w = 4$ and $b = 8$.

The 1D Kaiser-Bessel function $KB(k)$ (Figure 13.12a) is defined by:

$$KB(k) = (1/w)I_0\left(b(1 - 2k/w)^2\right) \text{RECT}\left(\frac{2k}{w}\right) \tag{13.19}$$

where I_0 is the zero-order modified Bessel function of the first kind, w is the compactly supported width of the kernel, b is a scaling parameter, and $\text{RECT}(u)$ is the rectangle function defined by:

$$\text{RECT}(u) = \begin{cases} 1 & |u| \leq 1 \\ 0 & |u| > 1 \end{cases} \tag{13.20}$$

The IFT of $KB(k)$ (Figure 13.12b) is given by:

$$\text{FT}^{-1}[KB](x) = \frac{\sin(\sqrt{\pi^2 w^2 x^2 - b^2})}{\sqrt{\pi^2 w^2 x^2 - b^2}} \tag{13.21}$$

For the Kaiser-Bessel kernel, $g(k)$ and $G(x)$ correspond to $KB(k)$ and $FT^{-1}[KB](x)$, respectively. Note that the scaling factors of $g(k)$ and $G(x)$ are not important as long as they are consistent with one another. Alternatively, a scaling inconsistency can also be compensated for by changing the final image scale factor after reconstruction (Section 13.1).

Although $g(k)$ is usually chosen to be a Kaiser-Bessel function, any smoothly varying, compactly supported function will work reasonably well. The difference in image quality due to choice of gridding kernel is usually relatively minor for MRI data. Even a triangle function has been found to give acceptable results with MR data. Gridding has also been used with CT and positron emission tomography (PET) data. Perhaps due to the higher SNR of CT data, image quality is somewhat more sensitive to gridding kernel selections.

The gridding kernel width w is usually chosen to be a few k-space samples (two to four is common). Increasing w causes $G(x)$ to fall off more rapidly, resulting in more suppression of aliasing artifacts, but correspondingly increases the computation time. If the Kaiser-Bessel function is used for the gridding kernel, the b parameter can be adjusted to change the fall-off of $G(x)$ for a fixed choice of w. Because the final image is divided by $G(x)$, care must be taken that it does not go to zero within the final FOV. The minimum values of b to avoid such a problem are shown in Table 13.2 for various values of w and ξ.

13.2.4 DENSITY COMPENSATION

The density compensation is, in effect, the area surrounding each k-space sample for the 2D case. It can be approximated by the differential area expression (numerical or analytic) for the k-space trajectory. If the original

TABLE 13.2
Minimum Kaiser-Bessel b Parameters[a]

			w		
ξ	2	3	4	5	6
1	0	3.51	5.44	7.30	8.89
2	0	0	0	2.36	3.51

[a] The b parameters are designed to avoid a zero in the Fourier transform of the Kaiser-Bessel function within the display FOV. The parameters ξ and w are the k-space oversampling factor and the Kaiser-Bessel compact support width, respectively, both in k-space sampling units.

sample spacing is uniform over k-space, as with rectilinear spacing, then in 2D, $\Delta k_j^{(s)} = \Delta k_x \Delta k_y$ is the same for all input samples and can be omitted because it simply contributes to an overall scale factor.

In 2D polar coordinates, the differential area element is $k \, dk \, d\theta$. The density compensation is therefore given by $\Delta k_j^{(s)} = k_j \, \Delta k_j \, \Delta \theta_j$, where $k_j \geq 0$ and $0 \leq \theta_j < 2\pi$. With radial projection acquisition, each spoke is acquired at fixed θ and all spokes have fixed increments Δk and $\Delta \theta$. If Δk_j and $\Delta \theta_j$ are the same for all samples they can be omitted. The density compensation then reduces to $\Delta k_j^{(s)} = k_j$.

For a 2D spiral scan, the polar coordinate density compensation $\Delta k_j^{(s)} = k_j \, \Delta k_j \, \Delta \theta_j$ can also be used. For an Archimedean spiral (Section 17.6) with uniform radial density, $k_j = A\theta_j$ and $\Delta k_j = 2\pi\lambda$, where $\lambda = N_{shot}/(2\pi L)$, and N_{shot} and L are the number of interleaves and FOV, respectively. For an efficient constant-velocity spiral, $\Delta \theta_j$ is not constant but must be calculated numerically or approximated. Hoge et al. (1997) has a more extensive discussion of spiral density compensations.

Trajectories That Cross   Some nonrectilinear k-space trajectories sample points in k-space multiple times. For example, rosette trajectories (Noll 1997), stochastic trajectories (Scheffler and Hennig 1996), and spiral trajectories have been designed that sample points (other than the origin) multiple times. It can be difficult to estimate $\Delta k_j^{(s)}$ when this happens. Also, for trajectories that cannot be expressed analytically, estimating the density compensation can be difficult. For such cases, gridding itself can be used for the estimation as follows. The density compensation can be thought of as a function of k-space location, for example, in two dimensions, $\Delta k_j^{(s)} = \Delta k(k_{xj}, k_{yj})$. Estimating the density compensation at an arbitrary location (k_x, k_y) from gridding yields:

$$\Delta k^{(s)}(k_x, k_y) \approx \sum_j \Delta k^{(s)}(k_{xj}, k_{yj}) g(k_x - k_{xj}) g(k_y - k_{yj}) \Delta k_j^{(s)} \quad (13.22)$$

Using $\Delta k^{(s)}(k_{xj}, k_{yj}) \equiv \Delta k_j^{(s)}$ gives:

$$\Delta k^{(s)}(k_x, k_y) \approx \sum_j (\Delta k_j^{(s)})^2 g(k_x - k_{xj}) g(k_y - k_{yj}) \quad (13.23)$$

For the typical situation in which $\Delta k_j^{(s)}$ is slowly varying, we can use the approximation $\Delta k_j^{(s)} \approx \Delta k^{(s)}(k_x, k_y)$ within the summation in Eq. (13.23). This factor can then be pulled out of the summation, resulting in:

$$\Delta k^{(s)}(k_x, k_y) \approx \frac{1}{\sum_j g(k_x - k_{xj}) g(k_y - k_{yj})} \quad (13.24)$$

Equation (13.24) can be used to estimate $\Delta k_j^{(s)}$ at the original sample locations (k_{xj}, k_{yj}), as shown in Jackon et al. (1991). Alternatively, for slowly varying $\Delta k_j^{(s)}$, the density compensation can be pulled out of the summation in Eq. (13.18), resulting in:

$$S^{(c)}(m\Delta k_x, n\Delta k_y) = \frac{\sum_j S(k_{xj}, k_{yj}) g(m\Delta k_x - k_{xj}) g(n\Delta k_y - k_{yj})}{\sum_j g(m\Delta k_x - k_{xj}) g(n\Delta k_y - k_{yj})}$$

(13.25)

The denominator in Eq. (13.25) can be thought of as the normalization needed to get $S^{(c)} = 1$ when $S = 1$ for each input data point.

As yet another alternative, if an estimated density compensation $\Delta k_j^{(s)} \approx \Delta k_j^{(e)}$ is available, the estimation can be improved (Meyer et al. 1992), resulting in a better estimation of $S^{(c)}$ by using a straightforward extension of Eq. (13.25). The result is:

$$S^{(c)}(m\Delta k_x, n\Delta k_y) = \frac{\sum_j S(k_{xj}, k_{yj}) g(m\Delta k_x - k_{xj}) g(n\Delta k_y - k_{yj}) \Delta k_j^{(e)}}{\sum_j g(m\Delta k_x - k_{xj}) g(n\Delta k_y - k_{yj}) \Delta k_j^{(e)}}$$

(13.26)

Equation (13.26) may be valuable for trajectories that cross, but that otherwise have an accurate estimate of $\Delta k_j^{(s)}$.

For k-space trajectories that cannot be expressed analytically or that cross, an iterative algorithm for estimating the density compensating has also been developed (Pipe and Menon 1999). For such trajectories, yet another method for estimating the density compensation is the Voronoi diagram (Rasche et al. 1999).

13.2.5 MATHEMATICAL DETAILS OF GRIDDING

The following section describes the mathematics of gridding in more detail. This section shows more clearly the origin of gridding aliasing artifacts and also applies this insight to derive a method of optimizing the gridding kernel. Readers who are not interested in these details can skip this section.

Reconstructed Image   Let the ideal continuous k-space data be $S(\vec{k})$, where $\vec{k}$ is the 2D or 3D k-space vector. The details of gridding are connected to problems stemming from the sampling of continuous functions. The symbol *III* (called the picket fence function) is sometimes used to mathematically represent sampling by multiplication with the function to be sampled. With uniform sampling in one dimension:

$$III(k) = \sum_j \delta(k - j\Delta k)\Delta k \qquad (13.27)$$

The factor Δk in Eq. (13.27) represents the distance between samples. Although this factor is sometimes omitted, it is necessary to make the sampling function dimensionless because the units of a Dirac delta function are the inverse of the units of its argument. This ensures that the original continuous function and the sampled function resulting from multiplication by III have the same units. Here we generalize the notation to the case of sampling at arbitrary locations in two or three dimensions. Let the k-space sampling function for the pulse sequence be $III^{(s)}(\vec{k})$ defined by:

$$III^{(s)}(\vec{k}) = \sum_j \delta(\vec{k} - \vec{k}_j^{(s)})\Delta\vec{k}_j^{(s)} \qquad (13.28)$$

where $\vec{k}_j^{(s)}$ and $\Delta\vec{k}_j^{(s)}$ are the k-space sample locations and the N-dimensional area around each sample respectively. (We discuss $\Delta\vec{k}_j^{(s)}$ in more detail later.) The sampled k-space $S^{(s)}(\vec{k})$ is given by:

$$S^{(s)}(\vec{k}) = S(\vec{k})III^{(s)}(\vec{k}) \qquad (13.29)$$

To get uniform rectilinear samples, $S^{(s)}(\vec{k})$ is first convolved with the gridding kernel $g(\vec{k})$. The convolved k-space data $S^{(c)}(\vec{k})$ are given by:

$$S^{(c)}(\vec{k}) = \left[S^{(s)}(\vec{k})\right] \otimes \left[g(\vec{k})\right] = \int S^{(s)}(\vec{k}')g(\vec{k} - \vec{k}')d\vec{k}' \qquad (13.30)$$

The convolved k-space data are then resampled to a rectilinear grid by multiplying by the rectilinear sampling function:

$$III^{(r)}(\vec{k}) = \sum_j \delta(\vec{k} - \vec{k}_j^{(r)})\Delta\vec{k}_j^{(r)} \qquad (13.31)$$

where $\vec{k}_j^{(r)}$ and $\Delta\vec{k}_j^{(r)}$ are the uniform rectilinear k-space sample locations and area around each sample, respectively. In two dimensions, $III^{(r)}(\vec{k})$ is given by:

$$III^{(r)}(\vec{k}) = \sum_p \delta(k_x - p\Delta k_x)\Delta k_x \sum_q \delta(k_y - q\Delta k_y)\Delta k_y \qquad (13.32)$$

where p and q are integers. The k-space sampling distances are given by:

$$\Delta k_x = \Delta k_y = 1/(\xi L) \qquad (13.33)$$

where ξ is the k-space oversampling factor ($\xi \geq 1$), and L is the final FOV, assumed to be the same in both directions. The rectilinearly sampled data $S^{(\mathrm{r})}(\vec{k})$ are therefore:

$$S^{(\mathrm{r})}(\vec{k}) = III^{(\mathrm{r})}(\vec{k})S^{(\mathrm{c})}(\vec{k}) \tag{13.34}$$

The rectilinearly sampled data are then inverse Fourier transformed using FFTs to give an image $I^{(\mathrm{r})}(\vec{x})$:

$$I^{(\mathrm{r})}(\vec{x}) = \mathrm{FT}^{-1}\left[S^{(\mathrm{r})}(\vec{k})\right] \tag{13.35}$$

Using the convolution theorem and Eqs. (13.30) and (13.34), gives:

$$I^{(\mathrm{r})}(\vec{x}) = \mathrm{FT}^{-1}\left[III^{(\mathrm{r})}(\vec{k})\right] \otimes \left\{\mathrm{FT}^{-1}\left[S^{(\mathrm{s})}(\vec{k})\right]\mathrm{FT}^{-1}\left[g(\vec{k})\right]\right\} \tag{13.36}$$

We define $I^{(\mathrm{s})}(\vec{x})$ as the image that results from a conjugate phase reconstruction of the original k-space data $S^{(\mathrm{s})}(\vec{k})$:

$$I^{(\mathrm{s})}(\vec{x}) = \mathrm{FT}^{-1}\left[S^{(\mathrm{s})}(\vec{k})\right] \tag{13.37}$$

We also define the IFT of the gridding kernel:

$$G(\vec{x}) = \mathrm{FT}^{-1}\left[g(\vec{k})\right] \tag{13.38}$$

Equation (13.36) becomes:

$$I^{(\mathrm{r})}(\vec{x}) = \mathrm{FT}^{-1}\left[III^{(\mathrm{r})}(\vec{k})\right] \otimes \left\{I^{(\mathrm{s})}(\vec{x})G(\vec{x})\right\} \tag{13.39}$$

We note that the FT of a 1D picket fence function is another picket fence (Bracewell 1999):

$$\mathrm{FT}^{-1}\left[\sum_j \delta(k - j\Delta k)\Delta k\right] = \sum_j \delta(x - j\Delta x)\Delta x \tag{13.40}$$

where $\Delta x = 1/\Delta k$. Therefore $\mathrm{FT}^{-1}[III^{(\mathrm{r})}(\vec{k})]$ is also a picket fence function because $III^{(\mathrm{r})}(\vec{k})$ is separable into a product of 1D picket fence functions. For example, in two dimensions,

$$\mathrm{FT}^{-1}\left[III^{(\mathrm{r})}(\vec{k})\right] = \sum_p \delta(x - p\Delta x) \sum_q \delta(y - q\Delta y)\Delta x \Delta y \tag{13.41}$$

Convolution with a rectilinear picket fence function replicates the convolved function at the spacing of the delta functions. Equation (13.39) results in:

$$I^{(r)}(\vec{x}) = \sum_j I^{(s)}(\vec{x} - \vec{x}_j)G(\vec{x} - \vec{x}_j) \tag{13.42}$$

where the rectilinear image replication locations $\vec{x}_j$ form a grid with spacing ξL equal to the inverse of the rectilinear k-space sample spacing (see Eq. 13.33). (The notation $\vec{x}_j$ describes discrete rectilinear sampling of the spatial variable $\vec{x}$. For the 1D case, $\Delta \vec{x}_j = j\Delta x$, whereas, for the 2D case, the subscript j maps onto two integers that indicate x and y locations; that is, $\vec{x}_j$ is equivalent to the coordinates $(p\Delta x, q\Delta y)$ where p and q are integers as in Eq. 13.41.) The terms represented by the summation in Eq. (13.42) are aliased replicates created by the rectilinear resampling.

The center of the image (central $j = 0$ replicate) is extracted for final display, discarding any excess FOV at the edge that results from k-space oversampling. Mathematically, this step is represented by multiplying the image by an N-dimensional rectangle function, symbolically represented as $\mathrm{RECT}(2\vec{x}/L)$. For example, in two dimensions, the function is:

$$\mathrm{RECT}(2\vec{x}/L) = \mathrm{RECT}(2x/L)\,\mathrm{RECT}(2y/L) \tag{13.43}$$

The image weighting resulting from the FT of the gridding kernel is also removed. The final image $I_{\mathrm{final}}(\vec{x})$ is given by:

$$I_{\mathrm{final}}(\vec{x}) = \mathrm{RECT}\left(\frac{2\vec{x}}{L}\right) I^{(r)}(\vec{x})/G(\vec{x}) \tag{13.44}$$

Aliasing in Gridding   Next we discuss the origin of aliasing artifacts in gridding. The original k-space sampling always results in aliasing:

$$I^{(s)}(\vec{x}) = I_{\mathrm{ideal}}(\vec{x}) + A(\vec{x}) \tag{13.45}$$

where $I_{\mathrm{ideal}}(\vec{x})$ is the object without aliasing, and $A(\vec{x})$ is the aliasing pattern. If $III^{(s)}(\vec{k})$ is a rectilinear sampling pattern, $A(\vec{x})$ consists of replications of $I_{\mathrm{ideal}}(\vec{x})$ located on a rectilinear grid. If $III^{(s)}(\vec{k})$ is a spiral sampling pattern, $A(\vec{x})$ consists of swirls (Figure 13.9a). Equation (13.42) becomes:

$$I^{(r)}(\vec{x}) = \sum_j I_{\mathrm{ideal}}(\vec{x} - \vec{x}_j)G(\vec{x} - \vec{x}_j) + \sum_j A(\vec{x} - \vec{x}_j)G(\vec{x} - \vec{x}_j) \tag{13.46}$$

Ideally $III^{(s)}(\vec{k})$ is chosen using the Nyquist sampling criterion so that $A(\vec{x})$ lies outside $I_{\text{ideal}}(\vec{x})$. If the gridding kernel $g(\vec{k})$ is a SINC, then $G(\vec{x})$ is a rectangle function and there is no overlap between $I_{\text{ideal}}(\vec{x})$ and $A(\vec{x})$. This results in $A(\vec{x})G(\vec{x}) = 0$ and the second term in Eq. (13.46) vanishes. In that case, the central replicate ($j = 0$) extracted as the final image (Eq. 13.44) reduces to:

$$I_{\text{final}}(\vec{x}) = I_{\text{ideal}}(\vec{x}) \tag{13.47}$$

If, however, $g(\vec{k})$ is compactly supported, then $G(\vec{x})$ never goes to zero and the replicates are attenuated but still overlap. In this case $A(\vec{x})G(\vec{x}) \neq 0$ and the second term in Eq. (13.46) is nonvanishing and overlaps the central replicate, resulting in aliasing contamination.

Because $G(\vec{x})$ decreases with $|\vec{x}|$, the replicates farther from the origin are more attenuated at the central replicate. Therefore moving the noncentral replicates further away by oversampling k-space ($\xi > 1$) decreases the aliasing artifacts from rectilinear resampling. The excess FOV is discarded. The final image is:

$$I_{\text{final}}(\vec{x}) = I_{\text{ideal}}(\vec{x}) + \frac{\text{RECT}(2\vec{x}/L)}{G(\vec{x})} \sum_j A(\vec{x} - \vec{x}_j)G(\vec{x} - \vec{x}_j) \tag{13.48}$$

where the second term represents the aliasing artifacts.

One simple method of optimizing the gridding kernel is to consider the weighting applied to the first adjacent replicate of $A(\vec{x})$ evaluated at the central replicate. From Eq. (13.48), this weighting (given without loss of generality

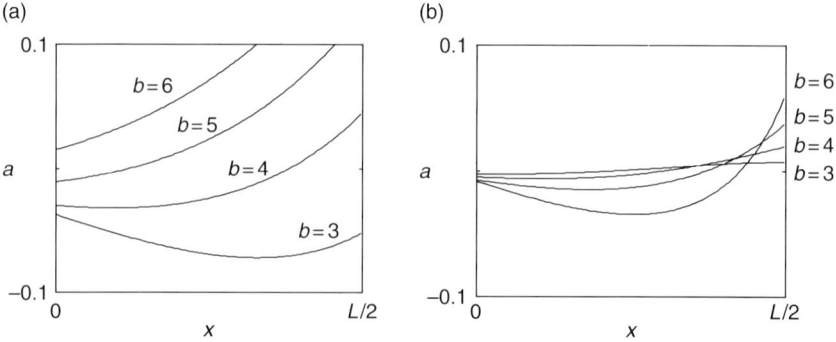

FIGURE 13.13 Plots of the gridding aliasing factor $a(x)$ given in Eq. (13.49) using a Kaiser-Bessel gridding kernel with $b = 3, 4, 5,$ and 6 (in units of k-space samples). The horizontal axis is the distance from the center to the edge of the displayed FOV. (a) $w = 2$. (b) $w = 4$. The k-space oversampling factor ξ is 2 for both cases.

for the first replicate in the x direction) is:

$$a(x) = G(x - rL)/G(x) \tag{13.49}$$

Choosing $G(\vec{x})$, or equivalently $g(\vec{k})$, to minimize $a(x)$ minimizes the weighting applied to the first adjacent aliasing replicate. Figure 13.13 shows plots of $a(x)$ for various Kaiser-Bessel function parameter choices.

SELECTED REFERENCES

Boada, F. E., Hancu, I., and Shen, G. X. 1999. Spherically symmetric kernels for improved convolution gridding. In *Proceedings of the 7th ISMRM*, p. 1651.

Bracewell, R. N. 1999. *The Fourier transform and its applications*. New York: McGraw-Hill.

Hoge, R. D., Kwan, R. K. S., and Pike, G. B. 1997. Density compensation functions for spiral MRI. *Magn. Reson. Med.* 38: 117–128.

Jackson, J. I., Meyer, C. H., Nishimura, D. G., and Macovski, A. 1991. Selection of a convolution function for Fourier inversion using gridding. *IEEE Trans. Med. Imaging* 10(3): 473–478.

Maeda, A., Sano, K., and Yokoyama, T. 1988. Reconstruction by weighted correlation for MRI with time-varying gradients. *IEEE Trans. Med. Imaging* 7(1): 26–31.

Matej, S., and Bajla, I. 1990. A high-speed reconstruction from projections using direct Fourier method with optimized parameters—An experimental analysis. *IEEE Trans. Med. Imaging* 9(4): 421–429.

Meyer, C. H., Hu, B. S., Nishimura, D. G., and Macovski, A. 1992. Fast spiral coronary artery imaging. *Magn. Reson. Med.* 28: 202–213.

Noll, D. C. 1997. Multishot rosette trajectories for spectrally selective MR imaging. *IEEE Trans. Med. Imaging* 16(4): 372–377.

Pipe, J. G., and Menon, P. 1999. Sampling density compensation in MRI: Rationale and an iterative numerical solution. *Magn. Reson. Med.* 41: 179–186.

Rasche, V., Proska, R., Sinkus, R., Bornert, P., and Eggers, H. 1999. Resampling of data between arbitrary grids using convolution interpolation. *IEEE Trans. Med. Imaging* 18(5): 385–392.

Rosenfeld, D. 1998. An optimal and efficient new gridding algorithm using singular value decomposition. *Magn. Reson. Med.* 40: 14–23.

Sarty, G. E., Bennett, R., and Cox, R. W. 2001. Direct reconstruction of non-cartesian k-space data using a nonuniform fast Fourier transform. *Magn. Reson. Med.* 45: 908–915.

Scheffler, K., and Hennig, J. 1996. Frequency resolved single-shot MR imaging using stochastic k-space trajectories. *Magn. Reson. Med.* 35: 569–576.

Van de Walle, R., Harrison, H. B., Myers, K. J., Altbach, M. I., Desplanques, B., Gmitro, A. F., Cornelis, J., and Lemahieu, I. 2000. Reconstruction of MR images from data acquired on a general nonregular grid by pseudoinverse calculation. *IEEE Trans. Med. Imaging* 19(12): 1160–1167.

RELATED SECTIONS

13.3 Parallel-Imaging Reconstruction

Parallel imaging is the use of phased array coils (sometimes called multicoil arrays) for the purpose of faster scanning. Phased array coils are most frequently used to improve SNR (Roemer et al. 1990). Except when imaging very small objects (e.g., tissue specimens) or at very low field strength (e.g., <0.2 T), the noise comes predominantly from the patient rather than from the measuring coils and electronics. The noise detected by a coil is induced by sources within the entire patient, but is weighted by the spatial sensitivity profile (receive B_1 field) of the coil. Phased array coils improve SNR by reducing the coil size (sensitive volume), thereby reducing the amplitude of the noise detected. Multiple coils, each with its own dedicated receiver channel, can be combined into an array, such that their sensitive volumes overlap slightly and cover the same volume as a single larger coil. When combined, these coils yield a signal with approximately the same amplitude as that of a single coil that covers the same larger volume. The noise, however, is greatly reduced, resulting in improved SNR.

Soon after the development of phased array coils, it was recognized that they could also be used to reduce scan time (Carlson 1987; Hutchinson and Raff 1988; Kelton et al. 1989; Ra and Rim 1993). The basis of all such parallel imaging methods is that scan time is linearly proportional to the number of phase-encoding lines in a Cartesian acquisition. Increasing the distance between phase-encoding lines in k-space by a factor of R, while keeping the maximal extent covered in k-space (spatial resolution) fixed, reduces the scan time (Figure 13.14) by the same factor. In parallel imaging, R is called the *reduction factor* or *acceleration factor*. Increasing the distance between phase-encoding lines also decreases the FOV. If the object extends outside the reduced FOV, aliasing or wrap-around artifact occurs (Section 8.2). In parallel imaging, the spatial dependence of the B_1 field of a receive coil array (also commonly called its *sensitivity*) is used to either remove or prevent the aliasing. SMASH (simultaneous acquisition of spatial harmonics) (Sodickson and Manning 1997) and SENSE (sensitivity encoding) (Pruessmann et al. 1999) are two well-known parallel-imaging strategies that prevent and remove the aliasing, respectively.

With SMASH, the spatial dependence of the sensitivities is used to synthesize missing k-space lines by approximating the corresponding sinusoidal phase twists produced by an encoding gradient. A single k-space data set is constructed and Fourier transformed to give the final unaliased image (Figure 13.15).

With SENSE, the individual receive coil k-space data sets are separately Fourier transformed, resulting in aliased images. The aliased images are then

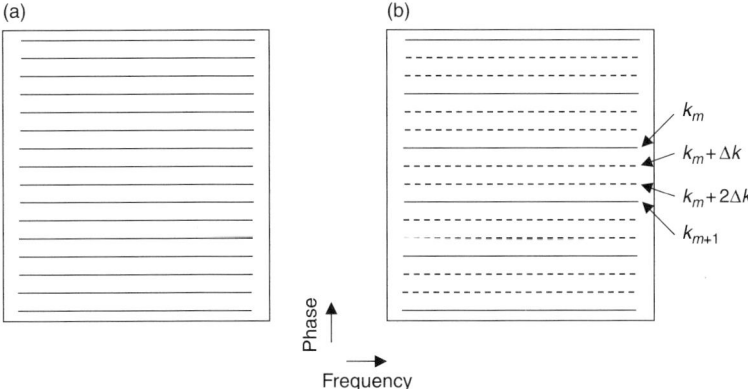

FIGURE 13.14 (a) Fully sampled k-space. (b) k-space for parallel imaging with an acceleration factor $R = 3$. Dashed lines represent k-space views that are not acquired. Two measured lines k_m and k_{m+1} are shown along with missing lines at locations $k_m + \Delta k$ and $k_m + 2\Delta k$, where Δk is the phase-encoding step size required for Nyquist sampling.

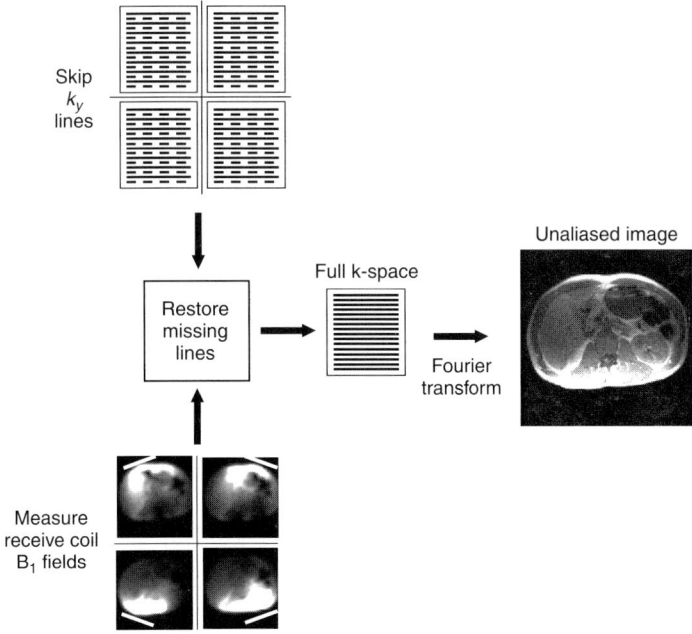

FIGURE 13.15 Schematic representation of the SMASH reconstruction with four receive coils. The dashed lines represent the skipped k-space lines.

combined using weights constructed from the sensitivities to give a single final image with the aliasing artifacts removed (Figure 13.16).

Parallel-imaging methods can generally be categorized as either k-space methods such as SMASH, in which missing k-space lines are restored prior to the Fourier transform, or image space methods such as SENSE, in which aliasing is removed in image space after the Fourier transform. The discussion in this section focuses on SENSE and SMASH. Other methods that do not fit into these categories are briefly mentioned later in this section. This section only covers parallel imaging for Cartesian (i.e., rectilinear) k-space trajectories that use phase-encoding. Parallel-imaging methods for nonrectilinear k-space trajectories such as spiral or projection acquisition have much greater computational complexity and are generally less practical with the computing hardware currently available on commercial scanners.

All parallel-imaging methods share several common features. SNR is always lower mainly due to reduced scan time, but there is usually an additional SNR penalty as well. In SENSE, unwrapping the image aliasing further magnifies the image noise. In SMASH, combining the data from individual coils in k-space can give partial signal cancellation and therefore reduce the SNR in some parts of the image. Usually, the noise variance in parallel imaging is also spatially varying.

Parallel-imaging methods require estimating the coil sensitivities. The sensitivities can be estimated using a separate calibration scan that covers

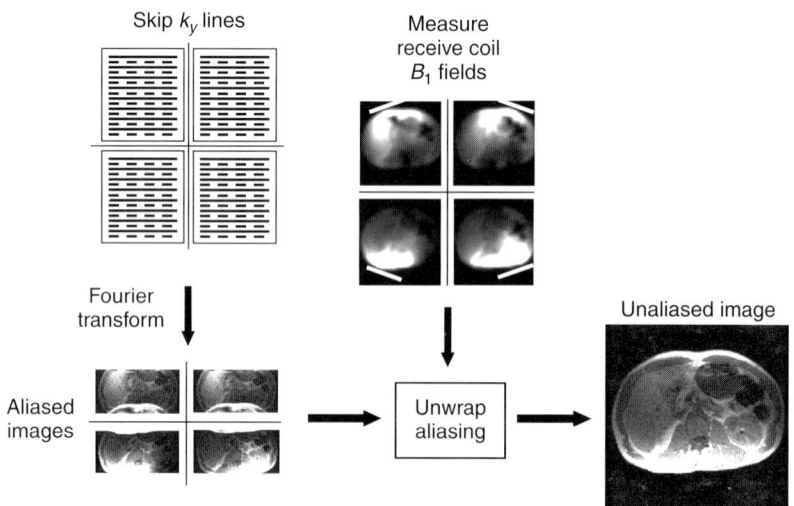

FIGURE 13.16 Schematic representation of the SENSE reconstruction with four receive coils. The dashed lines represent the skipped k-space lines.

the entire volume to be scanned with parallel imaging. Alternatively, a low-resolution sensitivity estimate can be built into the parallel-imaging sequence itself by measuring the central part of k-space with full Nyquist sampling while undersampling only the outer region of k-space.

The coils must have some sensitivity difference in the phase-encoded direction between object locations that alias to the same pixel in order to remove or prevent aliasing. Better separation of the sensitivity profiles gives better aliasing correction and less noise amplification, resulting in higher SNR. The optimal coil geometry for SMASH is probably an array of coils spaced along a line (a ladder array), although SMASH can produce high-quality images for any coil geometry. Parallel imaging can be applied to the secondary phase-encoding for 3D scans as well to the primary in-plane phase encoding. The object locations that produce aliased slices within a 3D slab are typically separated by much smaller distances than those that produce aliased pixels in the in-plane phase-encoded direction, assuming the same parallel-imaging acceleration factor R. This gives smaller coil-sensitivity differences between aliased replicates and worse image quality. Therefore parallel imaging in the slice-encoded direction has been found less useful. More discussion of this point is provided in Section 11.6.

Parallel imaging is most useful for applications that have abundant SNR. One of the most successful applications has been to contrast-enhanced MR angiography (Weiger et al. 2000). Reducing the scan time is beneficial for catching the peak of the bolus and for shorter breath-hold times. Figure 13.17 shows an example of contrast-enhanced MRA with SENSE.

Using steady-state free precession (SSFP) gradient-echo pulse sequences such as True FISP (Section 14.1) for cardiac scanning gives sufficient SNR to allow acceleration factors R of 2 or greater. This results in shorter breath-holding times, improved spatial resolution, or improved temporal resolution.

Another general way to use parallel imaging is for artifact reduction for echo train pulse sequences such as EPI (Section 16.1) or RARE (Section 16.4). EPI suffers from geometric distortion due to off-resonant spins, whereas RARE suffers from blurring due to T_2 decay. Parallel imaging reduces the total number of k-space lines, which in turn can reduce the echo train length. For a fixed echo spacing, the longer the echo train, the worse the artifacts, so greater benefits result from using parallel imaging. Thus parallel imaging is especially useful for single-shot pulse sequences such as HASTE (or single-shot RARE) and single-shot EPI, in which parallel imaging can substantially reduce the amount of geometric distortion (Bammer et al. 2002) or blurring (Figure 13.18).

An image can be reconstructed from undersampled k-space data with parallel imaging. Therefore, if full sampling (i.e., sampling that satisfies the Nyquist criterion) is used, parallel imaging provides a consistency check on

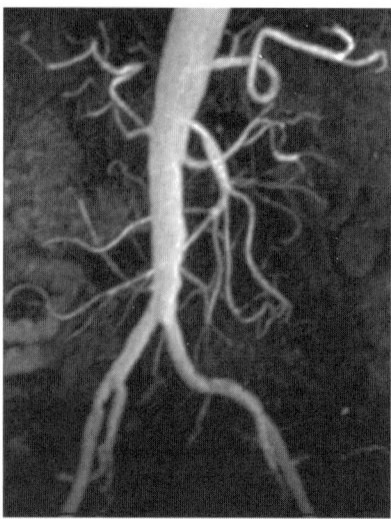

FIGURE 13.17 SENSE contrast-enhanced MRA of the abdominal aorta and branching vessels, with an acceleration factor of $R = 2$. A coronal maximum intensity projection is shown. (Courtesy Pr. Regent, Brabois Hospital, Nancy, France.)

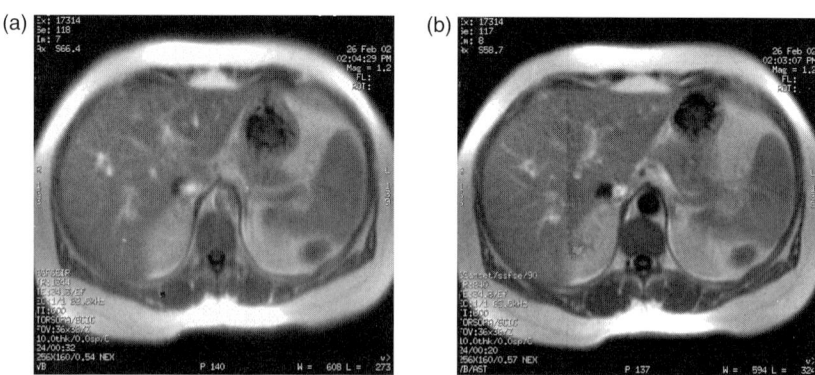

FIGURE 13.18 Single-shot RARE (HASTE) (a) without SENSE and (b) with SENSE. $R = 2$. The reduced echo train length with SENSE reduces image blurring. (Courtesy Larry Tanenbaum, M.D., Edison Imaging Associates, Edison, New Jersey.)

the data that can be used to correct for motion, Nyquist ghosting, or other artifacts (Kellman and McVeigh 2001; Bydder et al. 2003).

The next three subsections discuss the details of SENSE, SMASH, and their associated sensitivity calibration techniques, followed by an overview of other methods. Readers who are not interested in these mathematical details can skip these subsections.

13.3.1 SENSE

In MRI, the reconstructed image is weighted by the component of the receive coil B_1 field that lies in the transverse plane (Haacke et al. 1999), and this fact is key to parallel imaging. For 2D imaging, the image $I(x, y)$ is given by:

$$I(x, y) = B_{1\perp}(x, y)M_\perp(x, y) \qquad (13.50)$$

where $B_{1\perp}$ is the component of the receive B_1 field that lies in the transverse plane, and $M_\perp$ is the demodulated transverse magnetization, suitably defined to include relaxation, flow, diffusion, and transmit B_1 field nonuniformity effects. Note that this discussion assumes that we are using the rotating frame because $M_\perp$ is demodulated. In that frame, both $M_\perp$ and $B_{1\perp}$ appear static for on-resonance spins. In general, both $M_\perp$ and $B_{1\perp}$ are represented by complex numbers. (The magnetization and receive fields are vectors that we represent using complex notation, as described in Section 1.2.) To simplify the notation when discussing multiple coils, we drop the subscripts in Eq. (13.50) and introduce new subscripts that refer to each coil. Throughout this section we also denote the coil B_1 field or sensitivity as C. Thus, Eq. (13.50) can be rewritten:

$$I_j(x, y) = C_j(x, y)M(x, y) \qquad (13.51)$$

where the subscript j now refers to a particular receive coil.

With SENSE, the scan time is reduced by the acceleration factor of R by spreading the phase-encoded k-space lines by this factor (Figure 13.14). The FOV of the reconstructed image is therefore reduced by the same factor. If the object extends outside the reduced FOV, some pixels will be aliased, or wrapped. This means that the image signal at an aliased pixel is a superposition of signal from the desired location in the object plus pixels that are displaced by integer multiples of L/R, where L is the original (unreduced) phase-encoding FOV.

Without loss of generality, we take the phase-encoded direction to be the y direction in the image. We also drop any reference to the frequency-encoded direction because the following discussion holds for any frequency-encoded position x in the image. Let the total number of replicates due to aliasing at pixel location y be N_A. The value of N_A is pixel-dependent and is determined by R and by the size and shape of the object (Figure 13.19). For a square object with the same diameter in the phase-encoded direction as the original FOV, $N_A = R$ everywhere. If the object diameter is smaller, then some pixels will have $N_A < R$. If the object diameter is larger than L, some pixels will

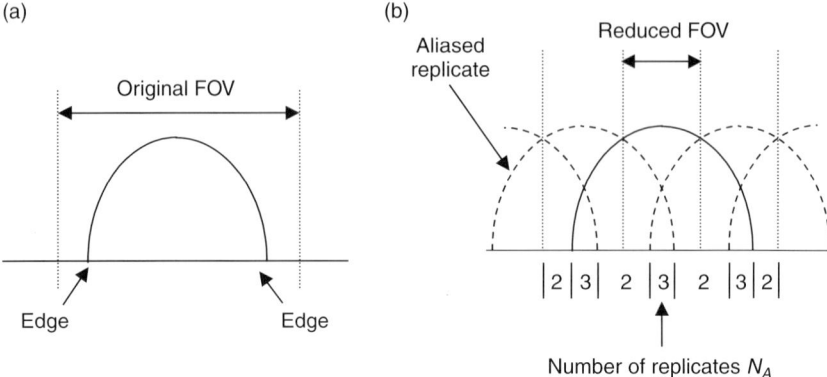

FIGURE 13.19 (a) Normal FOV. (b) Reduced FOV with $R = 3$ for parallel imaging. The number of aliased replicates N_A at each location y depends on the edge locations and the acceleration factor R.

have $N_A > R$ and there will be phase wrap even without the SENSE FOV reduction.

We can express the FOV reduction mathematically by saying that the R-fold FOV reduction results in an N_A-fold aliased image representation. For each location y, we can write the image signal $I_j(y)$ as a superposition of the original object and displaced replicates:

$$I_j(y) = \sum_{n=0}^{N_A-1} C_j(y + nL/R)M(y + nL/R) \qquad j = 0, 1, \ldots, N_c - 1$$

(13.52)

where N_c is the number of receive coils. Depending on the specific location of y, the number of replicates can vary. Thus, the range of summation is different, as schematically shown in Figure 13.20. If we assume that the coil sensitivities $C_j(y)$ can be measured, then for each value of y, Eq. (13.52) represents N_c simultaneous equations in N_A unknowns. The unknowns are the aliased magnetization values $M(y+nL/R)$. The $I_j(y)$ are known because they are simply the reconstructed aliased images. (Discussion of how to obtain the coil sensitivities is deferred until later in this section.) If $N_c \geq N_A$, the system of equations can be solved to obtain $M(y+nL/R)$. It is convenient to generalize Eq. (13.52) to a matrix equation. With N_c coils, we define appropriate matrices I, C, and M with dimensions $N_c \times 1$, $N_c \times N_A$, and $N_A \times 1$, respectively, and

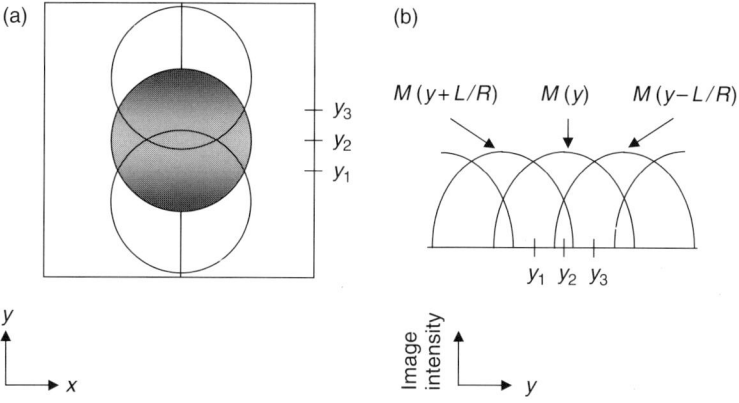

FIGURE 13.20 Aliased replicates for SENSE. (a) Image with original $M(y)$ (shaded) and two aliased replicates, $M(y + L/R)$ and $M(y - L/R)$. (b) Plot of image intensity along the vertical line in (a). At $y = y_1$, the overlapping replicates are $M(y)$ and $M(y + L/R)$, as in Eq. (13.52). At $y = y_2$, the overlapping replicates are $M(y + L/R)$, $M(y)$, and $M(y - L/R)$. At $y = y_3$, the overlapping replicates are $M(y)$ and $M(y - L/R)$.

rewrite Eq. (13.52) as:

$$I = CM \tag{13.53}$$

where:

$$I = \begin{bmatrix} I_0(y) \\ I_1(y) \\ \vdots \\ I_{N_c-1}(y) \end{bmatrix} \tag{13.54}$$

$$M = \begin{bmatrix} M(y) \\ M(y + L/R) \\ \vdots \\ M(y + (N_A - 1)L/R) \end{bmatrix} \tag{13.55}$$

and

$$C = \begin{bmatrix} C_0(y) & \cdots & C_0(y + (N_A - 1)L/R) \\ \vdots & \ddots & \vdots \\ C_{N_c-1}(y) & \cdots & C_{N_c-1}(y + (N_A - 1)L/R) \end{bmatrix} \tag{13.56}$$

If $N_c \geq N_A$, Eq. (13.53) can be inverted to find the estimated transverse magnetization $\hat{M}$. The most general solution that gives maximum image SNR is the pseudoinverse (Pruessmann et al. 1999):

$$\hat{M} = \left[\left(C^\dagger \psi^{-1} C \right)^{-1} C^\dagger \psi^{-1} \right] I \tag{13.57}$$

where ψ is the $N_c \times N_c$ coil noise correlation matrix in which a diagonal element represents noise variance from a single coil and an off-diagonal element represents a noise cross-correlation between two coils. (See Section 13.1 for the definition and a discussion of ψ.) If $N_c > N_A$, the inversion problem of Eq. (13.53) is overdetermined. The extra degrees of freedom are then used with the coil-noise correlation matrix ψ to improve the SNR. If $N_c = N_A$, there are no extra degrees of freedom available to improve the SNR. In that case, the coil-noise correlation matrix actually drops out of the solution. This can be seen by noting that for $N_c = N_A$, C is a square matrix and (assuming all inverses exist), $(C^\dagger \psi^{-1} C)^{-1} = C^{-1} \psi (C^\dagger)^{-1}$ so that Eq. (13.57) becomes:

$$\hat{M} = \left[(C^\dagger \psi^{-1} C)^{-1} C^\dagger \psi^{-1} \right] I = C^{-1} \psi (C^\dagger)^{-1} C^\dagger \psi^{-1} I = C^{-1} I \tag{13.58}$$

as we would expect from simply inverting Eq. (13.53).

Frequently the off-diagonal elements of ψ are negligible, and the diagonal elements are nearly equal to one another. In that case, ψ can be replaced by the identity matrix and Eq. (13.57) simplifies to:

$$\hat{M} = \left[(C^\dagger C)^{-1} C^\dagger \right] I \tag{13.59}$$

Usually, almost no difference in the SNR results from omitting the coil-noise matrix from the reconstruction algorithm for coils that are well decoupled.

With $R = 1$ (no scan time reduction), the SENSE reconstruction algorithm, Eq. (13.57), reduces to the optimal (maximal SNR) multicoil algorithm (Roemer et al. 1990). For the $R = 1$ case, the sensitivity matrix C is a column vector and the matrix product $C^\dagger \psi^{-1} C$ is a pixel-dependent number. Hence, $[C^\dagger \psi^{-1} C]^{-1}$ is just $1/(C^\dagger \psi^{-1} C)$. The reconstruction algorithm reduces to:

$$\hat{M} = \frac{C^\dagger \psi^{-1} I}{C^\dagger \psi^{-1} C} \tag{13.60}$$

This result is equivalent to that given in Section 13.1 for multicoil reconstruction (Eq. 13.10).

As we would expect, using SENSE always decreases the SNR because the scan time is reduced. The relationship between SNR with and without SENSE is:

$$SNR_{SENSE} = \frac{SNR_{NORMAL}}{g \sqrt{R}} \tag{13.61}$$

In Eq. (13.61), the normal scan has the optimal image combination given in Eq. (13.60). The factor $\sqrt{R}$ in Eq. (13.61) is the expected SNR loss that results from reducing the scan time by a factor of R (see Section 11.6). The factor g is called the *geometry factor* and represents noise magnification that occurs when aliasing is unwrapped. The geometry factor is determined by the diagonal elements of the matrix $C^\dagger \psi^{-1} C$ and its inverse. These diagonal elements are $[C^\dagger \psi^{-1} C]_{ii}$ and $[(C^\dagger \psi^{-1} C)^{-1}]_{ii}$, respectively for row (or column) i. The geometry factor is given by (Pruessmann et al. 1999):

$$g_i = \sqrt{\left[(C^\dagger \psi^{-1} C)^{-1}\right]_{ii} \left[C^\dagger \psi^{-1} C\right]_{ii}} \qquad (13.62)$$

Equation (13.62) applies to all pixels in the image with the same number N_A of aliased replicates. The subscript i refers to aliased replicate number i for that pixel and has the range $0, 1, \ldots, N_A - 1$. Equation (13.62) thus gives the geometry factor for all pixels that are related by aliasing at a particular location in the image.

In general, the geometry factor depends on the number of aliased replicates N_A and on the coil sensitivity difference between aliased pixels. The sensitivity difference depends on the coil conductor placement, the scan plane orientation, the phase-encoded direction within the scan plane, and the pixel location within the scan plane. In general, there must be some coil separation in the phase-encoded direction for aliasing unwrapping. Greater coil separation results in less noise magnification from the unwrapping. The geometry factor can therefore be thought of as a measurement of coil separation. It is useful to estimate the geometry factor when considering how to design a coil to be used with SENSE (Weiger et al. 2001). The geometry factor is a function of N_A and ranges from $g = 1$ for $N_A = 1$ to $g \sim 1.5$–2 for $N_A = 2$ with typical coil designs. SNR is spatially dependent in SENSE and changes abruptly as N_A varies within the image.

The noise amplification described by the geometry factor is also related to a property of the matrix $C^\dagger \psi^{-1} C$ that is inverted in Eq. (13.57), called its *conditioning*. A poorly conditioned matrix amplifies the noise in the unwrapped SENSE images. The noise amplification for a poorly conditioned matrix can be reduced by a process called *regularization*. Conditioning and regularization are explained in more detail in Press et al. (1992). There are several methods for regularizing a matrix. If the matrix $C^\dagger \psi^{-1} C$ is inverted using singular value decomposition (SVD), the matrix can be regularized by setting all eigenvalues that are below a certain threshold either to zero or to some appropriate lower limit. Alternatively, the matrix $C^\dagger \psi^{-1} C$ can be regularized by adding a term proportional to the unit matrix (King 2001). The amount of regularization can be adjusted to reduce noise at the expense of additional uncorrected aliasing. Regularization can be optimized for each pixel to give more uniform SNR.

13.3.2 SMASH

SMASH Reconstruction Algorithm	Data acquisition for a SMASH scan is the same as for SENSE—the phase-encoding line separation is increased by a factor of R, as shown in Figure 13.14. For simplicity, we assume here that R is an integer, although SMASH also works with noninteger acceleration factors. The concept underlying SMASH is that the coil sensitivities provide a spatial weighting of the received MR signal that is completely analogous to the spatial weighting provided by the sinusoidal (complex exponential) Fourier-encoding functions. In SMASH, linear combinations of the coil sensitivities are found that approximate the complex exponential functions corresponding to the omitted k-space phase-encoding lines.

As in the SENSE discussion, we take y to be the phase-encoded direction and drop reference to the frequency-encoded direction x. The desired k-space phase-encoding step size for a conventional (non-parallel-imaging) scan is:

$$\Delta k_y = 1/L_y \tag{13.63}$$

where L_y is the phase-encoding FOV. To reduce the amount of cumbersome notation, we henceforth drop the y subscript on k and introduce a subscript m that refers to the measured phase-encoding line number. The k-space data are therefore:

$$S_j(k_m) = \int C_j(y) M(y) e^{i2\pi k_m y} dy \tag{13.64}$$

where, as before, j refers to the coil number. Suppose the acceleration factor is $R = 3$, so $S_j(k_m)$ is measured for $m = 0$, $m = 3$, $m = 6$, and so forth. For a given measured k-space line m, we wish to construct the three new synthetic k-space lines:

$$\hat{S}(k_m) = \int M(y) e^{i2\pi k_m y} dy$$

$$\hat{S}(k_m + \Delta k) = \int M(y) e^{i2\pi k_m y} e^{i2\pi \Delta k y} dy \tag{13.65}$$

$$\hat{S}(k_m + 2\Delta k) = \int M(y) e^{i2\pi k_m y} e^{i2\pi (2\Delta k) y} dy$$

where the $\hat{S}$ notation denotes the new k-space data. Note that the new k-space lines $\hat{S}$ have no coil dependency (the subscript j is gone) and therefore there is no sensitivity weighting in the integrals on the right-hand side of Eq. (13.65). The goal is to synthesize the additional complex exponentials $e^{i2\pi p \Delta k y}$ (where $p = 0, 1, 2$) that appear in the integrals of Eq. (13.65) using combinations of the coil sensitivities. If we can find weighting factors that approximate the desired exponentials, then the synthesized k-space data in Eq. (13.65) can also be approximated. For example, let the coil weighting factors that give $e^{i2\pi p\Delta ky}$ be $a_{j,p}$:

$$\sum_{j=0}^{N_c-1} a_{j,p}C_j(y) = e^{i2\pi p\Delta ky} \qquad (p=0,1,2,\ldots,R-1) \qquad (13.66)$$

We can now obtain the new k-space data:

$$\hat{S}(k_m + p\Delta k) = \int M(y)\, e^{i2\pi k_m y}\, e^{i2\pi(p\Delta k)y}\, dy \qquad (13.67)$$

as follows. Inserting Eq. (13.66) into Eq. (13.67) gives:

$$\hat{S}(k_m + p\Delta k) = \int M(y)\, e^{i2\pi k_m y} \sum_{j=0}^{N_c-1} a_{j,p}C_j(y)\, dy \qquad (13.68)$$

Taking the summation outside the integral in Eq. (13.68) yields:

$$\hat{S}(k_m + p\Delta k) = \sum_{j=0}^{N_c-1} a_{j,p} \int C_j(y)M(y)\, e^{i2\pi k_m y}\, dy$$

$$= \sum_{j=0}^{N_c-1} a_{j,p}S_j(k_m) \qquad (p=0,1,2,\ldots,R-1) \qquad (13.69)$$

This is the desired result. The unmeasured k-space lines without coil sensitivity weighting are constructed as linear combinations of the measured lines (with a different weighting factor for each offset $p\Delta k$). New lines at the measured locations m are also constructed the same way without coil sensitivity weighting. Note that the coil weighting factors $a_{j,p}$ are independent of the measured k-space line location k_m.

To see graphically how to construct $a_{j,p}$, consider a ladder-geometry array of coils as shown in Figure 13.21a. A sample set of coil sensitivities is shown for the array in Figure 13.21b. For this oversimplified example, the sensitivities are shown as real functions, although in general they are complex. Most multiple coil arrays are deliberately designed so that the sum of the sensitivities is approximately constant (to give approximately uniform image homogeneity). Therefore, the first complex exponential $e^{i2\pi(0\times\Delta k)y}=1$ can be approximated as a scaled sum of the coil sensitivities (Figure 13.21c). The second complex exponential $e^{i2\pi\Delta ky}=e^{i2\pi(y/L)}$ (sine and cosine with one

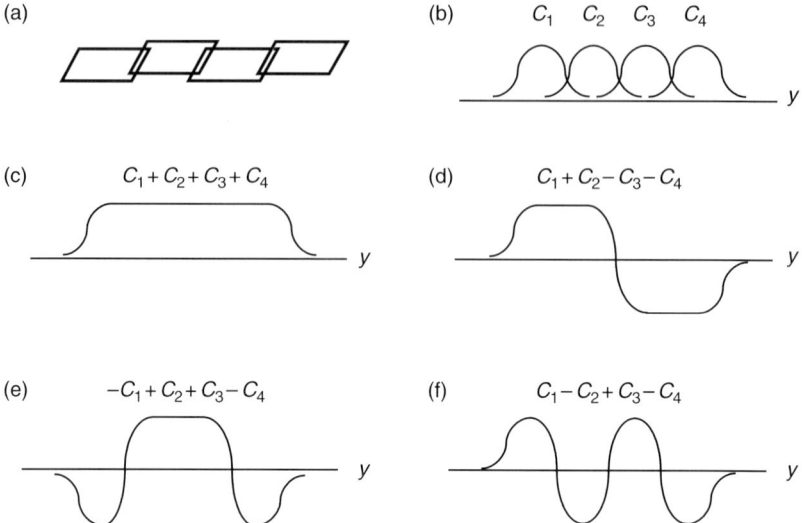

FIGURE 13.21 (a) Ladder array with four coils that could be used with SMASH. (b) Coil sensitivities. (c) Approximation of $e^{i2\pi(0\times\Delta k)y}=1$. (d) Approximation of $\sin(2\pi\,\Delta ky)$. (e) Approximation of $\cos(2\pi\,\Delta ky)$. (f) Approximation of $\sin(2\pi 2\Delta ky)$.

period over the FOV) can be approximated using scaled sums and differences of the coils as shown in Figure 13.21d–e. For the third complex exponential $e^{i2\pi 2\Delta ky}=e^{i2\pi(2y/L)}$ (two periods over the FOV), only the sinusoidal part can be well approximated as shown in Figure 13.21f. This illustrates an intrinsic problem with SMASH, namely that it is sometimes difficult to approximate harmonic orders comparable to the number of coils in the array.

This problem can be alleviated by generalizing the SMASH formalism (Sodickson and McKenzie 2001; Bydder et al. 2002; Sodickson 2000; McKenzie, Yeh, et al. 2001; McKenzie, Ohliger, et al. 2001). For example, for the $R=3$ case discussed earlier, we note that $\hat{S}(k_m+2\Delta k)$ is the same as $\hat{S}(k_{m+1}-\Delta k)$ (see Figure 13.14b). This means that instead of obtaining $\hat{S}(k_m+2\Delta k)$ as the second positive harmonic adjacent to line k_m, we can obtain it as the first negative harmonic adjacent to line k_{m+1}. The weighting factors to obtain $\hat{S}(k_{m+1}-\Delta k)$ from $S(k_m)$ will, in general, be different from those to obtain $\hat{S}(k_{m+1}-\Delta k)$ from $S(k_{m+1})$, but because a lower harmonic is being synthesized the synthesis may be more accurate.

Another generalization is the use of block reconstruction. Instead of synthesizing each missing harmonic $k_m+p\Delta k$ from a single measure k-space line k_m, as shown in Eq. (13.69), multiple measured lines are used. This is illustrated in Figure 13.22 where the six missing lines in each block of

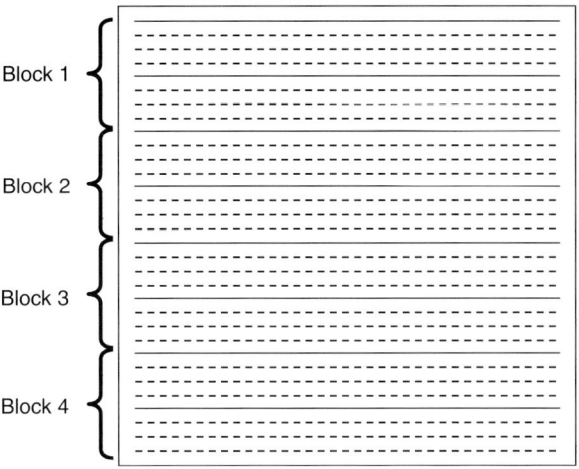

FIGURE 13.22 k-space for SMASH block reconstruction with $R=4$. Each block consists of eight k-space lines, two measured (solid) and six unmeasured lines (dashed). The six unmeasured lines in each block are synthesized from the two measured ones.

eight lines are synthesized from the two measured lines in the block. This generalization improves fitting accuracy, particularly for coil geometries for which complex exponentials are difficult to approximate by a linear combination of coil sensitivities. The block size can be chosen to trade reconstruction speed for image quality. Larger blocks give better image quality, but slower reconstruction.

The numerical procedure for determining $a_{j,p}$ is based on solving Eq. (13.66). To make the process clearer, we express the equation in matrix form. The matrix form is consistent with the use of discrete rather than continuous values of the variable y. Let:

$$f_{y,p} = e^{i2\pi(p\Delta k)y} \qquad (13.70)$$

where the values of y now correspond to discrete locations in the image and y can therefore be symbolically indicated by a subscript. Similarly we can write:

$$c_{y,j} = C_j(y) \qquad (13.71)$$

Equation (13.66) now becomes:

$$\sum_{j=0}^{N_c-1} c_{y,j}a_{j,p} = f_{y,p} \qquad (13.72)$$

which is a matrix equation of the form:

$$ca = f \tag{13.73}$$

where c, a, and f are matrices with dimensions $N_y \times N_c$, $N_c \times R$ and $N_y \times R$, respectively. The solution is:

$$a = c^{-1}f \tag{13.74}$$

Because c is not a square matrix in general, c^{-1} must be found either using the pseudoinverse such as $(c^{\dagger}c)^{-1}c^{\dagger}$ or using SVD. Because the pseudoinverse is the minimum-norm solution (Golub and Van Loan 1989) to Eq. (13.74), the resulting solution for $a_{j,p}$ satisfies Eq. (13.66) in the least-squares sense. Regularization can be helpful in reducing noise sensitivity of the fit.

SMASH scans have lower SNR than conventional scans (Sodickson et al. 1999; Madore and Pelc 2001). The SNR is dependent on the approximations used in the reconstruction algorithm (McKenzie, Yeh, et al. 2001; McKenzie, Ohliger, et al. 2001). Also, because of the approximations, the SNR dependency on the acceleration factor is more complicated than for SENSE. SMASH noise also varies spatially, but the variations are smooth rather than abrupt as with SENSE.

Variations of SMASH   In a method called generalized SMASH (Bydder et al. 2002), coil sensitivities are synthesized from Fourier harmonics instead of Fourier harmonics being synthesized from coil sensitivities. In AUTO-SMASH (Jakob et al. 1998), variable density (VD) AUTO-SMASH (Heidemann et al. 2001), and generalized autocalibrating partially parallel acquisition (GRAPPA) (Griswold et al. 2002), extra Nyquist-sampled k-space lines are acquired during the parallel-imaging scan and are used to calculate the weighting factors $a_{j,p}$ that determine the missing k-space data. More discussion of the latter three variations will be given next.

13.3.3 SENSITIVITY CALIBRATION

General Considerations   The image quality of all parallel imaging methods is determined by how well the coil sensitivities are characterized. Poor characterization results in uncorrected aliasing and low SNR. In general, it is better to measure the sensitivities from the imaged object rather than calculating them from the coil wire geometry using the Biot-Savart law or measuring them with a phantom. This is because the patient loading has an effect and also because coil placement is usually not predictable, especially with flexible coils.

There are two main calibration methods for measuring the sensitivity: direct and indirect measurement. In the direct method the sensitivity is explicitly calculated, whereas in the indirect measurement this step is skipped and the weighting factors $a_{j,p}$ for constructing k-space lines are computed from extra measured k-space lines. The latter method is only used with AUTO-SMASH, VD-AUTO-SMASH, and GRAPPA.

All practical calibration methods use low spatial resolution to save scan time. This generally works well because the sensitivities have rather slow spatial variation. When a separate calibration scan is used, the volume of image data acquired must encompass the entire region to be reconstructed with parallel imaging. Also when a separate calibration scan is used, the acquisition is usually a fast 2D or 3D gradient echo, and therefore has parameters that can differ from those of the parallel imaging scan. For example a low resolution 3D gradient echo calibration scan might use only a $32 \times 32 \times 32$ matrix over a $48 \times 48 \times 48$ cm^3 volume.

Sensitivity Normalization

Unnormalized Sensitivity   In the previous subsections, we have implied that the reconstructed images correspond to magnetization density without coil sensitivity weighting. In fact, all parallel-imaging techniques reconstruct images that have some type of coil sensitivity weighting. This is because a measurement of the pure coil sensitivity is not possible because all MR data are inherently weighted by the coil sensitivity.

Suppose that we use unnormalized complex surface coil image data to estimate the sensitivity. Let the surface coil calibration image data be $I_j^{\text{cal}}(y)$. Because of the reduced spatial resolution (and possibly different scan parameters), $I_j^{\text{cal}}(y)$ is generally different than the diagnostic image $I_j(y)$. We can define an effective calibration magnetization $M^{\text{cal}}(y)$ such that:

$$I_j^{\text{cal}}(y) = C_j(y)M^{\text{cal}}(y) \tag{13.75}$$

Using Eq. (13.75), we can rewrite the SENSE equation, Eq. (13.51), as:

$$I_j(y) = I_j^{\text{cal}}(y) \left(\frac{M(y)}{M^{\text{cal}}(y)} \right) \tag{13.76}$$

Using the unnormalized surface coil image $I_j^{\text{cal}}(y)$ as the sensitivity therefore results in a SENSE reconstruction of $M(y)/M^{\text{cal}}(y)$. The $M^{\text{cal}}(y)$ weighting in the image can be eliminated by multiplying the unwrapped magnitude image by a sum-of-squares calibration image given by:

$$\sqrt{\sum_{j=0}^{N_c-1} \left| I_j^{cal}(y) \right|^2} = \left| M^{cal}(y) \right| \sqrt{\sum_{j=0}^{N_c-1} |C_j(y)|^2} \qquad (13.77)$$

The resulting magnitude image is $|M(y)|\sqrt{\sum_{j=0}^{N_c-1} |C_j(y)|^2}$. The image is weighted by the sum-of-squares coil intensity $\sqrt{\sum_{j=0}^{N_c-1} |C_j(y)|^2}$ and therefore has the usual phased-array image shading. Therefore, if the intensity shading is acceptable or if a separate surface coil intensity correction is available (see Meyer et al. 1995, for example), the unnormalized calibration images can be used as a surrogate for the sensitivities in SENSE. As described in Sodickson and McKenzie (2001), a similar argument also holds for SMASH reconstruction, which can be shown by substituting Eq. (13.75) into Eq. (13.64).

Target Function Normalization   The final image intensity weighting for either SENSE or SMASH can be manipulated by appropriately normalizing the surface coil sensitivity data. As discussed in Sodickson (2000), it is useful to define a target sensitivity function $T(y)$. $T(y)$ can be a body coil sensitivity, a single-surface coil sensitivity $C_j(y)$, a surface coil sum-of-squares sensitivity $\sqrt{\sum_{j=0}^{N_c-1} |C_j(y)|^2}$, or a complex (phased) sum of surface coil sensitivities. The SENSE equation, Eq. (13.51) can be rewritten as:

$$I_j(y) = \left[\frac{C_j(y)}{T(y)} \right] [T(y)M(y)] = \left[\frac{C_j(y)M^{cal}(y)}{T(y)M^{cal}(y)} \right] [T(y)M(y)] \quad (13.78)$$

Thus, dividing the surface coil calibration image $C_j(y)M^{cal}(y)$ by the target calibration image $T(y)M^{cal}(y)$ gives a reconstructed SENSE image $T(y)M(y)$, in which the final image is weighted by the target sensitivity. For example, if $T(y)$ is a body coil sensitivity, then dividing the surface coil calibration image by the body coil calibration image gives a SENSE image with the body coil sensitivity weighting, which results in a relatively uniform image. Another common choice is $T(y) = \sqrt{\sum_{j=0}^{N_c-1} |C_j(y)|^2}$. Target-function normalization has no effect on the SNR in SENSE images. The target function multiplies both the image signal and noise, resulting in no change in the SNR.

A similar argument about target function normalization is also valid for SMASH. Equation (13.67) can be generalized to include a target function by writing it as

$$\hat{S}(k_{ym} + p\Delta k) = \int T(y)M(y)\,e^{i2\pi k_m y}\,e^{i2\pi(p\Delta k)y}\,dy \qquad (13.79)$$

The SMASH fitting equation, Eq. (13.66) is modified to be:

$$\sum_{j=0}^{N_c-1} a_{j,p}C_j(y) = T(y)e^{i2\pi p\Delta ky} \qquad (13.80)$$

The synthesized k-space lines are obtained, as before, using linear combinations of the measured k-space lines:

$$\hat{S}(k_m + p\Delta k) = \sum_{j=0}^{N_c-1} a_{j,p}S_j(k_m) \qquad (13.81)$$

Using a target function also improves the numerical conditioning of the SMASH fit, allowing more accurate results and better image quality. In particular, target-function normalization may produce fits with smaller $|a_{j,p}|$, resulting in lower noise and better SNR in the SMASH images (Sodickson 2000).

Note that the target function can be defined by the weights $a_{j,0}$ because by setting $p = 0$ in Eq. (13.80) we obtain:

$$\sum_{j=0}^{N_c-1} a_{j,0}C_j(y) = T(y) \qquad (13.82)$$

If we choose the weights $a_{j,0}$ to define the target function, then Eq. (13.82) holds exactly. However if we choose the target function rather than the $a_{j,0}$ (for example as a sum-of-squares of coil sensitivities), the coefficients $a_{j,0}$ are determined by fitting so that Eq. (13.82) holds in the least-squares sense.

Some SMASH variations have used the former method where the $a_{j,0}$ are chosen (rather than determined by fitting) so that the resulting $T(y)$ is a complex sum of coil sensitivities, as shown in Eq. (13.82). When this is done, partial cancellation in this sum can result in considerable shading or signal loss in the final image. Although the weights $a_{j,0}$ can be adjusted to minimize cancellation in a particular area, the shading can simply move to a different area of the image. This problem can be overcome by reconstructing N_c separate images, each with a target function equal to one of the coil sensitivities—that is, $T(y) = C_j(y)$ (coil-by-coil reconstruction). The resulting SMASH images are then combined either using the optimal phased array method (Eq. 13.60), or using a sum-of-squares (McKenzie, Ohlinger, et al. 2001). The resulting images are free of shading from cancellation, although the reconstruction time increases by a factor of N_c.

Direct Sensitivity Measurement   There are two general sensitivity measurement approaches currently used: acquiring a separate calibration scan and collecting extra data during the parallel-imaging scan itself to use for the calibration (self-calibration) (McKenzie et al. 2002). The latter method uses variable density sampling such that the lines near the center of k-space are sampled at the Nyquist frequency in order to reconstruct a low-resolution sensitivity map (Figure 13.23).

The main advantage of self-calibration is that it avoids the problem of patient motion between the calibration and parallel-imaging scans. Such motion, particularly respiration (or variation of inhalation position for breath-held scans), causes uncorrected aliasing and poor SNR. A disadvantage is longer scan time because of the fully sampled calibration lines (although the scan time can be shorter than the combined parallel-imaging time and a separate calibration scan). The overall acceleration factor can be recovered by increasing the acceleration factor in the outer part of k-space (outer reduction factor). The self-calibration lines can also be used in the parallel-imaging

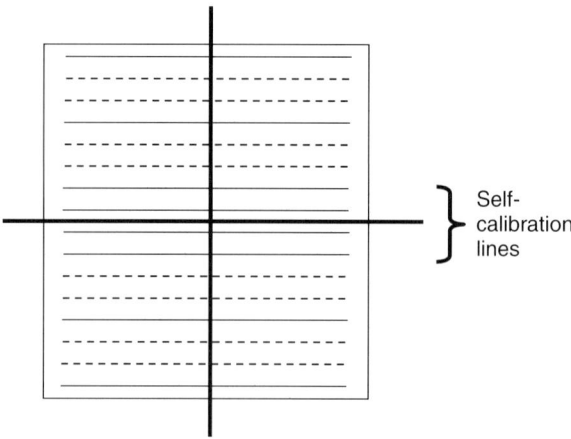

FIGURE 13.23 k-space for self-calibrated parallel imaging. The frequency- and phase-encoded directions are horizontal and vertical, respectively. The center four lines are sampled at the Nyquist frequency and are used to construct a low-resolution sensitivity map. Dashed lines are not acquired. The acceleration factor is $R = 3$ in the outer part of k-space.

reconstruction, thereby decreasing the amount of inherent aliasing that must be corrected and also giving higher SNR.

Indirect Sensitivity Measurement   In indirect sensitivity measurement method, one or more (extra) Nyquist-sampled lines are acquired near the center of k-space, similar to the self-calibration method described in McKenzie et al. (2002). The extra data are used to determine weighting factors $a_{j,p}$ for estimating the missing k-space lines, without explicitly computing coil sensitivity maps. The group of Nyquist-sampled lines are called the autocalibration signal (ACS) lines.

AUTO-SMASH   In AUTO-SMASH, $R-1$ extra lines are acquired (bold lines in Figure 13.24). The weighting factors $a_{j,p}$ are obtained by fitting the measured data using Eq. (13.81). A target coil weighting $T(y)$ is first created by choosing $a_{j,0}$ (Eq. 13.82). The ACS lines are then combined over coils using the $a_{j,0}$ to create composite ACS k-space lines that have the chosen target sensitivity:

$$\hat{S}^{ACS}(k_m + p\Delta k) = \sum_{j=0}^{N_c-1} a_{j,0} S_j^{ACS}(k_m + p\Delta k) \qquad (13.83)$$

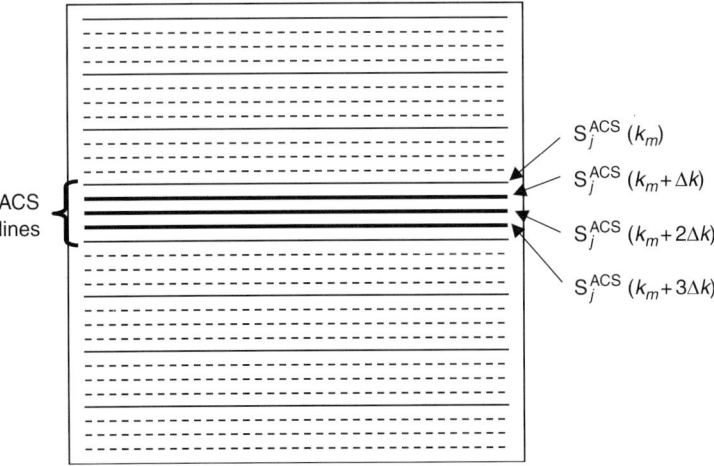

FIGURE 13.24   (a) k-space for AUTO-SMASH with $R=4$. Three extra k-space lines are acquired. The group of Nyquist sampled lines, or ACS lines, are used to determine weighting factors to synthesize the missing (dashed) lines. The frequency- and phase-encoded directions are horizontal and vertical, respectively.

Weighting factors $a_{j,p}$ can now be determined that will give $\hat{S}^{ACS}(k_m + p\Delta k)$ as linear combinations of $S_j^{ACS}(k_m)$:

$$\hat{S}^{ACS}(k_m + p\Delta k) = \sum_{j=0}^{N_c-1} a_{j,p} S_j^{ACS}(k_m) \qquad (p = 1, 2, \ldots, R-1)$$

$$(13.84)$$

Equation (13.81) can be written in matrix form and inverted to obtain the factors $a_{j,p}$. These same weighting factors can then be used to fill in missing k-space lines. As with conventional SMASH, instead of synthesizing missing lines as positive harmonics of k_m we can also synthesize them as negative harmonics of k_{m+1}.

In VD-AUTO-SMASH, additional sets of ACS lines are acquired to improve the fitting robustness and obtain more reliable $a_{p,j}$. The additional ACS lines are also included in the reconstruction, giving an improved SNR and reduced aliasing artifacts. Details of the fitting methods for AUTO-SMASH and VD-AUTO-SMASH are provided in Heidemann et al. (2001).

GRAPPA   GRAPPA is an improved version of AUTO-SMASH that uses two of the ideas previously discussed for better fitting accuracy and higher SNR. In the first enhancement, a coil-by-coil reconstruction is used in which N_c images are reconstructed, each with a target sensitivity equal to one of the coil sensitivities $T(y) = C_j(y)$. The images are then combined using the standard multicoil sum-of-squares algorithm.

In the second enhancement, instead of synthesizing a missing k-space line from a single measured line, the synthesis uses a group of nearby measured lines. The group of measured lines is moved depending on which k-space line is being synthesized (sliding block reconstruction). In general, multiple choices of group size and location are possible for any given missing k-space line. For the example in Figure 13.25 with $R = 2$, if four measured lines are used to synthesize each missing line, the bold dashed line can be constructed using measured line groups (0, 1, 2, 3), (1, 2, 3, 4), (2, 3, 4, 5), and so forth. If one or more ACS lines are acquired, the weighting coefficients can be determined for each such combination using the AUTO-SMASH method. Because each group of measured lines, in general, gives a different estimate of a missing line, the estimates can be combined in a weighted average. The weighting can be chosen to emphasize combinations that produce a higher SNR and better fits (Griswald et al. 2002).

Practical Considerations   The optimal sensitivity calibration may be application-dependent. If patient motion due to respiration is a concern, for

FIGURE 13.25 k-space for GRAPPA reconstruction with $R = 2$ and one extra (ACS) line. If four lines are used to synthesize each missing (dashed) line, the bold dashed line can be synthesized using measured lines $(0, 1, 2, 3)$, $(1, 2, 3, 4)$, and so on. The extra line (bold) allows the determination of the weighting factors. The frequency- and phase-encoded directions are horizontal and vertical, respectively.

example, with axial liver scans, self-calibration may be preferable to minimize the inconsistency between the calibration and parallel-imaging data. However, if motion inconsistency is less of a concern and scan time is very important, for example, with contrast-enhanced body MRA or real-time imaging, a separate calibration may be preferable. The same is true if relatively high acceleration factors are used (e.g., $R \geq 4$), because, as the acceleration factor increases, the self-calibration data becomes a greater percentage of the total scan time. GRAPPA and AUTO-SMASH are inherently restricted to using autocalibration. In this case, a trade-off between the number of ACS lines and scan time is made. Using more ACS lines generally results in better image quality at the cost of scan time. The optimal sensitivity normalization method may also be application-dependent. Using a body coil normalization gives a more homogeneous image, but requires extra calibration scanning. The extra scanning may be acceptable if an external calibration scan is used or if the image homogeneity would be unacceptable otherwise.

13.3.4 OTHER PARALLEL-IMAGING METHODS

Here we introduce methods that are either less widely used than SENSE and SMASH or in the early phase of development.

An algorithm called sensitivity profiles from an array of coils for encoding and reconstruction in parallel (SPACE RIP) formulates parallel-imaging MR reconstruction as a matrix inversion problem (Kyriakos et al. 2000). The algorithm requires inversions of very large matrices (e.g., inverting 256 matrices that have dimension 256×256) and hence can have a long reconstruction time. Its advantage is flexibility—any k-space sampling pattern can be accommodated.

An algorithm called parallel imaging with localized sensitivities (PILS) cuts away most of the aliased parts of the image for each coil and pastes together the remnants (Griswold et al. 2000). The cutting and pasting is done based on coil sensitivity weighting and coil separation distances. Sometimes also called the scissors method (Madore and Pelc 2001), the algorithm can work well if the coil sensitivities have little overlap. It is the computationally fastest method for reconstructing parallel-imaging data with nonrectilinear k-space trajectories such as spiral scans.

Parallel-imaging reconstruction with optimal image quality for spiral scans and other nonrectilinear k-space data requires the inversion of matrices that are two orders of magnitude larger than those arising for rectilinear trajectories. Such large matrices generally require iterative inversion methods (Pruessmann et al. 2001) such as conjugate gradient (Press et al. 1992). These methods are still generally too slow to be useful on current commercial scanners, but may become practical as computing hardware improves.

A method called unaliasing by Fourier encoding the overlaps using the temporal dimension (UNFOLD) (Madore et al. 1999) is a method for faster scanning, similar to parallel imaging. It is only applicable to a time series of images, for example, a functional imaging series, a dynamic imaging series, or a series of multiphase cardiac images. UNFOLD uses spatial aliasing to decrease scan time, similar to parallel imaging, but converts the spatial aliasing into temporal aliasing that is removed using a temporal filter. Unlike parallel imaging, UNFOLD does not require multiple coils. UNFOLD can also be combined with parallel imaging for even faster scanning or reduced artifacts (Madore 2002).

SELECTED REFERENCES

Bammer, R., Auer, M., Keeling, S. L., Augustin, M., Stables, L. A., Prokesch, R. W., Stollberger, R., Moseley, M. E., and Fazekas, F. 2002. Diffusion tensor imaging using single-shot SENSE-EPI. *Magn. Reson. Med.* 48: 128–136.

Bydder, M., Atkinson, D., Larkman, D. J., Hill, D. L. G., and Hajnal, J. V. 2003. SMASH navigators. *Magn. Reson. Med.* 49: 493–500.

Bydder, M., Larkman, D. J., and Hajnal, J. V. 2002. Generalized SMASH imaging. *Magn. Reson. Med.* 47: 160–170.

Carlson, J. W. 1987. An algorithm for NMR imaging reconstruction based on multiple RF receiver coils. *J. Magn. Reson.* 74: 376–380.

Golub, G. H., and Van Loan, C. F. 1989. *Matrix computations.* Baltimore: Johns Hopkins University Press.

Griswold, M. A., Jakob, P. M., Heidemann, R. M., Nittka, M., Jellus, V., Wang, J., Keifer B., and Haase, A. 2002. Generalized autocalibrating partially parallel acquisitions (GRAPPA). *Magn. Reson. Med.* 47: 1202–1210.

Griswold, M. A., Jakob, P. M., Nittka, M., Goldfarb, J. W., and Haase, A. 2000. Partially parallel imaging with localized sensitivities (PILS). *Magn. Reson. Med.* 44: 602–609.

Haacke, E. M., Brown, R. W., Thompson, M. R., and Venkatesan, R. 1999. *Magnetic resonance imaging: Physical principles and sequence design.* New York: John Wiley & Sons. p 99–101.

Heidemann, R. M., Griswold, M. A., Haase, A., and Jakob, P. 2001. VD-AUTO-SMASH imaging. *Magn. Reson. Med.* 45: 1066–1074.

Hutchinson, M., and Raff, U. 1988. Fast MRI data acquisition using multiple detectors. *Magn. Reson. Med.* 6: 87–91.

Jakob, P. M., Griswold, M. A., Edelman, R. R., and Sodickson, D. K. 1998. AUTO-SMASH: A self-calibrating technique for SMASH imaging. *MAGMA* 7: 42–54.

Kellman, P., and McVeigh, E. R. 2001. Ghost artifact cancellation using phased array processing. *Magn. Reson. Med.* 46: 335–343.

Kelton, J., Magin, R. M., and Wright, S. M. 1989. An algorithm for rapid acquisition using multiple receiver coils. In *Proceedings of the 8th Annual SMRM*, p. 1172.

King, K. 2001. SENSE image quality improvement using matrix regularization. In *Proceedings of the 9th ISMRM*, p. 1771.

Kyriakos, W. E., Panych, L. P., Kacher, D. F., Westin C.-F., Bao, S. M., Mulkern, R. V., and Jolesz, F. A. 2000. Sensitivity profiles from an array of coils for encoding and reconstruction in parallel (SPACE RIP). *Magn. Reson. Med.* 44: 301–308.

Madore, B. 2002. Using UNFOLD to remove artifacts in parallel imaging and in partial-Fourier imaging. *Magn. Reson. Med.* 48: 493–501.

Madore, B., Glover, G. H., and Pelc, N. J. 1999. Unaliasing by Fourier-encoding the overlaps using the temporal dimension (UNFOLD), applied to cardiac imaging and fMRI. *Magn. Reson. Med.* 42: 813–828.

Madore, B., and Pelc, N. 2001. SMASH and SENSE: Experimental and numerical comparisons. *Magn. Reson. Med.* 45: 1103–1111.

McKenzie, C. A., Ohliger, M. A., Yeh, E. N., Price, M. D., and Sodickson, D. K. 2001. Coil-by-coil image reconstructon with SMASH. *Magn. Reson. Med.* 46: 619–623.

McKenzie, C. A., Yeh, E. N., Ohliger, M. A., Price, M. D., and Sodickson, D. K. 2002. Self-calibrating parallel imaging with automatic coil sensitivity extraction. *Magn. Reson. Med.* 47: 529–538.

McKenzie, C. A., Yeh, E. N., and Sodickson, D. K. 2001. Improved spatial harmonic selection for SMASH image reconstructions. *Magn. Reson. Med.* 46: 831–836.

Meyer, C. R., Bland, P. H., and Pipe, J. 1995. Retrospective correction of intensity inhomogeneities in MRI. *IEEE Trans. Med. Imaging* 14: 36–41.

Press, W. H., Teukolsky, S. A., Vetterling, W. T., and Flannery, B. P. 1992. *Numerical recipes in C.* Cambridge, U.K.: Cambridge University Press.

Pruessmann, K. P., Weiger, M., Boernert, P., and Boesiger, P. 2001. Advances in sensitivity encoding with arbitrary k-space trajectories. *Magn. Reson. Med.* 46: 638–651.

Pruessmann, K. P., Weiger, M., Scheidegger, M. B., and Boesiger, P. 1999. SENSE: Sensitivity encoding for fast MRI. *Magn. Reson. Med.* 42: 952–962.

Ra, J. B., and Rim, C. Y. 1993. Fast imaging using subencoding data sets from multiple detectors. *Magn. Reson. Med.* 30: 142–145.

Roemer, P. B., Edelstein, W. A., Hayes, C. E., Souza, S. P., and Mueller, O. M. 1990. The NMR phased array. *Magn. Reson. Med.* 16: 192–225.

Sodickson, D. K. 2000. Tailored SMASH image reconstructions for robust in vivo parallel MR imaging. *Magn. Reson. Med.* 44: 243–251.

Sodickson, D. K., Griswold, M. A., Jakob, P. M., Edelman, R. R., and Manning, W. J. 1999. Signal-to-noise ratio and signal-to-noise efficiency in SMASH imaging. *Magn. Reson. Med.* 41: 1009–1022.

Sodickson, D. K., and Manning, W. J. 1997. Simultaneous acquisition of spatial harmonics (SMASH): Fast imaging with radiofrequency coil arrays. *Magn. Reson. Med.* 38: 591–603.

Sodickson, D. K., and McKenzie, C. A. 2001. A generalized approach to parallel magnetic resonance imaging. *Med. Phys.* 28: 1629–1643.

Weiger, M., Pruessmann, K. P., Kassner, A., Roditi, G., Lawton, T., Reid, A., and Boesiger, P. 2000. Contrast-enhanced 3D MRA using SENSE. *J. Magn. Reson. Imaging* 12: 671–677.

Weiger, M., Pruessmann, K. P., Leussler, C., Roeschmann, P., and Boesiger, P. 2001. Specific coil design for SENSE: A six-element cardiac array. *Magn. Reson. Med.* 45: 495–504.

RELATED SECTIONS

Section 8.2 Phase-Encoding Gradients
Section 13.1 Fourier Reconstruction

13.4 Partial Fourier Reconstruction

In partial Fourier acquisition, data are not collected symmetrically around the center of k-space. Instead, one-half of k-space is completely filled, while only a small amount of additional data in the other half is collected. Figure 13.26

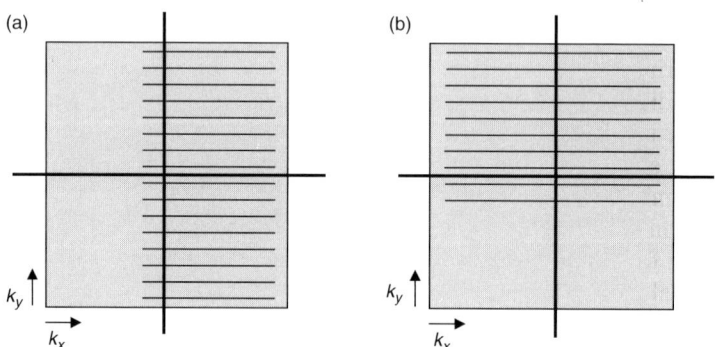

FIGURE 13.26 Two partial Fourier acquisition methods for 2D data sets. k_x and k_y represent the frequency- and phase-encoded directions, respectively. (a) Partial k_x or partial echo. (b) Partial k_y or partial NEX.

shows two examples of partially covered k-space along the frequency-encoded (Figure 13.26a) and phase-encoded (Figure 13.26b) directions. Partial Fourier acquisition in the frequency-encoded direction is also called *partial echo*, whereas partial Fourier acquisition in the phase-encoded direction is also called *partial NEX* because it is analogous to using less than one signal average. Partial Fourier acquisition is possible because, if the object is real, its Fourier transform is Hermitian (named for the French mathematician Charles Hermite, 1822–1901), meaning that the real part is symmetric and the imaginary part is antisymmetric around the center of k-space (Bracewell 1999). Mathematically, Hermitian 3D k-space data obeys:

$$S(-k_x, -k_y, -k_z) = S^*(k_x, k_y, k_z) \qquad (13.85)$$

where * denotes complex conjugation. Thus, only one-half of k-space is needed to reconstruct a real object. Unwanted phase shifts, however, resulting from motion, resonance frequency offsets, hardware group delays, eddy currents, and receive B_1 field inhomogeneity cause the reconstructed object to be complex, instead of being purely real. The additional data (sometimes called overscan data) collected in the incompletely filled half of k-space shown in Figure 13.26 are used to overcome this problem.

The primary advantages of partial Fourier acquisition in the frequency- and phase-encoded directions are reduced echo time (TE) and reduced scan time, respectively. Partial Fourier acquisition in the frequency-encoded direction also reduces gradient moments along that axis, which can reduce flow and motion artifacts. The spatial resolution, which is determined by the maximal extent in k-space, is not compromised and is equivalent to the corresponding full k-space acquisition case, although the SNR is reduced and some image artifacts can be introduced. More discussion of partial Fourier acquisition can be found in Sections 8.1 and 8.2.

In principle, partial Fourier acquisition can also be used in the slice-encoded direction (i.e., the secondary phase-encoding direction) for 3D scans, but this is not as commonly done. The relatively small number of slice phase-encoding steps (compared to the typical number of in-plane phase-encoding steps) combined with the need to acquire overscan data makes partial Fourier acquisition along the slice direction relatively less beneficial for saving scan time than for the in-plane phase-encoded direction.

Partial Fourier k-space acquisition can be characterized by a parameter known as the *partial Fourier fraction*, which is defined as the ratio between the partially acquired k-space data size and the full k-space data size with the same maximal extent in k-space (spatial resolution). According to this definition, we call the acquisition of exactly one-half of k-space a partial Fourier fraction of 0.5. This special case is sometimes called *half-Fourier acquisition*.

As overscan data are added, the partial Fourier fraction increases. Full k-space acquisition gives a partial Fourier fraction of 1.0. With this definition, most partial Fourier acquisitions use a fraction between 0.55 and 0.75.

Example 13.1   A partial Fourier acquisition in the phase-encoded direction uses a partial Fourier fraction of 0.625. The acquisition has spatial resolution equivalent to a full Fourier acquisition with a matrix size of 256. How many phase-encoding lines are acquired, and how many of these are overscan lines?

Answer   The number of acquired phase-encoding lines is

$$0.625 \times 256 = 160$$

The number of overscan lines is therefore

$$(0.625 - 0.5) \times 256 = 32$$

A number of different partial Fourier reconstruction algorithms have been developed. In this section we focus on three of the most commonly used algorithms: zero filling (also known as zero padding), homodyne processing, and iterative homodyne processing. These algorithms provide a good balance between computational simplicity and image quality. A comparison of several simple methods can be found in McGibney et al. (1993). More complicated algorithms give incremental image-quality improvement, but at a fairly high computational cost. A detailed evaluation of some of these methods can be found in Liang et al. (1992).

13.4.1 ZERO FILLING

Zero filling is implemented by substituting zeros for unmeasured k-space data, followed by conventional reconstruction (see Section 13.1). For full k-space acquisitions, zero filling of raw data is commonly used to interpolate the image and reduce partial volume artifacts. For partial Fourier acquisitions, zero filling can be used to replace unmeasured data. (Additional zeros can be padded if image interpolation is desired with the partial Fourier acquisition.) After zero filling, the standard FT-based full k-space reconstruction can be used. This usually results in some amount of Gibbs ringing near sharp edges due to the truncation of the k-space data. The advantage of zero filling is that it gives a relatively faithful representation of the object over the low-spatial-frequency overscan range. In contrast to homodyne processing, phase information is preserved for this low-spatial-frequency range. The phase of most large structures is therefore accurate and allows zero filling to be used for phase-sensitive reconstruction. Reasonable phase accuracy usually requires acquiring a relatively high fraction of k-space, for example 0.75 or greater.

13.4.2 HOMODYNE PROCESSING

Homodyne (from the Greek for "self-power") processing uses a low-spatial-frequency phase map generated from the data itself to correct for phase errors produced by the reconstruction of incomplete k-space data (Noll et al. 1991). Homodyne processing exploits the Hermitian conjugate symmetry of k-space data that would result if the reconstructed object were real. To simplify the discussion, we consider here a one-dimensional case. Let the k-space data be $S(k)$, where k is normally measured from $-k_{max}$ to k_{max} with full Fourier acquisition. In the partial Fourier acquisition, k-space data are acquired only from $-k_0$ to k_{max} where the parameter k_0 is positive and represents the overscan k-space cutoff. The k-space data can be thought of as symmetrically sampled around $k = 0$ over the low frequency range $(-k_0, k_0)$ and asymmetrically sampled over the high-frequency range (k_0, k_{max}). We discuss the algorithm in two steps: Hermitian conjugate replacement of missing data and compensation for the imaginary component of the reconstructed object.

Hermitian Conjugate Replacement We begin by assuming an ideal case—for symmetrically sampled k-space data the reconstructed image is real and is given by:

$$I(x) = \int_{-k_{max}}^{k_{max}} S(k)e^{i2\pi kx}\, dk \tag{13.86}$$

Data in the range $(-k_{max}, -k_0)$ then can be replaced by the complex conjugate of the data in the range (k_0, k_{max}), resulting in:

$$I(x) = \int_{-k_{max}}^{-k_0} S^*(-k)e^{i2\pi kx}\, dk + \int_{-k_0}^{k_{max}} S(k)e^{i2\pi kx}\, dk \tag{13.87}$$

In the first term in Eq. (13.87), we change variables by setting $k' = -k$. The result is:

$$I(x) = \left[\int_{k_0}^{k_{max}} S(k')e^{i2\pi k'x}\, dk' \right]^* + \int_{-k_0}^{k_{max}} S(k)e^{i2\pi kx}\, dk \tag{13.88}$$

The second term in Eq. (13.88) can be split into two terms by breaking the range of integration into $(-k_0, k_0)$ and (k_0, k_{max}). Combining the second of these two terms with the first term in Eq. (13.88) gives:

$$I(x) = \int_{-k_0}^{k_0} S(k)e^{i2\pi kx}\,dk + 2\,\mathrm{Re}\left[\int_{k_0}^{k_{max}} S(k)e^{i2\pi kx}\,dk\right] \tag{13.89}$$

where we have used the fact that the sum of any complex variable and its complex conjugate is twice its real part, that is, $z + z^* = 2\mathrm{Re}[z]$. The second term in Eq. (13.89) is real by definition, and, because we are assuming that $I(x)$ is real, the first term must also be real. Therefore, we can write Eq. (13.89) as:

$$I(x) = \mathrm{Re}\left[\int_{-k_0}^{k_0} S(k)e^{i2\pi kx}\,dk + 2\int_{k_0}^{k_{max}} S(k)e^{i2\pi kx}\,dk\right] \tag{13.90}$$

Eq. (13.90) can be further simplified by defining a function $H(k)$ (Figure 13.27a) given by:

$$H(k) = \begin{cases} 0 & k < -k_0 \\ 1 & -k_0 \le k < k_0 \\ 2 & k \ge k_0 \end{cases} \tag{13.91}$$

to give:

$$I(x) = \mathrm{Re}[I_H(x)] \tag{13.92}$$

where:

$$I_H(x) = \int_{-k_{max}}^{k_{max}} H(k)S(k)e^{i2\pi kx}\,dk \tag{13.93}$$

The function $H(k)$ is sometimes called the homodyne high-pass filter.

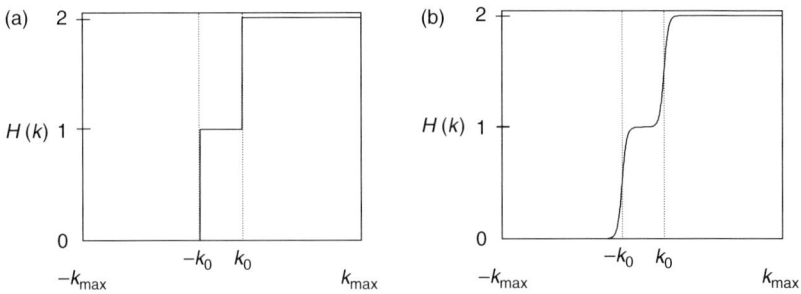

FIGURE 13.27 Homodyne high-pass filter. (a) Conceptual version. (b) Apodized version with smooth transitions.

Equations (13.92) and (13.93) imply that instead of using Hermitian conjugate symmetry, partial Fourier data can be reconstructed by using the homodyne high-pass filter, which zero-fills missing data and doubles the weighting of asymmetrically sampled data. The operation of taking the real part is required because doubling the asymmetrically sampled high frequencies generates an unwanted imaginary component. In practice, the abrupt transitions in $H(k)$ in Eq. (13.91) cause ringing. Therefore a function with smooth transitions is usually used for $H(k)$, as indicated in Figure 13.27b. The transition smoothing could be obtained by substituting an appropriate window, for example, a cosine taper window (see Section 13.1), to the sharp transitions of the function in Figure 13.27a:

$$H(k) = \begin{cases} 0 & k \leq -k_0 - w/2 \\ \cos^2\left(\dfrac{\pi(|k| - (k_0 - w/2))}{2w}\right) & -k_0 - w/2 < k < -k_0 + w/2 \\ 1 & -k_0 + w/2 \leq k \leq k_0 - w/2 \\ 1 + \cos^2\left(\dfrac{\pi(|k| - (k_0 + w/2))}{2w}\right) & k_0 - w/2 < k < k_0 + w/2 \\ 2 & k \geq k_0 + w/2 \end{cases}$$

(13.94)

where we assume $w/2 < k_0$.

Correction for the Imaginary Component   Because in practice $I(x)$ is not purely real, the operation of taking the real part in Eq. (13.92) discards some of the desired signal. This problem can be avoided by phase correction, that is, by unwinding the phase of $I(x)$ so that it resides entirely in the real component of the image prior to the operation of taking the real part in Eq. (13.92). In homodyne processing, the phase correction is derived from the symmetrically sampled k-space data. A low-frequency image $I_L(x)$ is reconstructed from:

$$I_L(x) = \int_{-k_0}^{k_0} S(k)e^{i2\pi kx}\, dk = \int_{-k_{max}}^{k_{max}} L(k)S(k)e^{i2\pi kx}\, dk \qquad (13.95)$$

where:

$$L(k) = \begin{cases} 1 & |k| \leq k_0 \\ 0 & |k| > k_0 \end{cases} \qquad (13.96)$$

is a low-pass filter, shown in Figure 13.28a. In practice a function with smooth transitions is used for $L(k)$, as indicated in Figure 13.28b.

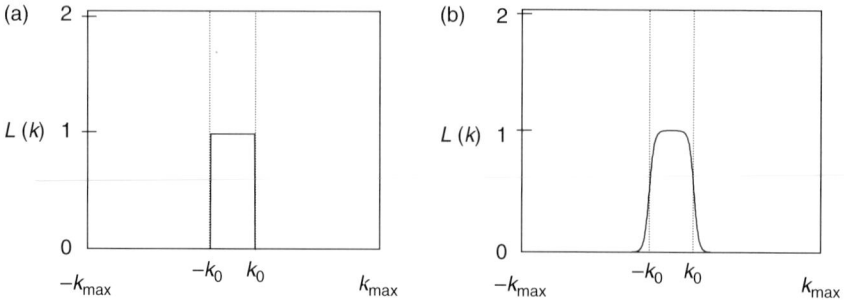

FIGURE 13.28 Homodyne low-pass filter. (a) Conceptual version. (b) Apodized version with smooth transitions.

For example:

$$L(k) = \begin{cases} 1 & |k| \leq k_0 - w/2 \\ \cos^2 \left(\dfrac{\pi(|k| - (k_0 - w/2))}{2w} \right) & k_0 - w/2 < |k| < k_0 + w/2 \\ 0 & |k| \geq k_0 + w/2 \end{cases}$$

$$(13.97)$$

We make the approximation that the phase of $I_L(x)$, denoted by $\phi_L(x)$, is a good approximation to the phase of $I(x)$. Then the phase-corrected image $I_H(x)e^{-i\phi_L(x)}$ has $I(x)$ registered to the real part of the image, allowing the removal of the undesired imaginary component that results from the homodyne high-pass filter (Figure 13.29). The entire homodyne reconstruction can therefore be compactly expressed by:

$$I(x) \approx Re[I_H(x)e^{-i\phi_L(x)}] \qquad (13.98)$$

To avoid phase wrapping from using an arctangent function, it is preferable to avoid calculating $\phi_L(x)$ explicitly. Instead, it is better to evaluate Eq. (13.98) using:

$$I_H(x)e^{-i\phi_L(x)} = I_H(x)\frac{I_L^*(x)}{|I_L(x)|} \qquad (13.99)$$

Note that from Eq. (13.98) the image phase is lost with homodyne reconstruction. This means that homodyne is unsuitable for applications that require the image phase such as shimming, phase contrast (reconstructed with phase difference), and phase-sensitive thermal imaging. Complex-difference phase contrast (Section 15.2), however, can use homodyne processing if the complex difference operation is performed in the k-space domain.

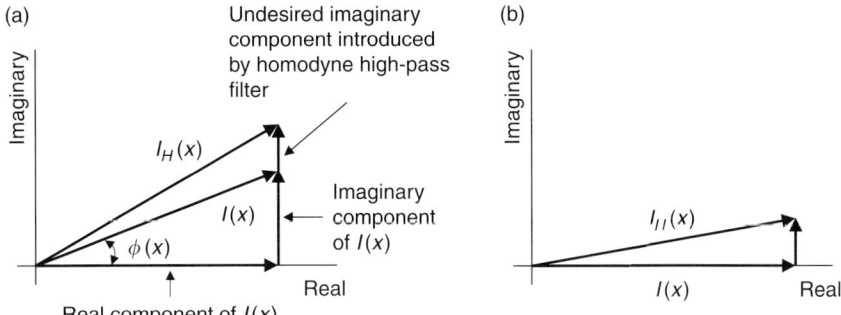

FIGURE 13.29 Complex image value at one pixel (a) before phase correction and (b) after phase correction. $I(x)$ has phase $\phi(x)$, which we approximate as $\phi_L(x)$, the phase of the low-pass-filtered image. The phase correction removes $\phi_L(x)$, thereby approximately registering $I(x)$ into the real part of the phase-corrected image $I_H(x)e^{-i\phi_L(x)}$. This allows the discarding of the imaginary image component introduced by the homodyne high-pass filter.

The approximation that the phase of the image can be represented by the low-frequency estimate $\phi_L(x)$ means that homodyne reconstruction performs relatively poorly in regions of rapidly varying phase caused, for example, by susceptibility changes. Iterative methods (discussed later) provide somewhat improved performance.

Extension to 2D and 3D k-Space   Hermitian conjugate symmetry can only be applied to a single axis in k-space. Consider the 2D version of Eq. (13.85):

$$S(-k_x, -k_y) = S^*(k_x, k_y) \tag{13.100}$$

Suppose that partial Fourier acquisition were used in both the k_x and k_y directions with a partial Fourier fraction of 0.5, thus acquiring only one of the four quadrants of 2D k-space. Using Eq. (13.100) will fill in only the diagonally opposed quadrant, leaving two other quadrants empty. Therefore, if partial Fourier acquisition is used in two orthogonal directions (assuming the partial acquisition fraction is larger than 0.5), one direction can be processed with homodyne reconstruction but the second direction must use zero filling.

Conversely, if partial Fourier acquisition is used in only one direction, the other k-space directions must be processed first with the normal (i.e. full k-space) algorithm. As an example, consider the 2D case again in which full Fourier acquisition is used in the k_x direction and partial Fourier acquisition is used in the k_y direction (Figure 13.26b). Taking the 1D Fourier transform with respect to the fully sampled k_x direction results in the partially transformed data $S_p(x, k_y)$ given by:

$$S_p(x, k_y) = \int S(k_x, k_y)e^{i2\pi k_x x} \, dk_x \qquad (13.101)$$

where $S_p(x, k_y)$ is sometimes called the signal in *hybrid* space. The Hermitian conjugate of $S_p(x, k_y)$ with respect to k_y is given by:

$$S_p^*(x, -k_y) = \int S^*(k_x, -k_y)e^{-i2\pi k_x x} \, dk_x \qquad (13.102)$$

Using the Hermitian conjugate relationship $S^*(k_x, -k_y) = S(-k_x, k_y)$ yields:

$$S_p^*(x, -k_y) = \int S(-k_x, k_y)e^{-i2\pi k_x x} \, dk_x \qquad (13.103)$$

Finally, making the variable substitution $k_x' = -k_x$ gives:

$$S_p^*(x, -k_y) = S_p(x, k_y) \qquad (13.104)$$

Because the partially transformed data in Eq. (13.104) obeys the same Hermitian conjugate relationship as 1D k-space data, the 2D data is first processed normally in the full Fourier (i.e., k_x) direction, followed by partial Fourier processing in the k_y direction. The extension to three dimensions is straightforward. Figure 13.30 shows the reconstruction steps modified to include homodyne processing. Note that if multiple coils are used, the input to the sum-of-squares algorithm is the real part of the homodyne reconstruction of the data from each coil.

13.4.3 ITERATIVE HOMODYNE PROCESSING

A drawback of the homodyne method is that the low-frequency phase map used in Eq. (13.99) cannot accurately depict rapidly varying phase. To address this problem, iterative partial Fourier methods have been developed, including a method proposed by Cuppen (1989). The method uses homodyne reconstruction to estimate a magnitude image while the phase is estimated from the low-frequency phase map. Combining the estimated magnitude and phase images gives a complex image that can be Fourier transformed to obtain estimated k-space data. The original measured k-space data in the range $(-k_0, k_{max})$ are combined with the newly estimated k-space data in the range $(-k_{max}, -k_0)$ and a new complex image I' is calculated. A new magnitude image is formed by applying the low-frequency phase correction to I' and taking the real component, as in noniterative homodyne reconstruction. This magnitude image is input to the next iteration. (See the flowchart in Figure 13.32 later in the chapter)

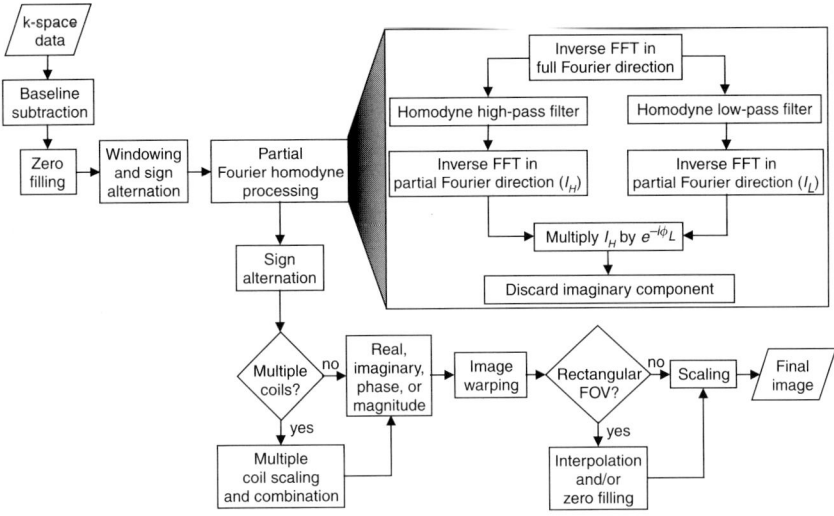

FIGURE 13.30 Flowchart for partial Fourier reconstruction with homodyne processing. The box for homodyne processing is expanded to show the steps involved.

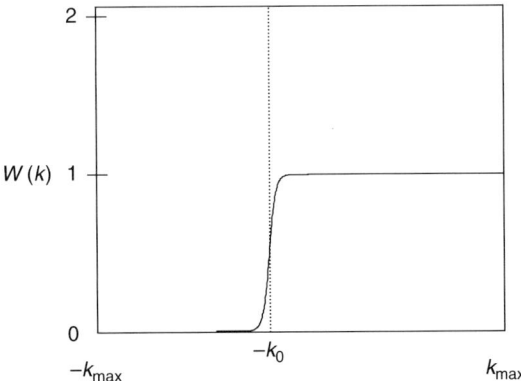

FIGURE 13.31 Plot of a merging function given by Eq. (13.107) for iterative homodyne reconstruction.

For the mathematical description, we again consider a 1D case. Let the original k-space data measured in the range $(-k_0, k_{max})$ be $S(k)$. Let $I_j(x)$ be the real image estimated at step j. (Note that with homodyne reconstruction, the real and magnitude images resulting from each step are the same because the imaginary component is discarded.) For the first iteration, $I_0(x)$ is given

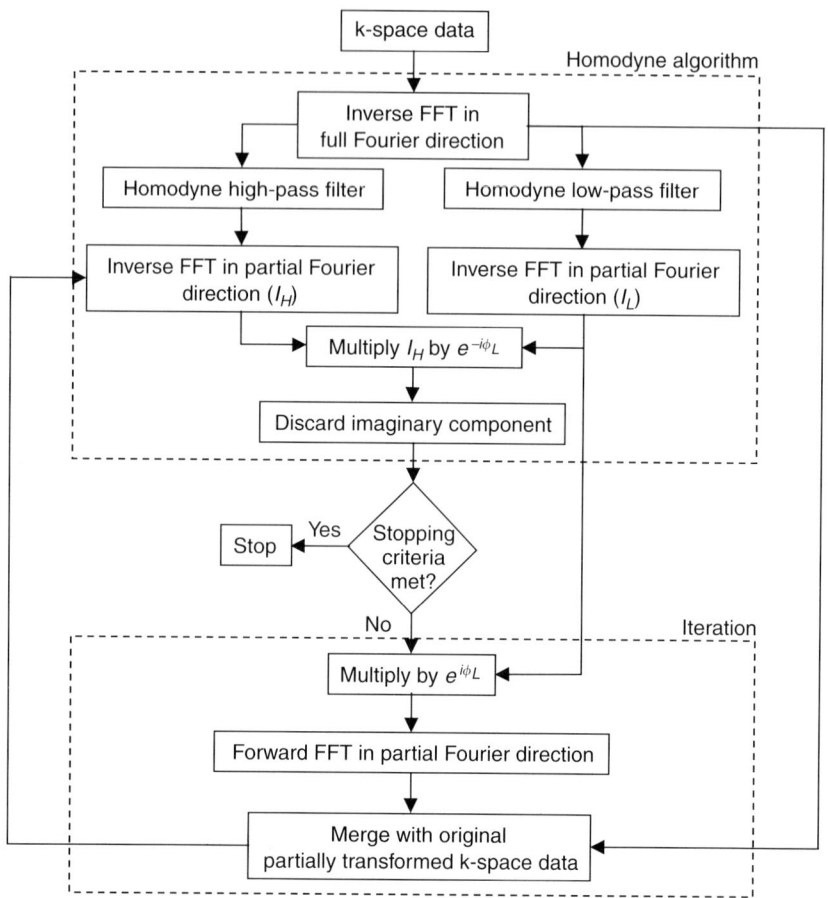

FIGURE 13.32 Flowchart for an iterative homodyne reconstruction. If iterative reconstruction is used, this flowchart replaces the contents of the partial Fourier homodyne processing box in Figure 13.30. The upper dashed box is the normal (noniterative) homodyne algorithm, and the lower dashed box represents the iterative process.

by Eq. (13.98). Let $S_j(k)$ be the complex k-space data estimated at step j. Iteration starts by computing $S_0(k)$. At each step:

$$S_j(k) = \mathrm{FT}[I_j(x)e^{i\phi_L(x)}] \tag{13.105}$$

The function $S_j(k)$ is an estimate of the k-space values for all values of k. However, in the range $(-k_0, k_{\max})$, the measured values $S(k)$ are assumed to be more accurate. Therefore, a combination of $S(k)$ in the range $(-k_0, k_{\max})$

and $S_j(k)$ in the range $(-k_{max}, -k_0)$ should yield a better-estimated image (with more accurate high frequencies) for the next iteration step. Simply concatenating the two data sets, however, will most likely create a discontinuity at $k = -k_0$. Therefore, it is better to smoothly blend the two data sets to obtain the estimated k-space data for the next iteration:

$$S_{j+1}(k) = W(k)S(k) + [1 - W(k)]S_j(k) \qquad (13.106)$$

where $W(k)$ is a merging function, such as:

$$W(k) = \begin{cases} 0 & k \le -k_0 - w_m/2 \\ \cos^2\left(\dfrac{\pi(|k| - (k_0 - w_m/2))}{2w_m}\right) & -k_0 - w_m/2 < k < -k_0 \\ & \qquad\qquad + w_m/2 \\ 1 & k \ge -k_0 + w_m/2 \end{cases}$$

$$(13.107)$$

where w_m is the merging width (Figure 13.31). The image for the next iteration $I_{j+1}(x)$ is given by:

$$I_{j+1}(x) = \text{Re}\left\{e^{-i\phi_L(x)}\text{FT}^{-1}[S_{j+1}(k)]\right\} \qquad (13.108)$$

Many choices for stopping criteria are possible. The algorithm can continue either for a fixed number of iterations or until a measure of the difference between successive images becomes sufficiently small. The measure could be the maximum of $|I_j(x) - I_{j-1}(x)|$ or a mean-squared error such as the average over x of $|I_j(x) - I_{j-1}(x)|^2$. In practice, most of the additional image-quality improvement comes after only a single additional iteration, except in regions of very rapidly varying phase. Figure 13.32 shows the flow chart for iterative reconstruction. As with noniterative homodyne reconstruction, $\phi_L(x)$ for the phase correction in Eq. (13.108) is not explicitly computed. Instead, the phase correction is performed as indicated in Eq. (13.99). Extension to 2D and 3D data sets is similar to the noniterative homodyne algorithm—normal reconstruction is performed first in the fully sampled Fourier directions.

A very similar iterative algorithm that uses zero filling instead of homodyne reconstruction is shown in Haacke et al. (1999).

SELECTED REFERENCES

Bracewell, R. N. 1999. *The Fourier transform and its applications.* New York: McGraw-Hill.

Cuppen, J. J. 1989. Method of reconstructing a nuclear magnetization distribution from a partial magnetic resonance measurement. U.S. patent 4,853,635.

Haacke, E. M., Brown, R. W., Thompson, M. R., and Venkatesan, R. 1999. *Magnetic resonance imaging, physical principles and sequence design.* New York: John Wiley & Sons.

Liang, Z.-P., Boada, F. E., Constable, R. T., Haacke, E. M., Lauterbur, P. C., and Smith, M. R. 1992. Constrained reconstruction methods in MR imaging. *Rev. Magn. Reson. Med.* 4: 67–185.

McGibney, G., Smith, M. R., Nichols, S. T., and Crawley, A. 1993. Quantitative evaluation of several partial Fourier reconstruction algorithms used in MRI. *Magn. Reson. Med.* 30: 51–59.

Noll, D. C., Nishimura, G. D., and Macovski, A. 1991. Homodyne detection in magnetic resonance imaging. *IEEE Trans. Med. Imaging* 10: 154–163.

RELATED SECTIONS

Section 8.1 Frequency-Encoding Gradients
Section 8.2 Phase-Encoding Gradients
Section 13.1 Fourier Reconstruction

13.5 Phase Difference Reconstruction

MRI, unlike CT, is a phase-sensitive imaging modality. After the Fourier reconstruction of the MR raw data, each pixel in the complex image has both a magnitude and a phase. The phase of the MR image is discarded when the standard magnitude reconstruction is performed. There can be, however, very useful information encoded into the phase. For example, the phase map can yield information about B_0 homogeneity, which is used for shimming, or about fluid flow, as described in Section 15.2 on phase contrast angiography. Emerging applications such as MR temperature mapping (Ishihara et al. 1995) and MR elastography (Muthupillai et al. 1995) also use the phase information.

In day-to-day MR acquisitions there are invariably unwanted contributions to the image phase, which can arise from system imperfections such as gradient eddy currents (Section 10.3) or from unavoidable physical effects such as chemical shift, magnetic susceptibility variations, and the concomitant (i.e., Maxwell) field (Section 10.1). These unwanted contributions make a phase map more difficult to interpret because the desired information is often overwhelmed by the unwanted phase. Acquiring two independent data sets and then forming a *phase difference* map can address this problem. As the name implies, the phase difference map is obtained by displaying the difference between a pair of phase images on a pixel-by-pixel basis (Moran et al. 1985). The goal is to accentuate the desired phase while canceling the unwanted phase. For example, to produce a B_0 map for shimming, two gradient-echo data sets are acquired with identical parameters, except that the TE is varied. The phases of the two complex images are subtracted to

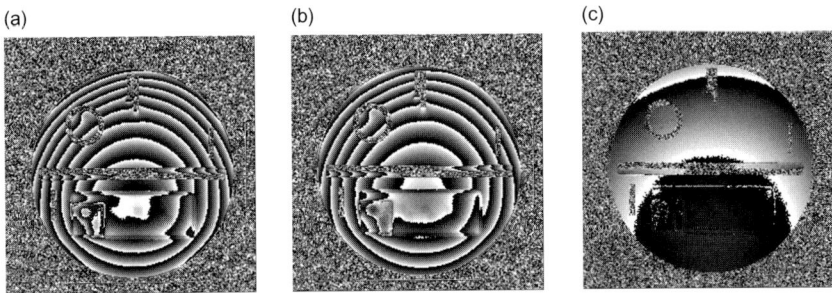

FIGURE 13.33 Phase difference reconstruction. The phase images (a) and (b) are subtracted on pixel-by-pixel basis to yield the phase difference map (c). The phase difference operation can cancel unwanted phase errors while accentuating useful phase information (e.g., about B_0 or flow). Note how the outline of the phantom is more easily discernable on (c). In practice, the intermediate step of reconstructing the individual phase images (a) and (b) is generally not necessary, and an algorithm such as Eq. (13.113) is used instead.

yield the phase difference map (Figure 13.33). Similarly, for phase-contrast angiography, the flow-encoding gradient (Section 9.2) is modified between the two acquisitions and a phase difference map is reconstructed, as described in Section 15.2.

13.5.1 QUANTITATIVE DESCRIPTION

The heart of any phase difference reconstruction is the per-pixel arctangent operation that yields the phase map. The tangent function is periodic and has discontinuities at $(n + 1/2)\pi$, ($n = 0, \pm1, \pm2, \ldots$), so the output of arctangent function is defined over a limited range, for example, $-\pi/2 < \arctan(x) < \pi/2$. (The range of the phase is increased to $[-\pi, \pi]$ when a four-quadrant arctangent function is used, as described later in this section.) In any case, the values of the phase outside the primary range are represented by a value in the primary range, or *alias*. Aliasing in the phase map is accompanied by discontinuities called *phase wraps*, which are abrupt transitions, for example, between π and $-\pi$ when the four-quadrant arctangent is used. For computational efficiency, and to minimize the number of phase wraps, an optimal phase difference reconstruction should employ only a single arctangent operation per pixel. Also, because of the discontinuities, it is desirable to perform operations such as the phased-array multiple coil combination and the concomitant-field phase correction *prior* to calculating that arctangent. The steps involved in a phase difference reconstruction, described next, are summarized in Figure 13.34.

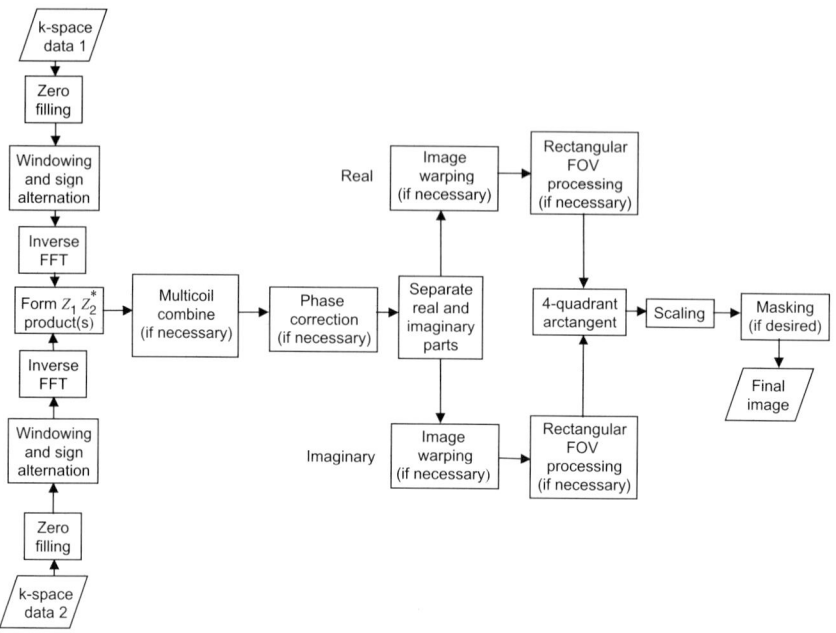

FIGURE 13.34 Flowchart for phase difference reconstruction steps.

Arctangent Operation   Suppose two k-space raw data sets are acquired, and we want to form a phase difference map from them. The data sets are first sign alternated and zero-filled, as described in Section 13.1, and then separately Fourier transformed to yield two independent complex images. We consider a particular pixel and denote its complex value in the first image by:

$$Z_1 = x_1 + iy_1 = \rho_1 e^{i\phi_1} \tag{13.109}$$

and in the second image by:

$$Z_2 = x_2 + iy_2 = \rho_2 e^{i\phi_2} \tag{13.110}$$

The phase difference for this pixel can be calculated by:

$$\Delta\phi = \arctan\left(\frac{y_1}{x_1}\right) - \arctan\left(\frac{y_2}{x_2}\right) = \phi_1 - \phi_2 \tag{13.111}$$

but Eq. (13.111) uses two arctangent operations per pixel, which is computationally costly and can introduce extra phase wraps. Instead, it is preferable to form a complex ratio and then extract the phase:

$$\Delta\phi = \angle\left(\frac{Z_1}{Z_2}\right) \equiv \arg\left(\frac{Z_1}{Z_2}\right) = \angle(\rho_1\rho_2 e^{i(\phi_1-\phi_2)}) = \arctan\left(\frac{\text{Im}\,(Z_1/Z_2)}{\text{Re}\,(Z_1/Z_2)}\right)$$

$$\tag{13.112}$$

Because the complex conjugate and the inverse of the complex number Z_2 both have the same phase (i.e., $-\phi_2$), Eq. (13.112) can be recast into a somewhat simpler form:

$$\Delta\phi = \angle(Z_1 Z_2^*) \equiv \arg(Z_1 Z_2^*) = \arctan\left(\frac{\text{Im}\left(Z_1 Z_2^*\right)}{\text{Re}\left(Z_1 Z_2^*\right)}\right) \tag{13.113}$$

Substituting Eqs. (13.109) and (13.110) into Eq. (13.113) yields an expression for the phase difference in terms of the real and imaginary components of the two complex values (O'Donnell 1985):

$$\Delta\phi = \arctan\left(\frac{x_2 y_1 - x_1 y_2}{x_1 x_2 + y_1 y_2}\right) \tag{13.114}$$

Whenever Eq. (13.113) or (13.114) is evaluated on a digital computer or array processor, it is useful to use the four-quadrant arctangent function, which is generically known as ATAN2 in several programming languages, including C (Kernighan and Ritchie 1998). The four-quadrant arctangent function takes two input arguments: the numerator and the denominator of the arctangent function. For example, Eq. (13.113) can be rewritten as:

$$\Delta\phi = \arctan\left(\frac{\text{Im}(Z_1 Z_2^*)}{\text{Re}(Z_1 Z_2^*)}\right) = \text{ATAN2}\left[\text{Im}\left(Z_1 Z_2^*\right), \text{Re}\left(Z_1 Z_2^*\right)\right] \tag{13.115}$$

The four-quadrant arctangent function tests the signs of its two individual arguments before forming their ratio. For example, if the numerator and denominator are both positive, then ATAN2 returns a value in first quadrant, but, if they are both negative, then it returns a value in third quadrant. In this way, the dynamic range is extended from $(-\pi/2, \pi/2)$ to $[-\pi, \pi]$, that is, to all four quadrants in the complex plane. Any phase difference value that lies outside the range $[-\pi, \pi]$ will be aliased back into the primary range by adding or subtracting multiples of 2π. For example, if the true phase difference value is 3.5π, then $-0.5\pi = 3.5\pi - 4\pi$ will be displayed. (Aliasing in phase-contrast angiography is discussed in more detail in Section 15.2.) Note that use

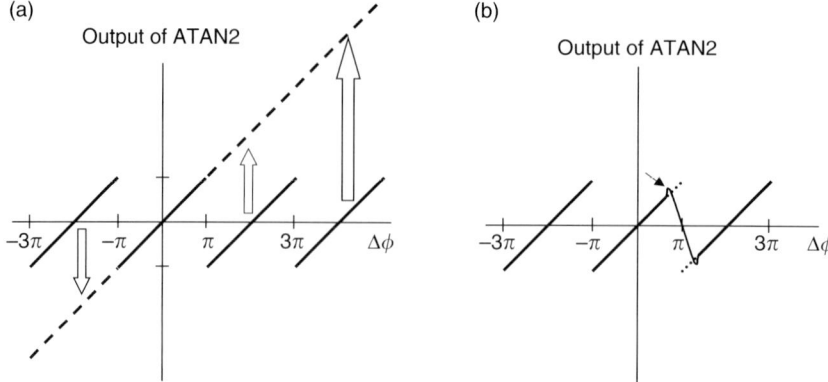

FIGURE 13.35 A plot of the output of the four-quadrant arctangent function versus the true phase difference. (a) When the true phase difference is in $[-\pi, \pi]$, the two are equal. When the true phase difference lies outside $[-\pi, \pi]$, the two differ by an integer multiple of 2π. This is phase aliasing, and the sharp transitions are phase wraps. Phase aliasing can be unwrapped by adding or subtracting the proper multiple of 2π (hollow arrows), so the output of the arctangent function and the true phase difference are equal over a longer stretch (dashed line). (b) A pitfall of interpolating phase images. If the phase image is interpolated (e.g., for image warping or for minification for rectangular field of view), overshoot (arrow) can occur at the aliasing boundary. Then the interpolated phase image can never be properly unwrapped. Instead, it is preferable to interpolate the real and imaginary images prior to the arctangent operation.

of the ATAN2 function compared to the conventional arctangent function can reduce the occurrence of phase wraps simply because of its increased range.

The process of restoring the phase difference values in the range $[-\pi, \pi]$ back to their true values is called *phase unwrapping* and is illustrated in Figure 13.35a. A detailed description of the postprocessing step of phase unwrapping is beyond the scope of this section, but several effective algorithms have been described for medical images (e.g., see Liang 1996 and Section 17.3).

Another advantage of the ATAN2 function is that instead of reporting a divide-by-zero error when the second argument is zero, it returns the correct value of $\pm\pi/2$, depending on the sign of the first argument. (It is always advisable to check the specific documentation for the ATAN2 function that is being used because some details can vary among implementations.)

Phased-Array Multiple Coil Data   Many acquisitions use multiple coils arranged in a phased array. The optimal acquisition and processing of these data requires multiple receivers, which produce multiple channels of MR data.

An algorithm to reconstruct a phase difference map from this multichannel data is described here.

Adopting the notation of Section 13.1, we denote the receiver channels by the index j and define σ_j^2 to be the measured noise variance for the jth channel, as explained in Section 13.1. Then the phase difference map can be calculated (Bernstein et al. 1994) from the expression:

$$\Delta\phi = \measuredangle\left(\sum_j \frac{Z_{1j}Z_{2j}^*}{\sigma_j^2}\right) = \text{ATAN2}\left(\text{Im}\sum_j \frac{Z_{1j}Z_{2j}^*}{\sigma_j^2}, \text{Re}\sum_j \frac{Z_{1j}Z_{2j}^*}{\sigma_j^2}\right)$$

(13.116)

Note that any spatially dependent phase contribution from an individual coil receive B_1 field is cancelled in Eq. (13.116) when the phase difference is formed.

Performing the multiple-coil combination prior to the arctangent operation, as in Eq. (13.116), has an advantage that is illustrated in the following example. Suppose the true phase difference $\Delta\phi$ is near the aliasing boundary of π (or 180°) and there are two receiver channels. Suppose further that because of noise, the individual phase differences that would be extracted from the two receivers straddle the aliasing boundary:

$$\Delta\phi_1 = \pi - \varepsilon$$
$$\Delta\phi_2 = -\pi + \varepsilon$$

(13.117)

where $\varepsilon \ll 1$. Simply averaging the phases gives the incorrect result, because the sum:

$$\Delta\phi = \Delta\phi_1 + \Delta\phi_2 = \pi - \varepsilon + (-\pi + \varepsilon) = 0 \qquad (13.118)$$

If, however the multiple-receiver combination is made before the arctangent operation according to Eq. (13.116), a better estimate to the correct value of $\Delta\phi = \pi$ is obtained. From Eq. (13.116), the phase difference for this two-receiver case can be written:

$$\Delta\phi = \measuredangle\left(\sum_{j=1}^{2} \frac{\rho_{1j}\rho_{2j}e^{i\Delta\phi_j}}{\sigma_j^2}\right) \qquad (13.119)$$

Assuming that the noise variances and image magnitudes have only weak dependence on the index j, it is a good approximation to remove the ρs and σs from the sum, and substituting Eq. (13.117) into Eq. (13.119) yields:

$$\Delta\phi \approx \measuredangle(e^{i(\pi-\varepsilon)} + e^{i(-\pi+\varepsilon)}) = \measuredangle(e^{i\pi}(e^{-i\varepsilon} + e^{-2\pi i}e^{i\varepsilon}))$$
$$= \measuredangle(e^{i\pi}2\cos\varepsilon) = \pi \qquad (13.120)$$

(Depending on the implementation of the ATAN2 function, the value $-\pi$ may be obtained instead. The two are equivalent because $+\pi$ and $-\pi$ differ by 2π.) Since Eq. (13.120) is the correct result, this example illustrates the general rule that as many of the other operations as possible should precede the arctangent operation in a phase difference reconstruction. Another example of an operation in which this rule applies is described next.

Correction of Predictable Phase Errors and the Concomitant Field   Even after forming the phase difference image, unwanted phase errors often remain. A common example is the phase contamination due to gradient eddy currents (Section 10.3) that can plague phase-contrast angiography. Because eddy currents are dependent on the design and calibration of the MR hardware, it is usually difficult to predict the exact spatial dependence of the phase error that is produced. Therefore, this type of phase error is often corrected by empirical fitting on the final phase difference image. For example, the constant and linear phases could be determined with a polynomial fit (Bernstein et al. 1998) of the phase difference image in a region that should have zero phase difference, such as stationary tissue in a phase-contrast angiogram. Because presumably the fitted phase is due entirely to system imperfections such as eddy currents, it is then removed with postprocessing.

Other phase errors, however, such as those produced by the concomitant (i.e., Maxwell) field, can be predicted with great accuracy because they are fundamental physics effects (Section 10.1). In that case, it is advantageous to correct for these phase errors *before* calculating the arctangent. This procedure avoids phase wraps in the phase difference map, thereby reducing the need for later phase unwrapping. Also, because the concomitant field has nonlinear spatial dependence, removing its phase error at this stage makes it easier to fit the eddy-current phase errors later. If the calculated concomitant phase error at the pixel of interest is ϕ_e, then the phase-corrected version of Eq. (13.113) is:

$$\Delta\phi_{corr} = \angle(Z_1 Z_2^* e^{-i\phi_e}) = \text{ATAN2}\left[\text{Im}\left(Z_1 Z_2^* e^{-i\phi_e}\right), \text{Re}\left(Z_1 Z_2^* e^{-i\phi_e}\right)\right]$$

$$(13.121)$$

Because the phase error from the concomitant field is independent of the receiver channel number, the phase correction for the multiple coil case becomes:

$$\Delta\phi_{corr} = \angle\left(e^{-i\phi_e} \sum_j \frac{Z_{1j} Z_{2j}^*}{\sigma_j^2}\right) \qquad (13.122)$$

The details of this phase correction method can be found in Bernstein et al. (1998).

Image Warping   The image warping operation described in Section 13.1 that corrects for gradient nonlinearity can also be applied to phase difference images. As with the multiple-coil combination, it is preferable to apply the image warping prior to the arctangent operation. This is because image warping is a conformal mapping that uses an interpolation method such as cubic splines. If the image warping is applied after the arctangent operation, a phase wrap may be encountered and its sharp discontinuity can cause unwanted ringing in the image. Moreover, a phase difference image processed in this way cannot be properly unwrapped at a later time because the sharp transition between $-\pi$ and π has been distorted (Figure 13.35b).

Suppose the warping operation on an image I is denoted by the function $W(I)$. Then one strategy is to apply the warping operation separately to the real and imaginary components of the image. Thus Eq. (13.115) is modified:

$$\Delta\phi_{\text{warped}} = \arctan\left(\frac{W\left(\text{Im}\left(Z_1 Z_2^*\right)\right)}{W\left(\text{Re}\left(Z_1 Z_2^*\right)\right)}\right)$$
$$= \text{ATAN2}\left[W\left(\text{Im}\left(Z_1 Z_2^*\right)\right), W\left(\text{Re}\left(Z_1 Z_2^*\right)\right)\right] \qquad (13.123)$$

where W should be understood to act on the entire image, rather than a single pixel. Other variations on Eq. (13.123) have also been proposed (Bernstein and Frigo 1995). Another advantage of applying the image warp separately to the real and imaginary images before the arctangent operation, as in Eq. (13.123), is that any change in image intensity caused by the warping algorithm will not affect the phase difference map.

As mentioned in Section 13.1, including the minification step in the image warp is a convenient way to reconstruct rectangular FOV images. This is true for rectangular FOV phase difference images as well.

Image Scaling   The output of the ATAN2 function is a real, floating point (or double-precision floating point) number in the range from $-\pi$ to π. Often it is desirable to scale this output to a more convenient range by multiplying it by some constant. For example, in phase-contrast angiography, the output can be scaled so that the pixel values represent velocity in convenient units such as millimeters per second. Similarly for a B_0 map, we might want the pixel intensity to represent frequency offset δf in hertz, tenths of hertz, or a convenient fraction of parts per million.

Example 13.2   Suppose a B_0 map is obtained by forming the phase difference from two gradient-echo images with values of TE equal to 10 ms and 25 ms. How should the result of the phase difference map be scaled so that each intensity count represents a frequency offset of 0.1 Hz?

Answer To convert from radians to tenths of hertz, the phase difference map must be scaled according to:

$$\delta f \left[\frac{\text{Hz}}{10} \right] = \frac{10\,\Delta\phi}{2\pi\,\Delta\text{TE}} = \frac{10\,\Delta\phi}{2\pi\,(0.015\,\text{s})} = 106.10\,\Delta\phi \tag{13.124}$$

So, a constant multiplier of 106.10 is applied to the output of the four-quadrant arctangent function.

Noise Masking Sometimes after the phase difference reconstruction, a noise mask is applied. With the standard magnitude images, regions of no signal (e.g., air) appear dark in the image because the intensity is confined to the lowest values of the dynamic range. In phase difference images, however, the noise background covers the entire dynamic range of image intensities. Consequently, the noise in air has a characteristic salt-and-pepper pattern. If this background is distracting or makes the window-level operation difficult, the noise from air can be suppressed by any of several masking techniques.

The common noise-masking methods employ a magnitude image reconstructed from the same raw data as is used to reconstruct the phase difference map. Suppose M is the magnitude image corresponding to the phase difference map $\Delta\phi$. For example, in the multiple-coil case, M could be calculated with (Bernstein et al. 1994).

$$M = \sqrt{\left| \sum_j \frac{Z_{1j} Z_{2j}^*}{\sigma_j^2} \right|} \tag{13.125}$$

Then the phase difference map can be masked using a threshold M_0:

$$\Delta\phi_{\text{thresh}} = \begin{cases} \Delta\phi & M \geq M_0 \\ 0 & M < M_0 \end{cases} \tag{13.126}$$

The threshold value M_0 can either be a predetermined constant or extracted from a histogram of the pixel values in M.

An alternative noise-masking method is to multiply the phase difference image by the magnitude image on a pixel-by-pixel basis:

$$\Delta\phi_{\text{mult}} = M\,\Delta\phi \tag{13.127}$$

The threshold and multiplicative masking methods each has its own advantages and pitfalls. The threshold method does not alter the phase difference pixel values (unless they are zeroed), which is convenient for extracting quantitative information. The threshold method has the drawback that over-aggressive masking can zero out pixel values that are of interest and setting a proper threshold value can require operator intervention. Conversely, the multiplicative masking method retains all the pixel values, but the mask must be divided out later if the true phase difference information is desired, for example, for quantitative flow analysis. Finally, we note that not using any masking method at all is a viable alternative because with practice it is not too difficult for the viewer to adapt to high dynamic range of the noise from air in unmasked phase difference maps.

SELECTED REFERENCES

Bernstein, M. A., and Frigo, F. J. 1995. Gradient non-linearity correction for phase difference images. In *Proceedings of the 3rd Annual Meeting SMR*, p. 739.

Bernstein, M. A., Grgic, M., Brosnan, T. J., and Pelc, N. J. 1994. Reconstructions of phase contrast, phased array multicoil data. *Magn. Res. Med.* 32: 330–334.

Bernstein, M. A., Zhou, X. J., Polzin, J. A., King, K. F., Ganin, A., Pelc, N. J., and Glover, G. H. 1998. Concomitant gradient terms in phase contrast MR: Analysis and correction. *Magn. Res. Med.* 39: 300–308.

Ishihara, Y., Calderon, A., Watanabe, H., Okamoto, K., Suzuki, Y., Kuroda, K., and Suzuki, Y. 1995. A precise and fast temperature mapping using water proton chemical shift. *Magn. Reson. Med.* 34: 814–823.

Kernighan, B. W., and Ritchie, D. M. 1998. *The C programming language.* Upper Saddle Mountain: Prentice Hall.

Liang, Z. P. 1996. A model based phase unwrapping method. *IEEE Trans. Med. Imaging* 15: 893–897.

Moran, P. R., Moran, R. A., and Karstaedt, N. 1985. Verification and evaluation of internal flow and motion. True MRI by the phase gradient modulation method. *Radiology* 154: 433–441.

Muthupillai, R., Lomas, D. J., Rossman, P. J., Greenleaf, J. F., Manduca, A., and Ehman, R. L. 1995. Magnetic resonance elastography by direct visualization of propagating acoustic strain waves. *Science* 269: 1854–1857.

O'Donnell, M. 1985. NMR blood flow imaging using multiecho, phase contrast sequences. *Med. Phys.* 12: 59–64.

RELATED SECTIONS

13.6 View Sharing

View sharing (Riederer et al. 1988; Foo et al. 1995; Markl and Hennig 2001) is a reconstruction method that reuses some of the same k-space data in order to reconstruct two or more different images. Thus, some k-space views are shared among multiple raw data sets. View sharing reduces the amount of time needed to acquire a complete set of k-space views. This can increase the frame rate of a real-time acquisition or the number of reconstructed phases for a cardiac examination. View sharing does not interpolate the k-space data but instead copies selected views intact from one memory location to another for reuse. For this reason, we call the additional images reconstructed with view sharing *intermediate images* rather than interpolated images.

Examples of acquisition techniques that use view sharing during reconstruction include keyhole and related methods (Section 11.3), real-time imaging with partial k-space updating (Section 11.4), and segmented k-space cardiac acquisition (i.e., FASTCARD) (Section 11.5). View sharing is also used to reconstruct intermediate images with cardiac triggered phase-contrast examinations (Foo et al. 1995; Markl and Hennig 2001).

This section focuses on sliding window reconstruction for real-time imaging and multiphase cardiac exams with segmented k-space acquisition. In these two examples, image reconstruction with view sharing does not affect the image acquisition. However, in some other cases, such as keyhole (Section 11.3), the acquisition is specifically designed under the assumption that the reconstruction will use view sharing.

13.6.1 SLIDING WINDOW RECONSTRUCTION FOR REAL-TIME IMAGING

Sliding window reconstruction (Figure 13.36) is commonly used for real-time acquisitions, and is an example of view sharing. Suppose a series of views $(1, 2, 3, \ldots, N)$ are acquired repeatedly at the same slice location:

$$\text{View order} = 1, 2, 3, \ldots, N, 1, 2, 3, \ldots, N, 1, 2, \ldots \qquad (13.128)$$

Unless the object changes, all the reconstructed images will be identical, except for their noise texture. So the purpose of this type of acquisition is to detect changes within the object, such as, motion. As described in Section 11.4, the views in Eq. (13.128) could be the standard phase- and frequency-encoded readouts of a Cartesian acquisition, interleaves of a spiral acquisition, or spokes in a radial projection acquisition.

Suppose each view takes a time TR to acquire. After the first N views are acquired, there are enough raw data to completely fill k-space once and the first image can be reconstructed. We could wait a time $N \times$ TR until the second group of views is acquired and then use it to reconstruct an entirely new image. By using the sliding window reconstruction (Figure 13.36), however, we can

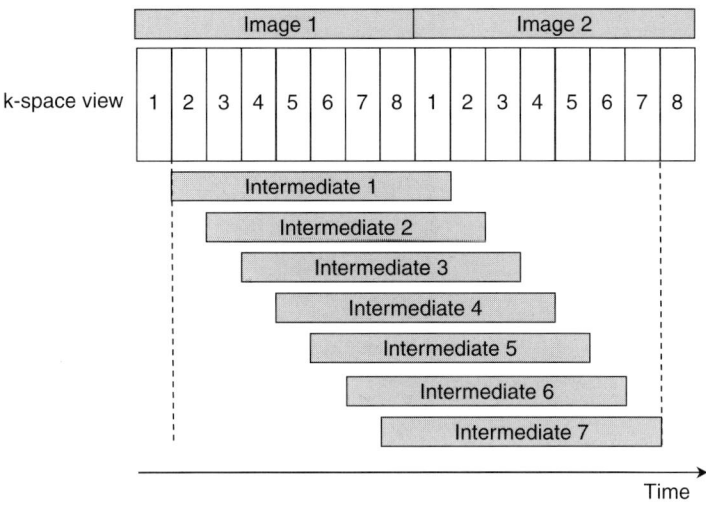

FIGURE 13.36 Sliding window reconstruction using view sharing. A slice location is repeatedly acquired with eight views, as in real-time imaging. Seven intermediate images (for a total of nine images) can be reconstructed with the sliding window reconstruction.

reconstruct an updated image after waiting only one TR interval (assuming NEX = 1). For example, an image can be reconstructed by dropping the first view, and replacing it with the refreshed view number 1, i.e., $(2, 3, \ldots, N, 1)$. The next updated image is reconstructed from views $(3, \ldots, N, 1, 2)$, and so on. In this way a total of $N - 1$ intermediate images can be reconstructed between any two.

Due to symmetry considerations, sliding window reconstruction can behave somewhat differently for interleaved multishot spiral and radial projection acquisitions compared to Cartesian acquisitions. For spiral and radial projection methods, all the views carry information from the center of k-space, so they are all on an equal footing. For Cartesian acquisitions, however, only selected views pass through the center of k-space. This means, for example, that if there is constant linear motion, the transition between some images reconstructed with view sharing can be more abrupt than for others. Suppose, for example, there are eight views for a k-space data set, and views 4 and 5 represent the center of k-space. Then the images reconstructed from views $(4, 5, 6, 7, 8, 1, 2, 3)$ and $(6, 7, 8, 1, 2, 3, 4, 5)$ can appear quite different from one another for a Cartesian acquisition. Even though the second image is reconstructed only $2 \times$ TR later, its center of k-space is acquired eight TR intervals after the previous one, again assuming NEX = 1.

13.6.2 SEGMENTED CARDIAC ACQUISITIONS AND VIEW SHARING

Multiphase cardiac-triggered images can be acquired in several ways. One method, called segmented cardiac or FASTCARD acquisition, is described in Section 11.5. The main purpose of segmented acquisitions is to reduce the total scan time by reducing the number of ECG triggers required to complete the data acquisition. The method divides the R-R interval into phases corresponding to k-space segments and acquires multiple k-space lines at each cardiac phase (Figure 13.37). As described in Section 11.5, the number of k-space lines acquired during each segment is called the views per segment (vps). Although segmenting reduces the scan time by a factor equal to the vps, it also degrades the true temporal resolution by the same factor. The total number of ECG triggers that is required to complete the acquisition of a single slice is the number of views divided by the vps, assuming NEX = 1. For example, if the acquisition in Figure 13.37 has a total of 100 views, then 25 heartbeats would be required because vps = 4. An image at each cardiac phase is reconstructed by pooling the data collected in all 25 heartbeats.

View sharing is commonly used to reconstruct segmented cardiac-triggered acquisition. By applying a sliding window reconstruction, up to (vps − 1) intermediate phases can be reconstructed (Figure 13.37) between any two. For example, phase 1.25 is reconstructed from views (2, 3, 4, 1) in

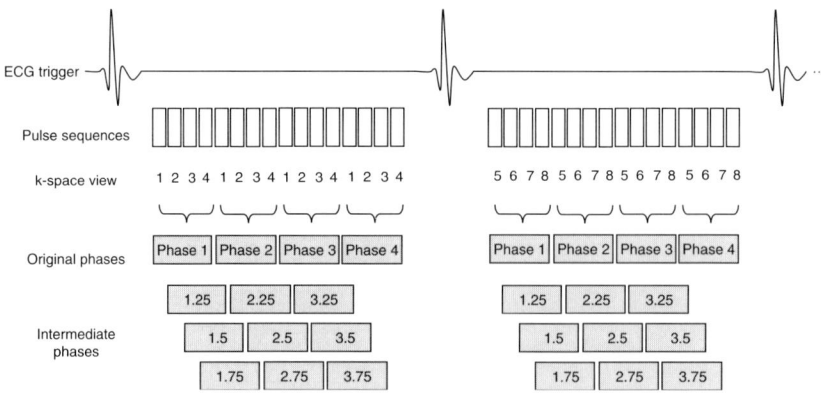

FIGURE 13.37 Segmented k-space multiphase cardiac acquisition with vps = 4 and four original phases for a single slice location. View sharing is used to reconstruct additional intermediate cardiac phases. In the first R-R interval k-space lines 1–4 are repeatedly acquired; in the second R-R interval k-space lines 5–8 are acquired, and so on, until the raw data matrix is completely filled. View sharing reconstruction allows up to (vps − 1) intermediate cardiac phases to be reconstructed between any two; for example, phases 1.25, 1.5, and 1.75 can be reconstructed between phases 1 and 2.

the first R-R interval, views (6, 7, 8, 5) in the second R-R interval, and so on. The intermediate reconstructed phases increase the apparent or effective temporal resolution by providing a more smoothly varying cine display. The true temporal resolution, however, is the time to acquire one k-space segment, vps times TR. View sharing does not increase the true temporal resolution because it does not add any new k-space data. Instead, it reuses existing data one or more times.

Even without view sharing, the number of reconstructed images in a cardiac-triggered acquisition can be quite large because it is the product of the number of slice locations and the number of cardiac phases (and echoes, for a multiecho scan). For this reason, sometimes only a single intermediate cardiac phase is reconstructed, instead of the maximal number (vps − 1). To obtain the greatest benefit from view sharing in that case, the intermediate cardiac phase halfway between the original phases is typically reconstructed. In Figure 13.37 this corresponds to phases 1.5, 2.5, and 3.5.

Although this discussion has focused on single-slice acquisitions, extension to multislice acquisitions is possible. Use of view sharing in real-time or multiphase cardiac studies acquired in 2D sequential mode is straightforward, because each slice location can be treated separately. Interleaved 2D multislice acquisition does not lend itself to view sharing, however, because views cannot be shared among different slice locations. View sharing has not been widely used in 3D volume imaging; for example, the TRICKS method described in Section 11.3 uses interpolation instead.

SELECTED REFERENCES

Foo, T. K. F, Bernstein, M. A., Aisen, A. M., Hernandez, R. J., Collick, B. D., and Bernstein, T. 1995. Improved ejection fraction and flow velocity estimates with use of view sharing and uniform repetition time excitation and fast cardiac techniques. *Radiology* 195: 471–478.

Markl, M., and Hennig, J. 2001. Phase contrast MRI with improved temporal resolution by view sharing: k-space related velocity mapping properties. *Magn. Reson. Imaging* 19: 669–676.

Riederer, S. J., Tasciyan, T., Farzaneh, F., Lee, J. N., Wright, R. C., and Herfkin, R. J. 1988. MR fluoroscopy: Technical feasibility. *Magn. Reson. Med.* 8: 1–15.

RELATED SECTIONS

PULSE SEQUENCES

Introduction

A pulse sequence is a series of events (or the computer program that initiates them) comprising RF pulses, gradient waveforms, and data acquisition. The purpose of the pulse sequence is to manipulate the magnetization in order to produce the desired signal. Pulse sequences play a central role in MR imaging. Many important concepts of MR are realized through pulse sequence design and implementation. Virtually every imaging application is enabled by one or more pulse sequences. Even after more than three decades of development, MRI pulse sequence design remains an active area of research and continues to extend the versatility of MRI compared to other imaging modalities. Based on the tools and pulse sequence components presented in the first four parts of this book, Part V describes a number of pulse sequences that are commonly used for both routine clinical diagnosis and advanced applications.

We have classified the pulse sequences into four categories: basic pulse sequences, angiographic pulse sequences, fast imaging pulse sequences utilizing echo trains, and pulse sequences for advanced applications. These classifications are not rigorous and are intended only for convenience based on some interrelationships among the pulse sequences.

Chapter 14 describes three families of basic pulse sequences: gradient echo or field echo (Section 14.1), inversion recovery (Section 14.2), and RF spin echo (Section 14.3). Many variations of these sequences, such as spoiled-gradient echo, STIR, FLAIR, and dual-echo spin echo, are also discussed in these sections. Pulse sequences described in Chapter 14 are the basis of many clinical and research applications.

Pulse sequences for MR angiography (MRA) are the subject of Chapter 15. Several commonly used MRA techniques are discussed: black blood angiography (Section 15.1), phase-contrast angiography (Section 15.2), and time-of-flight and contrast-enhanced angiography (Section 15.3). In accordance with the building-block organization of the book, Chapter 15 describes how these pulse sequences are used for MRA; the basics of these pulse sequences can be found in Chapters 14 and 16, as well as the earlier parts of the book. For example, two-dimensional time-of-flight angiography is described in Section 15.3, but detailed descriptions of gradient echoes, spatial saturation, and gradient moment nulling are found in their own sections. Also relevant image reconstruction and display techniques (e.g., complex difference reconstruction or maximum intensity projection) that are not discussed in Part IV of the book are explained in Chapter 15. Chapter 15 only provides an introduction to MRA, which is a subject with a very extensive literature. For more information the reader is referred to books dedicated solely to MRA, such as Anderson et al. (1993), Potchen and Haacke (1993), and Prince et al. (1999).

Chapter 16 focuses on fast imaging pulse sequences that employ an echo train, that is, multiple RF spin echo or gradient echoes following an RF excitation pulse. Echo planar imaging (EPI; Section 16.1) is one of the fastest imaging pulse sequences, capable of producing a 2D image in a few tens of milliseconds. This technique plays an essential role in many advanced MR applications, such as diffusion, perfusion, neurofunctional, and dynamic imaging. EPI techniques and applications span a very broad range. Interested readers are referred to Schmitt et al. (1998) for expanded discussions of subjects that cannot be thoroughly covered in Section 16.1. Rapid acquisition with relaxation enhancement (RARE; Section 16.4) and its variations (such as fast spin echo, FSE) rely on multiple RF spin echoes to sample k-space so that the total imaging time can be reduced several-fold compared to conventional spin echo pulse sequences. In this book, we use the term *RARE* to refer to all variations of such pulse sequences to avoid possible confusion with commercial names. RARE has virtually replaced conventional RF spin echo pulse sequences for T_2-weighted imaging, and its application is still expanding. A hybrid between EPI and RARE known as gradient and spin echo (GRASE) is discussed in Section 16.2. GRASE overcomes some of the limitations of EPI and RARE, but also inherits many of the problems of both. Section 16.3 is devoted to a pulse sequence known as principles of echo-shifting with a train of observations (PRESTO), in which a TE longer than TR can be achieved in an echo-train fast imaging sequence. This pulse sequence, although not as widely used as EPI and RARE, has found applications in neurofunctional, perfusion, and diffusion imaging.

The last chapter of the book, Chapter 17, includes several selected methods used for advanced applications and also two alternative k-space sampling strategies. Arterial spin tagging (Section 17.1) combines an inversion pulse with a fast imaging pulse sequence such as EPI or spiral to encode information about tissue perfusion into the MR signal. The section on diffusion imaging (Section 17.2) includes diffusion-weighted imaging (DWI), apparent diffusion coefficient (ADC) mapping, diffusion tensor imaging (DTI), and an introduction to q-space imaging. The diffusion-weighting gradient, central to all diffusion imaging techniques, is discussed in Section 9.1. Dixon's method (Section 17.3) is a technique for obtaining separate images from individual spectroscopic species using a limited number of acquisitions with different echo times. The ability to produce separate water and lipid images, even in the presence of B_0 inhomogeneity, makes Dixon's method particularly useful for lipid suppression, water suppression, and tissue–lipid content analysis. Driven equilibrium (Section 17.4) is a pulse sequence module that can be appended to the end of a pulse sequence to allow shorter TR while preserving the signal-to-noise ratio of tissues with long T_1 and T_2. Also described in that section is the driven equilibrium magnetization preparation module that can be appended to the beginning of a pulse sequence to achieve T_2-weighting. The last two sections of Chapter 17 focus on two alternative k-space sampling strategies: projection or radial acquisition (Section 17.5), which was the original method used to acquire MRI data, and spiral (Section 17.6), which has been increasingly used for fast imaging.

One continual source of confusion in the study of pulse sequences is that the various equipment manufacturers have called the same (or virtually the same) pulse sequence by completely different names. We have tried to list most of popular names for the pulse sequences as they are introduced in Part V. This situation is particularly confusing for the study of gradient echoes, so a table cross-referencing commercial names has been included in Section 14.1. Review articles such as Mugler (1999) and Nitz (1999) are also helpful for making sense of this acronym soup.

There are many other pulse sequences that are not covered in Part V of the book. The reader is referred to other books on the subject such as Haacke et al. (1999), Bradley and Bydder (1997), and Vlaardingerbroek and den Boer (2003), as well as the review articles cited earlier. Ongoing research efforts will continue to expand the scope of MR pulse sequences. We hope that the descriptions of the pulse sequences in Part V provide the reader with a basis to better appreciate the existing and future literature and aid the reader in implementing the existing pulse sequences and developing new ones.

SELECTED REFERENCES

Anderson, C. M., Edelman, R. R., and Turski, P. A., eds. 1993. *Clinical magnetic resonance angiography*. New York: Raven.

Bradley, W. G., and Bydder, G. 1997. *Advanced MR imaging techniques*. London: Dunitz.

Haacke, E. M., Brown, R. W., Thompson, M. R., and Venkatesan, R. 1999. *Magnetic resonance imaging: Physical principles and sequence design*. New York: Wiley-Liss.

Mugler, J. P, III. 1999. Overview of MR imaging pulse sequences. *Magn. Reson. Imaging Clin. N. Am.* 7: 661–697.

Nitz, W. R. 1999. MR imaging: Acronyms and clinical applications. *Eur. Radiol.* 9: 979–997.

Potchen, E. J., and Haacke, E. M. 1993. *Magnetic resonance angiography*. St Louis, MO: Mosby.

Prince, M. R., Grist, T. M., and Debatin, J. F. 1999. *3D contrast MR angiography*. Berlin: Springer.

Schmitt, F., Stehling, M. K., and Turner, R. 1998. *Echo planar imaging*. Berlin: Springer.

Vlaardingerbroek, M. T., and den Boer, J. A. 2003. *Magnetic resonance imaging*. Berlin: Springer.

14

BASIC PULSE SEQUENCES

14.1 Gradient Echo

Gradient echo (GRE) is a class of pulse sequences that is primarily used for fast scanning (Frahm et al. 1986). GRE is widely used in 3D volume imaging and other applications that require acquisition speed. Examples include vascular and cardiac imaging and acquisitions that require breath-holding. Gradient echoes are also called gradient-recalled echoes, gradient-refocused echoes, and field echoes. The term '*field echo*' refers to the magnetic field produced by the frequency-encoding gradient waveform that rephases the GRE.

GRE pulse sequences do not have the 180° RF refocusing pulse that is used to form an RF spin echo. Instead, gradient reversal on the frequency-encoded axis forms the echo. First a readout prephasing gradient lobe dephases the spin isochromats, and then they are rephased with a readout gradient that has opposite polarity. (This process is explained in detail in Section 8.1.) The peak of the GRE occurs when the area under the two gradient lobes is equal (see Figure 8.7). Partial-echo acquisition and reconstruction (Section 13.4) are commonly used in GRE and are implemented in the pulse sequence by reducing the gradient area of the readout prephasing lobe, as indicated on many of the pulse sequence diagrams in this section. Figure 14.1 shows a typical pulse sequence diagram for a GRE pulse sequence. The common features of GRE sequences are illustrated, including the gradient reversal on the frequency-encoding axis, the partial-echo acquisition, the phase-encoding lobe, and the rewinder. This

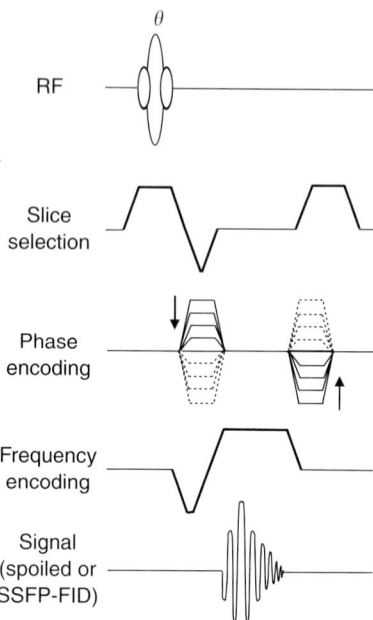

FIGURE 14.1 Pulse sequence used for spoiled GRE or SSFP-FID acquisitions.

pulse sequence (as well as several variations) is discussed in more detail later in this section, after a discussion of the response of the magnetization to a series of RF excitation pulses.

GRE acquisitions can be fast because the flip angle θ of the excitation pulse is typically less than 90°, so the longitudinal magnetization component is never inverted by an RF refocusing pulse (although sometimes a preparatory inversion pulse is applied, as described in Section 14.2). Therefore, no lengthy period of time is required for T_1 recovery, and GRE pulse sequences can use short TR (e.g., 2–50 ms). Even better, when low flip angles are used for the RF excitation pulse, an appreciable amount of transverse magnetization is created, leaving most of the longitudinal magnetization undisturbed. Figure 14.2, illustrates that the transverse magnetization that is gained is much greater than the longitudinal magnetization that is spent. This property is expressed by the relationship $M_\perp \gg (M_0 - M_z)$, which can be shown quantitatively by recalling that for values of $\theta \ll 1$ rad (approximately 57°), $\sin \theta \approx \theta$ is much larger than $1 - \cos \theta \approx \theta^2/2$.

Although acquisition speed is the main reason for using GRE pulse sequences, they have other useful features too. For example, GRE pulse sequences can provide images with bright (i.e., hyperintense) blood signal.

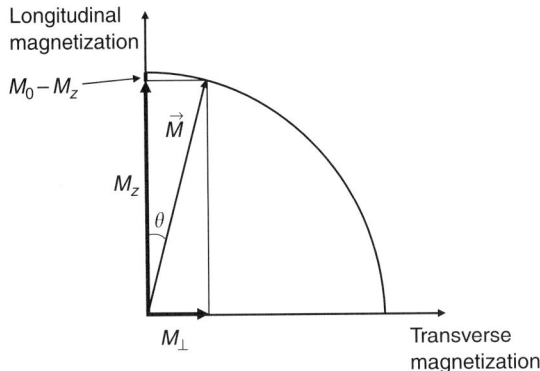

FIGURE 14.2 Response of fully relaxed magnetization to a small flip angle RF excitation pulse. The amount of transverse magnetization $M_\perp$ created by an RF excitation pulse is much greater than the loss of longitudinal magnetization ($M_0 - M_z$), which allows short TR and rapid acquisition with GRE.

This property is exploited in the time-of-flight and phase-contrast angiographic pulse sequences that are described in Chapter 15. GRE sequences also can provide susceptibility-weighted images because there is no 180° pulse to refocus the phase evolution caused by local variations in the magnetic field. The phase of the spin isochromats in the transverse plane continues to accumulate during the entire echo time. Consequently GRE images are contrast weighted by a factor $e^{-\text{TE}/T_2^*}$, instead of $e^{-\text{TE}/T_2}$ as in RF spin echo images. The parameter T_2^* (T_2 star) is sometimes called the apparent T_2 and is related to the spin-spin relaxation time T_2 by

$$\frac{1}{T_2^*} = \frac{1}{T_2} + \frac{1}{T_2'} \tag{14.1}$$

where T_2' is inversely proportional to the magnetic field inhomogeneity ΔB in each imaging voxel, that is, $T_2' \sim 1/(\gamma \Delta B)$. Whereas T_2 is an intrinsic property of the tissue, T_2' and T_2^* depend not only on external factors (e.g., susceptibility variations within the patient and how well the magnet is shimmed), but also on the prescribed imaging voxel size. Although a moderate amount of T_2^* weighting can be advantageous for some applications (e.g., to image hemorrhage), excessive T_2^* weighting causes signal-loss artifacts. For example, gradient-echo images are much more prone to signal loss than their RF spin-echo counterparts in regions near metallic implants. A signal-loss artifact specific to gradient-echo imaging is discussed in subsection 14.1.3. Finally note that the assumption of exponential dependence $e^{-\text{TE}/T_2'}$ is only true if the frequency distribution of the magnetic field inhomogeneity is the Fourier transform pair of an exponential (see Table 1.2), that is, a Lorentzian distribution.

Gradient echoes can be used with a variety of spatial-encoding methods. In this section we focus on two-dimensional Cartesian encoding. The extension to 3D volume acquisitions is straightforward, and the details are described in Section 11.6. GRE can also be used for other k-space coverage strategies such as radial projection acquisition, which is described in Section 17.5.

14.1.1 RESPONSE TO A SERIES OF RF EXCITATION PULSES

The excitation pulse is the only RF pulse in each TR interval, unless the GRE pulse sequence contains other modules (e.g., spatial saturation, magnetization transfer, spatial tagging, and magnetization preparation) that are described in other sections of the book. Even when some of those other modules are applied, they only affect selected magnetization (e.g., a spatial saturation band), so most of the magnetization in the imaging slice does not experience them. (An exception occurs for the MP-RAGE pulse sequence described in Section 14.2.) Therefore, much (if not all) of the magnetization in the imaging slice experiences a series of identical excitation pulses with flip angle θ, evenly spaced in time by TR (Figure 14.3). We assume that $\theta \neq 0, \pm 180°, \ldots$ This θ-TR-θ-TR-θ-TR $\ldots$ pulse sequence is the basis used to analyze GRE. (Note that many authors label the flip angle of the excitation pulse in a GRE pulse sequence by the Greek letter α and refer to the excitation pulses as alpha-pulses. To be consistent with the other sections of the book, however, we continue to use the symbol θ.)

The steady state is a concept that is repeatedly used in the study of gradient echoes. The steady state is also called *dynamic equilibrium*. If a system is not changing, and all of its parameters are constant, then the system is said to be in static equilibrium. A system that is continually changing can reach a steady state if the conditions are right. For example, if a bucket of water leaks but is

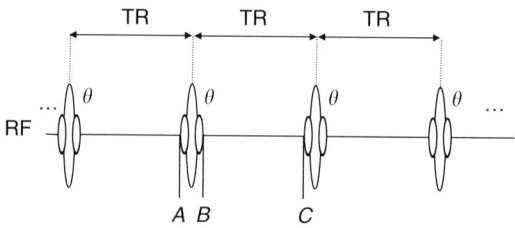

FIGURE 14.3 A train of RF excitation pulses that is used to analyze GRE.

being filled at exactly the same rate, the water level reaches a steady state. In GRE imaging, we consider steady states of both the longitudinal and transverse magnetization.

After a sufficient number of excitation pulses are applied, the longitudinal magnetization M_z reaches a steady state in GRE pulse sequences. That means that if we compare corresponding time points in adjacent TR intervals, the values of longitudinal magnetization M_z will be equal. GRE pulse sequences can be classified by the response of the transverse magnetization, $M_\perp$. If $M_\perp$ can be assumed to be zero just before each excitation pulse, then the GRE pulse sequence is said to be *spoiled*. If, however, the transverse magnetization reaches a (nonzero) steady state just before the application of each excitation pulse, then the pulse sequence is said to produce *steady-state free precession* (SSFP). The word *free* is used in the same sense as in free induction decay.

Spoiling Spoiled GRE pulse sequences can produce images with some T_1-weighted contrast (Figure 14.4). These sequences go by a variety of names including spoiled Fast Low-Angle Shot (FLASH), spoiled gradient echo (SPGR), and T_1 fast field echo (T1-FFE), as listed in Table 14.1.

Spoiling can be accomplished in a variety of ways. The simplest method is to select TR that is at least four to five times T_2, so that the transverse

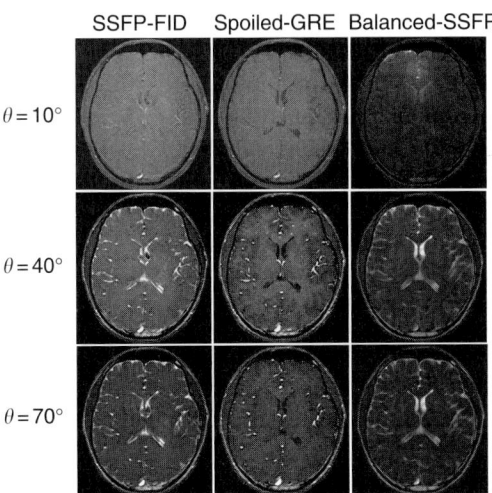

FIGURE 14.4 Axial brain images of a normal volunteer with three commonly used GRE pulse sequences at low, moderate, and high flip angles. TR = 14 ms, TE = 6 ms for the SSFP-FID and spoiled GRE images; and TR = 6 ms, TE = 3 ms for the balanced SSFP.

TABLE 14.1
Commercial Names of Common GRE Pulse Sequences Used by a Few MR Equipment Vendors[a]

Vendor	Spoiled Gradient Echo	SSFP-FID or Gradient Echo	SSFP-Echo, or CE-FAST	Balanced SSFP or True FISP	Multiacquisition SSFP or CISS	Dual-Echo SSFP or DESS
General Electric	SPGR	Gradient echo or GRASS	SSFP[b]	FIESTA	FIESTA-C	—
Philips	CE-FFE-T1 or T1-FFE	FFE	CE-FFE-T2 T2-FFE	Balanced FFE	—	—
Siemens	FLASH	FISP	PSIF	TrueFISP	CISS	DESS

[a]CE-FAST, contrast-enhanced Fourier-acquired steady state; CE-FFE, contrast-enhanced fast field echo; CISS, constructive interference in the steady state; DESS, dual-echo steady state; FFE, fast field echo; FID, free-induction decay; FIESTA, fast imaging employing steady-state acquisition; FIESTA-C, fast imaging employing steady-state acquisition with phase cycling; FISP, fast imaging with steady (-state free) precession; FLASH, fast low-angle shot; GRASS, gradient recalled acquisition in the steady state; PSIF, reversed fast imaging with steady (-state free) precession; SPGR, spoiled gradient echo; SSFP, steady-state free precession.
[b]SSFP-Echo pulse sequence not currently offered by General Electric.

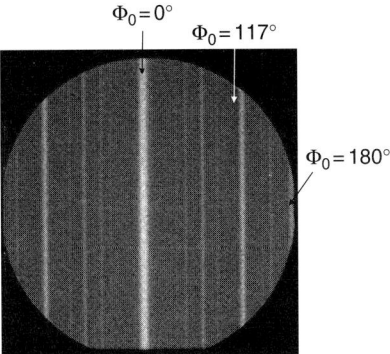

FIGURE 14.5 GRE image of a uniform, spherical phantom acquired with no phase-encoding rewinder gradient and TR = 20 ms, TE = 5 ms, and flip angle = 30°. The resulting stripe pattern provides insight into RF spoiling techniques.

magnetization decays nearly to zero by the end of the pulse sequence. Because the main advantage of using GRE is acquisition speed, this is not a very practical spoiling method, unless the interleaved multislice acquisition strategy is used to increase the number of slice locations per TR (Section 11.5). For 2D sequential or 3D volume acquisitions, however, a different spoiling strategy must be used. End-of-sequence gradient spoiler (Section 10.5) pulses can be applied, but they are not effective at spoiling the transverse steady state unless their gradient area varies from TR to TR interval. Even with time-varying spoilers, the spoiling will be spatially nonuniform because gradients produce spatially varying fields. This is illustrated by the stripe pattern in Figure 14.5, which is obtained by using the phase-encoding gradient as a spoiler, (i.e., no phase rewinding lobe is used). A better solution is to use RF spoiling (Crawley et al. 1988; Zur et al. 1991; Duyn et al. 1997) to phase cycle the RF excitation pulses according to a predetermined schedule. RF spoiling not only provides more spatially uniform results, but also avoids eddy currents that vary among the TR intervals. Several RF phase-cycling schemes that produce good results are described in the literature.

Let Φ_j be the phase of the B_1 field for the jth RF pulse in the rotating frame; $\Phi = 0$ for a θ_x pulse, and $\Phi = 90°$ for θ_y. One method is to use randomized phases Φ_j, but then the effectiveness of the spoiling can fluctuate from TR to TR interval. A more popular method is to use a phase-cycling schedule such as:

$$\Phi_j = \Phi_{j-1} + j\Phi_0, \quad j = 1, 2, 3, \ldots \tag{14.2}$$

so that the phases Φ_0, $\Phi_1 = 2\Phi_0$, $\Phi_2 = 4\Phi_0$, $\Phi_3 = 7\Phi_0, \ldots$, are applied. The starting value Φ_0 is an adjustable parameter. The value $\Phi_0 = 117°$ is recommended in Zur, Wood, and Neuringer (1991). Because the phase increment ($\Phi_j - \Phi_{j-1}$) in Eq. (14.2) is linearly proportional to j, the phase Φ_j varies quadratically with j. This quadratic dependence can be seen explicitly by solving the difference equation (14.2):

$$\Phi_j = \frac{1}{2}\Phi_0(j^2 + j + 2), \qquad j = 0, 1, 2, \ldots \tag{14.3}$$

With RF spoiling, the degree of spoiling depends strongly on the choice of Φ_0, but unlike random phase methods it is uniform among the TR intervals. Note that RF-spoiled GRE pulse sequences must apply a phase-encoding rewinder because the gradient area on any of the three logical axes must not vary from TR to TR interval or else the spoiling will be spatially dependent. Also, during each TR interval, the received MR signal must be shifted by a phase Φ_j, so that the k-space data are consistent.

Examining the structure of the stripes in Figure 14.5 can provide physical insight into RF spoiling and the choice of Φ_0. The linear increment of the phase represented by Eq. (14.2) is equivalent to the phase twist imparted by the phase-encoding gradient as it is stepped to Fourier-encode an image. Because images such as Figure 14.5 are obtained using the phase-encoding gradient as a spoiler, they have the remarkable property of providing a spatial map of the effect of many different values of Φ_0 between $+180°$ and $-180°$ in a single image. The bright stripes are unspoiled regions, corresponding to short phase cycles, such as $\Phi_0 = 360°/n$, where n is a small integer. A phase advance of $360°$ is equivalent to $\Phi_0 = 0°$, or $n = 1$ (i.e., no phase cycling) and corresponds to the bright stripe in the center. A value of $n = 2$ ($\Phi_0 = 180°$) corresponds to negating every other pair of pulses; that is, it sets up a short phase cycle (of length $4 \times$ TR) and produces the second brightest stripe, which is partially visible at the edge of the image. The dark regions are spoiled and correspond to phase cycles that have length much greater than T_2/TR. This explains why a phase increment of $117°$ works well—no small integer multiple of $117°$ is divisible by $360°$. Many other values of Φ_0 (e.g., $123°$) also produce good RF spoiling. Also note that the pattern of stripes is symmetric (on magnitude images) about the gradient isocenter; that is, choosing a phase increment of $-\Phi_0$ produces the same effect as $+\Phi_0$.

Steady State of the Longitudinal Magnetization for Spoiled Pulse Sequences   If we assume perfect spoiling, then $M_\perp$ is zero just before each RF pulse. Each excitation pulse converts longitudinal magnetization into transverse magnetization, which produces an FID that can be rephased into a GRE. Referring to Figure 14.3, if the longitudinal magnetization at point A is M_{zA}, then after the excitation pulse:

$$M_{zB} = M_{zA} \cos \theta \tag{14.4}$$

In the TR interval between points B and C, T_1 relaxation occurs, so according to the Bloch equations:

$$M_{zC} = M_{zB}e^{-TR/T_1} + M_0(1 - e^{-TR/T_1}) = M_{zA}\cos\theta E_1 + M_0(1 - E_1)$$
$$(14.5)$$

where $E_1 = e^{-TR/T_1}$. When a steady state for the longitudinal magnetization is reached:

$$M_{zA} = M_{zC} \qquad (14.6)$$

Eliminating M_{zC} from Eq. (14.5) yields:

$$\frac{M_{zA}}{M_0} = \frac{1 - E_1}{1 - \cos\theta E_1} \equiv f_{z,ss} \qquad (14.7)$$

where $f_{z,ss}$ is a dimensionless measure of the steady-state longitudinal magnetization. Returning to the bucket analogy of steady state, the longitudinal magnetization corresponds to the water level, the RF excitation pulse corresponds to the leak, and T_1 recovery corresponds to the water pouring in.

The signal S_{spoil} from a spoiled GRE acquisition is caused by the gradient rephasing of the FID at an echo time TE, so it is given by $M_{zA}\sin\theta e^{-TE/T_2^*}$. Writing the expanded form of E_1 yields the well-known result:

$$S_{spoil} = \frac{M_0\sin\theta(1 - e^{-TR/T_1})}{(1 - \cos\theta e^{-TR/T_1})}e^{-TE/T_2^*} \qquad (14.8)$$

The flip angle θ that maximizes the spoiled GRE signal in Eq. (14.8) is called the *Ernst angle*. Setting the first derivative to zero and verifying that the second derivative is negative yields:

$$\theta_E = \arccos E_1 = \arccos(e^{-TR/T_1}) \qquad (14.9)$$

The value of θ_E lies between 0 and $90°$, and monotonically increases as the ratio TR/T_1 increases. Physically, when the flip angle θ is less than the Ernst angle, it is an indication that the signal can be increased by further increasing the flip angle because the benefit of creating more transverse magnetization outweighs the further loss of longitudinal magnetization.

Equation (14.8) represents the signal from a perfectly spoiled GRE pulse sequence, provided that the longitudinal magnetization has reached a steady state. It also is useful to examine how the longitudinal magnetization responds to the first in the series of RF excitation pulses, the approach to steady state (Hänicke et al. 1990). If the magnetization experiences a total of j excitation

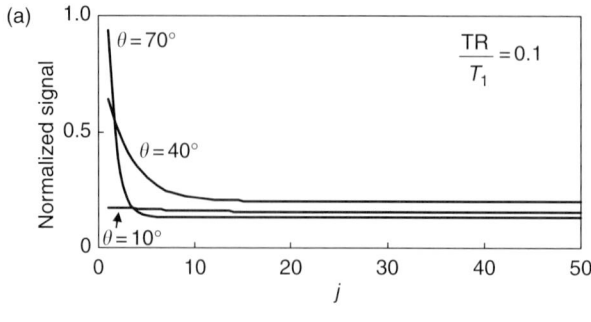

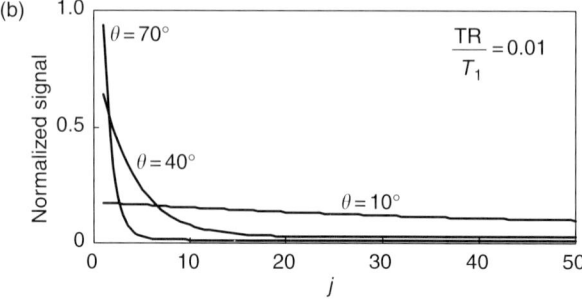

FIGURE 14.6 The approach to steady state for a spoiled GRE pulse sequence, plotted versus the number of excitation pulses that the magnetization experiences. (a) $TR/T_1 = 0.1$, which corresponds to an Ernst angle of 25.2°. (b) $TR/T_1 = 0.01$, with Ernst angle of 8.1°.

pulses ($j \geq 1$), then the steady-state expression for the spoiled GRE signal in Eq. (14.8) is replaced by the approach to steady state:

$$S_j = M_0 \sin \theta \left[f_{z,\text{ss}} + (\cos \theta e^{-TR/T_1})^{j-1}(1 - f_{z,\text{ss}}) \right] e^{-TE/T_2^*} \quad (14.10)$$

Figure 14.6 illustrates the approach to steady state for several values of the flip angles and for T_1 equal to 10 or 100 times the TR. Because of the factor $(\cos \theta)^{j-1}$ in Eq. (14.10), the approach to steady state is faster for larger values of the flip angle. This analysis has assumed perfect spoiling, which is difficult to attain in practice. The actual approach to steady state can have considerable deviations from the ideal case (Epstein et al. 1996).

When the flip angle is equal to the Ernst angle, $f_{z,\text{ss}}$ reduces to $(1 + E_1)^{-1}$, so the approach to steady state takes the form:

$$S_j = M_0 \sqrt{\frac{1 - E_1}{1 + E_1}} (1 + E_1^{2j-1}) e^{-TE/T_2^*} \quad (14.11)$$

Example 14.1 Verify Eq. (14.10) by using mathematical induction. That is, first show that it is true for $j = 1$. Then show that its truth for $j = m - 1$ implies its truth for $j = m$.

Answer When $j = 1$, Eq. (14.10) reduces to $S_1 = M_0 \sin\theta e^{-TE/T_2^*}$, which is true because it represents the FID response of the fully relaxed longitudinal magnetization to the first RF pulse that is applied. Now suppose that the longitudinal magnetization just before pulse $m - 1$ is:

$$M_{z,m-1}^- = M_0 \left(f_{z,ss} + (\cos\theta E_1)^{m-2}(1 - f_{z,ss}) \right) \qquad m \geq 2 \qquad (14.12)$$

Just after the pulse $M_{z,m-1}^+ = M_{z,m-1}^- \cos\theta$. Accounting for T_1 relaxation in between the pulses $m - 1$ and m yields:

$$M_{z,m}^- = M_{z,m-1}^- \cos\theta E_1 + M_0(1 - E_1) \qquad (14.13)$$

Substituting Eq. (14.12) into Eq. (14.13) yields:

$$M_{z,m}^- = M_0 \left(\cos\theta E_1 f_{z,ss} + (\cos\theta E_1)^{m-1}(1 - f_{z,ss}) + (1 - E_1) \right) \qquad (14.14)$$

Therefore to complete the inductive proof requires that $f_{z,ss} = \cos\theta E_1 f_{z,ss} + (1 - E_1)$, which can be readily verified with Eq. (14.7).

Equation (14.10) is used in the study of flow-related enhancement, as described in Section 15.3. It also allows us to predict how long it takes for the transient response to die away and the steady state to be established. This can be of practical importance, whether or not k-space data are collected during the approach to steady state. For example, Eq. (14.10) and knowledge about the view order can be used to estimate how many dummy pulse sequences (i.e., pulse sequences with the data acquisition disabled) to play. Also, several catalyzing methods have been developed to accelerate the approach to steady state. For example, a spatial saturation pulse can be applied, followed by a waiting period (Busse and Riederer 2001).

SSFP-FID and SSFP-Echo   SSFP-FID is a standard gradient-echo pulse sequence that provides greater signal than spoiled pulse sequences, but often at the cost of reduced contrast (Figure 14.4). It goes by a variety of commercial names (e.g., FISP) that are listed in Table 14.1. SSFP-echo is a less widely used pulse sequence, but is conceptually important for understanding the transverse steady state.

If the RF excitation pulses in the θ-TR-θ-TR-θ-TR... sequence are phase coherent and TR is less than or on the order of T_2, then an SSFP (Carr 1958;

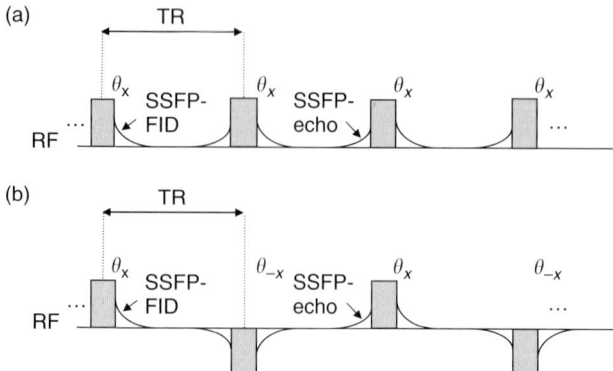

FIGURE 14.7 Schematic representation of the transverse steady state for (a) a standard train of RF pulses and (b) a sign-alternated pulse train. The magnitude of the SSFP signal is not affected by the sign alternation, but the polarity can be, as shown. The SSFP can have substantial oscillations (not shown), like any other FID or echo.

Ernst and Anderson 1966) is established. In this context, phase coherent means that the RF pulses all have the same phase in the rotating frame, (i.e., θ_x-TR-θ_x-TR-θ_x ...) or else a simple phase cycle such as sign alternation (θ_x-TR-θ_{-x}-TR-θ_x-TR-θ_{-x}-...). A further condition to avoid spoiling the steady state is that the phase accumulated by the transverse magnetization be the same in each TR interval. This condition requires that the gradient area in each TR interval be the same, so, for example, a phase-encoding rewinder lobe must be applied.

If these conditions are met, steady states for both the longitudinal magnetization and transverse magnetization will be established. The resulting SSFP of the transverse magnetization is schematically shown in Figure 14.7. It comprises two parts: an FID-like signal that forms just after each RF pulse and a time-reversed FID-like signal that forms just before each pulse. The former is called S^+ or SSFP-FID, and the latter is called S^- or SSFP-echo. If RF pulses are sign alternated, the amplitudes of the SSFP signals are unchanged, but their signs are reversed in every other TR interval, as shown in Figure 14.7b.

To calculate the strength of the SSFP-FID and SSFP-echo signals for GRE imaging, a two-step procedure is usually followed. (An alternative procedure is described in Gyngell 1988.) First, a recursion relation is set up that equates the magnetization in adjacent TR intervals, similar to Eq. (14.6). The procedure is more complicated than that used to derive Eq. (14.7), however, because both the transverse and longitudinal magnetization must be considered. Also, if sign alternation is used in the train of RF pulses, then the equality is assumed for every other TR interval. Details of the calculation are provided in Freeman and Hill (1971). Also a new parameter ϕ is introduced, which is the angle through which the transverse magnetization precesses during each TR interval. The second step is to recognize that in GRE the imaging gradients introduce a spread of ϕ across the voxel and to account for this spread by convolution (Zur et al. 1988). The final results of the calculation are presented in Hänicke and Vogel (2003):

$$\text{SSFP}_{\text{FID}} = M_0 \tan\left(\frac{\theta}{2}\right) \left(1 - \frac{(E_1 - \cos\theta)\left(1 - E_2^2\right)}{\sqrt{p^2 - q^2}}\right)$$

$$\text{SSFP}_{\text{ECHO}} = M_0 \tan\left(\frac{\theta}{2}\right) \left(1 - \frac{(1 - E_1 \cos\theta)\left(1 - E_2^2\right)}{\sqrt{p^2 - q^2}}\right) \tag{14.15}$$

where $E_2 = e^{-\text{TR}/T_2}$, and

$$\begin{aligned} p &= 1 - E_1 \cos\theta - E_2^2(E_1 - \cos\theta) \\ q &= E_2(1 - E_1)(1 + \cos\theta) \end{aligned} \tag{14.16}$$

The two lines in Eq. (14.15) are derived under the assumption that the SSFP-FID and SSFP-echo signals do not overlap substantially in the readout window.

Also note that, from Eq. (14.16), an alternative algebraic form can be derived:

$$\frac{1 - E_2^2}{\sqrt{p^2 - q^2}} = \sqrt{\frac{1 - E_2^2}{(1 - E_1 \cos\theta)^2 - E_2^2(E_1 - \cos\theta)^2}} \tag{14.17}$$

Although the SSFP signal formulas in Eq. (14.15) are more complicated than the spoiled case in Eq. (14.8), there are some simple limiting cases. For example, if $\text{TR} \gg T_2$, then E_2 is negligible, and $p \to (1 - E_1 \cos\theta)$ and $q \to 0$. Therefore $\text{SSFP}_{\text{ECHO}} \to 0$, and with the aid of the trigonometric identity $\tan(u/2) = \sin u/(1 + \cos u)$:

$$\text{SSFP}_{\text{FID}} \to M_0 \sin\theta \frac{(1 - E_1)}{1 - E_1 \cos\theta}, \qquad \text{TR} \gg T_2 \tag{14.18}$$

Equation (14.18) is the same as the expression for the spoiled case (Eq. 14.8), up to a factor of $e^{-\text{TE}/T_2^*}$. If the SSFP-FID is rephased as a GRE at time TE, the two expressions become identical. This limiting case indicates that prolonging the TR and waiting for the transverse magnetization to decay away is an effective spoiling method.

Another instructive case is $\theta \to 0$, that is, the small flip angle limit. After some algebra, we find that $\sqrt{p^2 - q^2} \to (1 - E_1)\left(1 - E_2^2\right)$. This in turn implies that:

$$\text{SSFP}_{\text{FID}} \rightarrow 2M_0 \tan\left(\frac{\theta}{2}\right) \approx M_0 \sin\theta, \qquad \theta \ll 1 \qquad (14.19)$$

that is the SSFP-FID becomes proton-density weighted at small flip angles, just like the spoiled signal in Eq. (14.8).

Despite the similarities between these two limiting cases, SSFP-FID and spoiled signals usually display substantially different contrast behavior. At intermediate and high flip angles, spoiled GRE provides considerable T_1-weighting and dark fluid, whereas SSFP-FID provides less contrast but bright fluid (Figure 14.4). It is useful to remember that at fixed acquisition parameters (TR, TE, flip angle, etc.) the signal from SSFP-FID is greater than the signal from spoiled GRE. In other words, spoiled GRE obtains increased contrast by removing signal, mostly from tissue with a long T_2, whereas SSFP-FID reuses transverse magnetization to increase signal.

The SSFP-echo signal can provide greater T_2-weighting compared to the SSFP-FID, especially at intermediate and high flip angles. Simplifying the algebra by setting $\theta = 90°$ so that $\cos\theta = 0$ and using Eqs. (14.15) and (14.17), we find the ratio of the two signals is:

$$\frac{\text{SSFP}_{\text{ECHO}}}{\text{SSFP}_{\text{FID}}} = \frac{1 - \sqrt{\left(1 - E_2^2\right)/\left(1 - E_1^2 E_2^2\right)}}{1 - E_1\sqrt{\left(1 - E_2^2\right)/\left(1 - E_1^2 E_2^2\right)}} \qquad (14.20)$$

Using Eq. (14.20) and the expansion $\sqrt{1+\varepsilon} \approx 1 + \varepsilon/2 + \cdots$, the interested reader can show that in the case of TR $\ll T_1$, as $E_1 \rightarrow 1$:

$$\frac{\text{SSFP}_{\text{ECHO}}}{\text{SSFP}_{\text{FID}}} \approx E_2^2 = e^{-2\text{TR}/T_2}, \qquad \text{TR} \ll T_1 \qquad (14.21)$$

A physical interpretation of Eq. (14.21) is that the SSFP-echo signal is primarily composed of the SSFP-FID signal refocused from the previous TR interval, that is, TE $= 2 \times$ TR. If the echo is shifted to the left by an amount Δ to form a GRE as shown in Figure 14.11 (later in the chapter), then Eq. (14.21) is modified to

$$\frac{\text{SSFP}_{\text{ECHO}}}{\text{SSFP}_{\text{FID}}} \approx e^{-(2\text{TR}-\Delta)/T_2}, \qquad \text{TR} \ll T_1 \qquad (14.22)$$

and T2′ weighting is introduced (see Example 14.5).

Balanced SSFP (True FISP)   To establish SSFP, the gradient area on any axis must not vary among the TR intervals. If a further condition is imposed that the total gradient area on any axis is zero during each TR interval, a very different steady state results. The peaks of the SSFP-FID and SSFP-echo will coalesce; that is, they rephase at the same time TE. Therefore the balanced SSFP signal is the coherent sum of the two signals (Oppelt et al. 1986; Duerk et al. 1998). Equation (14.15) is no longer valid because the analysis used to derive it assumes that the two signals are well separated in time. Also, unlike Eq. (14.15) the magnitude of the signal (and not just its sign as in Figure 14.7b) now strongly depends on whether the RF excitation pulses all have the same phase or are sign alternated. The result with sign alternation is:

$$\text{SSFP}_{\text{bal,alt}} = M_0 \sin\theta \frac{1 - E_1}{1 - (E_1 - E_2)\cos\theta - E_1 E_2} e^{-\text{TE}/T_2} \qquad (14.23)$$

and without sign alternation:

$$\text{SSFP}_{\text{bal,noalt}} = M_0 \sin\theta \frac{1 - E_1}{1 - (E_1 + E_2)\cos\theta + E_1 E_2} e^{-\text{TE}/T_2} \qquad (14.24)$$

Note the use of T_2 rather than T_2^* in the exponential in Eqs. (14.23) and (14.24). As shown in Scheffler and Hennig (2003), this is correct if the balanced SSFP signal is rephased in the center of the TR interval (i.e., TE = TR/2), in which case $e^{-\text{TE}/T_2} = \sqrt{E_2}$. As the peak of the balanced SSFP signal is moved away from the center of the TR interval, T_2' weighting is introduced. In practice, the amount of T_2' weighting is usually negligible because a very short TR is used and also because the homogeneity requirements are stringent in balanced SSFP imaging. But it is interesting to note that contrary to spoiled or SSFP-FID pulse sequences, decreasing TE can increase susceptibility weighting in balanced SSFP.

The signal in Eq. (14.23) is greater than (14.24), so in practice sign alternation is used. Physically, the effect of the sign alternation is analogous to the driven equilibrium methods discussed in Section 17.4. The RF pulses with negative flip angle help to drive the longitudinal magnetization back to its equilibrium position, increasing signal when TR is much less than T_1.

The effect of sign alternation is equivalent to a pulse sequence (without sign alternation) that has constant precession of the transverse magnetization by $\phi = 180°$ in each TR interval (Hinshaw 1976). Similarly, if a constant precession $\phi = 180°$ per TR interval occurs in a sign-alternated pulse sequence, it effectively removes the sign alternation, so that the lower signal represented by Eq. (14.24) results. A spatial region where this signal loss occurs is known as a band. Figure 14.8 shows a representative plot of signal versus ϕ with and without sign alternation. As described in Carr (1958), the shape of the curves in the plot depends on T_1, T_2, and θ. Because unwanted phase shifts are usually present in MRI, banding is a serious problem in balanced-SSFP

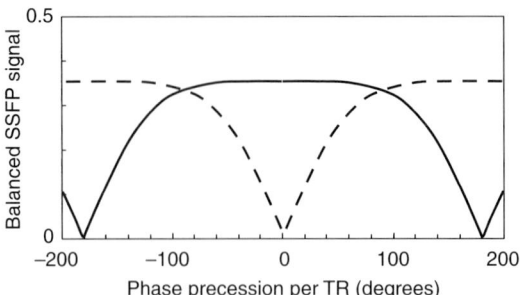

FIGURE 14.8 Representative plot of a balanced SSFP signal versus phase precession ϕ per TR interval of the transverse magnetization. When the RF pulses are sign alternated (solid line), strong signal results on resonance $\phi = 0$ and a minimum of the signal (a band) occurs at $\phi = \pm 180°$. When the RF pulses are not sign alternated (dashed line), the curve is shifted so that the minimum occurs on resonance. Both curves repeat with a period of 360°.

imaging. Assuming a constant resonance offset, the accumulated phase ϕ is proportional to the repetition time. Therefore short TR (e.g., 7 ms or less) is key to eliminating banding artifacts, especially because susceptibility variation is inevitable and can rarely be shimmed out completely. Technological strides in obtaining shorter TR (e.g., more powerful gradients), field homogeneity, and eddy-current compensation have allowed balanced SSFP to become a clinically important pulse sequence. Note that balanced SSFP becomes progressively more difficult to implement as the field strength B_0 increases, not only because of increased susceptibility variations (measured in hertz), but also because SAR becomes a concern with the use of very short TR.

For short TR (i.e., TR $\ll T_2 < T_1$), the signal formulas can be simplified because $E_1 \approx 1 - TR/T_1$, and $E_2 \approx 1 - TR/T_2$. In that case the signal from sign-alternated balanced SSFP can be expressed as a function of T_1/T_2:

$$\text{SSFP}_{\text{bal,alt}} \approx \frac{M_0 \sin\theta}{(T_1/T_2)(1-\cos\theta)+(1+\cos\theta)} e^{-TE/T_2}, \quad TR \ll T_2$$

$$(14.25)$$

Because the factor of T_1/T_2 is in the denominator of Eq. (14.25), balanced SSFP is sometimes said to have 'T_2/T_1' contrast weighting. This explains the hyperintense signal from fluids and fat often seen on balanced SSFP images. The signal in Eq. (14.25) is maximized when the flip angle is:

$$\theta_{\text{max}} = \arccos\left(\frac{T_1 - T_2}{T_1 + T_2}\right)$$

$$(14.26)$$

At flip angles near $90°$, $\cos\theta \approx 0$, so balanced SSFP becomes more highly T_2/T_1 weighted because Eq. (14.25) reduces to:

$$\text{SSFP}_{\text{bal,alt}}|_{\theta=90°} \approx \frac{M_0 T_2}{T_1 + T_2} e^{-\text{TE}/T_2}, \quad \text{TR} \ll T_2 \tag{14.27}$$

The signal in Eq. (14.27) reaches a maximum of nearly $M_0/2$ when $T_2 = T_1$, independent of TR. This is an extremely strong signal for a short TR pulse sequence, which helps to explain the popularity of balanced SSFP methods. Balanced SSFP methods have virtually replaced the use of SSFP-echo, which also provides images with bright fluid but which produces much less signal and has greater sensitivity to flow dephasing. That is why SSFP-echo is not emphasized in this book.

The approach to steady state in a balanced SSFP pulse sequence can take on the order of four to five times T_1. This is a long time to wait relative to TR, so accelerating or catalyzing (Scheffler 2003) the approach to steady state is an important practical problem. Moreover, once the steady state is established it often has to be interrupted, for example, for the periodic application of chemical saturation pulses or to resynchronize the pulse sequence with a detected cardiac trigger. A simple and relatively effective catalyzing method for sign-alternated balanced SSFP is to apply a half-flip angle pulse with a half-TR interval, that is, $(\theta_x/2) - (\text{TR}/2) - \theta_{-x} - \text{TR} - \theta_x \cdots$. More sophisticated catalyzing methods such as linearly ramping up flip angle are described in Le Roux (2003) and Hargreaves et al. (2001). Also the SSFP can be temporarily stored on the longitudinal axis (Scheffler et al. 2001) for the application of a chemical saturation or other magnetization-preparation pulse by ramping down the flip angle, for example, by applying the following train of RF pulses:

$$\cdots \theta_x - \text{TR} - \theta_{-x} - (\text{TR}/2) - (\theta_x/2) - (\text{Chemical saturation}) - (\theta_x/2)$$
$$- (\text{TR}/2) - \theta_{-x} \cdots$$

Multiple-Acquisition SSFP (CISS) In some applications such as imaging the structures of the inner ear, very small fields of view (10 cm or less) are desired. This necessarily increases the minimum TR, so that banding artifacts are unavoidable in balanced SSFP. Using a technique known as constructive interference in the steady state (CISS), or multiacquisition SSFP, can suppress the bands (Casselman et al. 1993). Two acquisitions are obtained sequentially, for example, one with sign alternation of the excitation pulses and the other without. The two images are separately reconstructed. Because of the phase cycling, the locations of the bands are shifted relative to one another by one-half the spatial period on the two corresponding images. Any given pixel can

(a)   (b)   (c)

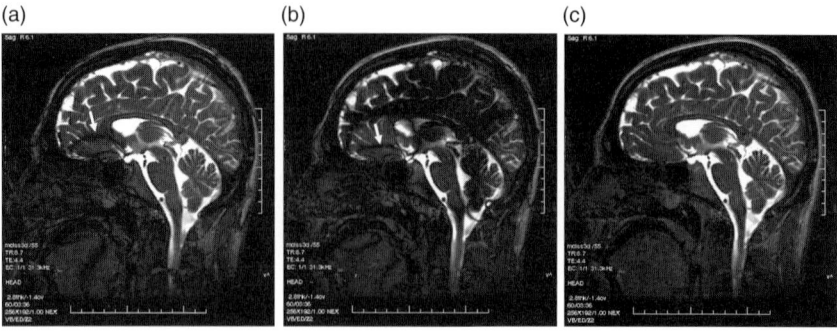

FIGURE 14.9 Sagittal head images of a healthy volunteer using a multiacquisition balanced SSFP technique known as CISS or FIESTA-C. (a) Balanced SSFP image displaying intense signal from fluid, but some banding artifact due to off-resonance effects (arrow) near the sinus cavities. (b) Balanced SSFP without sign alternation shifts the bands. (c) Maximum intensity calculation of the other two images removes the banding artifact. (Courtesy of Heidi Ward, Ph.D., GE Healthcare.)

lie within a band on one of the images, but unless there is extreme susceptibility variation, the pixel will not lie within a band on both images. Therefore, the bands can be suppressed on the final image by calculating a maximum intensity of the two magnitude images on a pixel-by-pixel basis, as shown in Figure 14.9.

Multiacquisition SSFP has several variations. For example, instead of two acquisitions, four can be used, each with a different phase cycle: $(\theta_x, \theta_x, \theta_x, \theta_x, \ldots)$, $(\theta_x, \theta_y, \theta_{-x}, \theta_{-y}, \ldots)$, $(\theta_x, \theta_{-x}, \theta_x, \theta_{-x}, \ldots)$, and $(\theta_x, \theta_{-y}, \theta_{-x}, \theta_y, \ldots)$. The bands are then shifted by one-quarter of the spatial period on each image. Four-acquisition can provide a smoother image appearance than two-acquisition, not only because of improved SNR but also because there should be three or four images on which any pixel does not lie in a band. A further variation is to replace the maximum intensity calculation with the square root of the sum of the squares, which can further improve the SNR (Bangerter and Nishimura 2003).

14.1.2 GRADIENT WAVEFORMS AND GRE PULSE SEQUENCE NAMES

As discussed, there are a variety of SSFP signals that can result from the application of a string of excitation pulses: SSFP-FID, SSFP-echo, and balanced SSFP. The desired signal is selected by applying the proper gradient

TABLE 14.2

Summary of the Gradient Waveforms, Radio Frequency Pulse Trains, and Contrast Formulas for Several Gradient Echo Pulse Sequences

Generic Name	Gradient Waveform	RF Pulse Train	Contrast Formula
Spoiled GRE	Forward (Fig. 14.1)	RF spoiled	Eq. (14.8)
SSFP-FID	Forward (Fig. 14.1)	Standard or sign alternated	Eq. (14.15)
SSFP-Echo	Reversed (Fig. 14.11)	Standard or sign alternated	Eq. (14.15)
Balanced SSFP	Balanced (Fig. 14.12 or 14.13)	Sign alternated	Eq. (14.23)
Multiacquisition SSFP	Balanced (Fig. 14.12 or 14.13)	Standard and sign alternated	Eqs.(14.23) with banding artifacts removed
Dual-echo SSFP	Balanced, but with extended readout (Fig. 14.14)	Standard or sign alternated	Eq. (14.15)
Dual-echo GRE	Two forward readouts: one with fat–water in phase and one out of phase (Fig. 14.10)	Usually RF spoiled	If spoiled Eq. (14.8) with TE_1 and TE_2

waveform. This is somewhat analogous to how crusher gradients are used to select the desired signal pathway, as discussed in Section 10.2. Also, the gradient waveform is necessary to rephase the FID into the desired GRE.

Gradient waveforms for GRE pulse sequences can be divided into three main groups: forward, reversed, and balanced. Table 14.2 lists which gradient waveforms are used with various GRE pulse sequences. Within each group, further divisions can be made, for example, whether or not gradient moment nulling or partial echo is used.

Figure 14.1 shows a forward gradient waveform with partial-echo sampling. This waveform is used to rephase a GRE from an SSFP-FID or a

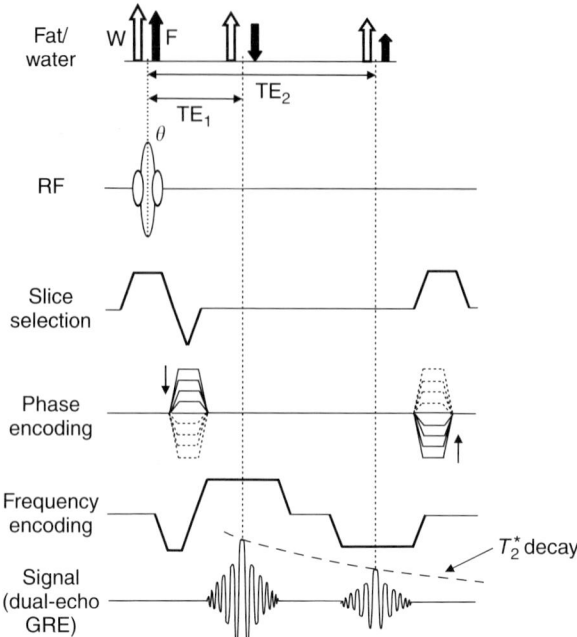

FIGURE 14.10 Dual-echo GRE pulse sequence. Often TE_1 and TE_2 are selected so that fat and water are out of phase on one echo and in phase on the other. This is indicated schematically by the solid and hollow arrows on the top row.

spoiled signal. The end of sequence spoiler pulse dephases any residual SSFP-echo signal. The spoiler pulse is shown on the slice axis, although it could be applied on any one, two, or all three of the logical axes. The pulse sequence can be extended to rephase two gradient echoes, as shown in Figure 14.10. Alternatively, the pulse sequence can be time-reversed as shown in Figure 14.11, in order to form an image from the SSFP-echo signal. The spoiler pulse at the beginning of the pulse sequence eliminates the SSFP-FID signal.

Figure 14.12 shows a typical gradient waveform used to acquire a full-echo, balanced SSFP signal. This same gradient waveform can be used regardless of whether the RF pulses are sign alternated or not. The key feature is the gradient area on any of the logical axes is zero when integrated over one TR interval. Any slight deviation from this requirement causes the SSFP-FID and SSFP-echo signals to separate from one another in the readout window and interfere, leading to banding artifacts in the image. Figure 14.13 shows how the gradient waveform is modified to acquire a partial-echo balanced SSFP signal. The readout prephasing lobe is reduced in area by the same amount as

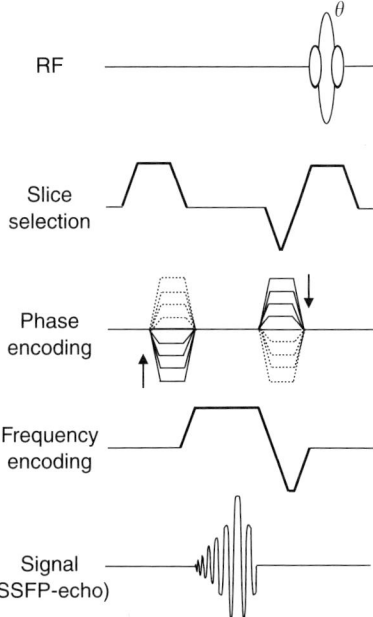

FIGURE 14.11 Pulse sequence used for SSFP-echo acquisitions. Note that it is a time-reversed mirror image of the pulse sequence used for SSFP-FID acquisitions. That is why we call it a reversed pulse sequence, as opposed to the forward sequence shown in Figure 14.1.

the readout lobe while the rephasing lobe is left unchanged, so that the total area on the frequency-encoding gradient waveform remains zero.

Sometimes the readout gradient is extended so that the SSFP-echo and SSFP-FID are intentionally separated enough not to interfere with one another and are collected as two distinct GREs (Bruder et al. 1988). This is called dual-echo steady state (DESS) free precession and representative gradient waveforms are shown in Figure 14.14. The readout gradient between the two echoes serves as a spoiler so that they do not interfere with one another. The two GREs have different contrast weightings, which can be seen from Eq. (14.15), and more easily from Eq. (14.21). They can be viewed as separate images or else combined with postprocessing, such as summing the two magnitude images. Note the differences between DESS and dual echo GRE (Figure 14.10), which rephases the same FID twice.

Various equipment manufacturers traditionally have given different names to equivalent or nearly equivalent pulse sequences (Elster 1993), which has

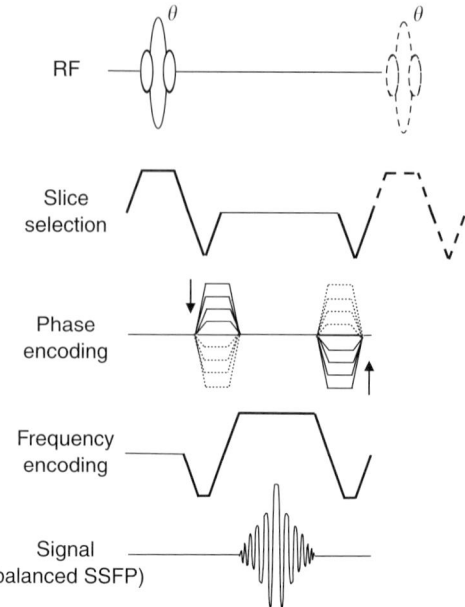

FIGURE 14.12 Pulse sequence used for balanced SSFP acquisitions. On any of the three gradient axes, the net gradient area is zero during one TR interval. That is why it is called a balanced pulse sequence, as opposed to the forward and reversed pulse sequences shown in Figures 14.1 and 14.11, respectively. The RF pulse and part of the slice-selection gradient for the next TR interval are shown (dashed lines), to emphasize the symmetry of the waveform.

complicated the study of GRE. Table 14.1 cross-references some of the commonly used names for GRE pulse sequences against the generic names that we have used.

14.1.3 PRACTICAL CONSIDERATIONS

GRE Pulse Sequence Selection   Because there are so many different GRE pulse sequences, it is not always clear which one to select for a particular application. If T_1 weighting is desired, then spoiled sequences are used. Spoiled GRE also has the greatest flexibility in the acquisition mode because sequential 2D, interleaved 2D, and 3D can all be used. The steady-state pulse sequences, however, require a short TR, so only the 3D or sequential 2D acquisition modes are practical. It is important to keep in mind that the signal formula for spoiled GRE (Eq. 14.8) is different from the signal formula for conventional RF spin

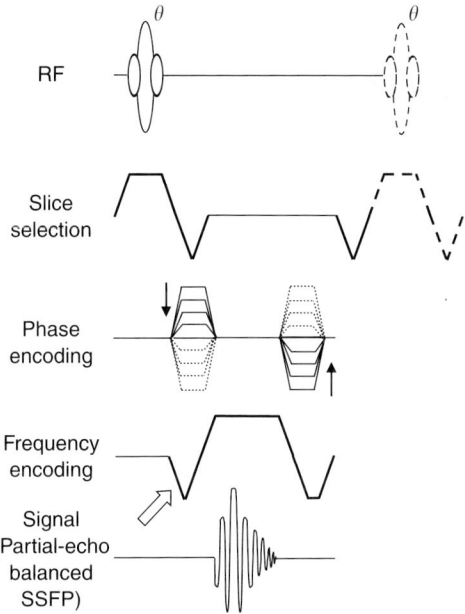

FIGURE 14.13 Pulse sequence used for partial-echo, balanced SSFP acquisitions. The net area on the readout gradient waveform remains zero. Because TE < TR/2, a slight amount of susceptibility weighting is introduced.

echo (Section 14.3), so quite different contrast behavior can be observed. These differences have been particularly noted in gadolinium-enhanced studies of the brain, as described in Mugler and Brookeman (1993).

As TR decreases for fast GRE acquisition, the Ernst angle (Eq. 14.9) for spoiled GRE also decreases. Attempts to obtain T_1 weighting by increasing the flip angle generally result in a poor SNR when TR is short (e.g., TR < 10 ms). Instead, the preferred strategy to obtain T_1 weighting with a short TR is to use magnetization preparation (e.g., inversion) followed by a series of GRE pulse sequences, as in MP-RAGE (Section 14.2). With MP-RAGE, the short TR becomes an advantage because the k-space lines are acquired closer in time, so there is less blurring introduced by the signal modulation of the inversion recovery curve.

Balanced SSFP with high flip angle provides the greatest SNR per unit time, so it is the method of choice if bright fluid signal is desired. Its two main drawbacks are banding artifacts in the region of susceptibility change, and a bright fat signal. To suppress the signal from lipids, the method in Scheffler et al. (2003) can be used. If banding artifacts are a problem, then

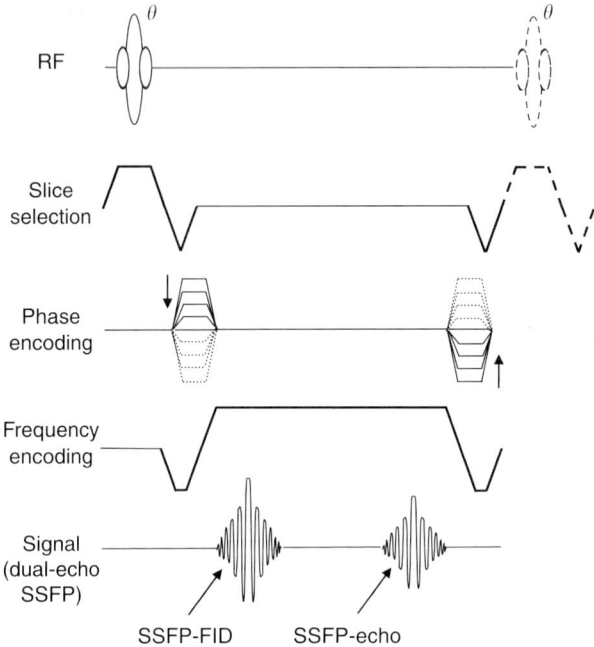

FIGURE 14.14 Pulse sequence used for dual-echo steady-state (DESS) acquisitions.

multiacquisition SSFP (i.e., CISS) is a good choice unless patient motion causes mis-registration artifacts. In that case, SSFP-FID is a robust alternative, although its acquisition efficiency per unit time is lower because the SSFP-echo signal is intentionally dephased.

With the multiple echo GRE sequences, DESS has found application to joint imaging because it can provide a good depiction of cartilage (Hardy et al. 1996). Dual-echo GRE is often used in a 2D mode with interleaved slice locations. The in-phase and out-of-phase images are particularly useful for body imaging because of the property described next.

Chemical Shift Artifact of the Second Kind and Dual-Echo GRE   The standard chemical shift artifact manifests itself as a spatial shift between fat and water in the frequency-encoded direction. It occurs both in RF spin-echo and in GRE images. If, however, fat and water are present in the same voxel, then at certain TE values GRE images display a second kind of chemical shift artifact. (That artifact is not seen on RF spin-echo images, although a similar artifact can occur when STIR is used; see Section 14.2.) This has been

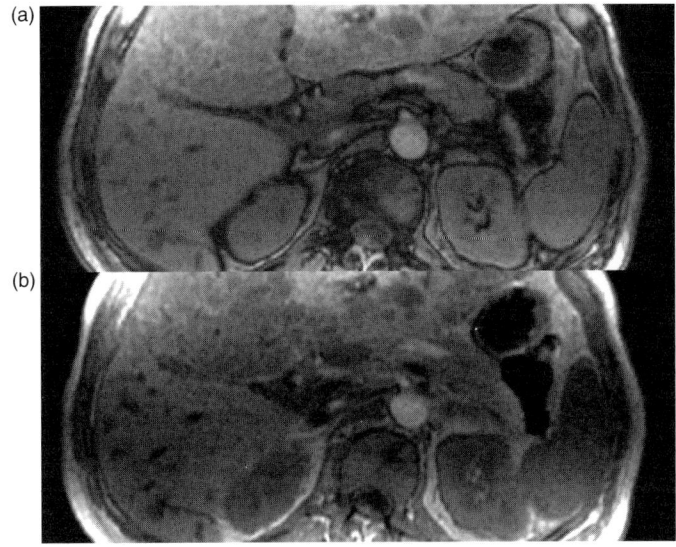

FIGURE 14.15 Axial dual-echo GRE images of the abdomen. Fat and water are out-of-phase in (a) and in-phase in (b).

called the phase cancellation artifact, the phase elimination artifact, the black boundary artifact, or the chemical shift artifact of the second kind.

Because the Larmor frequency of protons in water is approximately 3.3–3.5 ppm higher than protons in fat, the transverse magnetization of protons in water will continually accumulate phase relative to those in fat. In RF spin-echo pulse sequences, the 180° refocusing pulse negates the phase accumulated from 0 to TE/2, so that at the echo time TE fat and water are back in phase. In spoiled GRE and SSFP-FID, however, the phase accumulation from chemical shift is never negated. If a TE is selected so that the phase of the transverse magnetization of fat and water is opposed, signal cancellation will result. This process is explained in detail in Section 17.3 on Dixon's method and illustrated on Figure 14.10. Table 14.3 lists TE values at which fat and water are in- and out-of-phase for several field strengths, assuming a chemical shift of 3.4 ppm.

The effect of the chemical shift artifact of the second kind is to outline fat-banded anatomical structures (such as the kidneys). Although this is considered an artifact, it can be useful. Figure 14.15 shows an example of a dual-echo GRE image with $TE_1 = 2.2$ ms, and $TE_2 = 4.5$ ms, corresponding to fat and water out-of- and in-phase at 1.5 T, respectively. Because the information from the two echoes is complementary, dual-echo GRE pulse sequences have gained popularity, particularly for body imaging applications.

TABLE 14.3

Approximate Echo Times TE (ms)[a]

Field Strength, B_0 (T)	Fat–Water in Phase	Fat–Water Out of Phase
0.2	0, 34.5, 69.0, . . .	17.3, 51.8, . . .
0.5	0, 13.8, 27.6, . . .	6.9, 20.7, 34.5, . . .
0.7	0, 9.9, 19.7, . . .	4.9, 14.8, 24.6, . . .
1.0	0, 6.9, 13.8, 20.7, . . .	3.5, 10.4, 17.3, . . .
1.5	0, 4.6, 9.2, 13.8, . . .	2.3, 6.9, 11.5, . . .
3.0	0, 2.3, 4.6, 6.9, . . .	1.2, 3.5, 5.8, . . .

[a]The values are based on a fat–water chemical shift of 3.4 ppm.

Flow Effects For SSFP-echo and SSFP-FID, flow and motion can cause the precession of the transverse magnetization to experience inconsistent values of ϕ among the TR intervals, which can spoil the transverse steady state (Patz 1988). For this reason, spoiled GRE is generally preferred over SSFP-FID for time-of-flight angiography (Section 15.3). The signal obtained from flowing blood is usually the same as SSFP-FID, whereas the distracting signal from other fluids such as cerebrospinal fluid is attenuated. These properties are illustrated in the row of images obtained with 70° flip angle in Figure 14.4.

In balanced SSFP, flowing blood can set up a steady state because the net gradient area in any TR interval is zero (Haacke et al. 1990; Zur et al. 1990). Balanced SSFP generally works well as a bright-blood technique and already has found an important application in cardiac imaging. The contrast is excellent because the myocardium reaches steady state and has a low signal (due to its low T_2/T_1 ratio), whereas in-flowing blood shows a strong transient signal. One problem with balanced SSFP is that sometimes an anomalous enhancement of in-flowing blood occurs. These bright flashes occur when magnetization that is outside the imaging slice flows in and is rephased, effectively increasing the slice thickness (Markl et al. 2003).

SELECTED REFERENCES

Bangerter, N. K., and Nishimura, D. G. 2003. Artifact reduction and SNR comparison of multiple-acquisition SSFP techniques. In *Proceedings of the 11th meeting of the ISMRM*, p. 1017.

Bruder, H., Fischer, H., Graumann, R., and Deimling, M. 1988. A new steady-state imaging sequence for simultaneous acquisition of two MR images with clearly different contrasts. *Magn. Reson. Med.* 7: 35–42.

Busse, R. F., and Riederer, S. J. 2001. Steady-state preparation for spoiled gradient echo imaging. *Magn. Reson. Med.* 45: 653–661.

Carr, H. Y. 1958. Steady-state free precession in nuclear magnetic resonance. *Phys. Rev.* 112: 1693–1701.

Casselman, J. W., Kuhweide, R., Deimling, M., Ampe, W., Dehaene, I., and Meeus, L. 1993. Constructive interference in steady state-3DFT MR imaging of the inner ear and cerebellopontine angle. *Am. J. Neuroradiol.* 14: 47–57.

Crawley, A. P., Wood, M. L., and Henkelman, R. M. 1988. Elimination of transverse coherences in FLASH MRI. *Magn. Reson. Med.* 8: 248–260.

Duerk, J. L., Lewin, J. S., Wendt, M., and Petersilge, C. 1998. Remember true FISP? A high SNR, near 1-second imaging method for T2-like contrast in interventional MRI at .2 T. *J. Magn. Reson. Imaging* 8: 203–208.

Duyn, J. H. 1997. Steady state effects in fast gradient echo magnetic resonance imaging. *Magn. Reson. Med.* 37: 559–568.

Elster, A. D. 1993. Gradient-echo MR imaging: techniques and acronyms. *Radiology* 186: 1–8.

Epstein, F. H., Mugler, J. P., III, and Brookeman, J. R. 1996. Spoiling of transverse magnetization in gradient-echo (GRE) imaging during the approach to steady state. *Magn. Reson. Med.* 35: 237–245.

Ernst, R. R., and Anderson, W. A. 1966. Application of Fourier transform spectroscopy to magnetic resonance. *Rev. Sci. Instrum.* 37: 93–102.

Frahm, J., Haase, A., and Matthaei, D. 1986. Rapid NMR imaging of dynamic processes using the FLASH technique. *Magn. Reson. Med.* 3: 321–327.

Freeman, R., and Hill, H. D. W. 1971. Phase and intensity anomalies in Fourier transform NMR. *J. Magn. Reson.* 4: 366–383.

Gyngell, M. L. 1988. The application of steady-state free precession in rapid 2D FT NMR imaging: FAST and CE-FAST pulse sequences. *Magn. Reson. Med.* 6: 415–419.

Haacke, E. M., Wielopolski, P. A., Tkach, J. A., and Modic, M. T. 1990. Steady-state free precession imaging in the presence of motion: Application for improved visualization of the cerebrospinal fuid. *Radiology* 175: 545–552.

Hänicke, W., Merboldt, K. D., Chien, D., Gyngell, M. L., Bruhn, H., and Frahm, J. 1990. Signal strength in subsecond FLASH magnetic resonance imaging: The dynamic approach to steady state. *Med. Phys.* 17: 1004–1010.

Hänicke, W., and Vogel, H. U. 2003. An analytical solution for the SSFP signal in MRI. *Magn. Reson. Med.* 49: 771–775.

Hardy, P. A., Recht, M. P., Piraino, D., and Thomasson, D. 1996. Optimization of a dual echo in the steady state (DESS) free-precession sequence for imaging cartilage. *J. Magn. Reson. Imaging* 6: 329–335.

Hargreaves, B. A., Vasanawala, S. S., Pauly, J. M., and Nishimura, D. G. 2001. Characterization and reduction of the transient response in steady-state MR imaging. *Magn. Reson. Med.* 46: 149–158.

Hinshaw, W. S. 1976. Image formation by nuclear magnetic resonance: the sensitive point method. *J. Appl. Phys.* 47: 3709–3721.

Le Roux, P. 2003. Simplified model and stabilization of SSFP sequences. *J. Magn. Reson.* 163: 23–37.

Markl, M., Alley, M. T., Elkins, C. J., and Pelc, N. J. 2003. Flow effects in balanced steady state free precession imaging. *Magn. Reson. Med.* 50: 892–903.

Mugler, J. P., III, and Brookeman, J. R. 1993. Theoretical analysis of gadopentetate dimeglumine enhancement in T1-weighted imaging of the brain: Comparison of two-dimensional spin-echo and three-dimensional gradient-echo sequences. *J. Magn. Reson. Imaging* 3: 761–769.

Oppelt, A., Graumann, R., Barfuss, H., Fischer, H., Hartl, W., and Shajor, W. 1986. FISP: A new fast MRI sequence. 1986. *Electromedica* 54: 15–18.

Patz, S. 1988. Some factors that influence the steady state in steady-state free precession. *Magn. Reson. Imaging* 6: 405–413.

Scheffler, K., Heid, O., and Hennig, J. 2001. Magnetization preparation during the steady state: Fat-saturated 3D TrueFISP. *Magn. Reson. Med.* 45: 1075–1080.

Scheffler, K. 2003. On the transient phase of balanced SSFP sequences. *Magn. Reson. Med.* 49: 781–783.

Scheffler, K., and Hennig, J. 2003. Is TrueFISP a gradient-echo or a spin-echo sequence? *Magn. Reson. Med.* 49: 395–397.

Zur, Y., Stokar, S., and Bendel, P. 1988. An analysis of fast imaging sequences with steady-state transverse magnetization refocusing. *Magn. Reson. Med.* 6: 175–193.

Zur, Y., Wood, M. L., and Neuringer, L. J. 1990. Motion-insensitive, steady-state free precession imaging. *Magn. Reson. Med.* 16: 444–459.

Zur, Y., Wood, M. L., and Neuringer, L. J. 1991. Spoiling of transverse magnetization in steady-state sequences. *Magn. Reson. Med.* 21: 251–263.

RELATED SECTIONS

14.2 Inversion Recovery

Many biological tissues have distinct T_1 relaxation times. The differences in T_1 values are exploited in MRI to produce images with T_1-weighted contrast. In a spin-echo pulse sequence, for example, T_1-weighted contrast is achieved with relatively short TR and TE (e.g., 500 and 10 ms, respectively). Because the longitudinal magnetization of the tissue with longer T_1 has recovered less before the next RF excitation pulse is applied, it is hypointense in the image relative to the shorter T_1 components, whose longitudinal magnetization has experienced a more complete recovery.

Image contrast due to variations in T_1 relaxation time can be manipulated using an alternative method. In this method, an inversion pulse (Section 3.2) flips the longitudinal magnetization from the $+z$ axis to the $-z$ axis (see Figure 3.5). Before applying the RF excitation pulse of the subsequent pulse sequence, a time delay is provided to allow the inverted magnetization to recover toward its equilibrium value (i.e., returning from the $-z$ axis to the $+z$ axis). Tissues with different T_1 values recover at different rates, creating a T_1 contrast among them. The RF excitation pulse then converts the differences in the longitudinal magnetization into differences in the transverse magnetization. This produces signals that form an image with T_1-weighted contrast, although additional contrast may also be introduced by the remainder of the pulse sequence. Pulse sequences with an inversion pulse followed by a time delay prior to an RF excitation are known as *inversion recovery* (IR) pulse

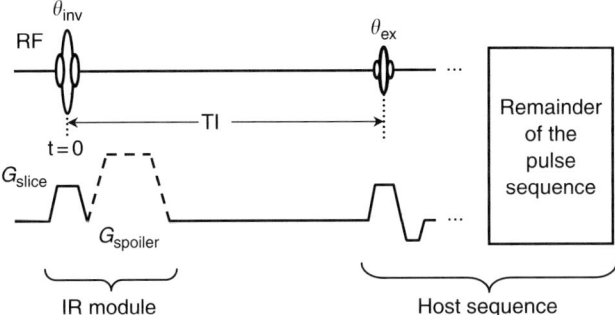

FIGURE 14.16 A generic IR pulse sequence consisting of an IR module and a host pulse sequence, separated by inversion time TI. θ_{inv} and θ_{ex} are the flip angles of the RF inversion and excitation pulses, respectively. The optional spoiler gradient (dotted line) dephases any residual transverse magnetization produced by the inversion pulse. A selective inversion pulse is shown, but a nonselective pulse can also be used. The host sequence can be RF spin-echo, gradient echo, RARE, EPI, spiral, or others.

sequences. The time delay between the inversion and the excitation pulses (Figure 14.16) is known as the *inversion time* (denoted by TI).

An inversion recovery pulse sequence consists of two parts (Figure 14.16). The first part includes an inversion pulse, an optional spoiler gradient after the pulse, and the associated slice-selection gradient, if the inversion pulse is selective. After a waiting time TI, the second part of the sequence is played out, which is typically a self-contained pulse sequence such as an RF spin-echo, gradient echo, RARE, EPI, GRASE, or spiral. In this section, we collectively refer the first part as an inversion recovery module, or IR module, and the second part as a host pulse sequence, or simply host sequence.

In many IR pulse sequences, one IR module is played for each host sequence. Under some circumstances, two or three IR modules are executed before a host sequence, such as in the case of a double or triple IR that is used for black-blood angiography (Section 15.1). Under other circumstances, a single IR module is followed by multiple host sequences, such as in spectral inversion at lipids (SPECIAL) (Foo et al. 1994) and magnetization-prepared rapid gradient echo (MP-RAGE) imaging (Mugler and Brookeman 1990). These IR variations are further discussed in subsection 14.2.4.

Most IR pulse sequences require a relatively long TR (e.g., TR = 2–11 s) to preserve the contrast established by the IR module. Because of this, 2D IR sequences are more frequently used than 3D and fast imaging techniques are usually used in the host sequence. Even with 2D IR imaging with a fast host sequence, the acquisition time can become prohibitively long.

Several strategies to improve the IR acquisition efficiency are discussed in subsection 14.2.2.

Although IR images are commonly reconstructed as magnitude images, they can benefit from real reconstruction (Park et al. 1986; Xiang 1996) due to the increased dynamic range. The longitudinal magnetization immediately before the excitation pulse can be either positive or negative, depending on the TI/T_1 ratio. Thus, the useful magnetization in a real image ranges from $-M$ to $+M$, instead of from 0 to $+M$ as in the case of a magnitude image. This implies that tissue contrast can be considerably increased in real images. Real IR images are also referred to as *phase-sensitive inversion recovery* (sometimes abbreviated PSIR) images, and the reconstruction process as phase-sensitive reconstruction. A few phase-sensitive reconstruction algorithms are discussed in subsection 14.2.3.

Inversion recovery pulse sequences have many applications and are widely used in clinical practice. In addition to producing images with a broad range of T_1-weighted contrast, IR is also used to generate T_1 maps. A prevalent IR application is selective signal attenuation, such as lipid suppression, fluid attenuation, and blood-signal nulling in black-blood angiography (Section 15.1). These applications are discussed in Section 14.2.4. The basic principles underlying the IR applications are described next.

14.2.1 PRINCIPLES OF IR

To demonstrate the principles of IR and to analyze its signal behavior, consider the generic IR pulse sequence shown in Figure 14.16. A selective inversion pulse is assumed, but the following discussion also applies to nonselective inversion pulses. Prior to the inversion pulse, the magnetization vector is at its equilibrium position along the $+z$ axis, that is, $\vec{M} = (0, 0, M_0)$. Immediately after the inversion pulse, the transverse ($M_\perp$) and longitudinal (M_z) magnetization components are:

$$M_\perp = M_0 \sin \theta_{\text{inv}} \tag{14.28}$$

$$M_z = M_0 \cos \theta_{\text{inv}} \tag{14.29}$$

where θ_{inv} is the flip angle of the inversion pulse. By applying a spoiler gradient after the inversion pulse, $M_\perp$ is dephased while M_z is not affected. During the time interval TI, the longitudinal magnetization experiences T_1 relaxation according to the following Bloch equation (see Section 1.2)

$$\frac{dM_z}{dt} = \frac{M_0 - M_z}{T_1} \tag{14.30}$$

Using the initial condition given by Eq. (14.29) at $t = 0$ (defined in Figure 14.16), the time-dependent longitudinal magnetization is found to be:

$$M_z(t) = M_0 \left[1 - (1 - \cos \theta_{\text{inv}}) e^{-t/T_1} \right] \tag{14.31}$$

Equation (14.31) assumes that TR is infinitely long. With a finite TR, $M_z(t)$ depends on the details of the host sequence. For example, $M_z(t)$ in RF spin-echo (SE) (Dixon and Ekstran 1982) and RARE (Rydberg et al. 1995) pulse sequences is given by:

$$M_z(t) = \begin{cases} M_0 \left[1 - (1 - \cos \theta_{\text{inv}}) e^{-t/T_1} + e^{-\text{TR}/T_1} \right] & \text{(for SE)} \\ M_0 \left[1 - (1 - \cos \theta_{\text{inv}}) e^{-t/T_1} + e^{-(\text{TR} - \text{TE}_{\text{last}})/T_1} \right] & \text{(for RARE)} \end{cases} \tag{14.32}$$

where TE_{last} is the echo time of the last echo in the echo train, and recovery from the transverse magnetization to $M_z(t)$ through the T_1-relaxation mechanism (as described in Section 17.4) is neglected. If $\theta_{\text{inv}} = 180°$, the magnetization experiences a complete inversion and Eq. (14.31) becomes:

$$M_z(t) = M_0 \left(1 - 2e^{-t/T_1} \right) \tag{14.33}$$

If $\theta_{\text{inv}} = 90°$, the magnetization is 'saturated' and its return to the equilibrium value is sometimes called *saturation recovery* (or SR), which is described by:

$$M_z(t) = M_0 \left(1 - e^{-t/T_1} \right) \tag{14.34}$$

Examples of an IR and an SR curve are shown in Figure 14.17.

Following an IR pulse, the longitudinal magnetization recovers along the z axis until being nutated by the excitation pulse (Figure 14.16). For TR $\gg T_1$, the available magnetization at the time of excitation is:

$$M_z(\text{TI}) = M_0 \left(1 - 2e^{-\text{TI}/T_1} \right) \tag{14.35}$$

The magnetization becomes zero (or nulled), when:

$$\text{TI}_{\text{null}} = \begin{cases} T_1 \ln 2 & \text{TR} \to \infty \\ T_1 \left[\ln 2 - \ln(1 + e^{-\text{TR}/T_1}) \right] & \text{for SE} \\ T_1 \left[\ln 2 - \ln(1 + e^{-(\text{TR} - \text{TE}_{\text{last}})/T_1}) \right] & \text{for RARE} \end{cases} \tag{14.36}$$

where the natural logarithm of 2 is approximately 0.693. The TI value that nulls the longitudinal magnetization is sometimes called the nulling time, or

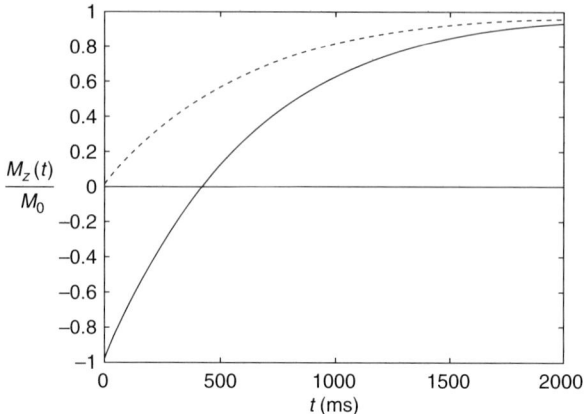

FIGURE 14.17 Inversion recovery (IR; solid line) and saturation recovery (SR; dashed line) curves for a tissue with T_1 of 600 ms. Longitudinal magnetization ranges from $-M_0$ to $+M_0$ in IR. The range is reduced to $(0, +M_0)$ in SR.

zero-crossing point. The selection of a proper nulling time to eliminate or attenuate tissues with a specific T_1 is the basis of STIR, FLAIR, and black-blood angiography, as discussed in subsection 14.2.4 and Section 15.1.

In IR, tissue contrast can be manipulated by varying TI. Consider two tissues with the same proton density (i.e., identical M_0s) but different T_1 values, T_{1a} and T_{1b}. Assuming TR $\gg T_1$ and TE $\ll T_2$, the tissue contrast is:

$$\Delta M = M_{z,a} - M_{z,b} = M_0 \left[(1 - \cos \theta_{\text{inv}}) \left(e^{-\text{TI}/T_{1b}} - e^{-\text{TI}/T_{1a}} \right) \right] \quad (14.37)$$

The absolute value of ΔM reaches a maximum when:

$$\text{TI} = \frac{\ln(T_{1a}/T_{1b})}{T_{1a} - T_{1b}} T_{1a} T_{1b} \quad (14.38)$$

The contrast between the tissues also depends on the flip angle of the inversion pulse. It can be readily seen from Eq. (14.37) that IR (i.e., $\theta_{\text{inv}} = 180°$) provides twice the contrast compared to SR (i.e., $\theta_{\text{inv}} = 90°$).

It is interesting to note that the excitation pulse in a T_1-weighted SE pulse sequence acts as an SR pulse. In that case, TI in Eqs. (14.37) and (14.38) is replaced by TR and the optimal image contrast becomes $M_0(e^{-\text{TR}/T_{1b}} - e^{-\text{TR}/T_{1a}})$ provided that TE $\ll T_2$ and TE $\ll$ TR. Assuming optimal TI for the IR sequence (with TR $\gg T_1$) and optimal TR for the SE sequence, the image contrast produced by IR doubles that of the SE sequence.

The contrast provided by IR sequences, however, is not always fully realized with magnitude reconstruction. Assuming $T_{1a} < T_{1b}$,

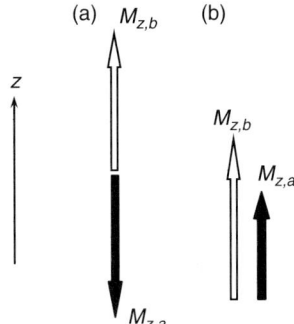

FIGURE 14.18 (a) Phase-sensitive reconstruction can increase tissue contrast compared to magnitude reconstruction when the longitudinal magnetization vectors point in opposite directions. (b) This advantage vanishes when both vectors point in the same direction.

if $T_{1a} \ln 2 < \text{TI} < T_{1b} \ln 2$, then for the infinite TR case $M_{z,a}$ has already recovered to the $+z$ axis whereas $M_{z,b}$ remains along the $-z$ axis. When $M_{z,b} = -M_{z,a}$, the two tissues become indistinguishable (i.e., zero contrast) on a magnitude image, despite the opposite polarity of $M_{z,a}$ and $M_{z,b}$. If the sign of the signal is maintained, as in phase-sensitive reconstruction, the available image contrast $\Delta M = 2M_{z,a}$ is realized (Figure 14.18a). In general, tissue contrast in phase-sensitive IR images is better than that of magnitude images if the longitudinal components of magnetization vectors of the two tissues point in opposite directions along the z axis (Figure 14.18).

14.2.2 INVERSION RECOVERY ACQUISITION STRATEGIES

IR modules can be added to 1D, 2D, or 3D pulse sequences. 1D IR sequences are rarely used, except for a few applications such as the measurement of inversion profiles. Because a relatively long TR is required in a majority of IR pulse sequences, the scan time of volumetric 3D IR can become prohibitively long, unless alternative strategies are used. 2D IR pulse sequences are more popular. Even with interleaved acquisition mode for 2D multislice imaging (Section 11.5), the long scan time can be problematic, especially when a long TI is required, such as in the case of fluid signal nulling (Hajnal, De Coene et al. 1992). In this subsection, we describe several acquisition strategies for multislice 2D and 3D IR sequences, with a special attention to their efficiency. Unless stated otherwise, we assume that each IR module is followed by a single host sequence, as shown in Figure 14.16.

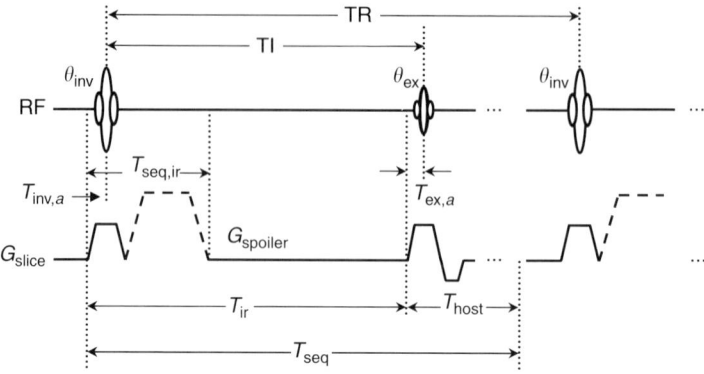

FIGURE 14.19 A timing diagram for a generic IR pulse sequence. A slice-selective IR module is assumed. The full host pulse sequence is not explicitly shown.

2D IR   Refer to Figure 14.19. Let us use $T_{\text{inv},a}$ to denote the interval from the beginning of an IR pulse (including the ascending ramp of the slice-selection gradient if the IR pulse is selective) to its isodelay point. $T_{\text{seq,ir}}$ is the duration of the IR RF and gradient waveforms (including the optional spoiler gradient), $T_{\text{ex},a}$ is the time from the beginning of the excitation pulse (also including the ascending slice-selection gradient ramp if the pulse is selective) to its isodelay point, and T_{host} is the host sequence length starting from the excitation pulse. For simplicity, we assume that there are no other preparatory pulses (e.g., spatial saturation pulses or tagging pulses) played before or after the IR pulse. Thus, the total sequence length is:

$$T_{\text{seq}} = T_{\text{inv},a} + \text{TI} + T_{\text{host}} - T_{\text{ex},a} \qquad (14.39)$$

We define T_{ir} (Figure 14.19) as the duration of the IR module:

$$T_{\text{ir}} = \text{TI} + T_{\text{inv},a} - T_{\text{ex},a} \qquad (14.40)$$

Equation (14.39) can be equivalently expressed as:

$$T_{\text{seq}} = T_{\text{ir}} + T_{\text{host}} \qquad (14.41)$$

To avoid partial saturation and preserve the contrast established by the IR module, TR is usually much longer than T_{seq}. In an interleaved 2D multislice acquisition, the maximal number of slices that can be accommodated by a TR is given by Eq. (11.34):

$$N_{\text{slice}} = \text{int}\left(\frac{\text{TR}}{T_{\text{seq}}}\right) \qquad (14.42)$$

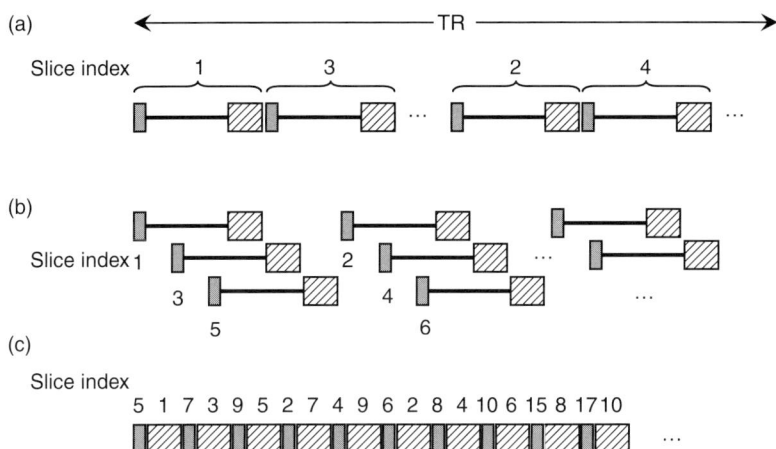

FIGURE 14.20 Three IR acquisition schemes for 2D multislice imaging: (a) sequential IR acquisition, (b) interleaved IR acquisition, (c) distributed (or optimal) IR acquisition. In all three cases, an interleaved 2D acquisition mode (see subsection 11.5.2) is assumed. The shaded and the cross-hatched boxes represent the IR module with duration $T_{seq,ir}$ and the host sequence with duration T_{host}, respectively. The solid line linking the two boxes denotes the idle time ($T_{idle,ir} = T_{ir} - T_{seq,ir}$) between the IR module and the host sequence.

These slices can be arranged in IR-module-host sequence pairs within a TR, as illustrated in Figure 14.20a, where an odd-even slice ordering has been assumed (Section 11.5). This acquisition scheme is sometimes called *sequential IR acquisition* (Park et al. 1985). Note that the sequential IR acquisition should be distinguished from the 2D sequential acquisition discussed in Section 11.5, in which data from only a single slice location are acquired during each TR. In fact, the *sequential* IR acquisition shown in Figure 14.20a belongs to 2D *interleaved* acquisition defined in Section 11.5.

When TI is short (i.e., TI $\approx T_{seq,ir}$, and $T_{seq} \approx T_{seq,ir} + T_{host}$), there is little idle time ($T_{idle,ir} = T_{ir} - T_{seq,ir}$) in the sequential IR grouping. In this case, a large number of slice locations can be acquired within a TR and the sequential IR acquisition operates at or close to its maximal efficiency. For longer TI (i.e., TI $\gg T_{seq,ir}$), however, considerable idle time is present, resulting in fewer slices per TR and reduced efficiency.

To improve efficiency, *interleaved IR acquisition* is preferred when long TI is required for an IR sequence. In this acquisition mode, the idle time for a given slice location is used to play out IR modules and/or host sequences for other slices, as shown in Figure 14.20b. During the first part of a TR, the scanner plays out a series of IR modules for N slices, whereas the host sequences for these slices are executed during a later part of the same TR interval (Park et al. 1985). Any remaining time in a TR interval can be used to accommodate additional slices, as shown in Figure 14.20b. In this way, the number of slices that can be acquired per TR is increased, resulting in scan-time reduction by reducing the number of acquisitions for the desired slice coverage.

Because T_{host} is almost always longer than $T_{seq,ir}$, the minimal separation between the IR modules is determined by T_{host}. Thus, the maximal number of slices that can be acquired in a TI interval is given by:

$$N_{slice} = \begin{cases} \text{int}\,[(TR - T_{ir})/T_{host}] & \text{if } TR \leq 2T_{ir} \\ 1 + \text{int}\,[(T_{ir} - T_{seq,ir})/T_{host}] & \text{if } TR > 2T_{ir} \end{cases} \quad (14.43)$$

If $TR \leq 2T_{ir}$, the maximal number of slice locations that can be accommodated within a TR interval is also given by Eq. (14.43). If $TR \gg 2T_{ir}$, however, more slices than predicted by Eq. (14.43) can be incorporated into a TR interval, as shown in Example 14.2 (also see Figure 14.20b).

Example 14.2   A 2D RARE IR pulse sequence with the following parameters is used to acquire 20 slices from the brain: $TR = 10$ s, $TI = 2.2$ s, $T_{host} = 110$ ms, $T_{seq,ir} = 72$ ms, $T_{inv,a} = 4$ ms, $T_{ex,a} = 2$ ms, $NEX = 1$, $N_{phase} = 160$, and echo train length (N_{etl}) $= 8$. (a) What is the total scan time when sequential IR acquisition is used? (b) Recalculate the total scan time for interleaved IR acquisition. (c) If the total number of slices is increased to 40, what is the total scan time for interleaved IR acquisition?

Answer

(a) The inversion duration and the sequence length can be obtained from Eqs. (14.40) and (14.41), respectively:

$$T_{ir} = TI + T_{inv,a} - T_{ex,a} = 2200 + 4 - 2 = 2202 \text{ ms}$$
$$T_{seq} = T_{ir} + T_{host} = 2202 + 110 = 2312 \text{ ms}$$

For sequential IR acquisition, the maximal number of slices for each TR is:

$$N_{slice} = \text{int}\left(\frac{TR}{T_{seq}}\right) = \text{int}\left(\frac{10,000}{2312}\right) = 4$$

Thus, five acquisitions are required to cover 20 slices. To sample 160 phase-encoding steps with an N_{etl} of eight, 20 shots are needed. The scan time can be obtained from Eq. (16.40):

$$T_{scan} = TR \times N_{shot} \times NEX \times N_{acq} = 10 \times 20 \times 1 \times 5 = 1000 \text{ s}$$
$$= 16.7 \text{ min}$$

(b) For interleaved IR acquisition, the number of slices that can be acquired in a TI interval can be calculated from Eq. (14.13) (TR $> 2T_{ir}$):

$$N_{slice} = 1 + int[(T_{ir} - T_{seq,ir})/T_{host}] = 1 + int[(2202 - 72)/110]$$
$$= 20$$

Therefore, all 20 slices can be acquired in a single acquisition. The total scan time becomes

$$T_{scan} = TR \times N_{shot} \times NEX \times N_{acq} = 10 \times 20 \times 1 \times 1 = 200 \text{ s}$$
$$= 3.3 \text{ min}$$

It can be seen that the interleaved acquisition reduces the scan time by a factor of 5 and makes it practical to use this sequence clinically.

(c) Within a TR interval, acquisition of 20 slices using the interleaved IR method takes $T_{ir} + 20 \times T_{host} = 2202 + 20 \times 110 = 4402$ ms. This leaves $10,000 - 4402 = 5598$ ms idle time, which can be used to acquire a second group of 20 slices (see Figure 14.20b). Thus, increasing the number of slices from 20 to 40 does not increase the total scan time.

In interleaved IR acquisition, each inversion module and its associated host sequence for a given slice location are acquired during the same TR. Due to this constraint, idle time can still exist. For example, when $T_{host} > T_{seq,ir}$, gaps exist between the inversion modules for different slices (Figure 14.20b). In addition, an idle time is present at the end of the inversion train if $T_{ir} > N_{slice}T_{host}$. Otherwise, an idle time may exist at the end of the host-sequence train if $T_{host} < T_{seq,ir}$. To further improve the efficiency by making use of the idle times, *distributed IR acquisition* (also known as optimized IR acquisition) has been developed (Oh et al. 1991). In this mode, the idle time is used to play out the inversion module or the host sequence for slices that may not be covered in the same TR. For example, the host sequence for a slice is played during the fifth TR, but its accompanying inversion module might be played during the fourth TR interval. (The inversion modules for the first few slices acquired during the first TR can be played in the preparatory dummy sequences that are used to drive the magnetization to a steady state.) Distributed IR acquisition can be thought of as a tightly packed, sequential IR acquisition with $T_{ir} = T_{seq,ir}$, except that the IR module and the adjacent host sequence do not correspond to the same slice location (Figure 14.20c). Idle time is maximally used, resulting in optimal acquisition efficiency. A drawback of this approach is that TR, TI, and the number of slices are tightly coupled together, which compromises the flexibility of independently choosing TR and TI. An optimization technique has been developed to search for the proper TR and TI values and number of slices within certain constraints (Listerud et al. 1996).

3D IR   Scan-time considerations often make it impractical to implement 3D IR sequences without using a fast imaging technique. 3D RARE IR sequences have been reported, but the secondary phase-encoded direction is typically limited to a small number (e.g., 8–16) of encoding steps to reduce the scan time (Barker 1998). In order to increase the coverage and obtain thinner slices, 3D IR can be implemented in multislab mode, in which each slab is treated as a slice. The acquisition order of the multiple slabs can be arranged analogously to 2D multislice IR imaging. Any one of the schemes shown in Figure 14.20 can be used, depending in the TR, TI, and number of slices. Another approach is to play out multiple host sequences, collecting multiple $k_y - k_z$ points following a single IR module to speed up acquisition. k-space data acquired by a series of host sequences, however, have different TIs. The desired TI time is typically reserved for the acquisition of the central k-space lines because the image contrast is predominantly determined by those lines. This approach is used in SPECIAL (Foo et al. 1994) and MP-RAGE (Mugler and Brookeman 1990).

14.2.3 PHASE-SENSITIVE IR

As discussed previously, T_1 contrast can be greatly enhanced if the sign of the longitudinal magnetization is preserved in an IR image by using real, or phase-sensitive, image reconstruction. Phase-sensitive image reconstruction entails much more than simply displaying the real part of a complex image. As soon as the longitudinal magnetization is nutated to the transverse plane by an excitation pulse, phase errors can begin to accumulate, obscuring the phase that would be used to determine the polarity of the longitudinal magnetization immediately before excitation. Many factors contribute to the phase error. Examples include magnetic susceptibility variations, receiver resonance offset, phase associated with the B_1 field, eddy currents, gradient group delays, mismatches of frequency-encoding gradient and data acquisition window timing, motion, and flow. With the inclusion of the phase error, the 2D complex IR image intensity $I(x, y)$ can be expressed by (Xiang 1996):

$$I(x, y) = I_{\text{mag}}(x, y)P(x, y)e^{-i\vartheta(x,y)} \tag{14.44}$$

where $I_{\text{mag}}(x, y)$ is the magnitude image intensity, $P(x, y)$ is a binary function (i.e., $P(x, y) = 1$ or -1) describing the polarity of the longitudinal magnetization immediately prior to the RF excitation pulse, and $\vartheta(x, y)$ is the phase error, which in general is spatially dependent. Thus, the goal of phase-sensitive reconstruction is to recover $I_{\text{mag}}(x, y)P(x, y)$ from $I(x, y)$.

One early approach (Bakker et al. 1984) to phase-sensitive reconstruction is to acquire a series of IR images (e.g., ≥ 4) with varying TI values. The magnitude image intensity is plotted as a function of TI on a pixel-by-pixel basis, and a search is made for the zero-crossing point. After determining the zero-crossing point T_{null}, the image intensity is negated if TI < TI_{null}. This method is equivalent to using a T_1 map to sort the signal polarity without invoking any phase calculations. The long data acquisition time for multiple IR images has limited the use of this method.

In Eq. (14.44), the polarity function and the phase error are coupled. If the phase error $\vartheta(x, y)$ is known, then it can be removed from Eq. (14.44) and a real image $R(x, y) = I_{mag}(x, y)P(x, y)$ is readily obtained. Along this line, two categories of techniques have been developed.

In the first category of methods, a spatial phase map $\vartheta(x, y)$ is produced by acquiring a separate data set. Although the phase map can be acquired using a large phantom covering at least the FOV of the image to be corrected, the phantom phase map does not contain the subject-dependent phase errors, such as those induced by magnetic susceptibility variations, motion, and flow. Because of this, a reference scan is typically performed on the imaged subject using a sequence similar to the actual IR sequence (Patk et al. 1986; Kellman et al. 2002). For example, the IR pulse sequence for actual data acquisition can be used for the reference scan by disabling the phase-encoding gradient and the inversion pulse (Patk et al. 1986), producing a single k-space line at $k_y = 0$. Because the inversion pulse is disabled, the phase of the k-space line is not influenced by the polarity function $P(x, y)$ but reflects the phase error term $\vartheta(x, y)$. This phase is then analyzed in the spatial domain using a linear model $\tilde{\vartheta}(x) = \alpha + \beta x$ and subtracted from the phase of the actual IR image. Another method is to acquire the reference scan data from the entire k-space without using the IR pulse or with a sufficiently long TI to ensure all spins have passed the nulling point. To minimize the spatial misregistration, the reference scan can be interleaved with the actual IR acquisition as described in Kellman et al. (2002). The spatial phase map $\vartheta(x, y)$, obtained from the reference image, is subtracted from the phase of the actual IR image on a pixel-by-pixel basis without assuming a specific spatial dependence. Phase mapping using reference scans typically increases the total scan time and reduces the acquisition efficiency.

In the second category of methods, phase correction is performed from the image data without the need of a reference scan. Most phase-correction methods are based on the assumption that the phase error $\vartheta(x, y)$ varies slowly in the image domain, whereas the polarity function $P(x, y)$ abruptly changes at tissue interface. This is generally a good assumption, except in areas with severe artifacts that cause the phase change between adjacent pixels to exceed π.

In one phase-correction method (Borrello et al. 1990), a small kernel $\mathbb{k}$ containing a cluster of pixels (e.g., 5 × 5) is selected from the complex IR

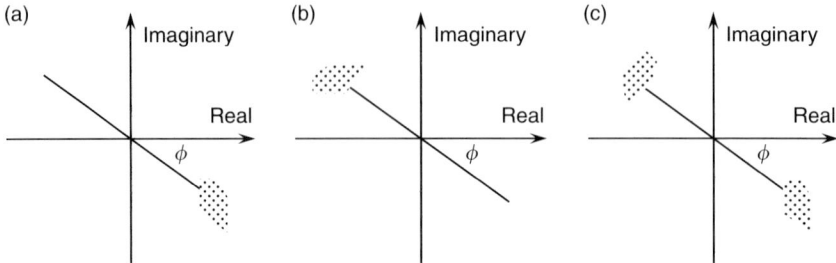

FIGURE 14.21 A diagram showing phase slope calculations as described in Borrello et al. (1990). The cluster of dots shows the complex points within a kernel $\mathbb{k}$. The solid lines represent the phase slope. (a) All complex points in the kernel have positive $P(x, y)$. (b) All complex points in the kernel have negative $P(x, y)$. (c) The complex points in the kernel have a mixture of positive and negative $P(x, y)$.

image $I(x, y)$. The phase slope (i.e., the slope of a line linking a complex data point to the origin in the complex plane) is calculated for each pixel within the kernel:

$$\phi(x, y) = \arctan\left(\frac{\mathrm{Im}I(x, y)}{\mathrm{Re}I(x, y)}\right), \qquad (x, y) \in \mathbb{k} \qquad (14.45)$$

In Eq. (14.45), a two-quadrant arctangent operation is used (Section 13.5) that gives $-90° \le \phi \le 90°$. The average of the phase slope $\bar{\phi}(x, y)$ can be obtained with a least-squares fit over $\mathbb{k}$. Within the kernel $\mathbb{k}$, there are three possibilities: all pixels have positive $P(x, y)$ (Figure 14.21a), all pixels have negative $P(x, y)$ (Figure 14.21b), and some pixels have positive $P(x, y)$ while other pixels have negative $P(x, y)$ (Figure 14.21c). Provided that the phase error within the kernel is small, all three cases give approximately the same phase slope $\bar{\phi}(x, y)$ (Figure 14.21) because a phase of $180° + \bar{\phi}(x, y)$—for example, associated with negative $P(x, y)$—is wrapped back to $\bar{\phi}(x, y)$ by the two-quadrant arctangent operation. In doing so, the contribution from $P(x, y)$ to Eq. (14.44) is eliminated, and a phase map $\bar{\phi}(x, y)$ is produced independent of the polarity function $P(x, y)$. Following a phase-unwrapping process on $\bar{\phi}(x, y)$ (Borrello et al. 1990), the unwrapped phase is compared with the original phase of $I(x, y)$ on a pixel-by-pixel basis to determine whether the vector representation of the complex numbers are parallel or anti-parallel. This can be done, for example, by evaluating the sign of the inner product of the two vectors in the complex plane. With this method, an ambiguity still exists because parallel vectors represented by $\bar{\phi}(x, y)$ and $I(x, y)$ can be associated with either positive or negative $P(x, y)$. To solve this problem, a positive (or negative) value is first assigned to $P(x, y)$ for parallel vectors, and a negative (or positive) value to $P(x, y)$ for anti-parallel vectors. After the operator reviews the image, the image polarity can be reversed, if necessary.

The phase-correction methods discussed so far all require phase unwrapping, which is a rather error-prone process (Section 17.3). Any error in phase unwrapping results in erroneous assignment of $P(x, y)$. This, along with the need for a reference scan or operator intervention, has greatly hindered the wide acceptance of phase-sensitive IR for routine clinical use.

Recently, a method that avoids these problems has been introduced (Xiang 1996). This method focuses on determining the simpler polarity function $P(x, y)$ instead of directly dealing with the more complicated phase error term $\vartheta(x, y)$. In this method, an orientation vector field is defined by combining the polarity function and the phase-error factor:

$$O(x, y) = P(x, y)e^{-i\vartheta(x,y)} \tag{14.46}$$

Equation (14.46) can be equivalently expressed in vector form (Section 1.2):

$$\vec{o}(x, y) = \begin{bmatrix} \mathrm{Re}\left(P(x, y)e^{-i\vartheta(x,y)}\right) \\ \mathrm{Im}\left(P(x, y)e^{-i\vartheta(x,y)}\right) \end{bmatrix} \tag{14.47}$$

A seed pixel is selected from the image, and its orientation vector $\vec{o}_1$ is calculated from Eq. (14.47). The dot product of this vector with its four nearest neighbors j ($j = 1, 2, 3, 4$) is then evaluated:

$$\eta_j = \vec{o}_1 \cdot \vec{o}_{1j} \tag{14.48}$$

When there is no phase error (i.e., the ideal case) or when $\vartheta(x, y)$ is the same for both pixels, $|\eta_j| = 1$. With a variation of phase errors between pixels, $|\eta_j| < 1$. As long as $|\eta_j|$ is larger than a predetermined threshold η_{thsh} (e.g., $\eta_{\mathrm{thsh}} = 0.96$), however, the relative orientation of the vectors is assumed to be predominantly determined by $P(x, y)$ rather than the phase error $\vartheta(x, y)$, noise, or artifacts. In this case, if $\eta_j > 0$, then the orientation of the jth neighbor is the same as the seed pixel. Otherwise, the orientation of the jth neighbor is opposite to that of the seed pixel. Once the relative orientations of the nearest neighbors are determined, they serve as the new seeds to probe their nearest neighbors. This region-growing algorithm proceeds as long as $|\eta_j| > \eta_{\mathrm{thsh}}$. If $|\eta_j| \le \eta_{\mathrm{thsh}}$, the pixel j is most likely to be in a region dominated by noise or severe artifacts and the region-growing algorithm stops. This process continues until all pixels in a connected region of the image are visited. In an image with multiple isolated regions (e.g., arms in an axial abdomen image, or cut-off due to low SNR or severe artifacts), multiple seeds can be selected, or a bridge filter can be used (Xiang 1996). Using this algorithm, either $+1$ or -1 is assigned to the polarity function everywhere in the image except for regions with noise and severe artifacts. The accurate determination of $P(x, y)$ in these regions, however, is not meaningful or critical because the image is already degraded. Their $P(x, y)$ values can be arbitrarily assigned $+1$ (or -1) to give a more natural appearance of the IR image.

The absolute determination of $P(x, y) = +1$ or $P(x, y) = -1$ for a given pixel depends on the choice of $P(x, y)$ of the initial seed. The polarity of the initial seed can be chosen so that the total magnetization in the tissue is non-negative (i.e., $\sum_{x,y} I_{mag}(x, y)P(x, y) \geq 0$). After $P(x, y)$ is fully determined, the final real IR image can be reconstructed using:

$$R(x, y) = I(x, y)\widetilde{O}^*(x, y)$$
$$= I_{mag}(x, y)P(x, y) \qquad (14.49)$$

where $\widetilde{O}^*(x, y)$ is the complex conjugate of the orientation vector after going through the region-growing algorithm that removes the contribution from the polarity function $P(x, y)$ (Xiang 1996). Equation (14.49) essentially rotates the signal to the real axis on a pixel-by-pixel basis, so that the imaginary part is zero. It can be seen that this method cleverly avoids the error-prone phase-unwrapping process, does not rely on a reference scan, and requires virtually no operator intervention. An excellent reliability has been reported. An example of this method is shown in Figure 14.22. Further details on this technique can be found in Xiang (1996).

14.2.4 IR APPLICATIONS

Contrast Manipulation   By varying TI, TR, and TE, a range of image contrast can be produced by an IR pulse sequence. When a long TR (e.g., a few seconds) and a short TE (e.g., a few milliseconds) are used, the image contrast is primarily determined by TI/T_1. The contrast behavior is very different in magnitude and real (or phase-sensitive IR) images.

First let us consider magnitude IR images by focusing on the contrast between two tissues, tissue A with a short T_1 and tissue B with a long T_1 (assuming both tissues have the same equilibrium magnetization M_0). The signals from these two tissues are denoted by S_A and S_B, respectively. At a relative short TI (e.g., 100 ms for gray and white matter in the brain), S_B experiences little recovery, whereas S_A recovers considerably. Assuming both S_A and S_B remain inverted (point a in Figure 14.23), tissue A will be hypointense relative to tissue B, giving an appearance resembling a T_2-weighted image (i.e., bright gray matter and dark white matter). After the nulling point for S_A, as long as S_A is not greater than the magnitude of S_B (point b in Figure 14.23), tissue A remains hypointense. At a specific time $TI = T_{iso}$, the amplitudes of S_A and S_B become identical (point c in Figure 14.23), and the two tissues

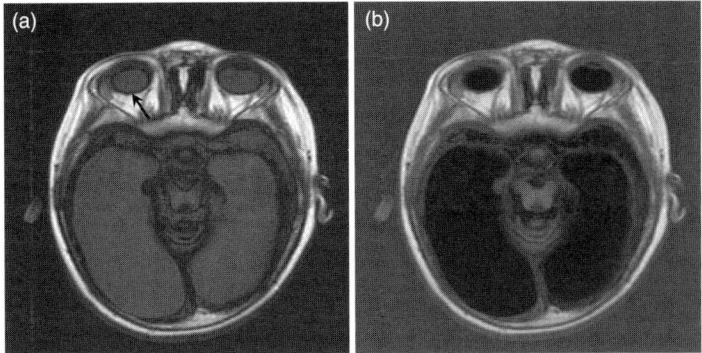

FIGURE 14.22 A pair of IR images from a pediatric patient with hydrocephalus: (a) magnitude image, and (b) real image reconstructed using the method in Xiang (1996). With magnitude reconstruction, the contrast between the fluid and the brain stem is unremarkable. The contrast, however, is greatly increased in the real image. The phase-sensitive IR reconstruction algorithm works well even with multiple unconnected regions and pulsatile flow artifacts in the image. The arrow in (a) points to the dark line due to the cancellation of water and lipid signals. TR/TI/TE = 2000/600/30 ms. Field strength = 1.5 T. (Courtesy of Q-S. Xiang, Ph.D., University of British Columbia, Canada.)

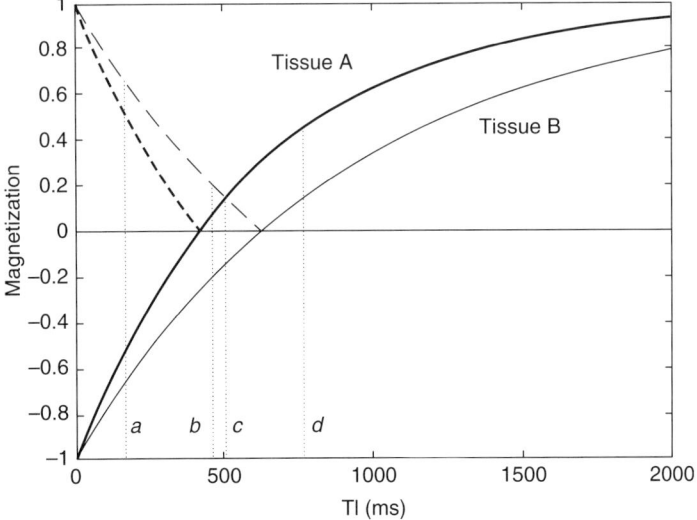

FIGURE 14.23 Signal intensity in an IR image as a function of TI for tissue A (thick lines) and tissue B (thin lines) in magnitude image (dotted lines) and phase-sensitive IR image (solid lines). Image contrast at four points a, b, c, and d is discussed in the text.

appear isointense in the image. When TI is longer than T_{iso} (e.g., TI = 650 ms for gray and white matter in the brain), the amplitude of S_B becomes smaller than that of S_A (point d in Figure 14.23), and the contrast between the two tissues reverses. Tissue A now appears hyperintense to tissue B, giving the appearance of a typical T_1-weighted image. For specific values of TI (e.g., TI = T_{iso}) when the magnetization vectors from the two tissues are opposed, signal cancellation occurs, producing a dark line in the image at the tissue interface as pointed by the arrow in Figure 14.22a.

Now consider the same example for phase-sensitive IR images. Assuming the equilibrium magnetization for both tissues A and B are the same, S_B is always smaller than S_A for the entire range of TI (i.e., $0 < \text{TI} < \infty$) (Figure 14.23). Although the contrast varies with TI, there will never be a contrast reversal, as in the case of a magnitude IR image. Partially for this reason, phase-sensitive IR images are much less sensitive to TI than are their magnitude counterparts and the dark lines at the tissue interface are not seen in the image (although the partial volume effect still exists).

T_1 Mapping Inversion recovery pulse sequences are often employed to produce quantitative T_1 maps. In this application, a series of IR images are acquired from the same location, each with a different TI while keeping all other parameters identical. To avoid signal saturation, a long TR time must be used. For example, a TR can be selected to satisfy TR $> 4T_{1,\text{max}}$, where $T_{1,\text{max}}$ is the longest T_1 value of interest. The pixel intensity from the series of images is plotted as a function of TI. For phase-sensitive IR images, a nonlinear fitting to Eq. (14.35) can be directly applied. For magnitude IR images, the zero-crossing point is first obtained and then the image intensities before the zero-crossing point are negated prior to fitting to Eq. (14.35). To avoid the step of negating the signals before the zero-crossing point, an SR pulse sequence can be used instead. The signals thus obtained are fitted to Eq. (14.34). For all these cases, a Levenberg-Marquardt nonlinear fitting method is typically used (Press et al. 1992).

T_1 mapping using IR (or SR) with a conventional spin-echo pulse sequence requires a very long acquisition time. To shorten this time, fast imaging sequences, such as EPI, are frequently used. Alternative methods have also been developed with much shorter TR times, such as the one described in Henderson et al. (1999).

Lipid Suppression—STIR An important clinical application of IR is to null the signal from lipids (Bydder and Young 1985; Bydder et al. 1985). A lipid signal appears bright in T_1-weighted and RARE T_2-weighted images (Section 16.4). Because many lesions also appear bright on postcontrast

T_1-weighted and RARE T_2-weighted images, suppression of the confounding hyperintense lipid signals can increase the conspicuity of lesions embedded in fat, such as edema in bone marrow, multiple sclerosis plaques in the optic nerve, lymph nodes, and metastases in the vertebral bodies.

The T_1 relaxation time of lipid is approximately 230 ms at 1.5 T, which is considerably shorter than most of the tissues in the human body (e.g., the white matter of the brain has a T_1 of $\sim$600 ms at 1.5 T). To null the lipid signal, an IR pulse is first applied to invert signals from both water and fat. If a TI is selected according to Eq. (14.36):

$$\text{TI}_{\text{null}} = T_{1,\text{lipids}} \ln 2 = 230 \times 0.69 \approx 159 \text{ ms}$$

the lipid signal is nulled. This technique is called *short TI inversion recovery*, or short tau inversion recovery (*STIR*) (Bydder et al. 1985). In practice, TI_{null} typically ranges from 150 to 170 ms to account for variability in host sequence timing parameters such as TR and TE.

Example 14.3 Liver parenchyma has a T_1 of $\sim$500 ms at 1.5 T. In a STIR sequence with a TI of 160 ms, and TR $\gg T_1$, how much is the water signal in the liver attenuated?

Answer According to Eq. (14.35), the water signal after a TI of 160 ms is

$$M_{\text{water}} = M_0 \left(1 - 2e^{-\text{TI}/T_1}\right) = M_0 \left(1 - 2e^{-160/500}\right) \simeq -0.45 M_0$$

This represents $\sim$55% loss of the signal compared to its maximal equilibrium value.

As indicated in Example 14.3, considerable water signal is also lost in STIR, especially for tissues with short T_1s. STIR substantially suppresses any tissue that has T_1 similar to that of fat, such as subacute hemorrhage, making it difficult to distinguish fat in teratoma from blood in an ednometrioma. This is one of the primary drawbacks of the STIR technique. Another drawback of STIR is the relatively long acquisition time even with the interleaved IR acquisition scheme discussed in Section 14.2.2. Because of this, STIR is most commonly used in combination with a fast imaging sequence, such as RARE. In addition, due to the use of short TI, the image contrast in STIR is reversed from what is seen in T_1-weighted spin-echo images, unless phase-sensitive IR is used. If a long TE is also used with STIR, the contrast can be further enhanced, making some lesions even brighter. Although this can be an advantage in T_2-weighted imaging, STIR is usually not a good pulse sequence for

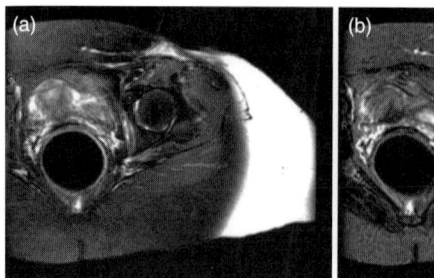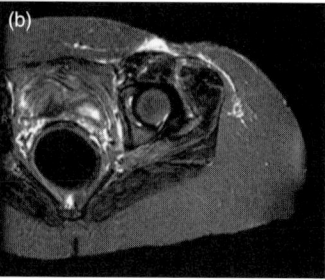

FIGURE 14.24 Lipid-suppressed pelvis images using (a) a spectrally selective pulse and (b) STIR. The B_0-field inhomogeneity on the left side of the patient renders lipid suppression with a spectrally selective pulse ineffective. This problem is avoided in the STIR image. A TI somewhat shorter than TI_{null} was used. Hence, the lipid signal is not completely nulled.

postcontrast T_1-weighted imaging because the water signal suffers more signal loss due to its T_1 shortening.

Despite these problems, STIR offers some advantages over other lipid-suppression techniques, such as spectrally selective lipid saturation, spatial-spectral pulses, and Dixon's method. STIR is based on the difference in T_1 relaxation times between water and lipid, not their chemical shift. Therefore, as shown in Figure 14.24, it is insensitive to B_0 field inhomogeneity. Also, STIR is quite effective for suppressing lipids at low magnetic field (e.g., < 1.0 T) in which the decreased chemical shift (in hertz) makes spectrally selective RF pulses difficult to use. When an adiabatic inversion pulse is employed, STIR also becomes insensitive to B_1-field variations. Compared to the Dixon technique (Section 17.3), STIR does not require phase correction and does not suffer from ambiguity in determining the relative signal polarity between water and fat. Due to these advantages, STIR remains a popular method for lipid suppression in clinical practice.

In some fast gradient-echo sequences, lipid suppression is desired, but a short TR must be used. A variation of the STIR technique is to invert the lipid signals using a spectrally selective, but not spatially selective, pulse. This pulse inverts the lipid signal within the active volume of the transmitting coil. After a certain inversion time (e.g., ~60 ms at 1.5 T) so that the lipid magnetization is substantially attenuated, multiple excitation RF pulses with a very short TR (e.g., a few milliseconds) are applied to acquire a number of k-space lines (e.g., 64). To maximize lipid-suppression efficiency, the central k-space lines are typically acquired when TI ≈ TI_{null}. This technique, known as SPECIAL (Foo et al. 1994), is used in a number of fast 3D gradient-echo pulse sequences.

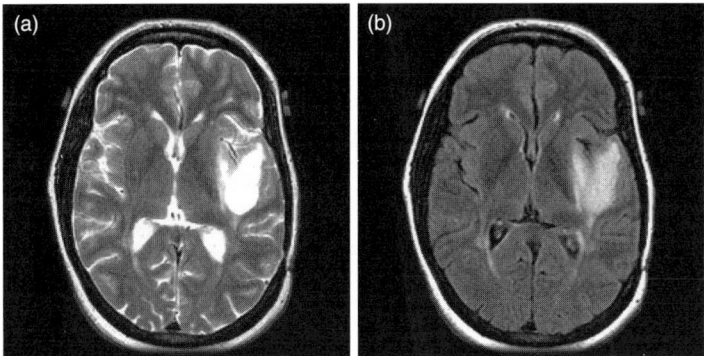

FIGURE 14.25 (a) Fast spin echo (FSE, or RARE) T_2-weighted image, and (b) FSE FLAIR image, both from a patient with a glioma. The presence of a bright CSF signal makes it difficult to assess the edema surrounding the tumor mass. The conspicuity of edema and the tumor mass is improved in FLAIR.

Fluid Attenuation—FLAIR   Just as the hyperintense lipid signal reduces the conspicuity of some lesions, the hyperintense fluid (e.g., cerebrospinal fluid, CSF) signal in T_2-weighted images causes problems in detecting lesions with long T_2s. For example, vasogenic edema surrounding a brain tumor (Figure 14.25a) and multiple sclerosis plaques within periventricular white matter are difficult to visualize in T_2-weighted images, primarily due to the hyperintense signals from the CSF.

Similar to STIR, CSF signals can also be nulled using an IR pulse sequence because its T_1 value is considerably longer than those of brain parenchyma as well as a majority of lesions. For example, at 1.5 T, the T_1 of CSF is $\sim$4200 ms, whereas the T_1 values of white and grey matters are only $\sim$600 and $\sim$950 ms, respectively. To null the fluid signal, a rather long TI value is required, as indicated by Eq. (14.36). If we use the typical T_1 value for CSF at 1.5 T and assume an infinitely long TR, the theoretical TI time for nulling fluid is approximately 2900 ms. In practice, the actual TI is somewhat shorter, as shown in Example 14.4. The technique of using an IR pulse sequence to null or substantially reduced the fluid signals is called *fluid-attenuated inversion recovery (FLAIR)* (Hajnal, De Coene et al. 1992; Hajnal, Brynat et al. 1992). This technique has been widely used in neuroradiologic diagnosis.

Example 14.4   A FLAIR sequence based on RARE is implemented at 1.5 T with the following parameters: TR $=$ 10 s and $TE_{last} =$ 300 ms. Assume the T_1 values of CSF, white and grey matter are 4200, 600, and 950 ms, respectively. (a) What TI should be used to null the CSF signal? (b) At this TI, what is the magnetization for the white matter and gray matter as a percentage of their equilibrium values, respectively?

Answer

(a) According to Eq. (14.36), TI_{null} is given by:

$$\text{TI}_{\text{null}} = 4200[\ln 2 - \ln(1 + e^{-(10000-300)/4200})] = 2514 \text{ ms}$$

which is shorter than what is calculated based on $\text{TI} = T_1 \ln 2$. In practice, a somewhat smaller TI_{null} is used (e.g., $\sim$2200 ms) to optimize the contrast for specific lesion detections as well as to compensate for variability in host sequence timing parameter selection.

(b) Using Eq. (14.32) with $\theta_{\text{inv}} = 180°$, the percentage of the magnetization for white and gray matter are:

$$\text{WM} = 1 - 2e^{-\text{TI}/T_1} + e^{-(\text{TR}-\text{TE}_{\text{last}})/T_1}$$

$$= 1 - 2e^{-2514/600} + e^{-(10000-300)/600} = 0.97$$

$$\text{GM} = 1 - 2e^{-\text{TI}/T_1} + e^{-(\text{TR}-\text{TE}_{\text{last}})/T_1}$$

$$= 1 - 2e^{-2514/950} + e^{-(10000-300)/950} = 0.86$$

With a long TI, magnetization of the brain parenchyma and most other tissues has already passed the zero-crossing points. This is quite different from the situation in STIR in which magnetization of most of the nonnulled tissues remains inverted. Even though the nonnulled tissues recover more completely in FLAIR than in STIR, some signal loss is inevitable, especially for tissues with long T_1s, as shown by Example 14.4. The long TI in FLAIR can also allow CSF to flow from an adjacent region into the imaged slice. Because the inflow CSF signal has not experienced inversion, it will not be attenuated in the image. To offset this effect, the slice profile of the IR pulse is sometimes thicker than that of the selective pulses in the host sequence.

The goal of FLAIR is to achieve T_2-contrast among tissues other than CSF. Thus, a long TR (e.g., 10 s) and long TE (e.g., 120 ms) are typically used. TE values in FLAIR are usually longer than those typically used in RARE T_2-weighted images to increase the contrast between lesions and normal tissues. This, in conjunction with the incomplete magnetization recovery, as shown in Example 14.4, gives a rather low SNR in FLAIR images. The optimal selection of TR/TI/TE depends on specific applications. An example is analyzed in Rydberg et al. (1995).

The extremely long TR can increase the total scan time considerably. In the initial implementation employing spin-echo as a host sequence, multiple spin-echo pulse sequences for different slice locations were used, following a single nonselective inversion pulse. Although the efficiency is improved, different slices have slightly different TIs, resulting in a varying degree in CSF suppression across the slices (Hajnal, De Coene et al. 1992). On clinical scanners, FLAIR is almost always implemented with a fast imaging pulse sequence, with RARE being most popular. To further increase efficiency, interleaved IR acquisition is usually implemented. More time-efficient distributed IR (Figure 14.20c) acquisition has also been used, such as the scheme used in optimized interleaved FLAIR (OIL FLAIR) (Listerud et al. 1996).

Constrained by the total acquisition time, FLAIR is typically used as a 2D sequence. It has been shown that 3D FLAIR can also be successfully implemented using techniques such as MP-RAGE (see below) (Epstein et al. 1995) and multislab interleaved acquisition (Barker 1998). So far, the 3D sequences have not been used as extensively as the 2D counterparts.

Although FLAIR is mainly used in T_2-weighted imaging, it has also found application in suppressing CSF in T_1-weighted images, such as images of the spine. A T_1-weighted FLAIR image of the spine is shown in Figure 14.26.

Magnetization Preparation in Fast Gradient-Echo Sequences   IR pulse sequences based on spin echo, RARE, and EPI typically play an IR module for

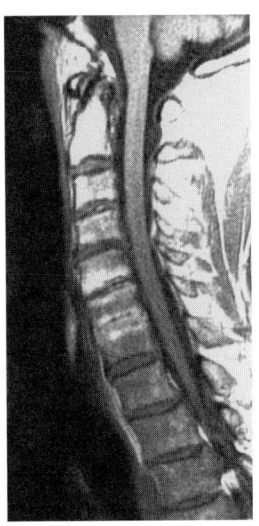

FIGURE 14.26 A T_1-weighted FLAIR image of the cervical spine. The key acquisition parameters are TR $= 2500$ ms, TI $= 860$ ms, TE ~ 15ms, FOV $= 22$ cm, slice thickness $= 3$ mm, and matrix $= 320 \times 224$.

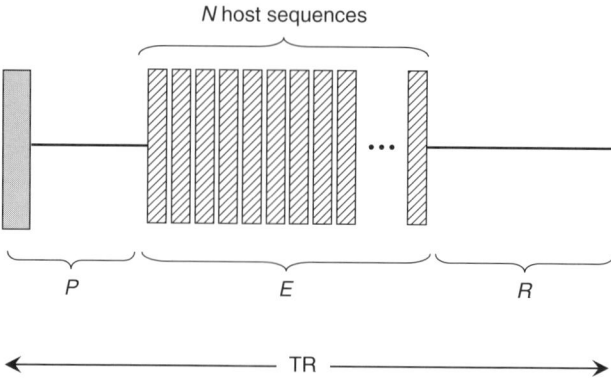

FIGURE 14.27 A generic magnetization prepared pulse sequence. A preparatory RF pulse (and its associated gradient, if any) is first applied (shaded vertical bar), followed by a series of excitation pulse sequences (hatched vertical bars) to acquire k-space data. After acquisition, a recovery time is provided for the magnetization. P, E, and R denote preparation, excitation, and recovery, respectively.

each host sequence. For fast gradient echo sequences, however, the short TR makes it difficult to play an IR module before each excitation pulse. Instead, a number of host sequences are grouped together to share the same IR module (Haase 1990). This type of sequence consists of a magnetization preparation period, a time interval when the magnetization is excited and multiple lines of k-space are acquired, and a delay period for signal recovery. These three periods are denoted by P, E, and R, respectively, in Figure 14.27. One example of this type of sequences is SPECIAL, discussed earlier. Another example is 3D MP-RAGE (Mugler and Brookeman 1990).

For T_1-weighted imaging, 3D MP-RAGE starts with a nonselective preparatory pulse whose flip angle typically ranges from 0 to 180°. (Technically, it is an inversion only if the flip angle exceeds 90°.) After a delay time TI, T_1 contrast is introduced into the longitudinal magnetization. This T_1-prepared magnetization is excited and then read out by a series of fast gradient-echo sequences to sample multiple k-space lines. The maximum number of k-space lines depends on the temporal nature of the imaged object, the TR time, and the degradation rate of the prepared contrast. The sequence shown in Figure 14.27 is repeated multiple times to fill the k-space required for 3D image reconstruction. It is not uncommon to sample all the secondary phase-encoded lines (i.e., all k_z values) for one or more k_y values following one magnetization preparation pulse.

The T_1 contrast in 3D MP-RAGE is determined by both the flip angle of the preparation pulse θ_{inv} and the flip angle of the excitation pulse θ_{ex}.

The preparatory pulse can increase the contrast by more than 50% when θ_{ex} is small. At larger θ_{ex}, (e.g., 15–20°) the contrast enhancement begins to diminish (Mugler and Brookeman 1991).

Multiple IR   Inversion recovery is also employed in black-blood MR angiography. To null the signal from the moving blood, two IR pulses are applied. The first IR pulse is spatially nonselective. This pulse is immediately followed by a second slice-selective IR pulse so that the static tissues in the slice experience virtually no net magnetization perturbation, whereas the flowing blood from the adjacent regions to the slice remains inverted. After a specific TI delay (e.g., 830 ms), the blood magnetization is nulled. The details of this double IR (DIR) technique are described in Section 15.1. Sometimes, it is desirable to null multiple tissues with differing T_1s. In this case, DIR or triple IR (TIR) can be used. Examples of TIR to null both blood and lipid signals are provided in Section 15.1.

SELECTED REFERENCES

Bakker, C. J. G., de Graaf, C. N., and van Dijk, P. 1984. Restoration of signal polarity in a set of inversion recovery NMR images. *IEEE Trans. Med. Imaging* 3: 197–202.

Barker, G. J. B. 1998. 3D fast FLAIR: A CSF-nulled 3D fast spin-echo pulse sequence. *Magn. Reson. Imaging* 16: 715–720.

Borrello, J. A., Chenevert, T. L., and Aisen, A. M. 1990. Regional phase correction of inversion-recovery MR images. *Magn. Reson. Med.* 14: 56–67.

Bydder, G. M., and Young, I. R. 1985. MR imaging: Clinical use of the inversion recovery sequence. *J. Comput. Assist. Tomogr.* 9: 659–675.

Bydder, G. M., Steiner, R. E., and Blumgart, L. H. 1985. MR imaging of the liver using short TI inversion recovery. *J. Comput. Assist. Tomogr.* 9: 1084–1089.

Dixon, R. L., and Ekstrand, K. E. 1982. The physics of proton NMR. *Med. Phys.* 9: 807–818.

Epstein, F. H., Mugler, J. P., Cail, W. S., and Brookeman, J. R. 1995. CSF-suppressed T_2-weighted 3-dimensional MP-RAGE MR imaging. *J. Magn. Reson. Imaging* 5: 463–469.

Foo, T. K. F., Sawyer, A. M., Faulkner, W. H., and Mills, D. G. 1994. Inversion in the steady-state-contrast optimization and reduced imaging time with fast 3-dimensional inversion-recovery–prepared GRE pulse sequences. *Radiology* 191: 85–90.

Haase, A. 1990. Snapshot FLASH MRI: Application to T_1, T_2 and chemical-shift imaging. *Magn. Reson. Med.* 13: 77–89.

Hajnal, J. V., De Coene, B., Lewis, P. D., Baudouin, C. J., Cowan, F. M., Pennock, J. M., Young, I. R., and Bydder, G. M. 1992. High signal regions in normal white matter shown by heavily T_2-weighted CSF nulled IR sequences. *J. Comput. Assist. Tomogr.* 16: 506–513.

Hajnal, J. V., Bryant, D. J., Kasuboski, L., Pattany, P. M., Decoene, B., Lewis, P. D., Pennock, J. M., Oatridge, A., Young, I. R., and Bydder, G. M. 1992. Use of fluid attenuated inversion recovery (FLAIR) pulse sequences in MRI of the brain. *J. Comput. Assist. Tomogr.* 16: 841–844.

Henderson, E., McKinnon, G., Lee, T. Y., and Rutt, B. K. 1999. A fast 3D Look-Locker method for volumetric T_1 mapping. *Magn. Reson. Imaging* 17: 1163–1171.

Kellman, P., Arai, A. E., McVeigh, E. R., and Aletras, A. H. 2002. Phase-sensitive inversion recovery for detecting myocardial infarction using gadolinium-delayed hyperenhancement. *Magn. Reson. Med.* 47: 372–383.

Listerud, J., Mitchell, J., Bagley, L., and Grossman, R. 1996. OIL FLAIR: Optimized interleaved fluid-attenuated inversion recovery in 2D fast spin echo. *Magn. Reson. Med.* 36: 320–325.

Mugler, J. H., III, and Brookeman, J. R. 1990. Three-dimensional magnetization-prepared rapid gradient-echo imaging (3D MP RAGE). *Magn. Reson. Med.* 15: 152–157.

Mugler, J. P., and Brookeman, J. R. 1991. Rapid three-dimensional T_1-weighted MR imaging with the MP-RAGE sequence. *J. Magn. Reson. Imaging* 1: 561–567.

Oh, C. H., Hilal, S. K., Mun, I. K., and Cho, Z. H. 1991. An optimized multislice acquisition sequence for the inversion-recovery MR imaging. *Magn. Reson. Imaging* 9: 903–908.

Park, H. W., Cho, M. H., and Cho, Z. H. 1985. Time-multiplexed multislice inversion-recovery techniques for NMR imaging. *Magn. Reson. Med.* 2: 534–539.

Park, H. W., Cho, M. H., and Cho, Z. H. 1986. Real-value representation in inversion-recovery NMR imaging by use of a phase-correction method. *Magn. Reson. Med.* 3: 15–23.

Press, W. H., Flannery, B. P., Teukolsky, S. A., and Vetterling, W. T. 1992. *Numerical recipes in C: The art of scientific computing.* New York: Cambridge University Press.

Rydberg, J. N., Riederer, S. J., Rydberg, C. H., and Jack, C. R. 1995. Contrast optimization of fluid-attenuated inversion-recovery (FLAIR) imaging. *Magn. Reson. Med.* 34: 868–877.

Xiang, Q. S. 1996. Inversion recovery image reconstruction with multiseed region-growing spin reversal. *J. Magn. Reson. Imaging* 6: 775–782.

RELATED SECTIONS

Section 3.2: Inversion Pulses
Section 6.2: Adiabatic Inversion Pulses
Section 10.5: Spoiler Gradients
Section 11.5: Two-Dimensional Acquisition
Section 14.3: Radiofrequency Spin Echo
Section 15.1: Black Blood Angiography
Section 16.4: RARE

14.3 Radiofrequency Spin Echo

Radiofrequency spin echo or simply spin echo (SE) is a fundamental pulse sequence in MRI. As described in Section 3.3 and Hahn (1950), an RF SE is formed by an excitation pulse and one or more refocusing pulses. Usually the flip angles of the excitation and refocusing pulses are set to 90 and 180°, respectively. SE images are typically obtained in the 2D mode, so that the interleaved multislice acquisition strategy that is presented in Section 11.5 can be used. The main advantage of an SE pulse sequence is its ability to obtain a specific contrast weighting, either T_1-, T_2-, or proton density–weighted (Hendrick 1999), with the combinations of TR and TE values listed in Table 14.4. The TE and TR values listed in the table are approximate because the optimal values

TABLE 14.4

Combinations of TE and TR Values Used to Generate Various Contrast
Weightings in Spin Echo Imaging

	Short TE ($\leq$ 20 ms)	Long TE ($\geq$ 80 ms)
Short TR ($<$ 700 ms)	T_1-weighted	Not commonly used
Long TR ($>$ 2000 ms)	Proton density–weighted	T_2-weighted

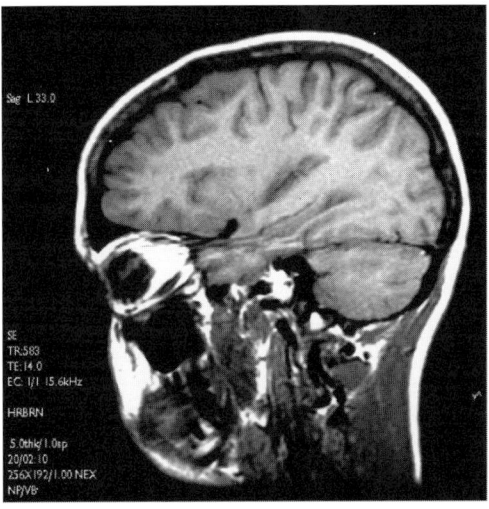

FIGURE 14.28 An image from a T_1-weighted sagittal SE exam at 1.5 T.

depend on the type of tissues being imaged and the B_0 field strength. An
example of a T_1-weighted SE image is shown in Figure 14.28. Another advantage of SE pulse sequences is robustness—they are less prone to blurring and
ghosting than RARE and EPI.

SE also offers greater immunity than gradient echoes (Section 14.1)
to artifacts arising from off-resonance effects such as main magnetic field
inhomogeneity and magnetic susceptibility variations. This is because the 180°
RF pulse in SE pulse sequences refocuses off-resonance effects, resulting in
fewer artifacts. Whereas gradient echoes are contrast weighted by the factor
$e^{-\text{TE}/T_2^*}$, SEs are weighted by the factor $e^{-\text{TE}/T_2}$. (A further discussion of
T_2 and T_2^* is provided in Section 14.1.) Because $T_2 \geq T_2^*$, RF SEs can use

longer echo delays, such as TE values greater than 80 ms to produce heavily T_2-weighted images without excessive signal loss due to T_2^*, even in the presence of moderate B_0 inhomogeneity. Also unlike gradient echoes, SE images are not prone to the type of chemical shift artifact that causes signal loss in a voxel that contains both water and lipids, acquired with a TE at which water and lipids are out of phase (see Sections 14.1 and 17.3). SE images, however, are still subject to the spatial chemical shift artifacts in the slice-selection and readout directions, as described in Sections 8.3 and 11.1, respectively.

SE images can be acquired with either a single-echo or a multiple-echo (Feinberg et al. 1985) pulse sequence, depending on the number of RF refocusing pulses that are applied in each TR interval. These options are described later in Section 14.3. Regardless of the number of echoes, data at only a single phase-encoding step are acquired in any TR interval. That is, k-space is filled one line at a time. This makes acquisition time for SE much longer than for echo-train pulse sequences such as RARE (Section 16.4). As described in Section 11.5, the acquisition time for a two-dimensional SE pulse sequence is given by:

$$T_{scan} = TR \times N_{phase} \times NEX \qquad (14.50)$$

The scan time calculated by Eq. (14.50) is the total for all the slices that are acquired in an interleaved fashion within a pass, but it can get quite long. For example, with 256 phase-encoding views, TR $= 3000$ ms, T_{scan} is nearly 13 min, even without signal averaging (NEX $= 1$). These long acquisition times have led to the increased popularity of echo-train pulse sequences such as RARE, particularly to acquire T_2-weighted images. Because their acquisition time is long and their SNR is relatively high, SE pulse sequences are a good application for the parallel imaging techniques described in Section 13.3. For T_1-weighted imaging, the acquisition time of an SE sequence is considerably less due to the reduced TR. For example, for the image shown in Figure 14.28 that has 192 phase-encoding views, 1 NEX, and a TR of 583 ms, the total acquisition time is only slightly over 2 min for 20 slices. Thus, SE pulse sequences are frequently used for T_1-weighted imaging.

SE pulse sequences are not limited to Fourier encoding with rectilinear k-space sampling. Other k-space sampling strategies, such as projection acquisition (Zhou and Lauterbur 1992), also use SE pulse sequences. This section focuses on Fourier-encoded SE.

14.3.1 SINGLE-ECHO SE

Basic Pulse-Sequence Considerations   A standard single-echo SE pulse sequence employs a 90° excitation and a single 180° refocusing pulse to form one RF SE per TR interval (per slice location). Ideally the slice profiles of

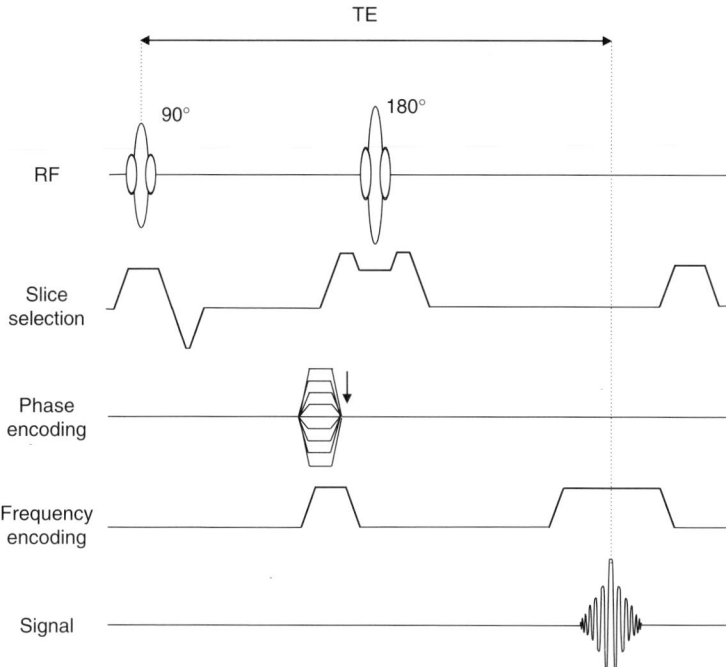

FIGURE 14.29 A single-echo RF SE pulse sequence. On the slice-selection wave-form, a crusher gradient pair straddles the refocusing pulse, and a spoiler gradient is played at the end of the waveform. The vertical arrow on the phase-encoding gradient indicates how the gradient changes for successive sequences to sample the k-space. (The details of these gradient waveforms are described in Sections 8.1, 8.2, 8.3, 10.2, and 10.5.)

the excitation and refocusing pulses are closely matched to one another so that the slice gap can be minimized. Figure 14.29 shows a typical 2D SE pulse sequence diagram used for Fourier encoding. Usually both of the RF pulses are spatially selective, so the acquisition of multiple slice locations can be interleaved within a TR interval. The echo is both phase- and frequency-encoded, as detailed in Sections 8.1 and 8.2. There are many variants to the basic pulse sequence, some of which are described later in this section.

In the absence of any imaging gradients, the temporal location of the peak of the echo is determined by when the RF pulses are played. In SE imaging pulse sequences, however, the gradient area on the frequency-encoding axis instead determines the temporal location of the peak of the echo. In single-echo SE, the peak of the echo occurs when the area under the readout gradient balances the area of the prephasing gradient lobe, as described in Section 8.1

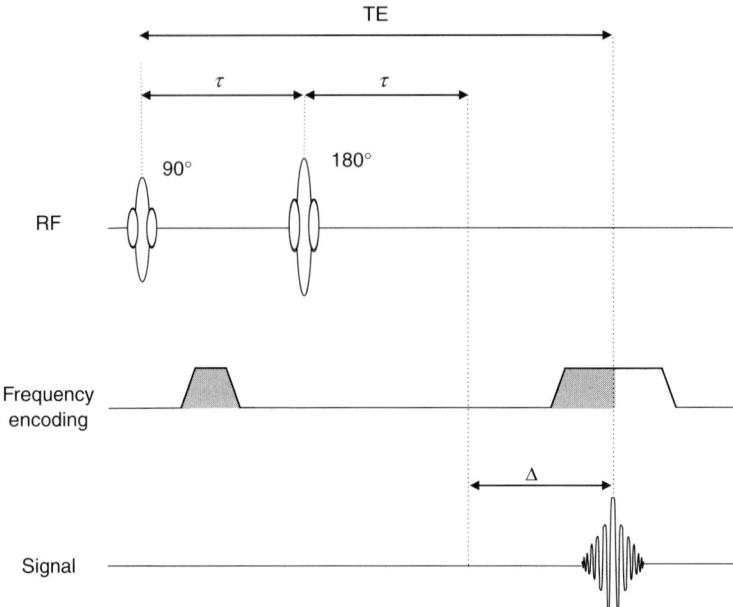

FIGURE 14.30 Pulse sequence diagram illustrating that the peak of the echo forms at TE, when the gradient area on the frequency-encoding waveform balances. If Δ is nonzero, then the resulting signal has some T_2^*-weighting.

and further illustrated in Figure 14.30. To minimize T_2^* weighting of the signal, the timing represented in Figure 14.30 with TE $= 2\tau$ (i.e., $\Delta = 0$) is used. In this case, the time between the isodelay point of the excitation pulse and the peak of the echo (i.e., TE) is equal to twice the distance from either point to the center of the refocusing pulse (i.e., 2τ). In other words, the gradient waveform on the frequency-encoding axis is designed so that the areas balance when the RF SE refocuses, in the absence of any imaging gradients.

Sometimes Δ is nonzero due to system imperfections, such as eddy currents, that can shift the point at which the total readout gradient areas before and after the refocusing pulse are equal. For some specialized applications such as GRASE (Section 16.2) and the Dixon method (Section 17.3), however, the pulse sequence is intentionally programmed to provide nonzero values of Δ.

Example 14.5   Suppose that $\Delta = $ TE $- 2\tau$ is nonzero. How is the standard contrast-weighting factor $W = e^{-\text{TE}/T_2}$ modified? Let T_2' be the contribution to the apparent T_2 from B_0 inhomogeneity (see Eq. 14.1).

Answer It is convenient to divide the problem into two cases: positive and negative Δ. For $\Delta > 0$, T_2 decay occurs over the entire echo delay, and the T_2' decay is refocused over the entire echo delay except Δ. Therefore:

$$W_{\Delta>0} = e^{-\text{TE}/T_2} e^{-\Delta/T_2'} = e^{-(2\tau+\Delta)/T_2} e^{-\Delta/T_2'} = e^{-2\tau/T_2} e^{-\Delta/T_2^*} \quad (14.51)$$

For $\Delta < 0$, T_2 decay also occurs during the entire echo delay, but T_2' is not refocused over the final $|\Delta|$. Therefore:

$$W_{\Delta<0} = e^{-\text{TE}/T_2} e^{-|\Delta|/T_2'} = e^{-(2\tau-|\Delta|)/T_2} e^{-|\Delta|/T_2'} \quad (14.52)$$

Single-Echo SE Pulse Sequence Variants There are many variations to the basic single-echo SE pulse sequence shown in Figure 14.29. As discussed in Section 8.3, the gradient areas of the slice-rephasing lobe and the left crusher are commonly combined. Also, as discussed in Sections 10.2 and 10.5, the crusher and spoiler gradients need not be played solely on the slice-selection axis. Each can be played on any one, two, or three of the logical gradient axes. If an end-of-sequence spoiler gradient is played on the frequency-encoding axis, that lobe is typically bridged with the readout.

First-order gradient moment nulling (i.e., velocity compensation) is often applied to SE pulse sequences. Figure 14.31 shows a representative pulse sequence design; additional gradient lobes are added to the frequency-encoding and slice-selection waveforms. The gradient lobes on each waveform are designed so that the zeroth and first gradient moments are nulled at the echo peak. As discussed in Section 10.4, gradients played before the peak of the refocusing pulse are effectively negated. (More details and methods for calculating the gradient lobe areas are presented in Section 10.4.)

Any SE pulse sequence can be augmented by adding modules to perform spatial saturation, chemically selective saturation, and magnetization transfer. Typically, the modules are played before the RF excitation pulse, but alternatively they can be played after the spoiler gradient pulse(s). The latter order is often preferred in conjunction with cardiac triggering in order to minimize the time between the detected R-wave and the excitation pulse, so that the true location of the heart is more accurately represented.

Another common pulse sequence variant is to acquire partial echo k-space data. To avoid T_2^* weighting of the signal, the frequency-encoding waveform is designed so that the peak of the echo (not the center of the readout) occurs when the RF spin would have refocused in the absence of imaging gradients, that is, 2τ. This is accomplished by reducing the area under the readout prephasing gradient lobe, as illustrated in Figures 14.32 and 8.7b. Additional discussion on partial-echo acquisition can be found in Section 8.1. The resulting data can be reconstructed with the partial Fourier methods detailed in Section 13.4.

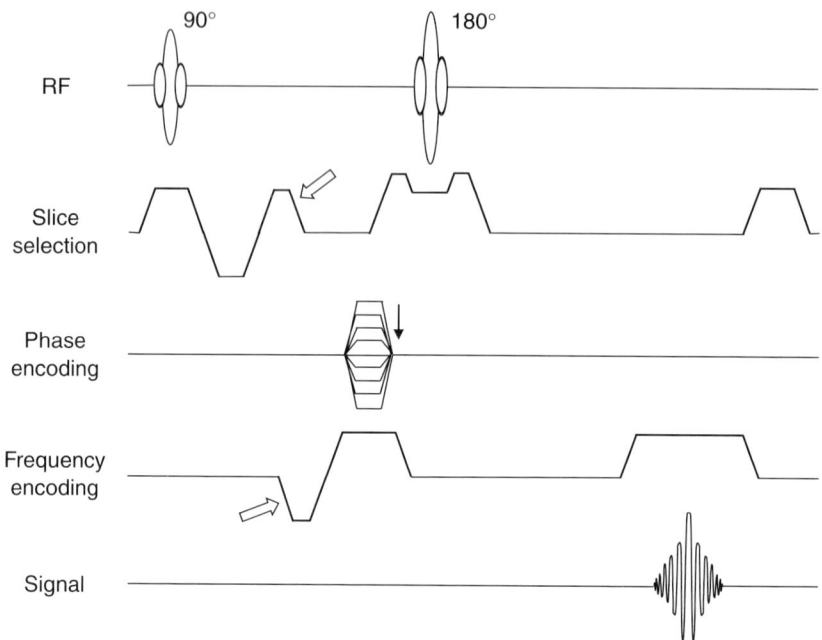

FIGURE 14.31 Example of a SE pulse sequence with first-order gradient moment nulling (i.e., flow compensation) on the slice-selection and frequency-encoding axes. Note the additional gradient lobes on those axes (arrow).

A less commonly used variant is to play the phase-encoding lobe after the RF refocusing pulse. This reduces spatial misregistration for oblique flow. Often, however, flowing blood produces no signal in RF SE images (see Section 15.1), so spatial misregistration of oblique flow is usually not a severe problem. Playing the phase-encoding lobe after refocusing pulse has the drawback that the residual FID following the imperfect 180° pulse is now phase encoded, so the artifact that it produces is no longer confined to a few image lines that can be phase cycled to edge of the FOV and discarded (Section 11.5).

If the transverse magnetization at the end of the pulse sequence is not negligible, playing a phase-rewinding gradient can help reduce artifacts. One situation in which this can occur is with the use of short TR (i.e., TR is not much longer than T_2). Another situation arises with view reordering to reduce respiratory motion artifact (Section 12.3), in which the acquisition of a very strong signal (i.e., a view with a small phase-encoding value) can immediately precede the acquisition of a very weak signal (i.e., a view with a large

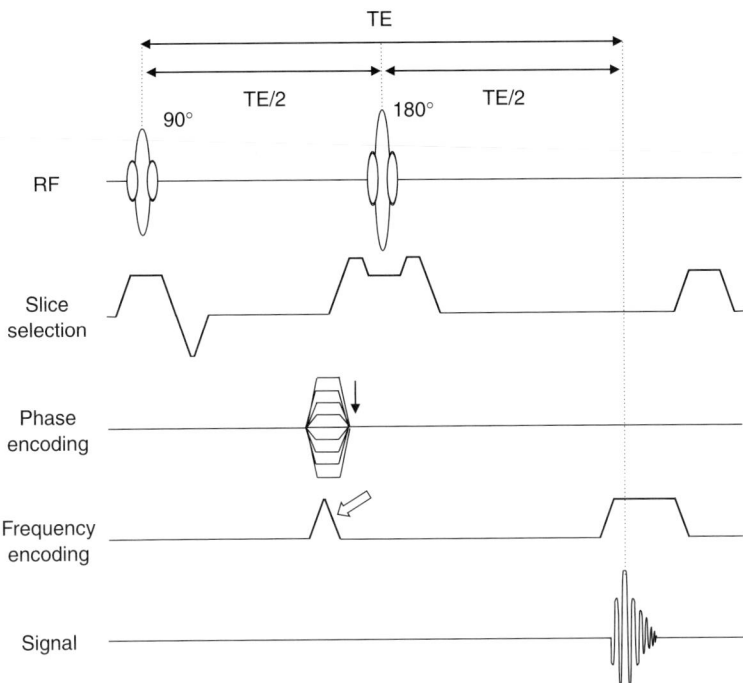

FIGURE 14.32 Pulse sequence diagram for a partial-echo SE acquisition. Note the reduced area of the readout prephasing lobe (hollow arrow).

phase-encoding value). When a rewinder is used, it can be advantageous to place the phase-encoding lobe after the refocusing pulse; otherwise the phase of the magnetization may not be fully rewound in areas where the refocusing flip angle is not ideal (e.g., in areas of B_1 inhomogeneity or in the transition band of the refocusing pulse).

Another interesting, but not widely used, variant of the SE pulse sequence is to play the slice-selection gradient for the RF refocusing pulse on the phase-encoding axis in order to limit aliasing (i.e., wraparound artifact). This method is called inner volume (Feinberg et al. 1985), zoom imaging, or local look (LoLo). The RF bandwidth and slice-selection gradient amplitude are chosen so that the passband of the slice profile matches the desired FOV in the phase-encoded direction. The major drawback of this method is the resulting pulse sequence is limited to single-slice acquisition. LoLo has found application in small-FOV imaging, such as that used for MR-guided biopsies (Buecker et al. 1998).

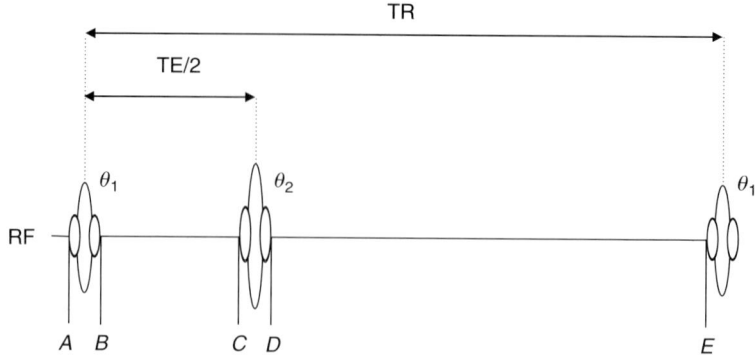

FIGURE 14.33 The timing points A–E used to calculate the signal intensity in an SE acquisition.

Signal Formula   The signal for a single-echo SE acquisition can be readily derived (Perman et al. 1984) by considering the longitudinal magnetization at various points within the pulse sequence, as shown in Figure 14.33. In the derivation we assume that the transverse magnetization at the end of the pulse sequence (point E) is negligible, either because TR $\gg T_2$ or because of an applied spoiler gradient. We also assume that $\theta_1 = 90°$ and $\theta_2 = 180°$. The more general case of arbitrary flip angles is considered in Example 14.6.

Let the equilibrium longitudinal magnetization be M_0, and let the longitudinal magnetization at point A be M_{zA}. Then at point B, neglecting T_1 relaxation during the RF excitation pulse (or equivalently, assuming the pulse has negligible width):

$$M_{zB} = M_{zA} \cos 90° = 0 \tag{14.53}$$

T_1 relaxation occurs for a time TE/2 during the interval between the excitation and refocusing pulses, so according to the Bloch equations (Section 1.2):

$$M_{zC} = M_0(1 - e^{-\text{TE}/2T_1}) \tag{14.54}$$

Again, neglecting T_1 relaxation during the refocusing pulse:

$$M_{zD} = M_{zC} \cos 180° = -M_0(1 - e^{-\text{TE}/2T_1}) \tag{14.55}$$

Accounting for the T_1 relaxation after the refocusing pulse:

$$M_{zE} = M_{zD}e^{-(\text{TR}-\text{TE}/2)/T_1} + M_0(1 - e^{-(\text{TR}-\text{TE}/2)/T_1})$$
$$= M_0(1 - 2e^{-(\text{TR}-\text{TE}/2)/T_1} + e^{-\text{TR}/T_1}) \tag{14.56}$$

According to Section 3.3, the signal S at the spin echo is given by:

$$M_{zE} \sin 90° \sin^2 \left(\frac{180°}{2}\right) e^{-\text{TE}/T_2}$$

and substituting Eq. (14.56) yields

$$S = M_0(1 - 2e^{-(\text{TR}-\text{TE}/2)/T_1} + e^{-\text{TR}/T_1})e^{-\text{TE}/T_2} \tag{14.57}$$

Calculating the difference between two expressions of the form Eq. (14.57), each with appropriate values of M_0, T_1, and T_2, provides a formula for image contrast.

Example 14.6   Generalize Eq. (14.57) to find the expression for the signal S when $\theta_1 \neq 90°$ and $\theta_2 \neq 180°$. Assume that a steady state for the longitudinal magnetization is reached, so that $M_{zA} = M_{zE}$, and use the notation $E_3 = e^{-\text{TE}/2T_1}$ and $E_4 = e^{-(\text{TR}-\text{TE}/2)/T_1}$.

Answer   We obtain:

$$M_{zB} = M_{zA} \cos \theta_1 \tag{14.58}$$

$$M_{zC} = M_{zA} \cos \theta_1 E_3 + M_0(1 - E_3) \tag{14.59}$$

$$M_{zD} = \cos \theta_2 M_{zC} \tag{14.60}$$

and

$$M_{zE} = M_{zD} E_4 + M_0(1 - E_4) \tag{14.61}$$

Using the steady state condition $M_{zA} = M_{zE}$, after some algebra we find:

$$M_{zE} = M_0 \frac{1 + (\cos \theta_2 - 1)E_4 - \cos \theta_2 E_3 E_4}{1 - \cos \theta_1 \cos \theta_2 E_3 E_4} \tag{14.62}$$

Finally we obtain:

$$S = M_0 \sin \theta_1 \sin^2\left(\frac{\theta_2}{2}\right) \frac{(1 + (\cos \theta_2 - 1)e^{-(\text{TR}-\text{TE}/2)/T_1} - \cos \theta_2 e^{-\text{TR}/T_1})}{1 - \cos \theta_1 \cos \theta_2 e^{-\text{TR}/T_1}}$$

$$\times \, e^{-\text{TE}/T_2} \tag{14.63}$$

If $T_1 \ll (\text{TR} - \text{TE}/2)$, then the signal in Eq. (14.63) is maximized by setting $\theta_1 = 90°$ and $\theta_2 = 180°$. Other values of the flip angles can be used with shorter TR to increase the signal or to maximize the contrast between a particular pair of tissue types. Sometimes a lower value of the flip angle of the refocusing pulse is used to reduce SAR, particularly at field strengths of 3.0 T and higher.

14.3.2 MULTI-ECHO SPIN ECHO

The transverse magnetization that forms an RF SE can be repeatedly refocused into subsequent SEs by playing additional RF refocusing pulses. The series of echoes obtained with this process is called an echo train. Usually Carr-Purcell-Meiboom-Gill (CPMG) phase cycling (i.e., $90x$, $180y$, $180y$, ...; see Sections 11.5 and 16.4) is used to reduce signal loss in the presence of B_1 inhomogeneity. We use here the notation that the series of RF spin echoes are refocused at times TE_1, TE_2, TE_3, and so on. Each echo number fills its own independent k-space, which is reconstructed with its own 2D Fourier transform. Because of the phase-reversal effect of the refocusing pulses, the images from even-numbered echoes have to be flipped in the phase-encoded direction, unless each readout is straddled by its own phase-encoding and rewinder pair.

Because the signal decays exponentially, the number of useful echoes in the echo train is limited by T_2 decay. For long-T_2 substances such as CSF, an echo-train length of 16 or more can be readily obtained, with the TE of the last echo in the train $\sim$100–200 ms. Sometimes, however, we are most interested in only two of the echoes, an early and a late one. According to Table 14.4, the two resulting images will be proton density–and T_2-weighted, respectively, provided a long TR is selected. To avoid the overhead associated with reconstruction, display, viewing, and archive of a larger number of images, sometimes only two echoes are acquired. This is called a two-echo, double-echo, or dual-echo acquisition. To achieve the desired proton density and T_2 contrast weighting, the second echo is usually delayed, $TE_2 > 2 \times TE_1$. This is sometimes called a variable echo acquisition. Note that the CPMG condition (see Section 16.4) cannot be met for this type of acquisition. Figures 14.34 and 14.35 show examples of dual-echo, variable echo acquisitions.

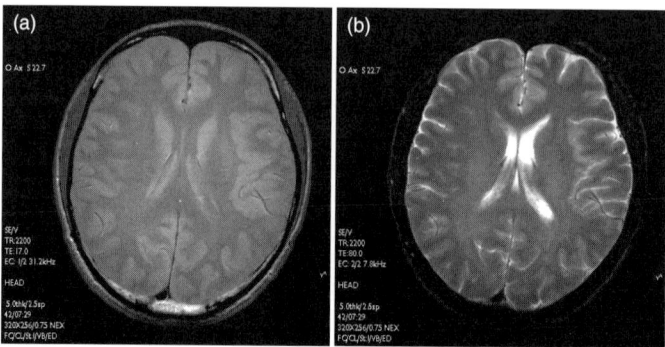

FIGURE 14.34 A dual-echo SE acquisition showing an oblique axial section of the brain of a healthy volunteer at 3.0 T. (a) Proton density–weighted (TE/TR = 17/2200 ms). (b) T_2-weighted (TE/TR = 80/2200 ms).

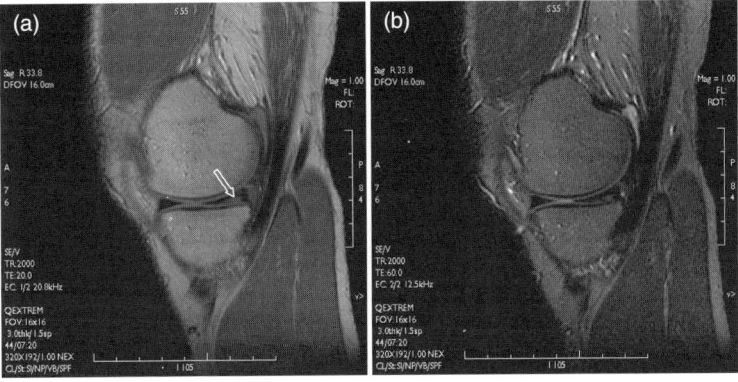

FIGURE 14.35 Sagittal dual-echo SE images of a knee at 1.5 T showing a tear of the posterior horn of the medial meniscus (arrow). (a) Proton density–weighted (TE/TR = 20/2000 ms). (b) T_2-weighted (TE/TR = 60/2000 ms). (Courtesy of Kimberly K. Amrami, M.D., Mayo Clinic College of Medicine.)

Even if two images are produced from echoes with the same TE value, their appearance can differ depending on the number of preceding refocusing pulses. This is because signal loss due to molecular diffusion, field inhomogeneity, and J coupling is reduced as the spacing between the refocusing pulses is decreased (Carr and Purcell 1954). The net result of using a dual echo instead of a long echo train to acquire T_2-weighted images is usually an attenuated lipid signal (due to the J coupling—see Section 16.4) and slightly increased T_2^* weighting. Both of these differences are usually well accepted clinically.

Dual Echo and Variable Echo   Figure 14.36 shows a dual-echo pulse sequence. Note that the crusher amplitudes associated with the first and second refocusing pulses are intentionally unequal. This is to avoid refocusing a stimulated echo (see Section 10.2) in the second readout window. This might be surprising, considering that the stimulated echo amplitude is proportional to $\sin\theta_1 \sin\theta_2 \sin\theta_3 = \sin 90° \sin^2 180° = 0$. When the crusher amplitudes are equal, however, at least a weak stimulated artifact is almost always seen because there are regions of its profile where the flip angle of the refocusing pulse is not exactly 180°.

The appearance of the stimulated echo artifact on the image is schematically depicted in Figure 14.37a. The stimulated echo can be thought of as arising from transverse magnetization that is rotated onto the z axis by the first 180° pulse and then rotated back into the transverse plane by the second 180° pulse (effectively experiencing a 90_x-90_{-y}-90_y pulse sequence). The phase

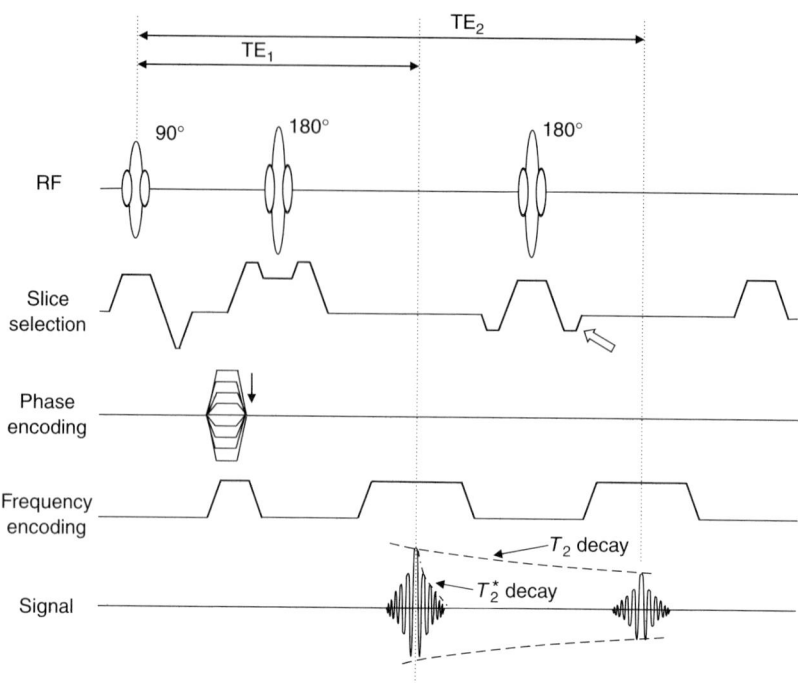

FIGURE 14.36 Pulse sequence for a dual-echo SE, variable echo acquisition. The second RF SE peaks at an echo time TE_2. Data from the second echo are independently reconstructed to form their own image. In order to avoid stimulated echo artifacts on the second echo, the amplitude of the second set of crushers (hollow arrow) must differ from that of the first set of crushers.

accumulated by stimulated echo magnetization from the phase-encoding gradient is negated relative to the phase accumulated by SE magnetization. The stimulated echo artifact is therefore the mirror-image reflection (in the phase-encoded direction) of the desired SE image. The stimulated echo artifact should not be confused with similar-looking artifacts arising from patient motion, system vibration or instability (Figure 14.37b), or quadrature imbalance (Figure 14.37c). (Quadrature imbalance means that the real part of the raw data is not demodulated exactly 90° out of phase relative to the imaginary part. With most modern receiver designs, the quadrature imbalance artifact has been eliminated because only a single digitizer per receiver channel is used. See Section 11.1.)

As in the single-echo case, to avoid T_2^* weighting, the gradient area on the frequency-encoding axis is designed to balance where the second SE would form, in the absence of any imaging gradients. Using Figure 14.36, we can

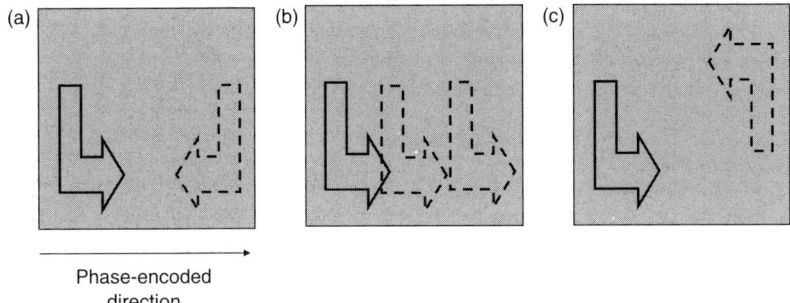

Phase-encoded
direction

FIGURE 14.37 (a) Schematic representation of a stimulated echo artifact, not to be confused with (b) artifacts arising from motion or system instability, or (c) artifacts due to imbalance in the quadrature detection.

readily show that TE_2 is equal to twice the spacing between the peaks of the two refocusing pulses. Using that relationship, Eq. (14.57) can be generalized to the variable-echo case. Assuming that the flip angles of the RF pulses are 90°, 180°, and 180°, the result for the signal intensity of the two echoes is:

$$
\begin{aligned}
S_1 = M_0\Big(1 &- 2e^{-(TR-(TE_1+TE_2)/2)/T_1} \\
&+ 2e^{-(TR-TE_1/2)/T_1} - e^{-TR/T_1}\Big)e^{-TE_1/T_2} \\
S_2 = M_0\Big(1 &- 2e^{-(TR-(TE_1+TE_2)/2)/T_1} \\
&+ 2e^{-(TR-TE_1/2)/T_1} - e^{-TR/T_1}\Big)e^{-TE_2/T_2}
\end{aligned}
\tag{14.64}
$$

Dual-Echo SE Pulse Sequence Variants   Frequently dual-echo pulse sequences use gradient moment nulling. The even-echo refocusing effect that is discussed in Section 10.4 automatically provides some flow compensation on the second echo, but it cannot be relied on for exact moment nulling. Instead, gradient lobes typically are added on the frequency-encoding and slice-selection waveforms to null the gradient first moment. To obtain shorter values of TE_1 and to minimize T_2-weighting in the proton density–weighted echo, sometimes only the second echo is moment nulled.

Because of T_2 decay, the second echo has lower signal than the first. Also, for variable-echo pulse sequences with $TE_2 > 2 \times TE_1$, the second echo has more time between the refocusing pulse and the readout gradient lobe. These two factors make dual-echo variable-echo an ideal application to reduce the receiver bandwidth $\Delta\nu$ for the second echo. This procedure is called matched bandwidth, optimized bandwidth, or variable bandwidth (Enzmann and Augustyn 1989). Reducing $\Delta\nu$ for the second echo implies that

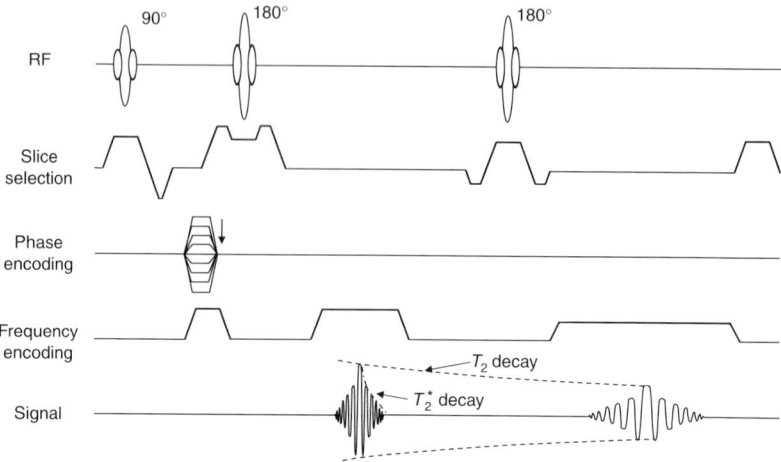

FIGURE 14.38 Pulse sequence for dual-echo acquisition with variable bandwidth. The bandwidth of the second echo is reduced, as reflected by the prolonged readout window.

its readout window has a longer duration. To preserve the FOV, the readout gradient amplitude is proportionately reduced (Figure 14.38). Because the gradient amplitude is reduced, the T_2^* during the readout of the second echo is longer and the echo envelope is dilated. Because the SNR is proportional to $1/\sqrt{\Delta \nu}$, variable bandwidth compensates for some of the SNR lost on the second echo from T_2 decay. The main drawback of variable bandwidth is the spatial chemical shift artifact in the frequency-encoded direction increases on the second echo because it is inversely proportional to $\Delta \nu$. For this reason, a lipid-suppression method for the second echo can be quite useful.

A pulse sequence module that performs chemically selective saturation can be added to nearly any pulse sequence, including dual-echo SE. At least partial suppression of the lipid signal, however, can be achieved in SE without chemical saturation, using a gradient reversal method (Gomori et al. 1988). This method is sometimes called classic. The pulse sequence modification used to suppress the lipid signal on the second echo is illustrated in Figure 14.39. (Gradient reversal fat suppression also can be used for the first echo if desired.) The polarity of the slice-selection gradient for the second refocusing pulse is reversed. To preserve the same slice location, the sign of the carrier frequency offset δf must also be negated. The net effect of these two actions is to reverse the direction of the spatial chemical shift in the slice-selection direction. If the carrier frequency is set to the Larmor frequency of water, then the water slice is unaffected, but the lipid slice is shifted (Figure 14.39b shows this

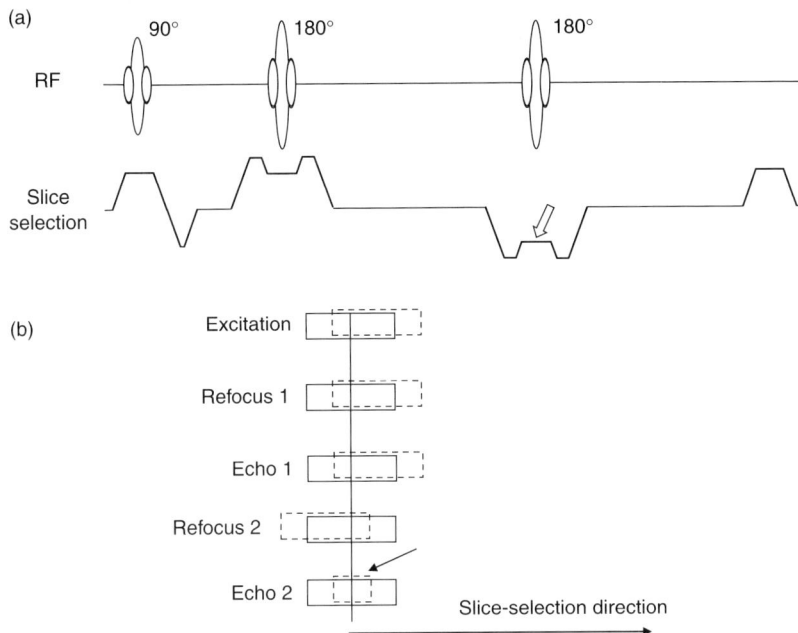

FIGURE 14.39 (a) Pulse sequence and schematic representation of second-echo lipid suppression. The gradient polarity of the slice-selection gradient for the second refocusing pulse is reversed (hollow arrow). (b) The box with solid lines represents the water slice, and the box with dashed lines represents the lipid slice. The second echo has reduced lipid signal intensity because the intersection of the slice profiles from the first and second refocusing pulses (arrow) decreases the lipid slice thickness for that echo.

effect, with the amount of shift exaggerated for purposes of illustration.) The second echo has reduced lipid signal because only the central portion of the slice experiences both refocusing pulses. The second echo images shown in Figures 14.34 and 14.35 use this type of lipid suppression.

T_2 Mapping Although not widely used in MRI, more than two echoes can be acquired per TR interval in an SE pulse sequence. A common application of acquiring longer echo trains is T_2 mapping. The goal of T_2 mapping is to provide a calculated image in which each pixel value quantitatively represents the average T_2 of the tissue within that voxel. Convenient units such as tenths of milliseconds can be used on the calculated image.

In principle, T_2 mapping is very simple. Acquire a long (e.g., 16) echo train of SEs and fit the signal intensity measured in each pixel to calculate T_2. In practice there are several systematic errors that can make T_2 mapping challenging

(Breger et al. 1989). First, if the CPMG condition (see Section 16.4) is not met, then the signal decays more rapidly than $e^{-\text{TE}/T_2}$. In addition to using CPMG phase cycling, sometimes a single-slice acquisition with hard RF refocusing pulses can be used to minimize systematic errors from variations in the flip angle across the slice profile. Second, contributions from the stimulated echoes can also introduce the unwanted T_1-weighting variations into the echo-train signals. This can make it difficult to perform curve fitting based on a monoexponential decay model. Third, if magnitude reconstruction is used, then the noise floor has a nonzero, positive mean, which incorrectly increases the measured T_2 values, especially for short T_2 tissues. To overcome this problem, a nonlinear fit to $S(\text{TE}) = N + Ae^{-\text{TE}/T_2}$ can be used, where S is the measured signal, and N, A, and T_2 are fitting parameters. (If the tissue of interest has multiple T_2 components, then a fitting function of the form $S(\text{TE}) = N + Ae^{-\text{TE}/T_{2A}} + Be^{-\text{TE}/T_{2B}} + \cdots$ can be used instead.) Nonlinear fitting is more computationally intensive than simply taking the natural logarithm of the measured signals and then using linear regression to extract T_2. The result of the linear regression can be used as a starting guess for the T_2 parameter for the nonlinear fit. Details about nonlinear fitting algorithms are in Press et al. (1992).

SELECTED REFERENCES

Breger, R. K., Rimm, A. A., Fischer, M. E., Papke, R. A., and Haughton, V. M. 1989. T_1 and T_2 measurements on a 1.5-T commercial MR imager. *Radiology* 171: 273–276.

Buecker, A., Adam, G., Neuerburg, J. M., Glowinski, A., van Vaals, J. J., and Guenther, R. W. 1998. MR-guided biopsy using T_2-weighted single-shot zoom imaging sequence (Local Look technique). *J. Magn. Reson. Imaging* 8: 955–959.

Carr, H. Y., and Purcell, E. M. 1954. Effects of diffusion on free precession in nuclear magnetic resonance experiments. *Phys. Rev.* 94: 630–638.

Enzmann, D., and Augustyn, G. T. 1989. Improved MR images of the brain with use of a gated, flow-compensated, variable-bandwidth pulse sequence. *Radiology* 172: 771–781.

Feinberg, D. A., Mills, C. M., Posin, J. P., Ortendahl, D. A., Hylton, N. M., Crooks, L. E., Watts, J. C., Kaufman, L., Arakawa, M., Hoenninger, J. C., and Brant-Zwadwaski, M. 1985. Multiple spin-echo magnetic resonance imaging. *Radiology* 155: 437–442.

Feinberg, D. A., Hoenninger, J. C., Crooks, L. E., Kaufman, L., Watts, J. C., and Arakawa, M. 1985. Inner volume MRI: Technical concepts and their application. *Radiology* 156: 743–747.

Gomori, J. M., Holland, G. A., Grossman, R. I., Gefter, W. B., and Lenkinski, R. E. 1988. Fat suppression by section-select gradient reversal on spin-echo MR imaging: Work in progress. *Radiology* 169: 493–495.

Hahn, E. L. 1950. Spin echoes. *Phys. Rev.* 80: 580–594.

Hendrick, R. E. 1999. Image contrast and noise. In *Magnetic resonance imaging*, Vol. 1, edited by D. D. Stark and W. G. Bradley, pp. 43–67. St. Louis, MO: Mosby.

Perman, W. H., Hilal, S. K., Simon, H. E., and Maudsley, A. A. 1984. Contrast manipulation in NMR imaging. *Magn. Reson. Imaging* 2: 23–32.

Press, W. H., Flannery, B. P., Teukolsky, S. A., and Vetterling, W. T. 1992. *Numerical recipes in C: The art of scientific computing*. New York: Cambridge University Press.

Zhou, X. J., and Lauterbur, P. C. 1992. NMR Microscopy using projection reconstruction, In *Magnetic resonance microscopy*, edited by B. Blumich and W. Kuhn, p. 1. Berlin: VCH Publishing.

RELATED SECTIONS

Section 3.1 Excitation Pulses
Section 3.3 Refocusing Pulses
Section 8.1 Frequency-Encoding Gradients
Section 8.3 Slice-Selection Gradients
Section 10.2 Crusher Gradients
Section 11.5 Two-Dimensional Acquisition
Section 16.4 RARE

CHAPTER

15

ANGIOGRAPHIC PULSE SEQUENCES

15.1 Black Blood Angiography

Some MR angiography methods produce images with suppressed (i.e., hypointense) blood signal. They are commonly referred to as dark or black blood angiographic methods, in distinction to the bright blood methods that are described in subsection 15.3. The terms *bright blood* and *black blood* refer to the pixel intensity and not to the image display. For example, vessels appear brighter than the background on a black blood angiogram if an inverse video display is used.

We discuss several mechanisms that can attenuate or eliminate the signal intensity from blood to make a black blood angiogram. First, spatial saturation (Section 5.3) can be added to virtually any pulse sequence. Second, any pulse sequence that uses at least one 180° RF refocusing pulse (e.g., RF spin echo or RARE) attenuates the signal of rapidly flowing blood by the mechanism illustrated in Figure 15.1. If the blood moves out of the imaging slice during the time between the RF excitation and refocusing pulses, then it does not experience both pulses and cannot form an RF spin echo (Bradley 1988). Third, IR magnetization preparation methods can be used, with the inversion time TI adjusted to null the signal from blood. Finally, the intrinsic T_2^* shortening of deoxygenated blood can be used to produce high-spatial-resolution black

648

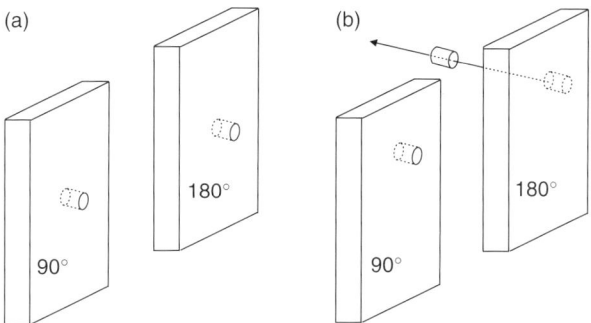

FIGURE 15.1 Signal loss from rapidly flowing blood in RF spin echo or RARE. (a) Stationary tissue experiences both a 90° RF excitation pulse and a 180° RF refocusing pulse so that its magnetization forms a spin echo. (b) Blood flows out of the imaging slice during the time interval between application of the two pulses so that no signal is obtained.

blood MR venograms, as in a method called susceptibility weighted imaging (SWI), described later in this section.

The main goal of black blood methods is to attenuate the signal of blood (ideally to zero) while preserving the signal from the surrounding stationary tissue. Frequently, two or more of the mechanisms are employed in the same pulse sequence. For example, RARE methods are often used in conjunction with IR magnetization preparation. The combination reduces the signal from very slowly flowing blood (e.g., a velocity of 2 cm/s). If a stack of contiguous black blood images is obtained, as in Alexander et al. (1998), then they can be postprocessed with a minimum intensity projection, which is analogous to the maximum intensity projection (Section 15.3), except only the minimum pixel values are retained.

One advantage of black blood methods is that intravoxel dephasing due to complex flow only further reduces the signal from blood, which in this case is helpful. Because regions of complex flow are often observed downstream from a stenosis, bright blood time-of-flight angiography can show signal voids that are a sensitive indicator of disease. Black blood angiography can then be used to improve specificity by providing a better depiction of the stenosis (Edelman et al. 1990). In recent years, however, contrast-enhanced MR angiography (CEMRA) (Section 15.3) has mainly supplanted black blood angiography in performing this role. Even though CEMRA is a bright blood method, it uses a short TE, and its signal enhancement is predominantly due to T_1 shortening caused by the contrast agent, so it is not very prone to signal loss in regions of complex flow. Black blood angiography is still widely used, however, and has become an important tool for cardiac imaging and for studying the vessel wall. Another advantage of black blood methods is that pulsatile flow does not produce ghosting on the image because the signal from blood is eliminated or substantially attenuated.

15.1.1   BLACK BLOOD PULSE SEQUENCE METHODS

RARE and Conventional RF Spin Echo   RARE and conventional RF spin echo can be relatively effective black blood angiographic methods, especially when spatial saturation pulses are added. The main signal loss mechanism is outflow of blood from the imaging slice in between the 90° excitation pulse and the 180° refocusing pulse(s) (Figure 15.1). The suppression of the blood signal becomes more effective as the echo time increases, and typically values in the range of TE $= 40-100$ ms are used. Consider a single-echo RF SE pulse sequence, in which the time between the 90° and 180° pulses is TE/2. There is complete outflow of the excited blood from the imaging slice (of thickness Δz) if the velocity component perpendicular to the slice exceeds:

$$v_\perp = \frac{2\Delta z}{\text{TE}} \tag{15.1}$$

For example, for a single-echo T_2-weighted image acquired with TE $= 80$ ms and a 4-mm slice thickness, good suppression of the blood signal is expected if the component of velocity perpendicular to the slice exceeds 10 cm/s. This condition is met in the major arteries in healthy human subjects.

The second echo image from a dual-echo RF spin echo (Section 14.3) can also be used for black blood angiography. The time gap between the two 180° refocusing pulses is $\text{TE}_2/2$, where TE_2 is the echo time for the second echo. Therefore the total time elapsed between the 90° and second 180° pulses is $(\text{TE}_1 + \text{TE}_2)/2$, and signal loss is expected when the perpendicular velocity component exceeds:

$$v_\perp = \frac{2\Delta z}{\text{TE}_1 + \text{TE}_2} \tag{15.2}$$

which is an easier criterion to meet than Eq. (15.1).

Example 15.1   Suppose a dual-echo T_2-weighted image is acquired with 3-mm-thick slices and $\text{TE}_1 = 30$ ms and $\text{TE}_2 = 80$ ms. If the axis of a vessel makes a 20° angle with the normal to the imaging plane, estimate the minimal blood velocity required to suppress the blood signal on the second echo.

Answer   From Eq. (15.2) the minimal perpendicular component of the velocity that produces black blood signal on the second echo is approximately:

$$v_\perp = \frac{2\Delta z}{TE_1 + TE_2} = \frac{2 \times 0.3}{(30 + 80) \times 10^{-3}} = 5.5 \text{ cm/s}$$

The minimal flow velocity in the vessel is $v = v_\perp / \cos\theta = 5.5/\cos 20° = 5.8$ cm/s.

RARE or fast spin echo acquisition can also provide black blood angiograms and is a preferred method because of its improved acquisition efficiency. To find the analog of Eqs. (15.1) and (15.2), recall that the center of k-space is acquired at an effective echo time TE_{eff} (Section 16.4). The time between the excitation pulse and the refocusing pulse played just before the acquisition of that view is $TE_{eff} - t_{esp}/2$, where t_{esp} is the echo spacing. Therefore signal loss from blood is expected when the perpendicular velocity component exceeds:

$$v_\perp = \frac{\Delta z}{TE_{eff} - t_{esp}/2} \tag{15.3}$$

Figure 15.2 shows an example of a T_2-weighted RARE image of an aneurysm, along with the corresponding bright blood time-of-flight image.

One advantage of using RARE or conventional RF spin echo methods is that the black blood angiograms are obtained for "free," provided the images are acquired anyway for their anatomical information. The main drawback of these

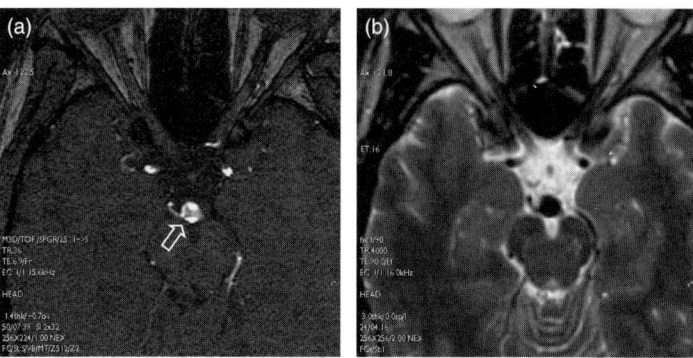

FIGURE 15.2 Basilar tip aneurysm (arrow) imaged in the axial plane. (a) Source image from a bright blood 3DTOF acquisition. (b) Corresponding image from a black blood acquisition, obtained with a RARE pulse sequence and a spatial saturation pulse placed inferior to the slice location. (Courtesy of John Huston, III, M.D., Mayo Clinic College of Medicine.)

methods is the incomplete suppression of blood signal for very slow or recirculating flow. Because an important application of black blood angiography is vessel-wall imaging and the flow speed tends to be lowest near the vessel wall, further refinements to black blood methods have been developed. This has led to an increased popularity of the IR black blood methods that are described next.

Inversion Recovery Black Blood Methods

Single Inversion Recovery Another method to suppress signal from blood is to apply an RF pulse to invert its longitudinal magnetization and then to image after a delay time TI, which is chosen so the inverted longitudinal magnetization recovers to approximately zero (Mayo et al. 1989). This is analogous to the short TI inversion recovery (STIR, Section 14.2) method used to make fat-suppressed images and to the fluid-attenuated inversion recovery (FLAIR, Section 14.2) method used to suppress signals from the CSF. One difference is that the inversion time for black blood methods is longer than that used for STIR but shorter than for FLAIR, because the T_1 of blood is approximately five times that of lipids (approximately 1200 ms vs. 230 ms at 1.5 T) and three to four times shorter than that of CSF. Methods that use only a single inversion pulse are not widely used, however, because the signal from nonflowing tissues that have T_1 values close to that of blood is also suppressed (see Example 14.3), which is undesirable. For example, the blood-myocardium contrast in the heart can be low when a single inversion pulse is used.

Double Inversion Recovery The unwanted suppression of myocardium and other tissue with single inversion recovery can be substantially reduced with the use of double inversion recovery (DIR). As its name implies, DIR uses two inversion pulses (Edelman et al. 1991). The first is a nonselective 180° RF pulse that inverts all of the magnetization within the active volume of the transmit coil; the second RF pulse, which immediately follows, is a selective 180° inversion pulse that is applied only to the imaging slice. The second pulse restores the magnetization to its original state within the imaging slice, while outside the imaging slice the longitudinal magnetization remains inverted.

The DIR magnetization preparation produces a black blood signal because the inverted magnetization flows into the imaging slice. TI is chosen so that the longitudinal magnetization of blood outside the slice recovers from its initial negative value to zero (Figure 15.3). At or near that time, the RF excitation pulse of the host sequence (i.e., the part of the imaging pulse sequence played after the inversion time, as defined in Section 14.2) is applied. A commonly used host sequence is RARE (fast spin echo), with one DIR module applied for each echo train (Simonetti et al. 1996; Fayad et al. 2000). Another option is to use a segmented k-space gradient echo (Edelman et al. 1991; Liu et al.

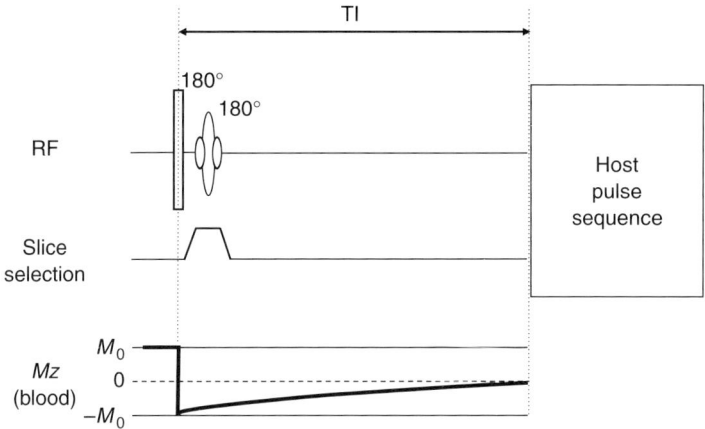

FIGURE 15.3 Magnetization preparation module for DIR. A selective inversion pulse immediately follows a nonselective inversion pulse. Just after the two inversion pulses, the tissue within the imaging slice experiences no net effect, but outside the imaging slice the magnetization is inverted. Blood flows into the imaging slice, but produces no signal because the inversion time TI is selected to null its signal. Adiabatic RF pulses can be used instead of the nonadiabatic pulses shown in this diagram.

1993; Sinha and Sinha 1996) to acquire multiple k-space views with each DIR module, similar to the procedure used in MP-RAGE (Section 14.2).

DIR relies on the inflow of blood into the imaging slice, whereas the non-inversion black blood methods such as RF spin echo rely on outflow. Naturally, inflow occurs at the same rate as outflow, and we could equally well say that DIR relies on the outflow of the noninverted blood from the imaging slice. Despite this similarity, DIR is more effective at suppressing slowly flowing blood because TI in DIR is much longer than TE (or TE_{eff}) in the spin-echo-based methods. Thus, there is more time for the outflow of slowly moving blood to occur. For DIR, the minimum velocity component in Eq. (15.1) is replaced by:

$$v_{\perp} = \frac{\Delta z}{TI} \tag{15.4}$$

A rough estimate of the inversion time TI required to null the blood signal at 1.5 T is:

$$TI \approx T_{1,blood} \times \ln(2) \approx 830 \text{ ms} \tag{15.5}$$

which is much longer than TE (typically 40–100 ms). Equation (15.5) represents an upper limit for the inversion time TI that is valid only when TR is greater than approximately $3 \times T_1$ (Dixon and Ekstrand 1982; Fleckenstein et al. 1991). When partial-saturation effects are accounted for, a more accurate representation of the inversion time that nulls the signal from the blood in an RF spin echo pulse (with TE $\ll$ TR) sequence is:

$$\text{TI} = T_{1,\text{blood}} \times \ln \left(\frac{2}{1 + e^{-\text{TR}/T_{1,\text{blood}}}} \right) \qquad (15.6)$$

(See Section 14.2 for a more complete discussion and similar formulas for other pulse sequences, such as RARE.) Still, TI values of at least 500–600 ms are typically used, so DIR is an effective method to suppress very slow flow.

The nonselective 180° RF inversion pulse in a DIR magnetization preparation module could be either a hard pulse (Section 2.1) or else an adiabatic inversion pulse (Section 6.2), if the B_1 homogeniety is a concern. The selective inversion pulse might be either an SLR inversion pulse (Section 2.3), or a slice-selective adiabatic pulse, such as a hyperbolic secant. The slice thickness of the second inversion pulse can be slightly greater than the thickness of the imaging slice to account for an imperfect slice profile and prevent signal loss. Often spoiler gradients (not shown on Figure 15.3) are applied after the selective inversion pulse to dephase any residual transverse magnetization.

The basic DIR pulse sequence has the drawback that it is limited to single slice-location acquisitions. In order to improve the acquisition efficiency of the method, several variations have been proposed. One method is to play multiple selective 180° inversion pulses during the DIR module, each corresponding to a different slice location. In addition, the slice locations can be interleaved to further increase the acquisition efficiency (Song et al. 2002; Parker et al. 2002). A different strategy (Yarnykh and Yuan 2003) is to use a single selective inversion pulse, but to increase its width so that it covers multiple (e.g., five) slice locations. This method gains acquisition efficiency at the expense of loss of suppression of very slow flow because the slice thickness Δz in Eq. (15.4) increases.

Triple Inversion Recovery　The DIR method can be extended to suppress a second tissue type, which is usually chosen to be the lipids. This is accomplished by adding one more selective 180° RF pulse to the magnetization preparation module (Simonetti et al. 1996), forming a triple inversion recovery (TIR). Figure 15.4 shows a comparison of DIR and TIR images. In the TIR image, both blood and lipid signals are suppressed, whereas only blood is suppressed in the DIR image.

A TIR magnetization preparation module has two inversion times: TI_a is adjusted to suppress blood that flows into the slice, whereas TI_b is adjusted to suppress fat, just like in a standard STIR pulse sequence. Because $T_{1,\text{blood}} > T_{1,\text{fat}}$, the second inversion time TI_b is shorter than the first. It is

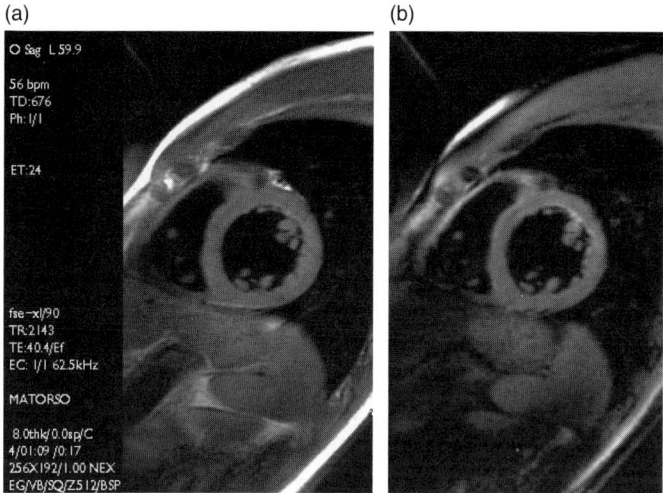

FIGURE 15.4 (a) DIR and (b) TIR short-axis images of the heart of a healthy volunteer. Both images display good suppression of blood signal, but fat is also suppressed on the TIR image. A single slice location is acquired during each 17-s breath-hold, and cardiac triggering is used. (Courtesy of Kiaran McGee, Ph.D., Mayo Clinic College of Medicine.)

usually true that by the time the second selective inversion pulse is played (point B in Figure 15.5), the inverted blood has flowed into the imaging slice. Therefore the inversion times TI_a and TI_b are selected assuming that the magnetization of blood has already crossed zero and is slightly positive at point B, because it will be re-inverted, and has time TI_b to further recover. The following simplified example illustrates some of the principles involved in selecting the two inversion times (also see Simonetti et al. 1996).

Example 15.2 If the T_1 of blood and fat are 1200 and 230 ms at 1.5 T, respectively, find the values of TI_a and TI_b that null both blood and fat. Referring to Figure 15.5, assume the longitudinal magnetization of fat has fully recovered at point B. Also assume that the longitudinal magnetization of blood completely recovers each TR interval (i.e., TR $\gg T_{1,\text{blood}}$).

Answer Because we assume that the longitudinal magnetization of fat has completely recovered to its equilibrium value at point B, the second inversion time TI_b satisfies the equation:

$$\left(1 - 2e^{-TI_b/T_{1,\text{fat}}}\right) = 0 \qquad (15.7)$$

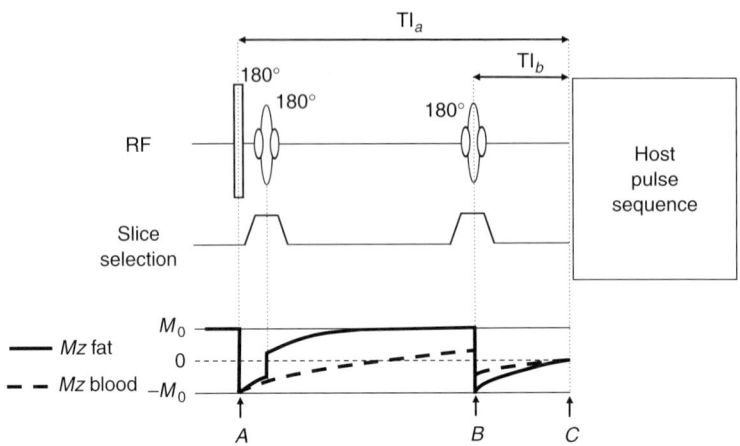

FIGURE 15.5 Magnetization preparation module for TIR. A second selective 180° pulse is added to null the signal from fat. The inversion times TI_a and TI_b are selected so that the longitudinal magnetization of both blood and fat are zero at point C.

or

$$TI_b = T_{1,\text{fat}} \ln(2) = 159 \text{ ms} \tag{15.8}$$

To ensure that the longitudinal magnetization of blood is also zero at point C, the solution to the Bloch equations gives:

$$0 = M_{z,B+} \, e^{-TI_b/T_{1,\text{blood}}} + M_0 \left(1 - e^{-TI_b/T_{1,\text{blood}}} \right) \tag{15.9}$$

where M_0 is the equilibrium longitudinal magnetization of blood, and $M_{z,B+}$ is the longitudinal magnetization of blood just after the second selective inversion pulse. Substituting Eq. (15.8) into (15.9), we find $M_{z,B+} = -0.1421 M_0$. That means that the longitudinal magnetization of the blood flowing into the slice must have recovered to $M_{z,B-} = +0.1421 M_0$ just before the inversion pulse. The T_1 relaxation of the magnetization of blood during the interval between points A and B yields:

$$0.1421 M_0 = M_0 \left(1 - 2e^{-(TI_a - TI_b)/T_{1,\text{blood}}} \right) \tag{15.10}$$

From Eq. (15.10), we obtain $TI_a = 1175$ ms. Because $TI_a - TI_b = 1016$ ms, or approximately 4.4 times the T_1 of fat, the assumption that the longitudinal magnetization of fat has recovered completely at point B is valid in this example. Note that the value of TI_a used for TIR is generally higher than the value of TI used in DIR because the longitudinal magnetization of blood recovers to a positive value at point B. When shorter values of TR are accounted for, for example, using Eq. (15.6), both TI and TI_a are also reduced.

Cardiac Triggering Strategy Because DIR and TIR are commonly used for cardiac and vessel-wall imaging, cardiac triggering is frequently used. A popular cardiac triggering strategy (Simonetti et al. 1996; Fayad et al. 2000) is depicted in Figure 15.6. Because the inversion time is relatively long (~500 ms), the inversion module and the host sequence usually will not fit into a single R-R interval, unless the patient's heart rate is very slow. Instead, the trigger window is open only for every other R-wave, so that the TR time is equal to twice the R-R interval. The inversion module (DIR or TIR) is played immediately after the trigger is detected. After waiting the necessary inversion time(s), the imaging sequence such as RARE or multiple views of a fast gradient echo sequence are played. In some cardiac applications, it is advantageous to restrict the playing of the imaging sequence to diastole, which is feasible at the cost of acquisition efficiency.

SWI Black blood MR venograms can be obtained by exploiting gradient-echo signal loss from the shortened T_2^* of deoxyhemogloblin. A 3D volume is acquired with a spoiled gradient-echo pulse sequence. The images are T_2^*

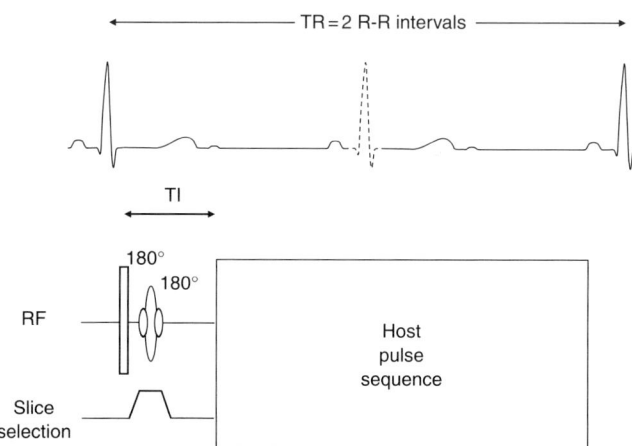

FIGURE 15.6 An acquisition scheme for DIR or TIR with cardiac triggering. Immediately after the detection of the R-wave, the inversion module is played (DIR is shown here). To allow sufficient time for TI and the host sequence, the next QRS complex (dotted line) is skipped, resulting in a TR that is twice the R-R interval.

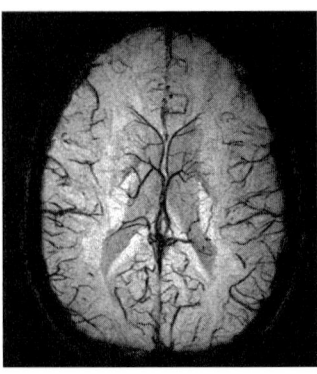

FIGURE 15.7 Axial SWI minimum intensity projection over 13 of the 48 contiguous 2-mm-thick slice locations, demonstrating the connectivity of the veins. The in-plane spatial resolution is 0.5×1 mm^2, and the TE, TR, and flip angle are 15 ms, 33 ms, and 12°, respectively. (Courtesy of E. Mark Haacke Ph.D. and Yingbiao Xu, M.S., Wayne State University, Detroit, Michigan.)

weighted because an echo delay of TE = 15–80 ms is used. Both magnitude and phase images are reconstructed from the same raw k-space data. The phase images are high-pass filtered to remove any slowly varying background phase that is not due to local susceptibility changes. Because the phase images are more sensitive to susceptibility variations than the magnitude images, they are used to calculate a mask image at each slice location, the details of which are described in Reichenbach et al. (1997). The mask images are then applied to the corresponding magnitude images to further accentuate the veins. Because the resulting images form a contiguous volume, they can be postprocessed with a minimum intensity projection. SWI has found applications in tumor evaluation and trauma imaging, as described in Tong et al. (2003). Figure 15.7 shows an example of a minimum intensity projection of a set of SWI images.

SELECTED REFERENCES

Alexander, A. L., Buswell, H. R., Sun, Y., Chapman, B. E., Tsuruda, J. S., and Parker, D. L. 1998. Intracranial black-blood MR angiography with high resolution 3D fast spin echo. *Magn. Reson. Med.* 40: 298–310.

Bradley, W. G., Jr. 1988. Flow phenomena in MR imaging. *Am. J. Roentgenol.* 150: 983–994.

Dixon, R. L., and Ekstrand, K. E. 1982. The physics of proton NMR. *Med. Phys.* 9: 807–818.

Edelman, R. R., Mattle, H. P., Wallner, B., Bajakian, R., Kleefield, J., Kent, C., Skillman, J. J., Mendel, J. B., and Atkinson, D. J. 1990. Extracranial carotid arteries: Evaluation with "black blood" MR angiography. *Radiology* 177: 45–50.

Edelman, R. R., Chien, D., and Kim, D. 1991. Fast selective black blood MR imaging. *Radiology* 181: 655–660.

Fayad, Z. A., Fuster, V., Fallon, J. T., Jayasundera, T., Worthley, S. G., Helft, G., Aguinaldo, J. G., Badimon, J. J., and Sharma, S. K. 2000. Noninvasive in vivo human coronary artery lumen and wall imaging using black-blood magnetic resonance imaging. *Circulation* 102: 506–510.

Fleckenstein, J. L., Archer, B. T., Barker, B. A., Vaughan, J. T., Parkey, R. W., and Peshock, R. M. 1991. Fast short-tau inversion-recovery MR imaging. *Radiology* 179: 499–504.

Liu, Y., Riederer, S. J., and Ehman, R. L. 1993. Magnetization-prepared cardiac imaging using gradient echo acquisition. *Magn. Reson. Med.* 30: 271–275.

Mayo, J. R., Culham, J. A., MacKay, A. L., and Aikins, D. G. 1989. Blood MR signal suppression by preexcitation with inverting pulses. *Radiology* 173: 269–271.

Parker, D. L., Goodrich, K. C., Masiker, M., Tsuruda, J. S., and Katzman, G. L. 2002. Improved efficiency in double-inversion fast spin-echo imaging. *Magn. Reson. Med.* 47: 1017–1021.

Reichenbach, J. R., Venkatesan, R., Schillinger, D. J., Kido, D. K., and Haacke, E. M. 1997. Small vessels in the human brain: MR venography with deoxyhemoglobin as an intrinsic contrast agent. *Radiology* 204: 272–277.

Simonetti, O. P., Finn, J. P., White, R. D., Laub, G., and Henry, D. A. 1996. "Black blood" T2-weighted inversion-recovery MR imaging of the heart. *Radiology* 199: 49–57.

Sinha, S., and Sinha, U. 1996. Black blood dual phase turbo FLASH MR imaging of the heart. *J. Magn. Reson. Imaging* 6: 484–494.

Song, H. K., Wright, A. C., Wolf, R. L., and Wehrli, F. W. 2002. Multislice double inversion pulse sequence for efficient black-blood MRI. *Magn. Reson. Med.* 47: 616–620.

Tong, K. A., Ashwal, S., Holshouser, B. A., Shutter, L. A., Herigault, G., Haacke, E. M., and Kido, D. K. 2003. Improved detection of hemorrhagic shearing lesions in children with post-traumatic diffuse axonal injury: Initial results. *Radiology* 227: 332–339.

Yarnykh, V. L., and Yuan, C. 2003. Multislice double inversion-recovery black-blood imaging with simultaneous slice reinversion. *J. Magn. Reson. Imaging* 17: 478–483.

RELATED SECTIONS

Section 3.2 Inversion Pulses
Section 5.3 Spatial Saturation Pulses
Section 6.2 Adiabatic Inversion Pulses
Section 14.2 Inversion Recovery
Section 14.3 Radiofrequency Spin Echo
Section 15.3 TOF and CEMRA
Section 16.4 RARE

15.2 Phase Contrast

Phase contrast (PC) (Moran 1982; Bryant et al. 1984; Moran et al. 1985) is a method that images moving magnetization by applying flow-encoding gradients. Although the primary use of PC is to image flow within blood vessels, it can also be used for a variety of other applications, such as to image the flow of CSF (Naidich et al. 1993) or to track motion (Drangova et al. 1998). In PC acquisitions, the flow-encoding gradient translates the velocity of the magnetization into the phase of the image. Typically a bipolar gradient (Section 9.2) is used, because it produces a phase that is linearly proportional to velocity. In other words, the flow-encoding gradient used in standard PC acquisitions is a velocity-encoding gradient.

The axis of the bipolar gradient determines the direction of flow sensitivity. Bipolar gradients can be added to any of the three logical gradient axes (slice-selection, frequency-encoding, or phase-encoding), as shown in Figure 15.8. Normally the bipolar gradient is applied to only one axis at a time, but by simultaneously applying them along two or more of the logical axes, flow sensitivity along any arbitrary axis can be achieved. PC pulse sequences are usually formed by adding the flow-encoding gradient lobes to a gradient-echo pulse sequence (usually without RF spoiling). Even faster PC pulse sequences can be obtained by adding flow-encoding gradients to EPI (Debatin et al. 1995) or spiral (Nayak et al. 2000), but to date these have been less widely used.

MR images in general, and gradient echo images in particular, contain other contributions to their phase (e.g., from B_0 inhomogeneity). For this

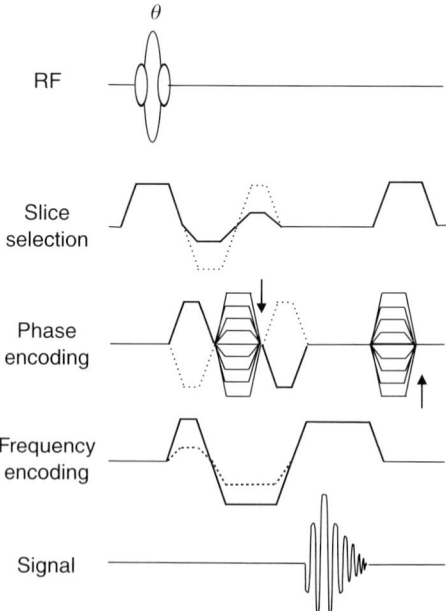

FIGURE 15.8 A typical PC pulse sequence. Toggling of the bipolar gradient (dotted lines) varies the gradient first moment m_1 of the waveforms and introduces flow sensitivity along that axis. Typically a bipolar gradient is added to only one of the three logical axes at a time.

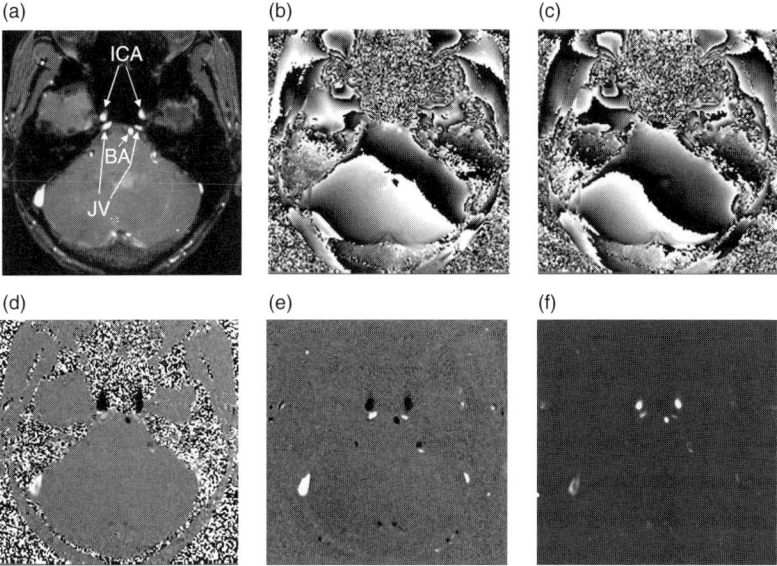

FIGURE 15.9 Axial images of the head of a healthy volunteer. (a) Magnitude reconstruction of the data showing the internal carotid arteries (ICA), jugular veins (JV), and basilar artery (BA). (b) Phase image acquired with the first setting of the bipolar gradient providing flow sensitivity in the superior-to-inferior direction. (c) Phase image with the toggled bipolar gradient. Note that phase errors in (b) and (c) obscure flow information. (d) Phase difference image reconstructed from (b) and (c). Inferior-to-superior flow such as that in the basilar artery is hypointense (black). (e) Magnitude-masked phase difference image obtained from (a) and (d). (f) Complex difference reconstruction.

reason, PC acquires two complete sets of image data with all the imaging parameters held fixed, except for the first moment of the bipolar gradient. Sometimes this is called toggling the bipolar gradient. The phases or the complex values of the two resulting images are subtracted on a pixel-by-pixel basis. The subtraction process accentuates flow while suppressing unwanted phase variation and the stationary tissue background, as illustrated in Figure 15.9. Two different subtraction methods are in common use: the phase difference and complex difference methods. The complex difference method is more robust against partial volume effects; it performs well even when a voxel contains an admixture of both stationary and moving magnetization. The phase difference method, on the other hand, is used to depict the direction of the flow and to quantify volume flow rate through a vessel, for example, in units of milliliters per minute. PC reconstructed with the phase difference reconstruction is also sometimes called velocity mapping or phase-velocity mapping.

Several building blocks of PC acquisition and reconstruction are discussed in other sections of this book, such as flow-encoding gradients (Section 9.2) and phase difference reconstruction (Section 13.5). In addition to describing how those pieces work together, this section also introduces other acquisition and reconstruction modes, including complex difference reconstruction and methods to produce PC images that are sensitive to flow in all three directions.

15.2.1 PHASE CONTRAST ACQUISITION AND RECONSTRUCTION

Bipolar Gradient and VENC The change in the gradient first moment Δm_1 between the two toggles of the bipolar gradient determines the amount of velocity encoding. Therefore, PC requires the operator to prescribe an additional parameter called the aliasing velocity (VENC), which is defined in Section 9.2. The parameter VENC is positive and is inversely related to the change in gradient first moment between the two toggles according to:

$$\text{VENC} = \frac{\pi}{|\gamma \Delta m_1|} \tag{15.11}$$

VENC has units of speed and is usually quoted in centimeters per second. The smaller the value of VENC, the greater is the sensitivity of the acquisition to slow flow. The principles of VENC selection are further discussed in subsection 15.2.2.

Even after the operator selects the value of VENC, there is still considerable latitude in the gradient waveform design. As discussed in Section 9.2, the bipolar gradient can be combined with the other lobes in the imaging waveform to reduce minimum TR and minimum TE. This combination is commonly performed for the frequency-encoding and slice-selection waveforms but not for phase encoding (see Figure 15.8). (For 3D PC pulse sequences, the secondary phase-encoding, bipolar, slab-selection, and slab rephasing gradients can be combined into a total of three lobes.) Also, according to Eq. (15.11), VENC determines the change in the gradient first moment between the two toggles, but not the values of m_1 on the individual waveforms. If we denote a velocity-compensated waveform by $m_1 = 0$, then two possible designs for the gradient waveform toggles are one-sided (i.e., $m_1 = 0$, $m_1 = -\Delta m$) and two-sided (i.e., $m_1 = \Delta m_1/2$, $m_1 = -\Delta m_1/2$), which are described further in Section 9.2 and again later in this section.

Regardless of the velocity-encoding strategy used, the toggling of the bipolar gradient is usually the innermost loop of the acquisition, as shown in Figure 15.10. Keeping the acquisitions for the two settings of the bipolar gradient closely spaced in time minimizes misregistration artifacts due to patient motion when the resulting data are subtracted.

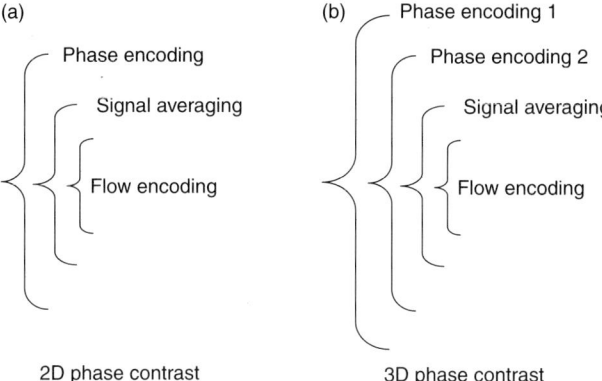

FIGURE 15.10 Looping orders that can be used to acquire PC data in two and three dimensions. The flow encoding (i.e., toggling the bipolar gradient) is the innermost loop to minimize the misregistration artifacts due to patient motion. The slice loop for 2D acquisition is not explicitly shown because it depends on whether we use sequential or interleaved mode (see Figure 11.18).

Example 15.3

(a) Consider the bipolar gradient consisting of two trapezoidal lobes (each with gradient area A) that is played as part of the phase-encoding waveform, as shown in Figure 15.8. Express the width w (including the duration of the ramps) of each trapezoidal lobe in the bipolar gradient in terms of VENC, the total width Δ of the phase-encoding lobe that separates them, the maximum gradient amplitude h, and rise time r. Use the relationship from Section 7.1 that for trapezoidal lobes $w = (A/h) + r$.

(b) If the two lobes in the bipolar gradient are placed next to one another (instead of separated by the phase-encoding lobe), explain why the width of each lobe must be increased if VENC is held fixed. By how much does the width of each lobe increase if VENC $= 10$ cm/s, $h = 30$ mT/m, $r = 0.200$ ms, and $\Delta = 1.15$ ms?

Answer

(a) From Section 9.2, the first moment of each bipolar pair is equal to the product of the area under one of the lobes and the lobe separation. In this case, $m_1 = A(w + \Delta)$. The change in first moment as the bipolar lobe is toggled is:

$$\Delta m_1 = 2m_1 = 2A(w + \Delta) = \frac{\pi}{\gamma \text{VENC}} \qquad (15.12)$$

Substituting $A = h(w - r)$ into Eq. (15.12) yields a quadratic equation for the lobe width w. The physically meaningful solution is:

$$w = \frac{r - \Delta + \sqrt{(r + \Delta)^2 + 2\pi/(\gamma h \text{VENC})}}{2} \tag{15.13}$$

(b) Bringing the two bipolar lobes closer together decreases their moment arm and consequently increases the gradient area necessary to produce a given first moment. We can use Eq. (15.13) with $\Delta = 0$ to calculate what the width of each lobe would be if they were adjacent:

$$w|_{\Delta=0}$$

$$= \frac{1}{2} \left(2 \times 10^{-4} \text{s} \right.$$

$$\left. + \sqrt{(2 \times 10^{-4}\text{s})^2 + \frac{1}{(30 \times 10^{-3} \text{ T/m})(42.57 \text{ MHz/T})(0.1 \text{ m/s})}} \right)$$

$$= 1.503 \text{ ms}$$

Similarly, from Eq. (15.13), $w|_{\Delta=1.15 \text{ ms}} = 1.078$ ms. So separating the lobes saves nearly one-half of a millisecond on the duration of each lobe. Finally, we note that if VENC is sufficiently high so that $w < 2r$, then Eq. (15.13) is no longer valid because triangular lobes are more time-efficient than trapezoids in achieving the desired gradient area. In this particular example, the transition occurs when VENC > 63.15 cm/s.

Phase-Difference Reconstruction Phase-difference reconstruction is performed in the image domain, as detailed in Section 13.5. PC images reconstructed with phase difference have two main applications: determining the flow direction and quantifying flow velocity and volume flow rate. The phase difference (in radians) of a pixel is given by:

$$\Delta\phi = \gamma \Delta m_1 v = \frac{v}{\text{VENC}} \pi \tag{15.14}$$

where v is the flow velocity. Because the dynamic range of phase-difference reconstruction is limited to $\pm\pi$ (i.e., $\pm180°$), we can only reliably determine the flow direction when $|v| \leq$ VENC, unless the phase is unwrapped with a postprocessing algorithm (see Sections 13.5 and 17.3). As long as VENC is sufficiently high, then we can extract the quantitative velocity from the measured phase difference by rearranging Eq. (15.14):

$$v = \left(\frac{\Delta\phi}{\pi}\right) \text{VENC} \qquad -\text{VENC} < v < \text{VENC} \qquad (15.15)$$

The sign of the phase difference tracks the sign of v, so we also can determine the flow direction from the sign of $\Delta\phi$.

If $|v| > \text{VENC}$ then it is said that velocity aliasing, flow-related aliasing, or flow aliasing occurs. Flow aliasing always results in the speed of the magnetization being incorrectly represented in the image as a lower value. On signed images reconstructed with phase-difference processing, flow aliasing also results in the incorrect representation of the direction of flow when:

$$1 < \left|\frac{v}{\text{VENC}}\right| < 2, \quad 3 < \left|\frac{v}{\text{VENC}}\right| < 4, \quad \dots \qquad (15.16)$$

as indicated on Figure 15.11. Therefore, if the primary goal of the exam is to determine flow direction, VENC should be chosen to be larger than the fastest speed expected in the vessel.

Sometimes, in order to suppress the background noise in air, phase difference images are magnitude-masked during image reconstruction (see Section 13.5). This is accomplished by multiplying (on a pixel-by-pixel basis) the phase difference $\Delta\phi$ by a magnitude image M reconstructed from the same raw data. For example, M can be obtained by averaging the two magnitude images obtained from the two k-space data sets used to make the phase-difference image. This is the preferred method for two-sided encoding because

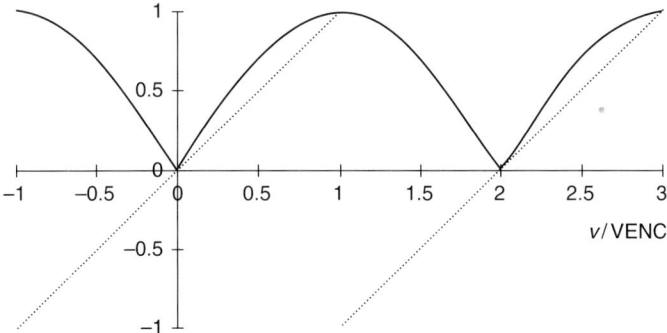

FIGURE 15.11 Plots showing the normalized phase-difference $\Delta\phi/\pi$ (dotted lines) and normalized complex-difference CD/(2M) signal, as calculated with Eqs. (15.14) and (15.25), respectively.

averaging improves the SNR of the magnitude mask. For one-sided encoding, however, the preferred magnitude mask is usually reconstructed solely from the velocity-compensated acquisition because it is expected to have the fewest flow artifacts. In addition to suppressing the noise background in air, magnitude masking can also increase the vessel conspicuity, especially if the magnitude image displays flow-related enhancement. Figures 15.9a, d, and e illustrate this point.

The SNR for phase-difference (as well as magnitude-masked phase-difference and complex-difference) images can be calculated, as detailed in Conturo and Smith (1990) and Bernstein and Ikezaki (1991). A representative result is that the SNR for a PC image using phase-difference reconstruction is:

$$\text{SNR}_{\Delta\phi} \propto \text{SNR}_{\text{mag}} \times \left(\frac{|v|}{\text{VENC}} \right) \qquad |v| < \text{VENC} \qquad (15.17)$$

where SNR_{mag} is the SNR that would be obtained if the k-space data (from either toggle of the bipolar gradient) were used to reconstruct a standard magnitude image.

Flow Quantification   The extraction of velocity and flow information with the postprocessing of PC images is called flow analysis, flow quantitation, or flow quantification. The flow velocity (in centimeters per second) can be obtained by using Eq. (15.15). If the voxel contains a distribution of velocity values, the measured value of v is not necessarily equal to the average velocity because the trigonometric functions used to calculate the phase difference (e.g., arctangent) are nonlinear. If the spread in velocities is small enough so that trigonometric functions can be well approximated by a linear function over that range, then the measured value of v will be close to the average velocity component within the voxel along the direction of the flow-encoding gradient. This is illustrated by the trigonometric identity:

$$\tan(x + \Delta x) = \frac{\tan(x) + \tan(\Delta x)}{1 - \tan(x)\tan(\Delta x)} \qquad (15.18)$$

For $\Delta x \ll 1$, the denominator is approximately equal to unity, and $\tan(x + \Delta x) \approx \tan(x) + \tan(\Delta x)$. In that case, the tangent function (and hence the arctangent function) is linear. An exception is when flow aliasing occurs, in which case even a small change in velocity produces an abrupt change in the phase difference.

The volume flow rates through a pixel Q_{pixel} (in milliliters per minute) are given by the product of the pixel area a (in square centimeters) and the average velocity (in centimeters per second):

$$Q_{\text{pixel}} = 60av \tag{15.19}$$

where the factor of 60 converts values from per second to per minute. To find the volume flow rate through an entire vessel, a region of interest (ROI) is placed over the vessel in the image, either manually or semiautomatically with the aid of a computer algorithm. The volume flow rate through all the individual pixels that cover the vessel is summed. Because all the pixels have the same area, a is a constant in the summation, and:

$$Q_{\text{tot}} = \sum_{i \text{ pixels}} 60a_i v_i = 60a \sum_{i \text{ pixels}} v_i \tag{15.20}$$

The acquisition used for flow quantification is usually thin-slice (e.g., $\Delta z = 3$ mm) PC with the scan plane oriented so that it cuts the vessel in cross section. The bipolar gradient is played on the slice-selection axis, that is, along the direction of the flow in the vessel. Fortunately the method works reasonably well even if the scan plane is not precisely perpendicular to the flow. As illustrated in Figure 15.12, the velocity component along the slice direction becomes $v \cos \beta$, while, for small values of β, the number of pixels in the intersection of the vessel and scan plane is increased by a factor $1/\cos \beta$. To a first-order approximation, the product of perpendicular velocity component and total cross-sectional area used in Eq. (15.20) is independent of β. The maximal acceptable value β increases as the slice thickness decreases, but values as high as 30° are usually tolerable.

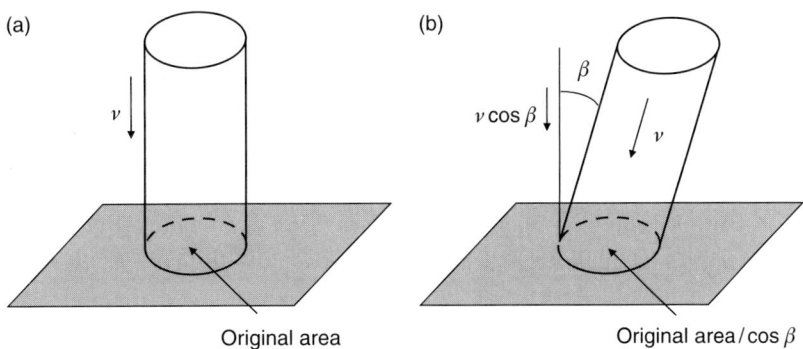

FIGURE 15.12 To a first-order approximation, the quantification of the volume flow rate docs not require the vessel to be precisely perpendicular to the imaging slice because the decrease in the velocity component is compensated for by an increase in the area of intersection.

It is often useful to obtain a time-resolved depiction of the flow (Nayler et al. 1986; Pelc, Herfkens et al. 1991), especially for quantifying pulsatile flow in arteries. In this case, PC is acquired with the retrospective ECG gating or prospective ECG triggering modes described in Section 11.5. Often segmented k-space acquisition and view sharing reconstruction (Section 13.6) are used to reduce the scan time and increase the number of reconstructed cardiac phases. If the heart rate is known, the total volume flow per cardiac cycle in milliliters can be calculated from the product of the time-averaged volume flow rate in milliliters per minutes and the R-R interval (expressed in minutes). In many cases an examination obtained without cardiac triggering can provide a good estimate of the average flow rate. Although the standard time-resolved acquisitions are 2D, 3D volume PC acquisitions have also been demonstrated (Markl, Chan et al. 2003).

Although in principle underlying flow quantification is relatively simple, it can be challenging in practice because there are several potential systematic errors. Flow quantification results that are within 10% of the true value are generally considered good. A few of the major systematic errors are mentioned here, and Wolf et al. (1993), Tang et al. (1993), and Pelc et al. (1994) contain more complete discussions.

The exact determination of the vessel boundary can be difficult because of partial volume effects for pixels that overlap the edge of the vessel. It is helpful to use a magnitude image reconstructed from the PC k-space data to help define the ROI boundary because the vessel wall is sometimes better delineated than on the corresponding phase-difference image. The volume flow rate for those edge pixels also tends to be systematically overestimated because the area a used in the calculation represents the entire pixel, but in reality only a fraction of the pixel contains flow. Using high spatial resolution can reduce this error. In this context, high spatial resolution means that approximately 16 or more isotropic pixels cover the vessel lumen. Lower flip angles (e.g., 30° instead of 60°) can also help because the use of higher flip angles suppresses stationary tissue, as in 2D time-of-flight angiography. When the stationary tissue is suppressed, the measured phase difference for the entire voxel is determined predominantly by flowing blood, even when it occupies only a small fraction of the voxel. The partial volume error tends to cause an overestimation of flow in that voxel.

Although partial volume often dominates, several other effects contribute to the errors in flow quantification. The concomitant field contributes an error to the phase, but fortunately this can be corrected for exactly during the phase-difference reconstruction, as described in Section 13.5. Generally more troublesome are phase errors from residual eddy currents that remain even after the waveform preemphasis techniques described in Section 10.3 are applied. Eddy currents depend on the specific hardware, so they cannot be easily predicted. Unlike phase errors from B_0 inhomogeneity, the phase error from eddy currents generally does not subtract out during the phase-difference reconstruction because the two toggles of bipolar gradient waveform produce different eddy-current patterns. Phase errors resulting from eddy currents have slow spatial variation, however, so they can be corrected for during the flow quantification postprocessing. Usually a small ROI is placed over a region that contains stationary tissue (*not* the air background) near the vessel of interest. If the concomitant-field phase error is properly removed and bulk motion is negligible, then a nonzero phase in that region can be assumed to be solely from eddy currents. A polynomial fit is applied in two dimensions, and the fitted phase is extrapolated to the vessel ROI, where it is subtracted from the measured phase.

If the gradient second (or higher) moment changes when the bipolar gradient is toggled, then acceleration (or higher derivatives of motion) can contaminate the measured phase difference. Usually this effect is small for typical physiological accelerations and commonly used gradient waveforms. Another effect of acceleration in PC is a spatial displacement artifact of the vessel location arising because spatial and velocity encoding have not been applied simultaneously (Fayne and Rutt 1995).

The spatial nonlinearity of the gradients causes yet another systematic error in flow quantification. This effect is usually negligible, but it becomes quite important far from the gradient isocenter. A further discussion of gradient nonlinearity effects in PC is provided in Markl, Bammer et al. (2003).

Complex-Difference Reconstruction   Complex-difference reconstruction is accomplished by subtracting the complex data obtained from the two toggles of the bipolar gradient. After the subtraction, a magnitude image is formed from the result. Figure 15.9f shows an example of an image reconstructed with complex difference. Because the inverse Fourier transform is a linear operation, the subtraction can be performed either in the k-space (Dumoulin et al. 1989) or in the image domain.

Performing the subtraction in the k-space domain can be simpler to implement because most scanners have existing data acquisition software that can add or subtract k-space data. Even if a scanner only has the capability to add k-space data together (e.g., for signal averaging) the subtraction can be implemented by negating the polarity of the RF excitation pulse when the bipolar gradient is toggled (i.e., chopping the RF to produce a negative signal). An advantage of performing the subtraction in the k-space domain is that the resulting complex difference can then be reconstructed with partial Fourier reconstruction methods such as homodyne (see Section 13.4), if desired.

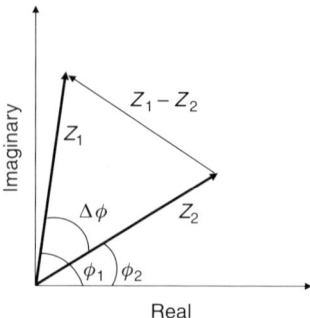

FIGURE 15.13 Diagram for the calculation of the complex difference in the image domain. The complex numbers Z_1 and Z_2 are depicted as vectors and represent the signal within corresponding voxels in the two images acquired with the two settings of the bipolar gradient.

The complex difference can be performed in the image domain instead. Complex image data from the two acquisitions can be directly subtracted on a pixel-by-pixel basis, but this is equivalent to k-space subtraction. Instead, consider the image domain subtraction suggested by Figure 15.13. Using the notation in Section 13.5, let Z_1 and Z_2 be the complex values for two corresponding pixels on images reconstructed from the k-space data corresponding to the two toggles of the bipolar gradient. Then if we denote the magnitude of the complex difference for a particular pixel by CD.

$$CD = |Z_1 - Z_2| = ||Z_1|e^{i\phi_1} - |Z_2|e^{i\phi_2}| \qquad (15.21)$$

Recalling that the phase difference is given by $\Delta\phi = \phi_1 - \phi_2$ and $|e^{i\phi_2}| = 1$:

$$CD = ||Z_1|e^{i\Delta\phi} - |Z_2|| = \sqrt{|Z_1|^2 + |Z_2|^2 - 2|Z_1||Z_2|\cos(\Delta\phi)} \qquad (15.22)$$

Equation (15.22) is equivalent to applying the law of cosines to the triangle represented in Figure 15.13. The main advantage of calculating CD in the image domain is the ability to apply phase correction, that is, to correct for the concomitant field and residual eddy currents (see Sections 10.1 and 13.5). Substituting a phase-corrected phase difference $\Delta\phi_{corr}$ into Eq. (15.22) provides a phase-corrected complex difference:

$$CD_{corr} = \sqrt{|Z_1|^2 + |Z_2|^2 - 2|Z_1||Z_2|\cos(\Delta\phi_{corr})} \qquad (15.23)$$

Usually the eddy-current phase correction used in Eq. (15.23) proceeds without the operator intervention described earlier in this section. One method is to magnitude-mask the phase-difference image to reduce noise (see Section 13.5) and then to fit the phase across the entire image with linear functions by minimizing the least-squares deviation.

Sometimes we can assume that the magnitude of corresponding pixels of the images reconstructed from the two toggles of the bipolar gradient are nearly equal, $|Z_1| \approx |Z_2|$. This is often true, especially for the two-sided encoding strategy mentioned earlier. If we assume that $|Z_1| = |Z_2| = M$ and apply the trigonometric identity $1 - \cos x = 2 \sin^2(x/2)$, Eq. (15.22) reduces to:

$$\text{CD} = \sqrt{2} M \sqrt{1 - \cos(\Delta\phi)} = 2M \left| \sin\left(\frac{\Delta\phi}{2}\right) \right| \qquad (15.24)$$

Using the definition of VENC, the complex difference becomes:

$$\text{CD} = 2M \left| \sin\left(\frac{\pi v}{2\,\text{VENC}}\right) \right| \qquad (15.25)$$

Unlike the phase difference, the complex difference does not display discontinuities and does not take on negative values. It does, however, have a discontinuous first derivative at $v = 0, \pm 2$ VENC, ± 4 VENC, ..., as illustrated in Figure 15.11. The discontinuity of the derivative generally does not cause any image quality problems, since the image intensity is zero.

Partial Volume Effects in PC   The phase- and complex-difference reconstruction methods perform quite differently when a voxel contains both stationary and flowing magnetization. The diagram in Figure 15.14 illustrates

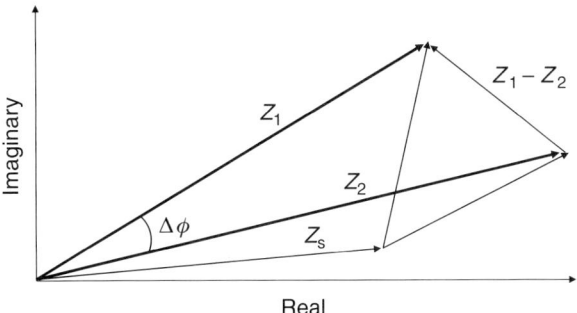

FIGURE 15.14 Modification to Figure 15.13 showing a stationary tissue contribution Z_s to the complex signal within a voxel. Unlike the phase difference $\Delta\phi$, the complex difference $|Z_1 - Z_2|$ is not affected by the presence of stationary tissue.

these effects by including a stationary tissue contribution Z_s, which in general can have an arbitrary phase. The complex difference CD $= |Z_1 - Z_2|$ is unaffected because Z_s is a common term and subtracts out. In the example shown in Figure 15.14, the phase difference $\Delta\phi$ is reduced compared to its value when $Z_s = 0$. The value of the phase difference can increase, decrease, become equal to zero, or change sign. A more complete discussion is provided in Bernstein and Ikezaki (1991). In practice, the sensitivity of the phase-difference reconstruction to partial volume effects means that the complex difference is usually preferred to reconstruct images, unless directional flow or quantitative information is required. In that case, the acquisition parameters are chosen so that partial volume effects are minimal (e.g., thin slices are used).

An effective way to deal with partial volume effects, is to increase the number of settings of the flow-encoding gradient beyond the standard number (two) used in phase contrast. Weber et al. (1993) describes one method to accomplish this, and the Fourier velocity-encoding method described in Section 9.2 is another. With Fourier velocity encoding, the stationary tissue contribution to the signal is placed in its own velocity bin, that is, the zero-frequency (DC) output of the discrete Fourier transform (DFT). It is interesting to recall from Section 1.1 that the DFT of a signal with two complex points (d_0, d_1) is given by the complex sum and difference: $(d_0 + d_1, d_0 - d_1)$. Thus the complex difference CD can be interpreted as the magnitude of the second element of the DFT. This interpretation helps to explain the complex-difference method's robustness against partial volume artifacts.

Image Sensitive to Flow in All Three Directions   The PC methods discussed so far are sensitive to flow along a single spatial direction. Sometimes an image that is sensitive to flow regardless of the direction of motion (Dumoulin et al. 1989) is desired. This type of phase-contrast image is sometimes called a speed or a three-direction image. A three-direction image is calculated by taking the square root of the sum of the squares of three PC images on a pixel-by-pixel basis. Each of the three individual PC images has the same acquisition parameters (matrix, field of view, slice location, etc.), but is sensitive to flow along a direction that is orthogonal to the other two. The values of VENC for the three logical directions need not be the same, resulting in what is sometimes called a multivenc acquisition. For simplicity, however, a common value of VENC is usually used, except for applications in which flow velocity is highly anisotropic, such as in the legs. Often the three individual images that make up the three-direction image are each reconstructed using the complex-difference method because three-direction images are not used to quantify flow and the signs of the individual flow-direction images are lost during the sum-of-squares operation anyway. A pixel value denoted by S in the three-direction image is calculated by:

$$S = \sqrt{CD_{Freq}^2 + CD_{PE}^2 + CD_{Slice}^2} \qquad (15.26)$$

where CD is a complex image reconstructed with Eq. (15.23), and the subscripts represent velocity encoding along one of the logical directions: frequency encoding, phase encoding, or slice selection. If desired, both complex-difference and phase-difference images can be reconstructed from the same k-space data set. For example, complex-difference images can be used to produce a three-direction image as in Eq. (15.26), while a separate set of phase-difference images can be reconstructed for each flow direction to provide directional and quantitative information. Information obtained from the complex-difference reconstruction can be used to reduce partial volume effects in the phase-difference images (Polzin et al. 1995).

A straightforward method for obtaining the data for the three-direction image is to acquire a total of six data sets, i.e., a pair with the bipolar gradient toggled for each of the three directions. Sometimes this is called a six-set or six-point acquisition. In order to minimize misregistration artifacts from patient motion, the toggling of the bipolar gradient is usually the innermost loop for this acquisition, followed by the three flow directions.

The scan time needed to acquire the data for a three-direction image can be reduced by 33% by using a common reference image for the three subtractions (Pelc, Bernstein et al. 1991, Hausmann et al. 1991; Conturo and Robinson 1992). This method is sometimes called a four-set or four-point acquisition. Similar to the six-point method, the toggling of the bipolar gradients is usually the innermost loop of the acquisition. One strategy for a four-point acquisition is to first obtain a reference view that, for example, could be velocity compensated (i.e., $m_1 = 0$) on all three axes. Then for the subsequent three views, the gradient waveforms are varied on one axis at a time to achieve the required change in first moment Δm_1 in each direction. For example, the second view would have first moments equal to $(-\Delta m_1, 0, 0)$, the third view $(0, -\Delta m_1, 0)$, and the fourth view $(0, 0, -\Delta m_1)$. (This is analogous to acquiring a common image with $b = 0$ in diffusion trace-weighted imaging and diffusion tensor imaging, as described in Section 17.2.) This strategy is sometimes called a simple four-point method. To obtain an image sensitive to flow in the readout direction, the data from the second view is subtracted from the reference view, and so on. The simple four-point method can also use two-sided encoding if the first moments of the reference scan equal to $\Delta m_1/2$ on each of the three gradient axes. In that case, the first moment on three axes for the second acquisition would be $(-\Delta m_1/2, +\Delta m_1/2, +\Delta m_1/2)$, respectively.

As an alternative to the simple four-point method, the bipolar gradients can be toggled on two axes at once. This is called a balanced-four point or

Hadamard velocity encoding. To obtain a phase-difference image proportional to velocity along a single axis, a Hadamard decoding reconstruction is used, which involves linear combinations of all four data sets. Despite this complexity, the Hadamard velocity-encoding strategy can offer some advantages in SNR and flow aliasing properties, as explained in Pelc, Bernstein et al. (1991).

15.2.2 PRACTICAL CONSIDERATIONS

A PC prescription requires the operator to select the VENC parameter. Equations (15.15) and (15.17) illustrate the dilemma: If VENC is too small, flow aliasing results; if VENC is too large, the sensitivity is poor, resulting in a poor SNR in the PC image. For PC images reconstructed by complex difference, some flow aliasing is more tolerable because there are no discontinuities when the signal is plotted versus velocity (Figure 15.11). The inverse dependence of the SNR on VENC also illustrates the value of phase unwrapping methods. Even if only one phase wrap can be removed, the dynamic range is doubled, and VENC can be cut in half. This doubles the SNR and allows the imaging time to be cut by a factor of four.

In practice, values selected for VENC depend on the vessel to be imaged and the reconstruction method. For example, to image the internal carotid artery VENC = 80–100 cm/s can be selected for phase-difference reconstruction, whereas VENC = 40–50 cm/s is more typical for complex-difference reconstruction. These are consistent with the range of peak velocities measured with Doppler ultrasound, 80–120 cm/s (De Witt and Wechsler 1999), keeping in mind that the average velocity over a voxel is smaller than its peak value and that some flow aliasing is usually acceptable in complex difference images. More discussion of VENC selection is provided in Turski and Korosec (1993).

Equation (15.17) also illustrates that the vessel SNR in PC can be improved by selecting image parameters that increase SNR_{mag}, such as selecting a good time-of-flight imaging protocol. An exception occurs for flow quantification in which, as mentioned earlier, too much flow-related enhancement can cause a systematic overestimation of the volume flow rate.

It is useful to minimize the echo time TE in phase-contrast acquisitions. This reduces signal loss from T_2^* dephasing and can also reduce higher-gradient moments (m_2, m_3, etc.) that introduce an error into Eq. (15.14) when the magnetization accelerates or experiences higher derivatives of motion. Therefore, PC acquisitions usually use partial echoes to minimize TE, as shown in Figure 15.8. A simple partial Fourier reconstruction such as zero-filling is used because (with the exception of k-space subtraction complex difference) more advanced methods such as homodyne are not compatible with PC. As explained in Section 13.4, using a fractional echo percentage that is too small in conjunction with zero-filling as a partial-echo reconstruction method degrades the image quality. A typical fractional echo percentage for PC is 70–80%.

In addition to thin-slice 2D and 3D volume acquisitions, PC can be acquired in 2D projection mode or thick-slab acquisitions. Whereas 3D PC images are often displayed using the maximum intensity projection (MIP, see Section 15.3), 2D thick-slab images acquire the entire volume of interest in a single slice and do not require MIP to show the path of a vessel. Due to the large amount of stationary tissue in the voxel, a twister (projection dephaser) gradient (Section 10.6) can be used to dephase the thick stationary slab while preserving signal from the vessels that are thinner. A four- or six-set acquisition gives flow sensitivity in all three directions. It is necessary to use complex-difference reconstruction to avoid severe partial volume artifacts. The twister gradient does not need to be played as a dedicated lobe because its area can be absorbed into any of the three existing lobes on the slice-selection axis that precede the readout, as shown in Figure 15.8.

Excellent stationary tissue suppression is an important advantage of PC. This is particularly valuable after the injection of gadolinium-based contrast agents, which can increase the signal of the stationary tissue background on time-of-flight images. Also, because time-of-flight images are essentially T_1-weighted fast scans, thrombus can appear bright (hyperintense) and be mistaken for flow. PC images can be used to show the true stationary nature of the thrombus. PC images can also be used to detect retrograde flow, for example in a subclavian steal (Figure 15.15). Although time-of-flight images can also be used to determine the direction of flow with the use of spatial saturation pulses, that method requires the prospective placement of the saturation pulses. PC can determine flow direction retrospectively, as long as VENC is set high enough to avoid flow aliasing in the vessel of interest.

Phase-contrast methods currently are not as widely used as time-of-flight and contrast-enhanced methods. One drawback of phase-contrast imaging is that the bipolar gradients can increase intravoxel dephasing because they necessarily increase minimum TE, diffusion-induced phase dispersion, and gradient moments. The main drawback of phase contrast, however, has been its relatively long acquisition time compared to time-of-flight imaging (twice as long for a single-direction flow image and at least four times as long for a three-direction image, if the TR is held fixed). 3D phase contrast, which is acquired without signal averaging (NEX = 1) is an excellent application for parallel imaging techniques such as SENSE. As phased array RF coils compatible with SENSE are more widely deployed, the use of 3D PC will probably increase. Figure 15.16 shows an example of a 3D PC image in which the acquisition time has been reduced from 42 to 7 min by using SENSE.

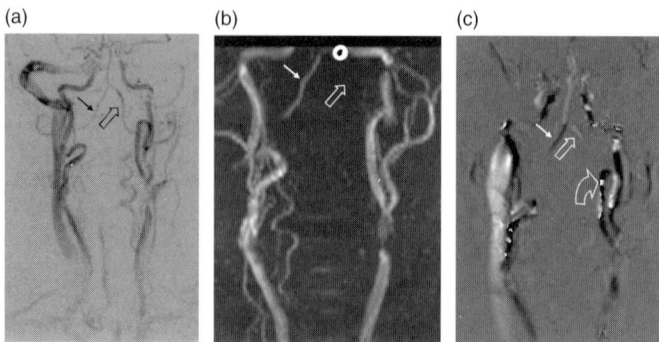

(a)   (b)   (c)

FIGURE 15.15 (a) Coronal thick-slab three-direction phase-contrast image reconstructed with complex difference. The major vessels of neck are visualized, including
the right and left vertebral arteries (thin and hollow arrows, respectively). (b) Coronal
2DTOF maximum intensity projection of the same patient. The hollow arrow indicates
a subclavian steal (i.e., retrograde flow in the left vertebral), which cannot be visualized
on this image due to the spatial saturation pulses that are applied superior to the 2DTOF
slices. (c) Magnitude-masked PC image with VENC = 50 cm/s, sensitive to flow in
the superior-to-inferior direction, confirming the retrograde flow in the basilar and left
vertebral arteries. Also note the abrupt transition between positive and negative pixel
values (curved arrow) indicating flow-related aliasing in the carotid arteries. (Courtesy
of John Huston, III, M.D., Mayo Clinic College of Medicine.)

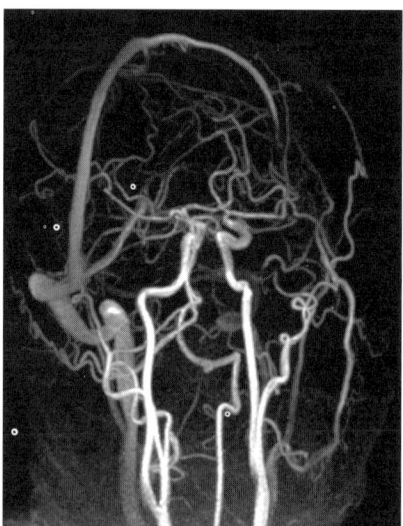

FIGURE 15.16 MIP projection of 3D PC acquisition of the whole brain using an eight-
element head coil and SENSE. No contrast agent is present, and complex difference
reconstruction is used. The voxel dimension is $1.0 \times 1.0 \times 1.2$ mm^3 prior to zero-filling.
TE, TR, flip angle, and VENC are 5.1 ms, 20 ms, 15°, and 40 cm/s, respectively. The
SENSE acceleration factor of 6 reduced the acquisition time from 42 to 7 min. (Courtesy
of Romhild M. Hoogeveen, Ph.D., Philips Medical Systems.)

Example 15.4 A 3D PC acquisition is acquired with flow sensitivity in all three directions, a TR = 15 ms, and a $256 \times 192 \times 192$ acquisition matrix. How long is the acquisition time?

Answer Assuming that four-point encoding is used, the imaging time is:

$$192^2 \times 4 \times 0.015 \text{ s} = 2212 \text{ s}$$

or nearly 37 min.

SELECTED REFERENCES

Bernstein, M. A., and Ikezaki, Y. 1991. Comparison of phase-difference and complex-difference processing in phase-contrast MR angiography. *J. Magn. Reson. Imaging* 1: 725–729.

Bryant, D. J., Payne, J. A., Firmin, D. N., and Longmore, D. B. 1984. Measurement of flow with NMR imaging using a gradient pulse and phase difference technique. *J. Comput. Assist. Tomogr.* 8: 588–593.

Conturo, T. E., and Robinson, B. H. 1992. Analysis of encoding efficiency in MR imaging of velocity magnitude and direction. *Magn. Reson. Med.* 25: 233–247.

Conturo, T. E., and Smith, G. D. 1990. Signal-to-noise in phase angle reconstruction: Dynamic range extension using phase reference offsets. *Magn. Reson. Med.* 15: 420–437.

Debatin, J. F., Leung, D. A., Wildermuth, S., Botnar, R., Felblinger, J., and McKinnon, G. C. 1995. Flow quantitation with echo-planar phase-contrast velocity mapping: In vitro and in vivo evaluation. *J. Magn. Reson. Imaging* 5: 656–662.

DeWitt, L. D., and Wechsler, L. R. 1988. Transcranial doppler. *Stroke* 19: 915–921.

Drangova, M., Zhu, Y., Bowman, B., and Pelc, N. J. 1998. In vitro verification of myocardial motion tracking from phase-contrast velocity data. *Magn. Reson. Imaging* 16: 863–870.

Dumoulin, C. L., Souza, S. P., Walker, M. F., and Wagle, W. 1989. Three-dimensional phase contrast angiography. *Magn. Reson. Med.* 9: 139–149.

Frayne, R., and Rutt, B. K. 1995. Understanding acceleration-induced displacement artifacts in phase-contrast MR velocity measurements. *J. Magn. Reson. Imaging* 5: 207–215.

Hausmann, R., Lewin, J. S., and Laub, G. 1991. Phase-contrast MR angiography with reduced acquisition time: New concepts in sequence design. *J. Magn. Reson. Imaging* 1: 415–422.

Markl, M., Bammer, R., Alley, M. T., Elkins, C. J., Draney, M. T., Barnett, A., Moseley, M. E., Glover, G. H., and Pelc, N. J. 2003. Generalized reconstruction of phase contrast MRI: Analysis and correction of the effect of gradient field distortions. *Magn. Reson. Med.* 50: 791–801.

Markl, M., Chan, F. P., Alley, M. T., Wedding, K. L., Draney, M. T., Elkins, C. J., Parker, D. W., Wicker, R., Taylor, C. A., Herfkens, R. J., and Pelc, N. J. 2003. Time-resolved three-dimensional phase-contrast MRI. *J. Magn. Reson. Imaging* 17: 499–506.

Moran, P. R. 1982. A flow velocity zeugmatographic interlace for NMR imaging in humans. *Magn. Reson. Imaging* 1: 197–203.

Moran, P. R., Moran, R. A., and Karstaedt, N. 1985. Verification and evaluation of internal flow and motion. True magnetic resonance imaging by the phase gradient modulation method. *Radiology* 154: 433–441.

Naidich, T. P., Altman, N. R., and Gonzalez-Arias, S. M. 1993. Phase contrast cine magnetic resonance imaging: Normal cerebrospinal fluid oscillation and applications to hydrocephalus. *Neurosurg. Clin. N. Am.* 4: 677–705.

Nayak, K. S., Pauly, J. M., Kerr, A. B., Hu, B. S., and Nishimura, D. G. 2000. Real-time color flow MRI. *Magn. Reson. Med.* 43: 251–258.

Nayler, G. L., Firmin, D. N., and Longmore, D. B. 1986. Blood flow imaging by cine magnetic resonance. *J. Comput. Assist. Tomogr.* 10: 715–722.

Pelc, N. J., Bernstein, M. A., Shimakawa, A., and Glover, G. H. 1991. Encoding strategies for three-direction phase-contrast MR imaging of flow. *J. Magn. Reson. Imaging* 1: 405–413.

Pelc, N. J., Herfkens, R. J., Shimakawa, A., and Enzmann, D. R. 1991. Phase contrast cine magnetic resonance imaging. *Magn. Reson. Q.* 7: 229–254.

Pelc, N. J., Sommer, F. G., Li, K. C., Brosnan, T. J., Herfkens, R. J., and Enzmann, D. R. 1994. Quantitative magnetic resonance flow imaging. *Magn. Reson. Q.* 10: 125–147.

Polzin, J. A., Alley, M. T., Korosec, F. R., Grist, T. M., Wang, Y., and Mistretta, C. A. 1995. A complex-difference phase-contrast technique for measurement of volume flow rates. *J. Magn. Reson. Imaging* 5: 129–137.

Tang, C., Blatter, D. D., and Parker, D. L. 1993. Accuracy of phase-contrast flow measurements in the presence of partial-volume effects. *J. Magn. Reson. Imaging* 3: 377–385.

Turski, P. A., and Korosec, F. R. 1993. Phase contrast angiography. In *Clinical magnetic resonance angiography* edited by C. M. Anderson, R. Edelman, and P. A. Turski, pp. 43–72. New York: Raven.

Weber, D. M., Wang, Y., Korosec, F. R., and Mistretta, C. A. 1993. Quantitative velocity images from thick slab 2D phase contrast. *Magn. Reson. Med.* 29: 216–225.

Wolf, R. L., Ehman, R. L., Riederer, S. J., and Rossman, P. J. 1993. Analysis of systematic and random error in MR volumetric flow measurements. *Magn. Reson. Med.* 30: 82–91.

RELATED SECTIONS

15.3 TOF and CEMRA

This section covers two families of MR vascular imaging methods: time-of-flight (TOF) and contrast-enhanced MR angiography (CEMRA). Both TOF and CEMRA produce magnitude images that display increased vessel signal intensity, but their mechanisms of signal enhancement differ. TOF methods rely on the inflow of blood into the imaging slice to increase vessel intensity compared to the stationary tissue background. This effect is known as wash-in, inflow enhancement, or flow-related enhancement (FRE). (Consequently, TOF is sometimes called inflow MRA.) CEMRA methods instead rely on an externally administered contrast agent to increase the signal from the blood. CEMRA is also called gadolinium infusion or gadolinium bolus MR angiography.

There are three main acquisition modes for TOF images. Two-dimensional time of flight (2DTOF) covers an imaging volume by acquiring a set of thin 2D slices sequentially, that is, one at a time (Section 11.5). The slices are either contiguous (zero slice gap) or overcontiguous (overlapped, i.e., acquired with a small negative slice gap). Three-dimensional time of flight (3DTOF) acquires the set of images in a single 3D volume (Section 11.6). The slices within the volume are also contiguous, unless overlapped slice locations are reconstructed using an interpolation method such as zero-filling in the slice-encoded direction. An advantage of 3DTOF is that thin (e.g., 1-mm) slices can be acquired with weaker imaging gradients than are required for 2DTOF, as illustrated in Example 11.8. This reduces the gradient moments and minimum TE, which reduces intravoxel dephasing. As described in Section 11.6, 3D acquisitions also have a substantial SNR advantage compared to 2D acquisitions that are obtained sequentially. The main drawback of 3DTOF is that it sacrifices some of the SNR advantage in vessels because FRE is reduced compared to 2DTOF, especially for slow flow. This is because the signal from blood is progressively attenuated as it traverses through the slab and repeatedly experiences RF excitation pulses. Several countermeasures have been developed to alleviate the signal saturation of slowly flowing blood in 3DTOF and to try to equalize the signal from the entry and exit slices of the imaging volume. One method is the ramp RF excitation pulse, which is the subject of Section 5.2. A second method is the third main TOF acquisition mode, multiple overlapping thin-slab acquisition (MOTSA). MOTSA is also known as sequential 3DTOF or multichunk MR angiography.

MOTSA is a hybrid of 2D- and 3DTOF and has many of the advantages of both. It uses 3D volume acquisition, so some SNR advantage is obtained relative to 2DTOF. The number of slices per slab, however, is restricted (e.g., 16–32) so that the slab thickness is no more than a few centimeters, and signal saturation of slow flow is limited to an acceptable level, even at the exit slices. By sequentially acquiring a series of slabs, the necessary spatial coverage is obtained. The main disadvantage of MOTSA is its slab boundary or venetian blind artifact, which is the discontinuity of the image intensity at the boundaries between adjacent slabs. Several countermeasures have been developed to alleviate the venetian blind artifact, and these are described in subsection 15.3.1.

CEMRA is the second family of angiographic methods covered in this section. The signal enhancement in CEMRA is flow-independent; that is, instead of relying on FRE its signal enhancement is due to the T_1-shortening effect of blood after an injection of contrast agent. An imaging volume is then covered with a fast 3D acquisition. CEMRA methods can be divided into those that are time-resolved and those that are not. Time-resolved methods repeatedly acquire the same imaging volume. They require less operator intervention, but usually sacrifice some spatial resolution and coverage. Another group of CEMRA techniques is called bolus chase or moving table methods.

Despite their differences, TOF and CEMRA share several common features. They are both widely used angiographic techniques, and both produce images with a bright (i.e., hyperintense) blood signal. TOF and CEMRA applications use variations of the same basic pulse sequences because fundamentally they both require T_1-weighted fast scans. The most commonly used pulse sequence is spoiled gradient recalled echo (Section 14.1), known as spoiled FLASH or SPGR. (SSFP-FID and balanced-SSFP gradient echo methods are also used, but spoiled methods are usually preferred because it is advantageous to suppress the signal from cerebrospinal and other fluids to avoid confusion with blood.) Also, both TOF and CEMRA methods cover an imaging volume to yield a stack of contiguous (or overcontiguous) slices, which are called source images. Unlike catheter-based x-ray angiography in which only a single arterial branch is visualized, MR angiography can show all the arteries within the MR imaging volume. The source images can be viewed one slice at a time or postprocessed a variety of ways, the most common being the maximum intensity projection (MIP), as discussed in subsection 15.3.3. Both TOF and CEMRA are commonly implemented using Fourier imaging (i.e., Cartesian k-space trajectories). Thus either 2D or 3D Fourier imaging is assumed for the pulse sequences discussed in this section, unless otherwise noted.

15.3.1 TIME OF FLIGHT

Partial Saturation and Flow-Related Enhancement   With the exception of a few single-shot acquisition techniques, the magnetization must be repeatedly excited once per TR to produce an MR image. Unless the longitudinal relaxation time $T_1 \ll$ TR, there is incomplete T_1 relaxation in between the RF excitation pulses, which causes attenuation of the signal. This effect is known as partial saturation, or simply saturation. (The former term is preferred by those who reserve the term *saturation* to describe a nonequilibrium state in which the magnetization is zero.) In general, saturation increases as the TR/T_1 ratio decreases.

For the spoiled gradient echo pulse sequences commonly used in TOF angiography, the T_1, TR, and flip angle dependence of the signal S is given by:

$$S = \frac{M_0 \sin\theta(1 - e^{-\text{TR}/T_1})}{(1 - \cos\theta e^{-\text{TR}/T_1})} e^{-\text{TE}/T_2^*} \equiv M_0 \sin\theta f_{z,\text{ss}} e^{-\text{TE}/T_2^*} \quad (15.27)$$

where $f_{z,\text{ss}}$ is a dimensionless measure of the steady-state longitudinal magnetization, and M_0 is the equilibrium longitudinal magnetization, which usually has a different value for blood than for other tissues. The signal S in

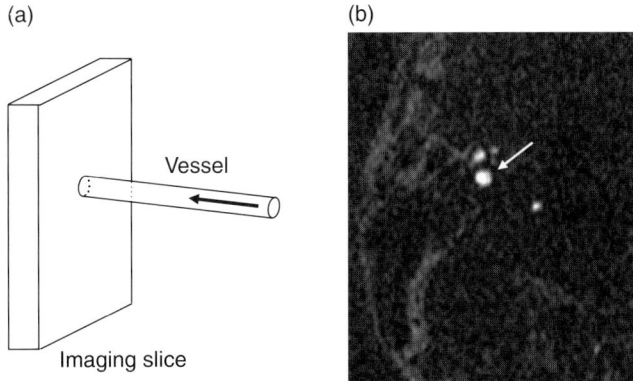

(a)

(b)

Vessel

Imaging slice

FIGURE 15.17 (a) Schematic representation of flow-related enhancement. Fully magnetized blood flows into an imaging slice. The signal from blood is enhanced relative to the stationary tissue background, which experiences partial saturation from exposure to repeated RF excitation pulses. (b) The right internal carotid artery (arrow) is hyperintense on an axial 2DTOF source image due to flow-related enhancement.

Eq. (15.27) monotonically decreases as the TR/T_1 ratio decreases, as expected. The maximal signal occurs when the flip angle is equal to the Ernst angle $\theta_E = \arccos(e^{-TR/T_1})$, implying that saturation is dominant over the creation of transverse magnetization for $\theta > \theta_E$.

FRE (Axel 1984) restores some of the signal intensity lost to partial saturation by the inflow of fully magnetized, or fresh, blood into the image slice (Figure 15.17). FRE increases with the flow velocity and as the flow trajectory becomes more perpendicular to the slice. FRE also increases as the slice thickness Δz is reduced. If, however, the perpendicular component of the velocity exceeds:

$$v_{max} = \frac{\Delta z}{TR} \tag{15.28}$$

then there is complete inflow replacement of magnetization in the slice during each TR interval. A further increase in velocity causes no further increase in FRE and might even begin to decrease the signal due to the intravoxel dephasing effects discussed in Section 10.4.

In 3DTOF and MOTSA imaging, the slices into which slowly flowing blood enters the slab generally have the greatest amount of FRE, and those from which it exits have the least. This is sometimes called the entry slice effect. We can try to generalize Eq. (15.28) to 3DTOF and MOTSA by replacing the slice thickness Δz with the slab thickness $N_z \Delta z$, where N_z is the number of slices per slab. If the path of the vessel is straight and perpendicular to the slices in the slab, then

$$v > \frac{N_z \Delta z}{\text{TR}} \tag{15.29}$$

implies complete inflow replacement, even at the exit slice. Often, however, the path of the vessel through the imaging volume is tortuous. To further complicate the situation, it is not uncommon for the speed of a small element of blood to change substantially while it traverses the slab as a vessel narrows, widens, or bends. Still, Eq. (15.29) can provide a useful estimate.

FRE can be mathematically modeled and quantified. If the magnetization experiences a total of j excitation pulses ($j \geq 1$), then the steady-state expression for the spoiled gradient echo signal in Eq. (15.27) is replaced by the approach to steady state:

$$S_j = M_0 \sin \theta \left[f_{z,\text{ss}} + (\cos \theta e^{-\text{TR}/T_1})^{j-1} (1 - f_{z,\text{ss}}) \right] e^{-\text{TE}/T_2^*} \tag{15.30}$$

(See Section 14.1.) Because $(\cos \theta e^{-\text{TR}/T_1}) < 1$, S_j approaches the steady-state value S for sufficiently large j. The amount of FRE in spoiled gradient recalled echo imaging is given by the difference:

$$\text{FRE} = S_j - S = M_0 \sin \theta (\cos \theta e^{-\text{TR}/T_1})^{j-1} (1 - f_{z,\text{ss}}) e^{-\text{TE}/T_2^*} \qquad j \geq 1 \tag{15.31}$$

A normalized measure of the enhancement is plotted versus flip angle θ in Figure 15.18. FRE increases monotonically as j decreases. Faster velocity implies decreasing j for a fixed TR and slice thickness. This trend continues until $v = v_{\text{max}}$, at which there is complete replacement of the magnetization in the slice, so it only experiences $j = 1$ RF pulse. In that case, the total signal given in Eq. (15.30) reduces to:

$$S_{j=1} = M_0 \sin \theta e^{-\text{TE}/T_2^*} \tag{15.32}$$

from which the effect of partial saturation is absent, as expected. Also note from Figure 15.18 that the fewer the number of RF pulses experienced, the higher the flip angle that maximizes FRE. Also, as the ratio TR/T_1 increases, the normalized FRE decreases. This is simply because, as TR/T_1 increases, the signal S in Eq. (15.31) increases.

The results presented here can be further refined by subdividing the imaging slice into multiple compartments and summing a geometric series that results. Also, when the velocity v is very small, FRE can be mathematically modeled as an apparent shortening of T_1 because both effects increase signal. The apparent T_1 shortening, however, is solely a mathematical construct because FRE has no physical effect on the T_1 of blood. A more complete discussion of these and other aspects of FRE can be found in Haacke et al. (1999).

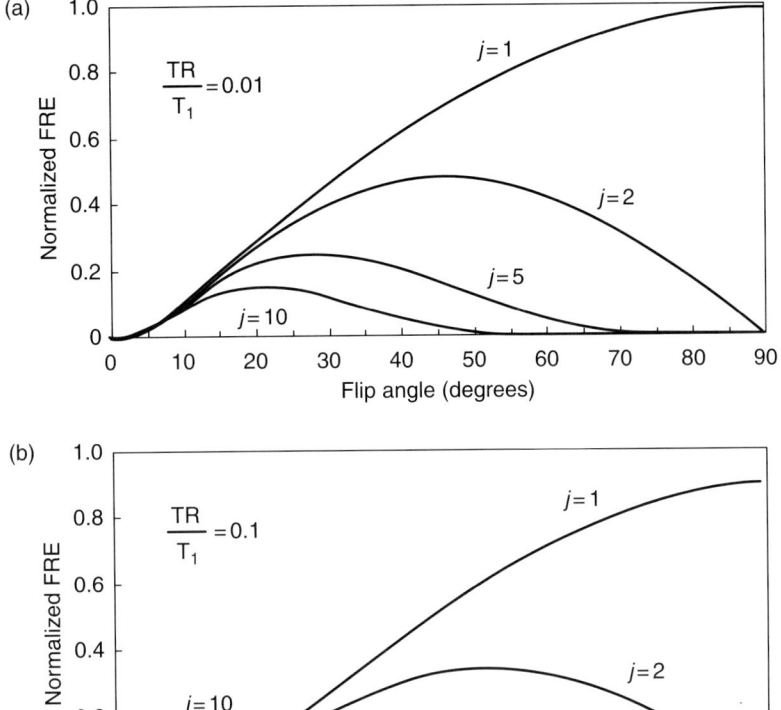

FIGURE 15.18 Plots of the normalized flow-related enhancement FRE/ $(M_0 \, e^{-\text{TE}/T_2^*})$, calculated from Eq. (15.31). The label j is the number of RF excitation pulses that the magnetization experiences. The value of TR/T_1 is 10 times shorter in (a) than in (b).

2DTOF   2DTOF (Keller et al. 1989) covers the imaging volume with a set of thin ($\Delta z = 1$–3 mm) slices that are acquired in 2D sequential mode. Because TR is typically 20–30 ms, the thin slices ensure that the number of RF pulses experienced by in-flowing blood is small, $j = 1$ (or at most 2) for typical arterial velocities ($v = 10$–100 cm/s). The flip angle is set to a relatively high value (e.g., 50–70°) in order to suppress the stationary tissue background and to maximize the vessel-to-background contrast. The imaging plane is selected to be perpendicular to the flow; for example, to image the carotid arteries the axial plane is typically used. In 2DTOF, spatial coverage and imaging time are the only considerations in choosing the number of slice locations, unlike 3DTOF in which SNR and FRE also depend on the number of slices.

Often nearby veins overlap the arteries of interest. The venous signal can be suppressed in 2DTOF by applying a spatial saturation pulse parallel to the imaging slice (see Section 5.3). A traveling saturation pulse with a fixed saturation gap is used so that venous suppression is uniform among all the slices. For example, to image the carotid arteries, the spatial saturation pulse is placed superior to each axial imaging slice to suppress the signal from the jugular veins (Figure 15.19).

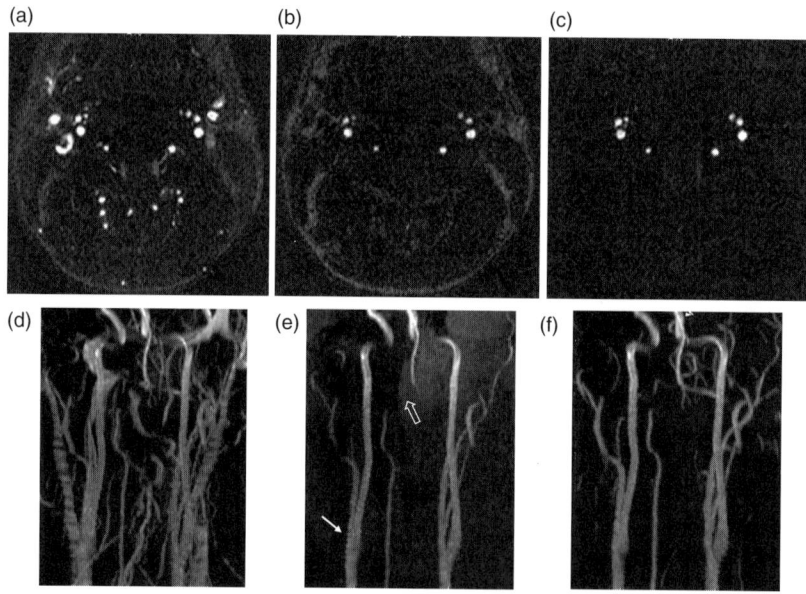

FIGURE 15.19 Axial 2DTOF acquisition of a healthy volunteer with TR = 28 ms, TE = 8.7 ms, and the flip angle is 50°. The matrix is 256 × 128, the FOV is 16 cm, and the acquisition time is 6 min for 100 2.2-mm-thick slices, overlapped by 0.7 mm to give a smoother vessel appearance on maximum intensity projections. (a)–(c) Axial source images acquired with no spatial saturation, traveling spatial saturation applied superior to the slice to suppress venous signal, and traveling spatial saturation using the SLIP technique to simultaneously suppress venous and lipid signal, respectively. (d)–(f) Corresponding coronal maximum-intensity projections. Note the jagged appearance of the right carotid artery on (e) due to vessel motion and pulsatile flow (arrow). Also note the signal loss between the right vertebral and the basilar arteries due to in-plane flow (hollow arrow).

It is important to remember that the saturation pulse distinguishes arteries from veins only by their direction of flow. If an artery has retrograde flow, the saturation pulse will suppress its signal. Conversely, venous signal will not be properly suppressed if its actual flow direction differs from the one that is presupposed when the saturation pulse is prescribed. Figure 15.15b (in Section 15.2 on phase contrast) shows an example of arterial suppression caused by the spatial saturation pulse and retrograde flow in the left vertebral artery.

Simultaneous venous and lipid suppression can be accomplished using the SLIP spatial saturation technique, which is described in Section 5.3, and illustrated on Figure 15.19. The use of the SLIP technique eliminates the need to use chemical saturation pulses on 2DTOF, which allows a shorter minimum TR.

Pulsatile flow and vessel motion can cause an irregular, jagged appearance on 2DTOF MIP images (see Figure 15.19e). Velocity compensation on the slice-selection and frequency-encoding gradient waveforms is helpful, and it is typically used because it reduces the inconsistent phase generated by pulsatile flow. Partial echo readout and low time-bandwidth product (i.e., $T \Delta f = 1$ to 2) RF excitation are also used to reduce gradient moments. Cardiac triggering can further reduce artifacts caused by pulsatile flow and vessel motion caused by pulsatile flow (Yucel et al. 1994). Even with cardiac triggering, however, artifacts from breathing, swallowing, or other bulk patient motion can remain problematic.

3DTOF   3DTOF (Masaryk et al. 1989; Lin et al. 1993) covers the desired imaging volume with a single slab of 3D slices. In order to maximize FRE, the volume is oriented (to the extent possible) so the slice planes are perpendicular to the flow. The axial imaging plane is often used to acquire intracranial 3DTOF (Figure 15.20). Depending on the vessel path, an oblique slab orientation sometimes improves FRE and allows the desired imaging volume to be covered by fewer slices, which reduces the scan time. A potential drawback of using an oblique imaging plane is that sometimes the minimum TE or TR must be increased to keep the gradient waveforms within hardware limitations, as described in Section 7.3. Typically, however, the increase is only a few milliseconds at most.

In order to shorten minimum TR, often spatial saturation is not used on 3DTOF because the venous signal is suppressed anyway due to slow flow, except on a few entry slices. Magnetization transfer (Section 4.2), however, is routinely used on 3DTOF to suppress the signal from stationary tissue. Unlike 2DTOF, low time-bandwidth-product RF excitation pulses generally cannot be used because they are not effective in eliminating slice wraparound artifacts.

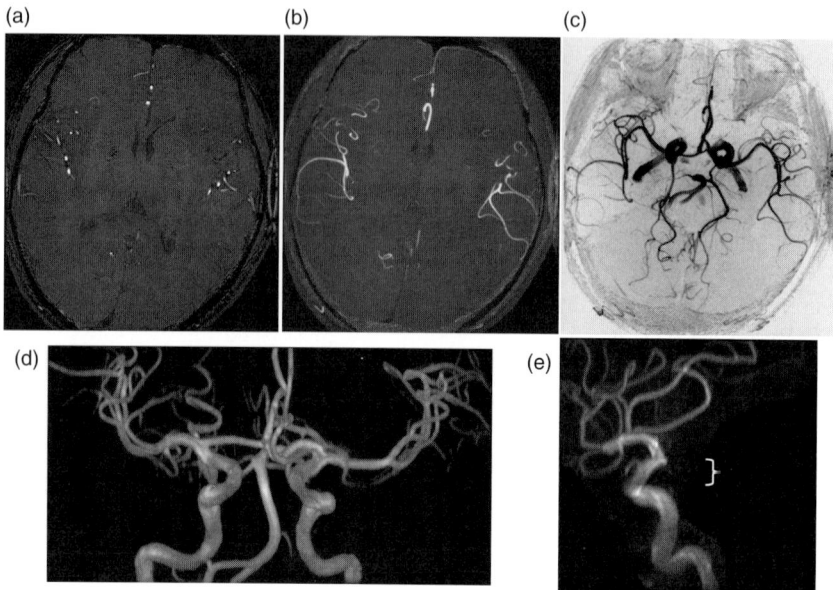

FIGURE 15.20 Axial two-slab MOTSA of a healthy volunteer at 3.0 T, along with several commonly used postprocessing displays. TR = 37 ms, TE = 4.6 ms, and flip angle = 25°. The matrix is 384 × 224, the FOV is 18 × 16 cm, and the acquisition time is 8 min for two slabs of 32 1.4-mm-thick slices. (a) A representative axial source image. (b) Thin-slab MIP from 10 axial source images. (c) Full-volume axial MIP displayed in inverse video. (d) Coronal volume rendering. (e) Targeted MIP showing only the right carotid artery in the sagittal plane; the bracket indicates the region of overlapped slices for the MOTSA acquisition.

To minimize gradient moments, 3DTOF pulse sequences use partial-echo acquisition and use RF excitation pulses with the shortest possible isodelay (e.g., minimum phase pulses, Section 2.3). 3DTOF pulse sequences commonly use ramp pulse RF excitation (Section 5.2) to partially equalize the blood signal across the slab. Either minimum TE is used, or dead time (i.e., delay) is added to gradient waveforms to increase TE, so that lipid and water transverse magnetization are out of phase (e.g., TE ≈ 2.3 or 6.9 ms at 1.5 T).

There is a variety of different gradient moment nulling strategies for 3DTOF, but at this time it appears that no clear consensus has emerged on which one is optimal. One strategy is not to use any flow compensation whatsoever in order to minimize TE and gradient moments of second order and higher. A second strategy is to use first-order moment nulling on all three axes, including velocity compensating each step of both the in-plane and slice phase-encoding gradient waveforms. Sometimes this strategy is called tri-directional flow compensation. Tridirectional flow compensation is the most gradient-intensive strategy, but it has the advantage of eliminating the mis-registration artifact if the flow is in a direction that is oblique relative to the logical gradient axes (Parker et al. 2003; Frank and Buxton 1993). A third, intermediate strategy is to null the first-order moments on the readout and slab-selection waveforms, but not the individual Fourier-encoding steps on the phase or slice axis. Higher-order gradient moment nulling (e.g., accelera-tion compensation) is seldom used because it prolongs the minimum TE and increases the higher-order moments that are not compensated.

Because 3DTOF acquisitions are phase encoded in two orthogonal directions, there is considerable flexibility in the $k_y k_z$ view order. Using a nonsequential view order such as elliptical centric (Section 11.6) can reduce the conspicuity of ghosts from pulsatile flow. The main mechanism behind this artifact reduction is to spread the ghosts evenly in two dimensions (phase and slice). With a sequential view order, the ghosts primarily propagate along a line that lies in the plane of the two phase-encoded directions (Frank et al. 1997) and can be conspicuous along the in-plane phase-encoded direction (Figure 15.21). Pulsatile ghost reduction is particularly important at 3.0 T because increased susceptibility changes aggravate pulsatile flow artifacts (Drangova and Pelc 1996). The increased SNR at high field also means that artifacts are more conspicuous because they are less likely to be obscured by noise.

Because each TR interval in a 3D acquisition corresponds to a specific value of k_y and k_z (assuming NEX = 1), there is additional latitude in the pulse

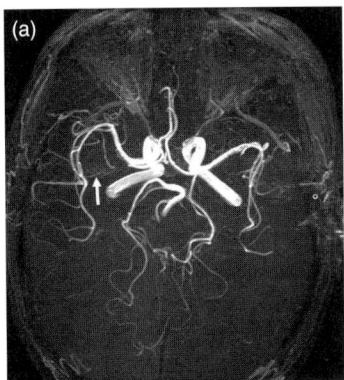 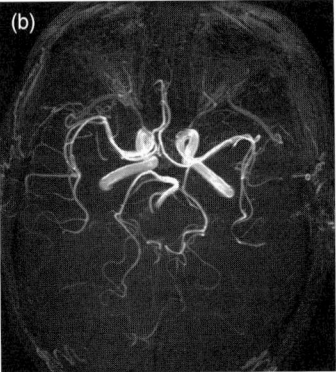

FIGURE 15.21 Axial MIP of 3DTOF acquisitions of a healthy volunteer at 3.0 T. (a) Sequential view order. (b) Elliptical centric view order. Notice how the ghost-ing (arrow) from pulsatile flow that propagates in the primary phase-encoded axis is reduced when the elliptical centric view order is used.

sequence design. Because the low-spatial-frequency information is acquired at the center of k-space, the pulse sequence can be altered to perform time-intensive tasks only for those views. Examples of this procedure include the restricted application of MT RF pulses (Section 4.2) and the prolonging of the TE to place fat–water out of phase (Lin et al. 1994).

MOTSA   MOTSA (Parker et al. 1991) covers the imaging volume with multiple, thin 3D slabs that are acquired sequentially. All the pulse sequence considerations mentioned for 3DTOF apply because MOTSA is composed of concatenated 3DTOF acquisitions. One exception is the use of spatial saturation, which is nearly always used on MOTSA to suppress venous signal at the slab boundaries. Figure 15.20 shows an example of MOTSA images and several widely used angiographic display formats.

The multiple thin slabs that make up a MOTSA acquisition reduce the signal saturation of slowly flowing blood compared to 3DTOF. To alleviate the resulting venetian blind artifact, the slabs can be overlapped; that is, slice locations in the overlap region can be acquired twice (Figure 15.22). In the overlap region, each slice location is acquired with an entry slice from one slab and an exit slice from the other. Taking the maximum of the two images on a pixel-by-pixel basis can moderate the variation of the final image intensity. Although this reduces the venetian blind artifact, it can introduce a "double exposure" misregistration artifact if the patient moves.

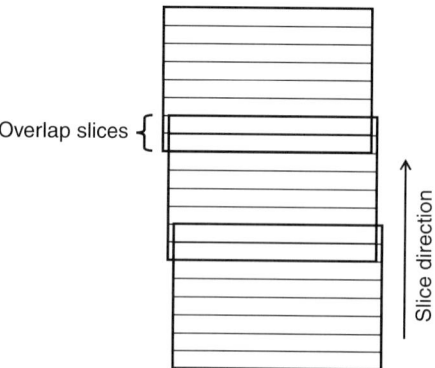

FIGURE 15.22 Schematic representation of a MOTSA acquisition with three slabs and eight slices per slab. There are two overlap slices at each boundary between the slabs. (To simplify the figure, any slices that are dropped at the ends of each slab to reduce slice wraparound artifacts are not shown. Also the slight horizontal offset between the slabs is solely for purposes of illustration.)

An alternative strategy to reduce the venetian blind artifact is called sliding interleaved k_y (SLINKY) (Liu and Rutt 1998). SLINKY is also known as the chunk acquisition and reconstruction method (CHARM). In regular MOTSA, the spatial offset of each RF slab excitation pulse is held fixed until all the k-space data for that slab are acquired. Once the data acquisition for that slab is complete, the next slab is acquired and the spatial offset of the RF slab excitation pulse is translated by one slab thickness (minus the total thickness of the overlap slices.) In SLINKY, the RF slab excitation pulse is translated every few views by one slice location. The net effect is to smooth out the venetian blind artifact over the entire imaging volume. A special reconstruction is used to obtain the entire volume of 3D slices. The implementation of SLINKY is simplified if the RF slab excitation pulse has a linear phase response that can be rephased by applying a gradient lobe. This gives SLINKY the minor drawback of being difficult to implement with minimum-phase RF excitation pulses, which generally provide the shortest isodelay, and reduces the minimum TE.

15.3.2 CONTRAST-ENHANCED MAGNETIC RESONANCE ANGIOGRAPHY

The Contrast Agent Bolus CEMRA (Prince et al. 1999) relies on an injected contrast agent that changes the relaxation time of blood. The most commonly used contrast agents shorten T_1 and are based on gadolinium (Gd) (Koenig 1991; Spinosa et al. 2002). Gadolinium is one of the more abundant of the rare earth elements and has atomic number 64 and atomic weight 157.25 g/mol. It is highly paramagnetic in its ionized state Gd^{3+} due to seven unpaired electrons in the $4f$ orbital shell, which is the maximum number allowed. Its electronic spin properties make gadolinium an effective T_1-shortening agent for protons. Gadolinium itself is toxic, but the approved contrast agents have excellent safety profiles because the gadolinium ion is chelated, or bound by a ringlike molecular cage. The term *chelate* is derived from the Greek word for "claw" (the gadolinium ion is held by ligands as if in the claw of a lobster). The contrast agents are often referred to as gadolinium chelates.

The gadolinium chelate is typically injected intravenously (e.g., into the anticubital vein) as a bolus, that is, over a short time (e.g., 5–10 s for a total volume of on the order of 20 mL). A power injector can be used to accurately control the dose and injection rate. Sometimes the injection of the contrast agent bolus is immediately followed by the injection of a volume (e.g., 10–20 mL) of saline, referred to as a saline flush. The main purpose of the saline flush is to create a tighter bolus—one that is more sharply peaked with respect to time. The saline flush accomplishes this by helping to push the contrast bolus through the vascular system.

After passage to the right ventricle, the pulmonary vessels, and the left ventricle, the contrast agent bolus remains partially intact as it makes its first pass into the arteries, but it is diluted. For example, if an undiluted gadolinium chelate solution has a concentration of 500 mM, a typical concentration when a 20 mL bolus reaches the carotid arteries is on the order of 1–10 mM. From Example 15.5, that concentration is sufficient to produce intense arterial enhancement. The main goal of CEMRA methods is to acquire a 3D imaging volume when the contrast agent is at (or near) its peak concentration during this first pass in the arteries of interest, but before nearby veins or stationary tissue enhance. (For this reason, sometimes CEMRA is referred to as a first-pass method.) Therefore, acquisition speed is the overriding design consideration for CEMRA pulse sequences. For example, the overlapping jugular veins enhance typically only 5–9 s after the carotid arteries.

T$_1$ *Reduction of Blood*   The T_1 of blood can be expressed as a function of the concentration [Gd] of the contrast agent:

$$\frac{1}{T_1} = \frac{1}{T_{1_0}} + R_1 \times [Gd] \tag{15.33}$$

where R_1 is the longitudinal relaxivity of the contrast agent, and T_{1_0} is the longitudinal relaxation time of blood in the absence of contrast agent, which is approximately 1200 ms at imaging field strengths (e.g., 1.5 T). A typical value for the longitudinal relaxivity of a gadolinium chelate is on the order of $R_1 = 5\ \text{mM}^{-1}\,\text{s}^{-1}$. The relaxivity of gadolinium chelates decreases slowly as the field strength is increased; for example, R_1 decreases by approximately 5–7% as B_0 is increased from 1.5 to 3.0 T (Koenig 1991; Bernstein et al. 2001).

Example 15.5   Use Eqs. (15.27) and (15.33) to estimate the concentration of gadolinium contrast agent necessary to increase the signal from blood by a factor of 10. Assume a spoiled gradient-echo pulse sequence, with TR = 5 ms, $\theta = 45°$, $T_{1_0} = 1200$ ms, $R_1 = 4.7\ \text{mM}^{-1}\,\text{s}^{-1}$, and that the TE is sufficiently short so that T_2^* decay is negligible.

Answer   According to Eq. (15.27), increasing the signal by a factor 10 implies that:

$$\frac{(1 - e^{-TR/T_1})}{(1 - \cos\theta e^{-TR/T_1})} = \frac{10(1 - e^{-TR/T_{1_0}})}{(1 - \cos\theta e^{-TR/T_{1_0}})} \tag{15.34}$$

Solving Eq. (15.34) by algebraic manipulation (or numerically) yields $e^{-TR/T_1} = 0.9543$, so $T_1 = 106.9$ ms or 0.1069 s. Equation (15.33) then yields the required concentration of [Gd] = 1.81 mM.

A very high concentration of gadolinium (e.g., on the order of 20 mM or higher) can be counterproductive because it causes signal loss from T_2^* decay (Neimatallah et al. 2000). To reduce the likelihood of that signal loss, moderate injection rates of the contrast agent are used, 2–3 mL/s being typical. Higher injection rates can also increase the risk of extravasation (i.e., leakage of contrast agent from the vein at the injection site into the surrounding tissues).

SNR and TR Considerations For most CEMRA applications, we can assume that TR $\ll$ T1 because even at peak enhancement the vessel T_1 is still on the order of 50 ms, whereas TR is only a few milliseconds with most modern gradient hardware. Assuming the use of a spoiled gradient-echo pulse sequence with the flip angle set to the Ernst angle, then $\cos \theta = e^{-TR/T_1} \approx (1 - TR/T_1)$. After some algebra, the signal in Eq. (15.27) can be expressed as:

$$S = M_0 \sqrt{\frac{1 - e^{-TR/T_1}}{1 + e^{-TR/T_1}}} e^{-TE/T_2^*} \approx M_0 \sqrt{\frac{TR}{2T_1}} e^{-TE/T_2^*} \tag{15.35}$$

Equation (15.35) implies that increasing TR increases the signal, but this can be misleading because it does not take into account the time-dependence of the bolus. A long TR increases imaging time, which means that data will be acquired when there is little or no contrast agent remaining in the vessel. These trade-offs can be quantified by first considering the rate Q of k-space area traversal per unit time for the 3D volume acquisition:

$$Q = \frac{\Delta k_y \Delta k_z}{TR} = \frac{1}{FOV_y FOV_z TR} \tag{15.36}$$

where Δk_y and Δk_z are the k-space step sizes for the phase- and slice-encoding directions, respectively. The point-spread function (PSF) for the resulting images can be calculated if the time-dependence of the contrast enhancement from the arterial bolus is parameterized (Fain et al. 1999), for instance, with a two-term gamma-variant model. The results of these calculations (assuming the elliptical centric view order) show that the FWHM of the PSF is inversely proportional to the square root of the rate k-space area traversal:

$$FWHM \propto \sqrt{\frac{1}{Q}} = \sqrt{TR \, FOV_y FOV_z} \tag{15.37}$$

Also, the peak amplitude of the PSF is directly proportional to Q:

$$PSF_{max} \propto Q = \frac{1}{TR \, FOV_y FOV_z} \tag{15.38}$$

Equation (15.37) for the FWHM illustrates the importance of minimizing TR and FOV in CEMRA to avoid loss of spatial resolution (i.e., blurring). Therefore, any method that reduces the acquired FOVs in either of the phase-encoded directions (or both) is of great value to CEMRA. Those methods include rectangular FOV, parallel imaging methods such as SENSE, and oblique orientation of the imaging volume to cover the vessels with fewer slices.

Equation (15.38) shows that the amplitude of the PSF increases as TR decreases (i.e., the signal of small structures, like most vessels, is increased). Decreasing TR also helps to suppress the signal from the tissue that surrounds the vessel. The increase in PSF amplitude more than compensates for the decrease in the signal indicated in Eq. (15.35). A longer TR, however, does allow the use of a narrower receiver bandwidth $\Delta \nu$, resulting in increased SNR because SNR $\propto 1/\sqrt{\Delta \nu}$. When these three effects are considered together, we expect the net SNR for small structures to be independent of TR, at least in the approximation that the entire TR interval can be used to readout data, and the model-based calculations for the PSF to apply.

To summarize, a short TR is valuable for CEMRA because it enables higher spatial resolution. There are, however, a number of practical limits to how fast the pulse sequence can be played. As TR $\rightarrow$ 0, Eqs. (15.37) and (15.38) are no longer necessarily valid because the bolus could be considered a constant over the duration of the acquisition. The receiver bandwidth and partial-saturation effects are then dominant, and the SNR approaches zero. Such a pulse sequence is not practical anyway because the RF bandwidth approaches infinity, as does the SAR. Finally, gradient hardware and regulatory limits on peripheral nerve stimulation are soon exceeded. Minimum TR, however, is nearly always used in practice, and it falls in the range of TR = 2–10 ms, depending on imaging protocol and scanner hardware. Additional discussion of the trade-off between SNR and TR in CEMRA can be found in Heid and Remonda (1997), Pelc et al. (1998), and Parker et al. (1998).

CEMRA Pulse Sequences Like TOF, CEMRA mainly uses spoiled gradient-echo pulse sequences. Because the signal enhancement does not rely on FRE, any imaging plane can be used. Often the coronal plane is preferred because aligning the frequency-encoding axis in the superior-to-inferior direction provides excellent coverage of many vascular structures with minimal wraparound artifacts.

Because speed is the primary design requirement for a CEMRA pulse sequence, a wide receiver bandwidth ($\Delta \nu = \pm 32$ to 128 kHz) is typically used in conjunction with partial-echo acquisition. In order to minimize TE and TR, gradient moment nulling is not used. To reduce minimum TE and simultaneously reduce the scan time, sometimes partial k-space acquisition is used in two or even all three directions. As described in Section 13.4, no partial Fourier reconstruction can recover all the missing data, so the spatial resolution is anisotropic for that type of acquisition. CEMRA acquisitions can be divided into two main groups: those that repeatedly acquire the imaging volume, called time-resolved methods, and those that do not, called here single-phase methods.

Single-Phase Methods   Single-phase CEMRA devotes the entire acquisition time to obtaining data for one set of 3D images. This strategy can increase spatial resolution and coverage. The drawback of single-phase methods is that they require a bolus timing method. The time between the injection and the peak enhancement of the vessel is called its circulation time. Methods to measure the circulation time include test bolus timing (Earls et al. 1997) and fluoroscopic triggering (Wilman et al. 1997), which are described in Section 11.4. Automatic triggering methods are also used, as described in Foo et al. (1997).

The elliptical centric view order (and related methods such as CENTRA) is commonly used for single-phase CEMRA. They are especially valuable when the venous enhancement follows quickly, as in the carotid-jugular system. If the center (i.e., approximately 10%) of $k_y k_z$ space is acquired during arterial (but before venous) enhancement, only the edges of the veins are apparent on the image (Figure 15.23). The total acquisition time can be extended to the entire duration of arterial enhancement. That duration is often on the order of 1 min or longer. When imaging the renal arteries or other structures in the abdomen and thorax, however, the length of the patient's breath hold usually limits the maximal useful acquisition time. One minor drawback of using the elliptical centric order is that there are no natural break points at which to periodically apply chemical saturation pulses.

Unlike CEMRA of arteries (arteriography), contrast-enhanced MR venography (Farb et al. 2003) does not place a premium on the speed of the acquisition. As long as the acquisition is started after the veins enhance, scan times of several minutes or more work well. This enables the acquisition of images with very high spatial resolution and SNR, as illustrated in Figure 15.24. The arterial signal is not suppressed in that image.

Time-Resolved Methods   Time-resolved CEMRA (Carr and Finn 2003) allows the visualization of various stages of vessel enhancement, including early, peak, and late arterial phases, as well as venous enhancement. Acquisition speed is at an even higher premium than in single-phase methods, so techniques such as SENSE are often used (Maki et al. 2002). Time-resolved methods are particularly valuable for applications such as the bilateral imaging of the vessels of the legs, in which the

(a) (b)

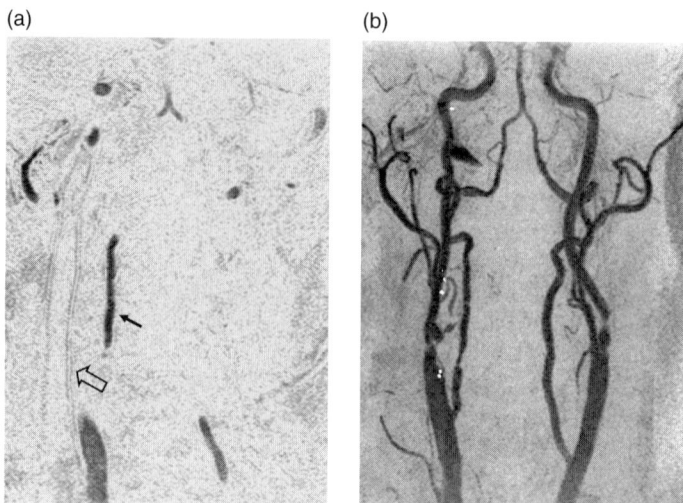

FIGURE 15.23 (a) Coronal CEMRA source image and (b) MIP, both displayed in inverse video. Note that only the edge of the jugular vein (hollow arrow) can be visualized on the source image because the elliptical centric view order is used. (Courtesy of John Huston III, M.D., Mayo Clinic College of Medicine.)

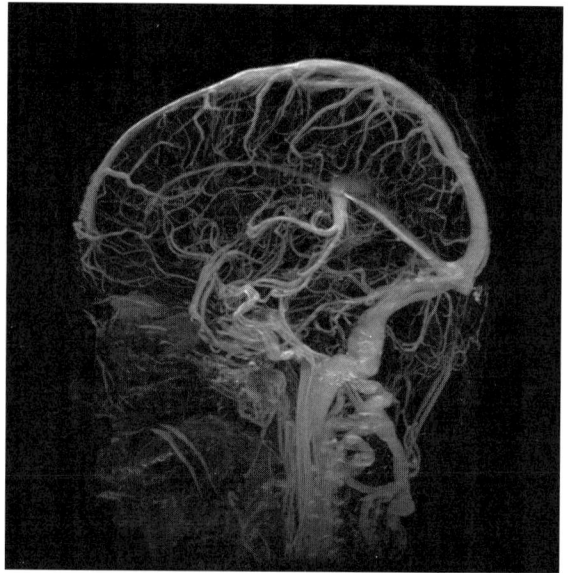

FIGURE 15.24 MIP of a contrast-enhanced MR venogram at 3.0 T. One hundred ten 1.4-mm-thick slices are acquired in 3 min 36 s in the sagittal plane with a 320×320 matrix and a 22-cm FOV. The TR = 5.3 ms, TE = 1.4 ms, and the flip angle is $25°$. (Courtesy of Norbert Campeau, M.D., Paul McGough, M.D., and Gary Miller, M.D., Mayo Clinic College of Medicine.)

arterial enhancement of different vessels often occurs at substantially different times. Unless breath-holding is required, time-resolved techniques also free the operator from the need to measure the circulation time because one of the phases will probably catch the peak arterial enhancement of the vessel. Stationary tissue can be suppressed by subtracting a precontrast mask image on a pixel-by-pixel basis. A convenient feature of time-resolved methods is that they automatically provide several sets of mask images for the subtraction. The main drawback of time-resolved methods is the intrinsic trade-off in MRI among acquisition time, spatial coverage, and spatial resolution. To optimize this trade-off, partial k-space updating methods such as keyhole or TRICKS (Section 11.3) can be used. TRICKS (Mistretta et al. 1998) has been preferred over keyhole for angiographic applications, because it periodically reacquires high-spatial-frequency data, which is important because the enhancing vessels are usually small. Another way to optimize the trade-off is to use angularly undersampled radial projection acquisition methods (Section 17.5). CEMRA is a particularly attractive application for these methods because the high contrast-to-noise ratio of the enhanced vessels makes the streak artifacts from the angular undersampling less objectionable (Peters et al. 2000).

Another method to increase the temporal resolution in time-resolved CEMRA is to use a 2D thick-slab acquisition (i.e., a 2D projection) rather than a 3D volume (Wang et al. 1996). Because there is no slice encoding, the temporal resolution can be dramatically increased. If mask subtraction is used, it is helpful to perform a subtraction on the complex data rather than magnitude images to minimize partial-volume effects.

Moving Table Methods   Moving table or bolus chase (Leiner et al. 2000; Goyen et al. 2002; Meaney 2003) methods are another class of CEMRA techniques that follow or chase the propagation of a single bolus a long distance (i.e., 1 m or more). The bed or table on which the patient lies is moved so that the imaging volume follows the course of the first pass of a single injection of contrast agent as it proceeds toward the feet. Moving table methods have found application in the imaging of the arteries of the abdomen, pelvis, legs, and feet. 3D volumes, usually in the coronal plane, are acquired at multiple locations, or stations. This technique is sometimes called step and shoot. Alternatively, the entire volume can be covered by continuously moving the table and acquiring one single volume (Kruger et al. 2002). The entire set of images is then reconstructed by appropriate interleaving of the data.

15.3.3 PRACTICAL CONSIDERATIONS

Signal-Loss Mechanisms   Both TOF and CEMRA images display a bright (hyperintense) signal from blood. The absence or reduction of the signal can indicate a narrowing of the vessel (i.e., a stenosis) or the presence of some other disease. Both TOF and CEMRA, however, can suffer from artifactual signal loss that is related to the imaging technique instead of disease.

There are two main mechanisms of signal loss for TOF images. The first is signal saturation, caused by slow, in-plane, or recirculating flow. Regions of recirculating flow are commonly found in aneurysms or in the carotid bulb. Decreasing the flip angle, increasing TR, or decreasing T_1 (by the injection of a contrast agent) can reduce signal saturation.

The second signal-loss mechanism for TOF imaging is intravoxel dephasing due to complex flow, often occurring distal to a stenosis (Figure 15.25a). Using smaller voxels, reduced TE, or gradient moment nulling can sometimes counteract it. Signal saturation and intravoxel dephasing are caused by very

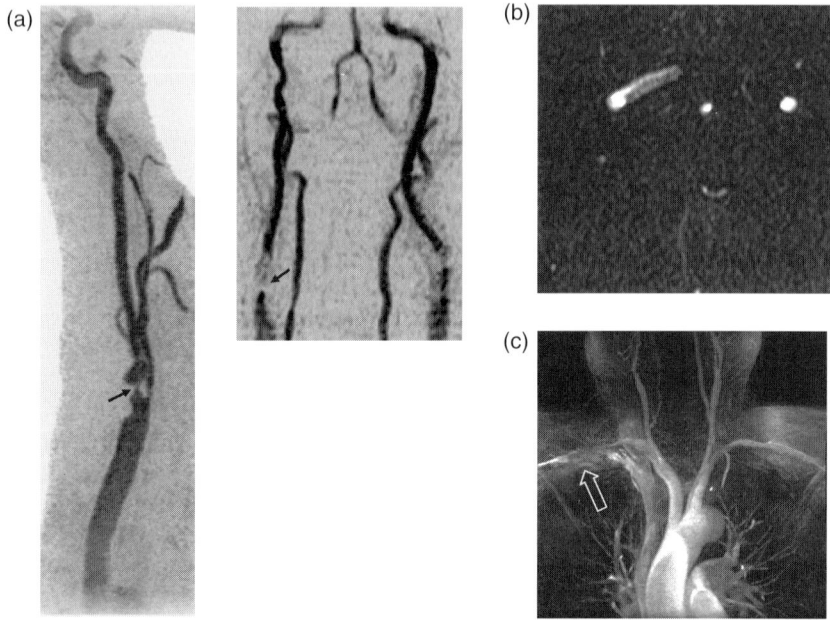

FIGURE 15.25 Examples of signal loss in MRA. (a) Intravoxel dephasing on 2DTOF coronal MIP (arrow) distal to a tight stenosis depicted on a targeted MIP of a CEMRA (left). (b) Central dark stripe due to signal saturation in the petrous portion of the carotid artery on a 2DTOF source image. (c) Coronal MIP of a CEMRA showing T_2^* dephasing in the right subclavian artery (hollow arrow) caused by its proximity to the right subclavian vein. The echo time is TE = 1.6 ms. (Courtesy of John Huston III, M.D., Mayo Clinic College of Medicine.)

different flow patterns, but it is not always clear which mechanism is causing signal loss on a TOF image. A well-known example is the dark center stripe image in the petrous portion of the internal carotid artery. It has been shown experimentally and with fluid dynamic calculations that the signal loss is caused by slow flow in the center of the vessel, resulting in signal saturation (Saloner et al. 1996). Figure 15.25b shows an example of this type of signal loss.

CEMRA can also suffer signal loss, but the most common mechanisms are different than for TOF. One mechanism of signal loss in CEMRA is improper bolus timing (Maki et al. 1996). If the value assumed for the circulation time is too small, the scan will be initiated too early and there will be little or no contrast agent in the artery when the center of k-space is acquired. The elliptical centric view order is particularly sensitive to this artifact, but with proper training and equipment, the technical reliability of single-phase CEMRA can be excellent (Riederer et al. 2000). The second common signal-loss mechanism in CEMRA is T_2^* dephasing. This artifact is commonly observed on part of the subclavian artery that overlaps the subclavian vein because the bolus is still relatively undiluted in the latter vessel (Figure 15.25c). T_2^* dephasing can be addressed by reducing TE or the voxel size. Also, the contrast agent can be prediluted or the injection rate reduced.

Table 15.1 summarizes some of the signal-loss mechanisms commonly experienced with TOF and CEMRA acquisitions while providing the typical ranges of the acquisitions parameters.

Angiographic Displays   The acquisition methods described in this section yield a stack of source images with a hyperintense vessel signal. Any single image shows only a small portion of the vessel. Postprocessing methods such as MIP (Laub 1990) and volume rendering are commonly used to follow the entire course of the vessel (Figure 15.20). For a detailed description of these methods see Cody (2002). Note that the same image-display postprocessing methods are used in both MRA and computed tomography angiography (CTA). One advantage of MRA is that the background tissue (fat, muscle, etc.) is usually easier to segment out than the surrounding bone on CTA images. Examples of a few of the commonly used angiographic displays are shown in Figure 15.20.

MIP is the most commonly used postprocessing technique. It projects a 3D data set onto a 2D image by forming rays through the stack of images. As its name implies, only the maximum pixel value along any ray is retained on the 2D display. Although MIP is very widely used, it has flaws. MIP does not provide any depth information; however, a series of MIP images from various projection angles can be played in a cine loop to give an impression of a spinning 3D display. Also an intense signal (e.g., from lipids or other vessels)

TABLE 15.1

Summary of Acquisition Parameters Used in TOF and CEMRA

MRA Technique	2DTOF	3DTOF	MOTSA	CEMRA
Typical TR range	20–30 ms	25–50 ms	25–50 ms	2–10 ms
Typical TE range	4–8 ms (minimum)	2–7 ms (minimum or fat–water out of phase)	2–7 ms (minimum or fat–water out of phase)	0.5–2 ms (minimum)
Flip angle range	50–70°	20–30°	20–40°	30–60°
Flow compensation	Frequency and slice	See text	See text	None
Spatial saturation	Yes	Optional	Yes	No
MT	No	Typically yes	Typically yes	No
Signal-loss mechanism(s)	In-plane or retrograde flow, intravoxel dephasing	Slow flow, intravoxel dephasing	Venetian blind artifact, very slow flow, intravoxel dephasing	Improper bolus timing, T_2^* dephasing

can obscure a vessel. For this reason, the source images are often preprocessed before MIP by carving away unwanted voxels. The result is called a subvolume or targeted MIP, and an example is shown on Figure 15.20e. Another useful method is a sliding thin-slab MIP (Napel et al. 1993), which forms the MIP from a limited number of source images (Figure 15.20b). It is important to remember that MIP discards all but the most intense pixel value in a ray, so it can artifactually narrow vessels, which can lead to the overestimation of stenosis (Anderson et al. 1990). For that reason, it is important to retain the source images for later review.

SELECTED REFERENCES

Anderson, C. M., Saloner, D., Tsuruda, J. S., Shapeero, L. G., and Lee, R. E. 1990. Artifacts in maximum-intensity-projection display of MR angiograms. *Am. J. Roentgenol.* 154: 623–629.
Axel, L. 1984. Blood flow effects in magnetic resonance imaging. *Am. J. Roentgenol.* 143: 1157–1166.

Bernstein, M. A., Huston, J., III, Lin, C., Gibbs, G. F., and Felmlee, J. P. 2001. High-resolution intracranial and cervical MRA at 3.0 T: Technical considerations and initial experience. *Magn. Reson. Med.* 46: 955–962.

Carr, J. C., and Finn, J. P. 2003. MR imaging of the thoracic aorta. *Magn. Reson. Imaging Clin. N. Am.* 11: 135–148.

Cody, D. D. 2002. AAPM/RSNA physics tutorial for residents: Topics in CT, Image processing in CT. *Radiographics* 22: 1255–1268.

Drangova, M., and Pelc, N. J. 1996. Artifacts and signal loss due to flow in the presence of B0 inhomogeneity. *Magn. Reson. Med.* 35: 126–130.

Earls, J. P., Rofsky, N. M., DeCorato, D. R., Krinsky, G. A., and Weinreb, J. C. 1997. Hepatic arterial-phase dynamic gadolinium-enhanced MR imaging: Optimization with a test examination and a power injector. *Radiology* 202: 268–273.

Fain, S. B., Riederer, S. J., Bernstein, M. A., and Huston, J., III. 1999. Theoretical limits of spatial resolution in elliptical-centric contrast-enhanced 3D-MRA. *Magn. Reson. Med.* 42: 1106–1116.

Farb, R. I., Scott, J. N., Willinsky, R. A., Montanera, W. J., Wright, G. A., and ter Brugge, K. G. 2003. Intracranial venous system: Gadolinium-enhanced three-dimensional MR venography with auto-triggered elliptic centric-ordered sequence — initial experience. *Radiology* 226: 203–209.

Foo, T. K., Saranathan, M., Prince, M. R., and Chenevert, T. L. 1997. Automated detection of bolus arrival and initiation of data acquisition in fast, three-dimensional, gadolinium-enhanced MR angiography. *Radiology* 203: 275–280.

Frank, L. R., and Buxton, R. B. 1993. Distortions from curved flow in magnetic resonance imaging. *Magn. Reson. Med.* 29: 84–93.

Frank, L. R., Buxton, R. B., and Kerber, C. W. 1993. Pulsatile flow artifacts in 3D magnetic resonance imaging. *Magn. Reson. Med.* 30: 296–304.

Goyen, M., Quick, H. H., Debatin, J. F., Ladd, M. E., Barkhausen, J., Herborn, C. U., Bosk, S., Kuehl, H., Schleputz, M., and Ruehm, S. G. 2002. Whole-body three-dimensional MR angiography with a rolling table platform: Initial clinical experience. *Radiology* 224: 270–277.

Haacke, E. M., Brown. R. W., Thompson, M. R., and Venkatesan, R. 1999. *Magnetic resonance imaging: Physical principles and sequence design.* New York: Wiley-Liss. p. 703–713.

Heid, O., and Remonda, L., 1997. Outer limits of contrast-enhanced 3D MRA. In *Proceedings of the 5th meeting of the ISMRM*, p. 254.

Keller, P. J., Drayer, B. P., Fram, E. K., Williams, K. D., Dumoulin, C. L., and Souza, S. P. 1989. MR angiography with two-dimensional acquisition and three-dimensional display: Work in progress. *Radiology* 173: 527–532.

Koenig, S. H. 1991. From the relaxivity of Gd(DTPA)2- to everything else. *Magn. Reson. Med.* 22: 183–190.

Kruger, D. G., Riederer, S. J., Grimm, R. C., and Rossman, P. J. 2002. Continuously moving table data acquisition method for long FOV contrast-enhanced MRA and whole-body MRI. *Magn. Reson. Med.* 47: 224–231.

Laub, G. 1990. Displays for MR angiography. *Magn. Reson. Med.* 14: 222–229.

Leiner, T., Ho, K. Y., Nelemans, P. J., de Haan, M. W., and van Engelshoven, J. M. 2000. Three-dimensional contrast-enhanced moving-bed infusion-tracking (MoBI-track) peripheral MR angiography with flexible choice of imaging parameters for each field of view. *J. Magn. Reson. Imaging* 11: 368–377.

Lin, W., Haacke, E. M., and Tkach, J. A. 1994. Three-dimensional time-of-flight MR angiography with variable TE (VARIETE) for fat signal reduction. *Magn. Reson. Med.* 32: 678–683.

Lin, W., Tkach, J. A., Haacke, E. M., and Masaryk, T. J. 1993. Intracranial MR angiography: Application of magnetization transfer contrast and fat saturation to short gradient-echo, velocity-compensated sequences. *Radiology* 186: 753–761.

Liu, K., and Rutt, B. K. 1998. Sliding interleaved kY (SLINKY) acquisition: A novel 3D MRA technique with suppressed slab boundary artifact. *J. Magn. Reson. Imaging* 8: 903–911.

Maki, J. H., Prince, M. R., Londy, F. J., and Chenevert, T. L. 1996. The effects of time varying intravascular signal intensity and k-space acquisition order on three-dimensional MR angiography image quality. *J. Magn. Reson. Imaging* 6: 642–651.

Maki, J. H., Wilson, G. J., Eubank, W. B., and Hoogeveen, R. M. 2002. Utilizing SENSE to achieve lower station sub-millimeter isotropic resolution and minimal venous enhancement in peripheral MR angiography. *J. Magn. Reson. Imaging* 15: 484–491.

Masaryk, T. J., Modic, M. T., Ross, J. S., Ruggieri, P. M., Laub, G. A., Lenz, G. W., Haacke, E. M., Selman, W. R., Wiznitzer, M., and Harik, S. I. 1989. Intracranial circulation: preliminary clinical results with three-dimensional (volume) MR angiography. *Radiology* 171: 793–799.

Meaney, J. F. 2003. Magnetic resonance angiography of the peripheral arteries: Current status. *Eur. Radiol.* 13: 836–852.

Mistretta, C. A., Grist, T. M., Korosec, F. R., Frayne, R., Peters, D. C., Mazaheri, Y., and Carrol, T. J. 1998. 3D time-resolved contrast-enhanced MR DSA: Advantages and tradeoffs. *Magn. Reson. Med.* 40: 571–581.

Napel, S., Rubin, G. D., and Jeffrey, R. B., Jr. 1993. STS-MIP: A new reconstruction technique for CT of the chest. *J. Comput. Assist. Tomogr.* 17: 832–838.

Neimatallah, M. A., Chenevert, T. L., Carlos, R. C., Londy, F. J., Dong, Q., Prince, M. R., and Kim, H. M. 2000. Subclavian MR arteriography: Reduction of susceptibility artifact with short echo time and dilute gadopentetate dimeglumine. *Radiology* 217: 581–586.

Parker, D. L., Goodrich, K. C., Alexander, A. L., Buswell, H. R., Blatter, D. D., and Tsuruda, J. S. 1998. Optimized visualization of vessels in contrast enhanced intracranial MR angiography. *Magn. Reson. Med.* 40: 873–882.

Parker, D. L., Goodrich, K. C., Roberts, J. A., Chapman, B. E., Jeong, E. K., Kim, S. E., Tsuruda, J. S., and Katzman, G. L. 2003. The need for phase-encoding flow compensation in high-resolution intracranial magnetic resonance angiography. *J. Magn. Reson. Imaging* 18: 121–127.

Parker, D. L., Yuan, C., and Blatter, D. D. 1991. MR angiography by multiple thin slab 3D acquisition. *Magn. Reson. Med.* 17: 434–451.

Pelc, N. J., Alley, M. T., Shifrin, R. Y., and Herfkens, R. J. 1998. Outer limits of contrast enhanced MRA Revisited. In *Proceedings of the 6th meeting of the ISMRM*, p. 98.

Peters, D. C., Korosec, F. R., Grist, T. M., Block, W. F., Holden, J. E., Vigen, K. K., and Mistretta, C. A. 2000. Undersampled projection reconstruction applied to MR angiography. *Magn. Reson. Med.* 43: 91–101.

Prince, M. R., Grist, T. M., Debatin, J. F. 1999. *3D Contrast MR Angiography*. Berlin: Springer.

Riederer, S. J., Bernstein, M. A., Breen, J. F., Busse, R. F., Ehman, R. L., Fain, S. B., Hulshizer, T. C., Huston, J., III, King, B. F., Kruger, D. G., Rossman, P. J., and Shah, S. 2000. Three-dimensional contrast-enhanced MR angiography with real-time fluoroscopic triggering: Design specifications and technical reliability in 330 patient studies. *Radiology* 215: 584–593.

Saloner, D., van Tyen, R., Dillon, W. P., Jou, L. D., and Berger, S. A. 1996. Central intraluminal saturation stripe on MR angiograms of curved vessels: Simulation, phantom, and clinical analysis. *Radiology* 198: 733–739.

Spinosa, D. J., Kaufmann, J. A., and Hartwell, G. D. 2002. Gadolinium chelates in angiography and interventional radiology: A useful alternative to iodinated contrast media for angiography. *Radiology* 223: 319–325.

Wang, Y., Johnston, D. L., Breen, J. F., Huston, J. 3rd, Jack, C. R., Julsrud, P. R., Kiely, M. J., King, B. F., Riederer, S. L., and Ehman, R. L. 1996. Dynamic MR digital subtraction angiography using contrast enhancement, fast data acquisition, and complex subtraction. *Magn. Reson. Med.* 36: 551–556.

Wilman, A. H., Riederer, S. J., King, B. F., Debbins, J. P., Rossman, P. J., and Ehman, R. L. 1997. Fluoroscopically triggered contrast-enhanced three-dimensional MR angiography with elliptical centric view order: Application to the renal arteries. *Radiology* 205: 137–146.

Yucel E. K., Silver, M. S., and Carter, A. P. 1994. MR angiography of normal pelvic arteries: Comparison of signal intensity and contrast-to-noise ratio for three different inflow techniques. *Am. J. Roentgenol.* 163: 197–201.

RELATED SECTIONS

16

ECHO TRAIN PULSE SEQUENCES

16.1 Echo Planar Imaging

Echo planar imaging (EPI) is one of the fastest MRI pulse sequences (Mansfield 1977). With modern gradient and RF hardware, EPI is capable of producing a 2D image in only a few tens of milliseconds (Figure 16.1).

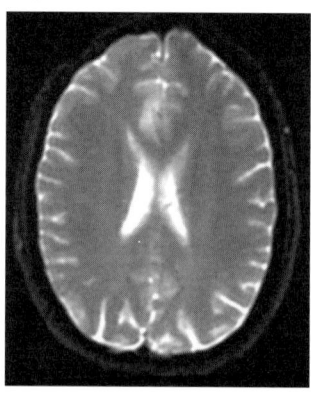

FIGURE 16.1 An example of a single-shot echo planar image of the brain. The acquisition time of this 128×128 image is 86 ms.

This ultrafast imaging speed has played an important role in the development of a number of challenging and exciting MR applications, such as diffusion imaging, perfusion imaging, neurofunctional brain mapping, cardiac imaging, dynamic studies, and real-time imaging.

An EPI pulse sequence differs from conventional pulse sequences (such as spin echo and gradient echo), mainly in the ways that the readout and phase-encoding gradients are applied. EPI employs a series of bipolar readout gradients to generate a train of gradient echoes. With an accompanying phase-encoding gradient, each gradient echo is distinctively spatially encoded so that multiple k-space lines can be sampled under the envelope of a free-induction decay (FID) or an RF spin echo. Unlike rapid acquisition with relaxation enhancement (RARE; Section 16.4), EPI uses a gradient-echo train, instead of an RF spin-echo train, to accelerate data acquisition. Because gradient echoes can be produced at a much faster rate than RF spin echoes, EPI generates an image in a considerably shorter time. For example, it is quite typical for an EPI pulse sequence to produce $\sim$100 gradient echoes so that a low-resolution 2D image can be constructed from a single RF excitation (i.e., single shot). Although segmented k-space acquisition is also possible with multiple excitations, EPI is often used as a single-shot technique to obtain a snapshot image in well under a second. The basic principles underlying EPI pulse sequence design are discussed in subsection 16.1.1, and three common EPI pulse sequences, spin-echo EPI, gradient-echo EPI, and inversion recovery EPI, are presented in subsection 16.1.2.

EPI pulse sequences can be used for either 2D or 3D acquisitions, but the vast majority of EPI applications are based on 2D sequences that use orthogonal readout, phase-encoding, and slice-selection gradient waveforms. The slice-selection gradient waveform is essentially the same as that employed in a conventional spin-echo or gradient-echo sequence. The characteristic readout and phase-encoding gradients, however, produce k-space trajectories that are different from conventional gradient waveforms. The resulting data require additional processing prior to image reconstruction using 2D Fourier transforms or gridding. Specific issues for EPI image reconstruction are briefly discussed in subsection 16.1.3.

Compared to conventional spin-echo and gradient-echo imaging, EPI is more prone to a variety of artifacts. A prominent EPI artifact is ghosting along the phase-encoded direction. Many system imperfections and physical phenomena (e.g., eddy currents, asymmetric anti-aliasing filter response, concomitant magnetic fields, mismatched gradient group delays, and hysteresis) can all lead to ghosts in EPI. These ghosts, often referred to as Nyquist ghosts, can be reduced or removed using a number of calibration, reconstruction, or postprocessing techniques. Chemical shift artifacts of the first kind (Section 11.1) have a unique appearance in echo planar images. Displacement due to chemical shifts is typically negligible along the EPI readout direction, but becomes very severe (e.g., 25% of the FOV) along the phase-encoded direction. To address this problem, lipid suppression is almost always required in EPI pulse sequences. Similar to chemical-shift-induced displacement, off-resonance effects arising from magnetic susceptibility variations (e.g., from tissue-air interfaces or metallic implants), B_0-field inhomogeneities, eddy currents, and concomitant magnetic fields (Section 10.1) can severely distort echo planar images and lead to signal loss. In addition, T_2^* decay during the formation of the gradient echo train causes image blurring. These commonly encountered artifacts and their cures are discussed in subsection 16.1.4.

EPI is an especially broad subject that involves many areas of MR imaging, including gradient and RF hardware design, image reconstruction, signal processing, safety considerations, applications, and pulse sequences. An exhaustive coverage of all these aspects is beyond the scope of this section. Instead, we focus on the basic principles in EPI pulse-sequence design and the associated issues with image reconstruction and artifact reduction. The interested reader is referred to Schmitt et al. (1998) for additional information.

16.1.1 PRINCIPLES OF ECHO PLANAR IMAGING

Conventional Gradient Echo versus EPI   First consider a simple gradient-echo pulse sequence shown in Figures 16.2a and b. Following the RF excitation pulse, the magnitude of the transverse magnetization $M_\perp$ decays according to

$$M_\perp(t) = M_\perp(0)e^{-t/T_2^*} \qquad (16.1)$$

where the decay constant T_2^* is defined as in Section 14.1. The half-lifetime of the transverse magnetization is given by $T_2^* \ln 2$. Suppose the transverse magnetization can be used to produce usable signals within 2 half-lifetimes. For a tissue with a T_2^* of $\sim$60 ms, the usable acquisition window is $2 \times T_2^* \times \ln(2) \approx 83$ ms. In the gradient-echo pulse sequence in Figure 16.2b, if a receiver bandwidth of $\Delta\nu = \pm 64$ kHz is used to sample 256 complex k-space data points, the acquisition time (i.e., the time when the A/D converter is sampling data) is $T_{acq} = 256 \times (1/(2 \times 64)) = 2$ ms per TR interval. Thus, a very small fraction (i.e., 2 ms) of the transverse magnetization lifetime (i.e., 83 ms) is actually used for data acquisition.

EPI is a technique that maximally uses the transverse magnetization without additional RF excitations. Unlike the conventional gradient-echo sequence, EPI produces a series of gradient echoes with a bipolar oscillating readout gradient before the transverse magnetization decays away due to T_2^* relaxation (Figure 16.2c). Each gradient echo in the echo train is individually phase-encoded so that multiple views (or k-space lines) can be covered

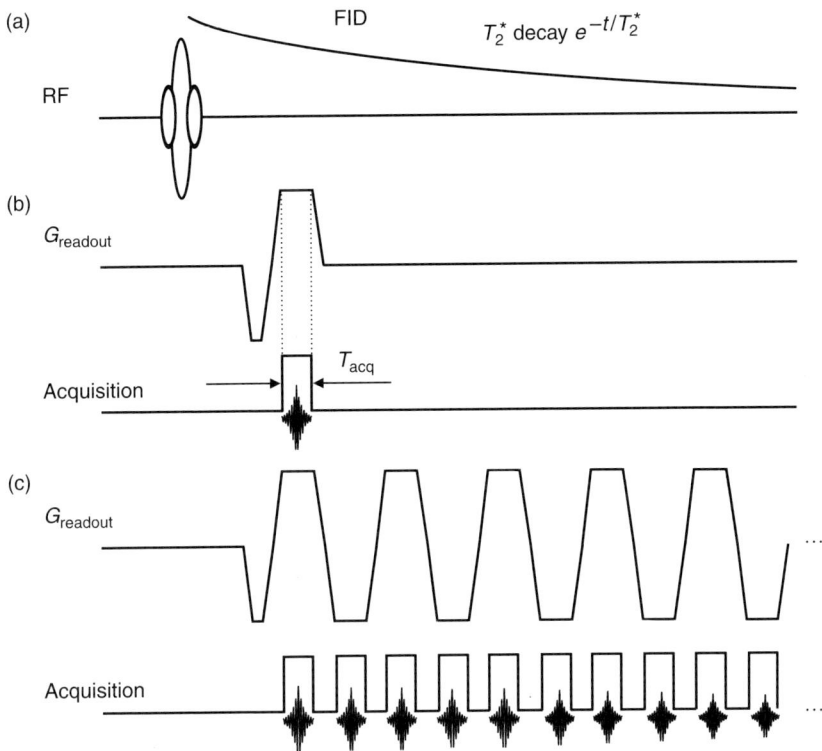

FIGURE 16.2 (a) An RF excitation pulse and comparison between (b) conventional gradient-echo acquisition and (c) EPI acquisition.

in a single RF excitation. The number of gradient echoes produced following an RF excitation is known as the *echo train length* (or ETL), denoted by N_{etl} here. Typically, the echoes in the echo train are evenly spaced. The interval between two adjacent echoes is known as the *echo spacing* (or ESP), denoted by t_{esp}. The concepts of ETL and ESP in EPI are very similar to those in RARE, except that gradient echoes are used instead of RF spin echoes. (For simplicity, we have used the same symbols to denote ETL and ESP as in Section 16.4 on RARE.)

As in RARE, ETL directly determines the scan-time reduction factor in EPI pulse sequences. Keeping the total sampling duration (as determined by the tissue T_2^*) fixed, the maximal ETL is inversely proportional to ESP. The minimal t_{esp} depends on many factors, such as the gradient slew rate, gradient amplitude, receiver bandwidth, and the k-space matrix size along the readout direction. On EPI-compatible scanners, t_{esp} is typically on the order of 1 millisecond or less, which is considerably shorter than t_{esp} in RARE sequences. Although T_2^* is shorter than T_2, the substantial reduction in t_{esp} generally outweighs the shortened transverse magnetization lifetime, leading to a longer ETL and making EPI faster than RARE.

Example 16.1 Consider a spin system with an average T_2^* relaxation time of 60 ms. If an EPI pulse sequence is used to acquire multiple gradient echoes prior to the time when the transverse magnetization $M_\perp(t) = 0.2 M_\perp(0)$, what is the maximal N_{etl} that can be acquired, assuming $t_{esp} = 1$ ms?

Answer The transverse magnetization decays according to Eq. (16.1). Substituting $M_\perp(t) = 0.2 M_\perp(0)$ and $T_2^* = 60$ ms into that equation, we obtain $t = 96.6$ ms. If $t_{esp} = 1$ ms, then the maximal $N_{etl} = \text{int}(t/t_{esp}) = \text{int}(96.6 \text{ ms}/1 \text{ ms}) = 96$. This ETL is considerably longer than the one calculated in Example 16.9 for RARE.

EPI Readout Gradient

The readout gradient waveform in EPI starts with a prephasing gradient $G_{x,p}$, followed by a series of readout gradient lobes $(G_{x,1}, G_{x,2}, G_{x,3}, \ldots)$ with alternating polarity, as shown in Figure 16.3. (As in many other sections of the book, we use subscripts x and y to denote the readout and phase-encoded

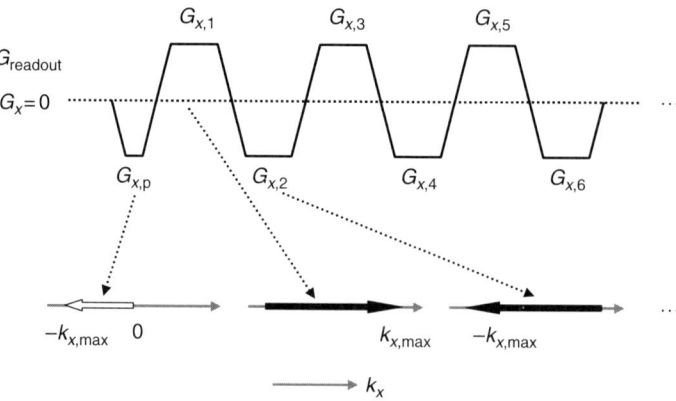

FIGURE 16.3 A bipolar EPI readout gradient waveform and its associated k-space trajectory. The dotted horizontal line shows zero gradient amplitude. $G_{x,p}$ is a prephasing gradient lobe. The readout gradient lobes are labeled as $G_{x,1}, G_{x,2}$, etc. The prephasing lobe k-space trajectory is represented by the hollow arrow. The solid arrows show the k-space trajectory of the readout gradient lobes.

directions, respectively.) The polarity of the prephasing gradient $G_{x,p}$ is opposite to that of the first readout gradient lobe $G_{x,1}$, unless $G_{x,p}$ occurs prior to the
RF refocusing pulse that negates the phase of the magnetization. The prephasing gradient area positions the k-space trajectory to $k_{x,\min}$ so that a k-space
line spanning from $k_{x,\min}$ to $k_{x,\max}$ can be acquired during the first readout
window. Typically, $k_{x,\min} = -k_{x,\max}$ as shown in Figure 16.3, although $k_{x,\min}$
can take other values in sequences such as mosaic EPI (see subsection 16.1.2).
When $k_{x,\min} = -k_{x,\max}$, the area of $G_{x,p}$ must be one-half the first readout
gradient area (see Figure 8.7a in Section 8.1). At the end of the $G_{x,1}$ lobe,
the k-space trajectory is placed at $k_x = k_{x,\max}$, which is opposite to that at
the end of the prephasing readout gradient (i.e., $k_x = -k_{x,\max}$). The second
half of $G_{x,1}$ lobe serves as a prephasing gradient for the second readout $G_{x,2}$,
provided that the polarity of $G_{x,2}$ is opposite to that of $G_{x,1}$. (This is why the
polarity of the readout gradient lobes must alternate throughout the echo train.)
With this prephasing gradient, a k-space line traversing from $k_{x,\max}$ to $-k_{x,\max}$
is acquired at the second readout (Figure 16.3). In general, the second half of
any readout gradient lobe functions as a prephasing gradient for the subsequent
readout gradient lobe. Thus, except for the first readout, prephasing gradient
lobes are not needed to produce a train of gradient echoes.

Recall the definition of k-space in Section 11.2, $\vec{k}(t) = (\gamma/2\pi) \int \vec{G}(t')dt'$.
With a bipolar readout gradient, the direction of the EPI k-space trajec-
tory alternates in accordance with the readout gradient, producing a set of
k-space lines with the following pattern: $(-k_{x,\max} \rightarrow k_{x,\max}, k_{x,\max} \rightarrow -k_{x,\max}, -k_{x,\max} \rightarrow k_{x,\max}, \ldots)$. The reversal of k-space trajectory direction for every other gradient echo must be corrected for prior to image
reconstruction (subsection 16.1.3).

To generate a series of gradient echoes centered at each readout window,
the area A_j of each gradient lobe in the readout gradient waveform is required
to satisfy Eq. (16.2)

$$
A_j = \begin{cases}
-A/2 & (j = 0; \text{ i.e., prephasing}) \\
A & (j = 1, 3, 5, \ldots, 2n - 1) \\
-A & (j = 2, 4, 6, \ldots, 2n)
\end{cases}
\tag{16.2}
$$

where j is the index of the gradient echoes. Although this condition does not
necessarily require all gradient lobes to have the same amplitude and the same
shape (see an example in skip-echo EPI discussed in subsection 16.1.5), the
EPI readout gradient typically consists of a series of identical readout gradient
lobes with alternating polarity. Three common readout gradient waveforms are
shown in Figure 16.4.

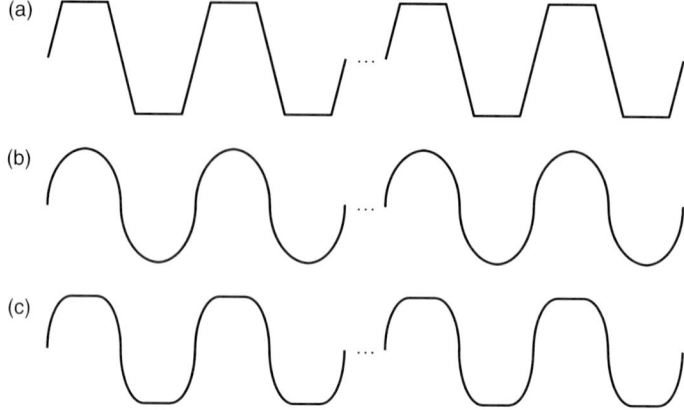

FIGURE 16.4 Three representative readout gradient waveforms: (a) trapezoid, (b) sinusoid, and (c) catch-and-hold.

Trapezoidal Readout Gradient   A trapezoidal gradient lobe in the readout gradient waveform in Figure 16.3a can be mathematically expressed as:

$$G_{\text{trap}}(t) = \begin{cases} S_R(t + t_2) & t \in [-t_2, -t_1) \\ G_x & t \in [-t_1, t_1) \\ S_R(t_2 - t) & t \in [t_1, t_2) \end{cases} \qquad (16.3)$$

where S_R is the slew rate for the gradient ramps, G_x is the gradient amplitude, and the timing parameters are defined in Figure 16.5a (assuming symmetry; i.e., that the ascending and descending ramps are of equal duration). Using the k-space definition given in Section 11.2 and assuming a prephasing gradient preceding $G_{\text{trap}}(t)$ with an area of $-G_x(t_1 + t_2)/2$, we can readily show that the readout k-space trajectory during this gradient lobe is:

$$k_x(t) = \frac{\gamma}{4\pi} \begin{cases} S_R(t + t_2)^2 - G_x(t_1 + t_2) & t \in [-t_2, -t_1) \\ 2G_x t & t \in [-t_1, t_1) \\ 2G_x t_1 + 2S_R t_2(t - t_1) + S_R(t_1^2 - t^2) & t \in [t_1, t_2) \end{cases}$$

$$(16.4)$$

which is graphically shown in Figure 16.5b. k-Space data acquisition can be performed either during the plateau portion of the trapezoid ($t \in [-t_1, t_1)$) or during the entire gradient lobe including the ramps ($t \in [-t_2, t_2)$). The latter approach is known as *ramp sampling* (Chen et al. 1986). Ramp sampling can be thought of as the data acquisition analog of variable-rate RF pulses, which are described in Section 2.4.

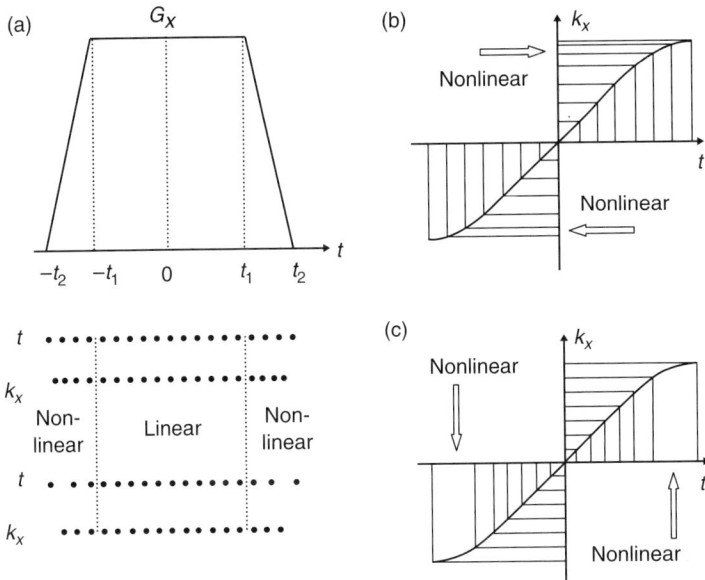

FIGURE 16.5 A trapezoidal gradient lobe (a) and the relationship between t and readout k-space variable k_x (b) and (c). When a constant sampling rate is used in the time domain, the k-space samples are nonlinear during the gradient ramps, (a) and (b). To achieve equidistant sampling in k-space, the dwell time becomes variable on the ramps, (a) and (c).

When data acquisition occurs only during the plateau of the trapezoid, k-space samples are linearly related to the time-domain signal (the second line of Eq. 16.4; also the central portion in Figures 16.5b and c). Thus, signals digitized with a constant dwell time (i.e., fixed bandwidth) can be directly used for fast Fourier transform without regridding. The acquisition time for a single echo is given by (see Eqs. 8.10 and 8.13):

$$T_{\mathrm{acq}} = \frac{n_x}{2\Delta v} = \frac{2\pi n_x}{\gamma L_x G_x} \tag{16.5}$$

where $2\Delta v$ is the full receiver bandwidth, n_x is the number of complex k-space data points along the readout direction, and L_x is the readout FOV. T_{acq} is a major contributor to ESP. To maximize the ETL within the lifetime of the transverse magnetization, the acquisition time for each echo must be minimized. Thus, according to Eq. (16.5), a wide receiver bandwidth should be used and the number of sampling points is often restricted to 64–128. Generally a wide receiver bandwidth results in decreased SNR (Recall that SNR $\propto 1/\sqrt{\Delta v}$, as discussed in Section 11.6). However, a wide receiver bandwidth also reduces the effect of T_2^*-induced signal decay, which can increase the SNR. The net effect on SNR depends on specific values of T_2^*, T_{acq}, and the bandwidth. Another implication of Eq. (16.5) is that the readout gradient amplitude must be increased to match the increased bandwidth. For most EPI applications on human subjects, a receiver bandwidth in the range of 100 kHz to 1 MHz generally can provide a good compromise among echo spacing, SNR, and the available gradient strength.

Without ramp sampling, the minimal ESP is given by (assuming ESP is solely determined by the readout gradient waveform):

$$t_{esp,min} = T_{acq} + 2(t_2 - t_1) = \frac{2\pi n_x}{\gamma L_x G_x} + \frac{2G_x}{S_R} \qquad (16.6)$$

Although T_{acq} can be reduced with a wide receiver bandwidth and an accompanying strong readout gradient G_x, time spent on the ramps, $2(t_2 - t_1)$, increases with the gradient strength and can cause a net increase in ESP for gradient systems with low slew rate, as shown in Example 16.2.

Example 16.2 An EPI scan without ramp sampling is performed with the following parameters: $\Delta v = \pm 62.5$ kHz, $n_x = 128$, $L_x = 22$ cm, and $S_R = 120$ T/m/s. (a) What is $t_{esp,min}$ as defined in Eq. (16.6)? (b) If Δv is increased to ± 125 kHz, what is $t_{esp,min}$? (c) If $S_R = 20$ T/m/s instead, recalculate (a) and (b).

Answer

(a) According to Eq. (16.5):

$$T_{acq} = \frac{n_x}{2\Delta v} = \frac{128}{2 \times 62.5} = 1.024 \text{ ms}$$

$$G_x = \frac{4\pi \Delta v}{\gamma L_x} = \frac{4\pi \times 62.5}{2\pi \times 4.257 \times 22} = 13.3 \text{ mT/m}$$

Thus:

$$t_{esp,min} = T_{acq} + \frac{2G_x}{S_R} = 1.024 + \frac{2 \times 13.3}{120} = 1.246 \text{ ms}$$

(b) If Δv is increased to ± 125 kHz, then T_{acq} is halved and G_x is doubled. Therefore:

$$t_{esp,min} = T_{acq} + \frac{2G_x}{S_R} = 0.512 + \frac{2 \times 26.6}{120} = 0.955 \text{ ms}$$

Because the slew rate is relatively high in this case, increasing the receiver bandwidth results in a reduction in $t_{esp,min}$.

(c) With a slower slew rate of 20 T/m/s and a bandwidth of $\pm 62.5\,kHz$, $t_{esp,min}$ is:

$$t_{esp,min} = T_{acq} + \frac{2G_x}{S_R} = 1.024 + \frac{2 \times 13.3}{20} = 2.354\,ms$$

When $\Delta\nu$ is increased to $\pm 125\,kHz$:

$$t_{esp,min} = T_{acq} + \frac{2G_x}{S_R} = 0.512 + \frac{2 \times 26.6}{20} = 3.172\,ms$$

In this case, increasing the receiver bandwidth does not lead to a shorter $t_{esp,min}$ because of the slower slew rate. Considerable time (2.66 ms) is wasted to ramp up and down the gradient, leading to a net increase in $t_{esp,min}$.

A longer ESP not only compromises the EPI data acquisition efficiency, but also exacerbates image artifacts such as distortion, chemical shift displacement, signal loss, and blurring (subsection 16.1.5). One way to shorten ESP is to increase the slew rate through gradient hardware design (e.g., increasing the driving voltage of the gradient amplifier or reducing the inductance of the gradient coils). Slew rates above certain thresholds, however, can cause a number of patient safety concerns, including pain, peripheral neurostimulation (e.g., muscle twitching), induced respiration, and even cardiac magnetostimulation (e.g., systolic excitation and fibrillations) (Shellock and Kanal 1994; Cohen et al. 1990). Another approach is to use ramp sampling so that the idle time on the ramps is eliminated by acquiring k-space data during the entire trapezoidal lobe.

To achieve the same spatial resolution with and without ramp sampling, the trapezoidal gradient area (i.e., the maximal extent of k-space) with ramp sampling must equal to $T_{acq}G_x$ given by Eq. (16.5). If the same acquisition time T_{acq} is used with and without ramp sampling, then the readout gradient amplitude must be increased to:

$$G_x{}' = \frac{T_{acq}}{T_{acq} - T_{ramp}} G_x \qquad (16.7)$$

where T_{ramp} is the ramp time (i.e., $T_{ramp} = t_2 - t_1$ in Figure 16.5a). Because $T_{ramp} = G_x{}'/S_R$, the gradient amplitude $G_x{}'$ for ramp sampling can be obtained by solving a quadratic equation:

$$\left(G_x{}'\right)^2 - T_{acq}S_R\left(G_x{}'\right) + T_{acq}S_R G_x = 0 \qquad (16.8)$$

For nonoblique scans, the increased gradient amplitude G_x' cannot exceed the maximal gradient strength h available on the scanner. For oblique scans, the maximal allowed value of G_x depends on both the oblique angles and h (Section 7.3). With the increased gradient amplitude, the receiver bandwidth must be increased accordingly to maintain the same FOV, resulting in a larger number of k-space samples n_x':

$$n_x' \geq \frac{G_x'}{G_x} n_x \tag{16.9}$$

where equality in Eq. (16.9) represents the minimally required number of data points to satisfy the Nyquist sampling criterion. In practice, the exact value of n_x' also relies on the clock rate of the A/D converter, as shown in Example 16.3.

Example 16.3 An EPI pulse sequence without ramp sampling has the following parameters: $n_x = 128$, $G_x = 15$ mT/m, and $T_{acq} = 0.512$ ms. When ramp sampling is used, the readout gradient must be increased to $G_x = 21$ mT/m. (a) What is the minimally required number of samples with ramp sampling? (b) If a digitizer with a 2-MHz clock is used for ramp sampling, determine the actual number of samples.

Answer

(a) According to Eq. (16.9), $n_x' \geq (G_x'/G_x)n_x = \frac{21}{15} \times 128 \approx 180$.
(b) For a digitizer with a 2-MHz clock, the dwell time must be integer multiples of 0.5 μs. Given that the total acquisition time is 0.512 ms, the number of points actually acquired is 205, which is the closest number to 180 with a dwell time of 2.5 μs.

With ramp sampling, the linear relationship between k-space variable and time does not hold any more (Eq. 16.4). An evenly sampled time-domain signal becomes unevenly spaced when mapped to k-space (Figure 16.5b). For example, using the first line of Eq. (16.4) to analyze the ascending ramp in Figure 16.5a, k-space sampling interval Δk_x is related to the dwell time Δt by:

$$\Delta k_x = \Delta t \sqrt{[\gamma S_R (k_x(t) - k_x(-t_2))]/\pi} \tag{16.10}$$

indicating Δk_x varies with k_x (or time t). The skewed k-space data can be restored to an evenly spaced linear array using one of the gridding techniques discussed in Section 13.2, prior to image reconstruction with a fast Fourier transform. The oversampled data points shown in Eq. (16.9) are typically interpolated (e.g., using a SINC kernel) to the uniformly spaced k-space grid of n_x. The major disadvantage of this approach is the longer computational time needed for gridding.

An alternative approach to addressing the nonlinear relationship between Δk_x and Δt is to sample the time-domain signal at a nonconstant rate so that the k-space samples are equally spaced (Figure 16.5c). This method is sometimes referred to as nonlinear sampling (Ordidge and Mansfield 1984). In nonlinear sampling, the gradient amplitude also needs to be scaled according to Eq. (16.7), but the number of k-space points n_x' can be kept the same as n_x if each Δt produces the same gradient area. For the ascending ramp in Figure 16.5a, this requirement can be explicitly expressed as:

$$\Delta t = \frac{2\pi}{\gamma L_x S_R(t+t_2)} \qquad t \in (-t_2, -t_1] \qquad (16.11)$$

Nonlinear sampling eliminates the need for gridding and allows the k-space data acquired to be directly used for fast Fourier transform; however, most receivers are not designed to sample data in this mode (see Section 11.1). Thus, nonlinear sampling is less commonly used then the fixed-rate sampling discussed previously.

Sinusoidal Readout Gradient   A sinusoidal gradient waveform (Figure 16.4b) is typically produced by resonant gradient coils, where the coil inductance and capacitance form an LC resonant circuit with a resonance frequency of $\Omega = 1/(2\pi\sqrt{LC})$ (Nowak et al. 1989). Typically Ω is $\sim 1\,\text{kHz}$. Due to resistive loss in the coil and cable, an external voltage source must be provided to maintain a constant amplitude of the sinusoidal current.

With a sinusoidal readout gradient lobe $G_x(t) = G_x\cos(2\pi\Omega t)$ (Figure 16.6a) and a prephasing gradient with an area of $-G_x/(2\pi\Omega)$, the k-space variable k_x becomes:

$$k_x(t) = \frac{\gamma G_x}{4\pi^2\Omega}\sin 2\pi\Omega t = \frac{\gamma G_x T_{\text{acq}}}{2\pi^2}\sin(\pi t/T_{\text{acq}}) \qquad (16.12)$$

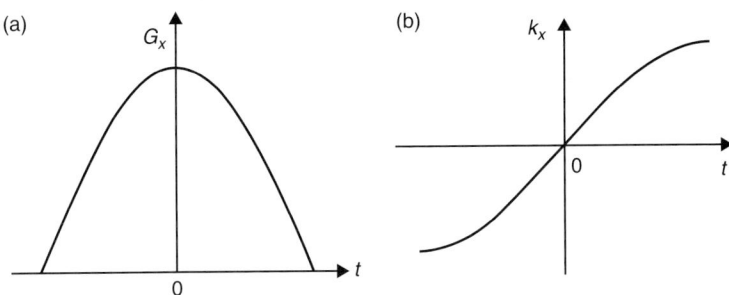

FIGURE 16.6 (a) A sinusoidal readout gradient lobe and (b) its k-space variable k_x as a nonlinear function of time t.

which is nonlinear with respect to time t during the entire gradient lobe (Figure 16.6b). The time-varying gradient amplitude makes ramp sampling the only option for a sinusoidal readout gradient. Either of the two ramp-sampling approaches (i.e., constant Δt or constant Δk) shown in Figure 16.5 can be adapted to sampling under a sinusoidal gradient. Compared to a trapezoidal readout gradient without ramp sampling, the sinusoidal readout gradient must increase its amplitude by a factor of $\pi/2$ if the same acquisition window is used. (The interested reader can derive this result based on conservation of the gradient area, as used in the derivation of Eq. 16.7.) When the sampling strategy with constant Δt is used, the number of k-space samples must also be increased by $\pi/2 \approx 1.57$ to maintain the same FOV and spatial resolution. For example, if a trapezoidal readout gradient without ramp sampling uses $n_x = 64$, n_x' should be increased to at least 101 when a sinusoidal readout gradient is employed. The k-space data are typically interpolated to an equidistance grid along the k_x direction. The interpolation algorithms are discussed in Zakhor et al. (1991) and Bruder et al. (1992), as well as in Section 13.2. Alternatively, a generalized transformation can be employed (Bruder et al. 1992).

Catch-and-Hold   A hybrid readout gradient that combines the features of trapezoidal and sinusoidal readout gradient waveforms is depicted in Figure 16.4c. The linear ramps of a trapezoidal gradient are replaced with one-quarter cycle of a sinusoidal function. This waveform is sometimes referred to as *catch-and-hold*. Similar to the trapezoidal waveform, the catch-and-hold waveform can be used with or without ramp sampling. Without ramp sampling, the situation is essentially identical to that described previously. With ramp sampling, data acquisition on the ramps is similar to that with two halves of sinusoidal lobes. Details on gradient amplitude, receiver bandwidth, and number of k-space points can be derived analogously.

EPI Phase-Encoding Gradient

Similar to the readout gradient, the EPI phase-encoding gradient also starts with a prephasing gradient lobe with an area of $A_{p,p}$ (Figure 16.7), prior to the generation of the EPI echo train. This prephasing gradient determines the initial position of k-space sampling along the phase-encoded direction. Any gradient lobe shape can be used, as long as the area satisfies a predetermined value (see Example 16.4). If an RF refocusing pulse is used in the sequence, the prephasing gradient lobe can be played before the refocusing pulse, but its polarity must be reversed to counteract the phase reversal effect by the refocusing pulse.

Following the prephasing gradient, an EPI phase-encoding gradient waveform can be played in one of two ways. In the first approach, a constant phase-encoding gradient G_y is used throughout the entire readout echo

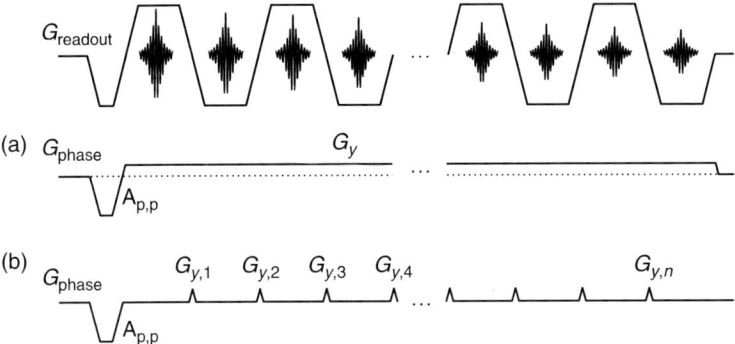

FIGURE 16.7 Two EPI phase-encoding waveforms: (a) constant gradient G_y, and (b) blip gradients $G_{y,1}, G_{y,2}, G_{y,3}, \ldots, G_{y,n}$. Both waveforms generally use a prephasing gradient with an area of $A_{p,p}$. To illustrate the relationship with readout gradient, a trapezoidal readout gradient waveform is also shown.

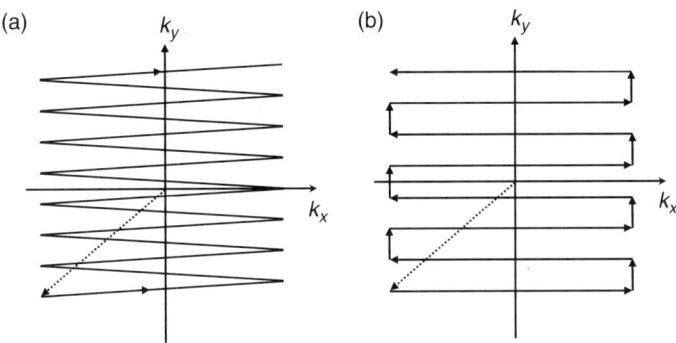

FIGURE 16.8 k-space trajectories (a) and (b) corresponding to the phase-encoding gradient waveforms (a) and (b) in Figure 16.7. The dotted diagonal lines show the trajectory of the prephasing gradients.

train (Figure 16.7a). Thus, the k-space variable along the phase-encoded direction (k_y) varies linearly with time. The phase-encoding gradient, in conjunction with the readout gradient, produces a zigzag k-space trajectory shown in Figure 16.8a. When the phase-encoding gradient area equals $A_{p,p}$, the center of k-space ($k_y = 0$) is sampled. Because the k-space data points do not fall onto a rectilinear grid, k-space regridding is required prior to image reconstruction. With the zigzag k-space trajectory in Figure 16.8a, the k-space sampling interval Δk_y is constant only at $k_x = 0$. This constant Δk_y can be used to determine the phase-encoding gradient amplitude G_y by using the relationship

$\Delta k_y = 1/L_y$ (where L_y is the FOV along the phase-encoded direction):

$$G_y = \frac{2\pi}{\gamma L_y t_{esp}} \tag{16.13}$$

Analogous to the dwell time during the readout (see Eq. 11.2), t_{esp} is the effective dwell time for the phase-encoding process because it represents the time between k_y sample points at $k_x = 0$. It corresponds to a full bandwidth of $\Delta \nu_{phase} \equiv 1/t_{esp}$, which is sometimes referred to as the *phase-encoding bandwidth* to distinguish it from the readout bandwidth discussed in Section 11.1. (Note that $\Delta \nu_{phase}$ is conventionally defined as the full bandwidth instead of half-bandwidth defined for the readout direction in Section 11.1.) Because t_{esp} is typically on the order of 1 ms, which is considerably longer than the readout dwell time (e.g., a few microseconds), the phase-encoding gradient amplitude is generally two to three orders of magnitude smaller than the corresponding readout gradient amplitude.

Example 16.4 An EPI pulse sequence with $t_{esp} = 1$ ms is used to form an image over a FOV of 20 cm. (a) If a constant phase-encoding gradient is used with a linear ramp at a slew rate of 50 T/m/s, what is the phase-encoding gradient amplitude? (b) If the sixteenth echo is used to sample the center of k-space, what is the prephasing gradient area along the phase-encoded direction?

Answer

(a) Using Eq. (16.13), the constant phase-encoding gradient amplitude is calculated to be:

$$G_y = \frac{2\pi}{2\pi \times 4.257 \times 20 \times 1} = 0.0117\,\text{G/cm} = 0.117\,\text{mT/m}$$

(b) With a slew rate of 50 T/m/s, the ramp time for the phase-encoding gradient is $T_{ramp} = 0.117/50 = 2.34\,\mu\text{s}$. The gradient area at the center of the sixteenth echo is:

$$A_{phase} = \frac{1}{2}T_{ramp}G_y + \left(\frac{1}{2} + 15\right)t_{esp}G_y$$

$$= \left(\frac{1}{2} \times 2.34 \times 10^{-3} + \left(\frac{1}{2} + 15\right) \times 1\right) \times 0.117$$

$$= 1.81\,\text{mT} \cdot \text{ms/m}$$

Thus, the prephasing gradient area should be $A_{p,p} = -A_{phase} = -1.81\,\text{mT} \cdot \text{ms/m}$, if the prephasing gradient is applied immediately before the phase-encoding gradient, as shown in Figure 16.7a. If the prephasing gradient is played before an RF refocusing pulse, then the gradient area should be $1.81\,\mathrm{mT}\cdot\mathrm{ms/m}$.

The second approach to applying the phase-encoding gradient is to use a series of blips $G_{y,j}$ with the same polarity and typically identical area A_{blip} (Chapman et al. 1987) (Figure 16.7b). Each blip is played before the acquisition of an echo, resulting in a k-space trajectory shown in Figure 16.8b. The phase-encoding gradient area is accumulated throughout the echo train. Thus, the k-space value (or the phase-encoding value) at the jth echo is given by:

$$k_{y,j} = \frac{\gamma}{2\pi}\left(A_{\mathrm{p,p}} + (j-1)A_{\mathrm{blip}}\right) \tag{16.14}$$

where $A_{\mathrm{p,p}}$ controls the starting position of the k-space trajectory (dashed gray line in Figure 16.8b), and the maximum value of j determines the final k-space location ($j = 1, 2, \ldots, n_y$). Using the relationship $\Delta k_y = 1/L_y$, A_{blip} can be calculated with:

$$A_{\mathrm{blip}} = \frac{2\pi}{\gamma L_y} \tag{16.15}$$

Any gradient lobe shape can be used for the blip phase-encoding gradient, as long as the gradient area requirement is satisfied. Because A_{blip} is generally very small, a triangular gradient lobe shape is frequently employed. It is worth noting that, unlike that in RARE, the phase-encoding gradient area can accumulate throughout the echo train without the need of a phase-rewinding gradient, because EPI pulse sequences are not subject to the CPMG conditions discussed in Section 16.4. With a blip phase-encoding gradient, k-space samples can be evenly spaced along the phase-encoded direction, which eliminates the need for gridding.

16.1.2 BASIC ECHO PLANAR IMAGING PULSE SEQUENCES

Gradient-Echo EPI   A representative 2D gradient-echo EPI (also known as GRE-EPI or GE-EPI) pulse sequence is shown in Figure 16.9. The pulse sequence starts with a selective excitation pulse to produce an FID signal. Under the envelope of the FID, a series of spatially encoded gradient echoes are produced using any combination of the readout and phase-encoding gradient waveforms described in subsection 16.1.1. Because the TR of EPI is typically much longer than that of a conventional gradient-echo pulse sequence, the flip angle of the excitation pulse is typically set to 90° to maximize the SNR (i.e., the Ernst angle $\theta_E \approx 90°$). To suppress the chemical shift artifacts (subsection 16.1.5) caused by lipid signals, the excitation pulse is often designed as a

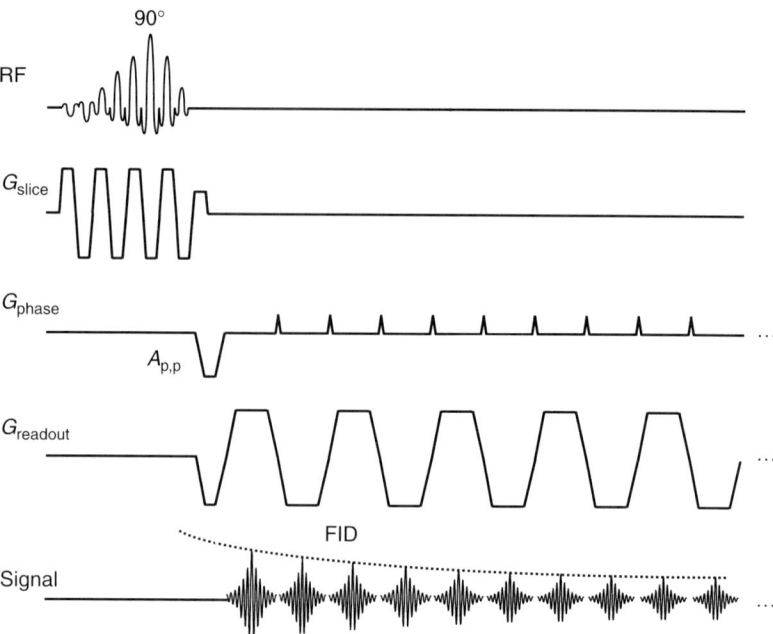

FIGURE 16.9 An example of a gradient-echo EPI pulse sequence. The spatial-spectral excitation pulse can be replaced by a slice-selection pulse preceded by a spectrally selective pulse to suppress lipid signals. For simplicity the optional spoiler gradient at the end of the sequence is not shown.

spatial-spectral pulse (Section 5.4), especially when a fast gradient slew rate is available so that the pulse width can be made short. Alternatively, a spectrally selective pulse (Section 4.3; not shown in Figure 16.9) is used before the excitation pulse to saturate the lipid signals. In that case, the excitation pulse typically has linear or minimum phase. The shorter isodelay of a minimum phase pulse can reduce the signal loss due to T_2^* decay, resulting in a slightly longer time window for echo train generation. The slice-selection gradients for a spatial-spectral pulse, a linear-phase excitation pulse, and a minimum phase excitation pulse are discussed in Sections 5.4 and 2.3. At the end of the pulse sequence, a spoiler gradient (not shown in Figure 16.9) is often employed to dephase any remaining transverse magnetization before the next excitation pulse is applied.

In gradient-echo EPI, each k-space line along the phase-encoded direction is acquired at a different TE. The amplitude of the corresponding gradient echo decays according to:

$$S(n) = S_0 e^{-\mathrm{TE}(n)/T_2^*} \tag{16.16}$$

where n is the echo index in the echo train and S_0 is the signal at time zero (i.e., the isodelay point of the excitation pulse). Because the image contrast is predominantly determined by the TE value when the central k-space lines are acquired, the effective TE (denoted by $\mathrm{TE}_{\mathrm{eff}}$) is defined as the TE that corresponds to the central k-space line, i.e., $\mathrm{TE}_{\mathrm{eff}} = \mathrm{TE}(k_y = 0)$. The position of the central k-space line in the echo train can be controlled by adjusting $A_{\mathrm{p,p}}$, as shown in Example 16.4. In gradient-echo EPI, the polarity of $A_{\mathrm{p,p}}$ is always opposite to that of the phase-encoding gradient. If $|A_{\mathrm{p,p}}|$ is increased, then it takes more time for the phase-encoding gradient to accumulate enough area to balance $A_{\mathrm{p,p}}$. Thus, a later echo in the echo train is used to sample the central region of k-space, resulting in an image with heavy T_2^* weighting. Conversely, if $|A_{\mathrm{p,p}}|$ is decreased, an image with less T_2^* contrast is produced.

The T_2^* contrast plays an important role in neurofunctional MRI (fMRI) because increased blood flow during neuronal activation results in an increase in the blood oxygenation level, which prolongs the local T_2^* value (Thulborn et al. 1982). The increase in image intensity due to the T_2^* change is detected and statistically analyzed to highlight the functional activation area. This contrast mechanism is known as blood oxygenation level dependent (BOLD) contrast (Kwong et al. 1992). At 1.5 T, a $\mathrm{TE}_{\mathrm{eff}}$ value of $\sim$40–60 ms is typically used to obtain an adequate BOLD contrast without considerably compromising the image SNR. At higher magnetic fields, the increased magnetic susceptibility effect shortens T_2^*. Thus, the $\mathrm{TE}_{\mathrm{eff}}$ must be adjusted accordingly (e.g., $\mathrm{TE}_{\mathrm{eff}} = 25$–30 ms at 3.0 T) to rebalance the contrast and SNR of the gradient-echo EPI.

Spin-Echo EPI   A 2D spin-echo EPI (SE-EPI) pulse sequence comprises two selective RF pulses, one excitation pulse with a typical flip angle of 90°, and a refocusing pulse with a flip angle of 180° (Figure 16.10). Similar to gradient-echo EPI, the excitation pulse can be a spatial-spectral pulse or a pulse with linear or minimum phase preceded by a spectrally selective pulse to suppress lipid signals. The refocusing pulse is typically a SINC pulse or linear phase SLR pulse. The two RF pulses generate a spin echo as described in Sections 3.3, 8.1, and 14.3. During a time window around the peak of the spin echo, EPI readout and phase-encoding waveforms are played to produce a series of spatially encoded gradient echoes. Like gradient-echo EPI, spin-echo EPI relies on gradient echoes to sample k-space lines, except that the gradient echoes are formed under the envelope of a spin echo instead of an FID. The slice-selection gradient waveform is essentially identical to that in a conventional spin-echo pulse sequence.

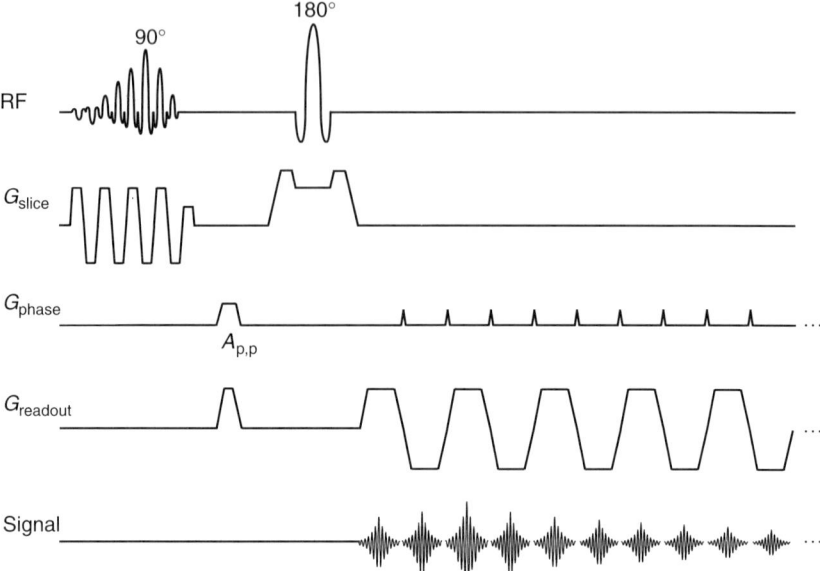

FIGURE 16.10 An example of a spin-echo EPI pulse sequence. The spatial-spectral excitation pulse can be replaced by a slice-selection pulse preceded by a spectrally selective pulse to suppress lipid signals. For simplicity the optional spoiler gradient at the end of the sequence is not shown.

With the use of a refocusing pulse, the prephasing gradient in either the readout or the phase-encoded direction does not have to be played immediately before the readout or the phase-encoding gradient. In many implementations, the prephasing gradients are placed between the excitation and the refocusing pulses (Figure 16.10) so that the time after the refocusing pulse can be more efficiently used to produce gradient echoes. With this strategy, the polarity of the prephasing gradient along the readout and the phase-encoded directions is the same as that of the first readout gradient lobe and the phase-encoding gradient, respectively, as discussed earlier. To dephase unwanted FIDs, spin-echo EPI often requires crusher gradients (shown in Figure 16.10) that straddle the refocusing pulse (see Section 10.2).

Similar to gradient-echo EPI, each gradient echo in spin-echo EPI is acquired at a different TE. The effective TE of the sequence is also defined as the TE when the central k-space line is acquired, $TE_{eff} = TE(k_y = 0)$. The TE of the spin echo, TE_{se}, may or may not correspond to TE_{eff}. When TE_{eff} coincides with TE_{se}, the sensitivity of the sequence to off-resonance effects is substantially reduced and the image becomes predominantly T_2

weighted, instead of T_2^* weighted (assuming TR $\gg T_1$ and $\text{TE}_{\text{eff}} \approx T_2$ or longer). This strategy is often implemented to improve EPI image quality, such as in diffusion-weighted and T_2-weighted EPI. When sensitivity to T_2^* or off-resonance effects is desired, however, TE_{eff} can be shifted away from TE_{se}.

Because off-resonance effects, such as magnetic susceptibility variation and magnetic field inhomogeneities, can be reduced or minimized in spin-echo EPI, the resulting images generally have fewer artifacts (e.g., decreased signal loss in regions with magnetic susceptibility variation) than the corresponding gradient-echo echo planar images. A major drawback of spin-echo EPI is its reduced sensitivity to BOLD contrast.

Inversion-Recovery EPI   Inversion-recovery EPI (IR-EPI) plays an inversion recovery (IR) module prior to a GE-EPI or SE-EPI pulse sequence (Stehling 1990). The pulse sequence can be used to attenuate cerebrospinal fluid as in FLAIR (Section 14.2), prepare a desired tissue contrast as in magnetization-prepared T_1-weighted imaging, measure tissue perfusion with arterial spin labeling (Section 17.1), or produce a T_1 map (Section 14.2). Reduced SNR limits the use of IR-EPI for lipid suppression. Alternative lipid-suppression techniques such as spectrally selective pulses and spatial-spectral pulses are generally adequate at the field strengths at which EPI is typically used (e.g., ≥ 1.5 T).

Single-Shot EPI   EPI was originally developed (and is still largely used) as a single-shot pulse sequence. In single-shot EPI, the entire 2D k-space data needed for image reconstruction are acquired using an echo train produced by a single RF excitation pulse. If a single slice is imaged without signal averaging, the total scan time is the same as the sequence length T_{seq}, irrespective of the TR value (which becomes undefined and irrelevant):

$$T_{\text{scan}} = T_{\text{seq}} = C + N_{\text{etl}} \times t_{\text{esp}} \tag{16.17}$$

where C is the interval between the start of the sequence and the beginning of data acquisition of the first echo. C is typically a few milliseconds in gradient-echo EPI and $\sim \text{TE}_{\text{se}}/2$ in spin-echo EPI. If we assume the following representative values for a single-shot EPI sequence: $C = 5$ ms, $N_{\text{etl}} = 80$, $t_{\text{esp}} = 1$ ms, then the total scan time is only 85 ms. For multiple slices (N_{slices}) without signal averaging, the scan time increases to:

$$T_{\text{scan}} = N_{\text{slices}} T_{\text{seq}} = N_{\text{slices}} (C + N_{\text{etl}} \times t_{\text{esp}}) \tag{16.18}$$

The acquisition time for each slice remains T_{seq}. With signal averaging, TR is defined and the scan time becomes:

$$T_{\text{scan}} = \text{TR} \times \text{NEX} \times N_{\text{acq}} \qquad (16.19)$$

where NEX is the number of signal averages (NEX > 1), N_{acq} is the number of passes required to image all prescribed slices (Section 11.5), and a 2D interleaved acquisition mode is assumed. Because the primary motivation of using a single-shot technique is to obtain snapshot images to freeze motion, signal averaging is not commonly used in single-shot EPI. In special applications such as diffusion-weighted imaging and diffusion tensor imaging (Section 17.2) with NEX > 1, signal averaging is typically performed by summing up the magnitude (i.e., modulus) images, instead of adding the k-space data, to avoid motion-induced phase errors.

Single-shot EPI provides excellent temporal resolution, but places more stringent requirements on the hardware and often produces images with compromised quality, such as low SNR, low spatial resolution, and pronounced artifacts. To maximize the ETL in single-shot EPI without prolonging the total acquisition window, the acquisition time for each echo must be kept to a minimum. As discussed in subsection 16.1.1, a wide receiver bandwidth is commonly used and the number of sampling points at each echo is often restricted to 64–128. A wide receiver bandwidth requires a strong readout gradient. For example, for a receiver bandwidth of $\pm 125\,\text{kHz}$ and a FOV of 20 cm, the required gradient strength is $\sim 29\,\text{mT/m}$ (Eq. 8.13). At a fixed slew rate, the higher gradient also requires a longer rise time to reach the targeted gradient value. This implies that the slew rate should also be increased to achieve the maximum possible echo train length. Even with these changes, the ETL allowed by the signal lifetime (see Example 16.1) may not be sufficient to acquire all phase-encoded k-space lines ranging from $-k_{y,\text{max}}$ to $k_{y,\text{max}}$. Partial k-space acquisition (Section 13.4) is often employed along the phase-encoded direction. (Although not commonly used, partial k-space acquisition can also be used along the readout direction to shorten ESP). The single-shot image can be reconstructed using one of the algorithms described in Section 13.4. For example, to reconstruct an image with a matrix of 128×128, the phase-encoded k-space index could range from -8 to $+63$ with an ETL of 72. The k-space lines with indices from -8 to -1 are sometimes called the EPI overscan lines. In this example, the eighth and the ninth echo in the echo train may be used to sample the two central k-space lines. The area of the prephasing gradient lobe can be determined in a way similar to Example 16.4.

Multishot EPI Multishot EPI acquires a fraction of the required k-space data with the echo train produced by each RF excitation. k-Space data from multiple nonredundant RF excitations (or shots) are combined prior to image reconstruction. Unlike single-shot EPI, the achievable spatial resolution (i.e., the extent of k-space) in multishot EPI is no longer limited by the ETL. A k-space matrix of 256×256 or even larger can be obtained. Because ETL does not have to be stretched to its maximum, multishot EPI can yield better image quality (i.e., better SNR, reduced blurring, less distortion, and lower ghost intensity) and have less stringent requirements on gradient and RF hardware (e.g., gradient amplitude, slew rate, and receiver bandwidth) compared to its single-shot counterpart. The major drawback is the increased scan time, which makes multishot EPI much more sensitive to motion.

Similar to multishot RARE, the number of required shots to acquire a total of n_y k-space lines is given by:

$$N_{\text{shot}} = \begin{cases} n_y/N_{\text{etl}} & \text{if } (n_y \bmod N_{\text{etl}}) = 0 \\ \text{int}(n_y/N_{\text{etl}}) + 1 & \text{if } (n_y \bmod N_{\text{etl}}) \neq 0 \end{cases} \qquad (16.20)$$

where the int function takes the integer part of its argument, and the modulo (mod) function gives the remainder of the integer division. In practice, n_y and N_{etl} are typically chosen to satisfy $(n_y \bmod N_{\text{etl}}) = 0$. The total scan time for a multishot EPI sequence is given by:

$$T_{\text{scan}} = \text{TR} \times N_{\text{shot}} \times \text{NEX} \times N_{\text{acq}} \qquad (16.21)$$

which represents an N_{shot}-fold increase in scan time as compared to Eq. (16.19).

k-Space data from multiple shots can be combined sequentially as a series of tiles (Figure 16.11a) or interleaved with one another along the phase-encoded direction (Figure 16.11b). The former approach is also known as *mosaic EPI*. Each tile is acquired within a single ETL in a manner equivalent to single-shot EPI. The position of the tile can be controlled by changing the prephasing gradient areas as well as the polarity of the readout or the phase-encoding gradients. For example, to sample any one of the four tiles in Figure 16.10a, the prephasing gradient area can be changed to 0 (assuming ramp sampling is used) along both the readout and the phase-encoded directions. Tile 1 is acquired when the readout gradient waveform starts with a negative lobe and the phase-encoding gradient has positive blips. The total number of the tiles required to cover k-space equals N_{shot}. A major problem with mosaic EPI is that each tile contains different phase errors, causing k-space data inconsistency that produces artifacts. One approach to correct for the phase error is to partially overlap the adjacent tiles and estimate the phase inconsistency based on the overlapped data. Another problem is that the phase-encoding bandwidth (i.e., $1/t_{\text{esp}}$) can be similar to that in a single-shot pulse sequence (e.g., when two tiles are used along the phase-encoded direction).

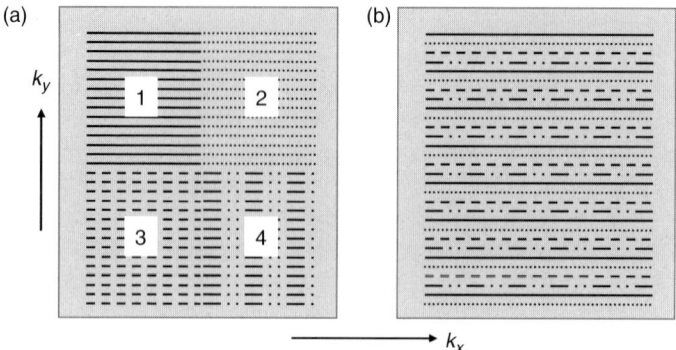

FIGURE 16.11 Representative multishot EPI sampling schemes using (a) mosaic and (b) interleaves. Four shots are assumed in both (a) and (b). The numbers in (a) indicate the shot index. The solid lines, dotted lines, dashed lines, and dash-dot lines represent the first, second, third, and fourth shots, respectively.

Thus, chemical shift artifacts, magnetic susceptibility effects, and Nyquist ghosts can be as bad as in single-shot EPI (subsection 16.1.4). Because of these problems, multishot mosaic EPI is not as commonly used as interleaved EPI on commercial scanners.

In interleaved multishot EPI (McKinnon 1993; Butts et al. 1994; Buonocore and Zhu 1998), the phase-encoding amplitude or the blip areas are increased so that the gap between k-space lines acquired within an ETL is also increased. The k-space lines from subsequent excitations are placed to fill up the gaps in an interleaved manner, as shown in Figure 16.11b. Because each shot produces the transverse magnetization anew (assuming efficient spoiling), any phase errors or amplitude modulation accumulated throughout the echo train are reset. If the directions of the k-space lines produced by each shot are parallel to one another (i.e., the readout gradient waveform is used for successive shots), both the phase and amplitude modulations are slowed down along the k_y direction of Figure 16.11b. Alternatively, if the directions of the k-space lines produced by multiple shots are anti-parallel for any two adjacent interleaves (i.e., the readout gradient alternates its polarity between successive shots), then only the amplitude modulation is slowed. The phase modulation is virtually the same as in single-shot EPI, provided that an odd number of interleaves is used (Buonocore and Zhu 1998). The parallel interleaf scheme is assumed in the following discussion.

The use of interleaved EPI has several implications for image quality. First, the reduced phase and amplitude modulations in k-space result in decreased spacing of the ghosts and lower ghost intensity. This situation is analogous to low-frequency view ordering used in respiratory compensation (Section 12.3). (Note that the use of the anti-parallel interleaf scheme is analogous to high-frequency view ordering.) Second, the T_2^* induced signal modulation described by Eq. (16.16) is slowed by a factor of N_{shot}. Consequently, imaging blurring is reduced because the entire k-space data are acquired within a much narrower time window. Third, the effective bandwidth along the phase-encoded direction is increased by a factor of N_{shot}:

$$\Delta \nu_{phase} = \frac{N_{shot}}{t_{esp}} \tag{16.22}$$

The increased bandwidth reduces chemical shift displacement and other off-resonance effects such as image distortion and signal loss. Additional discussion of these image artifacts is given in subsection 16.1.4.

With a frequency offset Δf, the nth echo in a multishot EPI sequence accumulates a phase given by:

$$\phi_n = 2\pi \int_0^{TE(n)} \Delta f \, dt \tag{16.23}$$

where TE(n) is the echo time for the nth echo. The amplitude attenuation of the nth echo can be obtained from Eq. (16.16). The phase accumulation and the amplitude attenuation do not depend on which shot is used to acquire the echo. Thus, stepwise phase and amplitude modulations are produced along the phase-encoded direction. The discontinuities can contribute to artifacts such as ghosting. An effective way to mitigate this problem is to slightly shift the echo train to the right (or left) in successive shots, so that the k-space modulation functions are smoothed (Figure 16.12). The amount of shift is given by t_{esp}/N_{shot}. This technique is known as echo time shifting or echo shifting (Butts et al. 1994; Feinberg and Oshio 1994) and is also sometimes used with GRASE (Section 16.2).

16.1.3 EPI IMAGE RECONSTRUCTION

In EPI, the k-space lines acquired with even echoes traverse in the opposite direction compared to those acquired with odd echoes. This requires that the k-space data be flipped along the readout direction for alternative k-space lines so that all the k-space lines point in the same direction. This operation is sometimes called *row flipping*. After row flipping, the k-space data usually will contain inconsistent phase errors caused by eddy currents, B_0-field inhomogeneity, receive chain and gradient amplifier group delays, concomitant magnetic fields, asymmetric anti-aliasing filter response, and so on. To

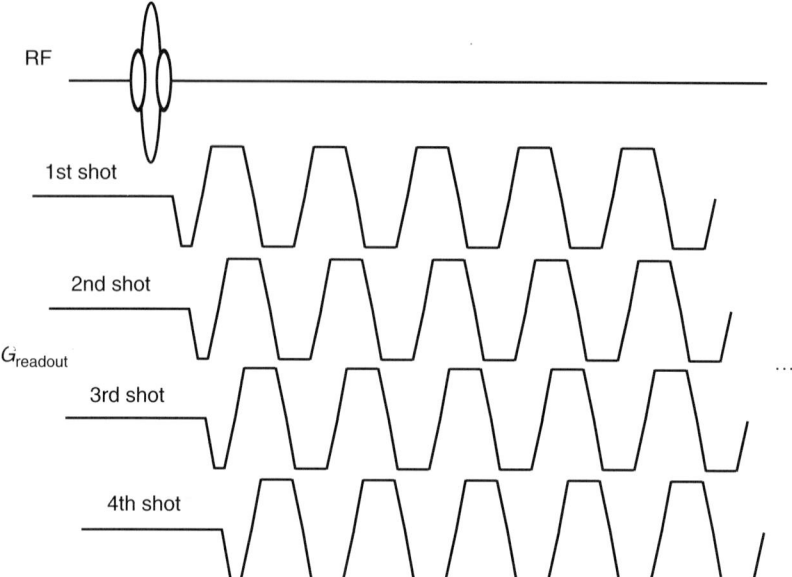

FIGURE 16.12 Echo timing shifting in multishot EPI. Four shots are assumed. The readout waveform for each successive shot is shifted by one-fourth of the echo spacing. For simplicity, only the readout gradient waveform is shown.

reduce the Nyquist ghosting artifacts, these errors must be corrected. A number of phase correction methods have been proposed, and several frequently used ones are discussed in subsection 16.1.4.

As discussed earlier, full k-space coverage is rarely obtained in single-shot EPI. Even in multishot EPI, full k-space coverage is not always achieved. To minimize artifacts while achieving the maximal possible resolution, many reconstruction algorithms have been developed for the partially covered k-space, as discussed in Section 13.4. Although advanced reconstruction techniques, such as parametric and nonparametric constrained reconstruction, have been developed (Liang et al. 1992), simpler algorithms such as the homodyne reconstruction method have also been shown to be computationally efficient and to give satisfactory results, especially with multiple iterations (Noll et al. 1991; McGibney et al. 1993).

16.1.4 ARTIFACTS

Nyquist Ghosts   One of the most common artifacts in EPI is *Nyquist ghosting* (Zakhor et al. 1991). Nyquist ghosts can originate from many sources that lead to signal amplitude modulation, phase inconsistency, or displacement of k-space data. These errors typically alternate between even and odd echoes. Consider, for example, a spatially independent phase error φ that alternates between odd and even echoes in a single-shot EPI sequence. The k-space signal can be expressed as:

$$S'(p,q) = \begin{cases} \sum_l \sum_m I(l,m) \exp\left(-\frac{i2\pi lp}{n_x}\right) \exp\left(-\frac{i2\pi mq}{n_y}\right) \exp(-i\varphi) & q = \text{even} \\[2ex] \sum_l \sum_m I(l,m) \exp\left(-\frac{i2\pi lp}{n_x}\right) \exp\left(-\frac{i2\pi mq}{n_y}\right) \exp(i\varphi) & q = \text{odd} \end{cases}$$

(16.24)

where I represents the ideal image intensity, p and q are the k-space indices along the readout and phase-encoded directions, respectively, and l and m are the corresponding indices in the image domain:

$$\begin{aligned} k_x &= p\Delta k_x \\ k_y &= q\Delta k_y \\ x &= l\Delta x \\ y &= m\Delta y \end{aligned}$$

(16.25)

Using the orthonormal properties of Fourier transforms (Section 1.1), it can be shown that an image I' reconstructed from S' is related to the ideal image I by:

$$I'(l,m) = I(l,m)\cos\varphi + iI\left(l, m - \frac{N_y}{2}\right)\sin\varphi$$

(16.26)

where N_y is the matrix size in the image domain along the phase-encoded direction. The first term represents the true image; its intensity is uniformly reduced by a factor of $|\cos\varphi| \leq 1$. The second term corresponds to the Nyquist ghost whose intensity is given by $I|\sin\varphi|$ and whose location is shifted by one-half of the FOV along the phase-encoded direction (Figure 16.13a). Because of the $N_y/2$ shift, the Nyquist ghost in single-shot EPI is also referred to as the N-over-two (N/2) ghost. Equation (16.26) indicates that the alternating phase error φ splits the ideal image into a "real" component $I(l,m)\cos\varphi$ and an "imaginary" component $iI(l, m - N_y/2)\sin\varphi$. (Note that because I is a complex function in general, neither $I(l,m)\cos\varphi$ nor $I(l, m - N_y/2)\sin\varphi$ is necessarily a real number. Thus, we put "real" and "imaginary" in quotations.) The brighter the ghost, the lower the image intensity of the object becomes. Two examples of sources of the spatially independent phase error φ are B_0 eddy currents (Section 10.3) and frequency mismatch in off-center FOV imaging

(a) (b) (c)

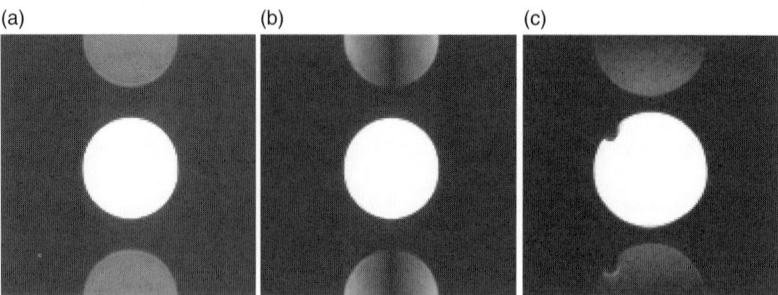

FIGURE 16.13 Examples of three types of Nyquist ghosts in single-shot EPI: (a) constant-phase ghost, (b) linear-phase ghost, and (c) oblique Nyquist ghost. (a) and (b) are simulated and (c) is the actual image from a water phantom.

(Maier et al. 1997). Because the phase error φ is spatially constant, the Nyquist ghost given by Eq. (16.26) is known as a constant-phase ghost, constant ghost, or even ghost.

If, after row flipping, the k-space data are alternatively shifted by $\delta k_x = u \Delta k_x$ between the odd and even echoes along the readout direction (e.g., all odd k-space lines are shifted by $u \Delta k_x$ and even k-space lines by $-u \Delta k_x$), a similar result to Eq. (16.26) can be derived:

$$I'(l, m) = I(l, m) \cos \left(\frac{2\pi u l}{N_x} \right) + i I \left(l, m - \frac{N_y}{2} \right) \sin \left(\frac{2\pi u l}{N_x} \right) \quad (16.27)$$

In this case, the image and the ghost are modulated by a cosine and a sine function, respectively, along the readout direction. At the center of the image ($l = 0$), the ghost is nulled, and all intensity is registered to the image (Figure 16.13b). Because a shift in k-space corresponds to a linear phase error in the image domain, the ghost described by Eq. (16.27) is sometimes called linear-phase ghost, or simply linear ghost. It is also called an odd ghost because the modulation function on the ghost is an odd function (i.e., $\sin(-x) = -\sin(x)$). The causes of the linear-phase ghost include (but are not limited to) spatially linear eddy currents along the readout direction, gradient group delays, and gradient amplifier hysteresis.

If the k-space data are alternatively shifted by $\delta k_y = \pm v \Delta k_y$ between the odd and even echoes along the phase-encoded direction, Eq. (16.27) becomes:

$$I'(l, m) = I(l, m) \cos \left(\frac{2\pi v m}{N_y} \right) + i I \left(l, m - \frac{N_y}{2} \right) \sin \left(\frac{2\pi v (m - N_y/2)}{N_y} \right)$$
$$(16.28)$$

In distinction to the ghost given by Eq. (16.27), the sine and cosine modulations are along the phase-encoded direction instead of the readout direction. At the edge of the FOV (i.e., $m = \pm N_y/2$), the ghost has a nodal line (i.e., is nulled) and all intensity is registered to the center of the image (i.e., $m = 0$) (Figure 16.13c). Because this ghost is typically observed in oblique EPI scans, it has been called the oblique Nyquist ghost (Zhou and Maier 1996; Zhou et al. 1997). Common sources for the oblique Nyquist ghosts include inconsistent eddy current characteristics and group delays among the physical gradient axes (also known as gradient anisotropy; Aldefeld and Bornert 1998) and cross-term eddy currents.

In addition to the scenarios already discussed, phase errors caused by higher-order eddy currents and concomitant magnetic fields can also produce Nyquist ghosts as discussed in Section 10.1 and in Du et al. (2002), Zhou et al. (1998), and Weisskoff et al. (1993). In practice, the ghost observed in an echo planar image is often a mixture of the ghosts discussed previously. For example, the combination of a constant-phase ghost and a linear-phase ghost will shift the vertical nodal line away from the image center. The combination of a linear-phase ghost and an oblique Nyquist ghost can produce a tilted nodal line. In multishot interleaved EPI with parallel readout direction, each ghost we have discussed is split into multiple ghosts with increased spatial frequency and decreased intensity.

Many techniques have been developed to reduce or remove the Nyquist ghosts. In one category of these methods, a reference scan is used to measure the inconsistent phase errors between odd and even echoes in the echo train (Bruder et al. 1992; Maier et al. 1992; Schmitt and Goertler 1992). The reference scan is commonly a separate single-shot acquisition with the phase-encoding gradient disabled (Figure 16.14), as discussed in Section 10.3. The non-phase-encoded echoes are individually inverse-Fourier-transformed along the readout direction to obtain a set of projections. Ideally, all projections should have the same phase because no phase-encoding gradient is applied. Any phase inconsistency can be calculated by comparing the phases among the projections. Typically, only the spatially constant and linear phase errors (α and β, respectively) are obtained by performing a linear regression or using the method described in Ahn and Cho (1987):

$$\Delta\phi = \alpha + \beta x \qquad (16.29)$$

To carry out phase correction, the EPI k-space data are first inverse-Fourier-transformed along the readout direction to produce a hybrid data set $P(x, k_y)$. The constant and linear phase errors, α and β, are removed from $P(x, k_y)$, followed by another 1D inverse Fourier transform along the phase-encoded direction k_y. Alternatively, a pixel-by-pixel phase correction can be performed along the x axis in the hybrid space (x, k_y) without being constrained to include only the constant and linear spatial variation in the phase errors (Bruder et al. 1992).

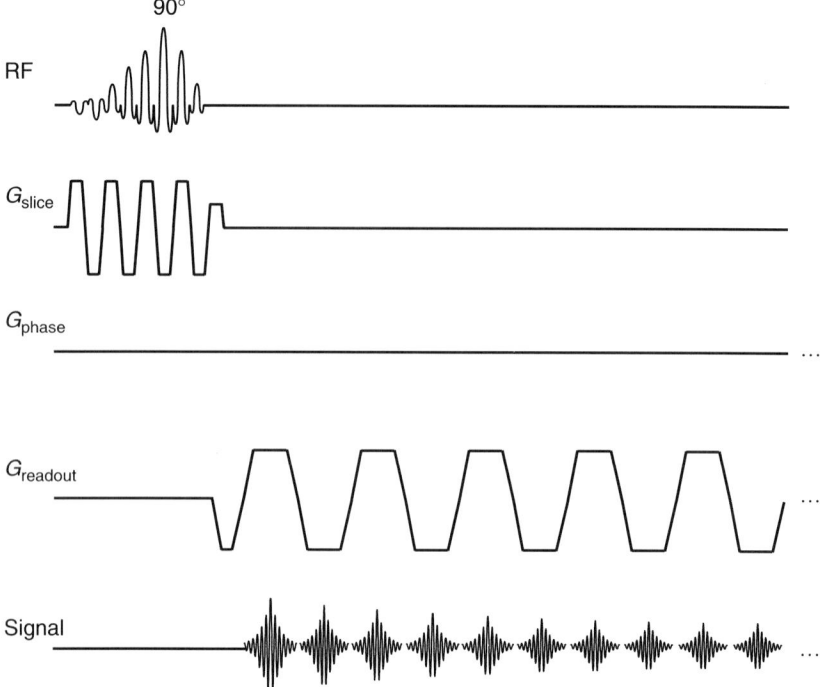

FIGURE 16.14 A reference-scan sequence for a gradient-echo EPI. The phase-encoding gradients are disabled, but all other gradients are identical to the gradient-echo sequence shown in Figure 16.9. The reference-scan sequence for spin-echo EPI can be designed analogously.

The reference scan can also be embedded in the EPI pulse sequence itself, eliminating the need for a separate reference scan. For example, in a spin-echo EPI, an odd and an even echo can be produced between the 90° and 180° pulses using a short ETL (i.e., $N_{etl} = 2$) and the same readout gradient amplitude and slew rate as the normal echo train. The phase errors α and β can be calculated from those two echoes. Another method is to acquire two adjacent echoes with zero phase encoding within the EPI echo train, producing two lines with $k_y = 0$ (Figure 16.15) (Jesmanowicz et al. 1993). These two k-space lines are used to estimate the phase inconsistency between the reference data and the nominal EPI data.

Although most reference scans are acquired without phase encoding the echoes, a reference scan can also be obtained from the phase-encoded data

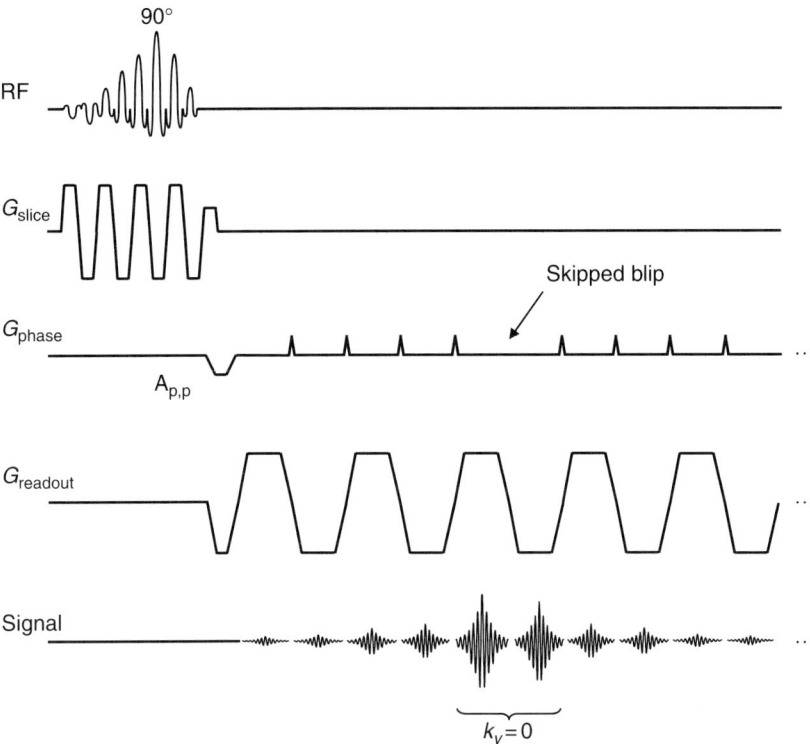

FIGURE 16.15 The reference scan can be embedded into the actual EPI sequence for k-space data acquisition. The central k-space lines are acquired twice, first with an odd echo and then with an even echo, as indicated. In this sequence, the prephasing gradient area $A_{p,p}$ equals four times the blip gradient area in order to give $k_y = 0$ at the fifth and sixth echoes.

(Hu and Le 1996). In this method, a reference scan is acquired by advancing the nominal EPI readout gradient waveform by one ESP while leaving the phase-encoding gradient waveform unchanged. In this way, the odd echoes in the reference scan have the same phase-encoding value as the corresponding even echoes in the nominal EPI scan (and vice versa). The phase inconsistency can be compared after each data set is inverse-Fourier-transformed along the readout direction, that is, in the hybrid space (x, k_y), and subsequently removed by performing a pixel-by-pixel correction. This method has been reported to yield better results than from reference scans acquired without the phase-encoding gradient (Hu and Le 1996). Similar to the reference-scan method shown in Figure 16.14, the method with phase-encoded reference scan increases the total scan time. This scan time increase, however, can be insignificant when the reference scan is repeatedly used to correct multiple EPI data sets, such as in the case of functional MRI or some dynamic studies.

Another category of ghost-reduction methods focuses on the image domain without using a reference scan (Buonocore and Gao 1997; Buonocore and Zhu 2001; Hennel 1998). Any data inconsistency, such as that caused by patient motion, between reference scan and the nominal EPI acquisition is thus eliminated. These methods typically require more intensive computation and may require operator interaction. Some algorithms rely on identifying nonoverlapping regions of the true image and the ghost, which may impose a constraint on the FOV relative to the size of the imaged object.

Many other ghost-reduction techniques have also been developed. For example, oblique Nyquist ghosts can be reduced by gradient waveform modification (Zhou et al. 1997). Ghosts caused by concomitant magnetic fields can be corrected by a higher-order phase correction (Du et al. 2002).

Chemical Shift Artifacts   In conventional spin-echo and gradient-echo imaging, chemical shift artifacts can be observed in the readout and slice-selection directions, but not along the phase-encoded direction. For EPI, chemical shift artifacts along the readout direction are effectively suppressed because the readout bandwidth Δv is considerably larger than that in conventional imaging. Along the phase-encoded direction, the full sampling bandwidth is given by Eq. (16.22), where interleaved k-space sampling is assumed if $N_{shot} > 1$. For spins with a chemical shift of Δf_{cs} (in hertz) relative to the receiver frequency, the chemical shift produces a spatial shift along the phase-encoded direction:

$$\Delta y_{cs} = \frac{\Delta f_{cs}}{\Delta v_{phase}} L_y = \frac{t_{esp} \Delta f_{cs}}{N_{shot}} L_y \qquad (16.30)$$

where L_y is the FOV. Because Δv_{phase} is typically only on the order of a 1 kHz, the shift along the phase-encoded direction can be substantial (see Example 16.5). Because of this, lipid suppression is almost always employed in EPI pulse sequences, as discussed earlier in this section.

Example 16.5   A gradient-echo EPI pulse sequence is used to image the human abdomen at 1.5 T without lipid suppression. The acquisition parameters are FOV $= 32 \times 32$ cm, matrix $= 128 \times 128$, $t_{esp} = 1$ ms, and the readout bandwidth $\Delta v = \pm 125$ kHz. (a) How much is the lipid signal shifted along the readout and phase-encoded directions in a single-shot sequence? (b) If k-space data are acquired with four interleaved shots, calculate the shifts in (a).

Answer

(a) At 1.5 T, the chemical shift difference between water and lipids is approximately $\Delta f_{cs} = 210\,\text{Hz}$. Thus, the shift along the readout direction is:

$$\Delta x_{cs} = \frac{\Delta f_{cs}}{2\Delta \nu}L_x = \frac{0.210}{2 \times 125} \times 32 = 0.027\,\text{cm}$$

Along the phase-encoded direction, the shift is obtained from Eq. (16.30):

$$\Delta y_{cs} = t_{esp}\Delta f_{cs}L_y = 1 \times 0.210 \times 32 = 6.72\,\text{cm}$$

For a 128×128 image, the shifts along the readout and the phase-encoding directions are 0.1 and 27 pixels, respectively.

(b) According to Eq. (16.30) the shift along the phase-encoded direction will be reduced by a factor of four, and the shift along the readout direction stays the same.

Image Distortion Due to the very low bandwidth in the phase-encoded direction, considerable image distortion can be produced in regions with off-resonance effects, such as field inhomogeneity, magnetic susceptibility variations, eddy currents with long time constants (e.g., $>100\,\text{ms}$), and concomitant magnetic fields. An example of image distortion is shown in Figure 16.16. When a nonzero baseline or background gradient exists on the

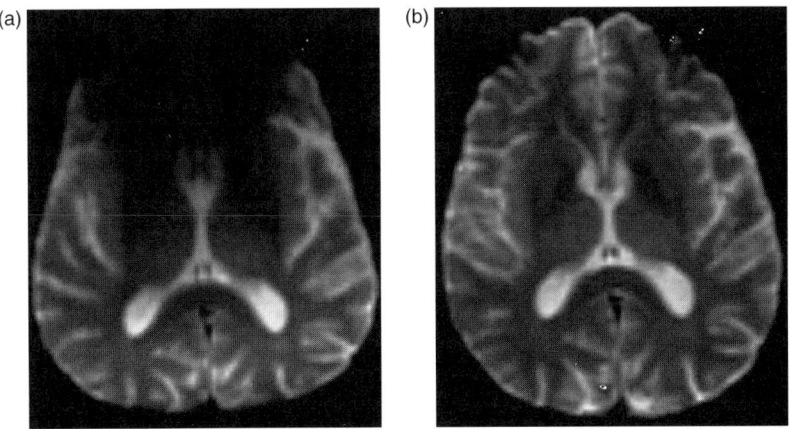

(a) (b)

FIGURE 16.16 (a) A denture remote from the imaging plane can cause substantial image distortion and signal loss in single-shot EPI due to the magnetic field perturbation. (b) After removing the denture, the image is considerably improved.

phase-encoding axis, the image will be either compressed or dilated along the phase-encoding direction. For a background gradient in the readout direction, the image is sheared. These image distortion artifacts are often observed in diffusion-weighted EPI where the background gradients are produced by eddy currents with long time constants (e.g., 100 ms) relative to $N_{etl} \times t_{esp}$ (Section 17.2). Visualizing the pattern of distortion can provide a good diagnosis of the system's B_0-field inhomogeneity problems, as well as detecting eddy-current gradients with long time constants. Image distortion caused by concomitant magnetic fields is typically much worse in nonaxial images, such as the sagittal and coronal planes (Du et al. 2002; Weisskoff et al. 1993). For axial images not located at isocenter, the concomitant magnetic fields produce image shift along the phase-encoded direction (Zhou et al. 1998). The shift is progressively larger as the off-center distance increases.

Image distortion can be effectively reduced by decreasing the echo spacing or the echo train length as in multishot EPI. Although the latter approach compromises the spatial resolution in single-shot sequences, this limitation can be overcome using parallel imaging techniques (Section 13.3). Another common solution to image distortion is to first acquire a B_0 map and unwarp the image through a phase correction (Jezzard and Balaban 1995).

T_2^*-*Induced Image Blurring*   Because the k-space lines in EPI are acquired at different times, each k-space line carries a different T_2^* weighting as shown by Eq. (16.16). This causes image blurring along the phase-encoded direction. The blurring becomes increasingly severe as T_2^* decreases. An effective way to address this problem is to restrict the k-space acquisition to a narrow time window in which the T_2^* decay is not substantial. This means that we either have to reduce the echo train length or shorten the interecho spacing. Changing from single-shot to multishot with interleaves can greatly alleviate image blurring. Typically, image blurring in single-shot EPI is less than in single-shot RARE. Thus, k-space amplitude correction discussed in Section 16.4 is rarely used.

Intravoxel Dephasing   SNR in single-shot EPI is generally low due to the use of high receiver bandwidth, long echo train, and introvoxel signal dephasing caused by off-resonance effects. Magnetic susceptibility variations at the tissue-air interface or near metallic implants often cause a signal void in these regions (Figure 16.16a). Although increasing the slice thickness generally improves the SNR of an image, a thicker slice in EPI does not always produce a higher SNR because intravoxel dephasing can be greater with thicker slices. When T_2^* dephasing is very severe, a thinner slice can even give a higher SNR than a thicker slice. This problem can be addressed by adjusting the slice-refocusing gradient lobe to offset the susceptibility effects as described in Yang et al. (1997, 1998).

16.1.5 VARIATIONS OF EPI PULSE SEQUENCES

Based on the basic pulse sequences described in subsection 16.1.1, many variations of EPI pulse sequences have been developed. A thorough review of these pulse sequences is beyond the scope of this book. Several selected EPI variations are discussed here. Additional variations can be found in Schmitt et al. (1998).

Skip-Echo EPI As the name implies, skip-echo EPI acquires every other echo in the EPI echo train. Thus, only half of the available echoes are used to sample k-space lines (Feinberg et al. 1990; Duerk and Simonetti 1991). Because the acquired echoes all correspond to the same readout gradient polarity, there is no need to flip every other row in k-space prior to image reconstruction. More important, any alternating phase error and amplitude modulation are eliminated from the k-space data, resulting in an image virtually free of Nyquist ghosts. To minimize echo spacing, the readout gradient that corresponds to the skipped echoes is often maximized to shorten its duration (the area must be conserved in gradient shape modification) (Figure 16.17). This effectively speeds up the return of k-space trajectory to the acquisition of the next echo. Skip-echo EPI pulse sequences using this strategy are sometimes called flyback EPI.

Circular EPI Because the data in the k-space corners are often apodized by a window function during image reconstruction to achieve an isotropic resolution, time spent on acquiring k-space corners reduces data acquisition efficiency. Circular EPI addresses this issue by designing gradient waveforms that produce a k-space trajectory confined to a circle (Figure 16.18). In this way, the acquisition time can be reduced compared to conventional EPI, as described by Pauly et al. (1995) and Kerr et al. (1997).

Balanced EPI EPI requires a high gradient amplitude to match the increased readout bandwidth. If each physical gradient cannot provide the required gradient strength, two physical gradient axes can be combined to synthesize a gradient vector $\vec{G}' = \hat{x}G + \hat{y}G$ whose amplitude is $\sqrt{2}$ times higher than the individual gradient amplitude G (see Section 7.3). This is equivalent to rotating the logical gradient axes by $45°$ with respect to the physical gradient axes so that the load on each physical gradient is more balanced (Kashmar and Nalcioglu 1991). After reconstruction, the image must be rotated back by $-45°$ to properly depict the orientation of the object. When the two physical gradient axes have different eddy-current characteristics or group delays, however, this method can produce oblique Nyquist ghosts. Additional calibration and correction are often needed to remove the ghost (Zhou et al. 1997).

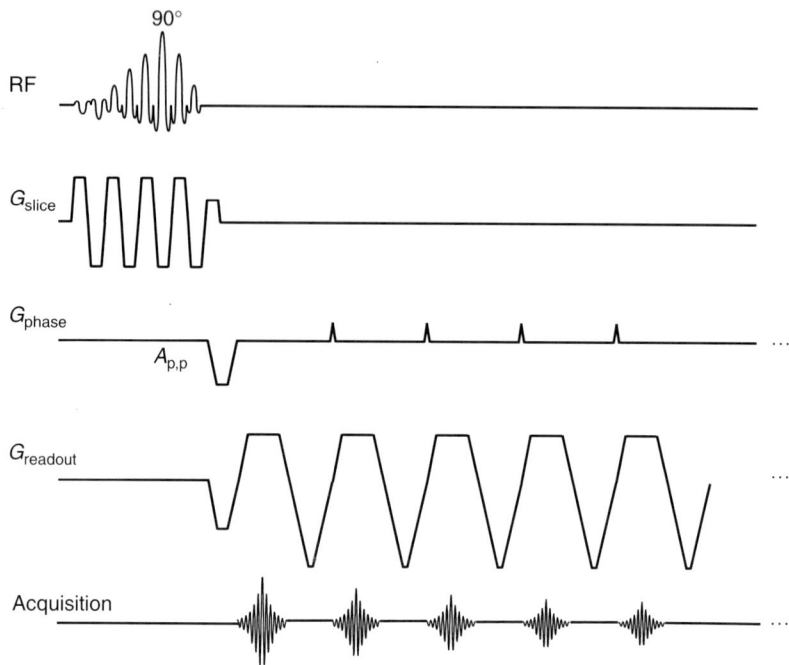

FIGURE 16.17 A skip-echo (or flyback) gradient-echo EPI sequence. Only the echoes corresponding to the positive readout gradient are acquired in this example.

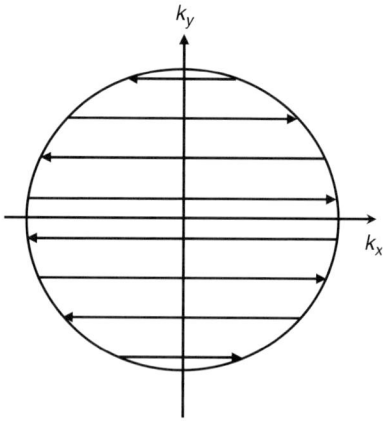

FIGURE 16.18 Circular EPI k-space trajectory. The k-space lines are confined to lie within a circle.

T_2^* *Mapping*   As discussed in Section 14.3, a multiecho spin-echo pulse sequence can be used for T_2 mapping. Similarly, a gradient-echo EPI pulse sequence can be modified to produce a T_2^* map. In this application, the EPI phase-encoding gradient waveform is replaced by a conventional phase-encoding waveform (i.e., one phase-encoding step per TR) that gives the same k_y for the entire echo train, as in gradient-echo pulse sequences. This is similar to a dual-echo gradient-echo pulse sequence (Section 14.1), except that a longer echo train is used. After data for all the required phase-encoding steps are obtained, a stack of images are generated with each image corresponding to a gradient echo. Because each gradient echo has its own distinctive TE value under the FID envelope, a pixel-by-pixel plot of the image intensity as a function of TE reveals the T_2^* decay curve. The T_2^* value can be readily obtained using a least-squares fitting algorithm.

3D EPI   Although EPI is predominantly used as a 2D sequence, 3D EPI has also been developed. A true 3D EPI, known as echo volume imaging (EVI), traverses k-space in 3D throughout the echo train (Song et al. 1994; Mansfield et al. 1995). Single-shot EVI has very low spatial resolution (e.g., matrix size $= 32 \times 32 \times 7$) and has not been widely used. Hybrid 3D EPI uses the EPI phase-encoding waveform to sample k-space along the primary (or the secondary) phase-encoded direction and conventional phase-encoding strategy along the remaining phase-encoded direction. 3D k-space is sampled in multiple shots, even though a single-shot 2D EPI phase-encoding waveform is often used. This is analogous to 3D RARE discussed in Section 16.4.

SELECTED REFERENCES

Ahn, C. B., and Cho, Z. H. 1987. A new phase correction method in NMR imaging based on autocorrelation and histogram analysis. *IEEE Trans. Med. Imaging* 6: 32–36.

Aldefeld, B., and Bornert, P. 1998. Effects of gradient anisotropy in MRI. *Magn. Reson. Med.* 39: 606–614.

Bruder, H., Fischer, H., Reinfelder, H.-E., and Schmitt, F. 1992. Image reconstruction for echo planar imaging with non-equidistant k-space sampling. *Magn. Reson. Med.* 23: 311–323.

Buonocore, M. H., and Gao, L. S. 1997. Ghost artifact reduction for echo planar imaging using image phase correction. *Magn. Reson. Med.* 38: 89–100.

Buonocore, M. H., and Zhu, D. C. 1998. High spatial resolution EPI using an odd number of interleaves. *Magn. Reson. Med.* 41: 1199–1205.

Buonocore, M. H., and Zhu, D. C. 2001. Image-based ghost correction for interleaved EPI. *Magn. Reson. Med.* 45: 96–108.

Butts, K., Riederer, S. J., Ehman, R. L., Thompson, R. M., and Jack, C. R. 1994. Interleaved echo planar imaging on a standard MRI system. *Magn. Reson. Med.* 31: 67–72.

Chapman, B., Turner, R., Ordidge, R. J., Doyle, M., Cawley, M., Coxon, R., Glover, P., and Mansfield, P. 1987. Real-time movie imaging from a single cardiac cycle by NMR. *Magn. Reson. Med.* 5: 246–254.

Chen, D. Q., Marr, R., and Lauterbur, P. C. 1986. Reconstruction from NMR data with imaging gradients having arbitrary time dependence. *IEEE Trans. Med. Imaging* 5: 162–164.

Cohen, M. S., Weisskoff, R. M., Rzedzian, R. R., and Kantor, M. L. 1990. Sensory stimulation by time-varying magnetic fields. *Magn. Reson. Med.* 14: 409–414.

Du, Y. P., Zhou, X. J., and Bernstein, M. A. 2002. Correction of concomitant magnetic field induced image artifacts in non-axial echo planar imaging. *Magn. Reson. Med.* 48: 509–515.

Duerk, J. L., and Simonetti, O. P. 1991. Theoretical aspects of motion sensitivity and compensation in echo-planar imaging. *J. Magn. Reson. Imaging* 1: 643–650.

Feinberg, D. A., Turner, R., Jakab, P. D., and Vonkienlin, M. 1990. Echo-planar imaging with asymmetric gradient modulation and inner-volume excitation. *Magn. Reson. Med.* 13: 162–169.

Feinberg, D. A., and Oshio, K. 1994. Phase errors in multi-shot echo planar imaging. *Magn. Reson. Med.* 32: 535–539.

Hennel, F. 1998. Image-based reduction of artifacts in multishot echo-planar imaging. *J. Magn. Reson.* 134: 206–213.

Hu, X. P., and Le, T. H. 1996. Artifact reduction in EPI with phase-encoded reference scan. *Magn. Reson. Med.* 36: 166–171.

Jesmanowicz, A., Wong, E. C., and Hyde, J. S. 1993. Phase correction for EPI using internal reference lines. *Proc. Soc. Magn. Reson. Med.* 3: 1239.

Jezzard, P., and Balaban, R. S. 1995. Correction for geometric distortion in echo planar images from B0 field variations. *Magn. Reson. Med.* 34: 65–73.

Kashmar, G., and Nalcioglu, O. 1991. Cartesian echo planar hybrid scanning with two to eight echoes. *IEEE Trans. Med. Imaging* 10: 1–10.

Kerr, A. B., Pauly, J. M., Hu, B. S., Li, K. C., Hardy, C. J., Meyer, C. H., Macovski, A., and Nishimura, D. G. 1997. Real-time interactive MRI on a conventional scanner. *Magn. Reson. Med.* 38: 355–367.

Kwong, K., Belliveau, J., Chesler, D., Goldberg, I., Weisskoff, R., Poncelet, B., Kennedy, D., Hoppel, B., Cohen, M., Turner, R., Cheng, H., Brady, T., and Rosen, B. 1992. Dynamic magnetic resonance imaging of human brain activity during primary sensory stimulation. *Proc. Natl. Acad. Sci. U.S.A.* 89: 5676–5679.

Liang, Z.-P., Boada, F. E., Constable, R. T., Haake, E. M., Lauterbur, P. C., and Smith, M. R. 1992. Constrained reconstruction methods in MR imaging. *Rev. Magn. Reson. Med.* 4: 67–185.

Maier, J. K., Vavrek, M., and Glover, G. H. 1992. Correction of NMR data acquired by an echo-planar technique. U.S. patent 5,151,656.

Maier, J. K., Ploetz, L. E., Zhou, X., Epstein, F. H., and Licato, P. E. 1997. A method for producing off-center images using an EPI pulse sequence. U.S. patent 5,689,186. November 18.

Mansfield, P. 1977. Multi-planar image formation using NMR spin echoes. *J. Phys. C: Solid State Phys.* 10: L55–58.

Mansfield, P., Coxon, R., and Hykin, J. 1995. Echo volume imaging of the brain at 3.0T: First normal volunteer and functional imaging results. *J. Comput. Assist. Tomogr.* 19: 847–852.

McGibney, G., Smith, M. R., Nichols, S. T., and Crawley, A. 1993. Quantitative evaluation of several partial Fourier reconstruction algorithms used in MRI. *Magn. Reson. Med.* 30: 51–59.

McKinnon, G. C. 1993. Ultrafast interleaved gradient echo planar imaging on a standard scanner. *Magn. Reson. Med.* 30: 609–616.

Noll, D. C., Nishimura, D. G., and Macovski, A. 1991. Homodyne detection in magnetic resonance imaging. *IEEE Trans. Med. Imaging* 10: 154–163.

Nowak, S., Schmitt, F., and Fischer, H. 1989. Method of operating a nuclear spin tomograph apparatus with a resonant circuit for producing gradient field. European patent EP 0429715B1.

Ordidge, R. J., and Mansfield, P. 1984. NMR methods. U.S. patent 4509015.

Pauly, J. M., Butts, K., Luk Pat, G. T., and Mackovski, A. 1995. A circular echo-planar pulse sequence. *Soc. Magn. Reson. Abstracts* 3: 106.

Schmitt, F., and Goertler, G. 1992. Method for suppressing image artifacts in a magnetic resonance imaging apparatus. U.S. patent 5138259.

Schmitt, F., Stehling, M. K, and Turner, R. 1998. *Echo planar imaging*. Berlin: Springer.

Shellock, F. G., and Kanal, M. 1994. *Magnetic resonance bioeffects, safety, and patient management*. New York: Raven.

Song, A. W., Wong, E. C., and Hyde, J. S. 1994. Echo-volume imaging. *Magn. Reson. Med.* 32: 668–671.

Stehling, M. K., Ordidge, R. J., Coxon, R., and Mansfield, P. 1990. Inversion-recovery echo-planar imaging (IR-EPI) at 0.5-T. *Magn. Reson. Med.* 13: 514–517.

Thulborn, K. R., Waterton, J. C., Matthews, P. M., and Radda, G. K. 1982. Oxygenation dependence of the transverse relaxation time of water protons in whole blood at high field. *Biochim. Biophys. Acta* 714: 265–270.

Weisskoff, R. M., Cohen, M. S., and Rzedzian, R. R. 1993. Nonaxial whole-body instant imaging. *Magn. Reson. Med.* 29: 796–803.

Yang, Q. X., Dardzinski, B. J., Li, S. Z., Eslinger, P. J., and Smith, M. B. 1997. Multi-gradient echo with susceptibility inhomogeneity compensation (MGESIC): Demonstration of fMRI in the olfactory cortex at 3.0 T. *Magn. Reson. Med.* 37: 331–335.

Yang, Q. X., Williams, G. D., Demeure, R. J., Mosher, T. J., and Smith, M. B. 1998. Removal of local field gradient artifacts in T_2^*-weighted images at high fields by gradient-echo slice excitation profile imaging. *Magn. Reson. Med.* 39: 402–409.

Zakhor, A., Weisskoff, R., and Rzedzian, R. 1991. Optimal sampling and reconstruction of MRI signals resulting from sinusoidal gradients. *IEEE Trans. Signal Proc.* 39: 2056–2065.

Zhou, X. J., and Maier, J. K. 1996. A new Nyquist ghost in oblique EPI. In *Proceedings of the International society of Magnetic Resonance in Medicine*, p. 386.

Zhou, X., Maier, J. K., and Epstein, F. H. 1997. Reduction of Nyquist ghost artifacts in oblique echo planar images. U.S. patent 5,672,969. September 30.

Zhou, X. J., Du, Y. P., Bernstein, M. A., Reynolds, H. G., Maier, J. K., and Polzin, J. A. 1998. Concomitant magnetic-field-induced artifacts in axial echo planar imaging. *Magn. Reson. Med.* 39: 596–605.

RELATED SECTIONS

16.2 GRASE

Gradient and spin echo or GRASE (also called turbo gradient spin echo, TGSE) pulse sequences use a train of RF refocusing pulses, each combined with a train of alternating polarity readout gradient lobes (Figure 16.19) to rephase a series of gradient and RF spin echoes (Feinberg and Oshio 1991; Oshio and Feinberg 1991). GRASE is a combination of EPI (Section 16.1) and RARE (Section 16.4) that overcomes some of the limitations of both pulse sequences, but also inherits most of the problems of both. Because more echoes can be collected per unit time using gradient reversal than using RF refocusing (see Examples 16.1 and 16.9), GRASE images can be acquired with higher spatial resolution than with RARE, for the same number of shots and the same echo train duration per shot. Alternatively, shorter T_2-weighted scans can be obtained for a given resolution. Because fewer RF refocusing pulses are

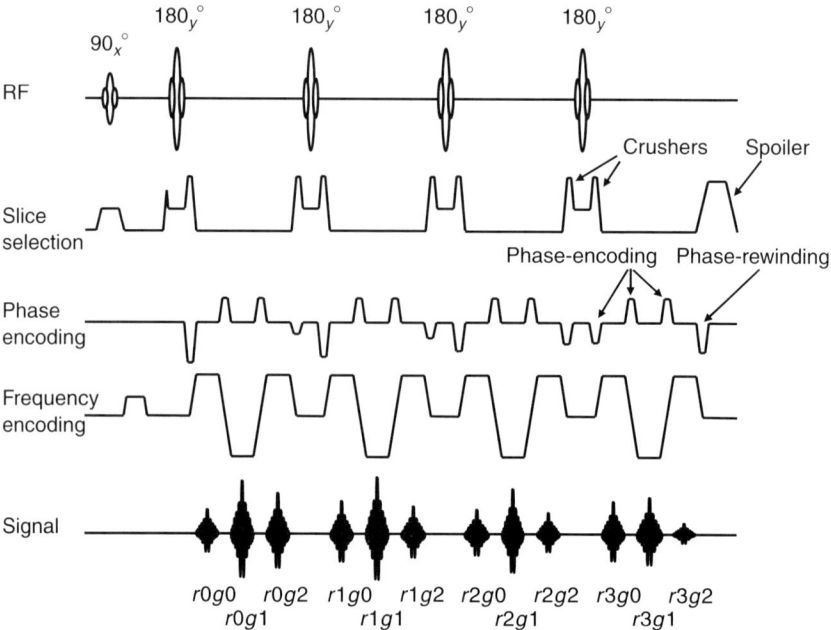

FIGURE 16.19 2D GRASE pulse sequence. This example shows four RF refocusing pulses ($N_{rf} = 4$), each followed by three gradient echoes ($N_{gre} = 3$) for a total echo train length of 12. The echoes are denoted by the RF refocusing pulse number and gradient echo number (starting from zero). For example, $r1g2$ is the third gradient echo associated with the second refocusing pulse.

needed to obtain a given number of echoes, the SAR is also considerably lower than for RARE, allowing more slices per TR, especially at high field strength (e.g., 3.0 T). The increased interval between refocusing pulses also results in a lipid signal that is more attenuated compared to RARE and is much closer to its intensity in conventional RF spin echo images. For a fixed number of echoes per excitation, GRASE has a shorter sequence length than RARE, leading to less image blurring (or edge enhancement). The use of RF refocusing pulses greatly reduces the phase accumulated by off-resonance spins, resulting in less geometric distortion and signal loss from intravoxel dephasing compared to EPI.

The k-space data acquired with GRASE have phase modulation from off-resonance spins similar to EPI, as well as amplitude modulation due to T_2 decay similar to RARE. There is also T_2^*-induced amplitude modulation, similar to EPI, that can be useful for increasing T_2^* weighting in BOLD fMRI. These combined modulations can cause severe ghosting artifacts, which can be minimized by carefully designing the phase-encoding order as well as using phase-correction techniques. Thus, most of this section describes various phase-encoding orders that have been proposed for GRASE. The ghosting amplitude also depends on the off-resonance frequency, T_2^* and T_2. For a fixed ETL, greater resonance offsets and shorter T_2s generate higher-amplitude ghosting. Even with a careful choice of phase-encoding order, it is usually beneficial to use fat saturation with GRASE to minimize ghosting from off-resonance magnetization. Although T_2^*-induced amplitude modulation can have an important effect on contrast, it is generally less important than amplitude modulation from T_2 effects when considering artifacts. Therefore for simplicity we ignore T_2^* decay when considering the k-space amplitude weighting.

With 2D GRASE, the phase and amplitude modulation are both in the phase-encoded direction. A variation of 2D GRASE called vertical GRASE distributes the phase and amplitude modulations on different k-space axes (frequency and phase, respectively), to improve image quality. With 3D GRASE (Figure 16.20), the phase modulation and amplitude modulation can also be placed on different Fourier encoding axes (slice and phase), giving somewhat better image quality.

Because gradient echoes are collected during both positive and negative polarity readout gradients, GRASE data are sensitive to eddy currents, mismatch between the gradient and receive chain group delays, and asymmetry in anti-aliasing filter response, just as in EPI. Phase corrections are necessary to remove inconsistency between echoes collected with the two gradient polarities. In addition, the spin echoes in GRASE are also subject to phase errors mainly induced by eddy currents, as in RARE. These phase errors must also be corrected.

GRASE has primarily been used for T_2-weighted imaging (Figure 16.21) in situations in which RARE provides insufficient spatial resolution, requires

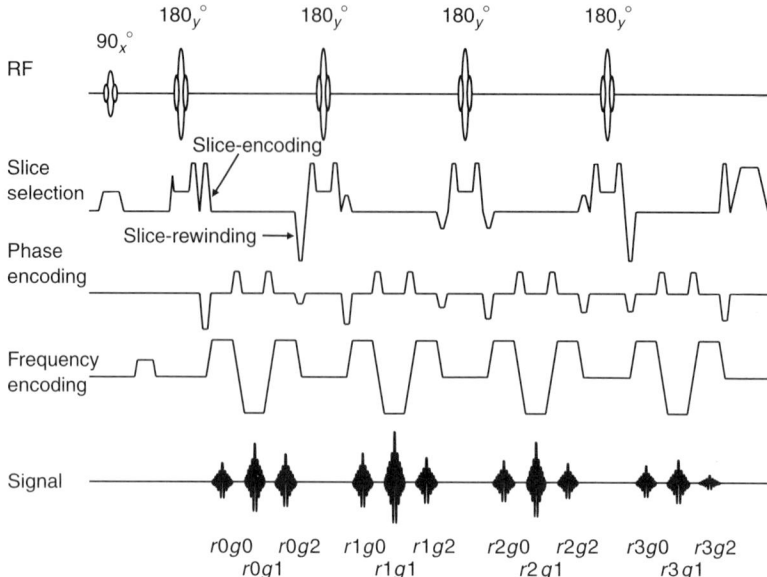

FIGURE 16.20 3D GRASE pulse sequence. The slice-encoding waveforms are rewound in each refocusing pulse interval. For clarity, the slice-encoding gradients are shown separately from the refocusing pulse crushers. In practice, the waveforms would be combined for improved efficiency.

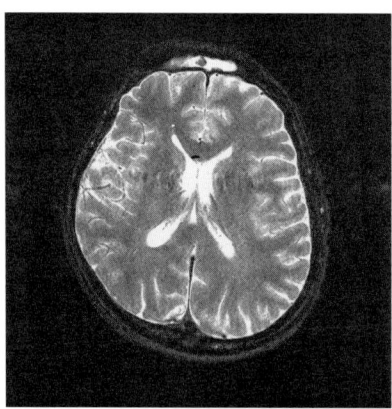

FIGURE 16.21 2D GRASE T_2-weighted image. Field strength $= 1.5$ T, TR/TE $= 3000/132$, 24-cm FOV, 5-mm slice, $N_{rf} = 5$, $N_{gre} = 3$, $N_{shot} = 28$, 512×420 acquisition, 512×512 reconstruction, ± 32-kHz receive bandwidth, two signal averages, scan time 3 min. The image asymmetry is due to the oblique orientation of the head, and is not artifactual. (Image courtesy of K. Oshio, M.D., Ph.D., Keio University, and Tetsuji Tsukamoto, M.S., GE Healthcare.)

excessive scan time, or produces unacceptable SAR. Because of the reduced k-space modulation artifacts, 3D GRASE has been used as an alternative to 2D and 3D RARE for reduced scan time. Imaging at 3.0 T or higher is particularly attractive with GRASE because of the reduced SAR compared to RARE. With proper phase-encoding view ordering, the gradient echoes also give more T_2^* weighting than with RARE, which can be advantageous for some applications such as imaging of small hemorrhagic lesions. Ghosting artifacts from residual k-space modulation and uncorrected system imperfections, however, are more difficult to remove than in EPI or RARE, which has slowed the introduction of GRASE into routine clinical practice (Patel et al. 1995).

16.2.1 GRASE PULSE SEQUENCE

We assume that there are N_{rf} RF spin echoes in each echo train and that each spin echo is split into N_{gre} gradient echoes. Because each RF spin echo corresponds to the preceding refocusing pulse, we also use N_{rf} to denote the number of refocusing pulses. GRASE scans can be single-shot or multishot, similar to RARE or EPI. Each gradient echo is labeled according to its shot number $s(s = 0, \ldots, N_{shot} - 1)$, RF refocusing pulse number $r(r = 0, \ldots, N_{rf} - 1)$, and gradient echo number $g(g = 0, \ldots, N_{gre} - 1)$. (Note that g and r should be distinguished from the eddy-current gradient g used in Section 10.3 and the spatial variable r used in the rest of the book.) To simplify the nomenclature, the first gradient echo from the first RF refocusing pulse is simply called $r0g0$, and so on. The number of echoes collected is $N_{shot} N_{rf} N_{gre}$. If all the echoes are separately encoded, the number of k_y lines for 2D scans is also $N_{shot} N_{rf} N_{gre}$. Because this number is usually not a power of two, zero filling of k-space is used in the reconstruction.

Each of the N_{gre} gradient echoes is Fourier encoded with a separate phase-encoding blip, similar to EPI. The net phase-encoding gradient area is completely rewound before the next RF refocusing pulse by a phase-rewinding lobe, similar to RARE (Figure 16.19). The net phase from the phase-encoding gradient is therefore zero over the interval between any two adjacent RF refocusing pulses. The rewinding is done for the same purpose as with RARE, to satisfy the CPMG conditions (Section 16.4). Imperfect flip angles for the 180° pulses, either due to slice profile degradation or B_1 inhomogeneity, creates stimulated echo magnetization that does not accumulate phase during the interval when it is stored along the z axis. If phase-rewinding lobes were not used, stimulated-echo and spin-echo magnetization (i.e., magnetization in the transverse plane) would accumulate different amounts of phase during the refocusing pulse interval, resulting in severe ghosting artifacts and reduced SNR.

The use of a constant phase-encoding gradient that produces a zigzag trajectory similar to ones used for EPI (see Section 16.1) is problematic for the same reasons. The phase-encoding area between all refocusing pulses will be the same, but the area will be nonzero, giving different phase-encoding values for stimulated-echo and spin-echo signals that occur in the same acquisition window.

Although the refocusing pulses normally use $180°$ flip angles, the use of variable flip angles within the echo train has also been investigated to reduce k-space echo amplitude modulation (sometimes called echo stabilization) (Schaffter and Leibfritz 1994). Although this technique has been widely used in RARE, it has not been used extensively with GRASE. In this section we assume that all refocusing pulses have $180°$ nominal flip angles.

For 3D scans, conventional phase-encoding gradients are also used in the secondary phase-encoded (i.e., slice) direction. The secondary phase-encoding gradients can use the same Fourier encoding value for all N_{rf} refocusing pulses. However, it can be advantageous for the slice Fourier encoding value to be different for each RF refocusing pulse (subsection 16.2.2) as shown in Figure 16.20. The secondary phase-encoding gradients are rewound for each RF refocusing interval.

As with RARE, the refocusing pulses used with GRASE are $90°$ out of phase with the excitation pulse; that is, a CPMG pulse train consisting of $90°_x$—τ—$180°_y$—2τ—$180°_y$—$\cdots$ is used (note that in this notation, the pulses are separated by dashes). Crushers are used before and after each RF refocusing pulse to dephase the FID resulting from nonideal refocusing pulses with flip angles differing from $180°$ due to B_1 inhomogeneity and to preserve the desired primary and stimulated echoes. The crushers are usually placed either on the slice-selection axis or the frequency-encoding axis. Crushers could also be used on both axes for greater effect. A spoiler gradient lobe at the end of the echo train is typically used to dephase any residual transverse magnetization.

If the artifacts caused by phase accumulated by off-resonance spins become problematic, GRASE can be used with some type of fat suppression, such as a spectrally selective saturation pulse that precedes the excitation pulse.

16.2.2 GRASE PHASE-ENCODING ORDER

We start by considering 2D acquisitions. Similar to RARE, there are many ways to choose the correspondence between k_y location and echo. The contrast is determined by the TE of the echoes that sample the central k-space lines. This TE is known as the effective echo time, denoted by TE_{eff}. The strategy for the phase-encoding order typically has three aims: to minimize the discontinuity of phase accumulation in k-space for off-resonance spins, to minimize the discontinuity of T_2 weighting in k-space, and to create the desired effective echo time. We start by considering the off-resonance phase accumulation. Figure 16.22

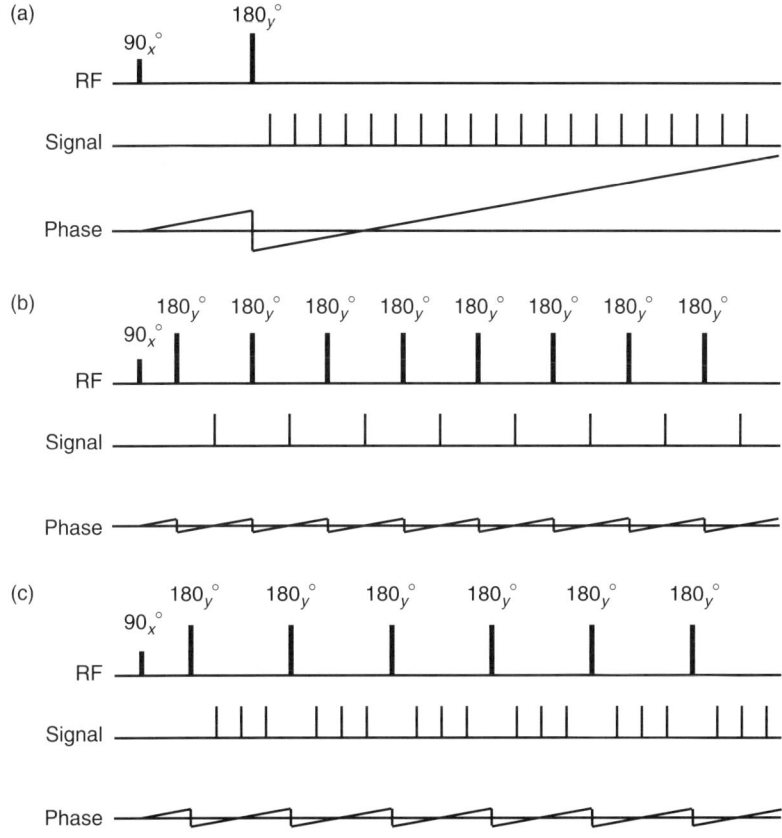

FIGURE 16.22 Phase accumulated by off-resonance spins for (a) EPI, (b) RARE, and (c) GRASE versus time (horizontal axes). For simplicity, only the RF pulses are shown for each pulse sequence. The center of each echo is represented by a vertical tick mark on the signal line.

compares the phase accumulation for an off-resonance spin isochromat for spin-echo EPI, RARE, and GRASE. For spin-echo EPI, the phase accumulates linearly throughout the echo train and is zero at the RF spin echo refocusing point. Consequently, each gradient echo (except one located exactly at the refocusing time) has a nonzero phase. A comparatively large phase accumulates by the end of the echo train. For RARE, the phase is repeatedly refocused by the train of 180° RF pulses. Therefore, at the center of each RF spin echo there is no net phase accumulation. GRASE is intermediate between the EPI and RARE cases. Off-resonance phase is periodically refocused midway between the 180° pulses, but evolves during the echoes collected using gradient reversal.

With GRASE, all echoes have off-resonance phase at the echo center, except for the echoes that are collected at the refocusing points of the 180° pulses.

T_2 decay is somewhat simpler than off-resonance phase accumulation and is simply monotonic throughout the echo train for EPI, RARE, and GRASE. Similar to RARE, either proton density or T_2 weighting can be achieved by properly ordering the phase encoding to give either short or long effective TE, respectively. T_1 weighting can be obtained by reducing TR combined with short effective TE. With GRASE, an odd number of gradient echoes are normally collected for each 180° refocusing pulse. Therefore the center echo of each gradient echo group has no net phase accumulation. The motivation behind collecting the odd number of gradient echoes is so that contrast devoid of T_2^* weighting (similar to a conventional RF spin echo) can be obtained by placing these center echoes at the center of k-space.

2D Linear Phase-Encoding Order   This method, also sometimes called sequential phase encoding, is almost never used in practice, and is only discussed here to motivate the descriptions of other variations. For a single-shot scan, the echoes are assigned sequentially or linearly in k-space in the temporal order in which they occur in the echo train. In the full k_y version of this method, the first echo in the echo train is assigned to the maximal phase-encoding value, the next echo is assigned to the adjacent phase-encoding value, and so on. For multishot scans, echoes from a given location within the echo train are grouped together in k-space for all shots (Figure 16.23a). Specifically the phase-encoding locations in k-space are given by:

$$k_y(s, r, g) = \left(-\frac{N_{\text{shot}} N_{\text{rf}} N_{\text{gre}} - 1}{2} + (s + r N_{\text{shot}} N_{\text{gre}} + g N_{\text{shot}}) \right) \Delta k_y$$

(16.31)

where Δk_y is the phase-encoding step size. (We assume a bottom-up phase-encoding order in which the maximal negative k_y value is filled first. A top-down order could just as easily be used, as long as the reconstruction program accounts for the resulting image flip in the phase-encoded direction.) A comparison of Eqs. (16.31) and (8.31) shows the similarity between the echo ordering and that of a non-echo-train pulse sequence. The phase accumulation and T_2-induced amplitude modulation are shown in Figure 16.23b and c, respectively, for the multishot case. The T_2 weighting contains N_{rf} monotonically decreasing steps across k-space. (If the echo amplitude variation due to T_2^* had not been ignored, a small amount of additional modulation would be present for each gradient echo within each step.) Although the k-space amplitude weighting from T_2 decay is relatively benign, the periodicity and discontinuities in the off-resonance phase accumulation cause severe ghosting.

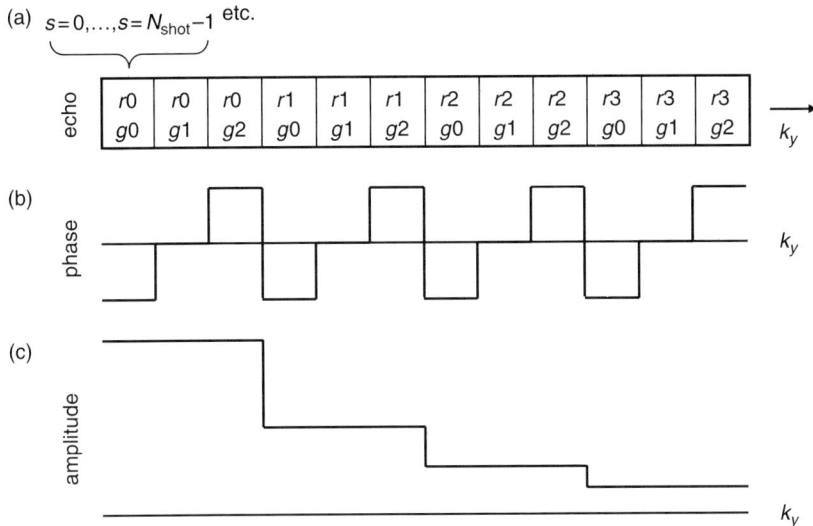

FIGURE 16.23 Linear (sequential) 2D GRASE phase-encoding order. (a) Echo number as a function of k_y. Each block is filled with one echo from all shots (N_{shot} values of k_y). (b) Off-resonance phase as a function of k_y. The phase has $N_{rf} = 4$ bands with $N_{gre} = 3$ monotonically changing steps within each band. (c) T_2-induced amplitude modulation as a function of k_y. The modulation function has $N_{rf} = 4$ monotonically decreasing steps. Each step is further modulated by T_2^* decay. For simplicity, the T_2^* modulation is not shown.

The effective TE is simply one-half the total echo train duration for full k-space acquisition.

2D Standard Phase-Encoding Order   To alleviate artifacts from the off-resonance phase accumulation, the original implementation of GRASE used the phase-encoding order illustrated in Figure 16.24. In the single-shot version of this method, the gradient echoes occurring at a given location after the RF refocusing pulses (i.e., $r0g0$, $r1g0$, etc.) are all grouped together at adjacent k_y lines. Adjacent gradient echoes are grouped at adjacent bands in k-space. For each gradient echo band, a linear phase-encoding order is used with respect to RF pulses; that is, echoes are grouped in order of increasing RF refocusing pulse number. For the multishot case, adjacent k_y lines can be filled with echoes from one RF pulse for all shots before advancing to the next RF pulse, similar to the interleaved case shown in Figure 16.44b in Section 16.4. Alternatively, adjacent k_y lines can be filled with echoes from one shot for all RF pulses before advancing to the next shot, similar to the case shown in Figure 16.44a

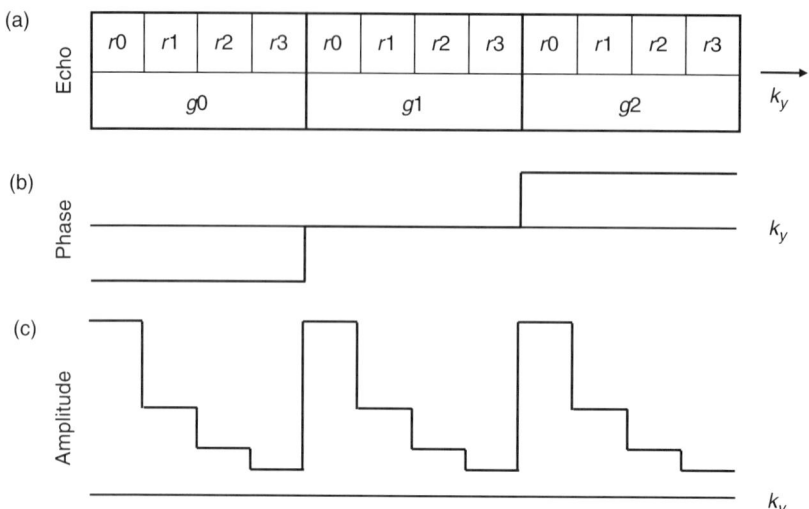

FIGURE 16.24 Standard 2D GRASE phase-encoding order. (a) Echo number as a function of k_y. (b) Off-resonance phase has $N_{gre} = 3$ bands with constant phase within each band. (c) T_2 weighting has $N_{gre} = 3$ bands with $N_{rf} = 4$ monotonically decreasing steps within each band.

in Section 16.4. We focus here on the former method, which is also shown in Figure 16.24 because it is more commonly used. For this case, the phase-encoding locations in k-space are given by:

$$k_y(s, r, g) = \left(-\frac{N_{shot} N_{rf} N_{gre} - 1}{2} + \left(s + r N_{shot} + g N_{shot} N_{rf} \right) \right) \Delta k_y$$

(16.32)

This phase-encoding order is usually called the standard GRASE phase-encoding order because it was used in most early GRASE work (Feinberg and Oshio 1991; Oshio and Feinberg 1991).

The off-resonance phase is a series of N_{gre} plateaus with linearly changing plateau amplitude as a function of k_y. Although the phase accumulation is much less problematic than with a linear phase-encoding order, the discontinuities in the phase still cause ghosting. The discontinuity and ghosting can be reduced using echo train shifting discussed in Section 16.1 and subsection 16.2.3.

The T_2 weighting in k-space has N_{gre} discontinuous bands with N_{rf} monotonically decreasing plateaus within each band. The width of each plateau is determined by N_{shot}. (For the single-shot case, each plateau becomes a single k_y point.) The discontinuities in T_2 k-space weighting also cause ghosting artifacts. Another problem is that the effective TE with the standard GRASE phase-encoding order is fixed at one-half the total echo train duration. Because the echo train duration is usually 200 ms or more for optimal time efficiency, the effective TE is 100 ms or more, limiting the pulse sequence to T_2-weighted contrast only.

Reversing the order of some of the echoes (Figure 16.25) can eliminate the worst discontinuities from T_2 modulation. Echoes from the RF refocusing pulses are placed in reverse order in k-space as a function of k_y for every other gradient echo. The phase weighting in k-space is the same as for the standard GRASE phase-encoding order, but the blip phase-encoding gradient amplitude is no longer constant within each group of gradient echoes with the same r value. Some of the required blip areas can be large and, depending on the imaging parameters and gradient hardware capabilities, they could increase the echo spacing compared to the standard order. This trade-off needs to be evaluated when deciding whether to use the reversed order.

Both the T_2 decay discontinuity and the inflexible effective echo time can be addressed by yet another variation that uses the same grouping of echoes from each RF refocusing pulse as that normally used for multishot RARE (Ishikawa et al. 1996, Gullapalli and Loncar 1996) (see Section 16.4). As an example, to achieve a short effective echo time, echoes from the earliest RF

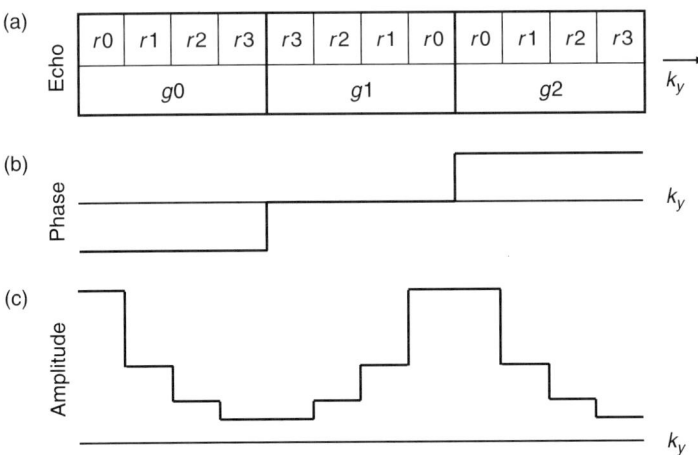

FIGURE 16.25 2D GRASE phase-encoding order with reversal of the direction in which echoes from RF refocusing pulses are placed in k-space for every other gradient echo. (a) Echo number, (b) off-resonance phase, and T_2-induced amplitude modulation as a function of k_y. In this example, echoes for the second gradient echo are ordered $r3, r2, r1, r0$ instead of $r0, r1, r2, r3$ as a function of k_y.

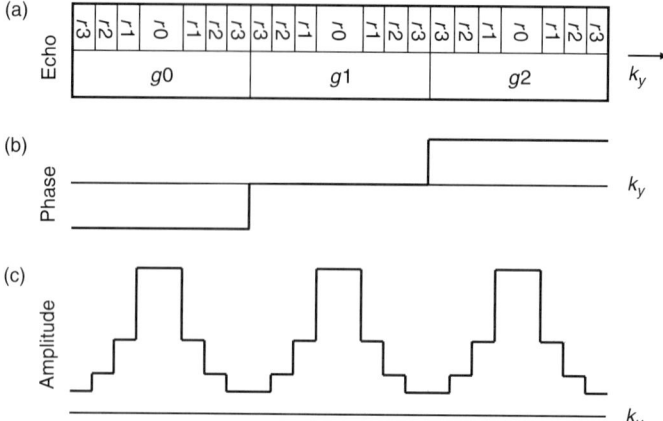

FIGURE 16.26 2D GRASE with echo ordering similar to that normally used for multishot RARE for short effective TE (rotated bands phase encoding). (a) Echo number, (b) off-resonance phase, and (c) T_2-induced amplitude modulation as a function of k_y.

refocusing pulse ($r0$) are assigned to the most central phase-encoding lines within each group of N_{rf} lines. Subsequent RF refocusing pulses are assigned to more negative or more positive phase-encoding lines moving out from the first (Figure 16.26). This strategy is sometimes called a centric GRASE phase-encoding variation (Johnson et al. 1996b). Longer effective TEs can be obtained by permuting or cyclically rotating the centric order (Figure 16.27). The off-resonance phase accumulation is the same as for the standard GRASE phase-encoding order. These variations are also sometimes called rotated bands phase encoding (Mugler 1999).

Example 16.6 A 2D GRASE pulse sequence uses $N_{gre} = 3$, $N_{rf} = 18$, $N_{shot} = 4$. The resulting minimum spacing between RF refocusing pulses is 10 ms. If the standard GRASE phase-encoding order illustrated in Figure 16.24 is used, what is the effective TE and how many phase-encoding lines are collected? Assume that subsequent shots are placed at adjacent k_y lines as illustrated in Figure 16.23 and that phase-encoding lines symmetrically straddle the $k_y = 0$ line.

Answer The standard GRASE phase-encoding order for this example places echo $g1$ (the center echo) at the middle of k-space (see Figure 16.24). Also by analogy with Figure 16.24, the $k_y = 0$ line is straddled by RF spin echoes from the ninth and tenth ($r = 8$ and $r = 9$) RF pulses. This can also be seen from Eq. (16.32). Setting $r = N_{rf}/2 - 1$, $s = N_{shot} - 1$, and $g = (N_{gre} - 1)/2$

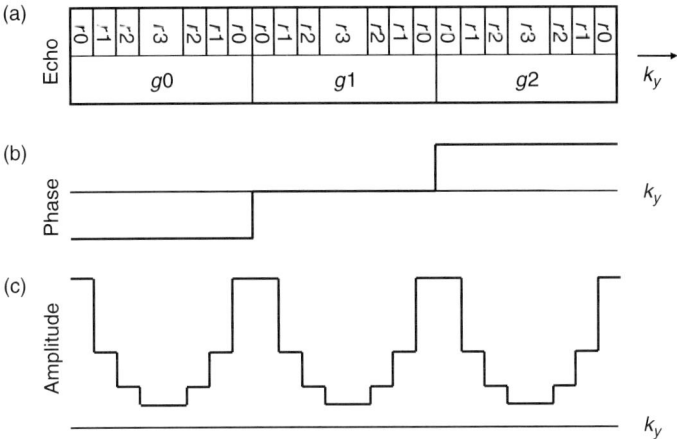

FIGURE 16.27 2D GRASE with echo ordering similar to that normally used for multishot RARE for long effective TE (rotated bands phase encoding). (a) Echo number, (b) off-resonance phase, and (c) T_2-induced amplitude modulation as a function of k_y.

gives $k_y = -\Delta k_y/2$. Setting $r = N_{rf}/2$, $s = 0$, and $g = (N_{gre} - 1)/2$ gives $k_y = +\Delta k_y/2$. The effective TE is approximately the average of the RF spin echo times for the ninth and tenth RF pulses. Therefore $TE_{eff} = 9.5 \times 10 \, ms = 95 \, ms$. The number of collected phase-encoding lines is $3 \times 18 \times 4 = 216$.

2D k-Banded Phase-Encoding Order The k-banded phase encoding (kbGRASE) was developed to alleviate some of the problems with the standard GRASE phase-encoding order (Feinberg et al. 1995). In this method, k-space is divided into bands, and each band is assigned to one continuous section of the spin echo train. Within each k-space band, one of the phase-encoding variations previously discussed is used. Figure 16.28 shows an example with $N_{rf} = 12$, $N_{gre} = 3$ in which k-space is divided into three bands labeled A, B, and C. Each band is filled with data from four consecutive RF refocusing pulses using the standard GRASE phase-encoding order shown in Figure 16.24. In this example, the earliest band in the echo train is assigned to the center of k-space, giving a short effective TE. kbGRASE was developed to decrease some of the T_2 weighting discontinuity that accompanies standard GRASE in exchange for increasing the off-resonance phase discontinuity. Another benefit of kbGRASE is that the effective echo time can be varied by simply changing which band is assigned to the center of k-space. Also, the bands are not necessarily constrained to be of equal width.

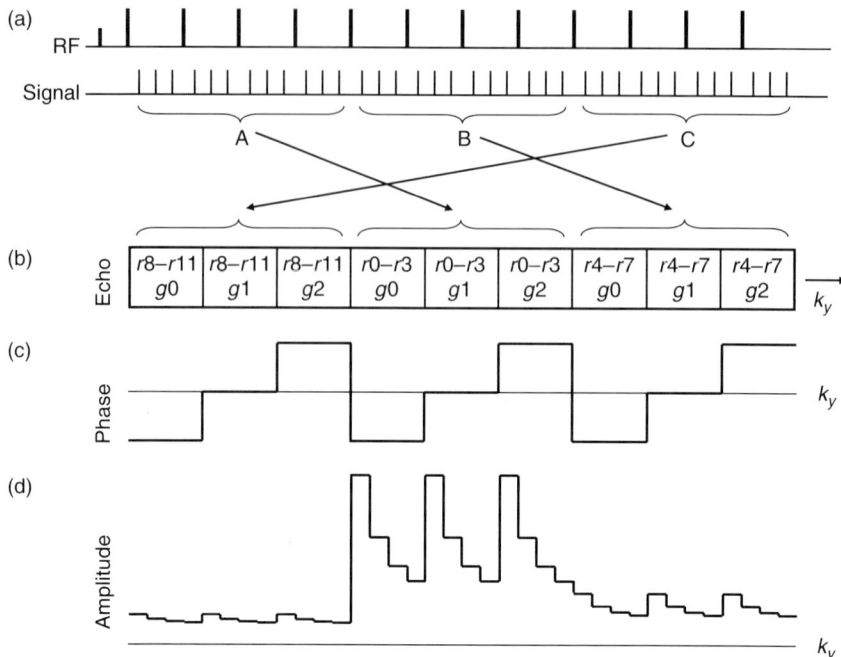

FIGURE 16.28 kbGRASE with standard GRASE phase-encoding order for each k-space band. (a) Pulse sequence using $N_{gre} = 3$ and $N_{rf} = 12$ with readout train divided into three bands A, B, and C. (b) Echo number as a function of k_y. (c) Phase modulation has three bands with three monotonically increasing steps per band. (d) T_2 weighting has three bands, each with three subbands and four monotonically decreasing steps per subband. (Adapted from Feinberg et al. 1995.)

Partial k_y processing is somewhat simpler with kbGRASE than with standard GRASE because a correspondence can be made between a contiguous group of RF refocusing pulses and a contiguous band in k-space; this is not possible with standard GRASE. For example, in Figure 16.28, a partial k_y acquisition could be obtained by simply omitting band C in the echo train. On the other hand, in the example in Figure 16.24, if the last RF refocusing pulse and associated gradient echoes were omitted, there would be three gaps in the k_y direction (echoes $r3g0$, $r3g1$, and $r3g2$), making partial Fourier reconstruction more difficult.

An important variation of kbGRASE reverses the order in which the gradient echoes are placed in k-space for every other k-space band. In the example shown in Figure 16.29, gradient echoes in band A (center of k-space) are placed in the order $g2$, $g1$, $g0$ instead of $g0$, $g1$, $g1$. This reduces discontinuity

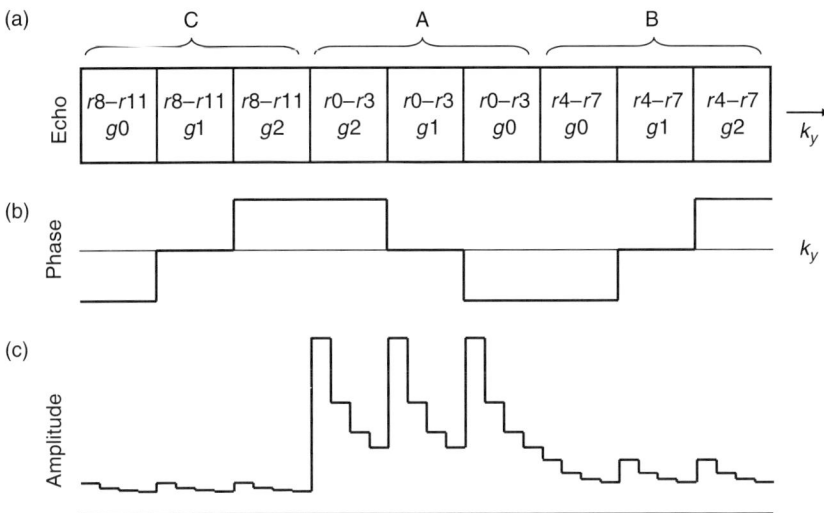

FIGURE 16.29 kbGRASE using reversed ordering of gradient echoes ($g2$, $g1$, $g0$ instead of $g0$, $g1$, $g2$) for band A (center third of k-space). (a) Echo number, (b) off-resonance phase, and (c) T_2-induced amplitude modulation as a function of k_y. Phase modulation has fewer discontinuities. Amplitude modulation is unchanged.

in the off-resonance phase accumulation, resulting in an increased ghosting frequency with reduced intensity. Further ghosting reduction is possible by varying the echo order within each k-space band (e.g., by using centric ordering).

A comparison of eleven 2D GRASE phase-encoding orders, including standard GRASE, kbGRASE, and a partially randomized order, is given in Johnson et al. (1996a). Artifacts depend on off-resonance frequency and T_2. For example, the linear order only works well when the resonance offset is zero because of the phase discontinuities, whereas the standard GRASE phase-encoding order works best when T_2 is long because of the reduced T_2-induced amplitude modulation. In this study, kbGRASE was found to be a good compromise and generally gave the least artifacts. Spatial resolution was found to be about the same for all phase-encoding orders for a fixed ETL. Contrast was also found to be fairly independent of all phase-encoding orders for a fixed effective TE. Increasing the number of gradient echoes was found to generally increase artifact levels in both standard GRASE and kbGRASE. Therefore, most 2D GRASE studies use $N_{gre} = 3$.

Example 16.7 A 2D GRASE pulse sequence uses $N_{gre} = 3$, $N_{rf} = 12$, $N_{shot} = 3$. The minimum spacing between RF refocusing pulses is 8 ms.

A k-banded phase-encoding order with three bands is used. The first band is chosen to sample the center of k-space as shown in Figure 16.28. If the standard GRASE phase-encoding order is used within each band, what is the effective TE and how many phase-encoding lines are collected?

Answer   Each k-space band has four RF pulses. The standard GRASE phase-encoding order places echo $g1$ (center echo) at the middle of k-space. The $k_y = 0$ line is straddled by RF spin echoes from the second and third ($r = 1$ and $r = 2$) RF pulses. The effective TE is approximately the average of the RF spin echo times these two RF pulses. Therefore, $TE_{eff} = 2.5 \times 8\,ms = 20\,ms$. The number of phase-encoding lines is $3 \times 12 \times 3 = 108$.

TIPE GRASE   Template interactive phase encoding (TIPE) attempts to make echo amplitude modulation maximally continuous as a function of k_y (Jovicich and Norris 1998). A scan without phase encoding (also called a template scan or reference scan) is used to determine echo amplitudes as modulated by T_2 and T_2^* decay. The phase-encoding order is then chosen to give continuity of the amplitudes for the desired echo time. Unfortunately, phase from off-resonance spin isochromats varies rapidly as a function of k_y with this method, giving significant ghosting. Although the point-spread function is narrower for this method than for other phase-encoding strategies when the resonance offset is zero, this advantage is almost never realized in practice. Other phase-encoding strategies work better (kbGRASE or standard GRASE), especially in areas of rapid susceptibility variation such as the sinuses.

TIPE GRASE has been used in neurofunctional MRI (fMRI) based on BOLD contrast (Jovicich and Norris 1999). The sensitivity to T_2^* effects is less than for gradient echo EPI (Section 16.1) but more than for spin-echo-based sequences such as spin-echo EPI (Bandettini et al. 1994) and RARE (Constable et al. 1994; Gao et al. 1995). The T_2^* contrast can be enhanced by T_2^* preparation (Jovicich and Norris 1999) as well as by assigning echoes with more T_2^* weighting to the k-space center.

2D Vertical GRASE   A problem with all 2D phase-encoding orders discussed so far is that both off-resonance phase accumulation and T_2 decay affect the k_y axis. Because both effects cannot be rendered continuous in k-space at the same time, some residual k-space discontinuity and ghosting result. Vertical GRASE (vGRASE) alleviates this problem by placing off-resonance phase accumulation along the k_x axis while leaving T_2-decay weighting along the k_y axis (Oshio 2000). The artifacts are effectively spread in two directions, resulting in lower overall artifact levels. The pulse sequence, shown in

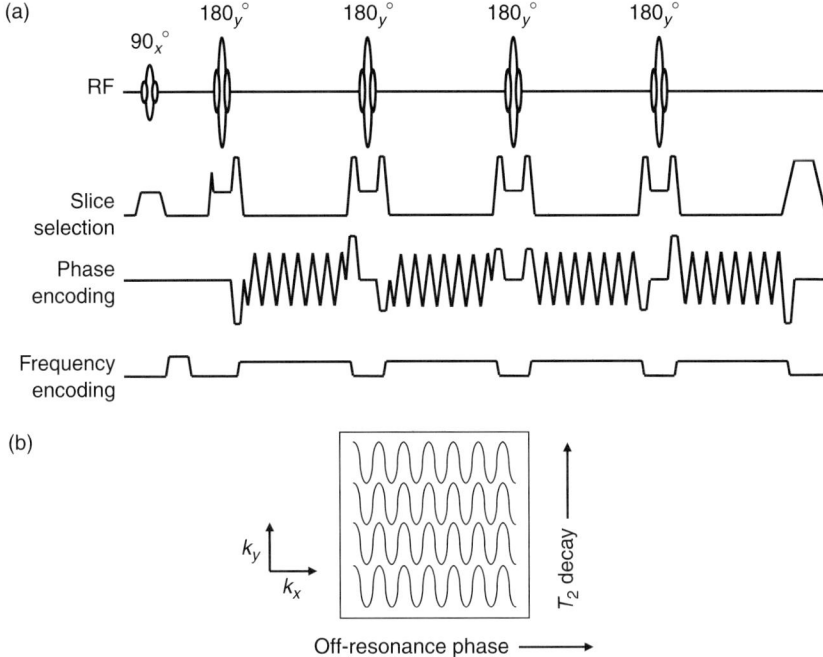

FIGURE 16.30 (a) Vertical GRASE pulse sequence that collects multiple gradient echoes per RF refocusing pulse using an oscillating gradient. (b) A k-space trajectory for one shot of a multishot scan. Phase and amplitude modulation affect different directions in k-space, reducing artifacts. (Adapted from Oshio 2000.)

Figure 16.30, has an oscillating gradient on one k-space axis and a constant gradient on the other axis. The resulting k-space trajectory is a series of zigzags (possibly curved depending on the type of oscillating gradient used), each one covering an adjacent k_y band. For maximal efficiency, sampling takes place continuously during the oscillating gradient. The images are typically reconstructed using gridding (Section 13.2). The method employing an oscillatory phase-encoding gradient and a constant readout gradient can also be employed in multishot EPI.

3D GRASE If the Fourier encoding in the secondary phase-encoded direction (slice) is the same for each echo in the echo train, off-resonance phase accumulation and T_2 decay are both placed along the k_y direction, the same as for a 2D scan (Figure 16.31a). The extra degree of freedom for 3D scans allows a Fourier-encoding order that separates off-resonance and T_2 effects,

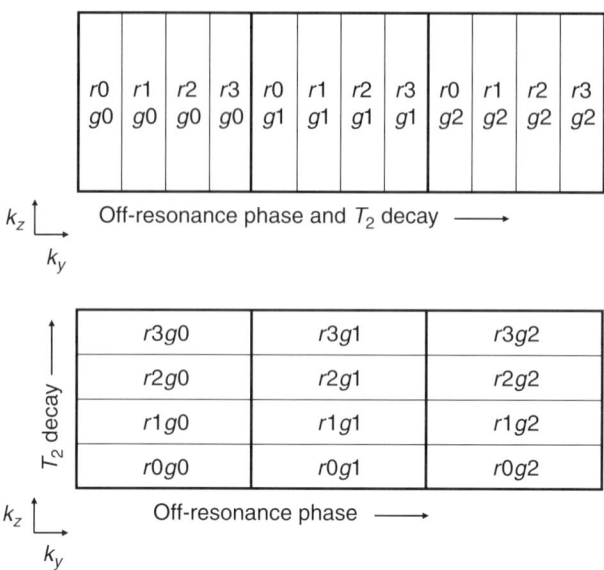

FIGURE 16.31 3D multishot GRASE k-space ordering. (a) The secondary Fourier-encoding step is the same for each RF refocusing pulse. (b) The secondary Fourier-encoding step varies for each RF refocusing pulse to place T_2 decay along the k_z direction. Each box contains data for the indicated echo from all shots. (Adapted from Mugler 1999.)

a method called SORT (Mugler 1999). By appropriately varying the secondary Fourier-encoding step for each RF refocusing pulse, the T_2 decay can be placed along k_z while phase accumulation remains along k_y (Figure 16.31b). As in vGRASE, the k-space modulation is spread over two directions instead of one, which reduces artifacts.

16.2.3 ECHO TIME SHIFTING

The stair steps or discontinuities in the phase accumulated by off-resonance spins (e.g., in the standard GRASE phase-encoding order, Figure 16.24) have been shown to cause ghosting artifacts. These discontinuities are also present in multishot EPI scans and can be decreased by using echo train shifting (ETS), also called a sliding window readout, echo time shifting, or echo shifting (Feinberg and Oshio 1992, 1994). Figures 16.32a and b show phase accumulated with the standard 2D GRASE phase-encoding order using $N_{gre} = 3$. Although phase accumulates linearly during each gradient

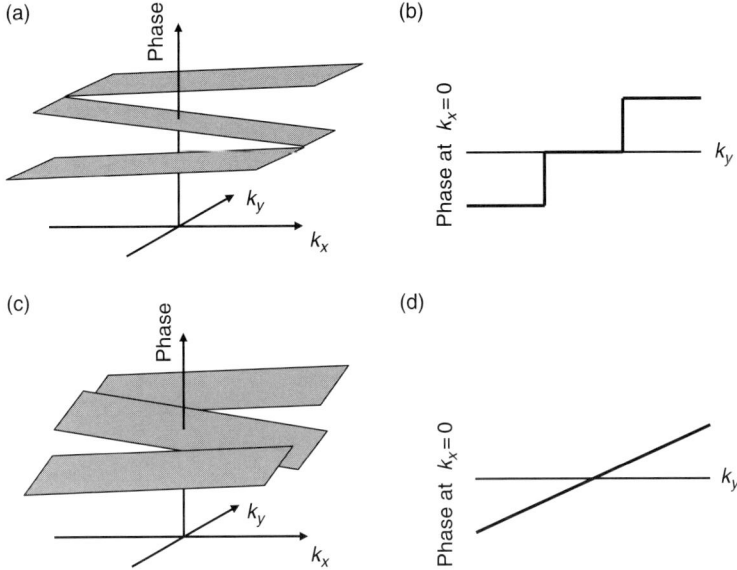

FIGURE 16.32 (a) and (b) Phase accumulation without echo train shifting for the standard GRASE phase-encoding order. Phase is discontinuous at $k_x = 0$ but continuous at alternately the $+k_x$ and $-k_x$ edges of k-space. (c) and (d) Phase accumulation with echo train shifting. Phase is linear at $k_x = 0$ but discontinuous at all other values of k_x. (Adapted from Mugler and Brookeman 1996.)

echo, time reversal on alternate echoes reverses the direction of phase accumulation in k_x for every other echo. The phase evolution is continuous at the $+k_x$ and $-k_x$ edges of k-space for alternate gradient echoes. However, the phase is discontinuous at all other k_x values. Because the image is dominated by the behavior at $k_x = 0$, the continuity causes ghosting. When ETS is used with GRASE, the train of bipolar readout gradients is either delayed or advanced slightly by a different amount for each RF refocusing pulse and each shot. Because the discontinuity between adjacent phase steps at $k_x = 0$ is due to the difference in phase accumulated between adjacent gradient echoes, distributing the echo times for all shots and RF pulses equally over the inter-echo duration T_{gre} removes the phase steps. For example, for the standard GRASE phase-encoding order, continuity at $k_x = 0$ is obtained when the frequency-encoding waveform shift $\Delta t(s, r)$ for each shot and RF pulse is given by:

$$\Delta t(s, r) = (r N_{\mathrm{shot}} + s) \frac{T_{\mathrm{gre}}}{N_{\mathrm{shot}} N_{\mathrm{rf}}} - \frac{T_{\mathrm{gre}}}{2} \tag{16.33}$$

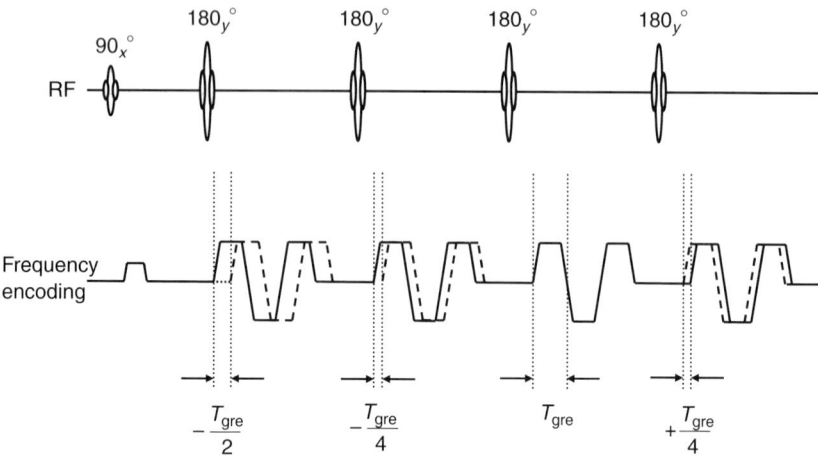

FIGURE 16.33 Frequency-encoding waveforms with echo train shifting (first shot of a multishot scan with $N_{rf} = 4$, $N_{gre} = 3$). Dashed lines show waveforms without echo train shifting. The frequency-encoding waveform for each RF pulse is shifted by T_{gre}/N_{rf} relative to the waveform for the previous RF pulse, as shown by the dotted lines. The waveforms for other shots are shifted by multiples of $T_{gre}/(N_{rf}N_{shot})$ relative to the waveform in the figure. (Adapted from Mugler and Brookeman 1996.)

where T_{gre} is the spacing between adjacent gradient echoes. The shift in Eq. (16.33) is relative to the waveform location without ETS. An example is shown in Figure 16.33 for the first shot ($s = 0$) of a multishot scan with $N_{rf} = 4$, $N_{gre} = 3$. The frequency-encoding waveform for the first RF pulse is shifted by $-T_{gre}/2$. Waveforms for subsequent RF pulses are shifted by an additional $+T_{gre}/4$ for each RF pulse. The waveform for the third RF pulse is therefore unshifted for this shot. Frequency-encoding waveforms for other shots are shifted by multiples of $T_{gre}/(N_{rf}N_{shot})$ relative to the waveforms shown in the figure For the standard phase-encoding order, the phase is converted from a series of steps into a linear function of k_y at $k_x = 0$. Although continuous at $k_x = 0$, the phase is now discontinuous at all other values of k_x (Figure 16.32c and d). According to the Fourier shift theorem, the lowest-order effect of the linear phase at $k_x = 0$ is a y-direction shift of the off-resonance magnetization in the image (misregistration). Ghosting of high-frequency information remains from discontinuity at $k_x \neq 0$.

A detailed study of ETS (Mugler and Brookeman 1996) shows that for relatively small resonance frequency shifts, ETS is beneficial by converting low-frequency ghosting into misregistration. As the resonance offset increases, however, there may be little benefit from ETS because of the increasing discontinuity at the edges of k-space in the k_x direction. The effect of the k-space discontinuity is somewhat object-dependent. More energy near the $+k_x$ and $-k_x$ edges of k-space results in higher ghosting. The discontinuity at the edges of k-space can be reduced by decreasing the total off-resonance phase accumulated during each gradient echo. For a fixed resonance frequency offset, this requires reducing the readout time for each gradient echo. If f_{cs} and T_{acq} are the resonance frequency offset and readout time per gradient echo, respectively, using a combination of ETS and T_{acq} such that $2\ f_{cs}T_{acq} \ll 1$ gives negligible off-resonance ghosting (Mugler and Brookeman 1996). For fat at 1.5 T, $f_{cs} = 210\,\mathrm{Hz}$, requiring $T_{acq} \ll 2.4\,\mathrm{ms}$. In practice, minimal artifacts have been observed for ETS combined with $T_{acq} \sim 1\,\mathrm{ms}$.

With 3D scans, the Fourier-encoding order can be chosen to give monotonically stepped phase evolution along k_y. In this case, ETS is only applied along k_y (i.e., the same echo shift is used for all slice encodings) to convert the stepped phase into a linear function of k_y.

When 2D phase-encoding orders other than the standard one are used (e.g., with kbGRASE), some phase discontinuity remains even with ETS and the benefit derived from ETS becomes less clear. One drawback of ETS is that it increases the minimum spacing between RF refocusing pulses by T_{gre} and increases the minimum effective echo time by $T_{gre}/2$. Many studies with GRASE do not use ETS but instead employ fat saturation to minimize the effects of off-resonance magnetization.

16.2.4 PHASE CORRECTION

In addition to the effort to reduce ghosting due to k-space discontinuity by using phase-encoding-ordering schemes, phase corrections similar to the ones used with EPI are almost always used with GRASE to further decrease ghosting artifacts associated with the bipolar readout gradients. Reference data acquired without phase encoding are typically used to remove the effects of linear and B_0 eddy currents and hardware group delays. Linear eddy currents and group delays shift the echo location as a function of k_x differently for the two gradient polarities. B_0 eddy currents shift the overall phase of the echo differently for the two gradient polarities. More extensive discussion of EPI phase correction methods is given in Section 16.1. With GRASE, the reference data consist of either a complete scan without phase encoding (Jovicich and Norris 1998) or an extra RF refocusing pulse and associated gradient echoes without phase encoding placed either at the beginning or end of the echo train. The processing of the reference data typically involves inverse Fourier transforming each echo to create a projection. The phase of the projection is then subtracted from the phase of the inverse Fourier transform of each phase-encoded echo along the readout direction. Fitting to the reference phase to remove only low-frequency components of the phase has also been used (Jovicich and Norris 1998).

In addition to the EPI-type phase errors associated with the bipolar readout gradients, GRASE also has phase errors of the type found in RARE pulse sequences. These phase errors have many of the same sources as with EPI (hardware group delays and eddy currents, for example). Because different coherence pathways (e.g., primary spin echoes and stimulated echoes) accumulate different phase errors, these phase errors cannot be corrected using postacquisition processing but must be corrected for as with RARE by changing the readout prephasing lobe area and refocusing pulse phase. More extensive discussion of RARE phase-correction methods is given in Section 16.4. The mixing of EPI-type and RARE-type phase errors makes the phase correction very difficult and has hindered the introduction of GRASE into routine clinical practice.

As mentioned previously, crushers for the refocusing pulse are usually placed on either the slice-selection or frequency-encoding axis. When the crushers are placed on the slice-selection axis, eddy currents from the crushers cause an echo amplitude shift that is difficult to measure with reference data due to the confounding effects of T_2^* and T_2 decay. When the crushers are placed on the frequency-encoding axis, eddy currents from the crushers cause a shift in the echo position that can be measured with reference data (Luk-Pat et al. 1999).

When ETS is used, some care must be taken with reference data to avoid making the artifacts worse. One study showed that reference data must be acquired with each individual echo shift $\Delta t(s, r)$; otherwise the phase correction could actually degraded the images (Mugler 1995).

16.2.5 VARIATIONS

Several variations of GRASE produce multiple images with different contrasts. A proton-density-weighted and a T_2-weighted image can be acquired in the same scan (Feinberg et al. 1994). The short effective TE echoes are collected with a higher receiver bandwidth that also allows more gradient echoes per RF refocusing pulse. For example, with four RF refocusing pulses, seven gradient echoes are collected for the first RF refocusing pulse and three gradient echoes are collected for each subsequent RF pulse. The first seven echoes are reconstructed into a short effective TE image whereas the nine subsequent echoes are reconstructed into a long effective TE image. Using $N_{shot} = 28$ allows the collection of 196 and 252 phase-encoding lines, respectively, for the two images.

An alternative GRASE acquisition and reconstruction method (altGRASE) (Keller et al. 1996) uses $N_{gre} = 3$ with the center echo (RF spin echo) phase-encoded for a short effective TE (e.g. 30 ms) to produce spin density contrast and the two adjacent echoes (outer echoes), both phase-encoded for a long effective TE (e.g., 120 ms) to produce T_2-weighted contrast. The two outer echoes are combined for better SNR and reconstructed separately from the center echo, resulting in two distinct images. The outer-echo images also have T_2^* weighting in addition to T_2 weighting. The spacing between gradient echoes is also chosen to place water and fat out of phase for the outer two gradient echoes, giving a partial cancellation of fat signal near water–fat interfaces for the long effective TE image. altGRASE overcomes some of the problems with conventional spin echo and RARE. Multiple contrast images are produced more efficiently than with conventional spin echo scans. Fat has low intensity on the long effective TE image, similar to a conventional RF spin echo. Susceptibility weighting is increased in the long effective TE image compared to RARE (more like a conventional RF spin echo). altGRASE also avoids many of the problems with normal GRASE. There is no phase modulation in k-space because the two outer gradient echoes are not combined with the center RF spin echo. The amplitude modulation in k-space is the same as for RARE. Because echoes from even and odd polarity readout gradients are reconstructed separately, there is no sensitivity to eddy currents or group delays. The disadvantage is that the acquisition is much less time efficient than for conventional GRASE.

GRASE has also been combined with projection acquisition (RAD-GRASE) and the PROPELLER k-space trajectory (turboprop). These variations are discussed in Section 17.5.

SELECTED REFERENCES

Bandettini, P. A., Wong, E. C., Jesmanowicz, A., Hinks, R. S., and Hyde, J. S. 1994. Spin-echo and gradient-echo EPI of human brain activation using BOLD contrast: A comparative study at 1.5T. *Nucl. Magn. Reson. Biomed.* 7: 12–20.

Constable, R. T., Kennan, R. P., Puce, A., McCarthy, G., and Gore, J. C. 1994. Functional NMR imaging using fast spin echo at 1.5T. *Magn. Reson. Med.* 31: 686–690.

Feinberg, D. A., Johnson, G., and Kiefer, B. 1995. Increased flexibility in GRASE imaging by k space-banded phase encoding. *Magn. Reson. Med.* 34: 149–155.

Feinberg, D. A., Kiefer, B., and Litt, A. W. 1994. Dual contrast GRASE (gradient-spin echo) imaging using mixed bandwidth. *Magn. Reson. Educ.* 31: 461–464.

Feinberg, D. A., and Oshio, K. 1991. GRASE (gradient- and spin-echo) MR imaging: A new fast clinical imaging technique. *Radiology* 181: 597–602.

Feinberg, D. A., and Oshio, K. 1992. Gradient-echo shifting in fast MRI techniques (GRASE imaging) for correction of field inhomogeneity errors and chemical shift. *Magn. Reson. Med.* 97: 177–183.

Feinberg, D. A., and Oshio, K. 1994. Phase errors in multi-shot echo planar imaging. *Magn. Reson. Med.* 32: 535–539.

Gao, J.-H., Xiong, J., Li, J., Schiff, J., Roby, J., Lancaster, J., and Fox, P. T. 1995. Fast spin-echo characteristics of visual stimulation-induced signal changes in the human brain. *J. Magn. Reson. Imaging* 5: 709–714.

Gullapalli, R., and Loncar, M. 1996. A new flexible phase ordering scheme for GSE. In *Proceedings of the 4th meeting of the International Society for Magnetic Resonance in Medicine*, p. 1470.

Ishikawa, A., Kohno, S., Iijima, N., and Fujita, A. 1996. Variable contrast GRASE using new phase encoding order. In *Proceedings of the 4th meeting of the International Society for Magnetic Resonance in Medicine*, p. 1469.

Johnson, G., Feinberg, D. A., and Venkataraman, V. 1996a. A comparison of phase encoding ordering schemes in T2-weighted GRASE imaging. *Magn. Reson. Med.* 36: 427–435.

Johnson, G., Feinberg, D. A., and Venkataraman, V. 1996b. Single-shot GRASE imaging with short effective TEs. *J. Magn. Reson. Imaging* 6: 944–947.

Jovicich, J., and Norris, D. G. 1998. GRASE imaging at 3 tesla with template interactive phase-encoding. *Magn. Reson. Med.* 39: 970–979.

Jovicich, J., and Norris, D. G. 1999. Functional MRI of the human brain with GRASE-based BOLD contrast. *Magn. Reson. Med.* 41: 871–876.

Keller, P. J., Karis, J. P., Fram, E. K., Heiserman, J. E., and Drayer, B. P. 1996. An alternative to GRASE: Toward spin-echo-like contrast with independent reconstruction of gradient-echo images. *Magn. Reson. Med.* 36: 804–808.

Luk-Pat, G. T., Gold, G. E., Olcott, E. W., Hu, B. S., and Nishimura, D. G. 1999. High-resolution three-dimensional in vivo imaging of atherosclerotic plaque. *Magn. Reson. Med.* 42: 762–771.

Mugler, J. P. 1995. Interference between echo time shifting and correction scans in multi-shot-EPI and GRASE pulse sequences. In *Proceedings of the 3rd meeting of the Society for Magnetic Resonance* p. 758.

Mugler, J. P. 1999. Improved three-dimensional GRASE imaging with the SORT phase-encoding strategy. *J. Magn. Reson. Imaging* 9: 604–612.

Mugler, J. P., and Brookeman, J. R. 1996. Off-resonance image artifacts in interleaved-EPI and GRASE pulse sequences. *Magn. Reson. Med.* 36: 306–313.

Oshio, K. 2000. vGRASE: Separating phase and T_2 modulations in 2D. *Magn. Reson. Med.* 44: 383–386.

Oshio, K., and Feinberg, D. A. 1991. GRASE (gradient- and spin-echo) imaging: A novel fast MRI technique. *Magn. Reson. Med.* 20: 344–349.

Patel, M. R., Klufas, R. A., and Shapiro, A. W. 1995. MR imaging of diseases of the brain: Comparison of GRASE and conventional spin-echo T_2-weighted pulse sequence. *Am. J. Roentgenol.* 165: 963–966.

Schaffter, T., and Leibfritz, D. 1994. PSF improvements in single shot GRASE imaging. In *Proceedings of the 2nd meeting of the Society for Magnetic Resonance*, p. 27.

RELATED SECTIONS

16.3 PRESTO

In many MRI applications it is desirable to minimize the effect that susceptibility variation has on images, for example, to reduce signal loss near metallic implants. This has helped to bolster the popularity of conventional RF spin echo and RARE methods for routine clinical imaging. Sometimes, however, T_2^* weighting is desired for applications such as perfusion imaging that use contrast agents, and fMRI based on the BOLD contrast (see Section 16.1). Because the T_2^*-weighting factor in gradient echoes is e^{-TE/T_2^*} (see Section 14.1), strong T_2^* weighting requires a long TE. In other applications, such as MR thermometry (i.e., temperature mapping), a long TE is also desirable to increase its sensitivity to proton resonance frequency offset. The main advantage of gradient echo pulse sequences, however, is their short TR, which provides acquisition speed. Because generally TE < TR, the use of conventional gradient echoes for these applications has been limited. By allowing TE to exceed TR, echo-shifted (ES) pulse sequences such as principles of echo shifting with a train of observations (PRESTO) (Liu, Sobering, Duyn, et al. 1993) enable the rapid acquisition of images that require a long TE.

Several other types of pulse sequences, such as gradient-echo EPI (Section 16.1) and reversed spiral (Section 17.6) also allow the rapid acquisition of T_2^*-weighted images. Because ES pulse sequences use gradient echoes (or an EPI readout with a relatively short ETL as in PRESTO), they are generally more robust against image-quality problems (e.g., blurring or distortion) than these other methods.

16.3.1 ECHO-SHIFTED GRADIENT ECHO

Basic ES Pulse Sequence   An ES gradient echo pulse sequence includes modified or additional gradient lobes that delay the echo formation by at least one TR interval (Moonen et al. 1992; Liu, Sobering, Olson, et al. 1993). A representative example of an ES gradient echo pulse sequence is shown in Figure 16.34. The modified gradient lobes are played on the slice-selection waveform in this example. The slice-selection rephasing gradient lobe has (negative) area $-2A$, which is equal to twice its normal value. (ES pulse sequences generally use a symmetric RF excitation pulse that has its isodelay point at the center of the slice-selection gradient lobe, so the modified slice-rephasing area is approximately equal to the area of the entire slice-selection gradient lobe.) The extra gradient area in the slice rephasing lobe (shaded) acts as a spoiler (Section 10.5) to dephase the transverse magnetization, so that no signal is observed in the first TR interval. After the first readout (during which data acquisition is skipped), a positive gradient lobe of area $+A$ is played on

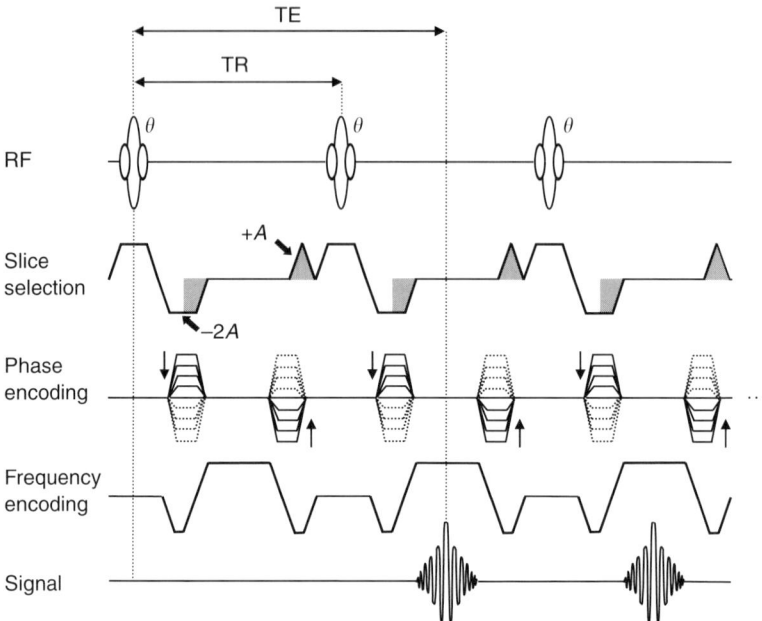

FIGURE 16.34 ES gradient echo pulse sequence. The slice rephasing lobe has area $-2A$, instead of its normal value $-A$. The extra gradient lobe of area $-A$ (shaded) dephases the MR signal in its own TR interval. The lobe of area $+A$ that is applied after the readout allows the transverse magnetization to be rephased into a gradient echo in the next TR interval, therefore giving TE > TR. (Only a single amplitude of the phase encoding and rewinder gradient is played in each TR interval. The stepped waveform is shown here to emphasize the similarity between the ES and standard gradient echo pulse sequences.)

the slice-selection axis so that the transverse magnetization is again in phase at the end of this gradient lobe. The next two lobes on the slice axis, the slice selection and rephasing for the next TR interval, have equal and opposite areas of $2A$ and $-2A$, respectively. After these two lobes are applied, the portion of the transverse magnetization that is produced by the first RF pulse (and is not perturbed by the second RF pulse) can be rephased in the center of the readout window, as shown on Figure 16.34. The transverse magnetization produced by the second RF pulse is dephased and does not contribute to the signal at the second readout window. Instead that magnetization is refocused at the third readout window. In general, the transverse magnetization created by the jth RF pulse is refocused at the $(j + 1)$th readout window. In this way, TE > TR is achieved.

The pulse sequence in Figure 16.34 shares several features in common with standard gradient echo sequences. For example, the frequency-encoding waveform shown is equivalent to that used in balanced SSFP (i.e., true FISP) because its net gradient area is zero in any TR interval. Also, as with most other gradient echo pulse sequences, a phase-encoding rewinder is applied. The RF pulses can be applied either in a coherent train (i.e., θ_x—TR—θ_x—TR—θ_x—$\cdots$) or with RF spoiling.

As described in Chung and Duerk (1999), there are many variations on the basic ES pulse sequence shown in Figure 16.34 which is only a representative example. One common variation is to use ES gradient echo with 3D acquisition mode. Pulse sequence diagrams for 3D ES gradient echo are shown, for example in Duyn et al. (1994) and Golay et al. (2000). Also, although almost all ES pulse sequences are gradient-echo-based, there is an RF spin echo analog called interlaced spin echo, as described in Duyn (2000). ES techniques can also be applied to stimulated echo acquisitions, as described in Mori et al. (1997).

More General Echo-Shifting Gradient Lobes   The basic ES pulse sequence shown in Figure 16.34 can be generalized by considering the ES gradient lobes independently from the rest of the pulse sequence. Three examples of design strategies are shown in Figures 16.35 to 16.37. In these figures, A' denotes an arbitrary gradient area that is sufficiently large to spoil the transverse magnetization. It is not necessarily equal to A, which is one-half the area of the entire slice-selection gradient lobe shown in Figure 16.34. Each of these three echo-shifting strategies can be applied to logical gradient waveform(s) that have zero net area in any TR interval. For example, the slice-selection, frequency-encoding, or phase-encoding waveforms of the balanced SSFP pulse sequence (Figure 14.12) can provide the basic waveforms to which the echo-shifting lobes are added.

One strategy to shift the echo by one TR interval is to apply gradient lobes of area $-A'$ and $+2A'$ before and after each readout, respectively, as shown in Figure 16.35. The slice-selection waveform of the standard ES pulse sequence shown in Figure 16.34 is a special case of this more general strategy. This can be verified by setting $A' = A$ and adding lobes as shown in Figure 16.35 to the balanced SSFP slice-selection waveform that has the characteristic $(-A, +2A, -A)$ gradient lobe grouping.

Figure 16.36 shows a second strategy that shifts the echo by one TR interval. The spoiler gradients, which are played before the readout, have equal area A', but their polarity alternates every TR interval. These spoiler gradients, which are also called crusher gradients in the literature, are often used in conjunction with RF spoiling to dephase the transverse steady state in ES pulse sequences. Both this strategy and the one shown in Figure 16.35 can

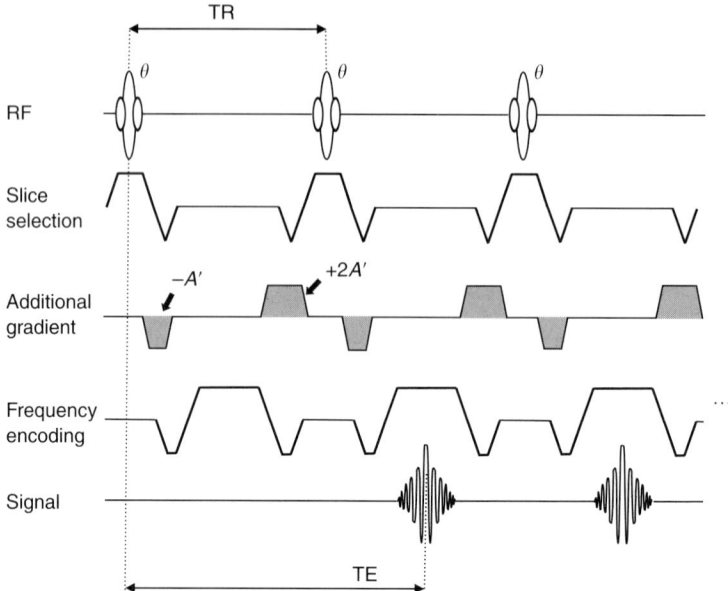

FIGURE 16.35 A general set of gradient lobes designed to delay the echo formation by one TR interval. The additional gradient can be added to the slice-selection or frequency-encoding waveforms shown or to the phase-encoding waveform (not shown) if a rewinding gradient is used.

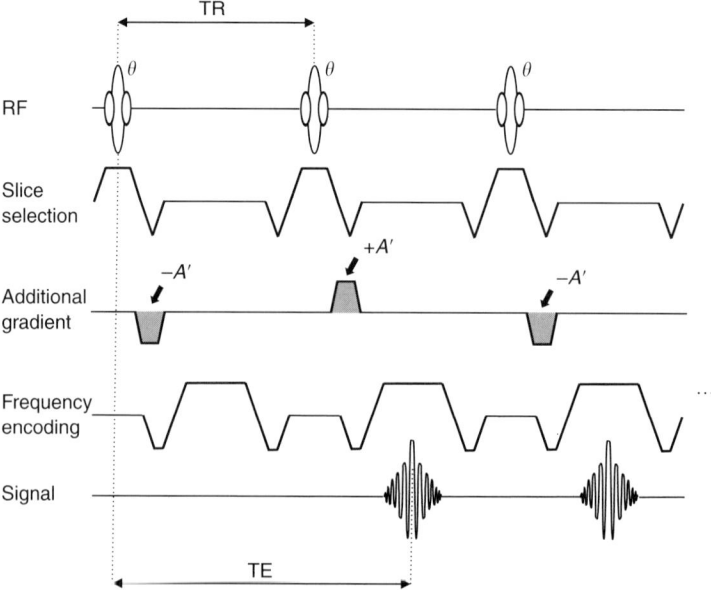

FIGURE 16.36 Another general strategy designed to delay the echo formation by one TR interval. The entire pulse sequence repeats with a period of two TR intervals.

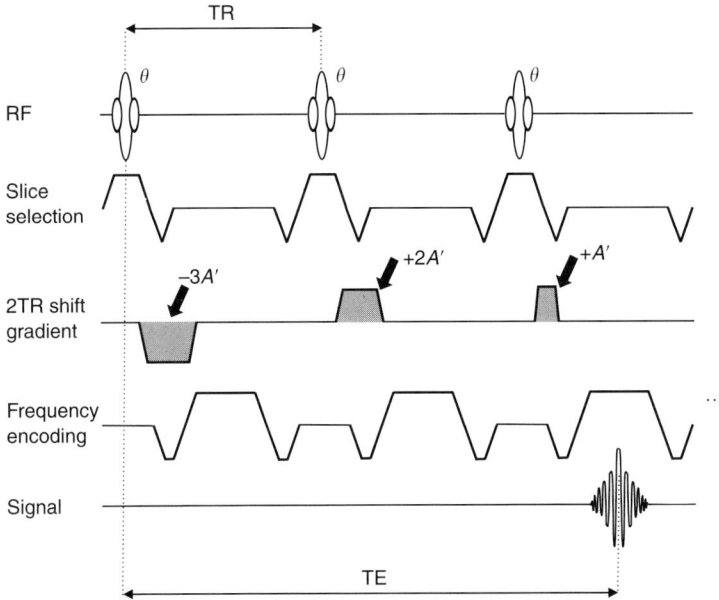

FIGURE 16.37 A set of gradient lobes designed to delay the echo formation by two TR intervals. The three-pulse sequence repeats with a period of three TR intervals.

be applied to the same pulse sequence because they both delay the echo by one TR interval. An advantage of using the strategy in Figure 16.36 is that the absolute value of the total spoiler gradient area per TR interval is reduced by a factor of three. A disadvantage of this strategy, however, is that the spoiler gradients are periodic every two TR intervals, so if there are uncompensated eddy currents, a half-FOV (i.e., Nyquist) ghost can result, as shown in Section 16.1.

Usually the echo is shifted by just one TR interval, so that, $TR < TE < 2 \times TR$. Values of TE greater than $2 \times TR$ further increase T_2^* weighting. These longer shifts are implemented with gradient lobes that vary periodically over a few TR cycles (Liu, Sobering, Olson, et al. 1993). For example, to shift the echo by two TR intervals, an additional gradient lobe with area $-3A'$ can be played before the readout in the first TR interval, $2A'$ in the second, and A' third TR interval (Figure 16.37). The entire cycle then repeats every three TR intervals, resulting in $2 \times TR < TE < 3 \times TR$.

It is useful to define n as the number of TR intervals by which the echo is shifted. Then:

$$TE = TE_0 + nTR \tag{16.34}$$

where TE_0 is the echo delay in the absence of shifting. From Eq. (16.34), the T_2^* weighting of the shifted echo is given by:

$$e^{-TE/T_2^*} = e^{-(TE_0+nTR)/T_2^*} = e^{-TE_0/T_2^*} e^{-nTR/T_2^*} \tag{16.35}$$

When $n = 2$, the factor of e^{-nTR/T_2^*} in Eq. (16.35) is reminiscent of the contrast weighting for the SSFP echo, which in some limits contains the factor e^{-2TR/T_2} (see Section 14.1). An important difference is the appearance of T_2^* in Eq. (16.35), rather than T_2.

Spoiling and Signal Considerations ES gradient echo pulse sequences can be designed either to establish a transverse steady state, or to be spoiled. Sometimes the spoiled gradient echo sequences are called ES-FLASH. Some of the early work on ES gradient echo pulse sequences (e.g., Moonen et al. 1992) did not apply a phase-rewinding lobe, so that the phase-encoding gradient itself served as a gradient spoiler. (When no rewinder is used, the area of each phase-encoding lobe must be reduced by a factor of $(n+1)$ to account for the multiple phase encodings that the transverse magnetization experiences.) As discussed in Chung and Duerk (1999), RF spoiling is more effective when the gradient waveform area is unbalanced (e.g., the additional spoiler gradient shown in Figure 16.36 is applied). As with standard gradient echoes, RF spoiling is usually the preferred method (if any spoiling is desired) to avoid image artifacts. The receiver phase used to demodulate the signal, however, is not matched to the phase of the RF excitation pulse in the same TR interval but instead to the phase of a previous one that depends on how many TR intervals the echo is shifted. For example, in the typical case of $n = 1$, the receiver phase is matched to the phase of the RF excitation pulse from the TR interval that immediately precedes it, because it generates the FID that is rephased into the ES signal.

When spoiling is used in conjunction with ES, the resulting signal is given by (Moonen et al. 1992; Chung and Duerk 1999):

$$S_{ES,spoil} = M_0 \sin\theta \cos^{2n}\left(\frac{\theta}{2}\right) \frac{(1 - e^{-TR/T_1})}{(1 - \cos\theta e^{-TR/T_1})} e^{-TE_0/T_2^*} e^{-nTR/T_2^*} \tag{16.36}$$

Equation (16.36) is very similar to the expression for a standard spoiled gradient echo pulse sequence (Section 14.1). One difference is the additional T_2^*-weighting factor e^{-nTR/T_2^*}, which originates from Eq. (16.35) and is the main benefit of ES pulse sequences. The other difference is the appearance of the extra factor $\cos^{2n}(\theta/2)$, which also attenuates the signal but does not provide any beneficial contrast. The origin of this cosine factor can be seen from the analysis of the coherence pathways in echo formation. In Section 3.3 on refocusing pulses, the response of the transverse magnetization is derived when RF pulses of flip angles θ_1 and θ_2 are applied. The resulting expression (Eq. 3.39) contains a term proportional to $\sin\theta_1 \cos^2(\theta_2/2)$, which represents the magnetization that remains in the transverse plane during the entire TE time. This term represents the signal that is rephased into the shifted gradient echo. Setting $\theta_1 = \theta_2 = \theta$ (to match the RF pulse train used in ES gradient echo) illustrates the origin of the factor $\sin\theta \cos^2(\theta/2)$ (instead of $\sin\theta$ alone) for an echo shifted by one TR interval ($n = 1$). With each additional TR period that the echo is shifted, the magnetization experiences another RF pulse, which introduces one more $\cos^2(\theta/2)$ factor. The product of all those factors explains the appearance of $\cos^{2n}(\theta/2)$ in Eq. (16.36).

Example 16.8 Suppose a standard spoiled gradient echo pulse sequence is acquired with TE = 5 ms, TR = 20 ms, and $\theta = 30°$. Assuming $T_2^* = 40$ ms, calculate the extra signal attenuation that the spoiled ES gradient echo pulse sequence experiences compared to a standard spoiled gradient echo. Consider shifts by one and two TR intervals (i.e., $n = 1$ and 2).

Answer The extra signal attenuation for a spoiled ES pulse sequence has two contributing factors: T_2^* dephasing and the cosine factor. For $n = 1$, Eq. (16.36) yields $e^{-20/40} = 0.607$ and $\cos^2(15°) = 0.933$. The product of the two factors is 0.566, so the net attenuation is increased by 43% compared to an unshifted spoiled gradient echo. For $n = 2$ both attenuation factors are squared, so the net additional attenuation is 68%.

One consequence of the cosine factor in Eq. (16.36) is that the flip angle is generally restricted to low values in spoiled ES pulse sequences, especially when $n > 1$. Otherwise, the factor of $\cos^{2n}(\theta/2)$ causes a substantial attenuation of the signal.

If RF spoiling is not used and the phase-encoding gradient is rewound, a steady state for the transverse magnetization is established with ES pulse sequences. In that case Eq. (16.36) is no longer valid. Sometimes this class of ES pulse sequences is called TR-periodic because even if $n > 1$ the pulse sequence repeats after a number of TR intervals. For example, the pulse sequence in Figure 16.37 has $n = 2$, but still repeats every three TR intervals. A detailed discussion of the mechanisms of signal formation in TR-periodic pulse sequences is provided in Chung and Duerk (1999), closed-form analytical expressions for the signal are derived in Hänicke and Vogel (2003), and further discussion is provided in Denolin and Metens (2004). From an image contrast standpoint, TR-periodic ES pulse sequences display higher signal fluid at moderate flip angles compared to their spoiled counterparts.

16.3.2 ECHO TRAIN ECHO-SHIFTED SEQUENCES

To further increase acquisition speed, ES pulse sequences are often combined with echo train imaging, as in PRESTO. Figure 16.38 shows a representative pulse sequence diagram for PRESTO. As in Figure 16.34, modified gradient lobes on the slice-selection waveform delay the echo formation by one TR interval. The frequency-encoding waveform now contains a train of EPI-type readouts (e.g., a train of six bipolar gradient lobes is shown here). A small positive gradient lobe is played on the frequency-encoding axis after the echo train. This ensures that the net gradient area in any single TR interval is zero because the frequency-encoding waveform is not contributing to the echo shift in this example. Before each readout window, a gradient lobe is played along the phase-encoding axis to produce an individually phase-encoded k-space line (Section 16.1). In this example, the use of the echo train reduces the number of TR intervals required to cover k-space and complete the acquisition (i.e., the number of shots) from $N_{phase} + 1$ to $(N_{phase}/6) + 1$, where N_{phase} is the number

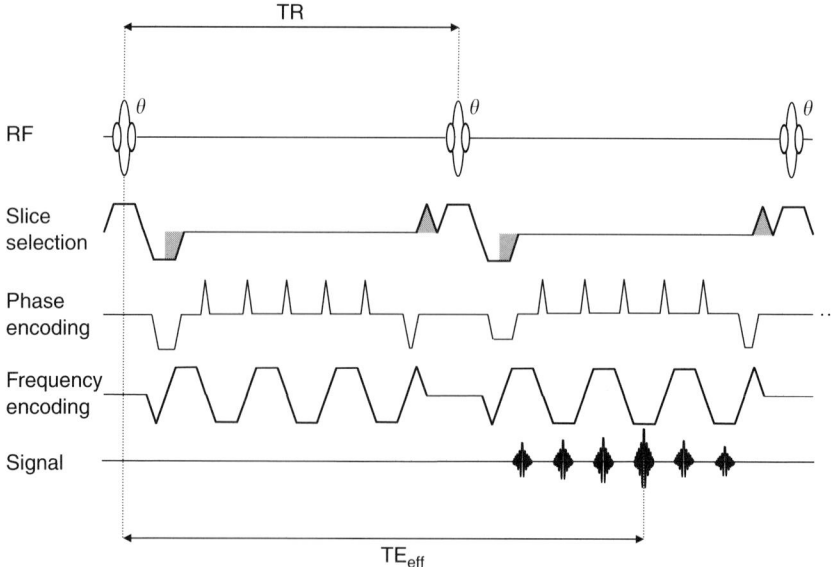

FIGURE 16.38 Pulse sequence diagram for PRESTO pulse sequence with an echo shift of one TR interval and an echo train length of six.

of phase-encoding steps. A more general expression for the number of shots required to cover k-space is:

$$
N_{\text{shot}} = \begin{cases} N_{\text{phase}}/N_{\text{etl}} + n & \text{if} (N_{\text{phase}} \bmod N_{\text{etl}}) = 0 \\ \text{int}(N_{\text{phase}}/N_{\text{etl}}) + n + 1 & \text{if} (N_{\text{phase}} \bmod N_{\text{etl}}) \neq 0 \end{cases} \quad (16.37)
$$

where the int function provides the integer part of its argument and the modulo (mod) function gives the remainder of integer division. (Equation 16.37 does not include any dummy acquisitions used to reach a steady state.) The echo train length N_{etl} in PRESTO is usually limited to 20 or shorter, which reduces the image distortion due to off-resonance effects as well as blurring artifacts that can occur in echo planar images in the presence of short T_2^* (Farzaneh et al. 1990). To further accelerate the PRESTO acquisition, partial Fourier (Brookes et al. 2000) and parallel imaging methods such as SENSE (Golay et al. 2000) can be used.

As shown on Figure 16.38, a negative phase-encoding prephasing lobe initializes the k-space trajectory away from $k_y = 0$. The amplitude of the prephasing lobe is incremented each TR interval. A series of positive blip phase encodings are then applied in between the readouts for k-space traversal in the k_y direction. At the end of the echo train, a negative rewinding lobe is applied so that the net area on the phase-encoding waveform is zero in any TR interval. A diagram that schematically depicts a typical interleaved traversal of k-space is shown in Figure 16.39, and additional discussion on the interleaved k-space trajectory is provided in Section 16.1. The echo with greatest amplitude

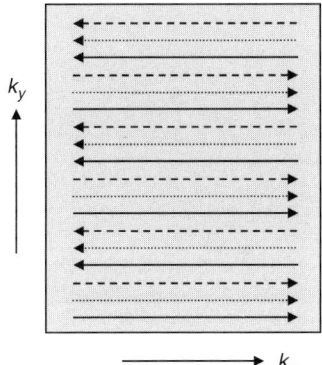

FIGURE 16.39 Schematic interleaved k-space traversal diagram for the PRESTO pulse sequence shown in Figure 16.38 with 18 views $N_{\text{etl}} = 6$ and $N_{\text{shot}} = 3$). The solid lines indicate the k-space trajectory obtained from the first echo train, the dotted lines from the second, and the dashed lines from the third.

occurs near the center of k-space, that is, where the accumulated blip area cancels (or most nearly cancels) the area of the prephasing lobe. That echo provides an effective echo time $TE_{eff} = TE_{eff,0} + nTR$, which replaces TE in Eq. (16.35).

As in other echo train methods, PRESTO is very sensitive to hardware imperfections such as inconsistent group delays or uncompensated eddy currents, especially when the polarity of the readout gradient alternates along the echo train. As described in Section 16.1, the flyback (i.e., skip-echo) method can be used to increase robustness at the cost of acquisition efficiency. The discussion in Section 16.1 about artifacts in EPI and corrections generally applies to PRESTO. An example of a calibration that uses a reference scan to minimize artifacts for 3D-PRESTO is described in Hoogduin et al. (2000).

16.3.3 APPLICATIONS

Applications of ES gradient echo and PRESTO include any imaging situation in which T_2^*-contrast weighting or a long TE is desired in conjunction with rapid acquisition. Perfusion imaging based on dynamic susceptibility changes induced by a bolus of gadolinium chelates (Moonen et al. 1992, 1994; van Gelderen et al. 2000) and fMRI based on the BOLD contrast (Duyn et al. 1994; Golay et al. 2000) are relatively well-established applications of PRESTO. One advantage that has been reported for using PRESTO in fMRI applications at 1.5 T is that confounding signal activation is less likely to occur in areas of the draining veins compared to standard gradient-echo EPI (Denolin et al. 2000) because the additional echo-shifting gradients tend to dephase moving spins.

Another application of ES pulse sequences is MR thermometry (de Zwart et al. 1996; Harth et al. 1997) using the dependence of proton resonance frequency (PRF) on temperature (De Poorter et al. 1995). Applications of PRF methods include *in vivo* temperature monitoring during procedures such as focused ultrasound tissue ablation. PRF methods calculate a temperature-difference map by forming a phase-difference image based on acquisitions obtained at two different temperatures. Because the change in PRF with temperature is very small (e.g., -0.01 ppm/°C for water; Hindman 1966), the sensitivity of the methods increases with TE. An excessively long TE, however, results in SNR loss due to T_2^* dephasing. This trade-off causes the optimal TE for PRF thermometry to be on the order of T_2^*, which is usually attainable with ES acquisition methods.

Diffusion imaging with PRESTO has also been demonstrated (Delalande et al. 1999). One diffusion-sensitizing gradient lobe is placed in each TR interval. The polarity of the lobes alternates between adjacent TR intervals, just like the additional spoiler gradient shown in Figure 16.36. Although a long TE is not usually considered to be an advantage in diffusion imaging, PRESTO allows the two lobes of the diffusion-weighting gradient to be separated by TR. Because the *b*-value is linearly proportional to the separation Δ of the two lobes (see Section 9.1), this allows high *b*-values to be obtained in a time–efficient manner. The efficiency of diffusion-weighted PRESTO is further improved by the fact that each diffusion-weighting gradient lobe serves a double function. That is, each lobe contributes to the diffusion weighting of the signal that is acquired in its own TR interval and also to the next one. Another advantage of diffusion imaging with PRESTO is that the image distortion often observed in single-shot EPI is avoided. As with other multishot diffusion techniques, however, the motion sensitivity can be problematic and often requires correction or compensation.

SELECTED REFERENCES

Brookes, J. A., Delalande, C., Ries M., Dilharreguy, B., Jones, R. A., and Moonen, C. T. W. 2000. Ultra-fast heavily weighted T_2^* weighted 3D brain imaging using a half k-space PRESTO acquisition. In *Proceedings of the 8th meeting of the International Society for Magnetic Resonance in Medicine*, p. 686.

Chung, Y. C., and Duerk, J. L. 1999. Signal formation in echo-shifted sequences. *Magn. Reson. Med.* 42: 864–875.

De Poorter, J., De Wagter, C., De Deene, Y., Thomsen, C., Stahlberg, F., and Achten, E. 1995. Noninvasive MRI thermometry with the proton resonance frequency (PRF) method: In vivo results in human muscle. *Magn. Reson. Med.* 33: 74–81.

de Zwart, J. A., van Gelderen, P., Kelly, D. J., and Moonen, C. T. 1996. Fast magnetic-resonance temperature imaging. *J. Magn. Reson. B.* 112: 86–90.

Delalande, C., de Zwart, J. A., Trillaud, H., Grenier, N., and Moonen, C. T. 1999. An echo-shifted gradient-echo MRI method for efficient diffusion weighting. *Magn. Reson. Med.* 41: 1000–1008.

Denolin, V., and Metens, T. 2004. On the calculation and interpretation of signal intensity in echo-shifted sequences. *Magn. Reson. Med.* 51: 123–134.

Denolin, V., Van Ham, P., and Metens, T. 2000. 3D techniques in BOLD fMRI: Comparison of PRESTO and standard EPI. In *Proceedings of the 8th meeting of the International Society for Magnetic Resonance in Medicine*, p. 939.

Duyn, J. H. 2000. High-speed interlaced spin-echo magnetic resonance imaging. *Magn. Reson. Med.* 43: 905–908.

Duyn J. H., Mattay V. S., Sexton R. H., Sobering G. S., Barrios F. A., Liu G., Frank J. A., Weinberger D. R., and Moonen C. T. 1994. 3-dimensional functional imaging of human brain using echo-shifted FLASH MRI. *Magn. Reson. Med.* 32: 150–155, 545 [erratum].

Farzaneh, F., Riederer, S. J., and Pelc, N. J. 1990. Analysis of T_2 limitations and off-resonance effects on spatial resolution and artifacts in echo-planar imaging. *Magn. Reson. Med.* 14: 123–139.

Golay, X., Pruessmann, K. P., Weiger, M., Crelier, G. R., Folkers, P. J., Kollias, S. S., and Boesiger, P. 2000. PRESTO-SENSE: An ultrafast whole-brain fMRI technique. *Magn. Reson. Med.* 43: 779–786.

Hänicke, W., and Vogel, H. U. 2003. An analytical solution for the SSFP signal in MRI. *Magn. Reson. Med.* 49: 771–775.

Harth, T., Kahn, T., Rassek, M., Schwabe, B., Schwarzmaier, H. J., Lewin, J. S., and Modder, U. 1997. Determination of laser-induced temperature distributions using echo-shifted TurboFLASH. *Magn. Reson. Med.* 38: 238–245.

Hindman, J. C. 1966. Proton resonance shift of water in the gas and liquid states. *J. Chem. Phys.* 44: 4582–4592.

Hoogduin, H., van Gelderen, P., van de Brink, J., and Ramsey, N. 2000. A slice encoded reference scan for 3D-PRESTO. In *Proceedings of the 8th meeting of the International Society of Magnetic Resonance in Medicine*, p. 1770.

Liu, G., Sobering, G., Duyn, J., and Moonen, C. T. 1993. A functional MRI technique combining principles of echo-shifting with a train of observations (PRESTO). *Magn. Reson. Med.* 30: 764–768.

Liu, G., Sobering, G., Olson, A. W., van Gelderen, P., and Moonen, C. T. 1993. Fast echo-shifted gradient-recalled MRI: Combining a short repetition time with variable T_2^* weighting. *Magn. Reson. Med.* 30: 68–75.

Moonen, C. T., Barrios, F. A., Zigun, J. R., Gillen, J., Liu, G., Sobering, G., Sexton, R., Woo, J., Frank, J., and Weinberger, D. R. 1994. Functional brain MR imaging based on bolus tracking with a fast T_2^*-sensitized gradient-echo method. *Magn. Reson. Imaging* 12: 379–385.

Moonen, C. T., Liu, G., van Gelderen, P., and Sobering, G. 1992. A fast gradient-recalled MRI technique with increased sensitivity to dynamic susceptibility effects. *Magn. Reson. Med.* 26: 184–189.

Mori, S., Hurd, R. E., and van Zijl, P. C. 1997. Imaging of shifted stimulated echoes and multiple spin echoes. *Magn. Reson. Med.* 37: 336–340.

van Gelderen, P., Grandin, C., Petrella, J. R., and Moonen, C. T. 2000. Rapid three-dimensional MR imaging method for tracking a bolus of contrast agent through the brain. *Radiology* 216: 603–608.

RELATED SECTIONS

Section 3.3 Refocusing Pulses
Section 10.5 Spoiler Gradient
Section 14.1 Gradient Echoes
Section 16.1 Echo Planar Imaging

16.4 RARE

Rapid acquisition with relaxation enhancement (RARE) is a fast imaging sequence that employs an RF excitation pulse followed by a train of refocusing pulses to produce multiple RF spin echoes (Hennig et al. 1986; Hennig 1988). Unlike the multiecho spin echo sequences discussed in Section 14.3, each echo in RARE is *distinctively* spatially encoded so that multiple k-space lines (or trajectories) can be sampled following each excitation pulse. This way, the total imaging time can be considerably reduced. For example, if 16 echoes are distinctively phase-encoded in RARE, the total acquisition time can be decreased by a factor of 16 compared to a single-echo spin echo sequence with otherwise identical parameters.

RARE is compatible with virtually all k-space sampling strategies, including (but not limited to) rectilinear Fourier imaging (Hennig et al. 1986), projection acquisition (Hall and Sukumar 1984; Trouard et al. 1999), PROPELLER (Pipe 1999), spiral (Pauly et al. 1993), and circular sampling (Zhou et al. 1998). In this section, we primarily focus on Fourier imaging (i.e., Cartesian k-space trajectories). Most of the discussion and analyses, however, can be readily generalized and adapted to other k-space sampling strategies.

RARE can be used in either 2D or 3D acquisition mode. In 2D RARE, the acquisition of multiple slice locations is almost always interleaved because the TR is typically much longer than the sequence length. In 3D RARE, phase encoding along one of the two phase-encoded directions is performed throughout the echo train while conventional phase encoding (i.e., one phase encoding step for each TR) is carried out along the other direction. The considerable time savings afforded by RARE make it possible to acquire 3D T_2-weighted images in clinical settings. 3D RARE is also useful in black blood MR angiography (Section 15.1). Further discussion of 2D and 3D RARE sequences is provided in subsection 16.4.1.

The primary advantage of RARE is the reduction in scan time compared to conventional spin echo sequences, especially for T_2-weighted imaging. Although similar or even better scan-time reduction can be achieved using EPI (Section 16.1) or GRASE (Section 16.2), RARE images are less sensitive to off-resonance effects, such as B_0-field inhomogeneity and tissue magnetic susceptibility variations. Its superior image quality makes RARE widely accepted for clinical diagnosis. For example, RARE has virtually replaced the conventional spin echo sequence for T_2-weighted imaging. The major drawbacks of RARE include increased RF power deposition, blurring, edge enhancement, ghosting, and altered image contrast due to increased lipid signal intensities and magnetization transfer effects. In addition, RARE has reduced signal loss from magnetic susceptibility effects. Although this can be advantageous when imaging the sinuses, skull base, or near artifact-producing metallic objects, it can be a slight disadvantage when imaging small hemorrhagic lesions or iron-containing tissue regions. These problems and some of their remedies are further discussed in subsections 16.4.4 and 16.4.5.

The reconstruction of RARE images is straightforward. For rectilinear k-space, Fourier reconstruction (discussed in Section 13.1) can be applied. Due to phase reversal of the transverse magnetization imposed by each refocusing pulse, all k-space lines sampled by a RARE sequence point in the same direction, provided that the readout gradient does not change its polarity. Thus, unlike EPI reconstruction, there is no need for row flipping (i.e., to reverse the k-space line for alternate echoes). For polar (including radial and circular) k-space data, either filtered back-projection or gridding can be used. For other non-Cartesian k-space data, gridding followed by Fourier reconstruction (Section 13.2) is often the method of choice.

Since the initial introduction of RARE (Hennig et al. 1986), a number of variations and modifications have been developed (Mulkern et al. 1990; Melki et al. 1991; Le Roux and Hinks 1993; Constable et al. 1992). Along with these developments, many names have also been proposed, including fast spin echo (FSE), turbo spin echo (TSE), fast acquisition interleaved spin echo (FAISE), and others. We will use RARE or FSE, in a general sense, for all these sequences.

16.4.1 RARE SEQUENCES

Echo Train Length   Let us first consider a conventional single-echo RF spin echo pulse sequence with a typical receiver bandwidth of $\Delta v = \pm 16\,\text{kHz}$ and a readout matrix size of 256. The acquisition time (i.e., the time when the A/D converter is sampling data) for this pulse sequence is $256 \times (1/(2 \times 16)) = 8\,\text{ms}$ per TR interval. Once the transverse magnetization is created, its lifetime is governed by the spin-spin relaxation time T_2, which is approximately 100 ms for many tissues. This example illustrates that the conventional spin echo pulse sequence acquires data only for a small fraction of the lifetime of the transverse magnetization; the considerable portion of signal that can be potentially acquired before or after the acquisition window is wasted.

After the acquisition of the spin echo shown in Figure 16.40, suppose that another 180° refocusing pulse is applied at time 3τ, where τ is the time interval between the 90° and the first 180° pulse shown in Figure 16.40. Then the dephased magnetization vectors are pancake-flipped about the axis of the 180° pulse, leading to another spin echo at 4τ. This echo can be used to sample a second view from k-space. Usually the second view provides another phase-encoded line in Fourier imaging, but it can also be used for a second frequency-encoded radial line in a projection acquisition, a second interleaf in a spiral scan, or an additional trajectory in other k-space sampling schemes. As long as the transverse magnetization does not substantially decay by T_2 relaxation, additional 180° refocusing pulses can be applied to form a train of spin echoes. The echo train, generated after a single excitation of the magnetization, can thus sample multiple k-space views. The number of primary spin echoes (i.e., spin echoes associated with each refocusing pulse; see additional discussion in subsection 16.4.2) produced by a RARE sequence is known as the echo train length (ETL; N_{etl}). N_{etl} is generally the same as the total number of RF refocusing pulses. If all echoes are distinctively phase-encoded, then N_{etl} equals the number of k-space lines acquired per TR interval.

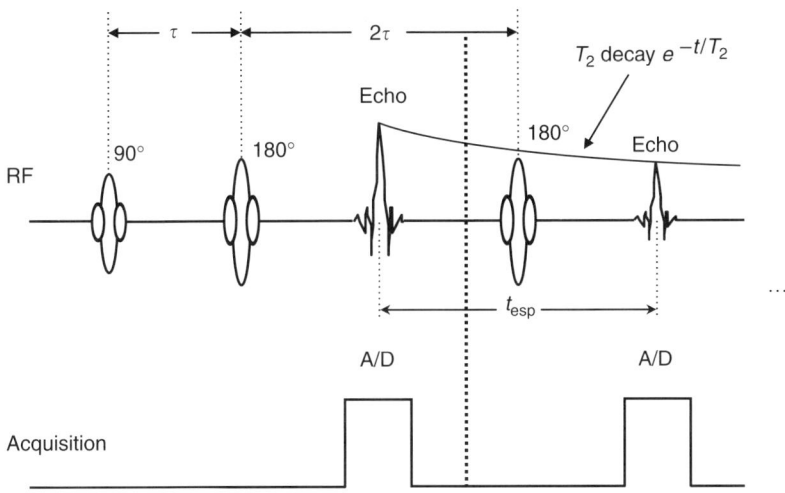

FIGURE 16.40 The relationship between a conventional RF spin echo pulse sequence and RARE. The spin echo sequence stops at the dashed vertical line, whereas RARE continues with additional refocusing pulses and echo acquisitions. A/D, analog-to-digital converter, signifying the actual data acquisition.

ETL is an important parameter of RARE sequences. It directly determines the scan-time reduction factor compared to conventional spin echo sequences. The longer the ETL, the more scan-time reduction. The maximal ETL that is practical is determined by two factors: tissue T_2 relaxation times (i.e., the lifetime of the transverse magnetization) and the interval between the peaks of two consecutive spin echoes. The latter is also known as echo spacing (ESP; denoted by t_{esp} and shown in Figure 16.40). If the refocusing pulses are evenly spaced in time, then t_{esp} is equal to 2τ, which is the interval between two adjacent refocusing pulses.

Example 16.9 Consider a spin system with an average T_2 relaxation time of 100 ms. If spin echoes are acquired prior to the time when the transverse magnetization decays to 20% of its peak value, what is the maximal N_{etl} that can be acquired when $t_{esp} = 8$ ms? If t_{esp} is shortened to 4 ms by reducing the refocusing pulse width, what is the new maximal N_{etl}?

Answer The transverse magnetization decays according to $S = S_0 e^{-t/T_2}$, where S_0 is the peak transverse magnetization immediately following the excitation pulse. Substituting $S = 0.2 S_0$ and $T_2 = 100$ ms into the signal equation, we obtain $t = 160.9$ ms. If $t_{esp} = 8$ ms, then the maximal N_{etl} is

$$N_{etl} = \frac{t}{t_{esp}} = \frac{160.9 \text{ ms}}{8 \text{ ms}} \approx 20$$

If $t_{esp} = 4$ ms, N_{etl} increases to 40.

2D RARE   A 2D RARE sequence starts with a 90° RF excitation pulse followed by a train of refocusing pulses. The phases of the refocusing pulses are shifted by 90° with respect to the phase of the excitation pulse (Figure 16.41) to improve the robustness of the sequence with respect to B_1-field nonuniformity (Meiboom and Purcell 1958). The interval between the refocusing pulses is typically twice as long as the time delay τ between the excitation and first refocusing pulse (Figure 16.41), although sequences that do not satisfy this condition

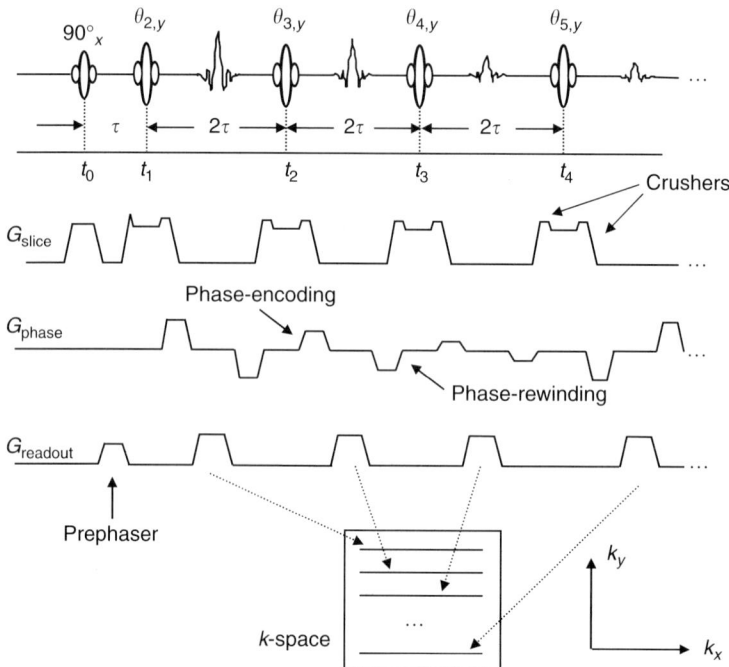

FIGURE 16.41 A 2D RARE sequence. The 90°_x is an excitation pulse and $\theta_{2,y}$, $\theta_{3,y}$, $\theta_{4,y}$, $\theta_{5,y}$, ... are the refocusing pulses. The subscripts x and y indicate the axis along which the RF pulse is applied in the rotating reference frame. The slice-rephasing gradient is combined with the left crusher gradient of the first refocusing pulse.

have also been developed. The timing and phase relationship of this RF pulse train, also called a Carr-Purcell-Meiboom-Gill (CPMG) train (Section 11.5), can be denoted by $(90_x^\circ - \tau - \theta_{2,y} - 2\tau - \theta_{3,y} - 2\tau - \theta_{4,y} - \cdots)$ where θ_2, θ_3, θ_4, ... are the flip angles of the refocusing pulses, and the subscripts x and y represent the phase of the corresponding pulse in the rotating reference frame. If every RF refocusing pulse has a flip angle of 180° the spin echo signals are maximized. In practice, this condition cannot always be satisfied throughout the entire imaging volume because of B_1-field nonuniformity and slice-profile imperfections, even when 180° flip angles are intended. In addition, practical considerations, such as RF power deposition, as measured by the SAR, often necessitate refocusing pulses with smaller flip angles (e.g., 130–160°) (subsection 16.4.5). Finally, the refocusing pulses need not have the same flip angle throughout the echo train. By adjusting the flip angles individually, signal variations can be regulated, in a procedure called echo stabilization (Le Roux and Hinks 1993).

For 2D RARE, the RF excitation pulse and refocusing pulses are usually both slice selective. Pulses with linear phase are most popular, although a minimum-phase SLR excitation pulse can be used to reduce τ. A slice-selection gradient is played out concurrently with each of these pulses. A slice-rephasing gradient is also needed following the excitation pulse. This gradient is often combined with other gradient lobes (e.g., a crusher) prior to the formation of the first echo. To select the desired signals while eliminating the unwanted ones (subsection 16.4.2), a pair of crusher gradients straddling each refocusing pulse is also required, as detailed in Section 10.2.

An identical readout gradient lobe is played to frequency-encode each echo. Prior to the first readout gradient lobe, a prephasing gradient (played between the excitation and first refocusing pulses) is required to center the echo in the first readout window. Additional prephasing gradient lobes are not required for the subsequent readouts because the second half of the preceding readout gradient serves this purpose. Although the readout window is most commonly centered on the peak of an echo to reduce sensitivity to off-resonance effects, the acquisition window can also be shifted with respect to the echo peak for applications such as two-point or three-point Dixon imaging (Section 17.3).

A phase-encoding gradient is played out after each refocusing pulse, but before the readout gradient. As discussed in subsection 16.4.2, an accompanying phase-rewinding gradient is necessary to ensure the signal coherence. All the phase-encoding and phase-rewinding gradient lobes typically have the same pulse width but varying amplitude throughout the echo train to produce multiple k-space lines as shown in Figure 16.41 (an exception is discussed in subsection 16.4.6). The assignment of the phase-encoding values to the echoes in the echo train determines the image contrast and influences the image artifacts. The details of how to distribute the echo signals in k-space are discussed in subsection 16.4.3.

For 2D Fourier imaging (assuming a single-slice acquisition), the total scan time of a RARE sequence is given by

$$T_{\text{scan, 2D}} = \text{TR} \times N_{\text{shot}} \times \text{NEX} \tag{16.38}$$

with

$$N_{\text{shot}} = \begin{cases} N_{\text{phase}}/N_{\text{etl}} & \text{if } (N_{\text{phase}} \bmod N_{\text{etl}}) = 0 \\ \text{int}\,(N_{\text{phase}}/N_{\text{etl}}) + 1 & \text{if } (N_{\text{phase}} \bmod N_{\text{etl}}) \neq 0 \end{cases} \tag{16.39}$$

where the int function takes the integer part of its argument, the modulo (mod) function gives the remainder of the integer division, N_{shot} is the number of shots, and N_{phase} is the number of required phase-encoding steps to reconstruct a 2D image. Comparing Eq. (16.38) with Eq. (14.50) in Section 14.3, the total scan time is reduced by approximately a factor of N_{etl} for the single-slice case. Equation (16.38) can also be adapted to non-Fourier imaging, such as projection acquisition and spiral scan with N_{phase} being replaced by the total number of radial lines and spiral interleaves, respectively.

For interleaved multislice 2D acquisition (Section 11.5), Eq. (16.38) remains the same when data from all the slice locations can be acquired within a TR. This generally implies that the following two conditions must be met simultaneously. First, the product of the number of slices N_{slice} and RARE sequence length T_{seq} must not exceed TR (i.e., $N_{\text{slice}} \times T_{\text{seq}} \leq \text{TR}$). Second, the SAR must be within predetermined limits. If either condition is not satisfied, the scan time in Eq. (16.38) increases to:

$$T_{\text{scan, 2D}} = \text{TR} \times N_{\text{shot}} \times \text{NEX} \times N_{\text{acq}} \tag{16.40}$$

where N_{acq} is the total number of acquisitions, as defined in Section 11.5.

The RARE sequence length is approximately given by:

$$T_{\text{seq}} \approx N_{\text{etl}} \times t_{\text{esp}} \tag{16.41}$$

Equation (16.41) neglects any preparatory pulses and end-of-sequence modules, such as spoiler gradients and driven equilibrium RF pulses. For 2D multislice imaging with acquisition greater than 1 (i.e., $N_{\text{acq}} > 1$), changing ETL does not necessarily affect the total scan time. Consider a 2D RARE acquisition where $N_{\text{acq}} = 2$, $N_{\text{etl}} = 64$, and $N_{\text{phase}} = 64$. If N_{etl} is reduced from 64 to 32, N_{shot} must be doubled to acquire the same number of phase-encoded k-space lines (Eq. 16.39). The sequence length T_{seq}, on the other hand, is halved (Eq. 16.41), which allows more slices (approximately twice as many when SAR is kept constant) to be incorporated into a TR. This reduces N_{acq} by a factor of two. The total scan time therefore remains unchanged according to Eq. (16.40). This is illustrated in Figure 16.42.

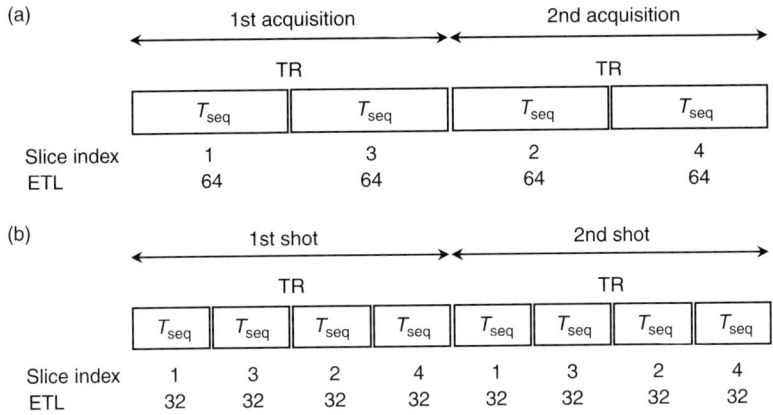

FIGURE 16.42 An example illustrating that reducing ETL does not necessarily increase the total scan time in 2D multislice imaging. (a) $N_{etl} = 64$, $N_{shot} = 1$; (b) $N_{etl} = 32$, $N_{shot} = 2$. A total of 64 phase-encoding steps are assumed in both cases.

3D RARE   3D volume RARE enables the acquisition of thin contiguous slices in a reasonable time while avoiding some of the image artifacts that can occur with gradient echo images (Hennig et al. 1987; Oshio et al. 1991). In principle, 3D volume RARE does not require selective RF pulses, but it is usually used to reduce slice wraparound (i.e., aliasing). When a single slab is imaged, the 90° excitation pulse is usually selective, but the refocusing pulses do not need to be (Figure 16.43). Nonselective refocusing pulses can shorten ESP, which allows a longer ETL to be used in the sequence. When multiple slabs are acquired, however, all RF pulses should be selective to allow slab interleaving.

The readout gradient waveforms of 2D and 3D RARE are identical (Figure 16.43). Phase encoding throughout the echo train can be performed along either the primary (i.e., k_y) or the secondary (i.e., k_z) phase-encoded directions. The phase encoding in the other direction (i.e., the one not performed along the echo train) is accomplished in the conventional manner—one phase-encoding step per TR interval.

A simple approach is to apply the conventional phase-encoding gradient between the excitation pulse and the first refocusing pulse. Because each refocusing pulse negates the accumulated phase of the spin echo, the phase-encoding values will alternate throughout the echo train (i.e., $-k_z$, k_z, $-k_z$, k_z, ...). Thus, an extra step is required to sort the 3D k-space data prior to image reconstruction. A more serious problem with this approach is that the phase-encoding value of the stimulated echoes does not always coincide with

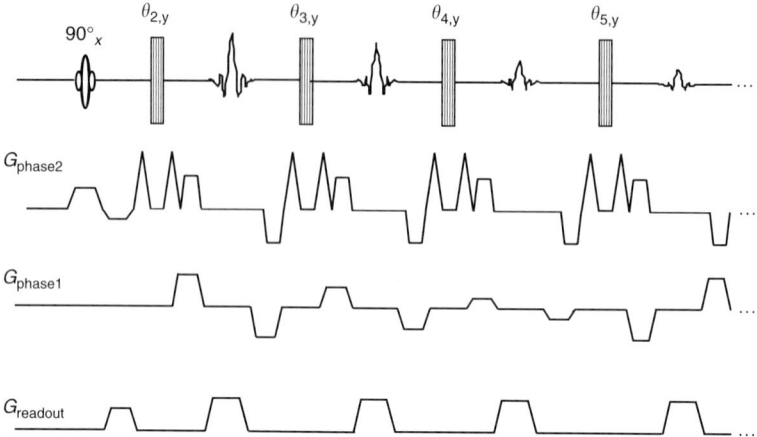

FIGURE 16.43 A 3D RARE sequence to image a slab selected by the 90° excitation pulse. The refocusing pulses are not selective, although selective pulses can also be used. The primary phase encoding (Phase 1 or k_y) is performed during the echo train. The secondary phase encoding (Phase2 or k_z) is performed in the conventional manner (i.e., one phase-encoding step per TR), but also has the phase-rewinding gradient analogous to the primary phase-encoding gradient axis. For clarify, each gradient lobe along the Phase2 direction is shown separately, although some of them can be combined in implementation.

that of the primary spin echoes (see subsection 16.4.2), causing image artifacts. To solve this problem, an alternative phase-encoding waveform is used along the k_z direction, as shown in Figure 16.43. The waveform contains a phase-encoding/phase-rewinding pair for each echo, similar to those used along the k_y direction, except that the gradient area of the phase-encoding (or phase-rewinding) lobes are the same throughout the echo train. This method not only confines all k_y lines acquired in a shot to the same k_z plane, but also produces the same phase-encoding value along the k_z direction for the spin echoes and the stimulated echoes. Another phase-encoding approach allows the k_z value (i.e., the phase-encoding gradient area along the k_z direction) to vary throughout the echo train, so that the associated RARE artifacts are more evenly distributed along both phase-encoded axes. This method has been called generalized k-space sampling scheme (Kholmovski et al. 2000).

The total acquisition time of 3D RARE (assuming a single-slab acquisition) is:

$$T_{\text{scan, 3D}} = \text{TR} \times N_{\text{shot}} \times N_{\text{phase2}} \times \text{NEX} \tag{16.42}$$

where N_{phase2} is the number of secondary phase-encoding steps.

Example 16.10   Calculate the total scan time of a 3D RARE sequence with the following parameters: TR=2000 ms, $N_{\text{phase}} = 192$, $N_{\text{etl}} = 64$, $N_{\text{phase2}} = 64$, and NEX = 1.

Answer   The number of shots needed to perform RARE phase encoding can be calculated using Eq. (16.39):

$$N_{\text{shot}} = N_{\text{phase}}/N_{\text{etl}} = 192/64 = 3$$

Thus, the total scan time is:

$$T_{\text{scan,3D}} = 2 \times 3 \times 64 \times 1 = 384\,\text{s} = 6.4\,\text{min}$$

Single-Shot versus Multishot   Depending on the number of the independent RF excitation pulses used to sample the required k-space data, RARE can be divided into single-shot and multi-shot sequences. Single-shot RARE, more commonly known as single-shot FSE (SS-FSE) or single-shot turbo spin echo (SS-TSE), has been used mostly for 2D imaging. It acquires the entire 2D k-space data needed for image reconstruction using a single echo train (i.e., $N_{\text{phase}} = N_{\text{etl}}$, resulting in $N_{\text{shot}} = 1$ according to Eq. 16.39). The primary applications of single-shot FSE are to freeze respiratory motion for abdominal imaging and to improve temporal resolution in dynamic studies.

In single-shot RARE, it is essential to maximize N_{etl} so that better spatial resolution can be achieved in the image. As shown in Example 16.9, for a fixed echo train duration, the maximal N_{etl} can be increased by shortening ESP. Increasing the receiver bandwidth, shortening the refocusing pulse width (often at the expense of degraded slice profile or reduced flip angle), and increasing the slew rate are the common strategies to minimize ESP. Even with these changes, N_{etl} is often inadequate to acquire the desired number of phase-encoding steps for full k-space coverage. Asymmetric k-space sampling is typically used, and the image can be reconstructed using a partial or half k-space reconstruction. An example of this technique is known as *half-Fourier acquired single-shot turbo spin echo* (HASTE), which is described in detail in Patel et al. (1997).

Single-shot RARE can also be incorporated into a 3D acquisition. In this case, RARE phase encoding is accomplished in a single shot along one spatial direction; conventional phase encoding is performed one step per TR (i.e., multishot mode) in the other direction. Sometimes, this sequence is referred to as 3D single-shot FSE, although 3D k-space is actually sampled in multiple shots.

Multishot RARE acquires a fraction of the k-space data with each shot. The k-space data from multiple shots are combined prior to image reconstruction.

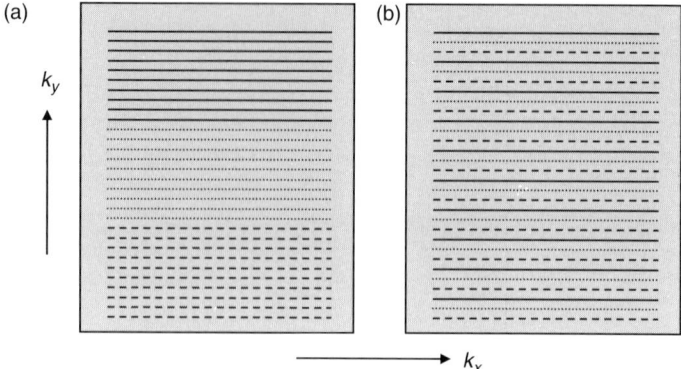

FIGURE 16.44 (a) Sequential and (b) interleaved k-space sampling in three-shot RARE. Solid line, first shot; dotted line, second shot; dashed line, third shot.

Because N_{etl} does not have to be stretched to its maximal value, multishot RARE offers better image quality (i.e., better SNR, reduced blurring, and higher spatial resolution) compared to its single-shot counterpart.

There are numerous ways to sample k-space in multishot RARE. For example, each shot can sequentially sample a segment of k-space (Figure 16.44a). Alternatively, the k-space lines can be interleaved with each shot (Figure 16.44b). The latter approach is almost always used because the T_2-induced signal amplitude decay and inconsistent phase errors (subsection 16.4.4) throughout the echo train modulate k-space data slowly, resulting in higher-frequency ghosts with less power. This situation is analogous to low-frequency view ordering used in respiratory compensation (Section 12.3).

16.4.2 Signal Pathways and the Carr-Purcell-Meiboom-Gill (CPMG) Condition

To limit the RF energy deposition into the imaged subjects, RARE is often implemented with reduced flip angles (i.e., $<180°$) for the refocusing pulses (Hennig 1988). In that case, the transverse magnetization is partially tipped onto the longitudinal axis (either $+z$ or $-z$ axis), partially refocused as usual, and partially left intact. Similarly, the longitudinal magnetization is partially excited to the transverse plane and partially inverted or left along the $+z$ or $-z$ axis. Each of these magnetization components is further divided following the subsequent non-180° refocusing pulse. The transverse magnetization component continues to accumulate phase until it is affected by the next RF pulse. The longitudinal magnetization, on the other hand, remains

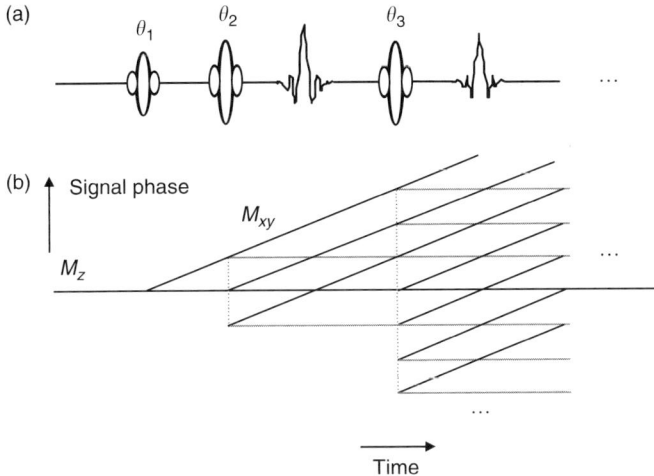

FIGURE 16.45 (a) RF pulse train and (b) its associated phase diagram. The effect of imaging gradients is not considered in the phase diagram. Thus, the phase accumulation may reflect B_0-field inhomogeneity. Whenever the phase of a coherence pathway crosses zero, an echo is formed. The gray horizontal lines represent longitudinal magnetization, the dotted vertical lines indicate phase reversal, and the solid diagonal lines denote the phase accumulation of the transverse magnetization.

constant unless a subsequent RF refocusing pulse changes it to the transverse plane (assuming the time scale is much less than T_1). The spatial dependence of the phase of the magnetization when it was previously in the transverse plane can be stored as the spatial dependence of the longitudinal magnetization. The phase evolution of the magnetization component is often depicted in a phase diagram (Hennig 1988) shown in Figure 16.45. Each line represents a particular pathway of a magnetization component. These pathways are often referred to as signal pathways, signal coherence pathways, or simply coherence pathways.

Whenever the phase of a coherence pathway crosses zero, an echo is produced. If a coherence pathway (solid lines in Figure 16.46b) experiences a phase reversal at *every* refocusing pulse, the echoes it generates are called primary spin echoes, or simply spin echoes (solid dots in Figure 16.46b). If a coherence pathway (dotted lines in Figure 16.46b) is excited by an imperfect refocusing pulse (thereby producing an FID, as denoted by the triangles in Figure 16.46b) and phase-reversed by subsequent refocusing pulses, it produces secondary spin echoes (the concentric circles in Figure 16.46b). If a coherence pathway (dashed lines in Figure 16.46b) is initially in the transverse plane, then returned to the longitudinal axis by an imperfect refocusing

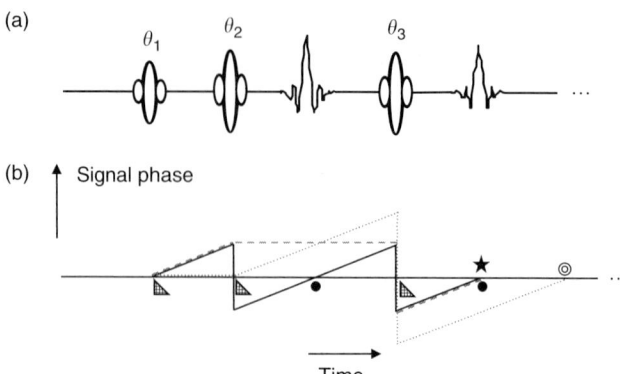

FIGURE 16.46 (a) RF pulse train and (b) phase diagram showing two primary spin echoes (solid dots), a secondary spin echo (concentric circles), a stimulated echo (star), and three FIDs (triangles) produced by three RF pulses. The signal pathways for the primary, secondary, and stimulated echoes are represented by solid lines, dotted lines, and dashed lines, respectively.

pulse, and reexcited by another imperfect refocusing pulse, it gives rise to stimulated echoes (the star in Figure 16.46b). Generation of a stimulated echo requires at least three RF pulses, as shown in Figure 16.46. As more refocusing pulses are incorporated into the RARE sequence, the number of echoes increases exponentially (see Eq. 10.34). Additional discussion of coherence pathways and their associated echoes can be found in Section 10.2.

In a multiecho pulse sequence, the echoes produced by various coherence pathways are generally not in phase, and their temporal positions do not necessarily coincide. When overlapping echoes are acquired within the same acquisition window (e.g., the second primary echo and the stimulated echo shown in Figure 16.46b), their phase inconsistency can cause signal cancellation and lead to ghosting artifacts and poor SNR. A goal in RARE sequence design is to ensure that echoes only occur at the desired positions in the pulse sequence *and* the signals at each temporal position have the same phase. The CPMG condition is a set of conditions to ensure that the two requirements are met. In the context of RARE pulse sequence design, the following two criteria are often used.

Condition 1. The refocusing RF pulses must be 90° out of phase with respect to the excitation RF pulse, and evenly positioned in the sequence with equal spacing (i.e., 2τ) between any two consecutive refocusing pulses. The spacing must be twice the time interval (i.e., τ) between the excitation RF pulse and the first refocusing RF pulse (Figure 16.41).

Condition 2. The phase accumulated by a spin isochromat between any two consecutive refocusing RF pulses must be equal:

$$\gamma \int_{t_1}^{t_2} B(t)dt = \gamma \int_{t_2}^{t_3} B(t)dt = \cdots = \gamma \int_{t_{N-1}}^{t_N} B(t)dt \qquad (16.43)$$

where the timing parameters are defined in Figure 16.41, and $B(t)$ includes every static magnetic field component (i.e., B_0 field, gradient field, and higher-order terms). For example, when the linear gradient is considered, Eq. (16.43) reduces to:

$$\int_{t_1}^{t_2} rG(t)dt = \int_{t_2}^{t_3} rG(t)dt = \cdots = \int_{t_{N-1}}^{t_N} rG(t)dt \qquad (16.44)$$

where $G(t)$ is a gradient along any axis, and r is a generalized spatial variable along the direction of $G(t)$. For static spins, Eq. (16.44) further reduces to:

$$\int_{t_1}^{t_2} G(t)dt = \int_{t_2}^{t_3} G(t)dt = \cdots = \int_{t_{N-1}}^{t_N} G(t)dt \qquad (16.45)$$

When conditions 1 and 2 are both satisfied, the primary and the stimulated echoes occur only at the mid-point between two consecutive refocusing RF pulses (Figure 16.41) and carry the same phase.

The CPMG conditions have several implications in RARE sequence design. First, they require that all of the crusher gradient pairs surrounding the refocusing pulses have the same area, as detailed in Section 10.2. A possible exception is the left crusher of the first refocusing pulse, when that crusher area is combined with the slice-rephasing gradient area. It is worth noting that combining the slice-rephasing gradient with the left crusher gradient of the first refocusing pulse does not violate the CPMG conditions. If the slice-rephasing gradient is combined with the right crusher gradient, however, the CPMG condition given by Eq. (16.45) is violated, unless the crusher gradients for all other refocusing pulses are also modified in the same fashion. If the crushers for subsequent refocusing pulses are not modified, it can be shown that the first stimulated echo (the star in Figure 16.46) carries a different phase than the primary echo at the same temporal position. Second, each phase-encoding gradient must be accompanied by a phase-rewinding gradient after the readout window, but prior to the next refocusing pulse. Third, RARE sequences that satisfy the CPMG conditions use both primary and stimulated echoes. The secondary spin echoes and the FIDs (triangles in Figure 16.46) following each refocusing pulse are eliminated by crusher gradients (see Section 10.2) so that they do not interfere with the desired signals. Fourth, if a nonuniform phase exists in the magnetization along the slice-selection direction, such as in the case of a minimum-phase excitation pulse, the CPMG conditions cannot be satisfied across the entire slice profile. When signal loss or image artifact due to this deviation becomes a concern, RF excitation pulses with a more uniform phase response should be sought. Fifth, moving spins can cause a violation of the CPMG conditions, if the gradients are designed based on Eq. (16.45) for static spins. This can be easily seen from Eq. (16.44). Finally, any correction gradient, such as a concomitant-field correction gradient, must be applied consistently throughout the echo train, as described in Section 10.1.

16.4.3 CONTRAST MANIPULATION

Assuming 180° refocusing pulses, the peak amplitude of the echoes decays according to

$$S(n) = S_0 e^{-nt_{esp}/T_2} \tag{16.46}$$

where n is the echo index ($n = 1, 2, \ldots, N_{etl}$). Each echo has its own TE value ($n \times t_{esp}$), resulting in k-space data with nonuniform T_2 weighting. Because the image contrast is predominantly determined by the low-spatial-frequency data in k-space (Mulkern et al. 1991; Constable et al. 1992), the TE of a RARE sequence is defined as the TE when the central k-space line is acquired (i.e., the echo acquired with the smallest phase-encoding gradient area). This TE is called the effective TE (TE_{eff}).

To produce a T_1-weighted or a proton-density-weighted image, earlier echoes in the echo train are used to sample the central k-space data so that TE_{eff} takes its minimal value (i.e., $TE_{eff} = t_{esp}$). Signals from the later echoes are used to fill the remaining k-space as shown in Figure 16.47a. For T_2-weighted imaging, a later echo can be assigned to the central region of k-space (e.g., $TE_{eff} = 12t_{esp}$). The rest of the echoes are used to sample the remaining k-space. The degree of T_2 weighting can be altered by assigning different echoes to the central k-space line, as shown in Example 16.11 and Figures 16.47b and c. The available effective TEs of a RARE sequence can only be integer multiples of t_{esp}. The maximal value of TE_{eff} is $N_{etl} \times t_{esp}$. For heavily T_2-weighted imaging such as in MR cholangiography, a long ETL is typically employed to achieve a long TE_{eff}. Examples of T_1-weighted and T_2-weighted RARE images are shown in Figure 16.48.

Example 16.11   A RARE sequence has an echo spacing of 8 ms and an ETL of 16. (a) What is the effective TE of the sequence for T_1-weighted imaging?

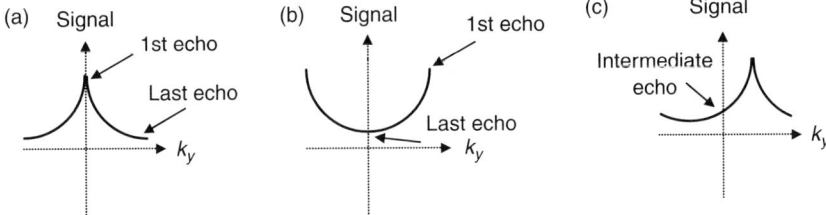

FIGURE 16.47 Sampling schemes to obtain (a) T_1-weighted (or proton-density-weighted) images, (b) heavily T_2-weighted images, and (c) moderately T_2-weighted images. The vertical axis shows the echo signal intensity for the various echoes described by Eq. (16.46). Two shots are assumed for all three cases with each exponential decay curve representing a shot. For more than two shots, k-space lines from successive shots can be interleaved, changing each curve to a stairwise function as in Figure 16.49a.

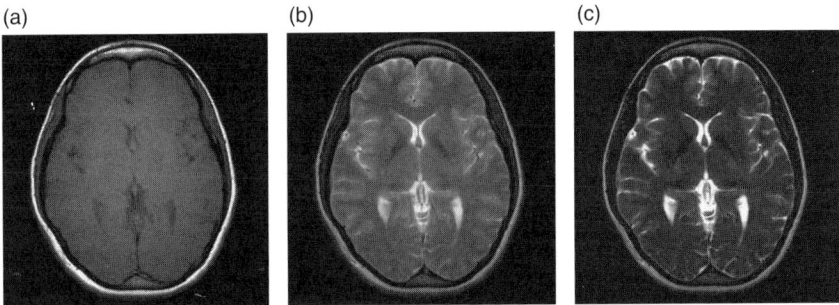

FIGURE 16.48 By using different echoes to sample the k-space center, considerably different image contrast can be obtained from a RARE sequence. (a) T_1-weighted image with TE = 11 ms, TR = 480 ms, and N_{etl} = 8. (b) Moderately T_2-weighted image with TE = 77 ms, TR = 4000 ms, and N_{etl} = 16. (c) Heavily T_2-weighted image with TE = 176 ms, TR = 4000 ms, and N_{etl} = 16.

(b) Which echo should be used to sample the k-space center for a T_2-weighted image with a TE of approximately 102 ms? (c) Suppose a heavier T_2-weighted image with TE=120 ms is needed; recalculate (b). (d) What is the longest TE_{eff} that the sequence can produce?

Answer

    (a) The first echo is used to sample k-space center. Therefore, TE_{eff} equals t_{esp}, which is 8 ms.

(b) The thirteenth echo has a TE value of 104 ms, which is the closest to
the desired TE. Thus, the thirteenth echo should be used to sample the
k-space center.
(c) The fifteenth echo should be used.
(d) The longest TE_{eff} is:

$$TE_{eff} = N_{etl} \times t_{esp} = 16 \times 8 = 128 \, ms$$

With its associated phase-encoding and phase-rewinding gradient pair,
each echo in RARE receives an independent phase-encoding value. This
provides great flexibility in assigning an echo to a particular k-space line for
both single-shot and multishot RARE. Although achieving the desired contrast
is the primary objective, minimizing the phase and amplitude discontinuities
of the k-space signal is also a goal when assigning the echoes to k-space lines.
In multishot RARE, for example, the total number of shots are first divided into
a few groups (e.g., two groups as shown in Figure 16.49). Each group covers a
specific region (or regions) in k-space. Within each group, echoes with the same
echo index in successive shots are placed next to one another, producing a stairwise amplitude and phase modulation in k-space (Figure 16.49a). This helps to
reduce artifacts by reducing k-space discontinuities (subsection 16.4.4). The
assignment of a particular echo to a k-space line can be accomplished using a
lookup table, which is sometimes called a view table.

Our discussion so far has assumed ideal refocusing pulses with flip angles
of 180°. With nonideal refocusing pulses, either as a result of B_1-field nonuniformity, slice-profile imperfection, or reduced flip angles due to RF energy
deposition considerations (see subsection 16.4.5), the acquired signal is a mixture of the primary and stimulated echoes. Although the primary spin echo

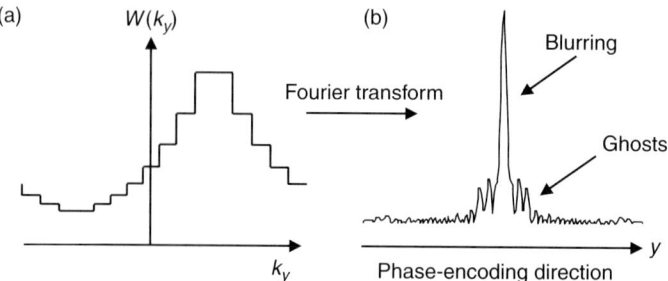

FIGURE 16.49 (a) A T_2-weighting function $W(k_y)$ and (b) its Fourier transform.
Blurring and ghosting arising from $W(k_y)$ are noted in (b).

signal can be described by Eq. (16.46), the stimulated echo signal does not experience T_2 decay while the magnetization is stored along the longitudinal axis. Instead, the stored magnetization undergoes T_1 relaxation, which introduces T_1 weighting into the signal. Therefore, the combined signal at each echo acquisition can no longer be expressed by Eq. (16.46), and some T_1-weighted contrast is inevitably contained in the image. This effect, however, is typically insignificant. The resultant image contrast arises predominantly from the T_2-weighting mechanism, even with low flip angles (e.g., 130°) of the refocusing pulses. Equation (16.46) is frequently employed to approximately describe the signal characteristics of RARE.

16.4.4 IMAGE ARTIFACTS

Blurring   The T_2-induced signal decay given by Eq. (16.46) produces a weighting function, $W(k_y)$, along the phase-encoded direction of RARE k-space data. This function (Figure 16.47) is sometimes called the T_2-weighting function. For a given tissue, $W(k_y)$ can be expressed as:

$$W(k_y) = e^{-n(k_y)t_{\text{esp}}/T_2} \qquad (16.47)$$

where the echo index n is a function of k-space index k_y and can be determined from the view table. With a nonuniform T_2-weighting function, the RARE k-space data become:

$$S(k_x,k_y) = S_0(k_x,k_y)W(k_y) \qquad (16.48)$$

Equation (16.48) indicates that the image obtained by taking the Fourier transform of $S(k_x, k_y)$ is the convolution of the ideal image (i.e., no T_2 blurring) and the Fourier transform of $W(k_y)$, which is a Lorentzian-like function (Figure 16.49). Therefore, the image is blurred. Image blurring by this mechanism does not occur with conventional spin echo and gradient echo pulse sequences because $W(k_y) = 1$ along the phase-encoded direction, although slight blurring can occur in the readout direction due to T_2 or T_2^* decay. Blurring (Figure 16.50a) artifacts are inherent to RARE images. Tissues with a shorter T_2 produce more blurring than those with a longer T_2. Blurring can also be aggravated with longer ETL or greater ESP. Depending on the specific values of these factors, blurring artifacts in single-shot RARE can be quite severe (Figure 16.50b).

If the T_2 value of each voxel is known, blurring can be reduced or even removed by deconvolution in the image domain. Such a method, however, requires a T_2, map, which can be rather time consuming to obtain. A less

(a)   (b)

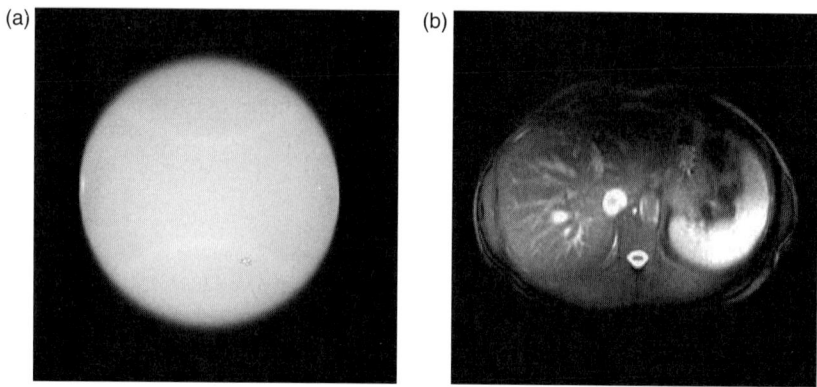

FIGURE 16.50 Single-shot RARE images acquired from (a) a phantom and (b) the abdomen of a patient. The blurring artifact is evident along the phase-encoded (vertical) direction.

accurate but simpler method is to use an average T_2 value along the phase-encoded direction to perform T_2 correction in the hybrid space (i.e., space defined by (x, k_y)) following a 1D Fourier transform along the readout direction; Zhou et al. 1993). This method requires a reference scan that can be acquired in a single TR. With a known average T_2 value (or values), deconvolution can be performed by dividing k-space data by $W(k_y)$ to remove the T_2-induced signal modulation (Zhou et al. 1993). This method works well when the estimated T_2 value is close to the actual value. Otherwise, the longer T_2 components are overcorrected, resulting in considerable edge enhancement, and the shorter T_2 components can suffer from substantial noise augmentation. To reduce the edge enhancement and noise amplification, a Wiener deconvolution filter can be used (Busse et al. 2000). This method gives good results over a broader range of T_2 values, although the deblurring correction for the T_2 component that matches the estimated T_2 value is not as effective as the approach with a simple exponential filter. Another method to reduce the T_2-induced image blurring requires at least two signal averages (NEX=2). The T_2-weighting function is reversed between the two averages, as demonstrated in Figure 16.51 for the case of NEX=2, so that the combined k-space signal has a flatter T_2-weighting function.

Edge Enhancement T_2-weighted RARE images use early echoes in the echo train to sample the edge of k-space, as shown in Figure 16.47b. The T_2-weighting function effectively imposes a high-pass filter on the k-space data along the phase-encoded direction, resulting in edge enhancement in the

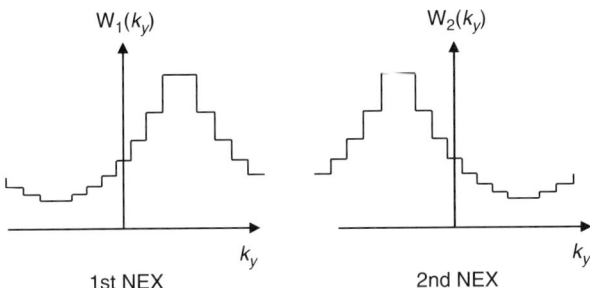

FIGURE 16.51 The T_2-weighting function can be modified between two signal averages. The signals are summed to compensate for the T_2-induced signal variations.

image. The problem can be partially alleviated with a monotonic T_2-weighting function that enhances the signal at one end of k-space while suppressing the signal at the other end. In addition, the methods that reduce blurring can also be adapted to reduce edge enhancement.

Ghosting   Ghosting along the phase-encoded direction is another common artifact in RARE images. Although both phase and amplitude modulations of the k-space data can produce ghosting artifacts, phase-induced artifacts are more common.

The k-space data almost always contain phase errors. If the phase error is consistent across k-space such as in the case of conventional RF spin echo imaging, it does not produce ghosting in the magnitude image. If the phase error varies along the phase-encoded direction as in the case of RARE, ghosts are generated. A high-frequency phase variation in k-space leads to ghosts with low frequencies in the image domain, and vice versa. To understand how a phase error can propagate throughout an echo train, consider a phase term ϕ that is accumulated during the first ESP. For the primary echo coherence pathway, each subsequent refocusing pulse changes the sign of this phase, resulting in an alternating phase pattern of (ϕ, $-\phi$, ϕ, $-\phi$, ...). With the aid of Figures 16.45 and 16.46, a different phase modulation pattern for stimulated echoes can be obtained analogously. The phase modulation on the echo train is converted by a view table to a phase modulation in k-space. As the echo train proceeds, new phase errors can accumulate and propagate further through the echo train. Thus, the actual phase modulation can be quite complicated.

The phase error ϕ can be fitted to a spatial polynomial:

$$\phi = \phi_0 + \phi_1 r + \phi_2 r^2 + \cdots \tag{16.49}$$

where r is a generic spatial variable. ϕ_0 is a spatially independent phase that can contain contributions from eddy currents and phase errors associated with RF pulses. Although resonance offsets such as magnetic susceptibility variations and B_0-field inhomogeneity also produce phase errors, they do not contribute to ϕ_0 because their phase errors are canceled at the peak of each echo. The cancelation occurs for both primary and stimulated echoes, provided that the CPMG conditions are met. The major contribution to the spatially linear phase is gradient waveform distortion caused by, for example, linear eddy currents, group delay, and gradient amplifier imperfection. Examples of the spatially quadratic phase term $\phi_2 r^2$ include the concomitant-field phase described in Section 10.1, and spatially quadratic eddy currents (Section 10.3).

Even on a well-calibrated scanner, the phase error in Eq. (16.49) can still be large enough to cause nonnegligible ghosting artifacts in RARE images. To reduce the artifacts in RARE, phase correction is often required. To compensate for ϕ_0 and $\phi_1 r$, a reference scan can be acquired using the same RARE sequence, but with all phase-encoding gradient amplitudes set to zero (Hinks et al. 1995). Each echo in the reference scan is then inverse-Fourier-transformed to obtain a set of projections along the readout direction. If no inconsistent phase errors were present, all projections should have the same phase. By comparing the phases of the projections, the inconsistent phase errors ϕ_0 and $\phi_1 r$ (where r is the spatial variable along the readout direction) can be obtained. Average phase errors for odd ($\Phi_{0,odd}$, $\Phi_{1,odd}$) and even echoes ($\Phi_{0,even}$, $\Phi_{1,even}$) are computed, respectively. To correct for the zeroth-order phase, the phase of the refocusing pulses is offset by ($\Phi_{0,even} - \Phi_{0,odd}$)/2. To compensate for the first-order phase, the area of the prephasing readout gradient is adjusted by an amount:

$$\Delta A = (\Phi_{1,odd} - \Phi_{1,even})/(2\gamma) \qquad (16.50)$$

This modified (or phase-compensated) RARE sequence is subsequently used in actual k-space data acquisition. An example of quadratic phase correction for concomitant phase errors can be found in Section 10.1.

After phase-induced ghosts have been substantially reduced, ghosts arising from the k-space amplitude modulation due to the discontinuous nature of the T_2-weighting function can become more conspicuous. A technique for reducing this kind of ghosting is to use the amplitude of reference-scan data to normalize the T_2-weighting function (Zhou et al. 1993). A drawback to this method is that the noise can be amplified. Stabilizing the echo train amplitude by adjusting the flip angles of the refocusing pulses also helps reduce the ghosting (as well as blurring) artifacts (Hinks and Listerud 1991).

16.4.5 PRACTICAL CONSIDERATIONS

Specific Absorption Rate   The SAR is defined as the total RF energy E dissipated in a sample over exposure time t_{exp} per unit mass M in kilograms:

$$\text{SAR} \equiv \frac{E}{t_{exp}M} \qquad (16.51)$$

SAR in RARE can be particularly high because multiple RF pulses are played out over a very short time. To operate the sequence within the regulatory limits, the number of slice locations per acquisition is often compromised. With the recent developments in very-high-field ($B_0 \geq 3\,\text{T}$) imaging, SAR management becomes a particularly important issue. To maximally use the time efficiency afforded by RARE without exceeding the regulatory limits on SAR, many techniques have been developed. For example, low-flip-angle (i.e., $<180°$) refocusing pulses can be employed (Alsop 1997; Hennig 1988; Hennig and Scheffler 2000, 2001). Because SAR is proportional to $(B_1)^2$, reducing the flip angle is an effective way to achieve a lower SAR. One approach is to use *hyperechoes*; this employs a $180°$ refocusing pulse in the center of the refocusing pulse train to antisymmetrically mirror the flip angles and phases of other refocusing pulses (Hennig and Scheffler 2001):

$$(\theta_1, \varphi_1)—\tau—(\theta_2, \varphi_2)—\cdots—(\theta_n, \varphi_n)—\tau—(180°, 0°)—\tau$$
$$—(-\theta_n, -\varphi_n)—\cdots—(-\theta_2, -\varphi_2)—\tau—(-\theta_1, -\varphi_1)$$

where θ_j and φ_j are the flip angles and the phase of the refocusing pulses, respectively. The low flip angles, for example, can range from 60 to $130°$. The echo produced at the end of this pulse train is equivalent to a primary spin echo generated simply by the $90°$ and the central $180°$ refocusing pulse, and it is dubbed a hyperecho. The hyperecho is typically used to sample the central k-space line, whereas other echoes are employed to sample other k-space lines. Using this method, SAR can be considerably reduced without compromising the SNR (Hennig and Scheffler 2001). Another method to decrease SAR is to use variable-rate RF pulses (Section 2.4), in which the amplitude of the refocusing pulses is reduced, leading to lower SAR (Conolly et al. 1988).

Bright Lipid Signals   Lipid signals appear brighter in RARE than in conventional RF spin echo sequences, especially in T_2-weighted images in which later echoes are used to sample the k-space center (Melki et al. 1991). This phenomenon can be explained by considering resonance frequencies of various proton groups in lipids and *spin-spin coupling* (also known as J-coupling) among the groups (Henkelman et al. 1992; Williamson et al. 1996).

J-coupling is an NMR phenomenon in which protons in adjacent groups of the same molecule interact with one another and split the resonance frequency into doublet, triplet, quadruplet, and so forth (Slichter 1989). Consider a segment of lipid molecule CH_3–CH_2–. The two groups of protons in methyl and methylene have slightly different resonance frequencies due to their different chemical shifts (~ 25 Hz at 1.5 T). J-coupling between the methyl and methylene groups splits each resonance peak into multiplets separated by $f_J \approx 7$ Hz. With J-coupling, the transverse magnetization decays according to:

$$S = S_0 e^{-t/T_2} \cos(n\pi f_J t_{esp}) \tag{16.52}$$

where n is the echo index. When multiple J-coupled groups are considered, as in the case of lipid molecules, beating of the cosine modulation functions results in a faster decay of the signal or a shortening of the apparent T_2. This effect of J-coupling, however, becomes negligible if the following condition is met:

$$t_{esp} \leq \frac{1}{2\sqrt{f_{cs}^2 + f_J^2}} \equiv t_c \tag{16.53}$$

where f_{cs} is the chemical shift difference of the coupled groups. If we take typical values of $f_{cs} = \sim 25$ Hz and $f_J = 7$ Hz, the critical time t_c is found to be approximately 20 ms. Because t_{esp} is less than t_c for most RARE sequences, additional signal decay induced by J-coupling is typically negligible. In T_2-weighted spin echo sequences, however, TE is much longer than t_c. Hence, J-coupling attenuates the lipid signals. This explains why lipids appear brighter in RARE images. Equations (16.52) and (16.53) also indicate that as t_{esp} is reduced, an enhanced bright lipid signal can be observed. If a shorter TE is used in spin echo sequences (e.g., for T_1 or proton-density-weighted images), the difference in lipid signal intensity between RARE and SE images diminishes. Unlike protons in lipids, water protons do not have J-coupling. Consequently, a water signal has similar intensity in RARE and SE images when the acquisition parameters are comparable.

Brighter lipid signals in T_2-weighted RARE images can obscure detection of lesions, such as metastases in the vertebral body. A remedy to this problem is to suppress lipid signals using a chemically selective pulse (Section 4.3) or short tau inversion recovery (Section 14.2). A drawback is reduced SNR because water signals can also be saturated or attenuated in these techniques.

Another technique to address the problem with bright lipid signal is to use dual-interval echo train (DIET), in which the first ESP is an odd-number multiple of the ESP for the rest of the echoes (Kanazawa et al. 1994; Stables et al. 1999).

Magnetization Transfer Effect   In 2D multislice interleaved RARE, the RF pulse train delivered to a given slice can serve as off-resonance magnetization transfer (MT) pulses for other slices, leading to MT-induced signal loss and altered image contrast (Melki and Mulkern 1992). Compared to spin echo sequences, the MT effect in RARE is particularly severe because of multiple refocusing pulses. As ETL is lengthened, the MT effect progressively increases. A practical solution to this problem is to reduce the number of slices acquired during each TR interval. Additional discussion of MT can be found in Section 4.2.

16.4.6 VARIATIONS OF RARE SEQUENCES

Dual-Echo RARE   Similar to the dual-echo RF spin echo pulse sequence discussed in Section 14.3, RARE can also be implemented in dual-echo mode. This is also known as shared-view acquisition using repeated echoes (SHARE) (Johnson et al. 1994) or a double contrast sequence. When two images with different TE_{eff} are desired, the echo train can be divided into two groups. The group with earlier echoes is used to sample k-space with a shorter TE_{eff}, and the group with later echoes is used to acquire an image with longer TE_{eff}. To increase the time efficiency, the two groups can partially overlap and the overlapped echoes are used in the high-spatial-frequency regions for both k-space data sets. Another strategy is to use two separate shots, one for the short TE_{eff} acquisition, and the other for the long TE_{eff} acquisition.

RARE with Other Pulse Modules   A number of preparatory pulses and modules can be appended to the basic RARE pulse sequences described in subsection 16.4.1. For example, an inversion pulse can be placed before a RARE sequence to form a fast inversion recovery sequence. Two applications are FLAIR and STIR, discussed in Section 14.2. Another example is to include spatially and/or chemically selective saturation pulses in a RARE sequence. Chemically selective saturation pulses are particularly useful to offset the bright fat effects in T_2-weighted images. In addition, velocity-compensation gradients (Section 10.4) are sometimes also used in RARE sequence to suppress flow-related artifacts, such as the CSF flow (Hinks and Constable 1994). In flow-compensated RARE, gradient moments of the primary spin echoes and the stimulated echoes must be both considered. The first level of compensation is accomplished by nulling the gradient moments at the isodelay point of each refocusing RF pulse. Additional compensation can be achieved by nulling gradient moments at both the RF pulse and at the echo (Hinks and Constable 1994). Moment nulling on both the slice and readout axes simultaneously is not possible because crushers are needed on at least one of those two axes. Finally, driven equilibrium pulses (Section 17.4) can also be used at the end of RARE echo trains to improve the efficiency and increase the SNR in RARE images.

Non-CPMG RARE Although a vast majority of RARE sequences are designed to satisfy the CPMG conditions, non-CPMG RARE sequences have also been developed. When the FOV is small and SAR is not a limiting factor (e.g., in the case of microscopic imaging), uniform 180° refocusing pulses can be delivered across the imaged object. Thus, the signal predominantly consists of primary spin echoes. Under these conditions, RARE sequences that do not satisfy the CPMG conditions have been found to work well, especially with the aid of crusher gradients to further filter out the stimulated echoes (Zhou et al. 1993). Another non-CPMG pulse sequence has also been developed that employs refocusing pulses with quadratic phase (Le Roux 2002).

RARE with Variable Encoding Time In the majority of pulse sequences, including RARE, the duration of the phase-encoding (and -rewinding) gradient lobes is held fixed from view to view, whereas their amplitudes vary. Alternatively, pulse sequences can be designed using constant phase-encoding gradient amplitude throughout the echo train and a variable gradient duration, provided that the phase-encoding gradient area is conserved. In a technique called variable encoding time (VET; Feinberg 1997), the durations of both the readout window (i.e., A/D window) and the phase-encoding (and phase-rewinding) gradient vary throughout the echo train. The total duration of the phase-encoding gradient, readout window, and phase-rewinding gradient, however, is held constant and is equal to the duration of a readout gradient (Figure 16.52). ESP is therefore the same for all echoes, satisfying one of the CPMG conditions. When the same receiver bandwidth is used for each echo, k-space lines with smaller $|k_y|$ values span a wider range along the k_x direction, resulting in nonrectangular k-space coverage, such as diamond (Figure 16.52), circular, or hexagonal raster. When $|k_y|$ is small, the time saved by reducing the phase-encoding and phase-rewinding gradient durations is used to increase the extent of k-space coverage along the k_x direction. Similarly, the extent along the k_y direction can also be increased by reducing the readout duration for large $|k_y|$ values. Thus, the spatial resolution along the readout and phase-encoded directions can be increased with VET, compared to that of a nominal RARE pulse

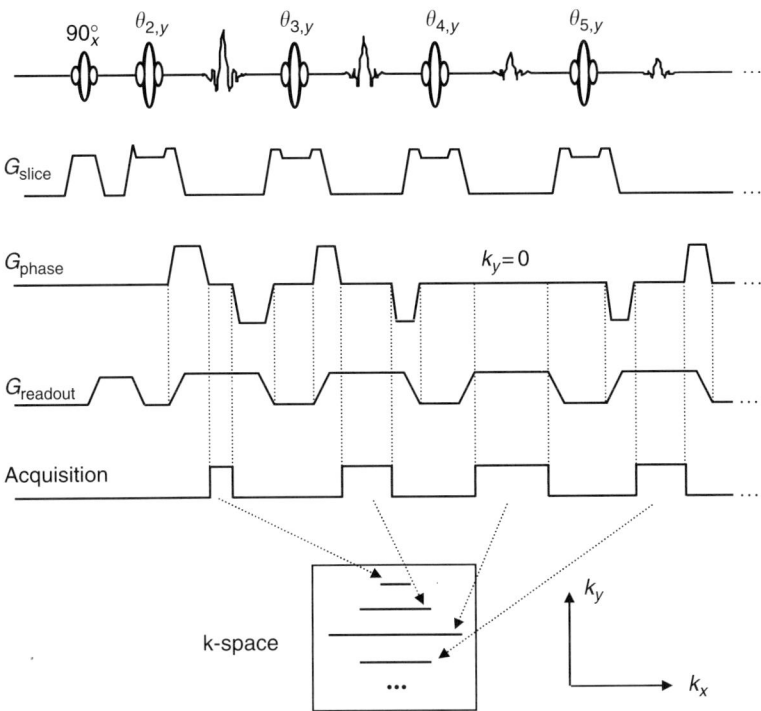

FIGURE 16.52 A RARE sequence with variable encoding time. The dotted vertical lines show the temporal relationship between the readout gradient, the phase-encoding gradient, the phase-rewinding gradient, and data acquisition window. All phase-encoding and phase-rewinding gradient lobes have the same amplitude. The length of the data acquisition window varies as a function of the phase-encoding gradient duration (i.e., k_y value), resulting in a variable length of k_x lines. When $k_y = 0$, the k_x line is the longest. As $|k_y|$ increases, the length of k_x lines decreases.

sequence (Feinberg 1997). Alternatively, when the diamond k-space coverage in Figure 16.52 is compared to a rectangular k-space coverage with the same extent along the k_x and k_y directions, the acquisition time is reduced because k-space data in the corners are not sampled.

SELECTED REFERENCES

Alsop, D. C. 1997. The sensitivity of low flip angle RARE imaging. *Magn. Reson. Med.* 37: 176–184.
Busse, R. F., Riederer, S. J., Fletcher, J. G., Bharucha, A. E., and Brandt, K. R. 2000. Interactive fast spin-echo imaging. *Magn. Reson. Med.* 44: 339–348.

Conolly, S., Nishimura, D., Macovski, A., and Glover, G. 1988. Variable-rate selective excitation. *J. Magn. Reson.* 78: 440–458.

Constable, R. T., Anderson, A. W., Zhong, J., and Gore, J. C. 1992. Factors influencing contrast in fast spin-echo MR imaging. *Magn. Reson. Imaging* 10: 497–511.

Feinberg, D. A. 1997. VET imaging: Magnetic resonance imaging with variable encoding time. *Magn. Reson. Med.* 38: 7–14.

Hall, L. D., and Sukumar, S. 1984. Rapid data acquisition technique for NMR imaging by the projection reconstruction method. *J. Magn. Reson.* 56: 179–182.

Henkelman, R. M., Hardy, P. A., Bishop, J. E., Poon, C. S., and Plewes, D. B. 1992. Why fat is bright in RARE and fast spin-echo imaging. *J. Magn. Reson. Imaging* 2: 533–540.

Hennig, J. 1988. Multiecho sequences with low refocusing flip angles. *J. Magn. Reson.* 78: 397–407.

Hennig, J., Friedburg, H., and Ott, D. 1987. Fast three-dimensional imaging of cerebrospinal fluid. *Magn. Reson. Med.* 5: 380–383.

Hennig, J., Nauerth, A., and Friedburg, H. 1986. RARE imaging: A fast imaging method for clinical MR. *Magn. Reson. Med.* 3: 823–833.

Hennig, J., and Scheffler, K. 2000. Easy improvement of signal-to-noise in RARE-sequences with low refocusing flip angles. *Magn. Reson. Med.* 44: 983–985.

Hennig, J., and Scheffler, K. 2001. Hyperechoes. *Magn. Reson. Med.* 46: 6–12.

Hinks, R. S., and Constable, R. T. 1994. Gradient moment nulling in fast spin-echo. *Magn. Reson. Med.* 32: 698–706.

Hinks, R. S., Kohli, J., and Washburn, S. 1995. Fast spin echo prescan for artifact reduction. *Soc. Magn. Reson. Abstracts* 3: 634.

Hinks, R. S., and Listerud, J. 1991. Approach to steady state in fast spin echo imaging. *Soc. Magn. Reson. Med. Abstracts* 10: 1235.

Johnson, B. A., Fram, E. K., Drayer, B. P., Dean, B. L., Keller, P. J., and Jacobowitz, R. 1994. Evaluation of shared-view acquisition using repeated echoes (SHARE)—a dual-echo fast spin-echo MR technique. *Am. J. Neuro Radiol.* 15: 667–673.

Kanazawa, H., Takai, H., Machida, Y., and Hanawa, M. 1994. Contrast naturalization of fast spin echo imaging: A fat reduction technique free from field inhomogeneity. *Soc. Magn. Reson. Abstracts* 2: 474.

Kholmovski, E. G., Parker, D. L., and Alexander, A. L. 2000. A generalized k-sampling scheme for 3D fast spin echo. *J. Magn. Reson. Imaging* 11: 549–558.

Le Roux, P., and Hinks, R. S. 1993. Stabilization of echo amplitudes in FSE sequences. *Magn. Reson. Med.* 30: 183–190.

Le Roux, P. 2002. Non-CPMG fast spin echo with full signal. *J. Magn. Reson.* 155: 278–292.

Meiboom, S., and Purcell, E. M. 1958. Modified spin-echo method for measuring nuclear relaxation times. *Rev. Sci. Instrum.* 29: 688–691.

Melki, P. S., and Mulkern, R. V. 1992. Magnetization transfer effects in multislice RARE sequences. *Magn. Reson. Med.* 24: 189–195.

Melki, P. S., Mulkern, R. V., Panych, L. P., and Jolesz, F. A. 1991. Comparing the FAISE method with conventional dual SE images. *J. Magn. Reson. Imaging* 1991: 319–326.

Mulkern, R. V., Wong, S. T. S., Winalski, C., and Jolesz, F. A. 1990. Contrast manipulation and artifact assessment of 2D and 3D RARE sequences. *Magn. Reson. Imaging* 8: 557–566.

Mulkern, R. V., Melki, P. S., Jakab, P., Higuchi, N., and Jolesz, F. A. 1991. Phase-encode order and its effect on contrast and artifact in single-shot RARE sequences. *Med. Phys.* 18: 1032–1037.

Oshio, K., Jolesz, F. A., Melki, P. S., and Mulkern, R. V. 1991. T_2-weighted thin-section imaging with the multislab 3-dimensional RARE technique. *J. Magn. Reson. Imaging* 1: 695–700.

Patel, M. R., Klufas, R. A., Alberico, R. A., and Edelman, R. R. 1997. Half-Fourier acquisition single-shot turbo spin-echo (HASTE) MR: Comparison with fast spin-echo MR in diseases of the brain. *Am. J. Neuro Radiol.* 18: 1635–1640.

Pauly, J. M., Spielman, D., Meyer, C. H., and Mackovski, A. 1993. A RARE-spiral pulse sequence. *Soc. Magn. Reson. Med. Abstracts* 12: 1258.

Pipe, J. G. 1999. Motion correction with PROPELLER MRI: Application to head motion and free-breathing cardiac imaging. *Magn. Reson. Med.* 42: 963–969.

Slichter, C. P. 1989. *Principles of magnetic resonance.* Berlin: Springer-Verlag.

Stables, L. A., Kennan, R. P., Anderson, A. W., Constable, R. T., and Gore, J. C. 1999. Analysis of J coupling-induced fat suppression in DIET imaging. *J. Magn. Reson.* 136: 143–151.

Trouard, T. P., Theilmann, R. J., Altbach, M. I., and Gmitro, A. F. 1999. High-resolution diffusion imaging with DIFRAD-FSE (diffusion-weighted radial acquisition of data with fast spin-echo) MRI. *Magn. Reson. Med.* 42: 11–18.

Williamson, D. S., Mulkern, R. V., Jakab, P. D., and Jolesz, F. A. 1996. Coherence transfer by isotropic mixing in Carr-Purcell-Meiboom-Gill imaging: Implications for the bright fat phenomenon in fast spin-echo imaging. *Magn. Reson. Med.* 35: 506–513.

Zhou, X., Cofer, G. P., Suddarth, S. A., and Johnson, G. A. 1993. High-field MR microscopy using fast spin-echoes. *Magn. Reson. Med.* 30: 60–67.

Zhou, X., Liang, Z.-P., Cofer, G. P., Beaulieu, C. F., Suddarth, S. A., and Johnson, G. A. 1993. Reduction of ringing and blurring artifacts in fast spin-echo images. *J. Magn. Reson. Imaging* 3: 803–807.

Zhou, X., Liang, Z. P., Gewalt, S. L., Cofer, G. P., Lauterbur, P. C., and Johnson, G. A. 1998. A fast spin echo technique with circular sampling. *Magn. Reson. Med.* 39: 23–27.

RELATED SECTIONS

Section 3.3 Refocusing Pulses
Section 4.2 Magnetization Transfer Pulses
Section 8.2 Phase-Encoding Gradients
Section 10.1 Concomitant-Field Correction Gradients
Section 10.2 Crusher Gradients
Section 10.3 Eddy-Current Compensation
Section 11.5 Two-Dimensional Acquisition
Section 11.6 Three-Dimensional Acquisition
Section 14.3 Radiofrequency Spin Echo

ADVANCED PULSE SEQUENCE TECHNIQUES

17.1 Arterial Spin Tagging

Tissue function depends heavily on perfusion, a process that brings nutritive blood supply to the tissue through the arterial system and drains the metabolic by-products into the veins. Abnormalities or disruption in this process can have profound effects. For instance, the cessation of blood flow to the brain tissue results in unconsciousness in only 5–10 s and can lead to permanent brain damage if the condition persists.

Perfusion measurement using MRI has been an active area for more than a decade. In general, perfusion MR techniques can be divided into two categories: those employing exogenous agents as a tracer and those using water protons in arterial blood as an endogenous label. Among many exogenous tracers that have been used in perfusion MR, gadolinium chelates (e.g., Gd-DTPA) are most prevalent. In a perfusion imaging technique known as dynamic susceptibility contrast (DSC) or bolus tracking (Rosen et al. 1990; Villringer et al. 1988), a bolus of gadolinium chelate (or other contrast agent) is intravenously injected, immediately followed by the acquisition of a series of snapshot images at a given slice location. The pixel image intensity is plotted as a function of time, which reveals the dynamic changes as the agent passes through the tissue. This curve is then fitted to a model from which quantitative or semiquantitative perfusion parameters can be extracted (Ostergaard et al. 1996). In a technique that relies on an endogenous tracer, the magnetization of water molecules in arterial blood is labeled so that it causes an NMR signal change as the arterial blood perfuses into the tissue (Detre et al. 1992). This method is called *arterial spin labeling* (ASL) or *arterial spin tagging* (AST).

AST labels the magnetization by saturation (Detre et al. 1992) or, more commonly, by inversion (Williams et al. 1992; Edelman et al. 1994). The technique is generally divided into pulsed AST and continuous AST. In pulsed AST, a bolus of arterial blood is labeled and passes through the tissue as a transient. In continuous AST, the labeled arterial blood establishes a steady state in the tissue of interest, which typically requires a much longer tagging time. Continuous AST has higher SNR than pulsed AST and can provide quantitative perfusion information using a simpler model. Pulsed AST, on the other hand, features a higher labeling efficiency and less RF power deposition. The general principles that are common to both techniques are described in subsection 17.1.2; issues specific to these two AST methods are discussed in more detail in subsections 17.1.3 and 17.1.4.

Although AST can be performed in 2D or 3D, 3D AST has not been commonly used, primarily due to its long data acquisition time. Hence, we limit our discussion to 2D single-slice and multislice acquisitions. Unlike most other pulse sequences, the extension from 2D single-slice to 2D multiple slices in AST is not straightforward due to several theoretical and practical considerations, such as the MT effect, accuracy in perfusion quantification, SAR, and imaging time. To simplify the discussion, we focus on 2D single-slice AST first and delay the discussion of 2D multislice AST until subsection 17.1.5.

Perfusion is a complicated phenomenon that can be characterized by numerous parameters. Although these parameters provide multiple avenues to studying tissue perfusion, they can often become a source of confusion, partially due to the inconsistent definitions and interchangeable use of various parameters in the literature. We start by briefly providing the definitions that we adopt for several perfusion parameters used in this section.

17.1.1 KEY PERFUSION PARAMETERS

Perfusion, Perfusion Rate, and Blood Flow   A common measure of perfusion is given by:

$$P \equiv \frac{F}{W} \qquad (17.1)$$

where F is the blood flow rate in milliliters of blood per minute (mL/min) and W is the tissue mass in 100 g. Thus, the nominal unit for perfusion is milliliters per minute per 100 grams [mL/(min · 100 g)]. This definition is inherited from perfusion measurements that use radioactive tracers. Because tissue mass is not directly measured in MRI, an alternative definition of perfusion, sometimes called perfusion rate f in the MR literature, is given by:

$$f \equiv \rho P \qquad (17.2)$$

where ρ is the tissue density in 100 g/mL. Although f is measured in per-minute (min^{-1}), it is more precisely expressed as milliliters per milliliter per minute [mL/(mL · min)] to distinguish the blood volume in the numerator from the tissue volume in the denominator. In the literature, both perfusion P and perfusion rate f have been loosely called perfusion or blood flow, although the blood flow rate is given by F in Eq. (17.1). In the context of brain perfusion, both P and f have been referred to as cerebral blood flow (CBF) or regional cerebral blood flow (r-CBF). Sometimes, CBF or r-CBF is expressed as a percentage of perfusion with respect to a reference tissue (such as the tissue exhibiting the largest CBF) and is referred to as relative CBF (sometimes also denoted by r-CBF in the literature). In healthy brain tissue, the perfusion of gray matter is ~ 2.6 times of that of white matter. The gray and white matter averaged perfusion is approximately 50–60 mL/(min · 100 g) for healthy adults. (Healthy female adults have a higher CBF than healthy male adults). Assuming a brain mass of 1.5 kg, the blood flow, according to Eq. (17.1), amounts to 750–900 mL/min for the entire brain. Note that the total blood flow to the brain can be measured noninvasively with phase contrast techniques (Section 15.2) as described in Marks et al. (1992).

Blood Volume   Blood volume V is defined as the subvolume occupied by blood within a volume of interest or in 100 g of tissue. With the former definition, the volume of interest is often chosen as the volume of a voxel V_0. Because the blood volume is typically measured using a tracer, V can be replaced by the volume of distribution of the tracer (e.g., an intravascular agent) within the tissue. The blood volume is sometimes expressed as a dimensionless volume fraction q:

$$q \equiv V / V_0 \qquad (17.3)$$

In the context of brain perfusion, blood volume is often referred to as cerebral blood volume (CBV), or regional cerebral blood volume (r-CBV) if CBV is evaluated within a region of interest.

Mean Transit Time   Another important parameter to describe tissue perfusion is the mean transit time (MTT), which is the average time required for a tracer to pass through the tissue (Weisskoff et al. 1993). For agents that remain in the blood pool, the MTT is typically a few seconds. For freely diffusible tracers (e.g., D_2O or $H_2{}^{17}O$), the MTT is much longer. In perfusion measurement using a contrast agent, the MTT (denoted by T_{mtt}) is related to the blood flow rate and the blood volume by:

$$F = \frac{V}{T_{mtt}} = \frac{q V_0}{T_{mtt}} \tag{17.4}$$

Equation (17.4) is based on mass conservation and is known as the central volume theorem. MTT is used more frequently in perfusion measurement using exogenous tracers than endogenous AST.

Tissue-Blood Partition Coefficient   When a tracer passes through tissue from the arterial blood supply, its concentration distributes between the blood pool and the tissue. If a constant concentration C_b is maintained in the arterial blood supply and the equilibrium concentration in the tissue is C_t, then the ratio of the two concentrations is called tissue-blood partition coefficient, λ:

$$\lambda \equiv \frac{C_t}{C_b} \tag{17.5}$$

For tracers that remain in the blood pool, C_t (including microvasculature) and C_b are given by m/V_0 and m/V, respectively, where m is the mass of the tracer in moles. In this case, λ reduces to q, as can be seen in Eqs. (17.3) and (17.5). For freely diffusible tracers, such as labeled arterial water, the tracer diffuses into the tissue, and as a result λ is close to 1. For instance, the partition coefficient of water in brain tissue is ~ 0.9 (Herscovitch and Raichle 1985).

17.1.2 BASIC PRINCIPLES OF ARTERIAL SPIN TAGGING

Arterial spin tagging uses the magnetization of water protons in the arterial blood stream as an endogenous, freely diffusible tracer for perfusion measurements (Figure 17.1). Any perturbation to the magnetization of the arterial blood that feeds the tissue can serve as a magnetic tracer. The perturbation is typically introduced by an RF inversion pulse (Section 14.2) at a location proximal (i.e., upstream) to the tissue of interest (Figure 17.1a), although an RF saturation pulse (Section 14.2) can also be used. After a time delay that allows the magnetically labeled arterial blood to reach the tissue capillary bed, the labeled water molecules exchange with the water molecules in the tissue, causing a change in the NMR signal. (Note that the exchange process involves both physical molecular exchange and magnetization exchange.) At this point, a pulse sequence is played to acquire an image or partial image data at a location

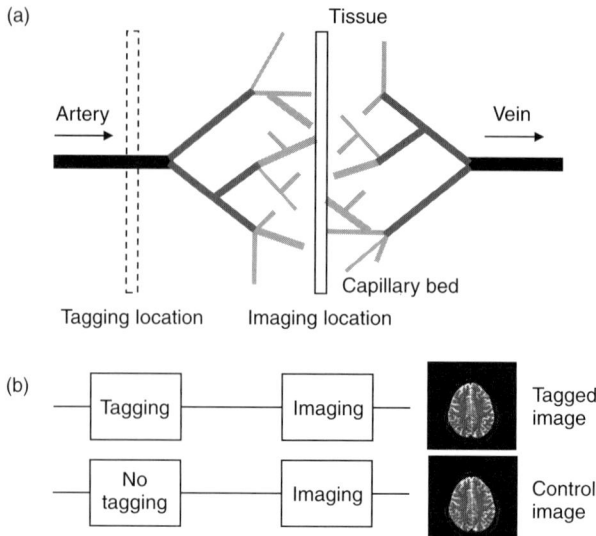

FIGURE 17.1 A schematic diagram showing (a) the principles of AST and (b) an associated conceptual pulse sequence. Water in arterial blood flows from an artery to the capillary bed, exchanges with tissue water, and drains to the vein. In (a) magnetization of the arterial blood is labeled at a location (dashed box) proximal to the imaging plane (box with solid lines). The two images in (b), acquired using the conceptual pulse sequence with and without AST, are subtracted. The arrows in (a) indicate the direction of blood flow.

distal (i.e., downstream) to the tagging position. The spatially resolved signal change is measured by subtracting the two images, acquired with and without labeling, as shown in a conceptual pulse sequence in Figure 17.1b. In the context of this section, we refer to these two images as the tagged image M_t and the control image M_c, and we refer to the pulse sequences that produce them as tagging and control pulse sequences, respectively. The signal-intensity change between M_c and M_t is fitted to a model, from which a quantitative perfusion map of f or P is obtained. The difference image $|M_c - M_t|$ can also be viewed directly as a qualitative perfusion-weighted image.

AST is essentially an inversion recovery pulse sequence with an inversion (or saturation) module and a host sequence (both defined in Section 14.2) that are applied at different locations. AST pulse sequences also resemble black blood angiographic techniques that employ inversion pulses (Section 15.3), except that the focus is on signal changes in the tissue instead of the arteries.

Perfusion quantification relies on the signal change between control and tagged images. Typically, this signal change is only 1–2%. Thus, other factors that can cause signal variation must be avoided or compensated for. A common source of error is the MT effect discussed in Section 4.2. In the presence of a gradient, the RF pulse delivered to the tagging position can serve as an off-resonance irradiation with respect to the imaging location. The MT effect can cause signal loss substantially larger than the perfusion-induced signal change. Hence, it is important to adequately equalize the MT effect between the tagged and the control images. The very small signal change in AST also makes perfusion quantification very sensitive to random noise, necessitating signal averaging to increase the SNR. Because of the need for signal averaging, imaging pulse sequences (e.g., EPI and spiral) that offer fast acquisition are highly desirable in AST, especially for studies involving human subjects.

17.1.3 PULSED ARTERIAL SPIN TAGGING

In pulsed AST or pulsed arterial spin labeling (PASL), an RF inversion pulse is applied to produce a *bolus* of labeled magnetization at a tagging location. The bolus travels from the artery to the capillary bed and exchanges the labeled magnetization with the unlabeled magnetization of the tissue water. The labeled magnetization in the tissue experiences T_1 relaxation and eventually becomes indistinguishable from the unlabeled magnetization. Because the bolus is transient, so is the AST signal, $|M_c - M_t|$.

Pulsed AST is a family of pulse sequences, all sharing the same basic principles, but differing from one another in the strategies by which the tagged and control images are acquired. In this subsection, we describe two categories of pulsed AST techniques, followed by a discussion on how quantitative perfusion information can be extracted from the pulsed AST images.

EPISTAR

EPISTAR stands for echo-planar imaging and signal targeting with alternating radiofrequency (Edelman et al. 1994). An EPISTAR pulse sequence is shown in Figure 17.2. The pulse sequence alternates between acquiring a tagged image (Figure 17.2a) and a control image (Figure 17.2b).

The tagging pulse sequence begins with a 90° slice-selective saturation pulse applied at the location (narrow gray band in Figure 17.2c) where the perfusion measurement is sought. This pulse saturates the spins in the slice location of interest (i.e., the imaging slice), providing some immunity to any perturbation that can be caused by the subsequent tagging pulse, such as side lobes in its spatial profile. Following the saturation pulse, a spoiler gradient is typically used to dephase the magnetization. (Note that the spoiling gradient lobe is bridged with the slice-selection gradient lobe in Figure 17.2.) After the saturation pulse and its associated spoiler, a spatially selective inversion pulse (i.e., a tagging pulse) inverts spins within a thick slab (e.g., 9 cm, shown as a

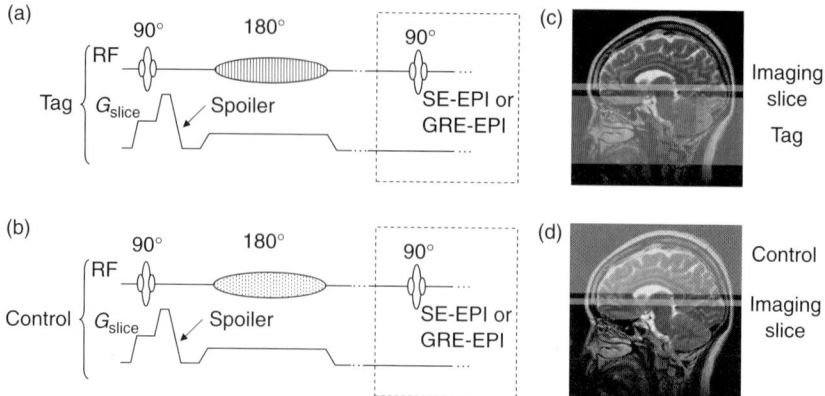

FIGURE 17.2 An EPISTAR pulse sequence. The tagging pulse sequence in (a) produces a tagged image in (c), and the control pulse sequence in (b) generates a control image in (d). The 90° pulses at the beginning of the sequences are spatial saturation pulses applied at the imaging slice location (uniform gray areas in (c) and (d)). The spoiler gradient can be played along any axis. The 180° pulses in (a) and (b) invert the spins in the boxed area in (c) (filled with vertical lines; labeled tag) and in (d) (i.e., filled with vertical dashed lines; labeled control), respectively. The two filled areas are symmetrically placed with respect to the imaging slice. The EPI pulse sequence is enclosed in the dashed box. SE and GRE denote spin echo and gradient echo, respectively. The RF pulses (without any filling pattern) are applied to the imaging plane. For simplicity, the readout and phase-encoding gradients are not shown.

shaded area with vertical lines in Figure 17.2c) proximal to the imaging slice. A hyperbolic secant adiabatic inversion pulse (Section 6.2) is most frequently used, although other adiabatic inversion pulses (Yongbi et al. 1998) or nonadiabatic inversion pulses can also be employed. To reduce the effect of the nonideal profile of the tagging pulse on the imaging slice, a gap (e.g., ~ 1 cm) is typically prescribed between the inverted slab and the imaging slice. At the end of the tagging pulse, a long delay time (e.g., 1 s) is introduced to allow the inverted arterial spins to travel from the tagged slab to the imaging plane and to perfuse into the tissue. Because the tagged arterial blood carries inverted magnetization, it causes a signal reduction (discussed later). The reduced magnetization is imaged using a GRE-EPI or SE-EPI pulse sequence, as denoted by the dashed box in Figure 17.2a.

The control image without arterial tagging can be acquired by simply repeating the sequence without the tagging pulse (Edelman et al. 1994). However, the tagging pulse is an off-resonance irradiation with respect to the imaging slice, resulting in MT effect in the tagged image that masks the subtle signal change due to perfusion. To balance the MT effect, an inversion pulse identical to that in the tagging sequence is also played prior to the acquisition of the control image, except that its carrier frequency is chosen to place the tagging slab (the shaded area filled with vertical dashed lines in Figure 17.2d) distal to the imaging plane by an equal distance (Figure 17.2d). If the imaging slice has a frequency offset of f_0, then the carrier frequency for the tagging and control inversion pulses should be $f_0 - f_{\text{epistar}}$ and $f_0 + f_{\text{epistar}}$, respectively, where f_{epistar} is given by:

$$f_{\text{epistar}} = \frac{\gamma}{2\pi} G \Delta r \qquad (17.6)$$

In Eq. (17.6), G is the tagging gradient and Δr is the center-to-center distance between the imaging slice and the tagging slab. As long as the MT effect is symmetric with respective to positive and negative off-resonance irradiation (i.e., $\pm f_{\text{epistar}}$), it cancels after image subtraction. We define the subtracted signal for EPISTAR as:

$$\Delta M_{\text{epistar}} = M_c - M_t \qquad (17.7)$$

where $\Delta M_{\text{epistar}}$ is a positive quantity because M_t carries the inverted magnetization.

The long inversion time (e.g., TI $\approx$ 1 s) and the need to minimize saturation of the arterial blood in successive excitations both require a long TR (e.g., 2 s or longer). The long TR, in conjunction with a large number of signal averages (e.g., 60), necessitates a fast imaging sequence to make pulsed AST practical. For this reason, single-shot EPI is used in EPISTAR. The single-shot RARE version of EPISTAR, known as STAR-HASTE, has also been developed (Chen et al. 1997). Single-shot acquisition not only reduces the total scan time, but also minimizes image misregistration due to patient bulk motion or system instability, provided that the acquisitions of the tagged image and the control image are interleaved.

Proximal inversion with a control for off-resonance effects (PICORE) (Wong et al. 1997) is a variation of EPISTAR. The tagging sequence is the same as that in EPISTAR, but an off-resonance inversion pulse in the control sequence is played without an accompanying slab-selection gradient (Figure 17.3). The carrier frequency of the inversion pulse is the same between the control and the tagging pulse sequences, so the MT effect can be subtracted out. The magnetization of the imaging slice is virtually unperturbed due to the large resonance offset (e.g., 5 kHz). The signal difference can be defined similarly to Eq. (17.7)

$$\Delta M_{\text{picore}} = M_c - M_t \qquad (17.8)$$

Compared to EPISTAR, the subtraction image ΔM_{picore} rejects the inflow from the distal side of the imaging slice, whereas the inflow causes a reduction

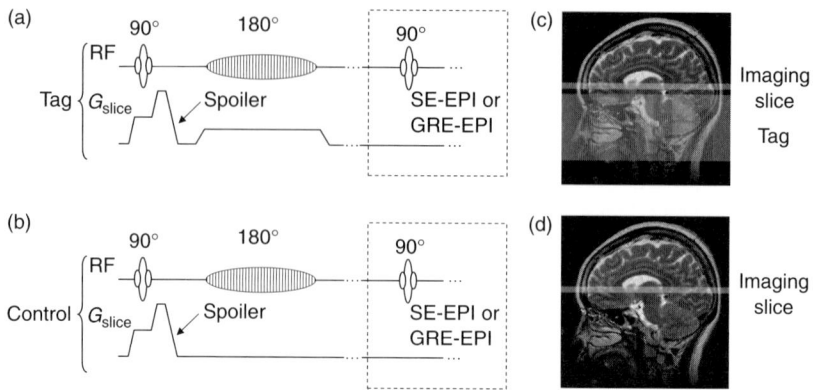

FIGURE 17.3 A PICORE pulse sequence. The tagging sequence (a) is identical to that in Figure 17.2a and produces the tagged image in (c). The control sequence (b) differs from that in (a) only in that the slice-selection gradient during the inversion pulse is not played. The resulting control image (d) does not experience any inversion because the carrier frequency of the inversion pulse is off-resonance.

in $\Delta M_{\text{epistar}}$. Another advantage is that asymmetry in MT effects is compensated in PICORE, but not in EPISTAR. A disadvantage of PICORE is, however, that it is less robust against eddy-current effects than EPISTAR because the control sequence uses a different gradient waveform from the tagging sequence.

Another variation of EPISTAR is known as transfer-insensitive labeling technique (TILT), in which the inversion pulse in EPISTAR is replaced by two consecutive 90° spatially selective pulses (Golay et al. 1999). To obtain the tagged image, the two 90° pulses have the same phase, effectively producing a 180° magnetization inversion at the tagging location. To acquire the control, the phase of the second 90° pulse is changed by 180° with respect to the phase of the first 90° pulse (i.e., the two pulses perform a 90° rotation and then a −90° rotation, respectively). Thus, the magnetization experiences no net nutation. Because the pulses for both tagged and control images are applied in the same proximal location, the MT effect is canceled in image subtraction, even in the presence of asymmetry in MT (subsection 17.1.6). Compared to EPISTAR (as well as FAIR, discussed next), TILT is also more robust against venous inflow.

FAIR

Flow-sensitive alternating inversion recovery (FAIR) (Kwong et al. 1995; Kim 1995) employs a frequency-selective inversion pulse with and without an accompanying slice-selection gradient to produce the tagged and the control

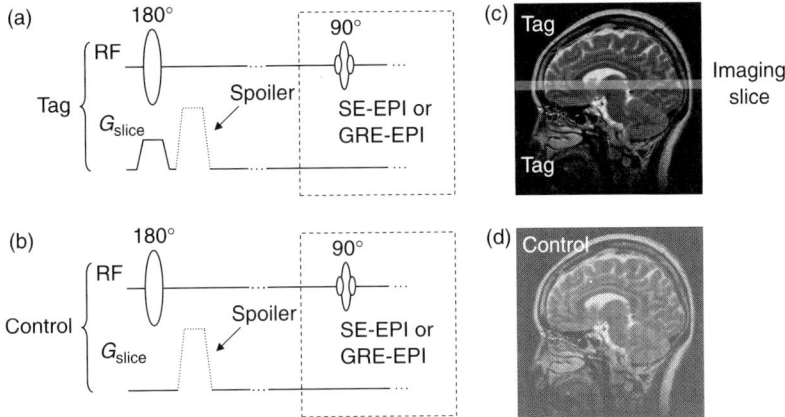

FIGURE 17.4 A FAIR pulse sequence. The tagging pulse sequence in (a) produces a tagged image in (c), and the control pulse sequence in (b) generates a control image in (d). The spatially selective 180° inversion pulse in (a) is applied to the imaging slice (uniform gray area in (c)). In the control sequence (b), the same inversion pulse is played without the slice-selection gradient, inverting the spins within the entire sensitive region of the RF coil (the gray area in (d)). The EPI pulse sequence is enclosed in the dashed box. SE and GRE denote spin echo and gradient echo, respectively. For simplicity, the readout and phase-encoding gradients are not shown.

images, respectively (Figure 17.4). Similar to EPISTAR, the inversion pulse is typically adiabatic with a bandwidth of approximately 1–5 kHz. Unlike EPISTAR, however, the inversion pulses for the control and tagged images have the same carrier frequency.

When the pulse is played with the slice-selection gradient (Figure 17.4a), it inverts the spins within the imaging slice while leaving spins elsewhere virtually unaffected. (In practice, the spatial profile of the inversion pulse is often made wider than the thickness of the imaging slice to minimize the impact of the side lobes and transition regions and to ensure a uniform inversion of the imaging slice.) After the pulse, an optional spoiler gradient can be applied, followed by a delay time, just as in EPISTAR. Finally, a single-shot EPI pulse sequence is played to produce the tagged image.

To acquire the control image, the slice-selection gradient can be either played with zero amplitude (Figure 17.4b) or played at a different time away from the slice-selection gradient (not shown in Figure 17.4b). The latter approach uses the slice-selection gradient as a spoiler (Kwong et al. 1995). By keeping the same gradient waveform, it also allows better cancelation of eddy-current effects between the tagged and the control images. In the absence of an accompanying slice-selection gradient, the inversion pulse inverts spins in the entire volume of the transmitting RF coil, provided that the bandwidth of the RF pulse is wide enough to encompass the resonance frequencies within the volume, a condition that is almost always satisfied. Because both the arterial blood and the tissue experience similar inversion recovery, and the T_1 of arterial blood is only slightly longer than that of gray matter, there is virtually no sensitivity to arterial inflow in the control image (Nishimura et al. 1987).

Unlike the situation in EPISTAR, the tagged magnetization in FAIR is not inverted and thus has a positive z component. The magnetization for the control image, on the other hand, is inverted and hence is negative. To maintain a positive sign for ΔM, we use the following definition for FAIR:

$$\Delta M_{\text{fair}} = M_{\text{t}} - M_{\text{c}} \tag{17.9}$$

(Note that some authors refer to the slice-selective inversion image as the control and nonselective image as the tag. Under that convention, the definition of ΔM is identical to that for EPISTAR given in Eq. 17.7; however, ΔM becomes negative.) Becuase the magnetization of the tagged region is not inverted, it does not fade away due to T_1 relaxation. However, the magnetization of the control image is inverted and experiences inversion recovery. Therefore, the net T_1-relaxation effect on ΔM_{fair} is similar to that in EPISTAR.

FAIR is more robust against the MT effect because no off-resonance irradiation is applied with respect to the imaging slice. This facilitates multislice imaging, as described in subsection 17.1.5. Another advantage of FAIR over EPISTAR is that arterial blood feeding the tissue from both proximal and distal sides of the imaging slice is tagged. When the flow direction is unknown or when the feeding arteries have tortuous paths, FAIR reduces underestimation of perfusion, because inflows from both directions are registered and contribute to the difference image.

Several variations of the FAIR pulse sequence have been developed. In a technique called uninverted flow-sensitive alternating inversion recovery (UNFAIR) (Helpern et al. 1997; Tanabe et al. 1999) or extraslice spin tagging (EST) (Berr and Mai 1999), two consecutive inversion pulses with the same carrier frequency are used in the pulse sequence. To acquire the tagged image, one of the inversion pulses is played with a slice-selection gradient to selectively invert the magnetization of the imaging slice while the other inversion pulse is nonselective (or very slightly selective with a much broader spatial profile than that of the selective inversion pulse) to invert all spins. As a consequence, the magnetization of the imaging slice experiences a 360° rotation and ends at a positive z axis. The inflow magnetization is affected by only one inversion pulse and thus is inverted. To acquire the control image, both inversion pulses are nonselective (or very slightly selective with the same spatial profiles), resulting in an uninverted image. With UNFAIR, the signal change is defined as:

$$\Delta M_{\text{unfair}} = M_{\text{c}} - M_{\text{t}}, \tag{17.10}$$

which is different from Eq. (17.9) for FAIR because the tagged image in UNFAIR caries negative magnetization. Compared to FAIR, UNFAIR does not invert the control image. Therefore, it is insensitive to the inversion time or the difference between blood and tissue T_1 s. This property also makes UNFAIR less sensitive to errors due to radiation damping (Zhou et al. 1998).

BASE is another variation of FAIR (Schwarzbauer and Heinke 1998). This technique acquires a basis (BA) image (i.e., a control) without any spin preparation and a tagged image with a selective (SE) inversion pulse applied at the imaging slice location. Because the nonselective inversion pulse is not used in the control image, BASE is more robust against a mismatch between the inversion profile and the imaging slice profile than FAIR. For example, if the inversion profile does not entirely contain the imaging slice, the noninverted stationary magnetization in the imaging slice contributes to ΔM in FAIR, but not in BASE. This property also makes BASE suitable when a small RF coil is used on a relatively large subject.

Another variation of FAIR is known as flow-sensitive alternating inversion recovery with an extra radiofrequency pulse (FAIRER) (Mai et al. 1999). As the name implies, FAIRER employs a slice-selective saturation pulse delivered to the imaging location immediately after the inversion pulse of a FAIR sequence. This technique was developed to reduce the TI sensitivity of the subtracted image and improve the robustness against TI values that are close to the nulling point of specific tissues.

Another technique, which is also called FAIRER (FAIR excluding radiation damping), addresses the problem of radiation damping (Zhou et al. 1998). In the presence of radiation damping, FAIR is subject to errors in perfusion quantification. In this FAIRER technique, the effect of radiation damping is suppressed by employing a very weak gradient (e.g., 0.6 mT/m) during the delays (e.g., the inversion delay and spin echo delays) in the pulse sequence.

Quantitative Perfusion Calculation

Apparent T_1   For simplicity, we first neglect the effects of transit delays from the tagging region to the imaged slice (this assumption is removed later). We then assume that (1) the effect of MT is completely compensated for and (2) the T_1 of blood is the same as the T_1 of tissue. With these assumptions, the Bloch equation for the longitudinal magnetization in the presence of perfusion can be modified to the following form (Detre et al. 1992):

$$\frac{dM}{dt} = \frac{M_0 - M}{T_1} + f M_b - \frac{f}{\lambda} M \tag{17.11}$$

where M is the longitudinal magnetization of the tissue with an equilibrium value of M_0, M_b is the longitudinal magnetization of the inflowing arterial blood, f is the perfusion rate defined in Eq. (17.2), and λ is the partition coefficient of water molecules between tissue and blood. Without these assumptions about transit delay and T_1-relaxation times, the Bloch equation can also be expressed in a form similar to Eq. (17.11) in which M_b is replaced with an apparent arterial blood magnetization. The first term of Eq. (17.11) is the nominal term that arises from T_1 relaxation, and the second and the third terms account for spins entering the tissue (inflow) and exiting the tissue (outflow), respectively, due to blood flow. From Eq. (17.11), it can be seen that the tissue T_1-relaxation rate (i.e., $1/T_1$) is effectively increased by f/λ, resulting in an apparent longitudinal relaxation time T_1' given by (Detre et al. 1992; Kwong et al. 1995):

$$\frac{1}{T_1'} \equiv \frac{1}{T_1} + \frac{f}{\lambda} \tag{17.12}$$

Because λ can be generally assumed to be a constant (~ 0.9 for brain tissue), one approach to quantifying perfusion is to obtain two T_1 maps (i.e., T_1' and T_1 maps). The T_1' map is computed from a series T_1-weighted *tagged* images with varying TI values, and the T_1 map from a set of T_1-weighted *control* images (Section 14.2). This simple model can also be modified to account for the difference between tissue and blood T_1-relaxation times (Kwong et al. 1995). Although this method has been employed for quantitative perfusion studies, its widespread use has been impeded largely due to the long acquisition times.

Perfusion Quantification by Image Subtraction   Once the arterial spins have been labeled, it takes time for them to travel from the tagging site to the imaging slice location. Assume that the arterial blood can be characterized as uniform plug flow at both the leading edge and the tailing edge and that the time origin is chosen to be the end of the tagging pulse. The labeled arterial magnetization (normalized to its maximal value) in the imaging location is proportional to:

$$c(t) = \begin{cases} 0 & 0 \le t < t_a \\ e^{-t/T_{1b}} & t_a \le t < t_a + \delta \\ 0 & t_a + \delta \le t \end{cases} \tag{17.13}$$

where t_a is the arrival time of the leading edge of the tagged spins, also known as the *transit delay*, $t_a + \delta$ is the departure time when the tailing edge of the tagged spins leaves the imaging slice, δ is the duration when the tag remains in the imaging slice, and T_{1b} is the T_1 relaxation time of the blood. Equation (17.13) has also assumed a thin slice at the imaging location. Thus, the discontinuities at $t = t_a$ and $t = t_a + \delta$ are completely caused by the plug flow. Using this model and assuming that the tagged water is completely extracted from the blood to the tissue under the well-mixed condition, it can be shown that ΔM in Eqs. (17.7)–(17.10) can be expressed as (Buxton et al. 1998; Yang et al. 1998):

$$\Delta M(t) = \begin{cases} 0 & 0 \leq t < t_a \\ 2\alpha \left(\dfrac{M_0}{\lambda}\right)(t - t_a) f e^{-t/T_{1b}} \vartheta(t) & t_a \leq t < t_a + \delta \\ 2\alpha \left(\dfrac{M_0}{\lambda}\right) \delta f e^{-t/T_{1b}} \vartheta(t) & t_a + \delta \leq t \end{cases} \qquad (17.14)$$

where α is the fraction of the achieved inversion over the maximal possible inversion of the magnetization (Zhang et al. 1993), and $\vartheta(t)$ is a dimensionless term that depends on t_a, δ, T_1', and T_{1b}. Alternative expressions of ΔM can also be found (e.g., Kwong et al. 1995; Kim 1995; Calamante et al. 1996). Note that Eq. (17.14) differs from that given by Buxton et al. (1998) because we have used M_0/λ to replace the equilibrium magnetization of the arterial blood. Eq. (17.14) also differs from the results in Yang (2002) because we have used the approximation $(1 - e^{-x}) \approx x$ that is valid for $x \ll 1$.

In Eq. (17.14), α can be experimentally determined or calculated with a theoretical model. $\vartheta(t)$ typically has a value close to 1 and can be dropped from Eq. (17.14). λ can be assumed to be a constant (e.g., 0.9 for brain tissue) (Herscovitch and Raichle 1985). T_{1b} is obtainable from a T_1 measurement ($T_{1b} \approx 1.2$ s at 1.5 T) or can be approximated by the tissue T_1 value. However, neither the transit delay t_a nor the bolus duration δ is known *a priori*. Therefore, perfusion quantification based on Eq. (17.14) requires measurements at least at two time points. Because t in Eq. (17.14) can be approximated by the inversion time TI of the sequence, the measurements can be performed at two different TI values. For example, the signal difference between the tag and the control images is first normalized with respect to M_0. The normalized signals ($\Delta M/M_0$) at two different TI values are used to calculate both f and t_a based on the second line of Eq. (17.14), provided that both TI values satisfy the condition $t_a \leq \text{TI} < t_a + \delta$. Alternatively, if data with multiple TI values are obtained, the normalized signal ($\Delta M/M_0$) can be plotted against TI and the perfusion rate f can be extracted by curve-fitting (Yang et al. 1998).

Lack of knowledge of the transit delay t_a makes perfusion quantification using pulsed AST difficult and time consuming. One technique used to address this problem is to employ one or more spatial saturation pulses during

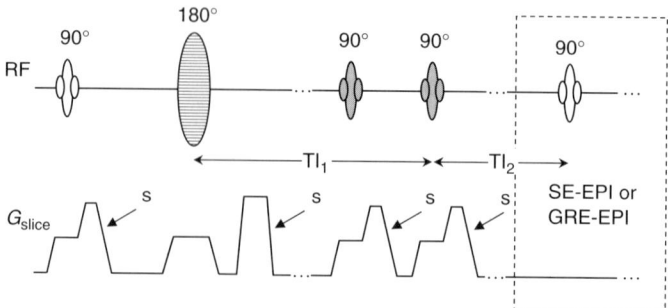

FIGURE 17.5 A QUIPPS or QUIPPS-II pulse sequence. The first 90° saturation pulse is applied to the imaging slice. The 180° inversion pulse can be played according to the strategies in EPISTAR, FAIR, or PICORE. The following two 90° saturation pulses (shaded) are applied to the imaging slice in QUIPPS or to the tagging slab in QUIPPS-II. More or fewer saturation pulses can be played. s indicates the spoiler gradient, which can be played along any axis. For simplicity, the readout and phase-encoding gradients are not shown.

the inversion time to saturate either the imaging slice or the tagging region (Figure 17.5). The former approach is known as quantitative imaging of perfusion using a single subtraction (QUIPSS) and the latter as QUIPSS-II (Wong et al. 1998). With the saturation pulses, the tagged bolus is shaved at either its leading or tailing edge. Compared to methods with a single saturation pulse, multiple saturation pulses applied to the same spatial location can improve the degree of saturation considerably. Because the time of the last saturation pulse can be experimentally controlled, the unknown transit delay in Eq. (17.14) can be replaced with a known pulse sequence timing parameter such as TI_1 and TI_2 in Figure 17.5, as detailed in Wong et al. (1998). For example, the elimination of the transit delay from the second line of Eq. (17.14) makes it possible to quantify perfusion with a data set acquired at a single TI value.

17.1.4 CONTINUOUS ARTERIAL SPIN TAGGING

Steady-state AST, also known as continuous arterial spin labeling (CASL) or continuous AST, was developed before pulsed AST (Detre et al. 1992; Williams et al. 1992). The early method employing multiple saturation pulses (Detre et al. 1992) has now largely been replaced by methods based on magnetization inversion (Williams et al. 1992). Unlike pulsed AST, adiabatic inversion in continuous AST relies on the flow-induced (also known as flow-driven or velocity-driven) fast adiabatic passage principle (Dixon et al. 1986) to provide a continuous supply of inverted arterial spins to the imaging location.

Flow-Induced Adiabatic Inversion Consider an arbitrary RF pulse $B_1(t) = Ae^{-i\omega_{rf}t}$ that has neither amplitude nor frequency modulation (i.e., both A and ω_{rf} are constants). According to Section 6.2, this pulse cannot behave as an adiabatic inversion pulse for stationary spins. For moving spins, however, the situation is quite different; the pulse can indeed produce adiabatic inversion if a magnetic field gradient G along the direction of motion is applied concurrently with the RF pulse. With such a gradient, spins located at $r_0 = \omega_{rf}/(\gamma G)$ along the gradient direction are on resonance (γ is the gyromagnetic ratio).

Consider a group of arterial spins moving from a remote location $r(t)$ toward the tagging plane at r_0, then passing through the imaging plane, and eventually flowing away from the plane (Figure 17.6a). The frequency offset of the spins relative to the RF carrier frequency is:

$$\Delta\omega(t) = \gamma Gr(t) - \omega_{rf} = \gamma G[r(t) - r_0] \qquad (17.15)$$

This frequency offset corresponds to a z component of the effective magnetic field $\vec{B}_{eff}$, defined in Section 1.2:

$$\vec{B}_{eff} = \frac{\hat{z}\Delta\omega(t)}{\gamma} + \hat{x}A \qquad (17.16)$$

where, without loss of generality, we have assumed that the RF pulse $B_1(t) = Ae^{-i\omega_{rf}t}$ is applied along the x axis in a B_1 rotating reference frame with a frequency of ω_{rf} (Section 1.2).

When $r(t)$ is far away from r_0 (e.g., $r(t) \ll r_0$), the effective field is approximately parallel (or anti-parallel) to the z axis because $|\Delta\omega(t)| \gg \gamma A$ (Figure 17.6b). As the spins approach the tagging plane at r_0, $\vec{B}_{eff}$ rotates to the transverse plane. As long as the adiabatic condition is satisfied (Sections 6.1 and 6.2), the magnetization $\vec{M}_{tag}$ of the moving spins follows $\vec{B}_{eff}$ and nutates toward the x axis (Figure 17.6c). When $r(t) = r_0$, the moving spins are on-resonance, and both $\vec{B}_{eff}$ and $\vec{M}_{tag}$ lie in the transverse plane (Figure 17.6d). As the spins move away from r_0, $|\Delta\omega(t)|$ increases, resulting in $\vec{B}_{eff}$ and $\vec{M}_{tag}$ turning toward the longitudinal axis (Figure 17.6e). Eventually, $\vec{B}_{eff}$ becomes anti-parallel (or parallel) to the z axis and $\vec{M}_{tag}$ is inverted from the $+z$ axis to the $-z$ axis (Figure 17.6f). Under the adiabatic condition described by Eq. (17.17), the magnetization of the moving spins is inverted irrespective of their velocity v:

$$\frac{1}{T_{2b}} \ll \frac{Gv}{\left|\vec{B}_{eff}\right|} \ll \frac{\gamma}{2\pi}\left|\vec{B}_{eff}\right| \qquad (17.17)$$

where T_{2b} is the T_2 relaxation time of the arterial blood. If the velocity is too fast, the inequality on the right side of Eq. (17.17) is violated. If the

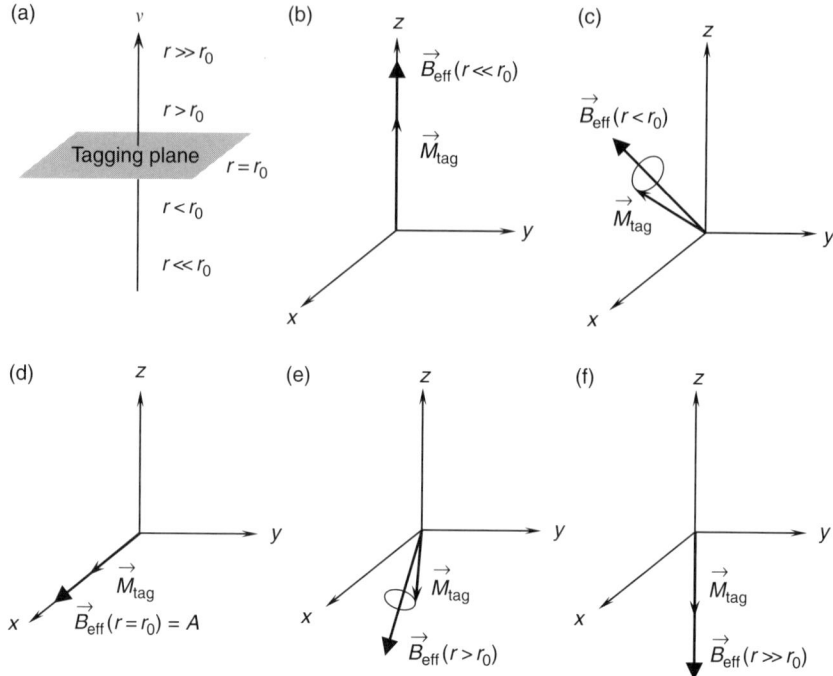

FIGURE 17.6 Flow-induced adiabatic inversion. (a) Arterial blood flowing from a location remote from the tagging plane ($r \ll r_0$), passing through the tagging plane ($r = r_0$), and eventually moving away from the tagging plane toward the imaging location ($r \gg r_0$). (b)–(f) Change in direction of the effective magnetic field $\vec{B}_{\text{eff}}$ together with the magnetization vector $\vec{M}_{\text{tag}}$ during the course of the arterial blood flow in (a). Under the adiabatic condition, the magnetization of arterial spins $\vec{M}_{\text{tag}}$ follows $\vec{B}_{\text{eff}}$. The conditions corresponding to (b)–(f) are $r \ll r_0$, $r < r_0$, $r = r_0$, $r > r_0$, and $r \gg r_0$, respectively. Although we have assumed $\vec{B}_{\text{eff}}$ is parallel to $\vec{M}_{\text{tag}}$ at $r \ll r_0$, adiabatic inversion of $\vec{M}_{\text{tag}}$ can also be achieved if $\vec{B}_{\text{eff}}$ is anti-parallel to $\vec{M}_{\text{tag}}$.

velocity is too slow, then the relaxation effect dominates and the inversion becomes ineffective. Because T_{2b} is not longer than T_{1b}, we have used $1/T_{2b}$ in Eq. (17.17) instead of $1/T_{1b}$. This is a more stringent condition than if T_{2b} were replaced by T_{1b}, which is used by some authors.

It is worth noting that the stationary spins at the tagging location r_0 do not satisfy the adiabatic condition and typically experience a very large flip angle (e.g., $1000°$). The stationary spins in the imaging slice, on the other hand, are virtually unaffected because the tagging pulse is off-resonance and has a narrow bandwidth. Similar to the case of EPISTAR, however, the tagging pulse does introduce MT effects to the imaging slice, which must be compensated for in the perfusion quantification.

Continuous AST Pulse Sequence   Similar to pulsed AST, a continuous AST pulse sequence also acquires at least two images, a tagged one and a control. The pulse sequence to acquire the tagged image begins with a flow-induced adiabatic inversion pulse and an accompanying gradient G along the direction of arterial flow. Although a rectangular RF pulse can be used, the extremely long pulse width (e.g., several seconds) needed to achieve a continuous arterial spin inversion often exceeds the RF amplifier capability or regulatory limits on SAR. Therefore, in practice, a rectangular pulse is approximated by a series of shorter hard pulses separated by a time delay, as shown in Figure 17.7. The typical duty cycle ranges from 70 to 90%. The carrier frequency f_{tag} of the pulse is adjusted so that the tagging location is a few centimeters proximal to the imaging slice. For a given value of f_{tag}, the tagging gradient G determines the tagging location. Note that G must also satisfy Eq. (17.17) for a range of velocities.

Example 17.1   A flow-induced adiabatic inversion pulse is used to tag spins at a location 3 cm proximal to the imaging slice. If a gradient of 4.5 mT/m is played with the RF pulse, what is the carrier frequency of the tagging pulse relative to an excitation RF pulse applied to the imaging slice?

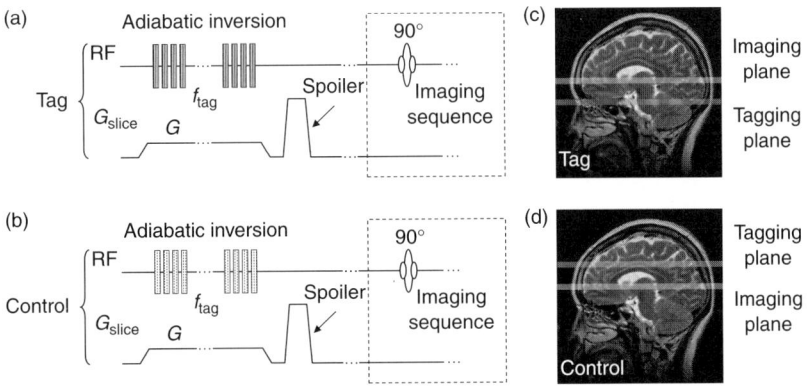

FIGURE 17.7 A continuous AST pulse sequence. (a) Pulse sequence to acquire a tagged image in (c). (b) Pulse sequence to acquire a control image in (d). In (a), the flow-induced adiabatic inversion pulse has a frequency offset f_{tag} relative to the excitation pulse, so that a tagging plane proximal to the imaging plane is selected. In (b), the flow-induced adiabatic inversion pulse has a frequency offset $-f_{tag}$ relative to the excitation pulse, which moves the tagging plane to the distal side of the imaging plane.

Answer   The resonance frequency offset for spins at the tagging location is:

$$f_{tag} = \frac{\gamma}{2\pi} G \Delta r = \frac{2\pi \times 42.57\,\text{MHz/T}}{2\pi} \times 4.5\,\text{mT/m} \times (-0.03\,\text{m})$$

$$= -5.75\,\text{kHz}$$

If the RF excitation for the imaging slice has a zero frequency offset, then the tagging pulse should be modulated by $-5.75\,\text{kHz}$.

Following the long tagging pulse, a spoiler gradient is often played out to dephase any transverse magnetization that might be produced by imperfections of the inversion pulse. After this inversion module and a time delay, an imaging pulse sequence (i.e., a host sequence as defined in Section 14.2) is executed to acquire a tagged image at the imaging slice location shown in Figure 17.7c. During the next TR, this pulse sequence repeats itself with the frequency of the tagging pulse changed to $-f_{tag}$, or with a negative tagging gradient $-G$ to obtain a control image (Figure 17.7b). The former approach ensures that the control and tagged images have the same eddy-current effects induced by the tagging gradient, whereas the latter method compensates for the MT effect more effectively (subsections 17.1.5 and 17.1.6). For multiple averages, the tagged and control images are almost always interleaved to improve robustness against patient bulk motion and system instability.

A number of pulse sequences can be used as the imaging pulse sequence following the inversion module. Examples include spin echo (Williams et al. 1992), gradient echo (Roberts et al. 1994), and EPI (Ye et al. 1996). Similar to the case of pulsed AST, single-shot EPI is a common choice due to its fast acquisition speed and robustness against misregistration in the subtracted images.

Perfusion Quantification   In continuous AST, the normalized labeled arterial magnetization (i.e., $\Delta M / M_0$) at the imaging location is proportional to:

$$c(t) = \begin{cases} 0 & 0 \leq t < t_a \\ e^{-t_a/T_{1b}} & t_a \leq t < t_a + \delta \\ 0 & t_a + \delta \leq t \end{cases} \tag{17.18}$$

All the timing parameters in Eq. (17.18) are defined analogous to those in Eq. (17.13), and the time origin is defined to be the end of the adiabatic inversion pulse. Unlike the case for pulsed AST, $c(t)$ now becomes a step function if a uniform plug flow is assumed. If we further assume that the kinetics of water exchange between tissue and blood is described by a single-compartment, well-mixed model (Buxton et al. 1998; Zhang et al. 1993) and water is completely extracted from the vascular space to the tissue immediately upon arrival at the tissue, then the magnetization difference ($\Delta M = M_c - M_t$) between the control image and the tagged image (on a pixel-by-pixel basis) is:

$$\Delta M(t) = \begin{cases} 0 & 0 \le t < t_a \\ 2\alpha\left(\frac{M_0}{\lambda}\right) f T_1' e^{-t_a/T_{1b}} \left(1 - e^{-(t-t_a)/T_1'}\right) & t_a \le t < t_a + \delta \\ 2\alpha\left(\frac{M_0}{\lambda}\right) f T_1' e^{-t_a/T_{1b}} e^{-(t-t_a-\delta)/T_1'} \left(1 - e^{-\delta/T_1'}\right) & t_a + \delta \le t \end{cases}$$

(17.19)

where, again, t can be approximated by the inversion time TI and T_1' is given by Eq. (17.12). Because the imaging pulse sequence is applied when $t_a < t < t_a + \delta$, we focus on the second line of Eq. (17.19). With a sufficiently long TI (i.e., $(\text{TI} - t_a) \gg T_1'$), $\left(1 - e^{-(t-t_a)/T_1'}\right) \approx 1$ and ΔM becomes independent of time. This condition can be satisfied by using a long TI value in the sequence, which is why a long delay time is necessary in continuous AST (Alsop and Detre 1996). With this approximation:

$$\Delta M = 2\alpha \left(\frac{M_0}{\lambda}\right) f T_1' e^{-t_a/T_{1b}} \qquad (17.20)$$

For rodent studies at high magnetic field (e.g., 4.7 T), the transit delay t_a is short relative to the blood T1 relaxation time T_{1b}. Under these conditions, Eq. (17.20) reduces to:

$$\Delta M = 2\alpha \left(\frac{M_0}{\lambda}\right) f T_1' \qquad (17.21)$$

ΔM, M_0, and T_1' can all be measured, α can be obtained by simulation or a calibration experiment (Zhang et al. 1993; Maccotta et al. 1997), and λ is known ($\lambda = 0.9$ for brain tissue). Thus, f can be determined from Eq. (17.21). Once f is known, perfusion in milliliters per 100 grams of tissue per minute (mL/100 g tissue/min) can be readily obtained from Eq. (17.2). Compared to the second line of Eq. (17.14), Eq. (17.21) is independent of the transit delay; therefore, perfusion quantification is easier with continuous AST than with pulsed AST.

For human studies performed at a lower magnetic field (e.g., 1.5 T), the contribution from the exponential factor in Eq. (17.20) is significant due to the increased ratio of t_a/T_{1b}. Ignoring this factor results in underestimation of f. If a delay time w (e.g., 1 s) is introduced between the end of the tagging pulse and the RF excitation pulse of the imaging sequence, then Eq. (17.20)

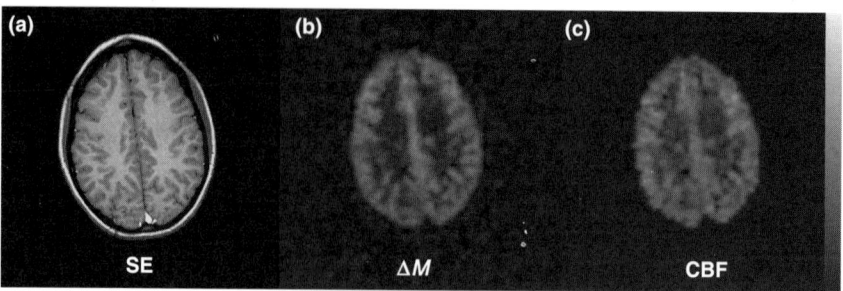

FIGURE 17.8 (a) A T_1-weighted spin echo brain image and (b) the corresponding perfusion-weighted image ΔM (b) and (c) the CBF map obtained at 1.5 T using continuous AST from a 22-year-old healthy female. Key acquisition parameters for the perfusion images are TR = 3.7 s, TE = 60 ms, FOV = 24 cm, in-plane matrix size = 64 × 64, delay time = 1 s, averages = 50 pairs (50 tagged and 50 control images), and the total acquisition time = 8.2 min. (Courtesy of Frank Q. Ye, Ph.D., National Institute of Mental Health, National Institute of Health)

becomes:

$$\Delta M = 2\alpha \left(\frac{M_0}{\lambda}\right) f T_1' \exp\left(-\frac{w}{T_1'}\right) \exp\left(\frac{t_a}{T_1'} - \frac{t_a}{T_{1b}}\right) \qquad (17.22)$$

provided that w is longer than t_a (Alsop and Detre 1996). By further assuming $T_{1b} \approx T_1'$, perfusion can be quantified from Eq. (17.22) without explicitly knowing the transit delay time t_a. This assumption holds well for gray matter because the difference between blood and gray matter T_1 s is rather small (e.g., within 10% at 1.5 T). For white matter, the T_1 difference is larger. The sensitivity to the transit delay, however, is still reduced by introducing a long delay time w.

To summarize, perfusion quantification with continuous AST involves (1) measuring the image intensity difference between the control and the tagged image; (2) normalizing the intensity to M_0, which is often approximated by the control image M_c; (3) obtaining a T_1 map (see Section 14.2); (4) determining α through calibration or simulation; (5) calculating f from Eq. (17.21) or Eq. (17.22); and (6) converting it to P if necessary. A perfusion map using the method outlined in this subsection is shown in Figure 17.8c, along with a qualitative perfusion-weighted image (Figure 17.8b).

17.1.5 MULTISLICE ARTERIAL SPIN TAGGING

Extending single-slice AST to multiple slice locations is not straightforward. If a tagging pulse is played for each slice using a 2D sequential acquisition mode (Section 11.5), the total acquisition time becomes prohibitively long because AST experiments require a long inversion time (or long tagging time) and consequently a long TR. Even with single-shot imaging pulse sequences such as EPI, the need for a large number of signal averages to increase the SNR still makes the total acquisition time problematic. For example, if 60 averages (30 control and 30 tagged images) are needed to achieve a sufficient SNR for the calculation of a reliable perfusion map at 1.5 T, the scan time for 10 slices will be 40 min using a single-shot EPI with a TR of 4 s. In addition, a T_1-mapping scan is also required, which exacerbates the already long imaging time. The scan time can be reduced if a single tagging pulse is played for a group of slices. This approach, however, faces other challenges.

In EPISTAR and continuous AST, each slice in the group receives a different off-resonance irradiation frequency f_1, f_2, f_3, ..., f_n (where n is the slice index) from the inversion pulse and hence experiences a different MT effect (Figure 17.9). When the inversion pulse in the control sequence is played, the order of the off-resonance irradiation reverses to f_n, ..., f_3, f_2, f_1 among the slices, and so does the MT effect. Subtracting the tagged image from the control image does not cancel the MT effect, except for the slice located at the center of the group, which experiences the same off-resonance irradiation between the tagged and the control images. One technique to address this problem is to apply the inversion pulse for the control image at the same location as in the tagged image (i.e., both inversion pulses are applied to a proximal location). In EPISTAR, this pulse is split into two back-to-back inversion pulses (Edelman and Chen 1998). The arterial spins experience a 360° rotation, as if there were no pulse applied, so a control image can still be obtained. The off-resonance irradiation on a given imaging slice in the group is equivalent

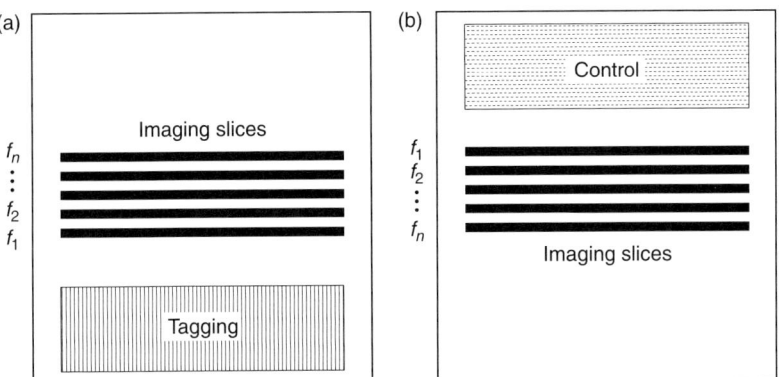

FIGURE 17.9 Magnetization transfer effect in multislice EPISTAR or continuous AST in (a) a tagged image and (b) a control image. The frequencies of off-resonance irradiation for the imaging slices are labeled on the left-hand side of each figure. For a given slice location, the off-resonance frequency is different between the tagged and the control images, unless the slice is located at the center of the group.

(or at least very similar) to that in the corresponding tagged image. The MT effect is thus compensated to a large extent. In multislice continuous AST, the inversion pulse for the control image can be amplitude-modulated with a cosine function (Alsop and Detre 1998). If the frequency of the cosine function is f_m (e.g., 200 Hz), then the original tagging position r_c is split into two locations $r_c \pm 2\pi f_m/(\gamma G)$. This is similar to the double sideband or Hadamard spatial saturation described in Section 5.3. Because f_m is much smaller than the frequency separation between the imaging slice and the tagging location, the two split locations are both near r_c. When the arterial spins pass through both locations en route to the imaging slice, they experience a 180° inversion at each location. Therefore, no net effect occurs on the magnetization (neglecting the relaxation effects) and the image can be used as a control. Because both control and tagging pulses are delivered to virtually the same location at or near r_c, the MT effect is compensated for. Another technique to compensate for the MT effect is to cosine modulate both the tagging inversion pulse and control inversion pulse with a *large* modulation frequency f_M (e.g., 15 kHz) (Talagala et al. 1998). The tagging pulse is applied in the presence of a tagging gradient so that the magnetization is inverted at both a proximal (e.g., with $-f_M$) and a distal location (e.g., with $+f_M$) symmetric to the imaging region of interest. The application of this double sideband RF irradiation produces an MT profile that is symmetric and reasonably flat over a range about the mid-point of the two RF bands. The control pulse is applied in the absence of a tagging gradient, producing an identical (or very similar) MT profile to that in a tagged image. The MT effect can then be canceled in the image subtraction for all slices within the region where the MT profile is symmetric and reasonably flat. In addition to techniques with pulse sequence design, the MT effect in multislice AST can also be addressed by using a small local RF coil to deliver the RF pulse for spin tagging while using another coil to perform imaging (Zhang et al. 1995; Zaharchuk et al. 1999). Because the RF irradiation is local, the MT effect at the imaging location can be substantially reduced.

In FAIR, PICORE, and TILT multislice imaging, the problem with the reversed MT effect shown in Figure 17.9 is avoided due to the ways that the control and the tagged images are acquired. The transit delay, however, varies among different slices. The same problem also exists in other pulsed AST techniques, including EPISTAR. Transit time has been modeled on a per-slice basis for quantitative multislice imaging (Yang et al. 1998; Kim et al. 1997). Figure 17.10 shows a set of six axial CBF maps acquired using a FAIR sequence and data processing outlined in subsection 17.1.3. The variable delay time for multiples slices has also been addressed using a technique known as simultaneous multislice acquisition with arterial flow tagging (SMART) (Kao et al. 1998). This technique relies on Hadamard encoding to simultaneously acquire multiple slices. The number of slices is, however, rather limited (e.g., two).

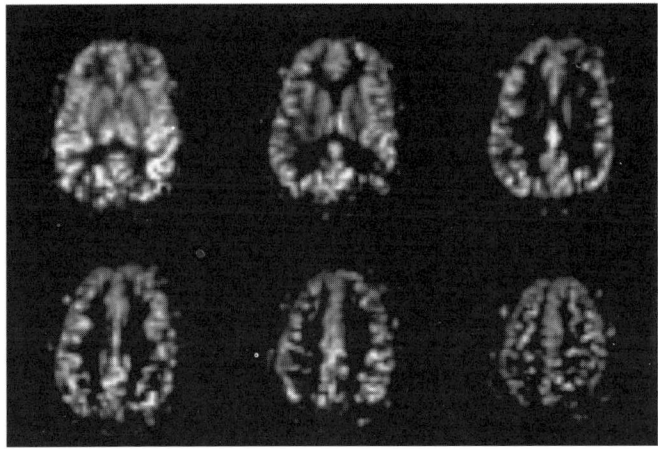

FIGURE 17.10 Six axial CBF maps obtained from a healthy human volunteer using a FAIR sequence on a 3.0T scanner. Key imaging parameters are TE = 7.6 ms, TR = 2000 ms, TI = 1200 ms, FOV = 22 cm, in-plane matrix size = 64 × 64, slice thickness = 5 mm, and averages = 50 pairs (50 tagged and 50 control images). (Courtesy of Yihong Yang, Ph.D., National Institute of Drug Abuse, National Institute of Health)

17.1.6 PRACTICAL CONSIDERATIONS

Asymmetric MT Effects   Signal loss due to MT is a major source of error in perfusion quantification. Several compensation schemes discussed earlier for single-slice imaging are based on the assumption that the MT effect is the same between positive (f_{tag}) and negative ($-f_{tag}$) off-resonance irradiation with respect to the water resonance frequency of the imaging slice. If the MT effect is different (i.e., asymmetrical), then it will not be canceled completely in the difference image ΔM. The techniques previously discussed for multislice imaging can be employed to address this problem. Alternatively, a four-step acquisition strategy (Pekar et al. 1996) can be used in a scan with $4N$ averages (where N is a positive integer). The frequency offset of the inversion pulse toggles between f_{tag} and $-f_{tag}$ as usual. At each frequency, the slab-selection gradient (for EPISTAR) or the tagging gradient (for continuous AST) alternates between $+G$ and $-G$, resulting in a total of four acquisitions. A difference image between (f_{tag}, G) and (f_{tag}, $-G$) compensates for the asymmetric MT effect, and a difference image between ($-f_{tag}$, G) and (f_{tag}, G) removes the eddy-current effect. Multiple difference images are combined to calculate ΔM. In this way, both asymmetric MT effect and the eddy-current effect induced by the tagging gradient are reduced.

Arterial Signal Elimination   One assumption we have made thus far is that the labeled arterial blood is completely extracted by the tissue. This assumption does not necessarily hold for all pixels (Silva et al. 1997). If the labeled spins remain in the arteries, the resulting ΔM image will appear hyperintense, leading to overestimation of perfusion. Because the arterial blood moves much faster than diffusion or perfusion, the arterial blood signal can be effectively suppressed by a small diffusion-weighting gradient without substantially affecting the desired signal. This gradient, also called a crusher in several papers on AST (Wong et al. 1998; Ye et al. 1997; Schepers et al. 2003), can be incorporated into either a gradient-echo- or a spin-echo-based imaging sequence, as detailed in Section 9.1.

Specific Absorption Rate   Continuous AST pulse sequences have high SAR in order to satisfy the adiabatic condition and to attain a steady state of the labeled spins in the imaging slice. This problem is worsened in multislice imaging or at higher main magnetic fields (e.g., 3.0 T). One approach to address this problem is to use a small coil (e.g., a surface coil) to transmit the inversion pulse locally to an artery, such as the carotid artery, while using a larger coil to transmit the RF pulses for imaging (Zaharchuk et al. 1999; Mildner et al. 2003). This approach can reduce SAR considerably as well as decreasing the MT effect discussed in subsection 17.1.5. A drawback of this method is that it involves additional hardware (i.e., two transmitters) as well a software control to switch between RF transmitters within a pulse sequence.

Slice Profile   It has been shown that imperfections in the spatial profile of the inversion pulse are a source of error in perfusion quantification with pulsed AST (Frank et al. 1997; Keilholz-George et al. 2001). For an adiabatic inversion pulse, the spatial profile imperfections can arise from off-resonance effects, relaxation (Frank et al. 1997), and flow (Zhan et al. 2002). The profile imperfection, if uncompensated, leads to substantial signal variation. This problem can be worsened in multislice AST, in which the broader slice coverage makes it more sensitive to the transition regions of the spatial profiles. To reduce this sensitivity, RF inversion pulses with reduced pulse width have been proposed (Frank et al. 1997). For example, the performance for multislice imaging with pulsed AST can be considerably improved simply by reducing the pulse width of a hyperbolic secant inversion pulse from 30 to 15 ms. Another solution is to employ a frequency offset corrected inversion (FOCI) pulse, which produces sharper transition regions than the hyperbolic secant pulse. The details of FOCI are described by Ordidge et al. (1996) and its applications to AST can be found in Yongbi et al. (1998, 1999).

SELECTED REFERENCES

Alsop, D. C., and Detre, J. A. 1996. Reduced transit-time sensitivity in noninvasive magnetic resonance imaging of human cerebral blood flow. *J. Cereb. Blood Flow Metab.* 16: 1236–1249.

Alsop, D. C., and Detre, J. A. 1998. Multisection cerebral blood flow MR imaging with continuous arterial spin labeling. *Radiology* 208: 410–416.

Berr, S. S., and Mai, V. M. 1999. Extraslice spin tagging (EST) magnetic resonance imaging for the determination of perfusion. *J. Magn. Reson. Imaging* 9: 146–150.

Buxton, R. B., Frank, L. R., Wong, E. C., Siewert, B., Warach, S., and Edelman, R. R. 1998. A general kinetic model for quantitative perfusion imaging with arterial spin labeling. *Magn. Reson. Med.* 40: 383–396.

Calamante, F., Williams, S. R., van Bruggen, N., Kwong, K. K., and Turner, R. 1996. A model for quantification of perfusion in pulsed labelling techniques. *Nucl. Magn. Reson. Biomed.* 9: 79–83.

Chen, Q., Siewert, B., Bly, B. M., Warach, S., and Edelman, R. R. 1997. STAR-HASTE: Perfusion imaging without magnetic susceptibility artifact. *Magn. Reson. Med.* 38: 404–408.

Detre, J. A., Leigh, J. S., Williams, D. S., and Koretsky, A. P. 1992. Perfusion imaging. *Magn. Reson. Med.* 23: 37–45.

Dixon, W. T., Du, L. N., Faul, D. D., Gado, M., and Rossnick, S. 1986. Projection angiograms of blood labeled by adiabatic fast passage. *Magn. Reson. Med.* 3: 454–462.

Edelman, R. R., and Chen, Q. 1998. EPISTAR MRI: Multislice mapping of cerbral blood flow. *Magn. Reson. Med.* 40: 800–805.

Edelman, R. R., Siewert, B., Darby, D. G., Thangaraj, V., Nobre, A. C., Mesulam, M. M., and Warach, S. 1994. Qualitative mapping of cerebral blood-flow and functional localization with echo-planar MR imaging and signal targeting with alternating radio-frequency. *Radiology* 192: 513–520.

Frank, L. R., Wong, E. C., and Buxton, R. B. 1997. Slice profile effects in adiabatic inversion: Application to multislice perfusion imaging. *Magn. Reson. Med.* 38: 558–564.

Golay, X., Stuber, M., Pruessmann, K. P., Meier, D., and Boesiger, P. 1999. Transfer insensitive labeling technique (TILT): Application to multislice functional perfusion imaging. *J. Magn. Reson. Imaging* 9: 454–461.

Helpern, J. A., Branch, C. A., Yongbi, M. N., and Huang, N. C. 1997. Perfusion imaging by un-inverted flow-sensitive alternating inversion recovery (UNFAIR). *Magn. Reson. Imaging* 15: 135–139.

Herscovitch, P., and Raichle, M. E. 1985. What is the correct value for the brain-blood partition coefficient for water? *J. Cereb. Blood Flow Metab.* 5: 65–69.

Kao, Y. H., Wan, X., and MacFall, J. R. 1998. Simultaneous multislice acquisition with arterial-flow tagging (SMART) using echo planar imaging (EPI). *Magn. Reson. Med.* 39: 662–665.

Keilholz-George, S. D., Knight-Scott, J., and Berr, S. S. 2001. Theoretical analysis of the effect of imperfect slice profiles on tagging schemes for pulsed arterial spin labeling MRI. *Magn. Reson. Med.* 46: 141–148.

Kim, S. G. 1995. Quantification of relative cerebral blood-flow change by flow-sensitive alternating inversion-recovery (FAIR) technique—application to functional mapping. *Magn. Reson. Med.* 34: 293–301.

Kim, S. G., Tsekos, N. V., and Ashe, J. 1997. Multi-slice perfusion-based functional MRI using the FAIR technique: Comparison of CBF and BOLD effects. *Nucl. Magn. Reson. Biomed.* 10: 191–196.

Kwong, K. K., Chesler, D. A., Weisskoff, R. M., Donahue, K. M., Davis, T. L., Ostergaard, L., Campbell, T. A., and Rosen, B. R. 1995. MR perfusion studies with T_1-weighted echo-planar imaging. *Magn. Reson. Med.* 34: 878–887.

Maccotta, L., Detre, J. A., and Alsop, D. C. 1997. The efficiency of adiabatic inversion for perfusion imaging by arterial spin labeling. *Nucl. Magn. Reson. Biomed.* 10: 216–221.

Mai, V. M., Hagspiel, K. D., Christopher, J. M., Do, H. M., Altes, T., Knight-Scott, J., Stith, A. L., Maier, T., and Berr, S. S. 1999. Perfusion imaging of the human lung using flow-sensitive alternating inversion recovery with an extra radiofrequency pulse (FAIRER). *Magn. Reson. Imaging* 17: 355–361.

Marks, M. P., Pelc, N. J., Ross, M. R., and Enzmann, D. R. 1992. Determination of cerebral blood-flow with a phase-contrast cine MR Imaging technique—evaluation of normal subjects and patients with arteriovenous-malformations. *Radiology* 182: 467–476.

Mildner, T., Trampel, R., Moller, H. E., Schafer, A., Wiggins, C. J., and Norris, D. G. 2003. Functional perfusion imaging using continuous arterial spin labeling with separate labeling and imaging coils at 3 T. *Magn. Reson. Med.* 49: 791–795.

Nishimura, D. G., Macovski, A., Pauly, J. M., and Conolly, S. M. 1987. MR angiography by selective inversion recovery. *Magn. Reson. Med.* 4: 193–202.

Ordidge, R. J., Wylezinska, M., Hugg, J. W., Butterworth, E., and Franconi, F. 1996. Frequency offset corrected inversion (FOCI) pulses for use in localized spectroscopy. *Magn. Reson. Med.* 36: 562–566.

Ostergaard, L., Weisskoff, R. M., Chesler, D. A., Gyldensted, C., and Rosen, B. R. 1996. High resolution measurement of cerebral blood flow using intravascular tracer bolus passages, 1: Mathematical approach and statistical analysis. *Magn. Reson. Med.* 36: 715–725.

Pekar, J., Jezzard, P., Roberts, D. A., Leigh, J. S., Frank, J. A., and McLaughlin, A. C. 1996. Perfusion imaging with compensation for asymmetric magnetization transfer effects. *Magn. Reson. Med.* 35: 70–79.

Roberts, D. A., Detre, J. A., Bolinger, L., Insko, E. K., and Leigh, J. S. 1994. Quantitative magnetic resonance imaging of human brain perfusion at 1.5-T using steady-state inversion of arterial water. *Proc. Natl. Acad. Sci. U.S.A.* 91: 33–37.

Rosen, B. R., Belliveau, J. W., Vevea, J. M., and Brady, T. J. 1990. Perfusion imaging with NMR contrast agents. *Magn. Reson. Med.* 14: 249–265.

Schepers, J., van Osch, M. J. P., and Nicolay, K. 2003. Effect of vascular crushing on FAIR perfusion kinetics, using a BIR-4 pulse in a magnetization prepared FLASH sequence. *Magn. Reson. Med.* 50: 608–613.

Schwarzbauer, C., and Heinke, W. 1998. BASE imaging: A new spin labeling technique for measuring absolute perfusion changes. *Magn. Reson. Med.* 39: 717–722.

Silva, A. C., Zhang, W. G., Williams, D. S., and Koretsky, A. P. 1997. Estimation of water extraction fractions in rat brain using magnetic resonance measurement of perfusion with arterial spin labeling. *Magn. Reson. Med.* 37: 58–68.

Talagala, S. L., Barbier, E. L., Williams, D. S., Silva, A. C., and Koretsky, A. P. 1998. Multi-slice perfusion MRI using continuous arterial spin water labeling: Controlling for MT effects with simultaneous proximal and distal RF. In *Proceedings of the 6th Meeting of the International Society of Magnetic Resonance in Medicine*, p 381.

Tanabe, J. L., Yongbi, M., Branch, C., Hrabe, J., Johnson, G., and Helpern, J. A. 1999. MR perfusion imaging in human brain using the UNFAIR technique. *J. Magn. Reson. Imaging* 9: 761–767.

Villringer, A., Rosen, B. R., Belliveau, J. W., Ackerman, J. L., Lauffer, R. B., Buxton, R. B., Chao, Y. S., Wedeen, V. J., and Brady, T. J. 1988. Dynamic imaging with lanthanide chelates in normal brain–contrast due to magnetic susceptibility effects. *Magn. Reson. Med.* 6: 164–174.

Weisskoff, R. M., Chesler, D., Boxerman, J. L., and Rosen, B. R. 1993. Pitfalls in MR measurement of tissue blood-flow with intravascular tracers—which mean transit-time? *Magn. Reson. Med.* 29: 553–559.

Williams, D. S., Detre, J. A., Leigh, J. S., and Koretsky, A. P. 1992. Magnetic resonance imaging of perfusion using spin inversion of arterial water. *Proc. Natl. Acad. Sci. U.S.A.* 89: 212–216.

Wong, E. C., Buxton, R. B., and Frank, L. R. 1997. Implementation of quantitative perfusion imaging techniques for functional brain mapping using pulsed arterial spin labeling. *Nucl. Magn. Reson. Biomed.* 10: 237–249.

Wong, E. C., Buxton, R. B., and Frank, L. R. 1998. Quantitative imaging of perfusion using a single subtraction (QUIPSS and QUIPSS II). *Magn. Reson. Med.* 39: 702–708.

Yang, Y. H. 2002. Perfusion MR imaging with pulsed arterial spin-labeling: Basic principles and applications in functional brain imaging. Concepts Magn. Reson. 14: 347–357.

Yang, Y. H., Frank, J. A., Hou, L., Ye, F. Q., McLaughlin, A. C., and Duyn, J. H. 1998. Multislice imaging of quantitative cerebral perfusion with pulsed arterial spin labeling. *Magn. Reson. Med.* 39: 825–832.

Ye, F. Q., Mattay, V. S., Jezzard, P., Frank, J. A., Weinberger, D. R., and McLaughlin, A. C. 1997. Correction for vascular artifacts in cerebral blood flow values measured by using arterial spin tagging techniques. *Magn. Reson. Med.* 37: 226–235.

Ye, F. Q., Pekar, J. J., Jezzard, P., Duyn, T., Frank, J. A., and McLaughlin, A. C. 1996. Perfusion imaging of the human brain at 1.5 T using a single-shot EPI spin tagging approach. *Magn. Reson. Med.* 36: 219–224.

Yongbi, M. N., Branch, C. A., and Helpern, J. A. 1998. Perfusion imaging using FOCI RF pulses. *Magn. Reson. Med.* 40: 938–943.

Yongbi, M. N., Yang, Y. H., Frank, J. A., and Duyn, J. H. 1999. Multislice perfusion imaging in human brain using the C-FOCI inversion pulse: Comparison with hyperbolic secant. *Magn. Reson. Med.* 42: 1098–1105.

Zaharchuk, G., Ledden, P. J., Kwong, K. K., Reese, T. G., Rosen, B. R., and Wald, L. L. 1999. Multislice perfusion and perfusion territory imaging in humans with separate label and image coils. *Magn. Reson. Med.* 41: 1093–1098.

Zhang, W. G., Silva, A. C., Williams, D. S., and Koretsky, A. P. 1995. NMR measurement of perfusion using arterial spin labeling without saturation of macromolecular spins. *Magn. Reson. Med.* 33: 370–376.

Zhang, W. G., Williams, D. S., and Koretsky, A. P. 1993. Measurement of rat brain perfusion by NMR using spin labeling of arterial water—*in vivo* determination of the degree of spin labeling. *Magn. Reson. Med.* 29: 416–421.

Zhou, J. Y., Mori, S., and van Zijl, P. C. M. 1998. FAIR excluding radiation damping (FAIRER). *Magn. Reson. Med.* 40: 712–719.

Zhan, W., Gu, H., Silbersweig, D. A., Stern, E., and Yang, Y. H. 2002. Inversion profiles of adiabatic inversion pulses for flowing spins: the effects on labeling efficiency and labeling accuracy in perfusion imaging with pulsed arterial spin-labeling. *Magn. Reson. Imaging* 20: 487–494.

RELATED SECTIONS

17.2 Diffusion Imaging

Diffusion is essentially a random walk of molecules in a medium. In the presence of a magnetic field gradient, diffusion of water molecules causes a phase dispersion of the transverse magnetization, resulting in the attenuation of the MRI signal (Carr and Purcell 1954; Stejskal and Tanner 1965). The degree of signal loss depends on tissue type, structure, physical and physiological state, as well as the microenvironment. MRI data acquisition methods that are designed to explore or exploit tissue diffusion properties are collectively called *diffusion imaging* pulse sequences.

To increase the sensitivity to diffusion, all diffusion imaging pulse sequences contain a diffusion-weighting gradient (Section 9.1). In principle, diffusion-weighting gradients can be incorporated into any pulse sequence, although sequences employing RF spin echoes are more popular than those based solely on gradient echoes. Examples of some diffusion imaging sequences include spin echo, spin-echo EPI, RARE (or fast spin echo), stimulated echo acquisition mode (STEAM), steady-state free precession (SSFP), spiral, and GRASE. Most of these pulse sequences are described in their respective sections. The incorporation of diffusion-weighting gradients into several pulse sequences is discussed in subsection 17.2.2. Depending on the imaging pulse sequence that is combined with the diffusion gradients, diffusion imaging can be performed in 1D, 2D, or 3D mode. This section focuses primarily on the 2D diffusion imaging techniques because they are used most frequently.

A diffusion-weighting gradient substantially increases the sensitivity of the sequence to molecular Brownian motion (named after Robert Brown 1773–1858, a British botanist), but it also introduces an undesirable sensitivity to other types of motion, such as bulk motion (Anderson and Gore 1994). To freeze bulk motion, single-shot pulse sequences, such as single-shot EPI, RARE, or spiral, are commonly used. The k-space matrix size of single-shot sequences, however, is limited (e.g., 128×128 or smaller), resulting in rather low spatial resolution (e.g., ~ 2 mm or worse). Multishot diffusion imaging sequences can considerably improve the spatial resolution, but require an accompanying motion correction technique, such as a navigator echo (Section 12.2).

Diffusion imaging is a family of techniques, including (but not limited to) diffusion-weighted imaging (DWI) (Le Bihan et al. 1986), quantitative mapping of diffusion coefficients, diffusion tensor imaging (DTI) (Basser et al. 1994), q-space imaging (Callaghan 1991), and other techniques to measure diffusion anisotropy such as diffusion spectroscopic imaging (DSI) (Tuch et al. 2002) and high-angular-resolution diffusion (HARD) imaging (Frank 2002).

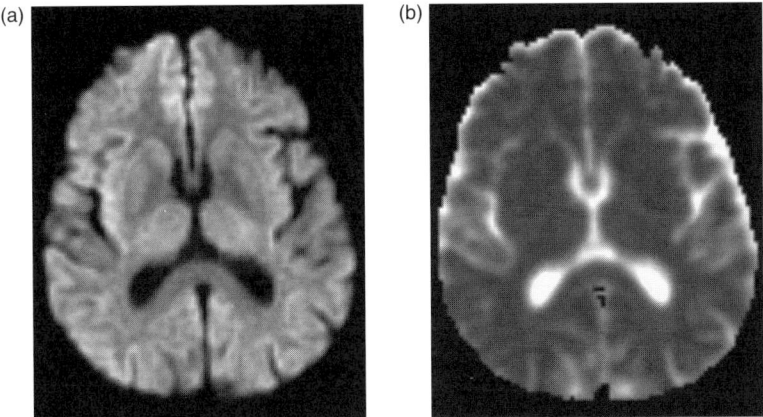

FIGURE 17.11 An example of (a) a DW brain image and (b) a corresponding quantitative ADC map. The DW image was acquired using a single-shot EPI pulse sequence with the following acquisition parameters: $b = 1000\,\text{s/mm}^2$, TR $= 6000\,\text{ms}$, TE $= 73\,\text{ms}$, FOV $= 22\,\text{cm}$, matrix size $= 128 \times 128$, and slice thickness $= 5\,\text{mm}$.

Diffusion-weighted imaging typically employs a single b-value (see Section 9.1) to produce an image. In this image, the intensity of each voxel is exponentially weighted by the average diffusion coefficient of the proton spins within that voxel (Figure 17.11a).

Quantitative diffusion coefficient mapping is based on at least two diffusion-weighted (DW) images, each acquired at the same location but with a different b-value to vary the degree of diffusion weighting. These images are processed to yield a quantitative map that displays the diffusion coefficients (Figure 17.11b). (In the context of this section, we use *map* to denote a calculated image that quantitatively reflects a physical or physiological parameter, and *image* to denote an image that is weighted by a physical or physiological property.) Because the calculated diffusion coefficients can be influenced by tissue perfusion, partial volume averaging, and other experimental errors, they are often referred to as apparent diffusion coefficients (ADCs) (Le Bilhan 1995). Quantitative diffusion coefficient mapping is thus also called ADC mapping. (Note that in the literature the abbreviation *ADC* is also used to denote the analog-to-digital converter hardware in the receiver chain. To avoid confusion, we abbreviate the name of that device by A/D.)

Diffusion tensor imaging is a technique that measures the spatial orientation dependence, or anisotropy, of the diffusion process. It requires not only at least two b-values, but also six or more independent diffusion gradient directions to produce a set of DW images. The independent directions are often referred to as noncollinear in the literature, although they cannot all lie in the same plane either. Through a series of mathematical calculations, the set of DW images can be converted to scalar and vector maps that describe a variety of tissue diffusion properties. Scalar diffusion anisotropy maps are used to visualize the location, size, and integrity of fibrous structures such as white-matter fiber tracts in the brain (Pierpaoli and Basser 1996). Vector anisotropy indices provide information on diffusion spatial orientation that can be used to infer fiber tract connectivity in three dimensions (Xue et al. 1999; Basser et al. 2000). In both cases, it is assumed that anisotropy in the diffusion process correlates to the structure of the tissue.

q-Space imaging (Cory and Garroway 1990; Callaghan et al. 1991) is less commonly used in MRI than the previously mentioned techniques, but has received renewed interest in recent years (Assaf et al. 2002; Basser 2002). It produces a diffusion displacement probability profile, from which translational displacement, diffusion coefficient, root-mean-squared spatial displacement, and the size of diffusion microenvironment can be measured. The spatial displacement that can be obtained from q-space imaging is typically much smaller than an imaging voxel dimension, which makes q-space imaging particularly attractive for microscopic studies (Callaghan et al. 1988).

17.2.1 BASICS OF DIFFUSION IN BIOLOGICAL TISSUES

Molecular diffusion is a stochastic thermal phenomenon characterized by Brownian motion. The behavior of the unrestricted diffusion is described by the equation:

$$r_{rms} = \sqrt{2Dt} \qquad (17.23)$$

which relates the 1D root-mean-squared displacement (r_{rms}) to the diffusion time (t) and the diffusion coefficient D. D is in distance squared per time (e.g., mm^2/s). Equation (17.23) is known as the Einstein equation, after Albert Einstein (1879–1955), the well-known German and American physicist.

In biological tissues, diffusion of water molecules is affected by the presence of macromolecules, organelles, cell membrane, and other cellular and subcellular structures (Le Bihan 1995). These structures manifest themselves as obstacles to molecular diffusion and can considerably reduce the diffusion coefficient of water. For example, intracellular space has a higher concentration of macromolecules and organelles than the interstitial space or extracellular space. Consequently, the diffusion coefficient in intracellular space is believed to be many times smaller than that in extracellular space (van Zijl et al. 1990; Inglis et al. 2001). The substantial difference between intracellular and extracellular diffusion coefficients has been exploited in several applications that relate diffusion measurements to cell-density changes during disease progression and regression (Sugahara et al. 1999; Zhou et al. 2002).

Generally, the restrictions on water diffusion imposed by macromolecules and tissue structures do not have spherical symmetry. The restriction in one direction can be considerably greater than that in other directions. This causes a phenomenon known as diffusion anisotropy, which means the diffusion varies with spatial orientation. Molecular diffusion in an anisotropic medium is described by multiple diffusion coefficients to account for the directional dependence. Mathematically, the directional dependence can be expressed as a second-rank tensor, known as the *diffusion tensor* (Basser et al. 1994), which is cast in a 3×3 matrix:

$$\overline{\overline{D}} = \begin{bmatrix} D_{xx} & D_{xy} & D_{xz} \\ D_{xy} & D_{yy} & D_{yz} \\ D_{xz} & D_{yz} & D_{zz} \end{bmatrix} \qquad (17.24)$$

Each of the six independent matrix elements in Eq. (17.24) represents a unique diffusion coefficient defined in a laboratory reference frame with x, y, and z being the spatial coordinates. (Without loss of generality, we have assumed that the physical axes, X, Y, Z, in the laboratory frame coincide with the logical axes, x, y, z, and have used lowercase x, y, and z for the subscripts of the diffusion coefficients in Eq. 17.24.) A matrix element along the diagonal corresponds to diffusion along that axis in the laboratory reference frame, and an off-diagonal element represents the degree of correlation between random motion in the two directions. The elements of the diffusion tensor are real, and the matrix in Eq. (17.24) is symmetric; that is, the matrix is unchanged when its elements are transposed. An intuitive description of the diffusion tensor is that the diffusion boundary at each spatial location is ellipsoidal, with three root-mean-squared (rms) spatial displacements r_1, r_2, and r_3, along the three axes, each obeying Eq. (17.23):

$$\begin{cases} r_1 = \sqrt{2D_1 t} \\ r_2 = \sqrt{2D_2 t} \\ r_3 = \sqrt{2D_3 t} \end{cases} \qquad (17.25)$$

where D_1, D_2, and D_3 are the corresponding diffusion coefficients along the axes of the diffusion ellipsoid shown in Figure 17.12. Note that here we use the term *diffusion boundary* to refer to the surface of the diffusion ellipsoid rather than the physical boundary that causes diffusion anisotropy or the boundary defined by the rms displacements.

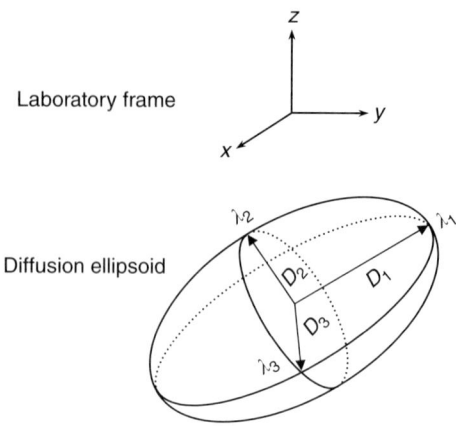

FIGURE 17.12 Anisotropic diffusion can be described by a diffusion ellipsoid with the semiaxes equal to the amplitude of the diffusion tensor eigenvalues D_1, D_2, and D_3. The directions of the three axes coincide with the directions of the eigenvectors $\vec{\lambda}_1$, $\vec{\lambda}_2$, and $\vec{\lambda}_3$.

In an isotropic diffusion medium, such as cerebrospinal fluid (CSF), the diffusion tensor described by Eq. (17.24) reduces to a single diffusion coefficient D (i.e, $D_{xx} = D_{yy} = D_{zz} = D$, and $D_{xy} = D_{yz} = D_{xz} = 0$). In an anisotropic diffusion medium, at least one of the three diffusion coefficients D_1, D_2, and D_3 is unequal to the other two. For example, in white-matter fiber tracts, the diffusion coefficient along the direction of the fiber tract is considerably larger than that of the other directions. This direction is often referred to as the principal diffusion direction. By characterizing the diffusion tensor at each spatial location, structures with varying degrees of diffusion anisotropy can be distinguished from one another. For fibrous tissues with a high degree of diffusion anisotropy, the fiber orientation and connectivity can also be revealed based on the principal diffusion directions, as further discussed in subsection 17.2.5.

17.2.2 DIFFUSION IMAGING PULSE SEQUENCES

Single-Shot Spin-Echo EPI　At the present time, single-shot spin-echo EPI is the most prevalent sequence for diffusion imaging due to its high acquisition speed (e.g., <100 ms per image) and motion insensitivity. Figure 17.13 shows a diffusion-weighted single-shot spin-echo EPI pulse sequence. In this pulse sequence, a pair of identical diffusion-weighting gradient lobes are placed on either side the 180° refocusing pulse. The gradient direction can be

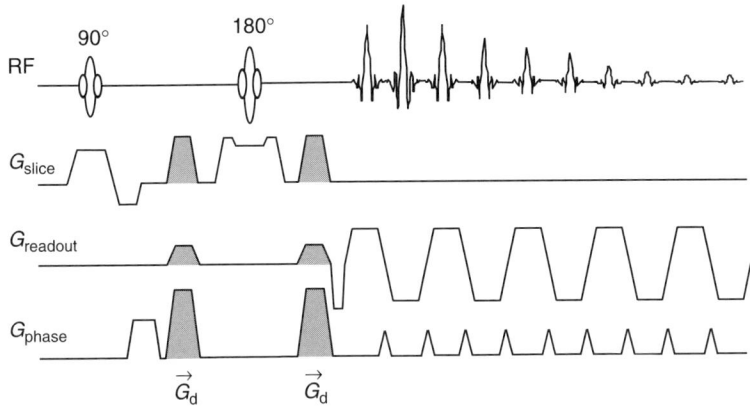

FIGURE 17.13 A diffusion-weighted single-shot spin-echo EPI pulse sequence. The diffusion-weighting gradient (shaded) can be applied in any arbitrary direction by varying the relative components along the three orthogonal gradient axes. For simplicity, only the positive gradient lobes are shown. (The diffusion-weighting gradient is not drawn to scale.)

controlled by varying its vector components (shown in shaded areas) along the three orthogonal axes. To minimize TE, the maximal gradient amplitude h is used to achieve the desired b-value. Although using the maximal slew rate S_R also reduces TE, its use can cause the pulse sequence to exceed regulatory limits for peripheral nerve stimulation. In addition, depending on the time constants, a faster slew rate can also cause more problems from eddy currents induced by the diffusion-weighting gradient.

Diffusion pulse sequences based on single-shot EPI inherit virtually all of the artifacts associated with EPI. For example, distortion caused by magnetic susceptibility variations is frequently observed in the frontal sinus and regions near the temporal bone. The susceptibility variations are difficult to correct even on a scanner equipped with resistive higher-order shimming coils. The susceptibility artifacts increase linearly with the field strength B_0. The recent advent of parallel imaging can help reduce susceptibility-induced artifacts by reducing the echo train length and thereby the amount of time that the off-resonant spins accumulate phase errors. Many system imperfections such as eddy currents and mismatches in hardware group delays can cause Nyquist ghosts in DW images by the mechanisms discussed in Section 16.1. The ghosts are typically less conspicuous than those in non-DW EPI images, primarily due to the reduced SNR. The image distortion caused by the eddy currents, however, is commonly seen in DW echo planar images. This artifact is further discussed in subsection 17.2.7.

RARE Sequences Incorporating a diffusion-weighting gradient into a RARE (or fast spin echo) pulse sequence is not straightforward. This is because adding a pair of diffusion-weighting gradient lobes that straddles the first RF refocusing pulse violates the CPMG conditions (see Section 16.4). This causes inconsistent phase errors between the spin echoes and the stimulated echoes, leading to signal loss and increased artifacts.

One approach that addresses this problem is to first prepare the transverse magnetization with proper diffusion weighting (Alsop 1997), then store the diffusion-prepared magnetization on the longitudinal axis, and finally recall this magnetization by employing stimulated echoes (Alsop 1997; Norris et al. 1992; McKinnon 2000). Because the signal from the primary echo is discarded, the images produced by this sequence suffer from low SNR. The signal loss can be substantially reduced by employing RF refocusing pulses with quadratic phase (i.e., non-CPMG fast spin echo), as described by Bastin and Le Roux (2002). An alternative approach is to play out the diffusion-weighting gradient around the first RF refocusing pulse in the refocusing pulse train and to use crusher gradients to eliminate signal from the stimulated echoes while preserving the spin echo signal (Beaulieu et al. 1993). (In this section, a spin echo means the primary spin echo as defined in Section 16.4.) Although this pulse sequence does not satisfy the CPMG conditions, as long as the B_1 field is homogeneous and the flip angles of the refocusing RF pulses are close to 180°, signal loss can be minimized. A pulse sequence employing this method is shown in Figure 17.14.

If the imperfect refocusing pulses are played out in the presence of an imbalanced readout gradient waveform (e.g., the readout gradient area is more than twice the prephasing gradient area), it has been shown that two families of echoes are produced in the echo train (Norris et al. 1992). Starting from the second refocusing pulse, each readout window can contain two echoes with different phases because of the violation of the CPMG conditions (i.e., the stimulated echo and the spin echoes are not in phase.). In a pulse sequence known as split acquisition of fast spin echo signals for diffusion imaging (SPLICE) each readout window is made sufficiently long so that the two echoes can be acquired separately (Schick 1997). Two separate DW images are reconstructed, one from each of the two echo families. The two magnitude (i.e., not complex) images are combined to improve the SNR. In this way, signals from both spin echoes and stimulated echoes can be used. A disadvantage of SPLICE is that the echo spacing must be prolonged by approximately 15–30%) to accommodate the acquisition of two echoes at each echo spacing interval, leading to increased image blurring or shorter echo train length. A SPLICE pulse sequence is shown in Figure 17.15, in which diffusion weighting is prepared using a stimulated echo (see additional discussion later).

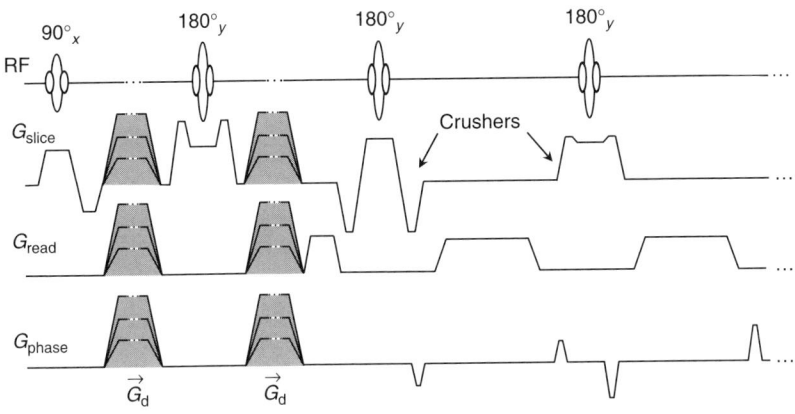

FIGURE 17.14 A diffusion-weighted RARE pulse sequence. The diffusion-weighting gradient pair (shaded) straddles the first refocusing pulse. The direction of the diffusion gradient is controlled by varying the relative components along the three orthogonal gradient axes. The diffusion gradients are shown as positive lobes, but any diffusion gradient lobe can be negative as well. Stimulated echo signal is dephased by varying the amplitude and (or) polarity of the crusher gradients. Coherence pathways based on spin echoes are used to produce the DW image. The refocusing pulses should have flip angles as close as possible to 180°. The phase of the RF pulses is indicated by the subscript of the flip angle for each pulse.

At the present time, diffusion pulse sequences based on RARE are still an active area of research and have not been as widely used as EPI.

Spin Echo Sequence Figure 17.16 shows a spin echo pulse sequence with a pair of diffusion gradients straddling the RF refocusing pulse. The implementation of this pulse sequence is straightforward, although a navigator echo (not shown in Figure 17.16) is typically required to monitor the motion-induced phase variations and correct the phase error during image reconstruction (Ordidge et al. 1994; de Crespigny et al. 1995). With proper motion correction, spin echo pulse sequences can yield high-quality high-resolution DW images with minimal artifacts. The data acquisition time, however, can be very long (10–20 min), which inhibits its widespread acceptance for clinical applications. Spin echo diffusion imaging is another area that can potentially benefit from parallel-imaging techniques.

Stimulated Echo Pulse Sequences A DW stimulated echo sequence is shown in Figure 17.17. Three 90° pulses with the same phase (e.g., all applied along the *x* axis in the rotating reference frame) are used to produce a stimulated

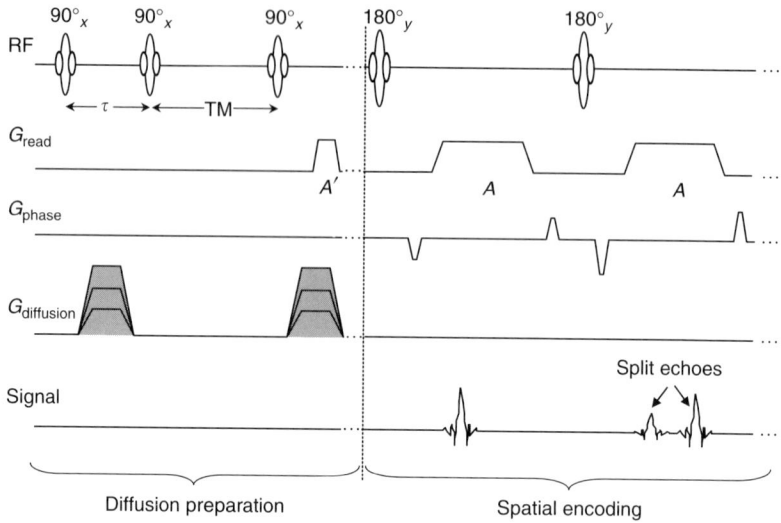

FIGURE 17.15 A SPLICE pulse sequence using RARE with a stimulated echo diffusion preparation. One diffusion gradient lobe is applied between the first two 90° pulses, and the other after the third 90° pulse (For simplicity, only the positive diffusion gradient lobes are shown as indicated by the shaded areas). The TM time allows a high b-value to be achieved without incurring the T_2^*- and T_2-induced signal decay because the magnetization is stored along the longitudinal axis. The readout gradient waveform is not balanced because the pre-phasing area A' is less than one-half of the readout area A. This produces two echo families when the refocusing pulses deviate from 180°. Two split echoes are acquired at each readout window. The slice-selection gradient waveform is not shown. The diffusion-weighting gradient can be applied to any axes.

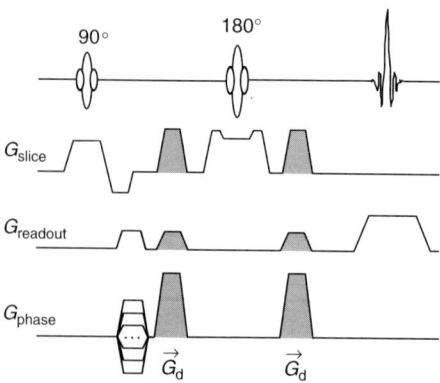

FIGURE 17.16 A diffusion-weighted spin echo pulse sequence. A navigator echo (not shown) is often required to detect and correct the phase errors due to motion.

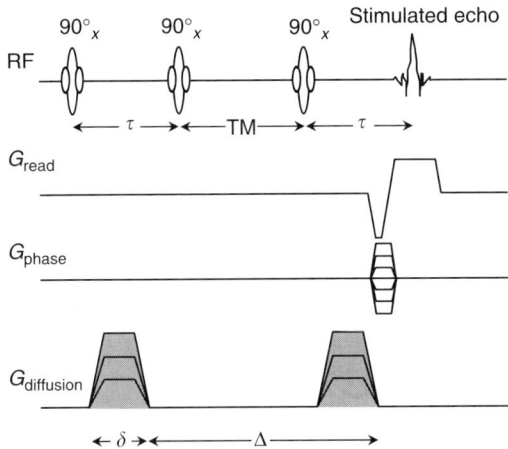

FIGURE 17.17 A diffusion-weighted stimulated echo (i.e., STEAM) pulse sequence. For simplicity, the slice-selection gradient waveform is not shown. The diffusion-weighting gradient can be applied to any axes.

echo. The first two pulses are separated by a time delay τ. After the same delay τ following the third pulse, a stimulated echo is produced. In order to introduce diffusion weighting into the stimulated echo, two identical diffusion gradient lobes are applied, one during the first and one during the second τ interval. Because the magnetization for the stimulated echo is stored along the longitudinal axis between the second and the third RF pulses, it does not experience any T_2^* or T_2 dephasing during the time interval TM. TM, however, does contribute to the diffusion gradient lobe separation Δ. Thus, a high b-value can be obtained without incurring the TE-induced signal loss, as compared to the spin echo and spin-echo EPI pulse sequences in Figures 17.16 and 17.14. The SNR of the stimulated echo pulse sequence, however, is less than that of the corresponding spin echo sequence with the same TE because the maximal amplitude of the stimulated echo is only one-half of that of a spin echo. The pulse sequence shown in Figure 17.17 is also known as a DW STEAM (stimulated echo acquisition mode) pulse sequence (Merboldt et al. 1985).

If the third pulse in Figure 17.17 is replaced by a series of low flip angle pulses separated by a short TR, a high-speed DW STEAM pulse sequence results (Merboldt et al. 1992). Similar to the SPLICE sequence shown in Figure 17.15, the stimulated echo produced by the first three RF pulses is used to prepare DW magnetization so that it can be used for subsequent spatial encoding with a fast gradient echo sequence. The high-speed DW STEAM pulse sequence has been used to produce single-shot diffusion images from the human brain with relatively low spatial resolution (Merboldt et al. 1992).

Other Diffusion Pulse Sequences In addition to the pulse sequences already discussed, many other sequences have been developed for diffusion imaging. Diffusion-weighted GRASE provides a good compromise between EPI and FSE, but problems inherent to both techniques must be dealt with (Liu et al. 1996). Diffusion-weighted spiral has a data acquisition speed comparable to EPI. For multishot spiral, multiple spiral interleaves all sample the center point in k-space, allowing zeroth-order phase correction to be performed without the need of additional navigator echoes (Chenevert et al. 1996; Tsukamoto et al. 1996). This concept of employing k-space data consistency is also used in DW projection acquisition and PROPELLER imaging (Section 17.5) to address the problem with motion sensitivity (Pipe et al. 2002). In DW projection acquisition, the motion-induced phase errors can also be removed by inverse Fourier transforming a radial k-space line to obtain a projection, followed by Fourier transforming the *magnitude* of the projection back to k-space. The resultant k-space data are regridded and inverse-Fourier-transformed to obtain the final image (Trouard et al. 1999). Diffusion-weighted line scan acquires a two-dimensional image one line at a time (Maier et al. 1998). Motion-induced inconsistent phase errors are removed prior to combining all the lines to form a 2D DW image. An example of a diffusion imaging pulse sequence using gradient echoes with echo shifting is discussed in Section 16.3. This sequence allows the two lobes of the diffusion-weighting gradients to be separated by one or more TR intervals (Delalande et al. 1999). Therefore, a high *b*-value can be achieved with a large gradient lobe separation Δ, analogous to the stimulated echo diffusion sequence discussed previously.

17.2.3 DIFFUSION-WEIGHTED IMAGING

In the presence of a gradient, molecular diffusion attenuates the MRI signal exponentially:

$$S = S_0 e^{-bD} \tag{17.26}$$

where S and S_0 are the voxel signal intensity with and without diffusion, respectively; D is the diffusion coefficient along the direction of the applied diffusion gradient; and b is the b-factor or b-value (see Section 9.1) that controls the degree of diffusion weighting in the image. The spatial dependence of D, S, and S_0 is not explicitly expressed in Eq. (17.26) to simplify the notation. At a given b-value, tissue with fast diffusion (e.g., CSF in the brain) experiences more signal loss, resulting in low intensity in the DW image, whereas tissue

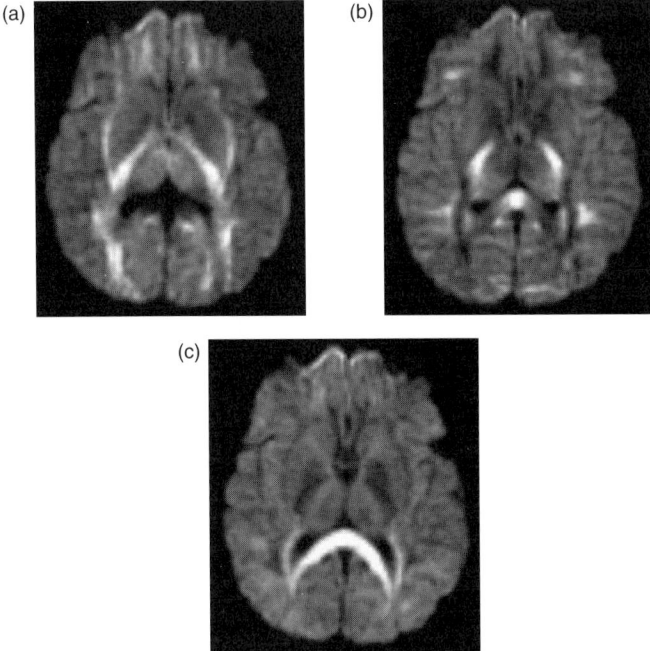

FIGURE 17.18 Three diffusion-weighted images acquired with the same b-value, but different gradient directions. Images are acquired with gradients along the (a) right-left, (b) anterior-posterior, and (c) superior-inferior directions.

with slow diffusion (e.g., gray matter) produces high intensity in the image (Figure 17.11a).

Equation (17.26) is valid for a diffusion-weighting gradient in any arbitrary direction. For a given diffusion gradient direction, contrast of the resultant DW image is specific to that gradient direction and can change with patient orientation. To remove the patient-orientation dependence, three DW images can be obtained, each with a diffusion-weighting gradient applied along one of the three orthogonal directions (e.g., physical X, Y, and Z gradient directions, or logical x, y, and z directions; Figure 17.18) (Sorensen et al. 1996). The corresponding MRI signal intensities for the general case of anisotropic diffusion are:

$$S_x = S_0 e^{-b_{xx} D_{xx}} \tag{17.27}$$

$$S_y = S_0 e^{-b_{yy} D_{yy}} \tag{17.28}$$

$$S_z = S_0 e^{-b_{zz} D_{zz}} \tag{17.29}$$

where b_{xx}, b_{yy}, and b_{zz} are the b-values associated with each diffusion gradient. Note that any nonzero off-diagonal matrix elements in the diffusion tensor do not contribute to Eqs. (17.27)–(17.29), provided that the diffusion-weighting gradient axes correspond to the axes of the coordinate system in which the diffusion tensor in Eq. (17.24) is defined. If the same b-value is used in all three directions (i.e., $b_{xx} = b_{yy} = b_{zz} \equiv b$), the geometric mean of the three signals is:

$$S_{xyz} \equiv \sqrt[3]{S_x S_y S_z} = S_0 e^{-b(D_{xx}+D_{yy}+D_{zz})/3} = S_0 e^{-bD_{\text{trace}}/3} \qquad (17.30)$$

where D_{trace} is the sum of the diagonal elements of the matrix in Eq. (17.24) and is known as the trace. The trace of a matrix is rotationally invariant; that is, it has the same numerical value if the matrix is expressed in a rotated coordinate system. Because of this property, the image intensity S_{xyz} is independent of patient orientation. The DW image obtained using this scheme is sometimes called the isotropic DW image or diffusion-trace-weighted image. Although the three diffusion gradient directions are most commonly selected to be along the orthogonal logical axes, any three directions can be used as long as they are mutually perpendicular to one another.

When a single-shot EPI pulse sequence is employed, the individual DW images used to produce the diffusion-trace-weighted image can contain inconsistent distortion, causing problems with image registration. To address this problem, a single DW image can be acquired with multiple diffusion-weighting gradient lobes along different axes in a single sequence (Mori and Zijl 1996; Wong et al. 1995). For example, a diffusion gradient lobe can be successively applied along each of the three gradient axes before a 180° refocusing pulse and again after the refocusing pulse. Although the resulting DW image is not exactly weighted by D_{trace}, the effect of diffusion anisotropy is notably reduced. By selecting a proper pattern of the diffusion gradient lobes in the pulse sequence, an image weighted by D_{trace} can also be obtained. A primary drawback of this technique is that it requires a higher diffusion gradient amplitude or a longer TE in order to achieve the same b-value compared to the simpler pulse sequence in Figure 17.13.

Clinically, the primary application of DWI has been for the early detection of cerebral ischemia (Warach et al. 1996). The regions under ischemic attack exhibit a hyperintense signal on DW images, with easily discernable contrast relative to normal brain tissue. It has been reported that the contrast between the early stage of stroke and the healthy tissue is typically not observed in conventional T_1- and T_2-weighted images, until damage at the cellular level considerably changes the tissue-relaxation properties.

17.2.4 QUANTITATIVE APPARENT DIFFUSION COEFFICIENT MAPPING

In quantitative ADC mapping, a series of DW images are acquired with multiple b-values, $S_1 = S_0 e^{-b_1 D}$, $S_2 = S_0 e^{-b_2 D}$, ..., $S_n = S_0 e^{-b_n D}$. Each signal can represent the geometric average of three DW images as described by Eq. (17.30) to remove the patient-orientation dependence. A linear fit between $\ln(S_0/S_i)$ and b_i is performed on a pixel-by-pixel basis, and the slope of a linear regression yields the apparent diffusion coefficient D. This process is very similar to T_2 mapping based on a series of T_2-weighted images with varying TE values (see Section 14.3). The pixel-by-pixel ADC values form an ADC map whose image contrast is inverted compared to a DW image (Figure 17.11). For example, tissues with a high diffusion coefficient appear hyperintense in an ADC map, but hypointense in a DW image.

When acquiring a series of DW images for ADC mapping, it is important to keep imaging parameters (other than the b-value) identical. To maintain a constant TE, b-values are typically changed by varying the diffusion-gradient amplitude instead of its duration. In addition, the contribution from imaging gradients should be included in the b-value calculation in order to avoid overestimation of the ADC value.

Example 17.2 In a diffusion pulse sequence, the diffusion-weighting gradient produces a b-value of $500\,\text{s/mm}^2$ and the imaging gradients contribute $40\,\text{s/mm}^2$ to the b-value. The measured DW signal is $S = 0.4S_0$. What is the ADC value if the contribution from the imaging gradients to the b-value is (a) neglected and (b) considered?

Solution

(a) Substituting $S = 0.4S_0$ and $b = 500\,\text{s/mm}^2$ into Eq. (17.26), we have:

$$D = \frac{\ln(0.4)}{-500} = 1.8 \times 10^{-3}\,\text{mm}^2/\text{s}$$

(b) Using $b = (500 + 40) = 540\,\text{s/mm}^2$, D is recalculated to be:

$$D = \frac{\ln(0.4)}{-540} = 1.7 \times 10^{-3}\,\text{mm}^2/\text{s}$$

Therefore, D is overestimated unless the imaging gradients are considered.

When an imaging gradient waveform G_{im} (G_{im} can be a readout, phase-encoding, or slice-selection gradient) is accounted for, the b-value has the following general form (Mattiello et al. 1994):

$$b = c_1 G_d^2 + c_2 G_d G_{im} + c_3 G_{im}^2 \tag{17.31}$$

where G_d is the diffusion gradient amplitude, and c_1, c_2, and c_3 are the coefficients that depend on the details of the pulse sequence. These coefficients can be analytically or numerically calculated using Eq. (9.5). The first term is expected from the diffusion-weighting gradient, as described in Section 9.1. The last term is independent of the diffusion gradient and, consequently, can be absorbed into S_0. The second term is known as the cross-term. Because the imaging gradient waveforms differ among the three logical (or physical) axes, the cross-term contribution varies with the direction of the diffusion gradient. This gives rise to false diffusion anisotropy, as well as overestimation of the ADC value. The cross-term can be compensated for during ADC mapping if the term $c_2 G_d G_{im}$ is known (Mattiello et al. 1994; Neeman et al. 1990). Because the phase-encoding gradient is changing during k-space space data acquisition, cross-term correction is typically used only for the readout and slice-selection gradient waveforms (Neeman et al. 1990; Eis and Hoehnberlage 1995).

When the b-value exceeds ~ 1500 s/mm^2, it has been shown that diffusion imaging signal of the brain tissue exhibits biexponential decay (Inglis et al. 2001; Mulkern et al. 1999; Clark et al. 2002), as described by:

$$S = S_0 \left(\xi e^{-bD_f} + (1 - \xi) e^{-bD_s} \right) \qquad (17.32)$$

where ξ and $(\xi - 1)$ are the diffusion compartmental fractions, and D_f and D_s are the ADCs for the fast and slow diffusion components, respectively. To produce maps of D_f, D_s, and ξ, nonlinear fitting algorithms such as Levenberg-Marquardt can be used (Press et al. 1992). Although it has been hypothesized that the two compartments could originate from the intracellular and the extracellular spaces, a good correlation between diffusion measurements and known cell-volume fraction has not been well established (Mulkern et al. 1999; Clark et al. 2002).

To minimize the effects of tissue relaxation in diffusion imaging, DW images should be acquired with sufficiently long TR (e.g., TR $> 4T_1$) and short TE (e.g., TE $< 3T_2$). Although long TR can be used in diffusion imaging pulse sequences, especially those based on echo trains, the time needed to play out the diffusion-weighting gradient can considerably prolong the minimum TE (e.g., TE$_{min}$ = 70 ms), which introduces T_2 or T_2^* contrast into the DW image. This effect can reverse (i.e., invert) the actual diffusion contrast in the brain tissue and is sometimes called T_2 *shine-through*.

Quantitative ADC mapping is an effective way to remove the T_2 shine-through effect. To reduce the scan time for ADC mapping, two b-values can be used, one at (or close to) zero to obtain S_0 and the other larger (e.g., $b = 1000$ s/mm^2) to measure S. Thus, ADC can be directly calculated from

Eq. (17.26) without a linear regression. If diffusion anisotropy is a concern, the image with nonzero b-value can be acquired three times, as described in subsection 17.2.3. An average ADC map (i.e., a map based on $D_{\text{trace}}/3$) can be calculated using Eq. (17.30).

Another approach to eliminate the T_2 shine-through effect is to calculate the ratio of the two images S and S_0 acquired with and without the diffusion-weighting gradient while keeping all other acquisition parameters identical. The ratio, evaluated on a pixel-by-pixel basis, yields an image weighted only by e^{-bD}, effectively eliminating any confounding T_2 effects without explicitly calculating ADC. An additional benefit of this approach is that the resultant image contrast is not reversed, as in the case of ADC mapping. This image is sometimes called an exponential diffusion image.

17.2.5 DIFFUSION TENSOR IMAGING

As discussed in Section 17.2.1, tissue structure imposes a nonspherical geometry on water diffusion boundaries, leading to diffusion anisotropy. A single, scalar diffusion coefficient D (or ADC) no longer suffices to describe diffusion in anisotropic media. Instead, a diffusion tensor given by Eq. (17.24) is used. DTI is a technique that maps diffusion anisotropy at each spatial location using the diffusion tensor formalism. Many types of images can be calculated from a DTI acquisition. Examples include scalar diffusion anisotropy indices, individual diffusion coefficients, ADC, trace, and vector maps of the principal diffusion direction.

Determination of Diffusion Tensor Elements   When diffusion anisotropy is considered, Eq. (17.26) is generalized to:

$$S_j = S_0 \exp\left(-4\pi^2 \int \vec{k}_j \cdot \overline{\overline{D}} \cdot \vec{k}_j^T \, dt\right) \qquad (17.33)$$

where

$$\vec{k}_j = \frac{\gamma}{2\pi} \int_0^t \vec{G}_j(t') dt' \qquad (17.34)$$

j is the index of the diffusion gradient orientation ($j = 1, 2, 3, \ldots, N$), and superscript T denotes transpose of the matrix representation of a vector. Neglecting the imaging gradients (i.e., $\vec{G}_j(t')$ is approximated by the diffusion gradient $\vec{G}_{dj}(t')$), we obtain:

$$S_j = S_0 \exp\left(-b \cdot \begin{bmatrix} u_j & v_j & w_j \end{bmatrix} \cdot \begin{bmatrix} D_{xx} & D_{xy} & D_{xz} \\ D_{xy} & D_{yy} & D_{yz} \\ D_{xz} & D_{yz} & D_{zz} \end{bmatrix} \cdot \begin{bmatrix} u_j \\ v_j \\ w_j \end{bmatrix}\right)$$

$$= S_0 e^{-bQ_j} \tag{17.35}$$

where u_j, v_j, and w_j are the direction cosines of the diffusion gradient vector $\vec{G}_{dj}(t')$:

$$\vec{G}_{dj}(t') = G_{dj}\begin{bmatrix} u_j & v_j & w_j \end{bmatrix} \tag{17.36}$$

The product Q_j of the vector transpose, matrix, and vector in Eq. (17.35) is known as the quadratic form of the diffusion tensor matrix. The quadratic form only takes on positive values and is a function of u_j^2, w_j^2, v_j^2, and hyperbolic terms such as $u_j w_j$. The elements of the matrix are the coefficients of this second-order polynomial. Geometrically, the quadratic form represents an ellipsoid when it is plotted in the $u_j w_j v_j$ coordinate system. If the axes of that coordinate system are aligned with the principal axes of the diffusion tensor, all the hyperbolic terms drop out, and the quadratic form simplifies to:

$$Q_j = D_1 u_j^2 + D_2 v_j^2 + D_3 w_j^2 \tag{17.37}$$

where D_1, D_2, and D_3 are defined in Eq. (17.25).

Similar to ADC measurement, the calculation of the diffusion tensor in Eq. (17.35) requires at least two b-values. Unlike the ADC measurement, however, the diffusion gradient must change its orientation along at least six noncollinear, noncoplanar directions at any b-value except for $b = 0$ (where the gradient directions are degenerate). Thus, the minimum number of images that must be acquired in DTI is seven: one with a zero b-value to yield S_0, and six with nonzero b-values to produce $S_1, S_2, \ldots, S_6$. . With this data set and known diffusion gradient directions, the six elements of the diffusion tensor can be evaluated by solving the following linear equation:

$$I_j \equiv \ln\left(S_0/S_j\right) = b \cdot \begin{bmatrix} u_j & v_j & w_j \end{bmatrix} \cdot \begin{bmatrix} D_{xx} & D_{xy} & D_{xz} \\ D_{xy} & D_{yy} & D_{yz} \\ D_{xz} & D_{yz} & D_{zz} \end{bmatrix} \cdot \begin{bmatrix} u_j \\ v_j \\ w_j \end{bmatrix}$$

$$= bQ_j \quad\quad j = 0, 1, 2, \ldots, N \tag{17.38}$$

When the number of gradient directions exceeds six, the tensor elements can be obtained using a least-squares fitting algorithm, such as singular value decomposition (SVD) (Arfken 1970).

The number of diffusion gradient directions (N) used in DTI data acquisition along with the spatial distribution of gradient directions at a given N are collectively referred to as the *diffusion gradient scheme*. Many diffusion gradient schemes have been published and evaluated in the literature (Jones et al. 1999; Skare et al. 2000; Papadakis et al. 1999; Poonawalla et al. 2000). Increasing N typically improves the precision of DTI tensor element calculation and produces diffusion anisotropy maps with superior quality. However, the gain in image quality becomes progressively less when the number of directions exceeds $\sim$25, provided that the total acquisition time is held constant by trading off the number of gradient directions N with the number of signal averages (Poonawalla and Zhou 2004).

For a specified value of N, there are infinite ways to distribute the N noncollinear gradient directions in the 3D space. The optimal distribution of gradient orientations is an active area of current research in DTI. The present consensus is to distribute the diffusion gradient directions as uniformly as possible across three dimensions (Jones et al. 1999; Skare et al. 2000; Papadakis et al. 1999; Batchelor et al. 2003). A common criterion in evaluating the diffusion gradient scheme is to minimize the condition number (Skare et al. 2000).

Scalar Diffusion Anisotropy Calculations　　The diffusion tensor elements (D_{xx}, D_{xy}, D_{yz}, ...) are defined in the laboratory coordinate system and thus are patient-orientation-dependent. To eliminate this dependency, the diffusion tensor matrix obtained from Eq. (17.38) can be diagonalized to the following form:

$$\overline{\overline{D'}} = \begin{bmatrix} D_1 & 0 & 0 \\ 0 & D_2 & 0 \\ 0 & 0 & D_3 \end{bmatrix} \tag{17.39}$$

This is equivalent to using a new coordinate system that is aligned along the three axes of the diffusion ellipsoid at each spatial location. The elements, D_1, D_2, and D_3, of Eq. (17.39) are known as the characteristic values or eigenvalues of the matrix. The sum of the three eigenvalues is the trace of the diffusion tensor, discussed in subsection 17.2.3. Each eigenvalue D_i ($i = 1, 2, 3$) corresponds to a characteristic vector or eigenvector $\bar{\lambda}_i$. If one eigenvalue is considerably larger than the other two (such as in the case of white-matter fiber tracts in the brain), the largest eigenvalue is referred to as the principal diffusion coefficient and its eigenvector is aligned along the principal diffusion direction. This scenario is graphically shown in Figure 17.12.

Once the eigenvalues are known, a number of diffusion parameters can be produced. For example, each eigenvalue can be used to form its own map to show the apparent diffusion coefficient along each axis of the diffusion ellipsoid. The sum of the eigenvalues can yield another map that is mathematically equivalent to a diffusion trace map described by Eq. (17.30). This map can be further used to synthesize a diffusion-trace-weighted image. To visualize the location of the fiber tracts, a diffusion anisotropy image is typically calculated based on one of several scalar anisotropy indices, such as relative anisotropy (RA), fractional anisotropy (FA), or volume ratio (VR) (Pierpaoli and Basser 1996; Ulug and van Zijl 1999):

$$RA = \frac{1}{\sqrt{3}D_{avg}} \sqrt{\sum_{i=1}^{3}(D_i - D_{avg})^2} \tag{17.40}$$

$$FA = \sqrt{1.5} \frac{\sqrt{\sum_{i=1}^{3}(D_i - D_{avg})^2}}{\sqrt{\sum_{i=1}^{3} D_i^2}} \tag{17.41}$$

$$VR = \frac{D_1 D_2 D_3}{D_{avg}^3} \tag{17.42}$$

where

$$D_{avg} = \frac{D_1 + D_2 + D_3}{3} \tag{17.43}$$

Both relative anisotropy and fractional anisotropy are based on the standard deviation of the eigenvalues, but they are normalized by different denominators and coefficients. Relative anisotropy ranges from 0 to $\sqrt{2}$ and is linear over a wide range of diffusion anisotropy found in the human brain tissues. Fractional anisotropy, which has values ranging from 0 to 1, has been found to be more sensitive than RA at low values of anisotropy. An FA map from a healthy human subject is shown in Figure 17.19.

Tractography Magnetic resonance tractography is a technique that maps the tissue fiber orientation and connectivity in three dimensions, guided by the principal diffusion directions (Xue et al. 1999; Basser et al. 2000). It is primarily used for tracking the white-matter fiber tracts in the brain, although applications to other tissues are also possible (Wedeen et al. 2001). A key assumption in tractography is that tissue fiber orientation at a location can be approximated by the principal diffusion direction at the same location. Let $\vec{\lambda}_1(r)$ be the eigenvector associated with the largest eigenvalue at location r.

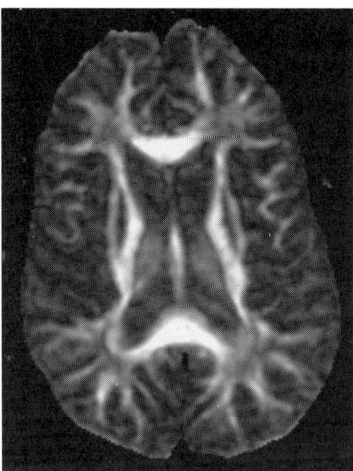

FIGURE 17.19 A fractional diffusion anisotropy map of the brain of a healthy human volunteer.

The fiber tract pathway, described by a 3D space curve $\vec{h}(r)$, can be calculated by solving the following equation:

$$\frac{d(\vec{h}(r))}{dr} = \frac{\vec{\lambda}(r)}{\left|\vec{\lambda}(r)\right|} \tag{17.44}$$

Solving Eq. (17.44) is analogous to mapping the trajectory of a moving object with known velocity at each spatial location. The details on how to solve Eq. (17.44) can be found in Basser et al. (2000).

Because $\vec{\lambda}_1(r)$ is typically measured with coarse spatial resolution (e.g., $2 \times 2 \times 5$ mm), interpolation is required to produce a visually continuous fiber pathway. With limited true spatial resolution, interpolation can introduce substantial errors. Also, when two fiber tracts with different orientations coexist in a voxel, the model based on a single tensor becomes inadequate. DSI (Tuch et al. 2002) and HARD imaging (Frank 2002) have been developed to address these problems.

The principal eigenvector can also be used to color-code a scalar diffusion anisotropy map, such as an RA or an FA map (Pajevic and Pierpaoli 1999). In this application, fiber orientation at a given voxel location is assumed to coincide with the direction of the principal eigenvector at the same voxel. By convention, orientations along left-right, anterior-posterior, and superior-inferior directions are represented by red, green, and blue, respectively.

For an arbitrary orientation that is not aligned with these orthogonal directions, a color is synthesized based on its relative vector components in the red, green, and blue channels. The intensity of the color-coded map is determined by the diffusion anisotropy value. A color-coded FA map from a healthy human brain is shown on the cover of this book.

17.2.6 Q-SPACE IMAGING

q-Space imaging is a diffusion NMR technique originally proposed to measure structures far smaller than the spatial resolution of an MR image (Callaghan 1991; Callaghan et al. 1991; Cory and Garroway 1990). This technique measures the displacement probability profile arising from molecular diffusion and relates the shape of the profile to the diffusion coefficient and the size of the molecular microenvironment. Earlier work on q-space measurement was largely focused on NMR microscopy. Recently, q-space imaging has been extended to localized MR spectroscopy and human brain imaging (Assaf et al. 2002; Neeman et al. 1990)

Consider a pair of rectangular Stejskal-Tanner gradient lobes with a gradient amplitude G_d and duration δ (see Figure 9.3). The q-space variable, also known as the *reciprocal spatial vector*, is defined as:

$$\vec{q} = \frac{1}{2\pi} \gamma \delta \vec{G}_d \tag{17.45}$$

or in scalar form

$$q = \frac{1}{2\pi} \gamma \delta G_d \tag{17.46}$$

With this definition and Eq. (9.8), Eq. (17.26) becomes:

$$S(q) = S_0 \exp\left[-4\pi^2 q^2 D(\Delta - \delta/3)\right] \tag{17.47}$$

where Δ is the center-to-center gradient lobe separation. In q-space imaging, $S(q)$ is measured at a number of q values (e.g., 16). A Fourier transform of $S(q)$ gives:

$$F(r) = FT[S(q)] = \alpha \exp(-\beta r^2) \tag{17.48}$$

where r is the Fourier conjugate of q, and α and β are parameters that depend on the diffusion properties. $F(r)$ is known as a displacement probability profile whose FWHM (Δr_{FWHM}) is related to the root-mean-squared displacement by (Callaghan 1991):

$$r_{rms} = \frac{\Delta r_{FWHM}}{2\sqrt{2\ln 2}} = 0.425\Delta r_{FWHM} \qquad (17.49)$$

Thus, for unrestricted diffusion, the diffusion coefficient can be readily obtained from Eqs. (17.49) and (17.23) by assuming $t \approx \Delta$. If diffusion is restricted within a sphere of diameter d, as long as $\Delta \gg d^2/8D$ (a condition known as long time-scale limit), the coefficient β of Eq. (17.48) becomes (Callaghan 1991):

$$\beta = \frac{5}{d^2}. \qquad (17.50)$$

Thus, the diameter of the sphere d can be obtained either by a Gaussian curve fitting or by measuring the FWHM of the displacement probability profile. For example, d as small as $\sim 10\,\mu m$ can be detected.

17.2.7 PRACTICAL CONSIDERATIONS

Achieving the highest possible SNR is pivotal for successful diffusion imaging. To reduce unnecessary signal loss due to relaxation effects, TE must be minimized at a given b-value while TR should be maximized within the total scan time constraint. The minimally achievable TE strongly depends on the gradient strength available on the scanner. The stronger the gradient strength, the shorter the minimum TE. Another important parameter that influences SNR is the b-value. For DW imaging of the human brain, the b-value typically ranges from 500 to 1000 s/mm². For spine and abdomen imaging, smaller b-values (e.g., 200–500 s/mm²) have been used, especially in non-EPI diffusion sequences (Zhou et al. 2002; Baur et al. 1998). For DTI with single-shot EPI, a recent study has suggested that the optimal b-value depends weakly on the number of diffusion-weighting gradient directions (Poonawalla et al. 2000). A larger number of directions allows a smaller b-value to be used without compromising the image quality.

In many quantitative applications, signal averaging is required to increase the SNR of the raw DW images. Due to the motion sensitivity of diffusion imaging pulse sequences, the k-space data can contain inconsistent phase errors across the individual data sets to be averaged. If signal averaging is performed in k-space, the phase errors can cause signal loss that varies across the image. To avoid this problem, the images to be averaged are first individually reconstructed. The magnitude images are then calculated and averaged to produce the final image. Alternatively, a phase correction can be applied prior to averaging the complex images (McKinnon et al. 2000).

When multiple diffusion images are used to calculate diffusion trace-weighted images, ADC maps, or diffusion tensor images, it is assumed that the raw DW images are all properly registered. This assumption is typically valid for diffusion pulse sequences based on spin echoes, stimulated echoes, and RARE. When single-shot EPI diffusion pulse sequences are used, however, considerable image misregistration can be observed primarily due to varying eddy currents produced by different diffusion-weighting gradient amplitudes and directions (Jezzard et al. 1998; Zhou and Reynolds 1997). It has been shown that eddy currents induced by the diffusion gradient produce B_0 fields and gradients along the readout, phase-encoding, and slice-selection directions. B_0 eddy currents can cause image shift along the phase-encoded direction. Gradient eddy currents along the readout and the phase-encoding axes lead to image shear and scaling (i.e., compression or dilation), respectively, also along the phase-encoded direction. Eddy-current gradients excited in the slice-selection direction reduce the overall image intensity due to imperfect slice rephasing, but do not cause geometric distortion. These image distortion and intensity-loss effects, collectively referred to as image misregistration, manifest themselves as image blurring in diffusion-trace-weighted images obtained from Eq. (17.30), errors on ADC maps, and false diffusion anisotropy in DTI images. For example, eddy currents can produce a bright rim (i.e., a false diffusion anisotropy in the regions with most image

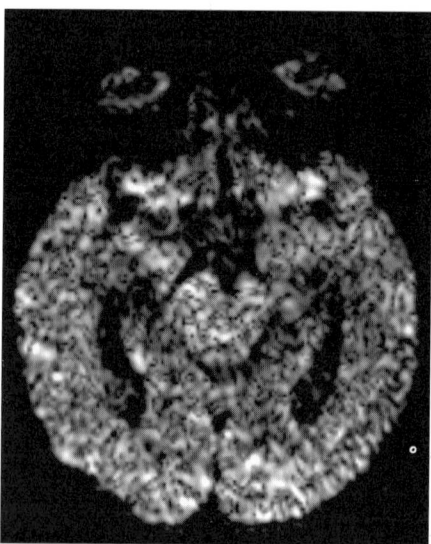

FIGURE 17.20 A diffusion-trace-weighted image showing the severe artifacts caused by gradient-induced vibration.

misregistration) at the edge of the brain and an increased intensity in gray matter in FA or RA maps. A number of techniques have been developed to address the eddy-current-induced distortion in diffusion imaging, such as pre-emphasis calibration (Calamante et al. 1999), employing twice-refocused RF spin echoes with two bipolar diffusion gradient pairs to better cancel eddy currents (Reese et al. 2003), real-time modification of pulse sequences to offset the eddy current effects (Zhou et al. 1999), and postacquisition image processing to reregister the diffusion images (Poupon et al. 2000).

Although diffusion pulse sequences based on single-shot EPI are rather insensitive to intrashot motion within an image, excessive intrashot motion as well as motion among different DW images can still degrade the diffusion image quality. Motion often arises from two sources: patient bulk motion and table vibration induced by the strong diffusion-weighting gradient. An example of artifacts caused by gradient-induced vibration is shown in Figure 17.20. The first problem can be addressed with improved patient cooperation or by using a patient-restraint device such as a face mesh. If the table cannot be mechanically stiffened, a solution to the second problem is to decrease the amplitude of the diffusion-weighting gradient. This can be done either by prolonging the diffusion gradient pulse width (while holding b-value fixed) or by reducing the b-value and maintaining the same gradient pulse width. It should be noted that the former approach also results in a longer TE, which degrades the SNR.

Selected References

Alsop, D. C. 1997. Phase insensitive preparation of single-shot RARE: Application to diffusion imaging in humans. *Magn. Reson. Med.* 38: 527–533.

Anderson, A. W., and Gore, J. C. 1994. Analysis and correction of motion artifacts in diffusion-weighted imaging. *Magn. Reson. Med.* 32: 379–387.

Arfken, G. 1970. *Mathematical methods for physicists.* New York: Academic Press.

Assaf, Y., Ben-Bashat, D., Chapman, J., Peled, S., Biton, I. E., Kafri, M., Segev, Y., Hendler, T., Korczyn, A. D., Graif, M., and Cohen, Y. 2002. High b-value q-space analyzed diffusion-weighted MRI: Application to multiple sclerosis. *Magn. Reson. Med.* 47: 115–126.

Basser, P. J. 2002. Relationships between diffusion tensor and q-space MRI. *Magn. Reson. Med.* 47: 392–397.

Basser, P. J., Mattiello, J., and LeBihan, D. 1994. Estimation of the effective self-diffusion tensor from the NMR spin echo. *J. Magn. Reson. B* 103: 247–254.

Basser, P. J., Pajevic, S., Pierpaoli, C., Duda, J., and Aldroubi, A. 2000. *In vivo* fiber tractography using DT-MRI data. *Magn. Reson. Med.* 44: 625–632.

Bastin, M. E., and Le Roux, P. 2002. On the application of a non-CPMG single-shot fast spin-echo sequence to diffusion tensor MRI of the human brain. *Magn. Reson. Med.* 48: 6–14.

Batchelor, P. G., Atkinson, D., Hill, D. L. G., Calmante, F., and Connelly, A. 2003. Anisotropic noise propagation in diffusion tensor MRI sampling schemes. *Magn. Reson. Med.* 49: 1143–1151.

Baur, A., Stabler, A., Bruning, R., Bartl, R., Krodel, A., Reiser, M., and Deimling, M. 1998. Diffusion-weighted MR imaging of bone marrow: Differentiation of benign versus pathologic compression fracture. *Radiology* 207: 349–356.

Beaulieu, C. F., Zhou, X., Cofer, G. P., and Johnson, G. A. 1993. Diffusion-weighted MR microscopy with fast-spin echo. *Magn. Reson. Med.* 30: 201–206.

Calamante, F., Porter, D. G. G, and Connelly, A. 1999. Correction for eddy current induced B_0 shifts in diffusion-weighted echo-planar imaging. *Magn. Reson. Med.* 41: 95–102.

Callaghan, P. T. 1991. *Principles of nuclear magnetic resonance microscopy.* Oxford: Oxford University Press.

Callaghan, P. T., Eccles, C. D., and Xia, Y. 1988. NMR microscopy of dynamic displacements: k-space and q-space imaging. *J. Phys. E Sci. Instrum.* 21: 820–822.

Callaghan, P. T., MacGowan, D., Packer, K. J., and Zelaya, F. O. 1991. Diffraction-like effects in NMR diffusion studies of fluids in porous solids. *Nature* 351: 467–469.

Carr, H. Y. and Purcell, E. M. 1954. Effects of diffusion on free precession in nuclear magnetic resonance experiments. *Phys. Rev.* 94: 630.

Chenevert, T. L., Brunberg, J. A., Tsukamoto, T., and King, K. F. 1996. Spiral diffusion studies of the human brain. *Radiology* 201: 511–511.

Clark, C. A., Hedehus, M., and Moseley, M. E. 2002. *In vivo* mapping of the fast and slow diffusion tensors in human brain. *Magn. Reson. Med.* 47: 623–628.

Cory, D. G., and Garroway, A. N. 1990. Measurement of translational displacement probabilities by NMR: An indicator of compartmentation. *Magn. Reson. Med.* 14: 435–444.

de Crespigny, A. J., Marks, M. P., Enzmann, D. R., and Moseley, M. E. 1995. Navigated diffusion imaging of normal and ischemic human brain. *Magn. Reson. Med.* 33: 720–728.

Delalande, C., de Zwart, J. A., Trillaud, H., Grenier, N., and Moonen, C. T. W. 1999. An echo-shifted gradient-echo MRI method for efficient diffusion weighting. *Magn. Reson. Med.* 41: 1000–1008.

Eis, M., and Hoehnberlage, M. 1995. Correction of gradient crosstalk and optimization of measurement parameters in diffusion MR imaging. *J. Magn. Reson. B* 107: 222–234.

Frank, L. R. 2002. Characterization of anisotropy in high angular resolution diffusion-weighted MRI. *Magn. Reson. Med.* 47: 1083–1099.

Inglis, B. A., Bossart, E. L., Buckley, D. L., Wirth, E. D., and Mareci, T. H. 2001. Visualization of neural tissue water compartments using biexponential diffusion tensor MRI. *Magn. Reson. Med.* 45: 580–587.

Jezzard, P., Barnett, A. S., and Pierpaoli, C. 1998. Characterization of and correction for eddy current artifacts in echo planar diffusion imaging. *Magn. Reson. Med.* 39: 801–812.

Jones, D. K., Horsfield, M. A., and Simmons, A. 1999. Optimal strategies for measuring diffusion in anisotropic systems by magnetic resonance imaging. *Magn. Reson. Med.* 42: 515–525.

Le Bihan, D. 1995. *Diffusion and perfusion magnetic resonance imaging: Applications to functional MRI.* New York: Raven Press.

Le Bihan, D., Breton, E., Lallemand, D., Grenier, P., Cabanis, E. A., and Laval-Jeantet, M. 1986. MR imaging of intravoxel incoherent motions: Application to diffusion and perfusion in neurologic disorders. *Radiology* 161: 401–407.

Liu, G., van Gelderen, P., Duyn, J., and Moonen, C. T. 1996. Single-shot diffusion MRI of human brain on a conventional clinical instrument. *Magn. Reson. Med.* 35: 671–677.

Maier, S. E., Gudbjartsson, H., Patz, S., Hsu, L., Lovblad, K. O., Edelman, R. R., Warach, S, and Jolesz, F. A. 1998. Line scan diffusion imaging: Characterization in healthy subjects and stroke patients. *Am. J. Roentgenol.* 171: 85–93. q

Mattiello, J., Basser, P. J., and Lebihan, D. 1994. Analytical expressions for the b-matrix in NMR diffusion imaging and spectroscopy. *J. Magn. Reson. A* 108: 131–141.

McKinnon, G. C. 2002. Fast spin echo pulse sequence for diffusion weighted imaging. U.S. patent 6,078,176.

McKinnon, G. C., Zhou, X. J., and Leeds, N. E. 2000. Phase corrected complex averaging for diffusion-weighted spine imaging. In *Proceedings of the 8th Meeting of the International Society for Magnetic Resonance in Medicine.* p. 802.

Merboldt, K. D., Hanicke, W., and Bruhn, H., Gyngell, M. L., Frahm, J. 1985. Diffusion imaging of the human brain *in vivo* using high-speed STEAM MRI. *Magn. Reson. Med.* 23: 179–192.

Merboldt, K.-D., Hanicke, W., and Frahm, J. 1985. Self-diffusion NMR imaging using stimulated echoes. *J. Magn. Reson.* 64: 479–486.

Mori, S., and van Zijl, P. C. 1996. Diffusion weighting by the trace of the diffusion tensor within a single scan. *Magn. Reson. Med.* 33: 41–52.

Mulkern, R. V., Gudbjartsson, H., Westin, C. F., Zengingonul, H. P., Gartner, W., Guttmann, C. R. G., Robertson, R. L., Kyriakos, W., Schwartz, R., Holtzman, D., Jolesz, F. A., and Maier, S. E. 1999. Multi-component apparent diffusion coefficients in human brain. *Nucl. Magn. Reson. Biomed.* 12: 51–62.

Neeman, M., Freyer, J. P., and Sillerud, L. O. 1990. Pulsed-gradient spin-echo diffusion studies in NMR imaging—effects of the imaging gradients on the determination of diffusion-coefficients. *J. Magn. Reson.* 90: 303–312.

Norris, D. G., Bornert, P., Reese, T., and Leibfritz, D. 1992. On the application of ultra-fast RARE experiments. *Magn. Reson. Med.* 27: 142–164.

Ordidge, R. J., Helpern, J. A., Qing, Z. X., Knight, R. A., and Nagesh, V. 1994. Correction of motional artifacts in diffusion-weighted MR images using navigator echoes. *Magn. Reson. Imaging* 12: 455–460.

Pajevic, S., and Pierpaoli, C. 1999. Color schemes to represent the orientation of anisotropic tissues from diffusion tensor data: Application to white matter fiber tract mapping in the human brain. *Magn. Reson. Med.* 42: 526–540.

Papadakis, N. G., Xing, D., Huang, C. L., Hall, L. D., and Carpenter, T. A. 1999. A comparative study of acquisition schemes for diffusion tensor imaging using MRI. *J. Magn. Reson.* 137: 67–82.

Pierpaoli, C., and Basser, P. J. 1996. Toward a quantitative assessment of diffusion anisotropy. *Magn. Reson. Med.* 36: 893–906.

Pipe, J. G., Farthing, V. G., and Forbes, K. P. 2002. Multishot diffusion-weighted FSE using PROPELLER MRI. *Magn. Reson. Med.* 47: 42–52.

Poonawalla, A., Karmonik, C., and Zhou, X. J. 2000. Optimization of B-value and gradient orientation for diffusion tensor MRI. In *Proceedings of the 8th Meeting of the International Society for Magnetic Resonance in Medicine*. p. 801.

Poonawalla, A. H., and Zhou, X. J., 2004. Analytical error propagation in diffusion anisotropy calculations. *J. Magn. Reson. Imaging.* 19: 489–498.

Poupon, C., Clark, C. A., Frouin, V., Regis, J., Bloch, I., Le Bihan, D., and Mangin, J. F. 2000. Regularization of diffusion-based direction maps for the tracking of brain white matter fascicles. *Neuroimage* 12: 184–195.

Press, W. H., Flannery, B. P., Teukolsky, S. A., and Vetterling, W. T. 1992. *Numerical recipes in C: The art of scientific computing*. Cambridge, UK: Cambridge University Press.

Reese, T. G., Heid, O., Weisskoff, R. M., and Wedeen, V. J. 2003. Reduction of eddy-current-induced distortion in diffusion MRI using a twice-refocused spin echo. *Magn. Reson. Med.* 49: 177–182.

Schick, F. 1997. SPLICE: Sub-second diffusion-sensitive MR imaging using a modified fast spin-echo acquisition made. *Magn. Reson. Med.* 38: 638–644.

Skare, S., Hedehus, M., Moseley, M. E., and Li, T. Q. 2000. Condition number as a measure of noise performance of diffusion tensor data acquisition schemes with MRI. *J. Magn. Reson.* 147: 340–352.

Sorensen, A. G., Buonanno, F. S., Gonzalez, R. G., Schwamm, L. H., Lev, M. H., Huang-Hellinger, F. R., Reese, T. G., Weisskoff, R. M., Davis, T. L., Suwanwela, N., Can, U., Moreira, J. A., Copen, W. A., Look, R. B., Finklestein, S. P., Rosen, B. R., and Koroshetz, W. J. 1996. Hyperacute stroke: Evaluation with combined multisection diffusion-weighted and hemodynamically weighted echo-planar MR imaging. *Radiology* 199: 391–401.

Stejskal, E. O., and Tanner, J. E. 1965. Spin diffusion measurements: Spin echoes in the presence of a time-dependent field gradient. *J. Chem. Phys.* 42: 288–292.

Sugahara, T., Korogi, Y., Kochi, M., Ikushima, I., Shigematu, Y., Hirai, T., Okuda, T., Liang, L., Ge, Y., Komohara, Y., Ushio, Y., and Takahashi, M. 1999. Usefulness of diffusion-weighted MRI with echo-planar technique in the evaluation of cellularity in gliomas. *J. Magn. Reson. Imaging* 9: 53–60.

Trouard, T. P., Theilmann R. J., Altbach M. I., and Gmitro A. F. 1999. High-resolution diffusion imaging with DIFRAD-FSE (diffusion-weighted radial acquisition of data with fast spin-echo) MRI. *Magn. Reson. Med.* 42: 11–18.

Tsukamoto, T., King, K. F., Foo, T. K., and Yoshitome, E. 1996. Spiral MR imaging for diffusion imaging with real-time motion monitoring and motion correction. *Radiology* 201: 146–146.

Tuch, D. S., Reese, T. G., Wiegell, M. R., Makris, N., Belliveau, J. W., and Wedeen, V. J. 2002. High angular resolution diffusion imaging reveals intravoxel white matter fiber heterogeneity. *Magn. Reson. Med.* 48: 577–582.

Ulug, A. M., and van Zijl, P. C. 1999. Orientation-independent diffusion imaging without tensor diagonalization: Anisotropy definitions based on physical attributes of the diffusion ellipsoid. *J. Magn. Reson. Imaging* 9: 804–813.

van Zijl, P. C. M., Moonen, C. T. W., Faustino, P., Pekar, J., Kaplan, O., and Cohen, J. S. 1990. Complete separation of intracellular and extracellular information in NMR spectra of perfused cells by diffusion weighted spectroscopy. *Proc. Natl. Acad. Sci. U.S.A.* 88: 3228–3232.

Warach, S., Dashe, J. F., and Edelman, R. R. 1996. Clinical outcome in ischemic stroke predicted by early diffusion-weighted and perfusion magnetic resonance imaging: A preliminary analysis. *J. Cereb. Blood Flow Metab.* 16: 53–59.

Wedeen, V. J., Reese, T. G., Napadow, V. J., and Gilbert, R. J. 2001. Demonstration of primary and secondary muscle fiber architecture of the bovine tongue by diffusion tensor magnetic resonance imaging. *Biophys. J.* 80: 1024–1028.

Wong, E. C., Cox, R. W., and Song, A. W. 1995. Optimized isotropic diffusion weighting. *Magn. Reson. Med.* 34: 139–143.

Xue, R., van Zijl, P. C., Crain, B. J., Solaiyappan, M., and Mori, S. 1999. In vivo three-dimensional reconstruction of rat brain axonal projections by diffusion tensor imaging. *Magn. Reson. Med.* 42: 1123–1127.

Zhou, X. J., Leeds, N. E., McKinnon, G. C., and Kumar, A. J. 2002. Characterization of benign and metastatic vertebral compression fractures with quantitative diffusion MR imaging. *Am. J. of Neuroradiol.* 23: 165–170.

Zhou, X., Maier, J. K., and Reynolds, H. G. 1999. Method to reduce eddy current effects in diffusion-weighted echo planar imaging. U.S. patent 5,864,233.

Zhou, X. J., and Reynolds, H. G. 1997. Quantitative analysis of eddy current effects on diffusion-weighted EPI. In *Proceedings of the 5th Meeting of the International Society for Magnetic Resonance in Medicine*, p. 1722.

RELATED SECTIONS

17.3 Dixon's Method

The suppression of lipid signal in MRI is very useful for improving contrast when imaging anatomy such as the breast or the optic nerve that contains (or is embedded in) fatty tissue. Because of its short T_1 (about 230 ms at 1.5 T), the bright (i.e., hyperintense) appearance of fat is especially problematic on T_1-weighted images with short TR and short TE. Suppression of fat signal is especially beneficial when T_1-shortening contrast agents such as gadolinium chelates are used to visualize contrast-enhancing lesions. In T_2-weighted RARE images, the bright fat signal intensity can also cause confusion when detecting lesions that exhibit hyperintensity. Because the NMR signal from the lipid protons is only second to that from water in human body, fat is a main contributor to chemical shift artifacts. At 1.5 T the fat-water chemical shift frequency difference is $f_{cs} \approx 210\,Hz$. Because typical RF bandwidths are on the order of 1–3 kHz, the selected slice for magnetization containing fat can be spatially shifted by an appreciable fraction of the slice width. Because typical readout bandwidths are on the order of 50–200 Hz/pixel, the chemical shift artifact for fat can be several image pixels. For pulse sequences employing a train of phase-encoded gradient echoes, such as single-shot EPI, the bandwidth along the phase-encoding direction is only ~1 kHz across the FOV. Thus, the chemical shift artifacts can be particularly severe. For example, in a 128×128 single-shot EPI image, lipid signals can be displaced by as many as 27 pixels along the phase-encoded direction, as shown in Example 16.5.

Methods for fat suppression include selective saturation of the lipid magnetization and selective excitation of water magnetization. Examples include spectrally selective RF pulses (Section 4.3), binomial RF pulses (Section 4.1), and spectral-spatial RF pulses (Section 5.4). Another fat suppression technique is short TI recovery (STIR), in which the water and fat magnetization is inverted, followed by a delay time TI that nulls the fat longitudinal magnetization (Section 14.2). Because water has longer T_1 than fat (unless contrast agents are present), the longitudinal magnetization of water is negative but nonzero at the time of the RF excitation pulse. The transverse magnetization and signal that result are primarily from water.

The use of spectrally selective RF pulses and STIR for fat suppression both have drawbacks. In general, spectrally selective RF pulses are sensitive to both B_1 nonuniformity and B_0 inhomogeneity, and they work poorly at low field strengths at which the fat-water frequency separation is small (e.g., f_{cs} is only approximately 70 Hz at 0.5 T). STIR is sensitive to B_1 nonuniformity (unless an adiabatic inversion pulse is used), prolongs scan time, and reduces the signal from other tissues in the process of nulling fat.

In addition to suppressing fat, it has been reported that determining the relative composition of fat and water in tissues can improve diagnosis for some diseases including bone marrow disease (Rosen et al. 1988), adrenal masses (Leroy-Willig et al. 1989) and some liver diseases (Lee et al. 1984). Imaging techniques that allow separation of magnetization components based on their chemical shifts are called spectroscopic imaging (SI) or chemical shift imaging (CSI) methods.

Many of these drawbacks of STIR and spectrally selective RF pulses can be addressed with a very simple SI method. The proton spectrum is approximated by a two-component model, in which the spectral peaks correspond to fat and water. In this method, separate images of the fat and water components are created, eliminating the need for fat saturation while still removing the contrast degradation from bright fat. Although in reality the fat spectrum can be composed of numerous spectral peaks, this simple model is adequate for many purposes (Figure 17.21).

Dixon's original method, also called two-point Dixon or 2PD, is an example of a two-component SI technique. The number of points refers to the number of images with distinct fat-water phase differences that are acquired per slice location. As we will see, the number of points is not necessarily the same as the number of spectral components to be separated. The original two-point method is sensitive to errors caused by B_0 inhomogeneity and has since been extended to deal with this problem. Even further robustness is provided by the three-point Dixon or 3PD method, which deals with B_0 inhomogeneity somewhat better than the extended two-point method. The Dixon method can be further extended to images with more than two spectral components, but the resulting acquisition times become rather long and other techniques can be more efficient (e.g., see Adalsteinsson et al. 1998). The Dixon method has primarily been used with 2D RF spin echo, gradient echo, and RARE pulse sequences, although some 3D gradient echo work has also been reported.

17.3.1 TWO-POINT DIXON

Original Two-Point Dixon Method   Consider the RF spin echo sequence shown in Figure 17.22. Magnetization with a nonzero but static resonance offset rephases at time τ after the 180° refocusing pulse. This is referred to as the RF spin echo or Hahn echo. B_0 inhomogeneity, chemical shift, or susceptibility variations can cause these resonance offsets. The phase accumulation caused by resonance offset due to the readout gradient, however, rephases at the point during the readout when the frequency-encoding gradient areas before and after the 180° pulse are equal ($k_x = 0$ point). In a conventional RF spin echo pulse sequence, $\Delta = 0$, so these two points coincide (see Section 14.3). If $\Delta \neq 0$, then isochromats with different chemical shifts will be out of phase

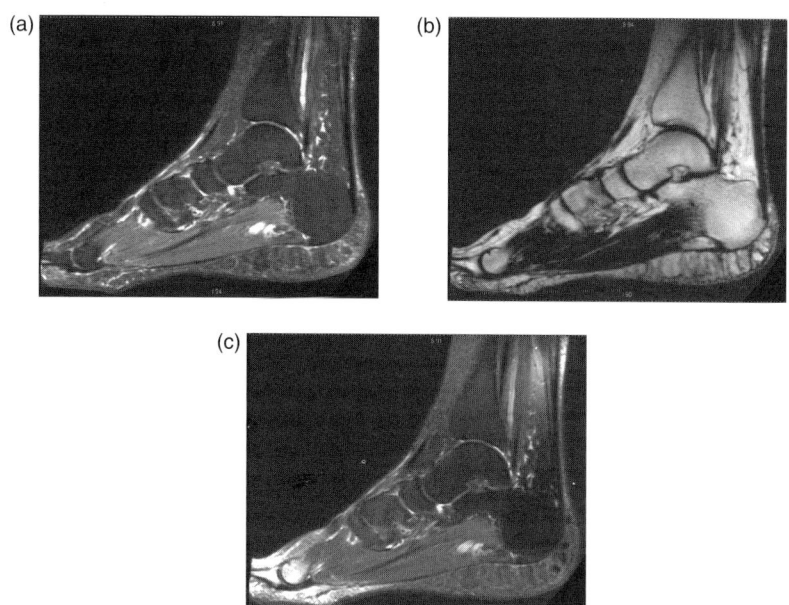

FIGURE 17.21 (a) Water and (b) fat (right) three-point Dixon images acquired with a four-channel transmit/receive coil using RARE (fast spin echo) with echo train length = 13, TR/TE = 4000/44, ±19.2-kHz bandwidth, 24 × 24 cm FOV, 3.5-mm slice thickness, 0.5-mm gap, 320 × 256 matrix, echo shifts Δ = 0, ±1.2 ms. (Courtesy Scott Reeder, M.D., Stanford University and Hubert Lejay, M.S., GE Medical Systems.) See Reeder et al. (2004) for more details about the processing algorithm. (c) Conventional fat saturation with a spectrally selective RF pulse using the same scan parameters plus 3 NEX. Nonuniform lipid suppression is evident across the image.

with one another at the point where $k_x = 0$, unless the phase shift happens to be an integer multiple of 2π. If the 180° pulse is delayed or advanced by $\Delta/2$, the RF spin echo is delayed or advanced by Δ relative to the location of $k_x = 0$. A spin isochromat with resonance frequency offset f_{cs} has phase $\phi = 2\pi f_{cs}\Delta$ at $k_x = 0$.

Consider two isochromats, one composed of fat and one of water proton spins, with each having a single spectral peak within a voxel and having a resonance frequency difference f_{cs}. Assume that the fat-water chemical shift is the only resonance frequency difference, that is, that there is perfect B_0 homogeneity and negligible magnetic susceptibility variations or other off-resonance effects. We acquire one RF spin echo image with $\Delta = 0$ using a normal acquisition and a second with $\Delta = 1/(2f_{cs})$ using an acquisition with

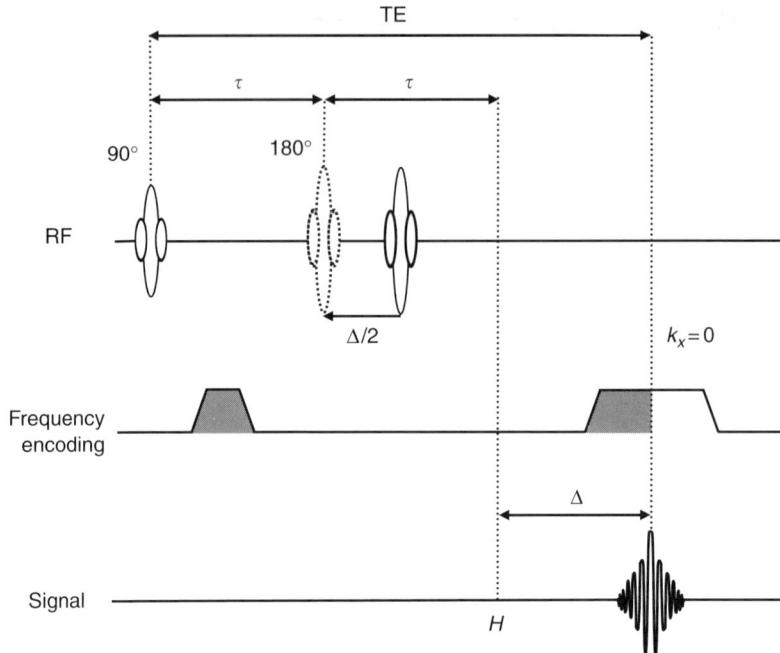

FIGURE 17.22 2PD RF spin echo pulse sequence. In the absence of gradients, the Hahn or RF spin echo would refocus at time τ after the 180° pulse, at point H when the refocusing pulse with the dotted line is used. The peak of the signal, however, refocuses at the point where the readout gradient has equal area (shaded) before and after the 180° pulse (i.e., the $k_x = 0$ point). The 180° refocusing pulse and associated echo that produce the in-phase image (normal RF spin echo image) are shown with a solid line; the RF pulse that produces the opposed-phase image is shown with a dotted line. Shifting the refocusing pulse by $\Delta/2$ shifts the RF spin echo by Δ. For simplicity, slice-selection and phase-encoding gradient waveforms are omitted.

the RF pulse either advanced or delayed by $\Delta/2 = 1/(4f_{\mathrm{cs}})$. To be definite, we assume the RF pulse is advanced as in Figure 17.22. An alternative design for the delayed case is to keep the refocusing pulse fixed and delay the readout gradient waveforms by Δ; however, this increases minimum TE and minimum sequence time, which can reduce the number of slice locations that can be acquired per unit time.

In the first image (called the in-phase image), fat and water magnetization are in phase at the $k_x = 0$ point of the readout. In the second image (called the opposed-phase image or out-of-phase image), fat and water magnetization are 180° out of phase at the $k_x = 0$ point (Figure 17.23a). Because image contrast

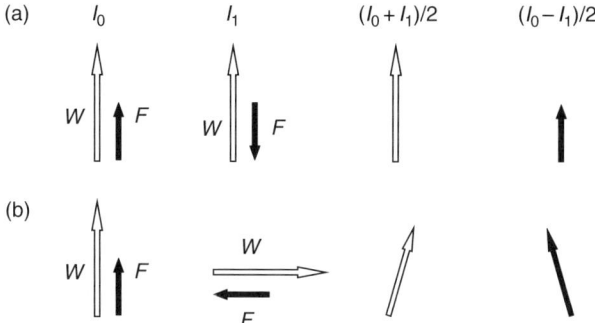

FIGURE 17.23 (a) Fat and water magnetization within a voxel for the in-phase image I_0, opposed-phase image I_1, and combined images assuming no B_0 inhomogeneity or magnetic susceptibility perturbation. The water magnetization is exactly on-resonance. The net magnetization within the voxel for I_0 and I_1 is the vector sum of the fat and water vectors. The magnetization in the combined images correctly estimates the fat and water magnetizations. (b) Fat and water magnetizations within a voxel assuming that B_0 inhomogeneity produces a 90° phase shift between the in-phase and opposed-phase images. The magnetization has the same magnitude in the resulting combined images, overestimating fat and underestimating water in this 2PD example.

is heavily determined by the peak signal amplitude that occurs at $k_x = 0$, the resulting complex images I_0 and I_1 are approximately given by:

$$I_0 = W + F$$
$$I_1 = W - F$$

(17.51)

where W and F are real, nonnegative, and proportional to the amount of water and fat magnetization in each voxel, respectively. Equation (17.51) ignores additional image weighting from T_2^* relaxation, diffusion, and flow and from other phase shifts that could arise from hardware group delays, eddy currents, and B_1 receive-field nonuniformity. We have also ignored the water-fat chemical shift separation in both the slice and readout directions in Eq. (17.51). Separate images of the water and fat magnetization can be reconstructed from:

$$W = \frac{1}{2}(I_0 + I_1)$$
$$F = \frac{1}{2}(I_0 - I_1)$$

(17.52)

The water image W can be used as a fat suppressed image, whereas W and F separately provide information about the relative water and fat contents of tissues.

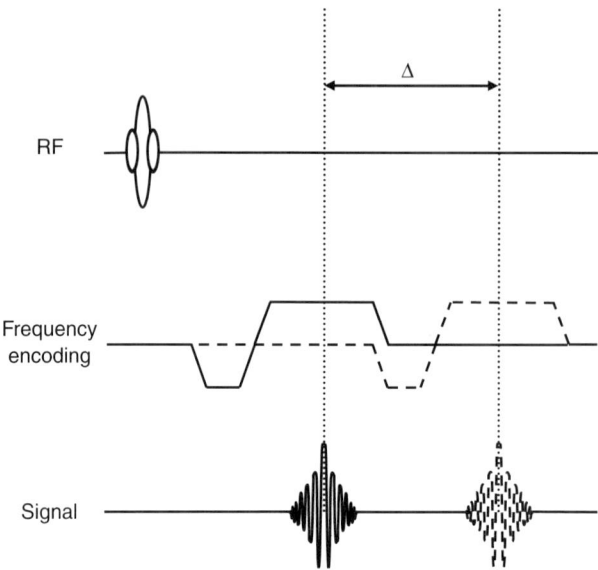

FIGURE 17.24 2PD gradient echo pulse sequence. The readout gradient waveform and echo that produce the in-phase image are solid lines; the gradient waveform and echo that produce the opposed-phase are dashed lines. For simplicity, slice-selection and phase-encoding gradient waveforms are omitted.

The in-phase and opposed-phase images can be acquired in two separate scans or as different echoes in one dual-echo scan. These options are discussed in more detail in subsection 17.3.4.

It is convenient to label the images acquired in Dixon acquisitions according to the relative water-fat phase shifts (in radians) at $k_x = 0$. In this nomenclature, the original Dixon method is denoted as a $(0, \pi)$ acquisition. In later subsections, generalizations using additional acquisitions and different phase angle combinations are discussed.

Instead of an RF spin echo, a gradient echo can be used for 2PD (Figure 17.24). For the gradient echo case, the readout gradient waveform is shifted by Δ from the desired TE. For the in-phase and opposed-phase images, the readout waveforms therefore have a relative shift $\Delta = 1/(2f_{cs})$.

Example 17.3 (a) For a RF spin echo 2PD acquisition, what is Δ at 1.5 T for the opposed-phase image, assuming $f_{cs} = 210$ Hz? How much is the refocusing pulse shifted for this case? If the gradient waveforms are shifted instead of the refocusing pulse, what is the required time shift? (b) For a gradient echo 2PD acquisition, what are the minimum echo times that can be prescribed to give in-phase and opposed-phase images, assuming that neither the duration of the gradient nor the RF waveform limits the echo times?

Answer

(a) $\Delta = 1/(2 \times 210\,Hz) = 2.38$ ms. The refocusing pulse is shifted by $\Delta/2$, which is 1.19 ms. Equivalently, the readout gradient waveforms can be shifted by 2.38 ms.

(b) The minimum echo times are TE $= 1/(210\,\text{Hz}) = 4.76$ ms for the in-phase and $1/(2 \times 210\,\text{Hz}) = 2.38$ ms for the opposed phase image. Finally, keep in mind that the lipid resonance is broad, so that no single value such as $f_{cs} = 210\,\text{Hz}$ completely describes the physical situation.

The main problem with the 2PD technique is that the assumption of perfect B_0 homogeneity and negligible susceptibility is never valid. With a main magnetic field shift ΔB_0, fat and water have accumulated an additional phase shift $\Delta \phi = \gamma (\Delta B_0) \Delta$ at the $k_x = 0$ point in I_1. Although fat and water spin isochromats in any given voxel are still anti-parallel in the opposed-phase image they might no longer be parallel or anti-parallel to the fat and water spins in the in-phase image (Figure 17.23b). Therefore the added and subtracted images in Eq. (17.52) contain admixtures of both fat and water.

An imperfect but workable solution is to use the magnitudes of I_0 and I_1 in Eq. (17.52). Although taking the magnitudes eliminates any relative phase shift between I_0 and I_1, it can result in fat and water being interchanged, that is, the fat signal being assigned to the water image and vice versa. For example, suppose we use the estimates $\widetilde{W} = (|I_0| + |I_1|)/2$ and $\widetilde{F} = (|I_0| - |I_1|)/2$, based on Eq. (17.52). Then, because $|I_0| + |I_1| \geq ||I_0| - |I_1||$, the resulting water image will always be brighter than the fat image. This is correct unless in reality $F > W$, in which case fat and water are interchanged in $\widetilde{W}$ and $\widetilde{F}$. To prevent this problem when magnitude images are used in 2PD, Eq. (17.51) is first written as:

$$W + F = |I_0|$$
$$W - F = p|I_1| \tag{17.53}$$

where

$$p = \begin{cases} +1 & W \geq F \\ -1 & W < F \end{cases} \tag{17.54}$$

is a binary sign factor that indicates whether fat or water is dominant within the voxel. The solution of Eq. (17.53) is:

$$W = \frac{1}{2}\left(|I_0| + p|I_1|\right)$$
$$F = \frac{1}{2}\left(|I_0| - p|I_1|\right) \tag{17.55}$$

Because the water and fat proportions are generally unknown a priori the correct determination of p can be difficult. This task is considered next.

Extended Two-Point Dixon Method   Extended 2PD attempts to address the B_0 homogeneity problem. We first consider a more general model that takes into account the phase errors that are ignored in Eq. (17.51):

$$I_0 = (W + F)e^{i\phi_0}$$
$$I_1 = (W - F)e^{i(\phi_0 + \phi)} \tag{17.56}$$

where W and F are again the water and fat magnetization in a given voxel (assumed to be real and nonnegative) and:

$$\phi = \gamma(\Delta B_0)\Delta \tag{17.57}$$

is the phase accumulated because of the B_0 inhomogeneity ΔB_0 during the echo shift Δ. Because W and F are real, all other phase errors are included in ϕ_0, which is a voxel-dependent phase that is the same for both images. For spin echo images, ϕ_0 is affected by gradient and receive chain group delays, eddy currents, concomitant fields, and the receive field B_1 phase. For gradient echo images, ϕ_0 includes the previous factors and also the phase accumulated from B_0 inhomogeneity during the echo time of the in-phase scan. Note that Eq. (17.56) has four unknown quantities (W, F, ϕ, and ϕ_0) and four independent equations (the magnitude and phase of I_0 and I_1) and is thus, in principle, exactly solvable.

To solve Eq. (17.56), we first eliminate ϕ_0 using:

$$|I_0| = W + F$$
$$I_1' = I_1 e^{-i\phi_0} = \frac{I_1 I_0^*}{|I_0|} = (W - F)e^{i\phi} \tag{17.58}$$

Next we need to eliminate ϕ, but simply calculating the phase of I_1' will not work because the phase of $W - F$ could be either 0 or π (i.e., the sign of $W - F$

could be either $+1$ or -1) and is not known in general. However, squaring I_1' eliminates the sign of $W - F$:

$$\left(I_1'\right)^2 = \left|W - F\right|^2 e^{i2\phi} \tag{17.59}$$

We can sometimes determine ϕ by taking one-half of the phase of $(I_1')^2$ and eliminating it from I_1'. Unfortunately because of phase wrapping, the direct use of the real and imaginary parts of $(I_1')^2$ to obtain 2ϕ does not necessarily give an accurate phase correction of I_1'. We can see this from:

$$\exp\left\{\frac{i}{2}\arctan\left[\frac{\mathrm{Im}\left((I_1')^2\right)}{\mathrm{Re}\left((I_1')^2\right)}\right]\right\} \neq \exp(i\phi) \tag{17.60}$$

if phase wrapping is present (see Section 13.5). An accurate determination of the phase of a 2D or 3D complex data set in the presence of both noise and phase wrapping is a difficult problem, and a complete discussion is beyond the scope of this book. Some of the methods that have been used in Dixon processing are discussed in subsection 17.3.3. For now we assume that 2ϕ can be accurately determined from $(I_1')^2$ and ϕ subsequently is removed from I_1'. We then have:

$$\begin{aligned} W + F &= |I_0| \\ W - F &= I_1' e^{-i\phi} = p|I_1| \end{aligned} \tag{17.61}$$

where for convenience we have reintroduced the sign factor p defined in Eq. (17.54). The solution of Eq. (17.61) is now given by Eq. (17.55), where p is determined by the sign of $I_1' e^{-i\phi}$. Note that the phase $I_1' e^{-i\phi}$ is either 0 or π, depending on the sign of $W - F$ (sign of p). When moving from a pixel that predominantly contains water to one that predominantly contains fat, the phase of $I_1' e^{-i\phi}$ flips from 0 to π (p flips from $+1$ to -1). From Eq. (17.55), this interchanges the assignment of $|I_0|+|I_1|$ and $|I_0|-|I_1|$ in water and fat images. To maintain a more continuous image appearance, it can be advantageous to use a continuous approximation of p (Glover and Schneider 1991):

$$p_c = \cos\left(\angle(I_1' e^{-i\phi})\right) = \frac{\mathrm{Re}(I_1' e^{-i\phi})}{|I_1'|} \tag{17.62}$$

where $\angle(z)$ denotes the phase of the complex variable z. Note that $p_c = p$ when $\angle(I_1' e^{-i\phi})$ is either 0 or π, but p_c also varies continuously between $+1$ and -1 if $\angle(I_1' e^{-i\phi})$ deviates from these ideal values due to noise or errors in the determination of ϕ. The final water and fat images for extended 2PD are given by:

$$W = \frac{1}{2}\left(|I_0| + p_c|I_1|\right)$$

$$F = \frac{1}{2}\left(|I_0| - p_c|I_1|\right)$$

(17.63)

Extended 2PD works well except in regions near water/fat boundaries where $W \approx F$ and I_1 therefore has low signal intensity (Skinner and Glover 1997; Coombs et al. 1997) The main problem with extended 2PD is that in these low signal areas, noise in I_1 can cause errors in the estimate of ϕ, which changes $\angle(I_1' e^{-i\phi})$ and causes the interchanged assignment of water and fat components. Another difficulty with extended 2PD is incomplete lipid suppression in the water image related to the fact that the two echoes have different amplitudes. These problems are alleviated by 3PD, which is considered in the next subsection.

We note that other definitions of p_c are possible (Chen et al. 1999) such as:

$$p_c = H_c\left(\cos\left(\angle\left(I_1' e^{-i\phi}\right)\right)\right)$$

(17.64)

where

$$H_c(x) = \begin{cases} +1 & \frac{1}{2} \le x \le 1 \\ 0 & -\frac{1}{2} < x < \frac{1}{2} \\ -1 & -1 \le x \le -\frac{1}{2} \end{cases}$$

(17.65)

Equation (17.64) gives $W = F = |I_0|/2$ for pixels that are likely to have an erroneous estimate of ϕ because $\angle(I_1' e^{-i\phi})$ deviates substantially from 0 or π.

The SNR in Dixon water and fat images can be calculated using the methods shown in Glover and Schneider (1991). Because Dixon's method uses multiple acquisitions, the SNR is generally higher than for conventional scans that do not signal-average. In Dixon's method, SNR is conveniently characterized by the effective number of signal averages (ENSA), the number of excitations or NEX that would give the equivalent SNR with a conventional scan. For extended 2PD, ENSA $= 2$ and the additional acquisition time is completely applied toward SNR improvement. As we see later, this is not true for some Dixon phase-angle choices or reconstruction methods.

17.3.2 THREE-POINT DIXON

Basic Three-Point Dixon Method In 3PD, images are collected at each of three different echo shifts Δ. The early 3PD work used $(0, \pi, -\pi)$ phase angles to obtain one in-phase and two opposed-phase images (Glover and Schneider 1991). The phase difference between the two opposed-phase images is due to B_0 inhomogeneity, and they are used to compute ϕ. The ϕ map is used to remove the B_0 inhomogeneity phase shift from one of the opposed-phase images and thereby determine the dominant species for each pixel (i.e., whether $W > F$, or vice versa). The magnitude in-phase and opposed-phase images are then combined as in to 2PD and extended 2PD. This approach has some of the same problems as the extended 2PD method because ϕ is estimated from opposed-phase images. For voxels with nearly equal amounts of fat and water, the signal in the two opposed-phase images is low and a reliable estimate of ϕ becomes difficult, causing incorrect water and fat assignments. 3PD with $(0, \pi, -\pi)$ phase shifts is still advantageous over the original 2PD method because B_0 inhomogeneity is taken into account and is advantageous over extended 2PD because of a better SNR.

An improved 3PD uses choices for Δ that give $(0, \pi, 2\pi)$ phase angles (Glover 1991; Chen et al. 1999). Water and fat are in-phase for the $\Delta = 0$ and 2π images, which are used to calculate ϕ. Because there is no water-fat cancellation on these images, the signal is higher than for an opposed-phase image, so the estimate of ϕ is more reliable. The opposed-phase image is the same as in the original 2PD method. The ϕ map is then used to remove the B_0 inhomogeneity phase shift from the opposed-phase image and thereby determine the relative water-fat admixture for each pixel, as is done with extended 2PD. The magnitude in-phase and opposed-phase images are combined to calculate fat and water images.

The images for the $(0, \pi, 2\pi)$ 3PD acquisitions are:

$$I_0 = (W + F)e^{i\phi_0}$$
$$I_1 = (W - F)e^{i(\phi_0 + \phi)} \qquad (17.66)$$
$$I_2 = (W + F)e^{i(\phi_0 + 2\phi)}$$

There are still four unknown quantities but now we have six equations constrained by:

$$\angle I_0 + \angle I_2 = \angle 2I_1 \qquad (17.67)$$

Equation (17.66) is therefore overdetermined, and two solutions exist that can be combined for an improved SNR. The solution presented next is valid for either spin echo or gradient echo images. A slightly different solution valid only for the gradient echo case is given in Wang et al. (1998). As before, we solve Eq. (17.66) by first removing ϕ_0:

$$I_0' = |I_0| = W + F$$

$$I_1' = I_1 e^{-i\phi_0} = \frac{I_1 I_0^*}{|I_0|} = (W - F)e^{i\phi} \tag{17.68}$$

$$I_2' = I_2 e^{-i\phi_0} = \frac{I_2 I_0^*}{|I_0|} = (W + F)e^{i2\phi}$$

Next 2ϕ is obtained from I_2'. Using I_2' instead of I_1' to determine ϕ avoids the problem of low signal due to the partial cancellation of W and F encountered in 2PD. Once the phase ϕ is removed from I_1' and I_2':

$$W + F = |I_0|$$

$$W - F = I_1' e^{-i\phi} = p|I_1| \tag{17.69}$$

$$W + F = |I_2|$$

There are two solutions, and we could use either the first or third line of Eq. (17.69) as the estimate of $W + F$. For an improved SNR we combine the two, either as an algebraic or geometric mean: $W + F = (|I_0| + |I_2|)/2$ or $W + F = \sqrt{|I_0||I_2|}$. Either way gives approximately the same SNR. Note that in the absence of noise, and ignoring echo amplitude differences, they are equivalent because $|I_0| = |I_2|$ and $\sqrt{|I_0||I_2|} = (|I_0| + |I_2|)/2$.) We use:

$$W + F = \sqrt{|I_0||I_2|}$$
$$W - F = p|I_1| = I_1' e^{-i\phi} \tag{17.70}$$

We finally obtain the solution:

$$W = \frac{1}{2}\left(\sqrt{|I_0||I_2|} + p_c|I_1|\right)$$
$$F = \frac{1}{2}\left(\sqrt{|I_0||I_2|} - p_c|I_1|\right) \tag{17.71}$$

As with the extended 2PD case, we have replaced p with p_c, defined either as in Eq. (17.62) or (17.64).

Three-Point Dixon including Echo Amplitude Modulation   Because Eq. (17.66) contains six equations (three for amplitude and three for phase) with the constraint in Eq. (17.67), we can determine five unknowns. In this case, we determine W, F, ϕ, and ϕ_0 and an additional piece of information about the echo amplitudes. Following the treatment in Glover (1991), we start with a more general analysis than in the previous subsection, taking into account echo amplitude factors that have been previously ignored. The 3PD images are described by:

$$I_0 = (A_{W0}W + A_{F0}F)e^{i\phi_0}$$

$$I_1 = (A_{W1}W - A_{F1}F)e^{i(\phi_0+\phi)} \qquad (17.72)$$

$$I_2 = (A_{W2}W + A_{F2}F)e^{i(\phi_0+2\phi)}$$

where the factors A_j in Eq. (17.72) describe the amplitude attenuation of the echoes that arises from three sources: diffusion, T_2^* decay, and spectral broadening. Diffusion attenuation occurs when water molecules diffuse through local magnetic field susceptibility gradients. The resulting phase dispersion within a voxel results in signal cancellation. T_2^* decay is also caused by local magnetic field susceptibility gradients that vary over the extent of a voxel. Even relatively static spins experience dephasing and intravoxel signal cancelation. Spectral broadening refers to the fact that the spectra of the water and lipid components are not delta functions as implicitly assumed. The width of the water spectrum is determined by T_2 for the water component, whereas the lipid spectrum is not a simple peak and has several overlapping resonances. The intravoxel dephasing caused by the multiple lipid resonances effectively results in a shorter T_2 for the lipid component as a whole.

In general, all the A_j are different. To solve Eqs. (17.72) we must make some simplifying assumptions that reduce the set of A_j to one unknown. Amplitude loss from diffusion can generally be ignored (Glover 1991). In the spin echo case, the spectral broadening and susceptibility dephasing effects are described by the amplitude factor $e^{-TE/T_2}e^{-j|\Delta|/T_2'}(j = 0, 1, 2)$ where T_2' is the field inhomogeneity loss component of T_2^* (see Example 14.5). The amplitude factor e^{-TE/T_2} is the same for all three images, but is different for fat and water because of different spectral broadening. The amplitude factor $e^{-j|\Delta|/T_2'}$ is the same for fat and water, but is different for the three images. In this section, we assume that the difference in spectral broadening between fat and water is negligible so that the amplitude factor e^{-TE/T_2} can be ignored. (Alternatively we can think of the spectral broadening amplitude differences as simply being absorbed into the definitions of F and W.) This allows the following simplification of Eqs. (17.72):

$$I_0 = (W + F)e^{i\phi_0}$$

$$I_1 = (W - F)Ae^{i(\phi_0+\phi)} \qquad (17.73)$$

$$I_2 = (W + F)A^2e^{i(\phi_0+2\phi)}$$

where $A = e^{-|\Delta|/T_2'}$. A similar simplification can be made for the gradient echo case.

To solve Eqs. (17.73), ϕ_0 is eliminated as before using:

$$I_0' = |I_0| = W + F$$

$$I_1' = I_1 e^{-i\phi_0} = \frac{I_1 I_0^*}{|I_0|} = (W - F)Ae^{i\phi}$$

$$I_2' = I_2 e^{-i\phi_0} = \frac{I_2 I_0^*}{|I_0|} = (W + F)A^2 e^{i2\phi}$$

(17.74)

The phase factor ϕ can now be obtained from the phase of I_2' and then eliminated from I_1' and I_2':

$$W + F = |I_0|$$

$$(W - F)A = I_1' e^{-i\phi} = p|I_1|$$

$$(W + F)A^2 = |I_2|$$

(17.75)

We can now obtain A using:

$$A = \sqrt{\frac{|I_2|}{|I_0|}}$$

(17.76)

The amplitude A is a susceptibility dephasing map and is useful for some applications such as blood oxygenation level–dependent (BOLD) brain functional imaging, the determination of iron concentration, or the assessment of trabecular bone structure. See, for example, Ma et al. (1997). The resulting equations:

$$W + F = |I_0|$$

$$W - F = \frac{I_1' e^{-i\phi}}{A} = \frac{p|I_1|}{A}$$

(17.77)

yield

$$W = \frac{1}{2}\left(|I_0| + \frac{p_c|I_1|}{A}\right)$$

$$F = \frac{1}{2}\left(|I_0| - \frac{p_c|I_1|}{A}\right)$$

(17.78)

where we have again replaced p with p_c. If we do not remove the amplitude A from the fat and water images, then using Eqs. (17.76) and (17.78) the solution is:

$$WA = \frac{1}{2}\left(\sqrt{|I_0||I_2|} + p_c|I_1|\right)$$
$$FA = \frac{1}{2}\left(\sqrt{|I_0||I_2|} - p_c|I_1|\right)$$
(17.79)

which is the same as Eq. (17.71). The equivalence of Eq. (17.71) and Eq. (17.79) shows that, under our assumptions, ignoring amplitude effects simply results in a multiplicative error in both water and fat components. This error is usually not serious and can be ignored. In fact, Eq. (17.78) has ENSA ≤ 2 (no better than the 2PD case), whereas Eq. (17.79) has ENSA $= 2.67$ (Glover 1991). Thus, there is a SNR penalty for the amplitude correction, and it is best avoided unless there is a specific need to compute A for the application of interest.

We now return briefly to 2PD and consider the effect of amplitude modulation. 2PD acquisitions do not have enough information to correct both the amplitude modulation A and B_0 inhomogeneity. Because the latter leads to more severe problems, amplitude modulation is usually not corrected with 2PD. We can understand the impact by considering the first two lines of Eq. (17.73), which are the same as the extended 2PD case, except now they include amplitude modulation. Eliminating ϕ_0 and ϕ as before yields the first two lines of Eq. (17.75). Substituting $|I_0|$ and $p|I_1|$ from the first two lines of Eq. (17.75) into the 2PD solution in Eq. (17.55) results in:

$$\left(|I_0| + p|I_1|\right) = W(1 + A) + F(1 - A)$$
$$\left(|I_0| - p|I_1|\right) = W(1 - A) + F(1 + A)$$
(17.80)

If $A = 1$, Eq. (17.80) reduces to Eq. (17.55), giving the correct values of water and fat. However, normally $A < 1$, resulting in the misrepresentation of water and fat in the two images. The water signal is slightly reduced in the water image, but, more important, spurious fat signal is also introduced, making the water image less useful as a fat-suppressed image. This problem is alleviated by using 3PD because the amplitude modulation cancels when the two in-phase echoes are combined, eliminating the water-fat mixing even when amplitude correction is omitted (Eq. 17.79). Using a $(\pi, 2\pi)$, 2PD acquisition also reduces the lipid contamination in the water image (Coombs et al. 1997).

Ideally we would like ENSA $= 3$ for 3PD to get the full benefit of the additional acquisition time. For phase angles $(0, \theta, 2\theta)$, the effective number of signal averages reaches its maximum value of ENSA $= 3$ when the three acquisitions are uniformly distributed around the circumference of a circle, that is, when $\theta = 2\pi/3$ (Glover 1991). For the phase choices $(0, \pi, -\pi)$ or $(0, \pi, 2\pi)$, ENSA $= 2.67$. Even though there is a slight SNR advantage to the uniform phase distribution $(0, 2\pi/3, 4\pi/3)$, two of the images can have a partial cancelation of fat and water. Thus, ϕ is always calculated from voxels that can have a low signal near water-fat boundaries because of the cancelation. The phase-angle choice for Dixon methods therefore involves a trade-off between the SNR and artifacts from errors in the phase determination.

Direct Phase Encoding   A generalization of 3PD, termed *direct phase encoding* (DPE) (Xiang and An 1997) uses the phase angle combination $(\theta_0, \theta_0 + \theta, \theta_0 + 2\theta)$. (Note that θ should be distinguished from the flip angle of RF pulses used in other sections of the book.) Ignoring amplitude modulation, the DPE images are:

$$
\begin{aligned}
I_0 &= (W + e^{i\theta_0} F) e^{i\phi_0} \\
I_1 &= (W + e^{i(\theta_0 + \theta)} F) e^{i(\phi_0 + \phi)} \\
I_2 &= (W + e^{i(\theta_0 + 2\theta)} F) e^{i(\phi_0 + 2\phi)}
\end{aligned}
\tag{17.81}
$$

The name DPE comes from an analogy with spatial phase encoding because the water and fat amplitudes are encoded into the DPE images through the phase angle combination $(\theta_0, \theta_0 + \theta, \theta_0 + 2\theta)$. Let X and Y be complex variables given by:

$$
\begin{aligned}
X &= W e^{i(\phi_0 + \phi)} \\
Y &= e^{i(\theta_0 + \theta)} F e^{i(\phi_0 + \phi)}
\end{aligned}
\tag{17.82}
$$

Equations (17.81) and (17.82) can be solved for X and Y. The fat and water components are then simply the magnitudes of X and Y for each voxel. The solution for X and Y is

$$
\begin{aligned}
X &= \frac{1}{2}(I_1 \pm \Delta I) \\
Y &= \frac{1}{2}(I_1 \mp \Delta I)
\end{aligned}
\tag{17.83}
$$

where

$$
\Delta I = \frac{\sqrt{(e^{i\theta} + 1)^2 - 4e^{i\theta} I_0 I_2}}{e^{i\theta} - 1}
\tag{17.84}
$$

The sign choice in Eq. (17.83) is ambiguous because of uncertainty about the absolute phase of X and Y. However, as long as $\theta_0 + \theta \neq 0, \pm\pi, \pm 2\pi, \dots$ (i.e. $e^{i(\theta_0 + \theta)} \neq \pm 1$), an unambiguous sign choice is possible without direct

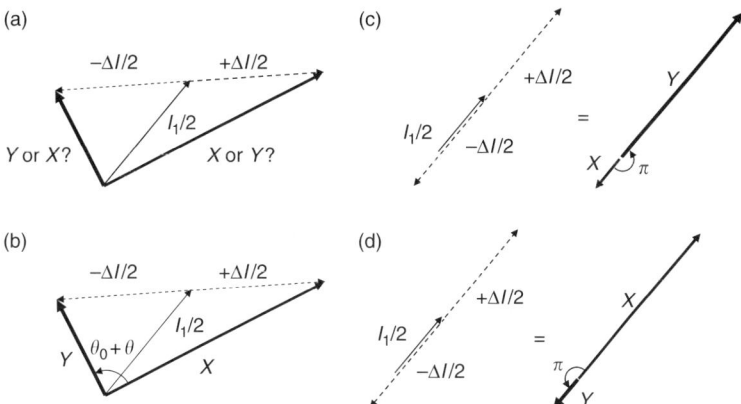

FIGURE 17.25 Direct phase encoding 3PD with phase angles $(\theta_0, \theta_0 + \theta, \theta_0 + 2\theta)$. (a) The correct sign in Eq. (17.83) to determine X and Y is ambiguous in general. (b) When $\theta_0 + \theta \neq 0, \pm\pi, \pm 2\pi, \ldots$, the correct sign can be chosen based on the phase relationship between X and Y. (c–d) When X and Y are parallel or anti-parallel ($\theta_0 + \theta = \pi$ in this example), either sign choice is consistent and the ambiguity must be resolved by determining the absolute phase of X and Y (thereby requiring phase unwrapping).

determination of the absolute phase of X and Y. (Note also that the constraint $\theta \neq 0, \pm 2\pi, \ldots$ is required or else the denominator in Eq. (17.84) becomes zero.) From Eq. (17.82), the relative angle between the vector representations of the complex numbers X and Y is known to be $\theta_0 + \theta$, and this is determined by the pulse sequence. The correct sign choice in Eq. (17.83) is therefore the one that is consistent with a relative angle of $\theta_0 + \theta$. As long as X and Y are not parallel or anti-parallel, the sign can be correctly determined (Figure 17.25a and b). When X and Y are parallel or anti-parallel, either sign choice is consistent and the absolute phase of X and Y must be determined to establish the correct sign (Figure 17.25c and d). Thus, for $\theta_0 + \theta \neq 0, \pm\pi, \pm 2\pi, \ldots$, the phase unwrapping problems associated with the 3PD phase choice $(0, \pi, 2\pi)$ are cleverly avoided.

Although phase-wrapping problems are avoided with this method, several additional countermeasures must still be taken to prevent the occasional interchange of fat and water signals. Voxels where one component is much smaller than the other can be difficult to assign correctly. If either X or Y has a much smaller magnitude than the other does (e.g., less than 10%), then the voxel may actually have only one true component and the other component is due to noise. The dominant component is likely to be water because voxels containing 100% fat are not expected to be present in living tissues (Xiang and An 1997). The longer vector is assigned as water in this case.

To further prevent the interchange of water and fat assignment, an elaborate set of local and global orientation filters are used in this technique (Xiang and An 1997). The filters are based on the assumption that the phase factor $e^{i(\phi_0+\phi)}$ in X and Y is expected to be slowly varying. An orientation field O, defined as $O = X + Ye^{-i(\theta_0+\theta)}$, ideally has phase $e^{i(\phi_0+\phi)}$ (see Eq. 17.82). The local orientation filter compares the orientation field for a voxel to that of its filtered neighbors (e.g., using a 5×5 or 7×7 filter) and swaps X and Y for the voxel if necessary to get better agreement. The global orientation filter computes the orientation field at each voxel by repeated region growing from randomly distributed seed voxels. The values of X and Y are swapped for the voxel if it results in a better agreement with the majority of the grown results. A complete discussion of the orientation filters is found in Xiang and An (1997). A similar orientation filter has been used for phase correction in phase sensitive inversion recovery (Section 14.2).

Once X and Y are determined for the voxel, Eq. (17.81) can be used to determine the phase factors $e^{i\phi_0}$ and $e^{i\phi}$, which can then be eliminated from the equations. Equation (17.81) can be solved again and the resulting multiple solutions for W and F combined for a better SNR.

The optimal choice for θ_0 and θ involves a trade-off between the SNR and solution stability (i.e., the immunity from interchange of water and fat). As mentioned before, the SNR is maximal (ENSA $= 3$) for $\theta = 2\pi/3$. However, as in the original 3PD case, a more stable solution is obtained when $\theta = \pi$. In addition, the correct determination of the sign in Eq. (17.83) is most probable when $\theta_0 + \theta = \pm\pi/2$ (i.e., when X and Y are orthogonal). Thus, the phase choices $(-3\pi/2, -\pi/2, \pi/2)$ and $(-\pi/2, \pi/2, 3\pi/2)$ are optimal for solution stability while giving ENSA $= 2.67$, which is close to the maximal SNR case.

Correction for Chemical Shift Misregistration   Once the water and fat images have been separately determined, the chemical shift of water and fat in the readout direction for Cartesian k-space trajectories can be eliminated. The water-fat chemical shift in pixels is:

$$\Delta x = \frac{N_x f_{cs}}{2\Delta\nu} \tag{17.85}$$

where $\pm\Delta\nu$ is the readout bandwidth and N_x is the image matrix size in the readout direction. One of the two component images (water or fat) can be shifted in the readout direction by Δx by Fourier transforming the image in that direction, multiplying the image by the appropriate linear phase ramp, and Fourier transforming it back to the image domain. If the fat image is shifted, for example, it can then be added to the water image to obtain a completely registered image showing both water and fat components. The cancelation of water and fat signals due to intravoxel dephasing is eliminated in the resulting composite image with all Dixon methods. As previously noted, however, some methods are more prone to interchange of the water and fat signals. Unfortunately, the resulting SNR efficiency of the composite image is rather poor. For small shifts with the $(0, \pi, 2\pi)$ or $(0, \pi, -\pi)$ 3PD methods, ENSA $= 1.33$ (Glover 1991). In summary, 3PD can offer images without the chemical shift artifact in the frequency direction, but at a substantial SNR cost.

17.3.3 Phase Determination Methods

The determination of the phase of noisy 2D or 3D complex data is a problem that has arisen in many fields. A completely satisfactory solution for all applications is still not available, prompting the continuing development of new methods. Some methods calculate the phase using the arctangent operation and then attempt to remove the phase wraps. Other methods do not use phase unwrapping and determine the phase either directly or indirectly using consistency criteria, for example with the orientation filters discussed in subsection 17.3.2 or the interecho phase consistency used in Wang et al. (1998). Most phase determination methods use some simplifying assumption about the phase behavior. If that assumption is violated, the phase is incorrectly calculated, resulting in incorrect estimates of the fat and water signals. Such errors are most common when the phase estimate is very noisy due to low signal amplitude. Problems with the robustness of phase unwrapping algorithms have slowed the introduction of Dixon techniques into routine clinical practice.

A brief description of two methods that have been reported in the literature with Dixon processing is presented here. These two methods are applicable to both gradient echo and spin echo acquisitions. Both methods are described with reference to 3PD, although they can also be used with 2PD data. For simplicity, the following discussion is based on 2D acquisition, although the methods can also be extended to 3D.

Polynomial Fitting   This method assumes that ϕ varies slowly over the image (not including the background noise in air) and can be described by a relatively low-order polynomial such as a quadratic or cubic, for example:

$$2\phi = ax + bx^2 + cy + dy^2 + exy + f \qquad (17.86)$$

where 2ϕ is the phase of I_2' in Eq. (17.68), x and y are coordinates on the 2D image plane, and a, b, c, d, e, and f are coefficients to be determined by fitting. Suppose an arctangent is used to calculate 2ϕ, resulting in a wrapped estimate $(2\phi)_w$:

$$(2\phi)_w = \arctan\left[\frac{\text{Im}(I'_2)}{\text{Re}(I'_2)}\right] \tag{17.87}$$

In Eq. (17.87), a four-quadrant arctangent (defined in Section 13.5) is used to minimize phase wraps. Phase wrapping precludes fitting $(2\phi)_w$ directly to Eq. (17.86). If the derivative of $(2\phi)_w$ is taken in the x and y directions, the phase wraps, which are discontinuities in $(2\phi)_w$, appear as spikes in the derivative and are easily detected using a threshold. The derivatives can then be fit to the appropriate x and y derivatives of the polynomial in Eq. (17.86) while excluding the phase wrap points from the fit. For example, $\partial(2\phi)_w/\partial x$ and $\partial(2\phi)_w/\partial y$ (excluding wrapped points) are fit to $a+2bx+ey$ and $c+2dy+ex$, respectively, giving estimates of a, b, c, d, and e (f can be defined as the mean of $(2\phi)_w$). Subtracting $a + 2bx + ey$ from $\partial(2\phi)_w/\partial x$ and $c + 2dy + ex$ from $\partial(2\phi)_w/\partial y$ gives new data that can be thresholded to further exclude noisy data from the fit. The process can be iterated to give improved estimates of a, b, c, d, e, and f. Once the polynomial in Eq. (17.86) is determined, it is subtracted from $(2\phi)_w$. Phase wraps in the difference $(2\phi)_w - (ax + bx^2 + cy + dy^2 + exy + f)$ now appear as discontinuities that are multiples of 2π. The phase wrapping can be detected by another threshold process and removed by shifting the difference by the nearest correct multiple of 2π. Once the data have been shifted, the polynomial in Eq. (17.86) is added back to obtain the unwrapped final phase 2ϕ. More details of this method can be found in Glover and Schneider (1991) and Chen et al. (1999).

One possible drawback with this method is poor unwrapping in regions where the phase varies rapidly due to local susceptibility changes. In such areas, the assumption of low-order phase variation (Eq. 17.86) is likely to be violated. The problem is alleviated by iterating the fitting as discussed in Chen et al. (1999), but if the phase wraps multiple times within a single voxel, no unwrapping method will be effective. The phase unwrapping algorithm described in this subsection is frequently used for phase-contrast image data to extract quantitative flow information (see Section 15.2). That application is much less demanding than 3PD, however, when the spatial region that needs to be unwrapped is limited to a small operator-placed region of interest that covers only a single vessel.

Region Growing   In this method, a four-quadrant arctangent is also used to calculate 2ϕ (Eq. 17.87), resulting in a wrapped estimate $(2\phi)_w$. A region of unwrapped pixels and a set of pixels to have their neighbors tested for phase wrapping are maintained. It is assumed that nearest neighbor pixels have at most one phase wrap. First, a threshold is applied to the image to

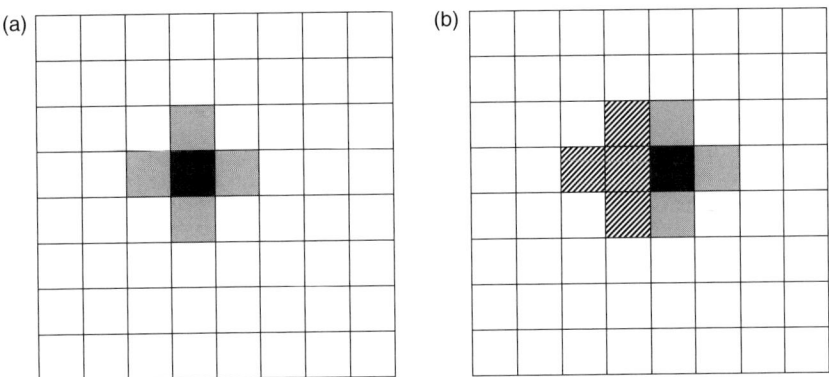

FIGURE 17.26 Phase unwrapping by region growing. (a) Starting seed pixel (dark) and the four nearest neighbors (gray) being tested for phase wraps. (b) After unwrapping, the nearest neighbors of the seed pixel are added to the region of unwrapped pixels (diagonal hatched lines). Each of the unwrapped pixels is used as a new seed pixel (dark) and tested against neighbors (gray).

eliminate regions of low signal intensity (e.g., regions where the magnitude image is less 10% of its maximum are eliminated). A seed pixel in a region of high signal is taken as the starting point. The four nearest neighbor pixels are unwrapped (Figure 17.26) by first testing whether the absolute value of the difference exceeds a threshold $\Delta\xi$ (e.g. $\Delta\xi \sim \pi/8$). Only neighbor pixels with magnitudes above the threshold are tested. If the difference is less than $\Delta\xi$, the neighbor pixel phase is not changed and the neighbor is added to the region of unwrapped pixels and to the set to pixels to have their neighbors tested. Otherwise, the neighbor phase is shifted by 2π in the appropriate direction and the new difference is checked against the threshold $\Delta\xi$. If the new difference is greater than $\Delta\xi$, the original neighbor pixel phase is maintained and the pixel is not added to the unwrapped region or set of pixels to check. Neighbor pixels that are already in the unwrapped region are not added to the set for testing. The process ends when there are no more pixels on the stack to be tested. This method is summarized in Figure 17.27 and described in more detail in Szumowski et al. (1994).

One possible problem with this method is wrapping by more than one multiple of 2π in regions of high susceptibility. Another possible drawback is that areas of low signal will not be unwrapped because of the initial amplitude thresholding, which could lead to isolated islands of unwrapped pixels. An example of this situation can be found in images consisting of multiple unconnected regions, such as an axial abdomen image with arms in the FOV. This problem can be alleviated by running the algorithm multiple times with seed

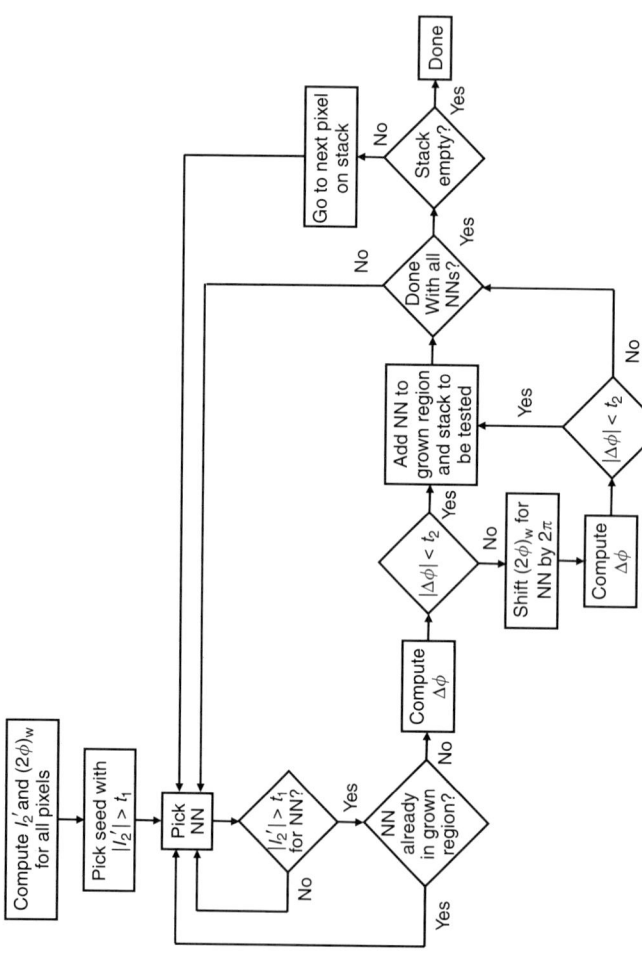

FIGURE 17.27 Flow chart showing a simple region growing phase unwrapping algorithm. NN, nearest neighbor voxel; t_1, a threshold to exclude points with low signal amplitude; $\Delta\phi$, the difference in wrapped phase $(2\phi)_w$ between adjacent voxels; $t_2 = \Delta\xi$, a threshold to detect phase-wrapped pixels.

points in different locations. Other types of region growing methods are possible. Two more variations are described in Zhang et al. (1996) and Akkerman and Mass (1995).

Other Methods   A method for determining ϕ that works for $(0, \pi, 2\pi)$ gradient echo acquisitions based on consistency of the phase between the in-phase images is given in Wang et al. (1998). This method does not require phase unwrapping, but requires that the absolute value of the phase in the first in-phase image be less than 270°.

Another method that is very general solves the Poisson equation:

$$\nabla^2 \phi = \nabla \cdot \left(\text{Wrap}[\nabla \psi] \right) \tag{17.88}$$

where ϕ is the true phase, ψ is the wrapped phase, and Wrap is the phase-wrapping operator, defined by:

$$\psi = \text{Wrap}[\phi] = \phi + 2\pi k \tag{17.89}$$

for some integer k such that $-\pi \leq \psi < \pi$ (Song et al. 1995). This method has also been used extensively in published 3PD work. Song et al. (1995) also has citations for numerous other phase-unwrapping methods.

A review of the MRI phase-unwrapping problem along with a general discussion of some mathematical properties of phase maps and literature citations of phase-unwrapping methods is given in Chavez et al. (2002). This reference also presents an unwrapping method based on the presence of dipoles within the phase map. (Dipoles are 2×2 pixel loops around which the phase is inconsistent.)

17.3.4 PULSE SEQUENCE ENHANCEMENTS AND VARIATIONS

Single-Point Dixon   The underlying idea of the single-point Dixon method is to acquire a single scan, either gradient echo or RF spin echo, with a water-fat phase shift of $\pi/2$. If there were no other phase shifts present, water would correspond to one component of the complex data (the real part for example) and fat would correspond to the other component (Paltiel and Ban 1985; Patrick and Haacke 1985). Instead, the phase errors discussed in previous subsections cause the real and imaginary components to be mixtures of water and fat. The image is given by:

$$I = (W + iF)e^{i\phi_0} \tag{17.90}$$

There is not enough information in a single scan to remove ϕ_0 because there are three unknown variables (W, F, and ϕ_0) and two equations (the magnitude and phase of I represent two independent equations). This can be especially problematic for gradient echoes in which B_0 inhomogeneity creates a large contribution to ϕ_0 due to phase accumulation during the entire echo time (for spin echoes, the B_0 inhomogeneity accumulates net phase only during the echo shift Δ). Fitting the image phase to a low-frequency polynomial in order to estimate ϕ_0 has met with some success (Hajal and Young 1995). So far, however, this technique has not been used very much clinically.

Four-Point Dixon   With four acquisitions, additional information about the echo amplitude modulation can be obtained and used (Glover 1991). Amplitude loss from fat spectral broadening as well as susceptibility dephasing can be included. A four-point phase increment method $(0, \theta, 2\theta, 3\theta)$ has an optimal SNR when $\theta = \pi/4$, but the equations are difficult to solve. The equations for a simpler 4PD method using $\theta = \pi$ can be written:

$$
\begin{aligned}
I_0 &= (W + F)e^{i\phi_0} \\
I_1 &= (W A_W - F A_F)e^{i(\phi_0 + \phi)} \\
I_2 &= (W A_W^2 + F A_F^2)e^{i(\phi_0 + 2\phi)} \\
I_3 &= (W A_W^3 - F A_F^3)e^{i(\phi_0 + 3\phi)}
\end{aligned}
\tag{17.91}
$$

where A_W and A_F are echo amplitude exponential decay factors for water and fat, respectively. Both A_W and A_F include signal loss from susceptibility dephasing as well as spectral broadening. For the special case:

$$
\begin{aligned}
A_W &\approx 1 - \varepsilon_W \\
A_F &\approx 1 - \varepsilon_F
\end{aligned}
\tag{17.92}
$$

with $\varepsilon_W \ll 1$ and $\varepsilon_F \ll 1$ Eq. (17.91) can be solved to obtain W, F, A_W, and A_F (Glover 1991). The solution for W and F has ENSA $= 1.14$, although ENSA $= 4$ for A_W and A_F. The low ENSA for W and F is due to the nonoptimal choice of phase increment $\theta = \pi$.

Multiple Spectral Components—Water, Fat and Silicone Imaging   Silicone implant rupture and leakage are potential problems with patients who have had reconstructive or cosmetic surgery (e.g., for the breast). At 1.5 T, the silicone resonance frequency is only approximately 105 Hz below that of lipid. This small difference makes the selective excitation of silicone or suppression of fat using spectrally selective RF pulses difficult. The discrimination of silicone from fat can be achieved with an extension of 3PD that exploits the fortuitous fact that the silicone-lipid frequency difference is approximately one-half of the lipid-water frequency difference (Schneider and Chan 1993). In this technique, silicone is placed on resonance and a 3PD acquisition with phases $(0, \pi, 2\pi)$ is used. However, the echo shift Δ is calculated for the silicone-lipid frequency difference, instead of the lipid-water frequency difference; that is, $\Delta = 1/(2 \times 105 \text{ Hz})$ at 1.5 T for the opposed-phase image. This places silicone and fat in phase on the first and third image and out of phase on the second image. Because the lipid-water frequency difference is approximately 210 Hz at 1.5 T, water and fat are approximately in phase (i.e., 0, 2π, and 4π) on all three images. Processing the data therefore gives a silicone-only image and a combined water-fat image, thereby enabling silicone detection without fat contamination.

An extension of DPE called chemical shift imaging with spectrum modeling (CSISM) is an efficient method for spectroscopic imaging with multiple spectral peaks (An and Xiang 2001). This method assumes that all spectral peaks can be modeled as delta functions with known resonance frequency differences. Images $I_0, I_1, \ldots, I_{K-1}$ are acquired with phase shifts $(0, \theta, 2\theta, \ldots, (K-1)\theta)$. A nonlinear system of equations for the complex image values as a function of spectral peak amplitudes results for each pixel in the image. If N spectral components are present, the system of equations can be solved for the spectral amplitudes if $2K - 1 \geq N + 1$. For example, with $N = 3$ spectral components, $K = 3$ separate phase shifts are sufficient to solve for the spectral peaks. The algorithm has been successfully applied to separating lipid, water, and silicone spectral components.

A method for dealing with an arbitrary number of spectral components with known chemical shifts, but with arbitrary phase angles $(0, \theta_1, \theta_2, \ldots)$ uses an iterative least-squares method to solve the resulting system of complex equations (Reeder et al. 2004). The B_0 inhomogeneity phase shift is not explicitly calculated but instead iteratively estimated starting from an initial guess, thus avoiding problems with phase unwrapping. This method has been successfully applied to separating lipid, water, and silicone spectral components, as well as lipid-water separation with RARE and SSFP where it is advantageous to use small echo shifts Δ in order to minimize increases to the echo spacing and TR. Another advantage is that the method is easily extendable to include multiple receive coils.

Scan Time Considerations One of the drawbacks of Dixon's method is its increased scan time. Although the longer acquisition time also improves SNR, misregistration artifacts can result from patient motion. This problem can be alleviated by interleaving the acquisition so that data with all desired temporal shifts Δ are acquired at a given Fourier-encoding step before moving on to the next one (Wang et al. 1998).

Scan time can be reduced by using multiple echoes of an RF spin echo pulse sequence with different shifts on the various echoes. The echo shifts could be incorporated in several different ways (Yeung and Kormos 1986; Williams et al. 1989; Szumowski et al. 1995). For example, one acquisition could use $\Delta = 0$ for all echoes, whereas a second one could use $\Delta = 1/(2f_{cs})$ for the first echo and $\Delta = 1/f_{cs}$ for the second echo. One potential problem with this method is the introduction of additional amplitude modulation into the in-phase and opposed-phase images due to differences in TE. (In Eq. 17.73, we assumed that with RF spin echo acquisitions, all echoes were acquired with the same TE and the resulting amplitude modulation A came from the RF refocusing pulse shift Δ, i.e., $A = e^{-|\Delta|/T_2'}$.) Depending on the TEs of the in-phase and opposed-phase echoes, the resulting amplitude modulation could introduce substantial mixing of the fat and water signals.

Another way to reduce scan time in an RF spin echo acquisition is to use a train of gradient echoes (also sometimes called sandwich echoes) to acquire data with multiple values of Δ with a single RF excitation (Zhang et al. 1996). The gradient echoes can be acquired after one 180° RF pulse or with multiple 180° pulses, like a GRASE pulse sequence (Section 16.2). Figure 17.28 shows a $(-\pi, 0, \pi)$ acquisition in which the center echo is in-phase and the other two are opposed-phase. Because all values of Δ are acquired within the same Fourier-encoding step, problems with patient motion are minimized. The time

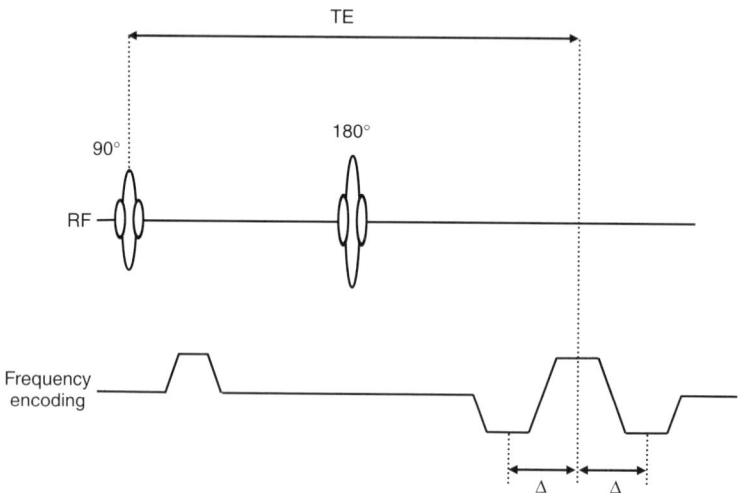

FIGURE 17.28 Dixon's method using a train of three gradient echoes (sandwich echoes) with alternating readout polarity. The second echo refocuses at the Hahn or RF echo time. The echo spacing Δ is chosen to give water-fat phase shifts $(-\pi, 0, \pi)$. Only the frequency-encoding gradient waveform is shown for simplicity.

between adjacent gradient echoes decreases with increasing field strength (e.g., adjacent echoes are approximately 7.1 ms apart at 0.5 T, but only about 2.4 ms apart at 1.5 T). Therefore scanners with relatively weak gradient hardware may only be able to apply this technique at low field strengths or with very low spatial resolution. If sufficient slew rate and amplitude are available, all echoes can be collected with the same frequency-encoding gradient polarity, otherwise the polarity must alternate, as in EPI. Alternating the readout polarity causes fat to be chemically shifted in opposite directions in the in-phase and opposed-phase images, which must be corrected by resampling (e.g., as described in subsection 17.3.2) unless the shift is substantially less than one pixel. Another problem with alternating the readout polarity is that RF and gradient group delays and eddy currents shift the echoes in the k_x direction. After time reversal to correct the gradient polarity reversal, the in-phase and opposed-phase echoes are misaligned in k-space, giving linear phase shifts that are inconsistent between in-phase and opposed-phase images. Correction methods similar to those used in EPI are necessary (Section 16.1).

Perhaps the ultimate use of echo train acquisition to acquire multiple echo shifts within one Fourier-encoding step is gradient echo sampling of FID and echo (GESFIDE) (Ma et al. 1997). This pulse sequence uses a 90° pulse followed by a train of gradient echoes, followed by a 180° pulse and another train of gradient echoes (Figure 17.29). The echoes are alternately in-phase and opposed-phase. This method was developed to image T_2 and T_2', as well as water and fat components. The echoes are first processed in groups of three to determine water and fat components. For example, in Figure 17.29 twelve echoes are collected that are processed in the groups (S_0, S_1, S_2), (S_2, S_3, S_4), and so on. Each group generates water and fat images, which are then averaged to improve the SNR. The T_2 and T_2' components can be obtained by linear regression fitting of the in-phase (for a higher SNR) echo amplitudes before and after the refocusing pulse to exponential curves.

RARE (fast spin echo) has replaced conventional RF spin echo for many imaging applications because of its speed. Fat is especially problematic with T_2-weighted RARE because it is brighter than on conventional T_2-weighted RF spin echo images. If Dixon's method were incorporated into RARE by simply time shifting the refocusing pulses by $\Delta/2$, as with an RF spin echo, the CPMG conditions (Section 16.4) would not be met, resulting in signal loss and artifacts.

One alternative is to shift the entire readout gradient waveform by Δ (Szumowski et al. 1995). Unfortunately, this increases the minimum echo spacing by 2Δ. At 1.5 T, $\Delta = 2.4$ ms, giving a minimum echo spacing increase of approximately 4.8 ms. Depending on the prescription parameters, this could be a large fraction of the minimum echo spacing, leading to blurring and reduced slice coverage for a given imaging time. The increase in echo spacing can be reduced by using a value of Δ smaller than the one required for opposed-phase

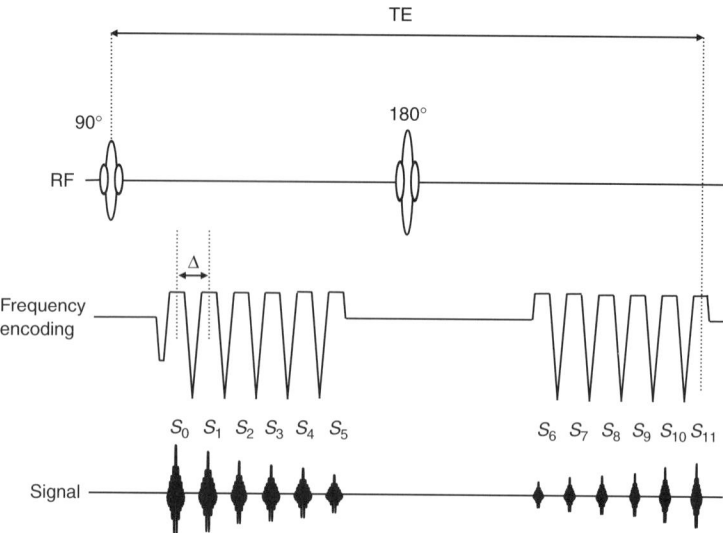

FIGURE 17.29 Dixon's method using GESFIDE. The echoes are alternately in-phase and opposed-phase. In this example, all twelve echoes are collected with the same readout gradient polarity. Only the frequency-encoding gradient waveform is shown for simplicity.

images (Reeder et al. 2004). For example, a 3PD acquisition with phase shifts $(0, \theta, -\theta)$ can be used, where $\theta < \pi$. Figure 17.21 shows a 1.5-T example of FSE with $\Delta = 0, \pm 1.2$ ms. The echo spacing was increased by only 2.4 ms in this case. Because of the arbitrary phase shifts, the data must be processed as described previously.

An alternative method is to keep the readout gradient lobe location held fixed, but to add a readout prephasing gradient lobe that shifts the point where each echo peak refocuses (Ma et al. 2002a). In order to maintain the CPMG condition, another gradient lobe of opposite polarity to the prephaser is added after the readout lobe (Figure 17.30). The shifted echo is truncated at the beginning (i.e., partial or fractional echo) because of the prephasing gradient. Because the two additional gradient lobes can be overlapped with the slice crusher gradient lobes and phase-encoding/rewinding lobes, there is not necessarily an increase in minimum echo spacing.

The echo for the first in-phase scan with $\Delta = 0$ is symmetric because there is no time shift. The second in-phase echo has the lowest echo fraction because Δ is greatest. Partial echo data are normally processed using partial-Fourier reconstruction algorithms such as homodyne reconstruction (Section 13.4). The homodyne algorithm removes the image phase information that would be

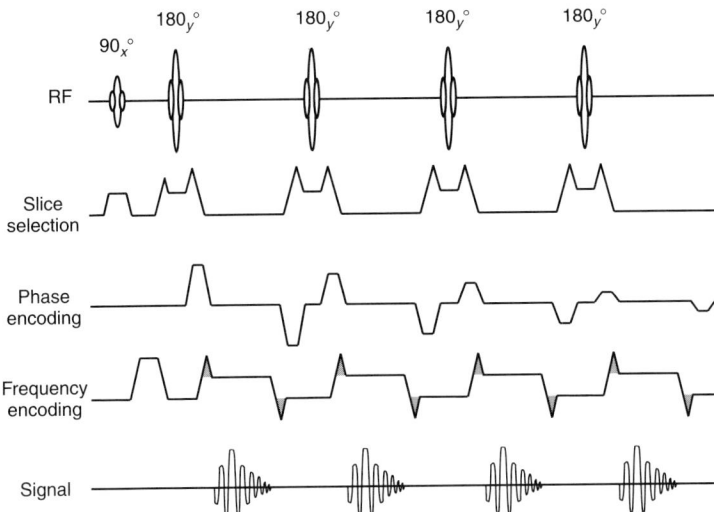

FIGURE 17.30 Pulse sequence for using Dixon's method with RARE. A readout gradient prephaser is added to shift each echo peak (positive gray area). To maintain the CPMG condition, a lobe of opposite polarity is also added after the readout lobe (negative gray area). This shifted echo is a partial echo because its beginning is truncated.

used to determine 2ϕ from I_2 (see Eq. 17.66). However, the low-frequency component of phase information that would normally be used in the homodyne algorithm can also be used in 3PD (Rybicki et al. 2001). This low-frequency phase information can be calculated from a portion of echo data that is symmetric around $k_x = 0$. The phase ϕ can be determined from low-frequency phase maps using the region-growing algorithm previously discussed. The magnitude images $|I_1|$ and $|I_2|$ can then be reconstructed using the homodyne algorithm. A simplification of this is to reconstruct $|I_1|$ using zero filling if the readout time is long enough that echo truncation is small (e.g., 15%). 3PD RARE data have been acquired using conventional 3PD phase choices as well as DPE phase choices and reconstructed using this algorithm with good image quality.

Multiple Coils The SNR improvement inherent with multiple coil arrays is desirable, especially with fast pulse sequences that use high bandwidth readout and gradient echoes. The magnetization in the reconstructed image is multiplied by the coil receive B_1 field or sensitivity. The phase of the sensitivity is therefore contained in the image phase. Because the receive coils generally each have different sensitivities and because phase information is used in Dixon processing for water-fat separation, some care must be taken when multiple coil data are combined. Reeder et al. (2004) and Ma et al. (2002b) show two methods for such a combination.

Finally, we note that parallel-imaging methods can lessen the scan time increase inherent to Dixon's method. The SNR increase from the multiple acquisitions necessary for Dixon processing is partially offset by the SNR loss inherent in parallel-imaging methods, but a net SNR benefit can still result in some cases (Ma et al. 2003).

SELECTED REFERENCES

Adalsteinsson, E., Irarrazabal, P., Topp, S., Meyer, C., Macovski, A., and Spielman, D. M. 1998. Volumetric spectroscopic imaging with spiral-based k-space trajectories. *Magn. Reson. Med.* 39: 889–898.

Akkerman, E. M., and Maas, M. 1995. A region-growing algorithm to simultaneously remove dephasing influences and separate fat and water in two-point Dixon. In *Proceedings of the 3rd meeting of the Society for Magnetic Resonance*, p. 649.

An, L., and Xiang, Q.-S. 2001. Chemical shift imaging with spectrum modeling. *Magn. Reson. Med.* 46: 126–130.

Brown, T. R. 1992. Practical applications of chemical shift imaging. *Nucl. Magn. Reson. Biomed.* 5: 238–243.

Chavez, S., Xiang, Q.-S., and An, L. 2002. Understanding phase maps in MRI: A new cutline phase unwrapping method. *IEEE Trans. Med. Imaging* 21: 966–977.

Chen, Q.-S., Schneider, E., Aghazadeh, B., Weinhous, M. S., Humm, J., and Ballon, D. 1999. An automated iterative algorithm for water and fat decomposition in three-point Dixon magnetic resonance imaging. *Med. Phys.* 26: 2341–2347.

Coombs, B. D., Szumowski, J., and Coshow, W. 1997. Two-point Dixon technique for water-fat signal decomposition with B0 inhomogeneity correction. *Magn. Reson. Med.* 38: 884–889.

Dixon, W. T. 1984. Simple proton spectroscopic imaging. *Radiology* 153: 189–194.

Glover, G. H. 1991. Multipoint Dixon technique for water and fat proton and susceptibility imaging. *J. Magn. Reson. Imaging* 1: 521–530.

Glover, G. H., and Schneider, E. 1991. Three-point Dixon technique for true water/fat decomposition with B0 inhomogeneity correction. *Magn. Reson. Med.* 18: 371–383.

Hajnal, J. V., and Young, I. R. 1995. Use of spatial phase distribution models to produce water and fat only images from single echo shifted data sets. In *Proceeding of the 3rd meeting of the Society for Magnetic Resonance*, p. 650.

Hardy, P. A., Hinks, R. S., and Tkach, J. A. 1995. Separation of fat and water in fast spin-echo MR imaging with the three-point Dixon technique. *J. Magn. Reson. Imaging* 5: 181–185.

Lee, J. K. T., Dixon, W. T., Ling, D., Levitt, R. G., and Murphy, W. A. 1984. Fatty infiltration of the liver: Demonstration by proton spectroscopic imaging. *Radiology* 153: 195–201.

Leroy-Willig, A., Bittoun, J., Luton, J. P., Louvel, A, Lefever, J. E., Bonnin, A., and Roucayrol, J. C. 1989. In vivo MR spectroscopic imaging of the adrenal glands: Distinction between adenomas and carcinomas larger than 15 mm based on lipid content. *Am. J. Roentgenol.* 153: 771–773.

Ma, J., Bankson, J. A., and Stafford, R. J. 2003. Multipoint Dixon imaging using sensitivity encoding. In *Proceedings of the 11th Meeting of the International Society for Magnetic Resonance in Medicine*, p. 1069.

Ma, J., Singh, S. K., Kumar, A. J., Leeds, N. E., and Broemeling, L. D. 2002a. Method for efficient fast spin echo Dixon imaging. *Magn. Reson. Med.* 48: 1021–1027.

Ma, J., Singh, S. K., Kumar, A. J., Leeds, N. E., and Broemeling, L. D. 2002b. Phased array coil compatible T2-weighted fast spin echo Dixon imaging. In *Proceedings of the 10th meeting of International Society for Magnetic Resonance in Medicine*, p. 735.

Ma, J., Wehrli, F. W., Song, H. K., and Hwang, S. N. 1997 A single-scan imaging technique for measurement of the relative concentrations of fat and water protons and their transverse relaxation times. *J. Magn. Reson.* 125: 92–101.

Paltiel, Z., and Ban, A. 1985. Separate water and lipid images obtained by a single scan. In *Proceedings of the 4th meeting of the Society for Magnetic Resonance in Medicine*, p. 172.

Patrick, J. L., and Haacke, E. M. 1985. Water/fat separation and chemical shift artifact correction using a single scan. In *Proceedings of the 4th meeting of the Society for Magnetic Resonance in Medicine*, p. 174.

Reeder, S. B., Wen, Z., Yu, H., Pineda, A. R., Gold G. E., Markl, M., and Pelc, N.J. 2004. Multicoil Dixon chemical species separation with an iterative least-squares estimation method. *Magn. Reson. Med.* 51: 35–45.

Rosen, B. R., Fleming, D. M., Kushner, D. C., Zaner, K. S., Buxton, R. B., Bennet, W. P., Wismer, G. L., and Brady, T. J. 1988. Hematologic bone marrow disorders: Quantitative chemical shift MR imaging. *Radiology* 169: 799–804.

Rybicki, F. J., Mulkern, R. V., Robertson, R. L., Robson, C. D., Chung, T., and Ma, J. 2001. Fast three-point Dixon MR imaging of the retrobulbar space with low-resolution images for phase correction: Comparison with fast spin-echo inversion recovery imaging. *Am. J. Neuroradiol.* 22: 1798–1802.

Schneider, E., and Chan, T. W. 1993. Selective MR imaging of silicone with the three-point Dixon technique. *Radiology* 187: 89–93.

Sepponen, R. E., Sipponen, J. T., and Tanttu, J. I. 1984. A method for chemical shift imaging: Demonstration of bone marrow involvement with proton chemical shift imaging. *J. Comput. Assist. Tomogr.* 8: 585–587.

Skinner, T. E., and Glover, G. H. 1997. An extended two-point Dixon algorithm for calculating separate water, fat and B0 images. *Magn. Reson. Med.* 37: 628–630.

Song, S. M.-H., Napel, S., Pelc, N. J., and Glover, G. H. 1995. Phase unwrapping of MR phase images using Poisson equation. *IEEE Trans. Image Processing* 4: 667–676.

Szumowski, J., Coshow, W., Li, F., Coombs, B., and Quinn, S. F. 1995. Double-echo three-point-Dixon method for fat suppression MRI. *Magn. Reson. Med.* 34: 120–124.

Szumowski, J., Coshow, W. R., Li, F., and Quinn, S. F. 1994. Phase unwrapping in the three-point Dixon method for fat suppression MR imaging. *Radiology* 192: 555–561.

Wang, Y., Li, D., Haacke, E. M., and Brown, J. J. 1998. A three-point Dixon method for water and fat separation using 2D and 3D gradient-echo techniques. *J. Magn. Reson. Imaging* 8: 703–710.

Williams, S. C. R., Horsfield, M. A., and Hall, L. D. 1989. True water and fat MR imaging with use of multiple-echo acquisition. *Radiology* 173: 249–253.

Xiang, Q.-S., and An, L. 1997. Water-fat imaging with direct phase encoding. *J. Magn. Reson. Imaging* 7: 1002–1015.

Yeung, H. N., and Kormos, D. W. 1986. Separation of true fat and water images by correcting magnetic field inhomogeneity in situ. *Radiology* 159: 783–786.

Zhang, W., Goldhaber, D. M., and Kramer, D. M. 1996. Separation of water and fat MR images in a single scan at .35T using "sandwich" echoes. *J. Magn. Reson. Imaging* 6: 909–917.

RELATED SECTIONS

Section 14.1 Gradient Echo
Section 14.3 Radiofrequency Spin Echo
Section 16.4 RARE

17.4 Driven Equilibrium

In T_2-weighted and proton-density-weighted RF spin echo and RARE pulse sequences, TR is usually relatively long to allow complete recovery of longitudinal magnetization. Reducing the scan time by using a shorter value of TR reduces the SNR of long T_1 tissues and introduces unwanted T_1 weighting. *Driven equilibrium* or DE (also known as driven equilibrium Fourier transform, DEFT; and fast recovery or FR) was first introduced into pulsed Fourier transform spectroscopy in order to increase the SNR for acquisitions with short repetition times (Becker et al. 1969).

In MRI, DE was originally applied to conventional RF spin echo pulse sequences (van Uijen and den Boef 1984; Maki et al. 1988) to allow TR to be decreased without SNR loss or increased T_1 weighting. With RF spin echo pulse sequences, DE is implemented by applying a 180° refocusing pulse after the echo is collected, followed by another 90° pulse at the refocusing point of the subsequent echo that results. This combination of RF pulses flips the transverse magnetization back to the longitudinal axis (Figure 17.31). Because the longitudinal magnetization is given a kick, it reaches a higher value by the time that the next excitation pulse is applied. This in turn yields more transverse magnetization and allows shorter TR without substantially compromising the SNR or introducing unwanted T_1 weighting. For RF spin echo imaging, both the 90° and 180° RF pulses added for DE are usually slice selective, although the 180° pulse can be nonselective as shown in Figure 17.31. The DE refocusing pulse is usually phase-shifted by $\pi/2$ with respect to the excitation pulse; that is, if the excitation pulse is 90°_x, the refocusing pulse is 180°_y. The flip-up pulse is then 90°_{-x}, giving the complete RF sequence $90^\circ_x - \tau - 180^\circ_y - 2\tau - 180^\circ_y - 90^\circ_{-x}$. (Recall that in this notation the pulses are separated by dashes, which should not be confused with minus signs. Recall also that in this notation 90°_{-x} is an RF pulse with a 90° flip angle that is applied along the negative x axis in the rotating frame. A 90°_{-x} pulse is equivalent to a -90°_x pulse.)

DE is also compatible with gradient echo pulse sequences when it is used in the form of a preparation pulse to increase T_2 weighting, without increasing TE (Haase 1990). A nonselective ($90^\circ_x - \tau - 180^\circ_x - \tau - 90^\circ_x$) or more commonly a ($90^\circ_x - \tau - 180^\circ_y - \tau - 90^\circ_{-x}$) sequence creates transverse magnetization that is refocused and flipped back to the longitudinal axis for repetitive use by a subsequent gradient echo pulse sequence (Figure 17.32). Because the transverse magnetization decays by spin-spin relaxation during the time between the DE 90° pulses, the amount of longitudinal magnetization after the preparation sequence depends on T_2. This use of driven equilibrium is also called T_2 preparation (T_2-prep). After the magnetization preparation, the gradient echo samples all or a fraction of 2D or 3D k-space. For example,

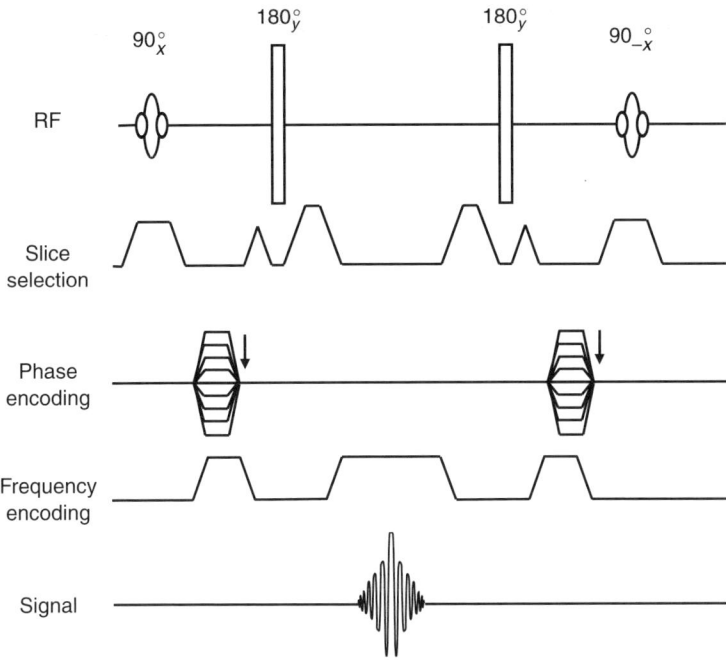

FIGURE 17.31 Driven equilibrium applied to an RF spin echo pulse sequence with nonselective refocusing pulses. The first 180° pulse produces the echo that is normally collected. The second 180° pulse refocuses the transverse magnetization so that it is flipped back to the longitudinal axis by the second 90° pulse. (Adapted from Maki et al. 1988.)

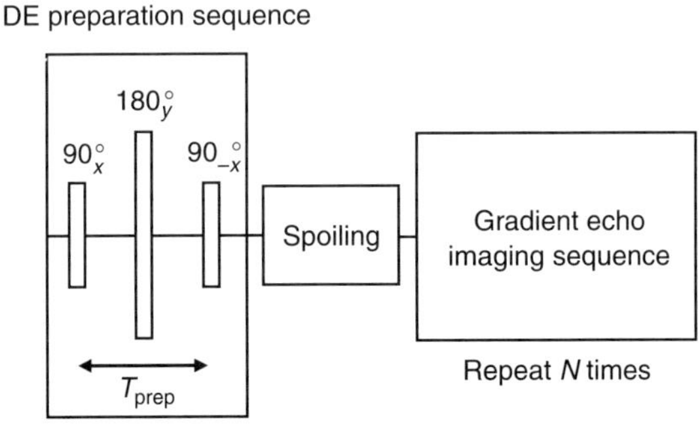

FIGURE 17.32 Driven equilibrium preparation sequence used with gradient echo imaging for T_2 weighting. The RF pulses are nonselective. The box labeled Spoiling represents gradient lobes on one or more axes that dephase any residual transverse magnetization. T_2 weighting is determined by the preparation duration T_{prep}.

in magnetization-prepared rapid gradient echo (MP-RAGE) imaging (Mugler et al. 1991), T_2-weighted longitudinal magnetization can be created and then used to sample a subset of the $k_y - k_z$ plane, followed by a recovery period. As long as the flip angle of the RF excitation pulse is kept small (e.g., $<10°$), then the T_2 prepared longitudinal magnetization can be reused many times, for example, to sample 32 $k_y - k_z$ values.

Although DE and FR originally had different meanings, the two terms have come to be used synonymously in many cases. The term *FR* now usually refers to the addition of a slice-selective 180° refocusing pulse followed by a slice-selective 90° flip-up pulse at the end of a RF spin echo or RARE pulse sequence. The term *DE* usually means either the same thing as FR or else refers to a nonselective ($90°_x$—τ—$180°_y$—τ—$90°_{-x}$) preparation sequence that precedes a gradient echo imaging sequence. To avoid confusion, we refer to these two uses as spin-echo FR sequences and gradient-echo DE preparation sequences, respectively. FR is also known by other commercial names, including RESTORE and DRIVE.

17.4.1 SPIN ECHO FAST RECOVERY

In addition to the conventional RF spin echo, FR has also been applied to RARE or fast spin echo (Melhem et al. 2001) and spin-echo EPI (Hargreaves et al. 1999) to reduce scan times as shown in Figures 17.33 and 17.34, respectively. Although scan time can also be reduced with RARE sequences by increasing the echo train length, this causes greater blurring. Reducing TR with RARE also reduces scan time but decreases signal from long T_1 tissues such as CSF. This can be detrimental in applications such as spine imaging in which cord-CSF contrast helps delineate pathology. FR provides an alternative scan-time reduction method with RARE, without increased blurring, and without decreased signal from long T_1 tissues. The long scan times of 3D RARE make FR especially beneficial.

The signal improvement with FR (compared to not using FR with shorter TR) is greatest for tissues that roughly satisfy TR $< 4T_1$; otherwise, the magnetization is fully relaxed after each TR anyway. The signal improvement is also greatest for tissues that roughly satisfy $T_{\text{seq}} < 4T_2$, where T_{seq} is the time to play one pulse sequence; otherwise, there is not much transverse magnetization remaining at the end of the sequence to flip back to the longitudinal axis. For RARE sequences, the latter requirement becomes $N_{\text{etl}} t_{\text{esp}} < 4T_2$, where N_{etl} and t_{esp} are the echo train length and echo spacing, respectively. FR allows reduced TR with maximum signal preservation for tissues with long T_1 and T_2, such as CSF. (For tissues with short T_1 and T_2, TR could be reduced without signal loss anyway.)

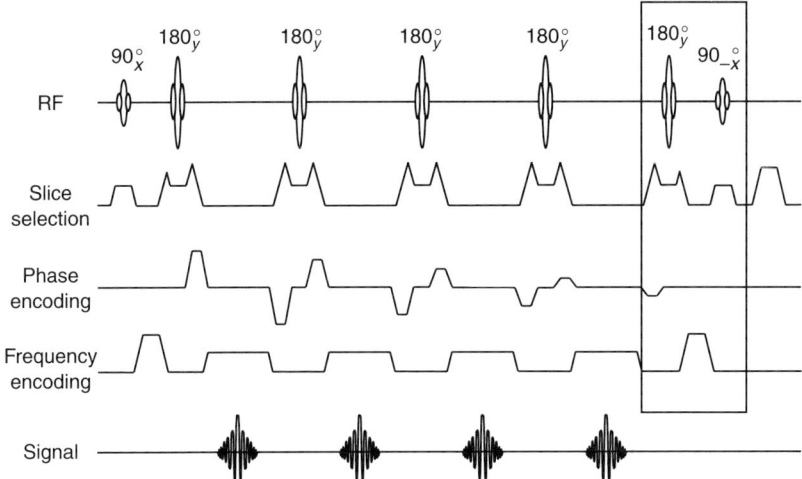

FIGURE 17.33 Fast recovery RARE sequence. Fast recovery waveforms are shown in the box. All gradients are rephased at the echo time for the fast recovery 180° pulse.

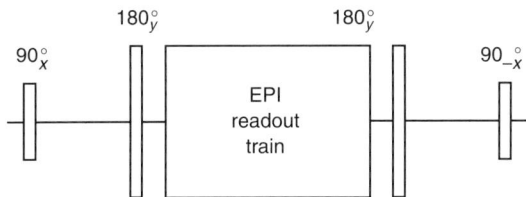

FIGURE 17.34 Fast recovery spin echo EPI sequence. The box represents an EPI echo train that collects multiple lines of k-space.

The FR method assumes that the additional 180° pulse properly refocuses the transverse magnetization, so that the 90° pulse can return it to the longitudinal axis. This is normally an excellent assumption, except in regions of extreme susceptibility variation, such as those caused by metallic implants. In this case, the incomplete refocusing caused by B_1 inhomogeneity and imperfect slice profiles results in a substantial phase shift of the transverse magnetization at the point where it is supposed to be refocused. If the transverse magnetization is very small or points in a different direction than expected, the final 90° pulse restores a reduced amount of magnetization to the longitudinal axis. The result is little signal improvement or even or signal loss compared to a non-FR pulse sequence.

Another possible mechanism for signal loss with FR in areas of high susceptibility is dephasing or T_2^* decay during the 90° flip-up pulse. In this case, the net transverse magnetization that reaches the z axis after the pulse can be substantially reduced, especially if the flip-up pulse has a long pulse width.

Figure 17.35 shows an example of a T_2-weighted sagittal thoracic spine image. The image, acquired with FR and gradient reversal lipid suppression (Section 14.3), generally has better cord-CSF contrast, except for the signal loss in the region of the metallic clip (arrow). (In these regions of very rapid susceptibility change, lipid suppression methods such as chemical saturation and slice selection gradient reversal are also ineffective.) For this reason, it is generally prudent to disable FR (and lipid suppression) in these situations.

When FR is used along with shorter TR, the contrast is generally somewhat different than with a non-FR pulse sequence. For tissues with $T_1, T_2 \gg$ TR, spin echo FR contrast is a function of T_2/T_1 similar to SSFP (van Uijen and den Boef 1984). Because most tissues have similar values of T_2/T_1, the resulting contrast is mostly determined by spin density (Maki et al. 1988). A notable exception is fluid, which can have a somewhat higher value of T_2/T_1 than most tissue. Spin echo FR therefore gives useful contrast for tissue-fluid

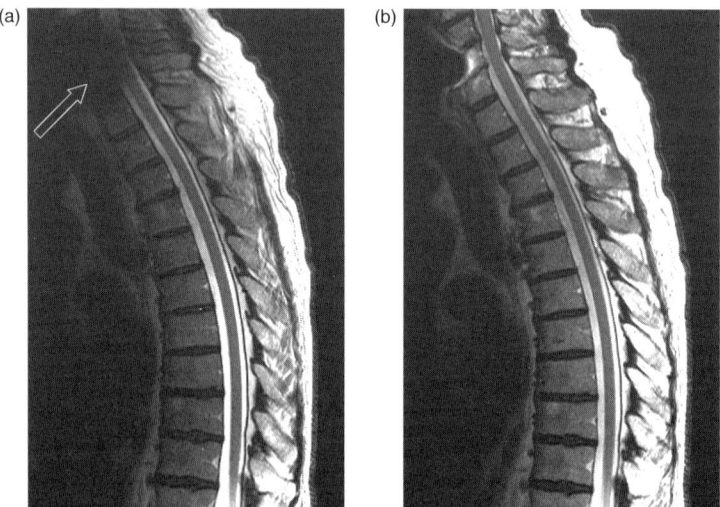

FIGURE 17.35 RARE images (a) with and (b) without fast recovery. TE = 105, TR = 2800, 3.5-mm slice, 0.5-mm gap, 256 × 512, four averages, receive bandwidth ±32 kHz, and echo train length 17. A metal clip (arrow) creates signal loss in the FR image due to incomplete rephasing by the FR refocusing pulse and T_2^* decay during the flip-up pulse. In other regions, FR improves the CSF-cord contrast.

combinations such as spine-CSF (Melhem et al. 1991) and cartilage-joint fluid (Hargreaves et al. 1999).

FR has been used with RARE to improve temporal resolution with real-time or interactive imaging (Busse et al. 2000; Makki et al. 2002). Another RARE application is simply to shorten scan time enough with T_2-weighted imaging that breath-holding can be used, reducing respiration artifacts (Schmalbrock 2000; Masui et al. 2001).

For a RARE sequence that satisfies the CPMG condition (Section 16.4), FR pulses refocus and restore signals from both spin echoes and stimulated echoes to the longitudinal axis. If the flip angles of the FR pulses deviate from the ideal values, residual transverse magnetization can be produced and interfere with the signals from the subsequent excitation. Crusher gradients surrounding the 180° refocusing pulse and a spoiler gradient following the 90° flip-up pulse are normally used to alleviate this problem.

17.4.2 GRADIENT-ECHO-DRIVEN EQUILIBRIUM PREPARATION

DE preparation can be used with either 2D or 3D sequences. The DE preparation RF pulses are followed by gradient spoiling lobes on one or more axes to dephase residual transverse magnetization, as shown in Figure 17.32. The duration of the preparation sequence T_{prep} determines the amount of T_2 weighting. If M_z is the longitudinal magnetization prior to the first 90° pulse, then assuming perfect flip angles for all three pulses, the longitudinal magnetization after the second 90° pulse is $M_z e^{-T_{prep}/T_2}$. In general, the longitudinal magnetization prior to the first 90° pulse must be calculated by taking into account steady-state conditions—it is not simply the equilibrium longitudinal magnetization. An example of the steady-state calculation is given in Parrish and Hu (1994). Typically $T_{prep} \sim 50$ ms. Greater T_2 weighting can be obtained by using multiple 180° pulses to prolong T_{prep} (Parrish and Hu 1994). Sometimes composite pulses are also used for the 90° or 180° pulses to decrease sensitivity to B_0 and B_1 inhomogeneity (also discussed in Parrish and Hu 1994).

One problem with DE preparation is degraded T_2 contrast caused by regrowth of longitudinal magnetization during the subsequent gradient echo imaging period. Using centric (or elliptical-centric for 3D) k-space acquisition can reduce the problem by acquiring the center of k-space before substantial regrowth occurs. Another problem is that if B_1 is inhomogeneous over the patient, the flip angle of the preparation pulses is not ideal. The result is that, after the preparation sequence, some longitudinal magnetization is present that is not directly determined by T_2 contrast.

These problems can be alleviated by applying a gradient dephasing lobe after the first 90° pulse and a corresponding rephasing lobe after each RF pulse

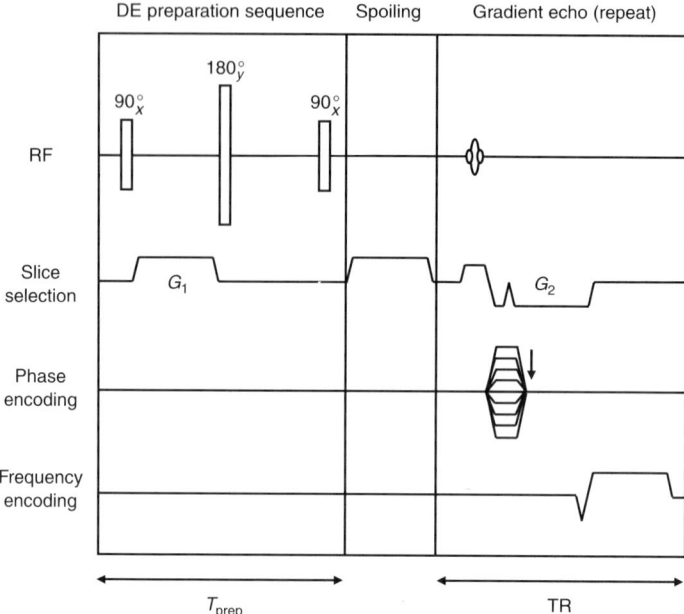

FIGURE 17.36 DE preparation pulse and gradient echo imaging pulse sequence using a dephasing lobe G_1 and subsequent rephasing lobe G_2 to eliminate signals unrelated to the preparation pulse. G_1 and G_2 have the same gradient areas. In practice G_2 is combined with the slice-selection rephaser gradient lobe. (Adapted from Parrish and Hu 1994.)

in the subsequent gradient echo imaging sequence (Parrish and Hu 1994), as shown in Figure 17.36. This scheme ensures that only the longitudinal magnetization that experiences the preparation sequence contributes to the signal. Transverse magnetization that either results from longitudinal magnetization regrowth after the preparation pulse or that results from residual longitudinal magnetization caused by B_1 inhomogeneity is dephased and does not contribute to the signal. A major drawback of this method is a reduced SNR from the elimination of the signal unrelated to the T_2 preparation. A minor drawback is a slight increase in the minimum TE and TR times.

DE preparation has been used for T_2-weighted head imaging with gradient echo pulse sequences (Mugler et al. 1991) and for cardiac imaging using T_2 shortening magnetic susceptibility contrast agents (Sakuma et al. 1994). When used with gradient echo imaging of heart, DE preparation increases blood-myocardial contrast (Brittain et al. 1995; Wiepolski et al. 1995).

Gradient lobes can be placed between the 90° and 180° preparation pulses, as shown in Figure 17.37 for the purpose of creating diffusion weighting in

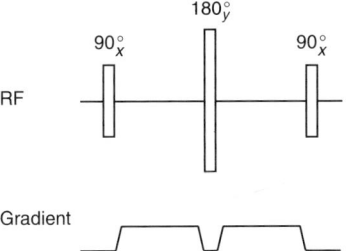

FIGURE 17.37 DE preparation pulse using gradient lobes to provide longitudinal magnetization with diffusion weighting. The gradient lobes can appear on any single axis or combination of several axes.

the resulting longitudinal magnetization. A discussion of the effects of such diffusion-weighting gradients can be found in Section 9.1. The resulting preparation sequence is also sometimes called a diffusion preparation sequence and has been used for diffusion imaging using gradient echo (Thomas et al. 1998) as well as RARE (Alsop 1997) pulse sequences. Eddy currents created by the diffusion-weighting gradient lobes prevent the complete rephasing of the transverse magnetization created by the first DE 90° pulse. As a result, only a fraction of the total transverse magnetization is returned to the longitudinal axis by the second DE 90° pulse. Because the eddy-current field is spatially dependent, the result is a nonuniform image intensity that does not reflect diffusion attenuation.

The problem can be alleviated by phase cycling the second 90° pulse at the expense of doubling the scan time (Pell et al. 2003). If θ is the angle between the magnetization vector in a voxel and the axis of the 180° pulse at the time of the 90° flip-up pulse, then the magnetization returned to the z axis is $M \cos \theta$. If the flip-up pulse is phase shifted by 90°, the orthogonal component $M \sin \theta$ is returned to the z axis. The first scan therefore uses $90^\circ_x - \tau - 180^\circ_y - \tau - 90^\circ_{-x}$, whereas the second uses $90^\circ_x - \tau - 180^\circ_y - \tau - 90^\circ_y$. The square root of the sum of the sum of the squares of the images restores the full signal.

DE preparation can also be used along with other preparation pulses such as fat saturation (Wiepolski et al. 1995) and adiabatic inversion (Pell et al. 2003).

SELECTED REFERENCES

Alsop, D. C. 1997. Phase insensitive preparation of single-shot RARE: Application to diffusion imaging in humans. *Magn. Reson. Med.* 38: 527–533.

Becker, E. D., Ferretti, J. A., and Farrar, T. C. 1996. Driven equilibrium Fourier transform spectroscopy—a new method for nuclear magnetic resonance signal enhancement. *J. Am. Chem. Soc.* 91: 7784–7785.

Brittain, J. H., Hu, B. S., Wright, G. A., Meyer, C. H., Macovski, A., and Nishimura, D. G. 1995. Coronary angiography with magnetization-prepared T_2 contrast. *Magn. Reson. Med.* 33: 689–696.

Busse, R. F., Riederer, S. J., Fletcher, J. G., Bharucha, A. E., and Brandt, K. R. 2000. Interactive fast spin-echo imaging. *Magn. Reson. Med.* 44: 339–348.

Hargreaves, B. A., Gold, G. E., Lang, P. K., Conolly, S. M., Pauly, J. M., Bergman, G., Vandevenne, J., and Nishimura, D. G. 1999. MR imaging of articular cartilage using driven equilibrium. *Magn. Reson. Med.* 42: 695–703.

Haase, A. 1990. Snapshot FLASH MRI: Applications to T_1, T_2, and chemical-shift imaging. *Magn. Reson. Med.* 13: 77–89.

Maki, J. H., Johnson, G. A., Cofer, G. P., and MacFall, J. R. 1988. SNR improvement in NMR microscopy using DEFT. *J. Magn. Reson.* 80: 482–492.

Makki, M., Graves, M. J., and Lomas, D. J. 2002. Interactive body magnetic resonance fluoroscopy using modified single-shot half-fourier rapid acquisition with relaxation enhancement (RARE) with multiparameter control. *J. Magn. Reson. Imaging* 16: 85–93.

Masui, T., Katayama, M., Kobayashi, S., Sakahara, H., Ito, T., and Nozaki, A. 2001. T2-weighted MRI of the female pelvis: Comparison of breath-hold fast-recovery fast spin-echo and nonbreath-hold fast spin-echo sequences. *J. Magn. Reson. Imaging* 13: 930–937.

Melhem, E. R., Itoh, R., and Folkers, P. J. M. 2001. Cervical spine: Three-dimensional fast spin-echo MR imaging—improved recovery of longitudinal magnetization with driven equilibrium pulse. *Radiology* 218: 283–288.

Mugler, J. P., Spraggins, T. A., and Brookeman, J. R. 1991. T_2-weighted three-dimensional MP-RAGE MR imaging. *J. Magn. Reson. Imaging* 1: 731–737.

Parrish, T., and Hu, X. 1994. A new T2 preparation technique for ultrafast gradient-echo sequence. *Magn. Reson. Med.* 32: 652–657.

Pell, G. S., Lewis, D. P., and Branch, C. A. 2003. Pulsed arterial spin labeling using turboFLASH with suppression of intravascular signal. *Magn. Reson. Med.* 49: 341–350.

Sakuma, H., O'Sullivan, M., Lucas, J., Wendland, M. F., Saeed, M., Dulce, M. C., Watson, A., Bleyl, K. L., LaFrance, N. D., and Higgins, C. 1994. Effect of magnetic susceptibility contrast medium on myocardial signal intensity with fast gradient-recalled echo and spin-echo MR imaging: Initial experience in humans. *Radiology* 190: 161–166.

Schmalbrock, P. 2000. Comparison of three-dimensional fast spin echo and gradient echo sequences for high-resolution temporal bone imaging. *J. Magn. Reson. Imaging.* 12: 814–825.

Thomas, D. L., Pell, G. S., Lythgoe, M. F., Gadian, D. G., and Ordidge, R. J. 1998. A quantitative method for fast diffusion imaging using magnetization-prepared turboFLASH. *Magn. Reson. Med.* 39: 950–960.

van Uijen, C. M., and den Boef, J. H. 1984. Driven-equilibrium radiofrequency pulses in NMR imaging. *Magn. Reson. Med.* 1: 502–507.

Wiepolski, P. A., Manning, W. J., and Edelman, R. R. 1995. Single breath-hold volumetric imaging of the heart using magnetization-prepared 3-dimensional segmented echo planar imaging. *J. Magn. Reson. Imaging* 4: 403–409.

RELATED SECTIONS

Section 14.1 Gradient Echo
Section 14.3 Radiofrequency Spin Echo
Section 16.4 RARE

17.5 Projection Acquisition

Projection acquisition (PA) was the first MRI k-space trajectory (Lauterbur 1973; Lai and Lauterbur 1981). It is also called projection reconstruction, projection imaging, or radial acquisition. PA fills in k-space data with radial spokes rather than a rectilinear raster as in Fourier imaging. There is a close connection between the PA k-space trajectory and parallel beam CT. The central slice theorem (also called the Fourier slice theorem), which is the basis of CT reconstruction (Kak and Slaney 2001), states that the Fourier transform of a line through the origin of k-space gives the projection of the object with beams perpendicular to that line in the image domain (Figure 17.38). In parallel-beam CT, 2D X-ray projections of a slice of the object are acquired through a range of projection angles. Fourier transformation of the projections results in measurements along radial spokes in 2D Fourier space (known as k-space in MR) at the same angles, which can then be reconstructed into images using either gridding (Section 13.2) or filtered backprojection (Kak and Slaney 2001; Liang and Lauterbur 2000). Filtered backprojection is used more commonly in CT than gridding because the aliasing artifacts from the latter are more prominent due to the higher SNR of CT. Both methods are used in MRI but gridding is preferred in many cases because the same algorithm can be used to reconstruct data acquired with any k-space trajectory. Filtered backprojection is employed

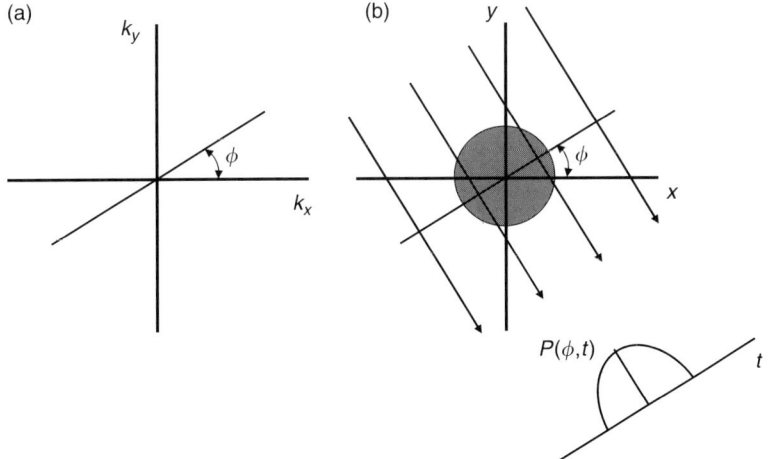

FIGURE 17.38 (a) A line of k-space that passes through the origin at angle ϕ is the Fourier transform of (b) the projection $P(\phi, t)$ of the object in image space with beams (arrows pointing to the lower right corner) perpendicular to a line at the same angle ϕ.

in MRI applications such as removing phase sensitivity in diffusion-weighted images (Trouard et al. 1999). Reconstruction methods for PA are discussed further in subsection 17.5.1.

Soon after the development of commercial MRI scanners, PA was largely replaced by rectilinear k-space trajectories to minimize artifacts related to B_0 inhomogeneity and gradient nonlinearity. With rectilinear k-space trajectories, these effects mainly shift the location and amplitude of the point-spread function (PSF), resulting in geometric and intensity distortion. With PA, they distort not only the location and amplitude, but also the shape of the PSF (O'Donnell and Edelstein 1985), causing blurring artifacts (Glover and Pauly 1992). Early MRI scanners had much worse B_0 homogeneity and gradient linearity than current commercial scanners. The blurring artifacts of PA were considered less tolerable than the geometric distortion accompanying rectilinear trajectories, and the use of PA was limited for a time. Improved B_0 homogeneity and gradient linearity, combined with a renewed appreciation of the advantages of PA for some applications, has led to its revival. These advantages are primarily shorter echo times, reduced sensitivity to motion, and improved temporal resolution for some applications.

The pulse sequences for 2D gradient and spin echo PA are shown in Figure 17.39. More discussion of the gradient waveforms is given in subsection 17.5.1. Although any of the gradient echo methods discussed in Section 14.1 can be used (Cremillieux et al. 1994), balanced SSFP has become

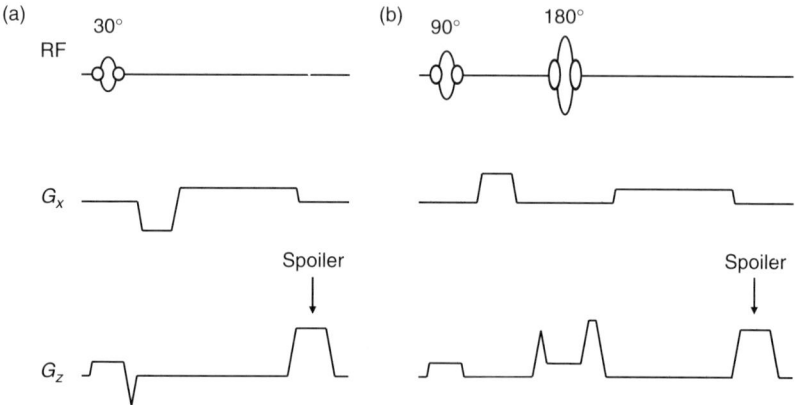

FIGURE 17.39 (a) 2D gradient echo PA pulse sequence. An example flip angle of 30° is shown. (b) 2D spin echo PA pulse sequence. For both (a) and (b), the logical readout gradient G_x is rotated in the XY plane for each view j (i.e., $\vec{G}_x(j) = \hat{X}G_X(j) + \hat{Y}G_Y(j)$, $j = 1, 2, \ldots, N_s$), where X and Y are the coordinates for the physical gradients and N_s is the number of spokes.

especially popular for cardiac imaging because of the high blood-myocardium contrast (Peters et al. 2002; Larson and Simonetti 2001; Larson et al. 2002; Shankaranarayanan, Simonetti, et al. 2001). Because no phase-encoding gradient is used, one of the advantages of PA is its shorter minimum TE when gradient echoes are acquired. If a half-Fourier readout is used in conjunction with ramp sampling and nonselective or half-pulse (Nielsen et al. 1999) RF excitation, the echo time can be as short as a few hundred microseconds. This has made PA particularly desirable for imaging very short T_2 nuclei, such as ^{23}Na (Ra et al. 1989; Boada et al. 1997) and ^{11}B (Glover et al. 1992) and tissues with short T_2^* such as lung parenchyma (Bergin et al. 1991) and cartilage (Brossmann et al. 1997).

Another advantage of PA is that artifacts from motion such as flow or respiration can be much less objectionable than for rectilinear trajectories (Glover and Pauly 1992). With rectilinear trajectories, motion results in ghosting artifacts that propagate throughout the entire (2D) image in the phase-encoded direction, regardless of the direction of object motion. The PA motion artifacts consist of streaks propagating perpendicular to the direction of object motion and are displaced from the image of the moving object itself. In addition, the inherent oversampling near the center of k-space with PA results in signal averaging that reduces motion artifacts at the expense of slightly increased blurring. One important example is reduction of motion artifacts in diffusion-weighted MRI (Jung and Cho 1991; Gmitro and Alexander 1993). When gradient echo PA starts data acquisition immediately after the RF pulse, the flow-induced displacement artifact that is sometimes present with rectilinear k-space trajectories is eliminated (Nishimura et al. 1991).

PA is somewhat self-navigating in the sense that consistency of the projections at different angles can be used to monitor and correct for motion. (Some of the navigator methods discussed in Section 12.2 use projections at one or more orthogonal angles). A discussion of several methods used to reduce motion artifacts with PA is given in subsection 17.5.2.

Another advantage of PA is that the aliasing artifacts from angular undersampling consist of streaks (similar to those of CT) instead of the wraparound that results from undersampled phase encoding with rectilinear trajectories (Scheffler and Hennig 1998) (Figures 17.40 and 17.41). This has allowed scan-time reduction with little spatial or temporal resolution loss and with minimal aliasing for some applications such as contrast enhanced MRA (Peters et al. 2000), cardiac imaging (Peters et al. 2001, 2002; Larson and Simonetti 2001; Larson et al. 2002; Shankaranarayanan, Simonetti, et al. 2001), and interventional imaging (Peters et al. 1993). More discussion of aliasing effects in PA is given in subsection 17.5.1.

One of the disadvantages of PA is increased scan time relative to rectilinear trajectories if the Nyquist criterion is satisfied. This is because Nyquist

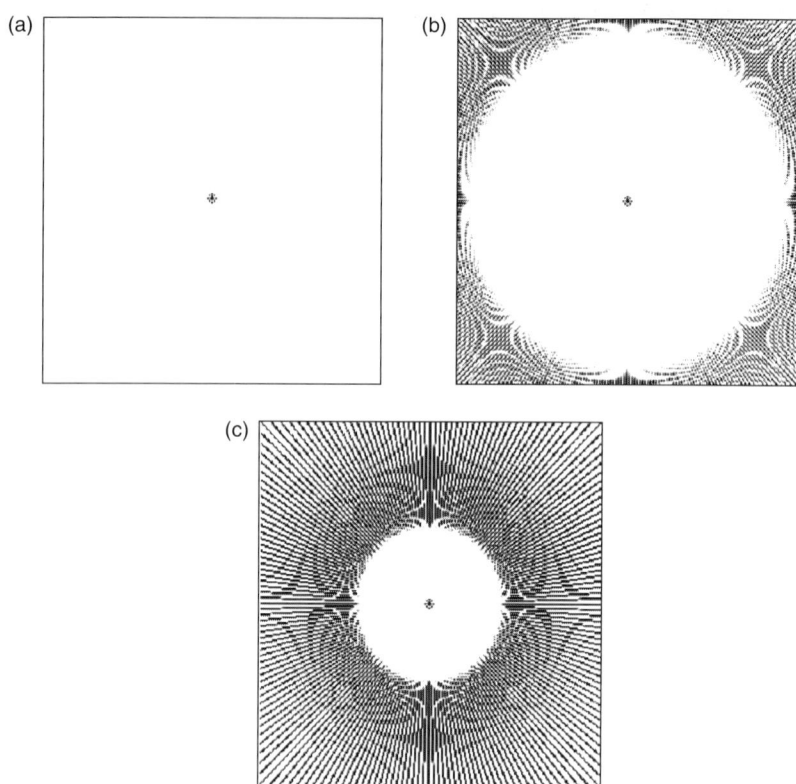

FIGURE 17.40 Simulated PA point-spread function with $0 \le \phi < \pi$ sampling and 256 readout points. (Note that the images are displayed in inverse video.) (a) 400 spokes, (b) 200 spokes, and (c) 100 spokes. Approximately 402 spokes are required to satisfy the Nyquist sampling criterion at the edge of k-space. Images were reconstructed using MATLAB (The Mathworks, Natick, MA) with filtered backprojection and an ideal ramp filter. The central lobe of the PSF is the central dark dot. The artifact-free area is the solid white region surrounding the central lobe.

sampling at the periphery of k-space causes the spokes to be angularly over-sampled closer to the center of k-space. As described in subsection 17.5.1, the use of partial Fourier acquisition (Section 8.1) allows scan-time reduction without reducing spoke sampling density. If aliasing artifacts can be tolerated, scan time can be reduced by also using angular undersampling near the periphery of k-space. Echo train acquisitions using either gradient echoes (Rasche et al. 1999; Larson and Simonetti 2001; Lu et al. 2003) or RF spin echoes (Rasche et al. 1994; Altbach et al. 2002; Trouard et al. 1999) have been developed to reduce scan time by acquiring multiple spokes per TR. A combination of

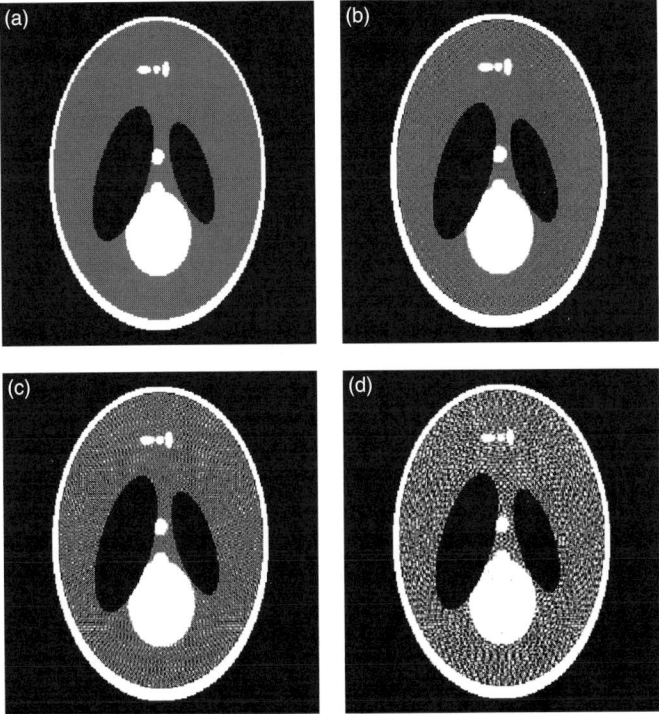

FIGURE 17.41 Simulated Shepp-Logan head phantom (Kak and Slaney 2000) with $0 \leq \phi < \pi$ sampling and 256 readout points reconstructed using MATLAB with filtered backprojection and an ideal ramp filter. (a) Ideal phantom, (b) 400 spokes, (c) 200 spokes, (d) 100 spokes.

gradient and spin echoes (RAD-GRASE, subsection 17.5.2) is also possible. A modified PA k-space trajectory, such as twisting radial line imaging (TWIRL; Section 17.6), that combines PA with spirals can also reduce scan time.

The k-space sampling raster produced by PA can alternatively be obtained by a set of concentric circular k-space trajectories (Matsui and Kohno 1986; Zhou et al. 1998). Although the net k-space raster can be the same between radial and angular (or circular) acquisitions, the PSFs can be quite different. If the number of samples per circle increases with the radius of the circle, the problem with angular undersampling in radial acquisition can be addressed, but this approach results in a reduced SNR for high spatial frequencies due to the increased receiver bandwidth.

Because PA is a type of k-space trajectory, it is compatible with many other MRI techniques. Both 2D and 3D PA methods have been developed. 3D imaging uses either a cylindrical k-space volume with a stack of 2D radial spokes combined with Fourier encoding in the slice direction (hybrid 3D PA) (Peters et al. 2000) or a spherical k-space volume with 3D radial spokes (Glover et al. 1992; Barger et al. 2002). PA can be used with preparation pulses such as flow-encoding gradients (Barger et al. 2000). The PA scan-time reduction with MRA can be further enhanced by combining it with segmented k-space acquisition methods such as TRICKS (Section 11.3) (Vigen et al. 2000). Temporal resolution for cardiac imaging can be improved by using view sharing (Section 13.6) with PA (Larson and Simonetti 2001; Shankaranarayanan, Simonetti, et al. 2001).

17.5.1 MATHEMATICAL DESCRIPTION

2D PA   For 2D acquisition we assume that the spoke angles ϕ are equally distributed, which is the usual case. See Scheffler and Hennig (1998) for a description of unequal angular sampling that is used to obtain an asymmetric FOV. For both 2D and 3D acquisitions, the maximum k-space radius k_{max} is determined by the desired spatial resolution Δx, which is assumed to be the same in all directions in the imaging plane:

$$k_{max} = \frac{1}{2\Delta x} \tag{17.93}$$

If we assume that a 2D PA is performed in the physical XY plane, the physical readout gradient waveform amplitudes for 2D PA are:

$$\begin{aligned} G_X &= G_0 \cos \phi \\ G_Y &= G_0 \sin \phi \end{aligned} \tag{17.94}$$

where $G_0 = G_x$ is the logical readout waveform amplitude (Figure 17.39). Although the basic PA k-space trajectory is very simple, many minor permutations are possible. Some of these permutations are discussed next for the 2D case.

2D PA k-space trajectories usually collect data either with $0 \leq \phi < 2\pi$ (Figure 17.42) or $0 \leq \phi < \pi$ (Figure 17.43). For a fixed angular sampling interval $\Delta\phi$, acquisition over π radians requires only one-half the number of views. Either full or partial (i.e., fractional) echo data collection can be used with either angular sampling method. Partial echo has the advantage of shorter minimum TE. Half-echo or FID acquisition is a variation of partial echo that starts collecting each spoke at $k = 0$ and is frequently used with angular sampling of $0 \leq \phi < 2\pi$. For example, an FID acquisition can be performed by turning on a readout gradient (without a prephasing gradient) either immediately following a nonselective RF excitation pulse or prior to the RF pulse.

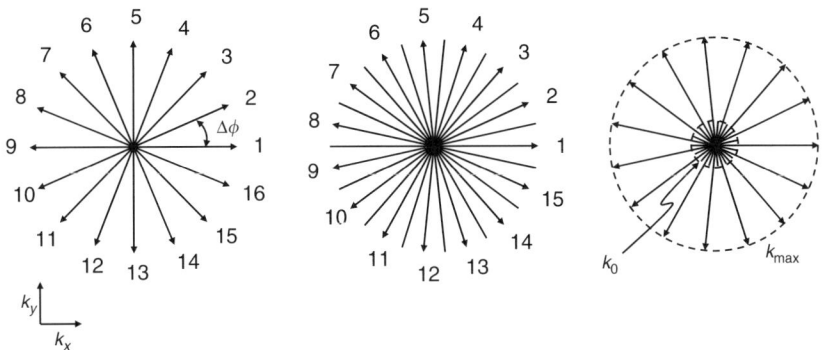

FIGURE 17.42 Data collection in the range $0 \leq \phi < 2\pi$. (a) $-k_{\max} \leq k \leq k_{\max}$ with 16 views, where $k_{\max}$ is the maximum k-space radius attained. (b) $-k_{\max} \leq k \leq k_{\max}$ with 15 views, (c) Same as (b) but with partial echo acquisition collecting $-k_o \leq k \leq k_{\max}$, where k_o is the partial echo overscan radius defined in Section 13.4.

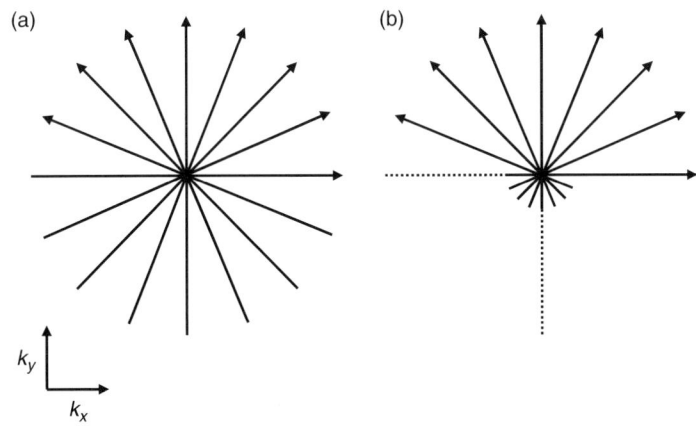

FIGURE 17.43 Data collection in the range $0 \leq \phi < \pi$. (a) $-k_{\max} \leq k \leq k_{\max}$ with 8 views, (b) partial echo acquisition collecting $-k_o \leq k \leq k_{\max}$, again with 8 views.

Figure 17.42a and b shows a full echo trajectory acquiring $-k_{\max} < k \leq k_{\max}$ for each radial spoke with $0 \leq \phi < 2\pi$. With an even number of spokes (Figure 17.42a) each angle is collected twice, whereas with an odd number (Figure 17.42b) the spokes are interleaved to improve the angular sampling density. Figure 17.42c shows a partial echo trajectory equivalent to Figure 17.42b that acquires data from $-k_o$ to $+k_{\max}$ for each spoke, where $k_o \geq 0$ is the overscan radius. The missing portions of each spoke in Figure 17.42c are compensated using partial-Fourier reconstruction (Section 13.4).

Figure 17.43 shows data collection over π radians with full echo and partial echo acquisitions. An even or odd number of spokes works equally well for this case.

Because the number of spokes acquired with PA is larger than the number of k-space lines acquired with a Cartesian trajectory, it is advantageous to collect multiple spokes within a single TR. Figures 17.44 and 17.45 show two examples. In Figures 17.44a and 17.45a, two spokes are acquired within the same TR using a bent-spoke trajectory (Noll et al. 1991; Boada et al. 1997). In this example, the two spokes are collected using a full echo. Each spoke moves inward starting at the periphery of k-space and bends slightly at the origin to collect a spoke adjacent to the one that would have been collected without the bend. The uncollected spokes are filled in using a homodyne reconstruction algorithm (Toropov and Block 2001). Note that bent-spoke acquisition is not the same as TWIRL. With bent-spoke acquisition, the spokes bend at the k-space origin, whereas with TWIRL the spokes become spirals away from the origin. The bend at the origin requires changing the readout gradient direction from angle ϕ to angle $\phi + \Delta\phi$. From Eq. (17.94), this requires a small but discontinuous change in the readout gradients. Because

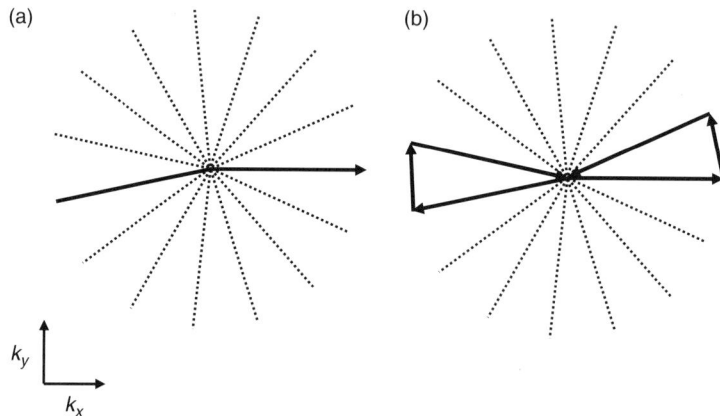

FIGURE 17.44 (a) Full-echo acquisition collecting two spokes per TR with bent projections. Angular sampling density is doubled with the same number of excitations compared to Figure 17.43b because the missing halves of each projection (spokes diametrically opposite to the collected one) can be filled in using homodyne reconstruction. (b) Half-echo acquisition beginning at the origin of k-space collecting four spokes per TR with bent-spoke projections.

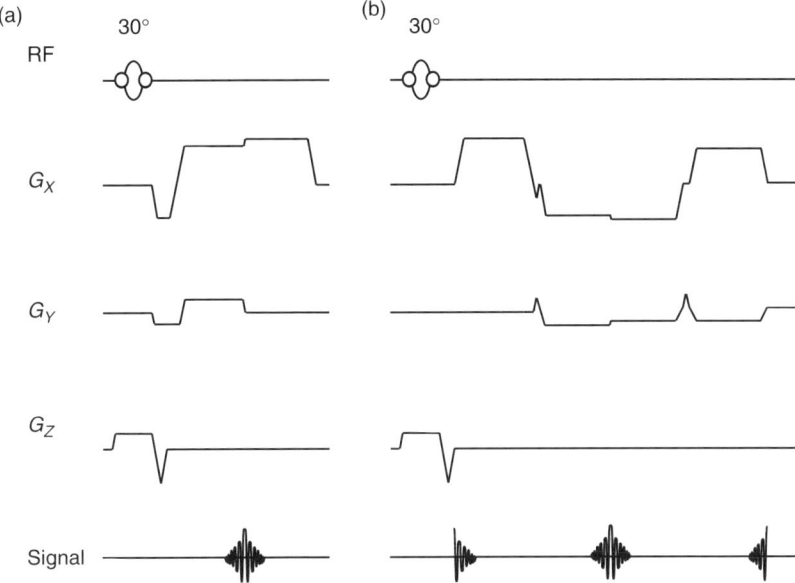

FIGURE 17.45 Pulse sequences for the k-space trajectories in Figure 17.44. An example flip angle of 30° is shown. (a) Two spokes collected within the same TR using a full echo bent projection acquisition. Note the change in physical readout gradient amplitudes at the origin of k-space to produce the bend. An optional spoiling or rewinding lobe (not shown) can be used. (b) Four spokes collected within the same TR with the first spoke using an FID acquisition. The small blips (or discontinuities) between readout trapezoids produce the shifts to neighboring spokes. An optional spoiling gradient lobe (not shown) can be used.

such a discontinuous change is not possible due to the restricted slew rate of gradient amplifiers, the trajectory is forced to deviate somewhat from the ideal one. In practice, some form of k-space trajectory measurement is frequently necessary to allow accurate reconstruction of the k-space data (see subsection 17.5.3).

Alternatively, the method depicted in Figures 17.44b and 17.45b can be used. Here the trajectory starts at the origin of k-space for each TR and collects four spokes. The first spoke in each TR uses an FID acquisition. The next two spokes are acquired with the left half and right half of a gradient echo (i.e., two back-to-back FIDs). The fourth spoke is sampled with a reversed FID. More or fewer spokes per TR could be collected than shown in this example. The acquisition of multiple spokes per TR is especially useful with 3D PA because the large number of spokes requires long scan times.

For 2D scans, there is no aliasing if the distance between spokes at the edge of k-space satisfies the Nyquist criterion:

$$k_{max} \Delta\phi \le \frac{1}{L} \tag{17.95}$$

where L is the FOV, which is assumed to be the same in all directions. For a 2D trajectory that samples over π rad, the number of spokes N_s required to satisfy the Nyquist criterion is:

$$N_s = \frac{\pi}{\Delta\phi} = \pi k_{max} L \tag{17.96}$$

For comparison, the number of phase encode lines N_{phase} in a Cartesian acquisition with the same FOV and resolution (i.e., the acquisition matrix size, not including zero filling) is:

$$N_{phase} = 2k_{max} L \tag{17.97}$$

Therefore, combining Eqs. (17.96) and (17.97):

$$N_s = \frac{\pi}{2} N_{phase} \tag{17.98}$$

Nyquist-sampled 2D PA therefore requires ~57% more views than a comparable rectilinear acquisition, even in the best-case scenario ($0 \le \phi < \pi$ sampling).

The 2D PA PSF has a central impulse response and an artifact-free region whose diameter is determined by the angular sampling density (Scheffler and Hennig 1998). Aliasing artifacts in the form of streaks appear outside this diameter. Figure 17.40 shows representative PSFs for different numbers of spokes. In Figure 17.40a, full Nyquist angular sampling is used, resulting in aliasing artifacts outside the reconstructed FOV. In Figure 17.40b and c, reduced angular sampling density reduces the PSF artifact-free radius to one-half and one-fourth of the reconstructed FOV, respectively. The PSF also depends on the reconstruction method (i.e., filtered backprojection or gridding); however, this dependency does not substantially change the angular sampling effects shown in the figure. Regardless of the number of spokes, k-space is fully sampled for some effective FOV L_{eff}. L_{eff} is the radius of the alias-free zone of the PSF and also the diameter of the alias-free zone of the FOV. From Eqs. (17.96) and (17.97) L_{eff} is given by:

$$L_{eff} = L \left(\frac{2N_s}{\pi N_{phase}} \right) \tag{17.99}$$

The reconstructed image is the magnetization density convolved with the PSF. Aliasing streaks are generated at a distance of L_{eff} from each pixel in the object (Figure 17.41). The amplitude of the aliased signal is proportional to the amplitude of the originating signal strength. Unless a very small value of N_s is used, if the highest intensity signal is near the center of the FOV, then the highest intensity aliasing appears near the periphery of the FOV. This makes PA useful for contrast-enhanced applications. The contrast-enhanced vessels are sometimes found near the center of the FOV in either direction, creating sparsely distributed aliasing streaks that usually do not interfere too severely with vessel conspicuity. The more intense the vessels are compared to background tissue (e.g., lipids) the better because those structures also create streaking artifacts of their own. Because spatial resolution is primarily determined by k_{max} and not angular sampling intervals, moderate angular undersampling enables scan-time reduction without sacrificing spatial resolution. The resulting improved temporal resolution can also be traded for additional spatial resolution. Although originally applied to contrast-enhanced vascular imaging, undersampled PA has been successfully extended to other applications (Peters et al. 1993, 2001, 2002).

3D PA   3D PA that uses Fourier phase encoding in the slice-selection direction (hybrid 3D PA) has the same general properties as 2D PA. Hybrid 3D PA is particularly useful for anatomy such as peripheral vessels that are confined to a thin slab. In this subsection we discuss 3D PA with radial spokes in all three directions (full 3D PA). One advantage of full 3D PA over hybrid 3D PA is its greater volume coverage and isotropic resolution for the same scan time. To simplify the discussion, we consider only sampling with an FID acquisition. For 3D PA, the physical readout waveforms are

$$G_X = G_0 \sin\theta \cos\phi$$
$$G_Y = G_0 \sin\theta \sin\phi \qquad (17.100)$$
$$G_Z = G_0 \cos\theta$$

where θ and ϕ are the polar and azimuthal angles, respectively (Figure 17.46a). (Note that θ should be distinguished from the flip angle of an RF pulse, a convention used in many other sections of this book.)

The data are sampled over the ranges $0 \leq \theta < \pi$ and $0 \leq \phi < 2\pi$. The most efficient strategy (Glover et al. 1992) is to use equal-solid-angle sampling. The sampling area on the surface of a k-space sphere with radius k_{max} is required by the Nyquist theorem to be $(\Delta k)^2 = 1/L^2$ (Figure 17.46b). If the solid-angle sampling interval associated with each k-space spoke is $\Delta\Omega$,

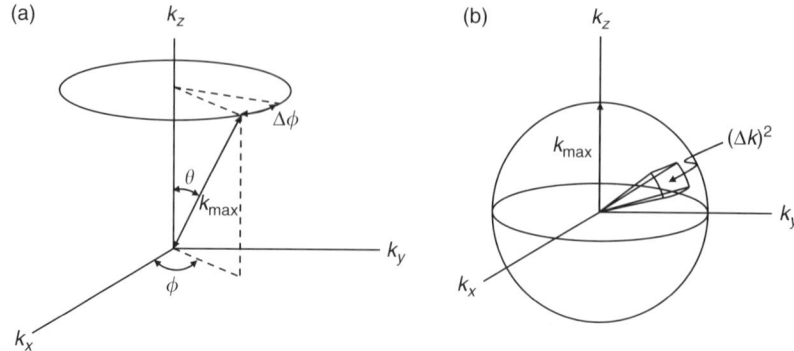

FIGURE 17.46 (a) Polar and azimuthal projection angles θ and ϕ for 3D PA. Azimuthal sampling interval is $\Delta\phi$. The maximum k-space radius is k_{max}. (b) 2D sampling area $(\Delta k)^2$ on the surface of a sphere.

the area subtended by each spoke on the sphere is required to be:

$$k_{max}^2 \Delta\Omega = (\Delta k)^2 = \frac{1}{L^2} \tag{17.101}$$

where the solid-angle sampling interval $\Delta\Omega$ is:

$$\Delta\Omega = \sin\theta\,\Delta\theta\,\Delta\phi \tag{17.102}$$

Using equidistant polar angle sampling at the Nyquist limit gives:

$$\Delta\theta = \frac{1}{k_{max}L} \tag{17.103}$$

Combining Eqs. (17.101), (17.102) and (17.103) gives:

$$\Delta\phi = \frac{1}{k_{max}L\sin\theta} \tag{17.104}$$

This strategy results in isotropic sampling on a circle perpendicular to the k_z axis (Figure 17.46). Because there are 4π sr in a sphere, Eq. (17.101) implies that the number of required spokes is:

$$N_s = \frac{4\pi}{\Delta\Omega} = 4\pi(k_{max}L)^2 \tag{17.105}$$

Because $k_{max}L$ is the number of image pixels in one dimension, N_s is typically two orders of magnitude larger than in the corresponding 2D case (see Eq. 17.96). For a 3D Cartesian k-space scan with isotropic resolution, the number of Fourier encoding steps $k_Y - k_Z$ is $(2k_{max}L)^2$ and is smaller than N_s by a factor of π. (Isotropic resolution is not necessarily used in 3D Cartesian k-space acquisitions, which allows them to be faster than 3D PA scans by a factor somewhat larger than π.) Similar considerations about aliasing artifacts that have been discussed for the 2D case also apply to the 3D case.

Example 17.4 Calculate the number of shots (i.e., RF excitations) required for 3D PA with a 40-cm FOV and matrix size of 256 if Nyquist sampling is used with (a) half-echo readout and (b) full echo readout with one echo per shot for both cases. Ignore sampling density improvements that are possible using homodyne reconstruction.

Answer Using Eqs. (17.105) and (17.93), the number of spokes is:

$$N_s = 4\pi \left(\frac{40}{2(40/256)} \right)^2 \approx 205{,}888$$

For case (a), the number of shots is the same as the number of spokes, 205,888. For case (b), the number of shots is $N_s/2 = 102{,}944$.

Reconstruction The methods of gridding or filtered backprojection both work about equally well to reconstruct PA data. The reader is directed to Kak and Slaney (2001) and Liang and Lauterbur (2000) for a complete description of filtered backprojection. Here we consider a few differences between the techniques.

A detailed comparison of reconstruction times between the two techniques is outside the scope of this book; however, gridding is generally somewhat faster than filtered backprojection. The most time-consuming step in gridding is the convolution and k-space resampling step. For 2D gridding, the computation time for this step for PA is proportional to $N_s N_{read} w^2$, where N_{read} is the number of readout points per spoke, and w is the gridding function width in pixels. The most time-consuming step in filtered backprojection is the backprojection step. For 2D filtered backprojection, the computation time for this step is proportional to $N_s N^2$, where N is the image matrix size. To simplify the comparison, we assume $N_{read} = N$. Because N is typically on the order of 256, whereas w is typically 2 to 4, gridding can be roughly an order of magnitude faster than filtered backprojection.

An analysis of gridding and filtered backprojection (Lauzon and Rutt 1998) has shown that the images produced are equivalent, with one major and a few minor exceptions. The major difference is that filtered backprojection produces minimal aliasing artifacts, provided the k-space data are sampled at the Nyquist limit. Gridding, however, can add aliasing artifacts from the rectilinear resampling. With a judicious choice of convolution kernel and k-space oversampling, however, the artifacts are usually acceptable, as discussed in Section 13.2.

A minor difference between filtered backprojection and gridding relates to resolution and noise. With gridding, the k-space data are weighted by a density compensation function prior to rectilinear resampling. For 2D PA data without ramp sampling, the density compensation function is proportional to the radial distance from the origin of k-space (radial ramp). With filtered backprojection, the k-space data are multiplied by the Fourier transform of the convolution filter, which is also a ramp in k-space. The ramp density compensation function of gridding and the ramp filter of filtered backprojection are equivalent and originate from the Jacobian of the coordinate transformation from rectilinear to polar coordinates.

With filtered backprojection, it is customary to roll off the ramp filter in k-space (i.e., to multiply it by a smoothly varying window that goes to zero at a k-space radius determined by the desired spatial resolution). With gridding, such windowing of the density compensation is not typically used. Data reconstructed using gridding without the windowed density compensation produce images with a higher spatial resolution and a correspondingly lower SNR than when reconstructed using filtered backprojection. In addition, during the backprojection step, it is necessary to interpolate the filtered projections in image space to obtain values at the exact pixel locations reconstructed in the image. This step arises because the sampled filtered projection locations needed for backprojection into each pixel at any given view angle do not in general correspond to the measured sample locations. For example, a linear interpolation is typically used, which is equivalent to convolving the filtered projections with a triangle function. In k-space, this is equivalent to multiplication by the square of a SINC function that further rolls off the ramp filter, increasing the SNR and decreasing the spatial resolution. Of course, it is possible to modify the two algorithms to match their k-space weightings, that is, to omit the roll-off window with filtered backprojection or to add a window that rolls off the density compensation ramp used with gridding. When this is appropriately done, the two methods produce images with the same resolution and SNR. More discussion of these points can be found in Lauzon and Rutt (1998).

Another minor difference is that when filtered backprojection is used, it is sometimes useful to discard the phase of the projection in the image domain to reduce artifacts from motion and flow (Jung and Cho 1991; Gmitro and Alexander 1993), eddy currents, and mismatched group delays. This is done by taking the magnitude of the inverse Fourier transform of each k-space spoke. The resulting real projections are then filtered and backprojected to obtain the final image. This operation compensates for translational (but not rotational) motion and can give slightly better results than gridding when motion effects are important.

In filtered backprojection, the convolution with the filter is done as a multiplication in k-space and is therefore a circular or periodic convolution in the image. In reconstruction of CT data using filtered backprojection, it is conventional to zero-pad each image space projection to twice its measured length. This step is done prior to Fourier transformation and multiplication by the filter in order to remove wraparound or interference effects from the periodic convolution. The interference causes image nonuniformity, or dishing. This step has also been shown to be beneficial when reconstructing equally spaced MR projections (i.e., non-ramp-sampled projections) using filtered backprojection and is equivalent to radial SINC interpolation of the k-space samples to twice their measured density (Lauzon and Rutt 1996; Joseph 1998).

In the reconstruction of CT data, it is also customary to use a slightly modified ramp filter that does not go to zero at the origin of k-space. This step is taken because, in the reconstruction of parallel-beam CT data, weighting the sample at the origin of k-space with a value of zero (the ideal ramp value) produces an image with distorted low spatial frequencies resulting in image nonuniformity, or dishing. This is sometimes called the '$k = 0$ problem'. The problem can be traced back to the fact that the filter must have infinite length in image space to have a value of zero at the origin of k-space. The CT filter is usually computed by truncating the ideal k-space ramp to the Nyquist frequency, apodizing it with an appropriate window if desired, inverse Fourier transforming to image space, and sampling at the correct Nyquist limit. The periodic convolution in image space uses only a finite length of the filter. When the resulting image space representation of the filter is then truncated to the length required for the convolution, zero-padded to prevent wraparound, and discretely Fourier transformed back into Fourier space, the values near the origin of Fourier space are slightly different from the ideal ramp, reflecting the fact that the filter no longer integrates to zero in image space (Kak and Slaney 2001; Joseph 1998).

Although the artifact improvement resulting from radial SINC interpolation and the modified filter can be easily demonstrated with a filtered backprojection of either ideal simulated data or real CT data, the improvement using real MR data is less clear. This is because the image nonuniformity artifacts that result can be much smaller than the image nonuniformity caused by transmit and receive B_1 inhomogeneity.

When gridding is used, the radial SINC interpolation step could be used if equally spaced radial samples are collected. However, the point of gridding is to avoid SINC interpolation, and the benefits are also less clear if the twofold k-space oversampling normally used with gridding is employed. The modified k-space ramp previously discussed has also been used as the density compensation for gridding of PA data instead of the ideal ramp (Peters et al. 2003). The benefit of this change, as well as possible extension to other nonuniform k-space sampling methods such as spiral, remains an unexplored nuance of reconstruction from sampled data.

When ramp sampling is used with PA, the samples are no longer uniformly spaced along radial spokes. In this case, a hybrid reconstruction algorithm that uses gridding to create equally spaced radial samples followed by filtered backprojection can be used. The benefit is reduced aliasing compared to a full gridding algorithm, but with a penalty of increased reconstruction time (Lauzon and Rutt 1998).

17.5.2 VARIATIONS AND ADVANCED TOPICS

Motion Correction   In one algorithm, called consistent projection reconstruction (CPR), the moments of the image space projections are used (Glover 1993). The zeroth moment or integral of any projection (also equal to the k-space echo peak) is the area of the 2D complex object and should therefore be the same for all projections. Similarly, the first moment of the projections (center of mass) should have sinusoidal variation as a function of projection angle. The angular variation of projection moments is related to a set of consistency conditions called the Ludwig-Helgason conditions (Helgason 1990; Natterer 2001). In general, each projection moment should have an angular variation related to the order of the moment. Angular variation that has higher order than expected for a given moment can be attributed to motion or other artifactual causes and can be eliminated. The use of projection first moments to correct for object translation has also been extended to 3D acquisitions (Wieben et al. 2001).

A self-navigating approach using moments has been used to compute cardiac phase information to enable retrospective gating without an ECG signal (Larson et al. 2004). Any variation of either the zeroth moment or first moment that deviates from the expected angular variation (constant or sinusoidal, respectively) for a slice that intersects the heart serves as an indicator of cardiac phase. The projection first moment or center of mass was first used for retrospective gating in CT, where it is referred to as a kymogram (Kachelriess et al. 2002). One limitation of this technique is that the resulting gating signals depend on slice plane orientation (e.g., long axis vs. short axis of the heart) because it is measuring changes in either the area of the object or its location. Consequently, it can give inconsistent information relative to the true cardiac phase for different slice planes.

Another approach to exploiting the self-navigating properties of PA takes advantage of the fact that through-plane translation of the object often gives a uniform phase shift for each spoke, whereas in-plane translation of the object along the spoke direction gives a linear phase shift of the k-space data (i.e., a phase shift proportional to k). A two-step correction uses the property that each spoke is expected to have the same phase at the origin of k-space ($k = 0$) because the linear phase shift is zero there. A uniform phase is first removed to force consistency of the $k = 0$ phase, followed by the removal of the linear phase component of each spoke (Shankaranarayanan, Wendt, et al. 2001). Because moving the object off-center would also produce a linear phase shift, the reconstructed object location is different in corrected and uncorrected images. Object rotations are not corrected by this method because rigid body rotation corresponds to rotating the k-space spokes.

Linogram Acquisition   *Linogram* acquisition (LA) is a variation of PA that samples k-space on a set of concentric squares in 2D k-space (Axel et al. 1990) or concentric cubes in 3D k-space (Herman et al. 1992), as shown in Figure 17.47 for the 2D case. The data are collected along a set of spokes similar to PA; however, with LA the spokes are unequally spaced in angle and the data sample spacing along a spoke varies with spoke angle. LA was originally developed for CT to enable faster image reconstruction without the need for specialized backprojection hardware because LA data can be reconstructed using only FFTs (Edholm and Herman 1987).

The term *linogram* is a variation on the word *sinogram*. For the 2D case, a point at location (X, Y) in the image is mapped to a sinusoidal curve:

$$t = X \cos \phi + Y \sin \phi \qquad (17.106)$$

in the (t, ϕ) space of Fig. 17.38b. The (t, ϕ) coordinates are also called Radon space, after Johann Radon (1887–1956), a Czech-born Austrian mathematician. An image in (t, ϕ) space is therefore sometimes called a sinogram. In linogram acquisition, the Radon space coordinates are transformed to a new coordinate system in which a fixed point in the image is mapped to a straight line, hence the term linogram. LA did not become popular in CT because it ideally requires a fanbeam detector with equidistant spacing between detector channels rather than the more commonly used equiangular spacing.

2D linogram data can be split into two "butterflies," one with uniform sampling in k_X and the second with uniform sampling in k_Y (Figure 17.47). The spokes for each butterfly can be acquired as either full echo or half echo. For simplicity, we consider only the full echo case that uses $-\pi/4 \le \phi < \pi/4$ for the first butterfly and $\pi/4 \le \phi < 3\pi/4$ for the second. The physical readout gradient waveform amplitudes for this case are given by:

$$\left.\begin{array}{l} G_X = G_0 \\ G_Y = G_0 \tan \phi \end{array}\right\} -\pi/4 \le \phi < \pi/4$$
$$\left.\begin{array}{l} G_X = G_0 \tan(\pi/2 - \phi) \\ G_Y = G_0 \end{array}\right\} \pi/4 \le \phi < 3\pi/4 \qquad (17.107)$$

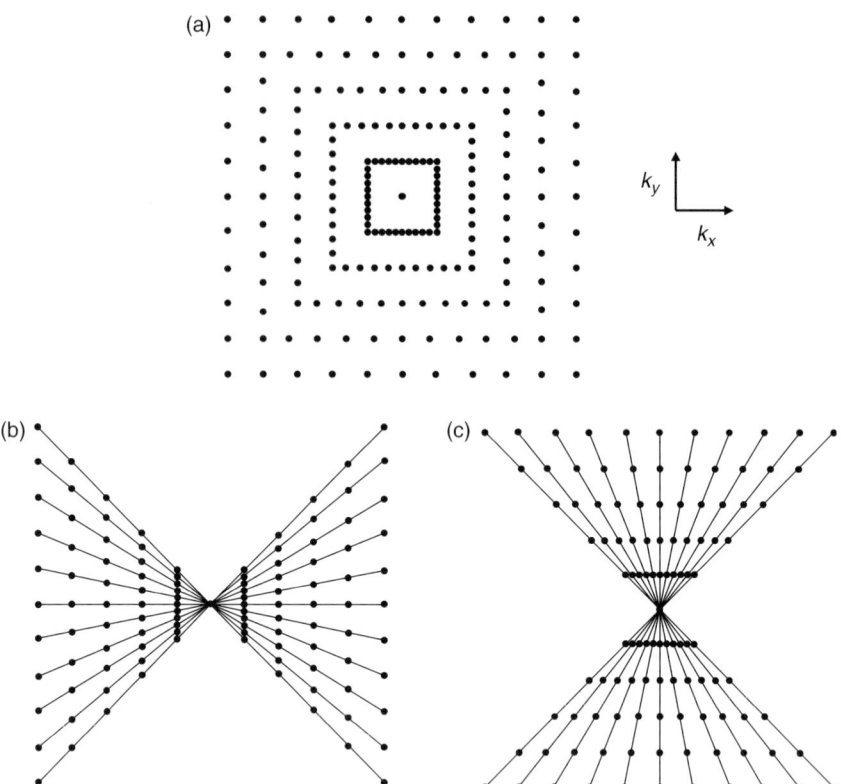

FIGURE 17.47 (a) k-space for linogram acquisition is composed of two orthogonal butterflies (b) and (c), each covering one-half of k-space. (Only the central portion of k-space is shown).

where the discrete angle for the nth spoke satisfies:

$$\tan \phi_n = \begin{cases} 4n/N_s - 1 & 0 \le n < N_s/2 \\ \frac{1}{3-4n/N_s} & N_s/2 \le n < N_s \end{cases} \tag{17.108}$$

where N_s is the total number of spokes. (Compare Eq. 17.107 to Eq. 17.94.) LA Nyquist sampling requires twice the number of views as Cartesian sampling:

$$N_s = 2N_{\text{phase}} \tag{17.109}$$

(compare also to Eq. 17.98 for PA). This can be seen by noting that each butterfly has the same k-space sample spacing as a Cartesian acquisition at the edge of k-space for Nyquist sampling and hence requires N_{phase} spokes.

The net readout gradient amplitude as a function of angle is given by:

$$G = \sqrt{G_X^2 + G_Y^2} = \begin{cases} G_0/\cos\phi & -\pi/4 \le \phi < \pi/4 \\ G_0/\sin\phi & \pi/4 \le \phi < 3\pi/4 \end{cases} \qquad (17.110)$$

To avoid aliasing, the readout bandwidth is ideally chosen to give Nyquist sampling along the spokes with the highest net gradient amplitude (i.e., spokes at $-\pi/4$, $\pi/4$ and $3\pi/4$). With this sampling density, the k_X samples for the first butterfly and the k_Y samples for the second butterfly have $\sqrt{2}$ smaller spacing than required for Nyquist sampling.

The data for the two butterflies are separately reconstructed and added to obtain the final image. Consider the first butterfly, which has uniform k_X spacing and k_Y spacing that changes from column to column but does not vary within a column. Because the k_Y sample spacing along each column is less than the Nyquist spacing (except for the outermost columns), the most computationally efficient method for evaluating the DFT of each column is the chirp-z transform, implemented as three FFTs (Oppenheim et al. 1999). Next, a FFT of each row gives the image for the first butterfly. Excess FOV due to k_X oversampling is discarded. The entire process is repeated for the second butterfly with the chirp-z transform in the row direction and FFT in the column direction. More discussion of the reconstruction steps can be found in Gai and Axel (1997b).

Because LA data are acquired as radial spokes, LA has many of the advantages of PA, including reduced sensitivity to motion due to oversampling near the center of k-space, short TE with FID acquisition, and azimuthal undersampling artifacts that are frequently less objectionable than with Cartesian acquisition. The self-consistency conditions inherent in PA (Ludwig-Helgason conditions) also apply to LA and can be exploited to reduce motion artifacts. For example, the zeroth, first, and second moments of the projections can be used in LA to correct for object scaling (i.e., dilation or stretching), rotation, and translation (Gai and Axel 1996). In addition, the degradation of the PSF with off-resonance spins is substantially different for LA than for PA. Whereas with PA off-resonant spins give rise to blurring in the PSF, with LA the degradation is similar to the geometric shift that results with Cartesian acquisition, except that the shift occurs in two directions rather than one (Gai and Axel 1997a). Because LA data can be reconstructed using only FFTs, the image quality might be better than for PA data reconstructed using gridding. LA has the disadvantage, however, of requiring even more spokes than PA. In general, the potential trade-offs of LA relative to PA and Cartesian acquisition have not been fully explored.

PROPELLER Periodically rotated overlapping parallel lines with enhanced reconstruction (PROPELLER) is a combination of rectilinear and

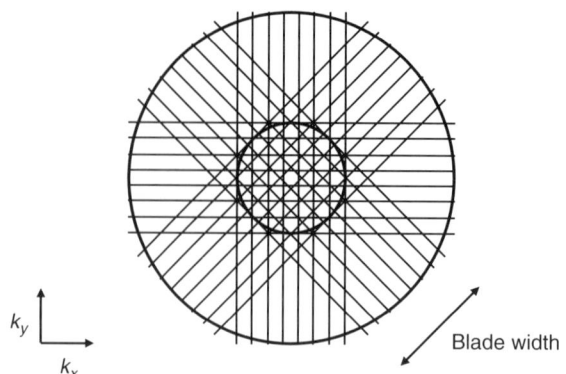

FIGURE 17.48 k-Space coverage for PROPELLER using four blades and eight lines per blade. The area inside the larger circle is covered by at least one blade everywhere. The area inside the smaller circle is sampled by each blade.

PA k-space trajectories (Pipe 1999). A rectilinear trajectory that samples a rectangular strip of k-space, or blade, is rotated about its center through a series of angles so that a disk in k-space is completely covered (Figure 17.48). PA can be thought of as PROPELLER with a blade width of one k-space line, whereas rectilinear sampling can be thought of as PROPELLER with a single blade wide enough to cover all of k-space. The lines that compose each blade can be collected in many ways, for example using a single RF excitation pulse per line or using echo train methods such as RARE or GRASE.

For the case in which the blade width is small compared to the diameter of k-space coverage, the number of k-space lines required by PROPELLER for Nyquist sampling is approximately the same as the number of spokes required for PA. This can be seen by noting that the sample spacing on a circle circumscribed at the periphery of k-space is determined by the Nyquist criterion and is therefore the same in both cases. For PA, each sample point is the end point of a spoke between the origin and the periphery of k-space. For PROEPLLER, each point on the circle is the approximate end point of one k-space line in one blade. The number of spokes required for PA is therefore apportioned equally among the PROPELLER blades. Using more blades allows fewer lines per blade. For a multishot RARE acquisition using N_{shot} blades and N_{etl} k-space lines per blade, Eq. (17.98) requires:

$$N_{shot} N_{etl} = \frac{\pi}{2} N \qquad (17.111)$$

for an effective matrix size N.

Example 17.5 A PROPELLER acquisition collected using a multishot RARE sequence has spatial resolution 0.5 mm and a 24-cm FOV. If the width of each blade is 28 lines, calculate the number of blades required for Nyquist sampling. If the TR is 6000 ms, calculate the total scan time, assuming only one pass is needed to collect all the slice locations.

Answer The effective matrix size is:

$$N = \frac{240\,\text{mm}}{0.5\,\text{mm}} = 480$$

Using Eq. (17.111) with $N_{\text{etl}} = 28$ gives:

$$N_{\text{shot}} = \frac{\pi}{2} \frac{480}{28} \approx 27$$

The scan time is $6 \times 27 = 162$ s, or 2 min 42 s.

PROPELLER usually requires a phase correction to remove echo-shift differences between the blades prior to combining them (see further discussion in subsection 17.5.3). A circular region near the center of k-space is sampled by every blade, whereas high spatial frequencies near the edge are sampled by only a single blade. The oversampling of the central disk of k-space reduces motion artifacts due to averaging and also allows correction for inconsistencies between blades caused by motion. Because rigid body rotation in image space produces an identical rotation in k-space, consistency of the gridded magnitude of the k-space data among blades within the central disk can be used to calculate the patient in-plane rotation error for each blade. After phase correction, the k-space magnitude data for each blade are compared to the average k-space magnitude data for all blades using a cross-correlation procedure. The resulting rotation error for each blade can be corrected using gridding during final reconstruction. Rigid body in-plane translation manifests itself as phase errors that can be calculated for each blade by comparing images reconstructed from the gridded complex k-space data within the central disk for the various blades. The complex low-resolution image for each blade is compared to the average for all blades using another cross-correlation. The resulting 2D translation error for each blade can be corrected by removing a 2D linear phase from the k-space data for the blade during final reconstruction.

Poor correlation between the data from different blades within the central disk indicates through-pane motion or other inconsistencies that cause artifacts in the image. Cross-correlation between blades within the central disk can be used to calculate a weighting factor that is applied to each blade during reconstruction. Blades that are highly correlated have a high weighting factor, whereas blades that correlate poorly with the rest of the data are assigned

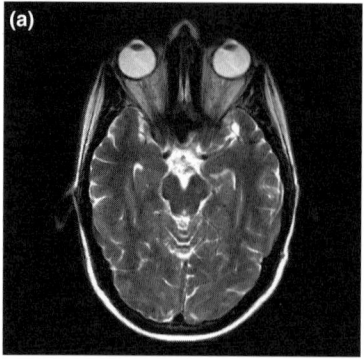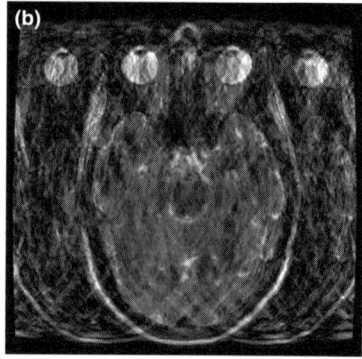

FIGURE 17.49 Comparison of the motion sensitivity of (a) PROPELLER and (b) RARE. A normal volunteer performed several large random head motions during the course of the scan to simulate uncooperative patient motion. PROPELLER scan parameters: 27 blades, blade width 28 k-space lines, TR/TE = 6000/134, ±50-kHz bandwidth, 24-cm FOV, 5-mm slice, 2-mm skip, 480 × 480 effective matrix size, scan time = 2 min 42 s. RARE scan parameters: 27 shots, ETL 10, TR/TE = 6000/102, ±16 kHz bandwidth, 24-cm FOV, 5-mm slice, 2-mm skip, 384 × 256, scan time = 2 min 42 s. (Images courtesy Emanuel Kanal, M.D., University of Pittsburgh Medical Center.)

a low weighting factor or are even discarded. The motion insensitivity of the PROPELLER k-space trajectory combined with the motion correction algorithm gives excellent robustness to even large-scale and rapid patient motion (Figure 17.49). More details about the motion correction algorithms can be found in Pipe (1999).

PROPELLER has been used for diffusion-weighted imaging and for diffusion tensor imaging with multishot RARE (Pipe et al. 2002), in which it has been found advantageous compared to single-shot EPI in areas of very high susceptibility because of PROPELLER's reduced signal loss in such areas. The scans are much longer than single-shot EPI, but also have a much higher SNR without the motion artifacts that accompany multishot EPI. PROPELLER has also been found useful for T_2-weighted head imaging, particularly for uncooperative patients or patients with involuntary head motion such as Parkinson's disease.

Although useful for reducing motion artifacts, PROPELLER with RARE requires long scan times and has high SAR. Scan time and SAR can be reduced by using a GRASE pulse sequence to acquire the PROPELLER k-space trajectory (Pipe 2002), which is a method known as turboprop. The phase-cycled refocusing pulse scheme required by PROPELLER cannot use flip angles substantially less than 180°. Turboprop is therefore especially useful for the

PROPELLER k-space trajectory at 3.0 T where the lower refocusing pulse flip angles used by conventional RARE acquisitions to reduce SAR are not feasible (Pipe et al. 2003).

VIPR Vastly undersampled isotropic projection reconstruction (VIPR) uses full 3D PA with spherical k-space coverage using radial spokes and a very high degree of angular undersampling (e.g., a factor of 3 to 10) to reduce acquisition time (Barger et al. 2002). With a very high degree of under-sampling, the undersampling artifacts become a nearly uniform background haze instead of discrete streaks. To further improve temporal resolution, the spokes are separated into interleaving subsets that each covers the full volume in k-space. To improve data collection efficiency, multiple spokes are collected per TR, as described in subsection 17.5.1, for example using a bent-spoke readout (Lu et al. 2003). To improve the effective temporal resolution and aliasing suppression, the data are reconstructed with a temporally sliding window (Section 13.6). Because the degree of undersampling increases with k-space radius, data at low k-space radii can be combined with a relatively narrow temporal aperture and achieve reasonable aliasing suppression. Data at high k-space radii, however, must be combined with a wider temporal aperture to achieve the same degree of aliasing suppression. The resulting sliding window gives high temporal resolution for low spatial frequencies and lower temporal resolution for high spatial frequencies. This is sometimes called a tornado filter because of the filter shape when the width is shown on a plot of radial distance in k-space versus time. Contrast bolus arrival and washout can be imaged with temporal and spatial resolution that are difficult to obtain with rectilinear acquisition (Figure 17.50).

RAD-FSE and RAD-GRASE PA combined with RARE (e.g., FSE and TSE) is also called radial FSE (RAD-FSE). So far, only 2D versions have been developed. The two main considerations with this technique are contrast behavior and view-angle ordering.

T_2 weighting in conventional RARE is adjusted by choosing which echoes in the echo train correspond to the central k-space lines (see Section 16.4). With RAD-FSE, the data from each echo pass through the center of k-space. Therefore, the center of k-space is acquired with multiple echo times. The result is that RAD-FSE images have T_2 weighting for an effective echo time $\mathrm{TE_{eff}}$ roughly equal to one-half the echo train length (Rasche et al. 1994):

$$\mathrm{TE_{eff}} \approx \frac{1}{2} N_{\mathrm{etl}} t_{\mathrm{esp}} \qquad (17.112)$$

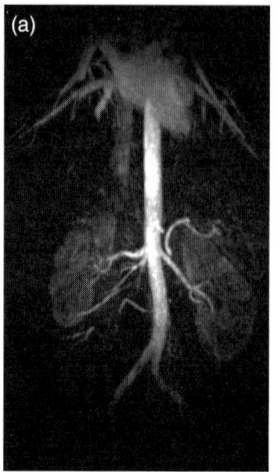
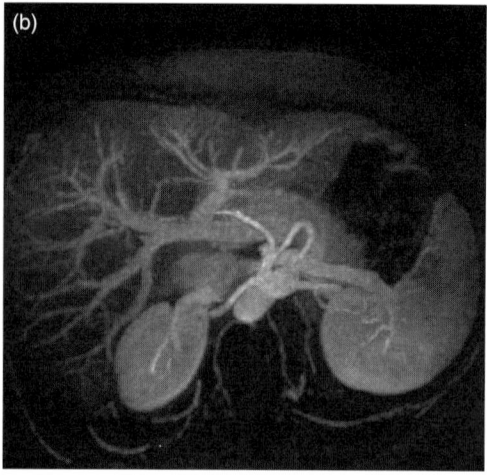

FIGURE 17.50 3D PA using VIPR. Field strength $= 1.5\,\mathrm{T}$, TR $= 4.4\,\mathrm{ms}$, 44-cm FOV, 1.7-mm isotropic resolution, 30-s scan, 2 s per frame, $N_s = 27{,}000$, four echoes collected per TR. (a) Coronal reformat of early arterial frame, (b) oblique reformat of late frame. (Images courtesy Walter Block, Ph.D., University of Wisconsin, Madison.)

where N_{etl} is the number of echoes in the echo train, and t_{esp} is the interecho spacing. Varying either N_{etl} or t_{esp} therefore, changes the image contrast. There is much less control over the contrast behavior than with conventional RARE.

The inability to control T_2 weighting with RAD-FSE can be overcome by using *k-space-weighted image contrast* (KWIC) (Song and Dougherty 2000). In this method, spokes from every echo in the echo train are distributed evenly over an angle π in k-space (Figure 17.51a). If azimuthal Nyquist sampling is used at the periphery of k-space, then spokes near the center of k-space are azimuthally oversampled. Therefore, azimuthal Nyquist sampling can be maintained near the center of k-space even if some spokes are omitted. Only those spokes for the echo with the desired TE are used near the center of k-space, out to some radius k_1. Beyond this radius, spokes from echoes for several TEs may be used (Figure 17.51b). Within the radius k_1, missing spokes can be filled in using interpolation. If Δk is the desired k-space sampling interval and $\Delta\phi$ is the angle between spokes within radius k_1 (Figure 17.51b), then:

$$k_1 = \frac{\Delta k}{\Delta\phi} = \frac{N_{shot}\,\Delta k}{\pi} \qquad (17.113)$$

where we have used the fact that the angular separation between spokes for the same echo in adjacent echo trains is π divided by the number of shots N_{shot}.

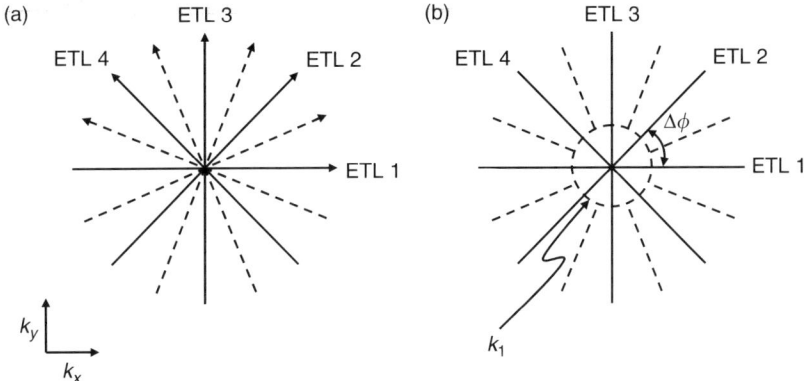

FIGURE 17.51 (a) RAD-FSE acquisition with four shots (ETLs) and two echoes per shot. The spokes for the first and second echoes are shown as solid and dotted lines, respectively. (b) KWIC reconstruction. The first echo from each shot is reconstructed within the circle of radius k_1. All echoes are reconstructed outside the circle.

Example 17.6 Calculate k_1 in k-space samples for a RAD-FSE pulse sequence that samples over π radians with $N_{etl} = 8$ and matrix size $N = 256$.

Answer From Eq. (17.98), the number of spokes is $N_s = \pi/2 \times 256$. Because each shot collects $N_{etl} = 8$ spokes, $N_{shot} = N_s/N_{etl} = (\pi/2 \times 256)/8 = 16\pi$. Using Eq. (17.113), $k_1 = 16\Delta k$ or approximately 16 k-space sample points.

View-angle ordering can be important in PA, even without the use of echo trains, in order to reduce the effects of patient motion (Glover and Pauly 1992). With RAD-FSE, the k-space modulation caused by T_2 decay also creates streaking artifacts. The artifacts get worse with longer echo trains or shorter T_2 because the intensity modulation over k-space increases. The choice of view ordering can have a substantial effect on T_2-related artifacts with RAD-FSE (Rasche et al. 1994; Altbach et al. 2002). In one view ordering scheme, streak artifacts are reduced by distributing the echoes within a single echo train over π radians in k-space in such a way that T_2 decay causes rapidly varying signal variation over any small angular section of k-space (Altbach et al. 2002).

Radial GRASE (RAD-GRASE) combines the GRASE pulse sequence (Section 16.2) with a PA k-space trajectory (Gmitro et al. 2002). Because all the echoes pass through the center of k-space, using all echoes in a normal reconstruction would result in a mixture of T_2 and T_2^* contrast. The KWIC algorithm for obtaining variable effective echo time with RAD-FSE can be adapted to increase or decrease T_2^* weighting with RAD-GRASE. For example, using only the RF spin echoes within radius k_1 and all echoes outside that radius gives an image with minimal T_2^* weighting (almost pure T_2 contrast). Similarly, using only the outer echoes of each gradient echo group within radius k_1 gives an image with increased T_2^* weighting.

Projection Acquisition with an Intrinsic Frequency Dimension   PA can also be used for spectroscopic imaging to create multiple images at different frequency offsets (Lauterbur et al. 1984; Bernardo et al. 1985). In addition to resolving chemical shift information, these images can be used to plot the B_0 field or combined to remove off-resonance effects such as those produced by B_0 inhomogeneity and magnetic susceptibility. In this method, a new view angle ψ is defined:

$$\psi = \arctan\left(\frac{\gamma G_0 r}{2\pi \zeta}\right) \tag{17.114}$$

where G_0 is the amplitude of the frequency-encoding gradient, r is a generic spatial variable along the direction of the gradient, and ζ is an intrinsic frequency variable (in Hz) that contains chemical shift, B_0 inhomogeneity, and other off-resonance effects. By varying the amplitude of G_0, data can be acquired at different view angles ψ. Thus, an additional dimension that contains the off-resonance information is sampled. Algorithms for image reconstruction are detailed in Lauterbur et al. (1984) and Stillman et al. (1986).

17.5.3 PRACTICAL CONSIDERATIONS

Gradient waveform infidelity, such as uncompensated eddy currents and mismatch in receive chain and gradient amplifier group delays, can distort the PA k-space trajectory causing artifacts (Peters et al. 2003). Because gradient waveform distortion and eddy-current effects are typically larger near gradient ramps, the distortion can be especially substantial if ramp sampling is used. If multiple spokes are collected per excitation or if bent-spoke sampling is used, the resulting k-space direction changes can result in inaccurate k-space locations if gradient fidelity is poor. Because the eddy currents and gradient amplifier group delays can differ on each physical axis (sometimes called gradient anisotropy), the effects depend on both the physical gradient waveforms and gradient axis (Aldefeld and Bornert 1998). Anisotropy of a few microseconds between axes has been found to be detrimental. The measurement and correction of these errors can substantially improve PA image uniformity and reduce streak artifacts.

To the lowest order, the distortion can be characterized as a time shift of the echo. This is because linear eddy currents with short time constants simply cause an apparent delay of the resulting physical gradient waveform to the lowest order (see Section 10.3). Therefore, gradient and receive chain group delays and short-time-constant linear eddy currents can be simultaneously corrected by adjusting the temporal location of the peak of the echo. One method of characterizing the echo shift uses a one-time phantom measurement with a generic 2D PA pulse sequence such as an SSFP that collects full echoes over a range of $0 \leq \phi < \pi$. Scans of axial, sagittal, and coronal planes allow the measurement of characteristic delays for each physical axis that are independent of projection angle and scan plane. These characteristic delays can then be combined using the rotation matrices to give appropriate delays for any oblique prescription and any projection angle. The delays are compensated for by adjusting the logical projection prephaser gradient areas. Typically delays for only the in-plane logical axes are corrected because the through-plane component of delay gives only a small signal loss, which can usually be ignored. More discussion of this method can be found in Peters et al. (2003).

Another correction first measures the k-space trajectory errors (Duyn et al. 1998) and follows this by gridding reconstruction. The k-space data are placed at the measured k-space locations during gridding instead of their nominal locations (Dale and Duerk 2002). This method is beneficial when the gradient waveform distortion is more complicated than a simple shift because of the use of ramp sampling, bent-spoke sampling, or collection of multiple echoes (Lu et al. 2003). Alternatively, the gradient prephasers can be adjusted for each spoke to remove the trajectory errors, at least to the lowest order (Wieben et al. 2003).

Because the gradient distortions approximately shift the echoes, according to the Fourier shift theorem the gradient errors become linear phase errors in the image space projections. Therefore, inverse Fourier transforming each k-space spoke and discarding the phase removes the gradient error effects to lowest order. This is easiest with data that is not ramp sampled, so that no gridding is required. Instead, the resulting real projections are then filtered and backprojected. A low-frequency phase correction in image space, followed by taking the real part of the image, similar to the method used for partial Fourier imaging with homodyne reconstruction, has been used with PROPELLER to remove the echo shifts for each blade prior to combining the blades (Pipe 1999).

Another method for characterizing the echo shifts is to compare projection data acquired with positive- and negative-polarity gradient readout amplitudes. This is similar to methods used in EPI that compute the temporal shift in k-space between echoes acquired with positive- and negative-polarity readout amplitudes using a reference scan (Section 16.1). With 2D PA, projections obtained with negated x and y readout gradient amplitudes are separated by

180°; that is, one projection is acquired at angle ϕ and the other at angle $\phi + \pi$. After flipping one echo in the frequency direction in k-space to compensate for the readout gradient polarity difference between the pair, the two echoes are shifted in opposite directions. One-half of the total shift difference between the pair gives the desired echo shift for angle ϕ. This method requires full echoes and data acquisition for $0 \leq \phi < 2\pi$ in order to have positive and negative polarities for every angle ϕ. Acquiring views at angles ϕ and $\phi + \pi$ is redundant from a sampling standpoint, but this disadvantage can be alleviated by using an odd number of spokes, which results in interleaved projections instead of redundant ones (see Figure 17.42a and b). Then the spoke at angle $\phi + \pi + \Delta\phi$ can be substituted as an approximation for a spoke at $\phi + \pi$ when estimating the echo shift. This method has been used in MR fluoroscopy with PA (Rasche et al. 1999).

For 3D PA, the echo shift due to eddy currents and gradient amplifier infidelity can also be addressed by turning on the gradients before the non-selective RF excitation pulse. By the time that the magnetization is nutated to the transverse plane, eddy currents with short time constants have already decayed away and the gradient amplifier has accurately settled to the requested currents. As long as the RF pulse width is short (e.g., 10 μs) and the gradient amplitude is not very large, spins within the desired volume can still be excited to form a 3D image. This approach can be used for either FID or spin echo acquisitions (Zhou and Lauterbur 1992).

SELECTED REFERENCES

Aldefeld, B., and Bornert, P. 1998. Effects of gradient anisotropy in MRI. *Magn. Reson. Med.* 39: 606–614.

Altbach, M. I., Outwater, E. K., Trouard, T. P., Krupinski, E. A., Theilmann, R. J., Stopeck, A. T., Kono, M., and Gmitro, A. F. 2002. Radial fast spin-echo method for T2-weighted imaging and T2 mapping of the liver. *J. Magn. Reson. Imaging* 16: 179–189.

Axel, L., Herman, G. T., Roberts, D. A., and Dougherty, L. 1990. Linogram reconstruction for magnetic resonance imaging (MRI). *IEEE Trans. Med. Imaging* 9: 447–449.

Barger, A. V., Block, W. F., Toropov, Y., Grist, T. M., and Mistretta, C. A. 2002. Time-resolved contrast-enhanced imaging with isotropic resolution and broad coverage using an undersampled 3D projection trajectory. *Magn. Reson. Med.* 48: 297–305.

Barger, A. V., Peters, D. C., Block, W. F., Vigen, K. K., Korosec, F. R., Grist, T. M., and Mistretta, C. A. 2000. Phase-contrast with interleaved undersampled projections. *Magn. Reson. Med.* 43: 503–509.

Bergin, C. J., Pauly, J. M., and Macovski, A. 1991. Lung parenchyma: Projection reconstruction MR imaging. *Radiology* 179: 777–781.

Bernardo, N. L., Lauterbur, P. C., and Hedges, L. K. 1985. Experimental examples of NMR spectroscopic imaging by projection reconstruction involving an intrinsic frequency dimension. *J. Magn. Reson.* 61: 168–174.

Boada, F. E., Christensen, J. D., Gillen, J. S., and Thulborn, K. R. 1997. Three-dimensional projection imaging with half the number of projections. *Magn. Reson. Med.* 37: 470–477.

Boada, F. E., Gillen, J. S., Shen, G. X., Chang, S. Y., and Thulborn, K. R. 1997. Fast three dimensional sodium imaging. *Magn. Reson. Med.* 37: 706–715.

Brossmann, J., Frank, L. R., Pauly, J. M., Boutin, R. D., Pedowitz, R. A., Haghighi, P., and Resnick, D. 1997. Short echo time projection reconstruction MR imaging of cartilage: Comparison with fat-suppressed spoiled GRASS and magnetization transfer contrast MR imaging. *Radiology* 203: 501–507.

Cremillieux, Y., Briguet, A., and Deguin, A. 1994. Projection-reconstruction methods: Fast imaging sequences and data processing. *Magn. Reson. Med.* 32: 23–32.

Dale, B. M., and Duerk, J. L. 2002. The use of measured k-space trajectory for reconstruction of radial MRI data. In *Proceedings of the 10th meeting of the International Society for Magnetic Resonance in Medicine*, p. 2334.

Duyn, J. H., Yang, Y., Frank, J., and van der Veen, J. W. 1998. Simple correction method for k-space trajectory deviations in MRI. *J. Magn. Reson.* 132: 150–153.

Edholm, P. R., and Herman, G. T. 1987. Linograms in image reconstruction from projections. *IEEE Trans. Med. Imaging* 6: 301–307.

Gai, N., and Axel, L. 1996. Correction of motion artifacts in linogram and projection reconstruction MRI using geometry and consistency constraints. *Med. Phys.* 23: 251–262.

Gai, N., and Axel, L. 1997a. Characterization and correction for artifacts in linogram MRI. *Magn. Reson. Med.* 37: 275–284.

Gai, N., and Axel, L. 1997b. A dual approach to linogram imaging for MRI. *Magn. Reson. Med.* 38: 337–341.

Glover, G. H. 1993. Consistent projection reconstruction (CPR) techniques for MRI. *Magn. Reson. Med.* 29: 345–351.

Glover, G. H., and Pauly, J. M. 1992. Projection reconstruction techniques for reduction of motion effects in MRI. *Magn. Reson. Med.* 28: 275–289.

Glover, G. H., Pauly, J. M., and Bradshaw, K. M. 1992. Boron-11 imaging with a three-dimensional reconstruction method. *J. Magn. Reson. Imaging* 2: 47–52.

Gmitro, A. F., and Alexander, A. L. 1993. Use of a projection reconstruction method to decrease motion sensitivity in diffusion-weighted MRI. *Magn. Reson. Med.* 29: 835–838.

Gmitro, A. F., Altbach, M. I., Theilmann, R. J., and Trouard, T. P. 2002. Simultaneous T2 and T2* imaging with RAD-GRASE. In *Proceedings of the 10th meeting of the International Society for Magnetic Resonance in Medicine*, p. 79.

Helgason, S. 1990. *The radon transform.* Boston: Birkhauser.

Herman, G. T., Roberts, D., and Axel, L. 1992. Fully three-dimensional reconstruction from data collected on concentric cubes in Fourier space: Implementation and a sample application to MRI. *Phys. Med. Biol.* 37: 673–687.

Joseph, R. M. 1998. Sampling errors in projection reconstruction MRI. *Magn. Reson. Med.* 40: 460–466.

Jung, K. J., and Cho, Z. H. 1991. Reduction of flow artifacts in NMR diffusion imaging using view-angle tilted line-integral projection reconstruction. *Magn. Reson. Med.* 19: 349–360.

Kachelriess, M., Sennst, D.-A., Maxlmoser, W., and Kalender, W. A. 2002. Kymogram detection and kymogram-correlated image reconstruction from subsecond spiral computed tomography scans of the heart. *Med. Phys.* 29: 1489–1503.

Kak, A. C., and Slaney, M. 2001. *Principles of computerized tomographic imaging.* Philadelphia: SIAM.

Lai, C.-M., and Lauterbur, P. C. 1981. True three-dimensional image reconstruction by nuclear magnetic resonance zeugmatography. *Phys. Med. Biol.* 26: 851–856.

Larson, A. C., and Simonetti, O. P. 2001. Real-time cardiac cine imaging with SPIDER: Steady-state projection imaging with dynamic echo-train readout. *Magn. Reson. Med.* 46: 1059–1066.

Larson, A. C., Simonetti, O. P., and Li, D. 2002. Coronary MRA with 3D undersampled projection reconstruction TrueFISP. *Magn. Reson. Med.* 48: 594–601.

Larson, A. C., White, R. D., Laub, G., McVeigh, E. R., Li, D., and Simonetti, O. P. 2004. Self-gated cardiac cine MRI. *Magn. Reson. Med.* 51: 93–102.

Lauterbur, P. C. 1973. Image formation by induced local interactions: Examples employing nuclear magnetic resonance. *Nature* 242: 190–191.

Lauterbur, P. C., Levin, D. N., and Marr, R. B. 1984. Theory and simulation of NMR spectro-scopic imaging and field plotting by projection reconstruction involving an intrinsic frequency dimension. *J. Magn. Reson.* 59: 536–541.

Lauzon, L. S., and Rutt, B. K. 1996. Effects of polar sampling in k-space. *Magn. Reson. Med.* 36: 940–949.

Lauzon, L. M., and Rutt, B. K. 1998. Polar sampling in k-space: reconstruction effects. *Magn. Reson. Med.* 40: 769–782.

Liang, Z.-P., and Lauterbur, P. C. 2000. *Principles of magnetic resonance imaging.* New York: IEEE Press.

Lu, A., Wieben, O., Grist, T. M., and Block, W. F. 2003. Vastly undersampled isotropic projection reconstruction imaging with multi-half-echo (VIPR ME). In *Proceedings of the 11th meeting of the International Society for Magnetic Resonance in Medicine*, p. 210.

Matsui, S., and Kohno, H. 1986. NMR imaging with a rotary field gradient. *J. Magn. Reson.* 70:157–162.

Natterer, F. 2001. *The mathematics of computerized tomography.* Phildelphia: SIAM.

Nielsen, H. T. C., Gold, G. E., Olcott, E. W., Pauly, J. M., and Nishimura, D. G. 1999. Ultra-short echo-time 2D time-of-flight MR angiography using a half-pulse excitation. *Magn. Reson. Med.* 41: 591–599.

Nishimura, D. G., Jackson, J. I., and Pauly, J. M. 1991. On the nature and reduction of the displacement artifact in flow images. *Magn. Reson. Med.* 22: 481–492.

Noll, D., Pauly, J., Nishimura, D., and Macovski, A. 1991. Magnetic resonance reconstruction from projections using half the data. *Proc. SPIE* 1443: 29–36.

O'Donnell, M., and Edelstein, W. A. 1985. NMR imaging in the presence of magnetic field inhomogeneities and gradient field nonlinearities. *Med. Phys.* 12: 20–26.

Oppenheim, A. V., Schaefer, R. W., and Buck, J. R. 1999. *Discrete-time signal processing.* 2nd ed. Upper Saddle River, NJ: Prentice-Hall.

Peters, D. C., Derbyshire, J. A., and McVeigh, E. R. 2003. Centering the projection reconstruction trajectory: Reducing gradient delay errors. *Magn. Reson. Med.* 50: 1–6.

Peters, D. C., Ennis, D. B., and McVeigh, E. R. 2002. High-resolution MRI of cardiac function with projection reconstruction and steady-state free precession. *Magn. Reson. Med.* 48: 82–88.

Peters, D. C., Epstein, F. H., and McVeigh, E. R. 2001. Myocardial wall tagging with undersampled projection reconstruction. *Magn. Reson. Med.* 45: 562–567.

Peters, D. C., Korosec, F. R., Grist, T. M., Block, W. F., Holden, J. E., Vigen, K. K., and Mistretta, C. A. 2000. Undersampled projection reconstruction applied to MR angiography. *Magn. Reson. Med.* 43: 91–101.

Peters, D. C., Lederman, R. J., Dick, A. J., Raman, V. K., Guttman, M. A., Derbyshire, J. A., and McVeigh, E. R. 1993. Undersampled projection reconstruction for active catheter imaging with adaptable temporal resolution and catheter-only views. *Magn. Reson. Med.* 49: 216–222.

Pipe, J. G. 1999. Motion correction with PROPELLER MRI: Application to head motion and free-breathing cardiac imaging. *Magn. Reson. Med.* 42: 963–969.

Pipe, J. G. 2002. Turboprop—an improved PROPELLER sequence for diffusion weighted MRI. In *Proceedings of the 10th meeting of the International Society for Magnetic Resonance in Medicine.*, p. 435.

Pipe, J. G., Farthing, V. G., and Forbes, K. P. 2002. Multishot diffusion-weighted FSE using PROPELLER MRI. *Magn. Reson. Med.* 47: 42–52.

Pipe, J. G., Han, E. T., and Busse, R. F. 2003. SAR reduction for PROPELLER DWI at 3T. In *Proceedings of the 11th meeting of the International Society for Magnetic Resonance in Medicine*, p. 2127.

Ra, J. B., Hilal, S.K., and Oh, C. H. 1989. An algorithm for MR imaging of the short T2 fraction of sodium using the FID signal. *J. Comput. Assist. Tomogr.* 13: 302–309.

Rasche, V., Holz, D., and Proska, R. 1999. MR fluoroscopy using projection reconstruction multi-gradient-echo (prMGE) MRI. *Magn. Reson. Med.* 42: 324–334.

Rasche, V., Holz, D., and Schepper, W. 1994. Radial turbo spin echo imaging. *Magn. Reson. Med.* 32: 629–638.

Scheffler, K., and Hennig, J. 1998. Reduced circular field of view imaging. *Magn. Reson. Med.* 40: 474–480.

Shankaranarayanan, A., Simonetti, O. P., Laub, G., Lewin, J. S., and Duerk J. L. 2001. Segmented k-space and real-time cardiac cine MR imaging with radial trajectories. *Radiology* 221: 827–836.

Shankaranarayanan, A., Wendt, M., Lewin, J. S., and Duerk, J. L. 2001. Two-step navigatorless correction algorithm for radial k-space MRI acquisitions. *Magn. Reson. Med.* 45: 277–288.

Song, H. K., and Dougherty, L. 2000. k-Space weighted image contrast (KWIC) for contrast manipulation in projection reconstruction MRI. *Magn. Reson. Med.* 44: 825–832.

Stillman, A. E., Levin, D. N., Yang, D. B., and Lauterbur, P. C. 1986. Back projection reconstruction of spectroscopic NMR images from incomplete sets of projections. *J. Magn. Reson.* 69: 168–175.

Toropov, Y. V., and Block, W. F. 2001. Increasing acquisition speed in undersampled 3D projection imaging. In *Proceedings of the 9th meeting of the International Society for Magnetic Resonance in Medicine*, p. 1809.

Trouard, T. P., Theilmann, R. J., Altbach, M. I., and Gmitro, A. F. 1999. High-resolution diffusion imaging with DIFRAD-FSE (diffusion-weighted radial acquisition of data with fast spin-echo) MRI. *Magn. Reson. Med.* 42: 11–18.

Vigen, K. K., Peters, D. C., Grist, T. M., Block, W. F., and Mistretta, C. A. 2000. Undersampled projection-reconstruction imaging for time-resolved contrast-enhanced imaging. *Magn. Reson. Med.* 43: 170–176.

Wieben, O., Barger, A. V., Block, W. F., and Mistretta, C. A. 2001. Correcting for translational motion in 3D projection reconstruction. In *Proceedings of the 9th meeting of the International Society for Magnetic Resonance in Medicine*, p. 737.

Wieben, O., Brodsky, E., Mistretta, C. A., and Block, W. F. 2003. Correction of trajectory errors in radial acquisitions. In *Proceedings of the 11th meeting of the International Society for Magnetic Resonance in Medicine*, p. 298.

Zhou, X., and Lauterbur, P. C. 1992. *NMR microscopy using projection reconstruction.* Edited by B. Blümich and W. Kuhn. Weinheim, Germany: VCH.

Zhou, X., Liang, Z.-P., Gewalt, S. L., Cofer, G. P., Lauterbur, P. C., and Johnson, G. A. 1998. A fast spin echo technique with circular sampling. *Magn. Reson. Med.* 39: 23–27.

RELATED SECTIONS

17.6 Spiral

Spiral or spiral echo planar imaging is a set of acquisition methods that follow a spiral k-space trajectory (Meyer 1998). Most other pulse sequences use a rectilinear (i.e., Cartesian) k-space raster (Figure 17.52a). In the gradient echo and spin echo pulse sequences discussed in Sections 14.1 and 14.3, each k-space line is acquired with its own RF excitation pulse. Acquiring a signal from a larger portion of k-space with each RF excitation (also called a shot) decreases scan time. Echo train pulse sequences, such as EPI (Section 16.1), GRASE (Section 16.2), and RARE (Section 16.4), can acquire multiple Cartesian lines with each shot. Spiral trajectories (Figure 17.52b) achieve higher data collection efficiency compared to Cartesian trajectories by requiring fewer shots for similar k-space coverage. More generally, pulse sequences such as RARE, GRASE, EPI and spiral allow a flexible trade-off between the number of shots, which determines scan time, and the amount of data collected per shot. Collecting more data per shot always poses additional potential image-quality challenges, for example, geometric distortion for EPI and blurring for RARE and spirals.

Sometimes only data within a central circular region of k-space are reconstructed, as shown by the dashed circle in Figure 17.52a (see Section 13.1 on Fourier reconstruction). The data outside this region are usually acquired with rectilinear k-space trajectories, but are sometimes apodized with a reconstruction window (i.e., a filter). Spiral sequences do not collect the unused data from the "corners" of k-space and therefore can be more time-efficient.

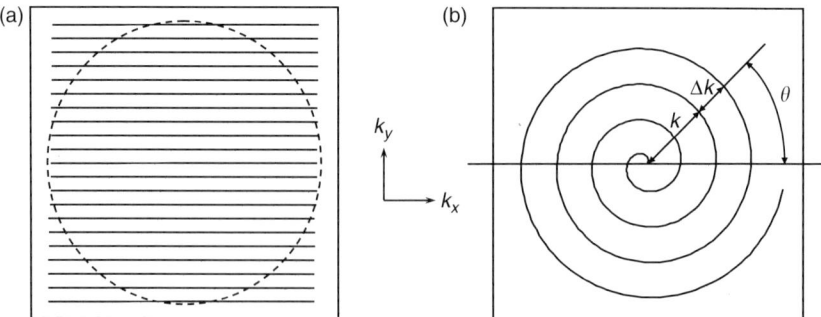

FIGURE 17.52 (a) Rectilinear k-space trajectory. The dashed circle shows the extent of a radial k-space window sometimes used for reconstruction. With such a window, data outside the circle are apodized and essentially discarded. (b) Spiral k-space trajectory. The radial and azimuthal coordinates are k and θ, respectively. The radial sampling interval is Δk.

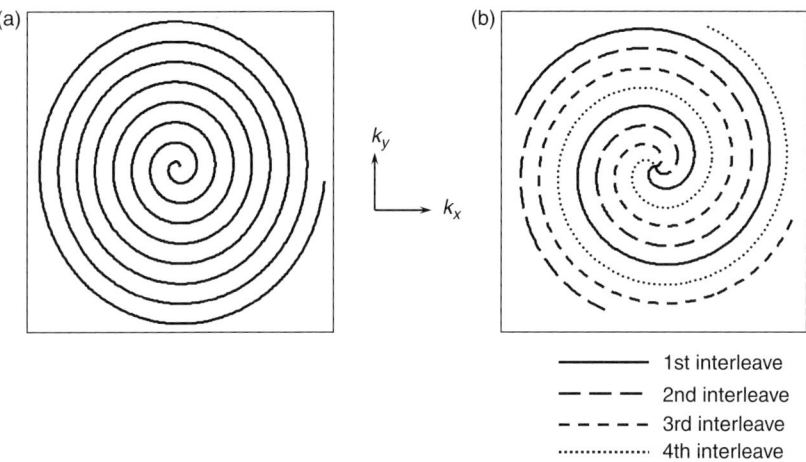

1st interleave
— — — 2nd interleave
— - — - — 3rd interleave
················· 4th interleave

FIGURE 17.53 (a) Single-shot spiral. (b) Interleaved multishot spiral.

Similar to EPI, GRASE, and RARE, spirals can acquire the entire k-space raw data set with either one or multiple shots. The k-space trajectories for adjacent shots of an interleaved multishot spiral are rotated by an angle $\pm 2\pi / N_{\text{shot}}$ with respect to one another (Figure 17.53), where N_{shot} is the total number of shots.

Because spiral acquisition is simply a method of traversing k-space, it can be combined with many other MRI techniques. For example, both FID and spin echo signal generation are compatible with a spiral readout (Figure 17.54). Spiral readout with an FID is often referred to as gradient-echo spiral. Spirals can be used in conjunction with diffusion gradients (Section 9.1), flow-encoding gradients (Section 9.2), or with RF preparation pulses such as magnetization transfer (Section 4.2) or inversion pulses (Section 6.2). In all these cases, spiral image data can be collected in either 2D or 3D acquisition mode, although 2D spirals are more commonly used.

Spirals can also be combined with RARE to acquire multiple spiral interleaves using a single RF excitation. We use the terms interleaves and shots interchangeably in this section, although for RARE spirals they are not necessarily the same. (A noninterleaved multishot spiral would collect nonoverlapping annuli for each shot, but such a trajectory is seldom used except for RARE spirals.) As the number of interleaves increases, the readout time for each interleaf T_{acq} decreases, assuming the spatial resolution and FOV are held fixed.

Spirals replace the independent frequency- and phase-encoding functions used in Cartesian k-space trajectories with a 2D readout function. The gradient

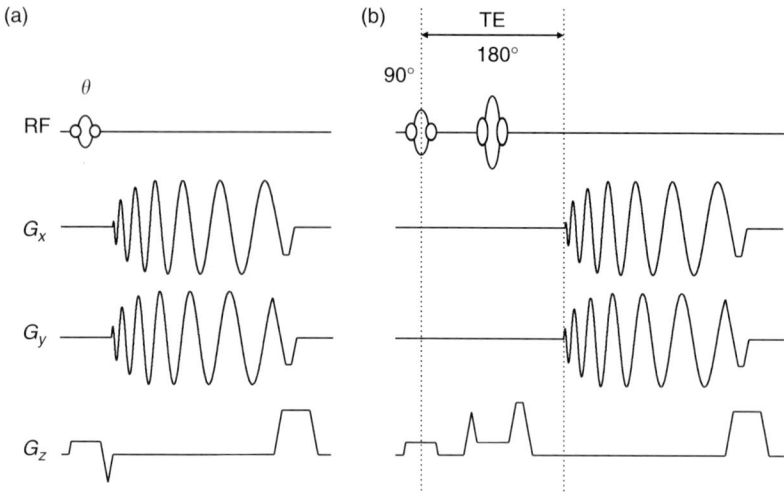

FIGURE 17.54 (a) 2D gradient echo spiral pulse sequence. (b) 2D spin echo spiral pulse sequence.

waveforms for spiral readouts are sinusoids that are usually both frequency and amplitude modulated. Most spiral trajectories begin by collecting data at the center of k-space for each interleaf. This results in gradient waveforms that start with an amplitude of zero at the beginning of the readout. As the readout progresses, the gradient amplitude increases while the sinusoid frequency decreases (Figure 17.55). Because of the restricted slew rate of all MR gradient amplifiers, the gradient amplitude cannot increase infinitely fast at the beginning of the readout. This results in data points near the center of k-space that are clustered closer than required by the Nyquist sampling theorem (Figure 17.56). This oversampling reduces the efficiency of spirals, but also reduces their sensitivity to motion.

Once the maximal k-space radius is reached, the spiral gradient is ramped to zero. The most commonly used variations of gradient echo spirals are spoiled, SSFP-FID, and balanced SSFP. A readout/rewinding lobe is usually applied to return the k-space trajectory to the origin for the same reason that most nonspiral gradient echoes use a rewinding lobe for the phase-encoding gradient (see Section 14.1). For example, for RF spoiled gradient-echo spirals, this results in a consistent phase on the readout axes for all interleaves, giving better image quality.

Another advantage of spirals is that the gradient moments oscillate periodically about zero because of the sinusoidal gradient waveforms (Figure 17.57). Because the readout waveforms start with zero amplitude, the data acquired in

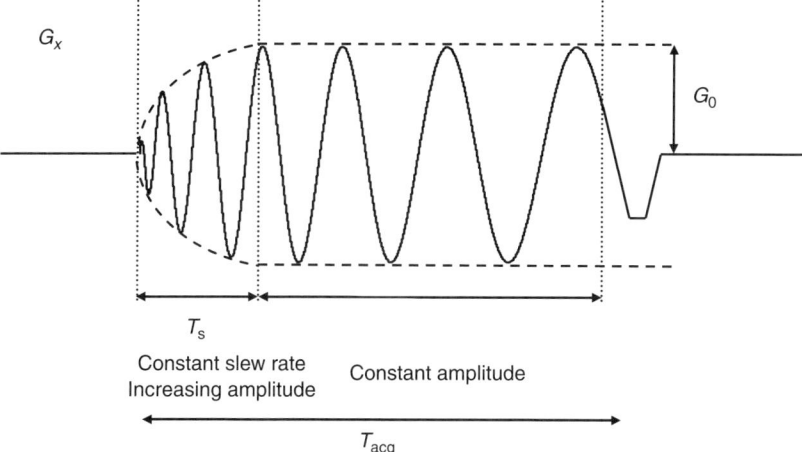

FIGURE 17.55 Sinusoidal gradient waveform for one of the readout axes for a typical 2D spiral prescription. The amplitude starts at zero and builds up at a constant slew rate to the final value G_0, which is determined by the FOV, bandwidth, and system gradient limit. The amplitude remains constant after G_0 is reached. As time progresses, the sinusoidal frequency decreases.

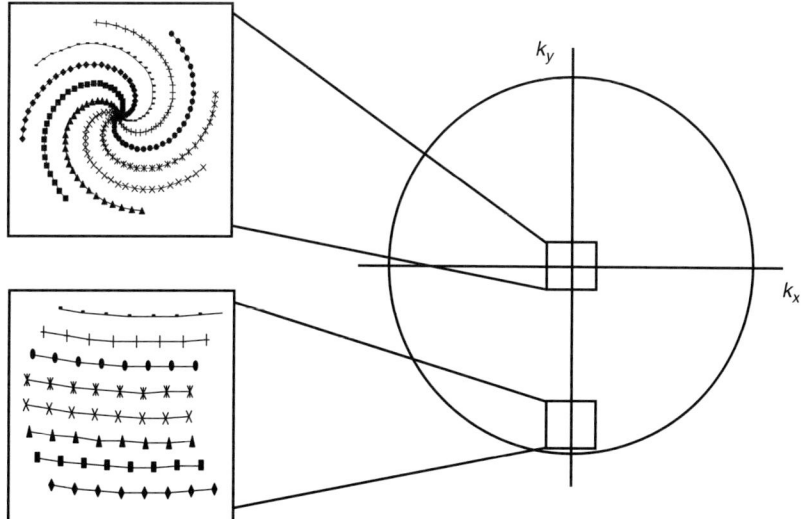

FIGURE 17.56 Distribution of data points in k-space for a spiral with eight interleaves. Near the center of k-space, the points are clustered much closer than required by the Nyquist sampling theorem. Near the edge of k-space, the points are spaced at the Nyquist sampling limit.

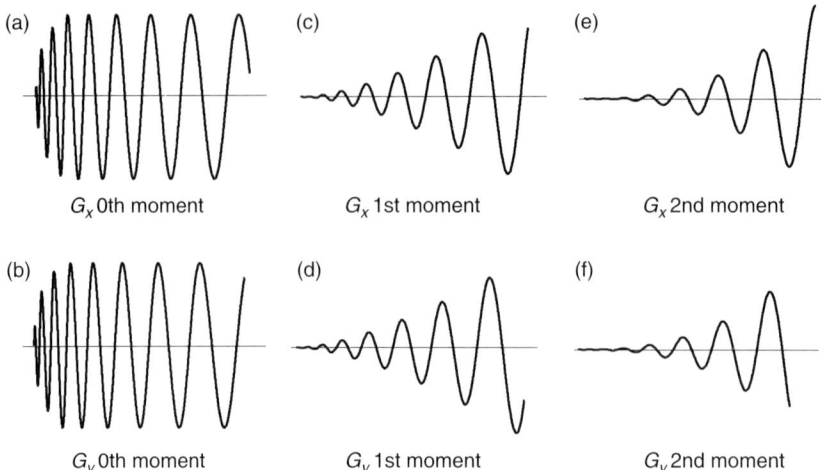

FIGURE 17.57 Gradient moments for a spiral readout waveform. (a) G_x zeroth moment, (b) G_y zeroth moment, (c) G_x first moment, (d) G_y first moment, (e) G_x second moment, (f) G_y second moment for a spiral with $N_{shot} = 16$, $L = 24\,cm$, $\Delta\nu = \pm112\,kHz$, and $N = 256$ pixels. Note that at the beginning of the readout, which corresponds to the center of k-space, all orders of the gradient moments are zero.

the center of k-space are gradient-moment-nulled to all orders along the two readout axes. This can result in less artifact and signal loss from intravoxel dephasing caused by flowing spins (Section 10.4).

Because spirals do not use phase-encoding gradients, spiral trajectories that start at the center of k-space can have very short echo times, a feature similar to projection acquisition with FID acquisition. Conversely, longer echo times to increase T_2^* sensitivity can be obtained by starting the trajectory at the edge of k-space and spiraling inward (i.e., reversed spiral, subsection 17.6.2).

The main disadvantage of spirals is image blurring from off-resonant spins. The blurring can be understood qualitatively from Figure 17.58. In a non-echo-planar rectilinear k-space acquisition, off-resonant spins appear displaced in the frequency-encoded direction of the image by a distance proportional to the resonance frequency offset. With a spiral acquisition, however, the readout direction is effectively rotating during the acquisition. Thus, the off-resonant spins are displaced in all directions in the image, causing a blurred appearance. (The actual amount of displacement at any time depends on the amplitude of the readout gradient at that point in the trajectory.) Blurring depends roughly on the total off-resonant phase accumulated at the completion of the readout. Thus, the longer the readout time, the worse the blurring. Uncorrected blurring has impeded the introduction of spirals into routine clinical practice. Even

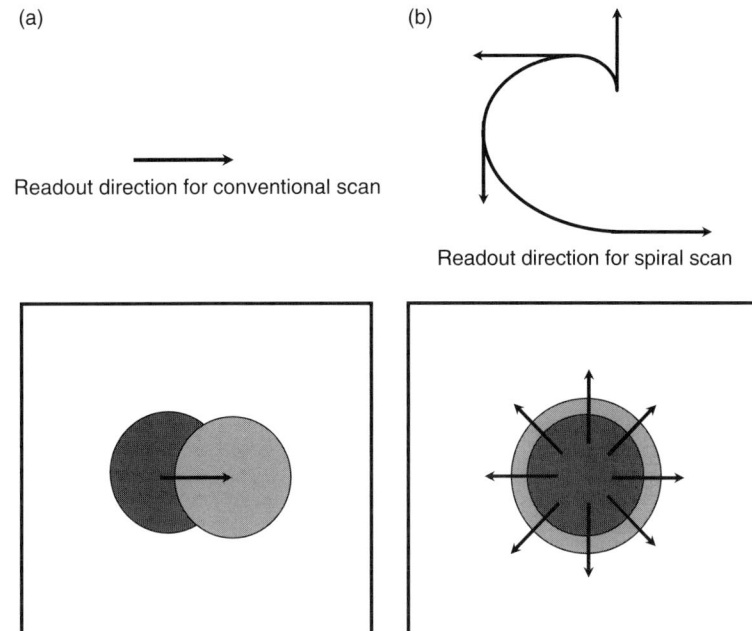

FIGURE 17.58 (a) Resonance offset in a conventional Fourier acquisition causes displacement in the frequency-encoded (i.e., readout) direction. (b) Resonance offset in a spiral acquisition causes displacement in all directions, which results in blurring.

small frequency offsets can cause substantial blurring for typical readout times (Figure 17.59). By contrast, T_2^* decay during the readout causes only a slight, spatially independent blurring and is not a significant problem. More discussion of off-resonance blurring and blurring corrections is given in subsection 17.6.3.

Another disadvantage of spirals is increased aliasing from objects that extend outside the FOV. With rectilinear k-space acquisition, signal from spins that are outside the FOV in the frequency-encoded direction is removed by the anti-aliasing filter. Signal from spins outside the FOV in the phase-encoded direction cannot be removed, so it aliases or wraps into the final image. With spirals, however, the frequency-encoded direction rotates throughout the scan. At any point during the readout, signal is acquired from spins outside the FOV in the direction orthogonal to the rotating readout gradient. This signal cannot be eliminated and causes aliasing artifacts.

A key difference between rectilinear trajectories and spirals is that aliased signal from rectilinear trajectories appears wrapped in the phase-encoded direction of the image, whereas aliased signal from spirals gives streaks and swirls

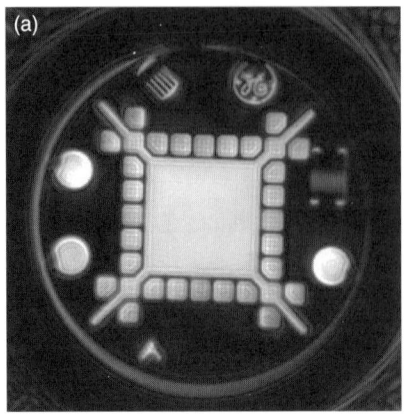
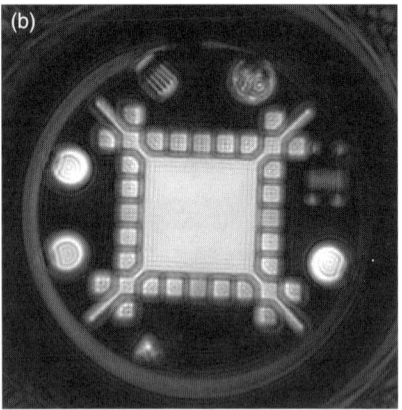

FIGURE 17.59 Spiral scan with $N_{\mathrm{shot}} = 16$, $L = 24\,\mathrm{cm}$, $\Delta\nu = \pm62.5\,\mathrm{kHz}$, $N = 200$ pixels, $S_{\mathrm{R0}} = 120\,\mathrm{T/m/s}$, $G_0 = 12.2\,\mathrm{mT/m}$, and $T_{\mathrm{acq}} = 16\,\mathrm{ms}$. (a) Transmit/receive on-resonance. (b) Transmit/receive 50 Hz off-resonance.

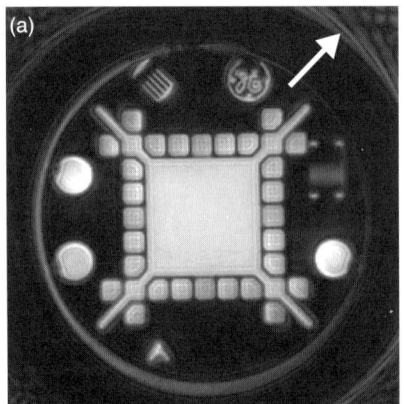
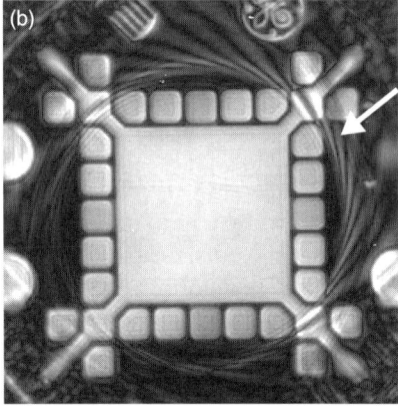

FIGURE 17.60 Aliasing artifacts (arrows) for spiral scans with $N_{\mathrm{shot}} = 16$, $\Delta\nu = \pm62.5\,\mathrm{kHz}$, $N = 200$ pixels, $S_{\mathrm{R0}} = 120\,\mathrm{T/m/s}$, $G_0 = 12.2\,\mathrm{mT/m}$, and $T_{\mathrm{acq}} = 16\,\mathrm{ms}$. (a) $L = 24\,\mathrm{cm}$ (object contained within the FOV), (b) $L = 16\,\mathrm{cm}$ (object larger than the FOV).

that bear no similarity to the anatomical region that generated the aliasing (Figure 17.60). Therefore more care must be taken in choosing the FOV for spiral scans than for conventional scans. More discussion of aliasing artifacts is given in subsection 17.6.1.

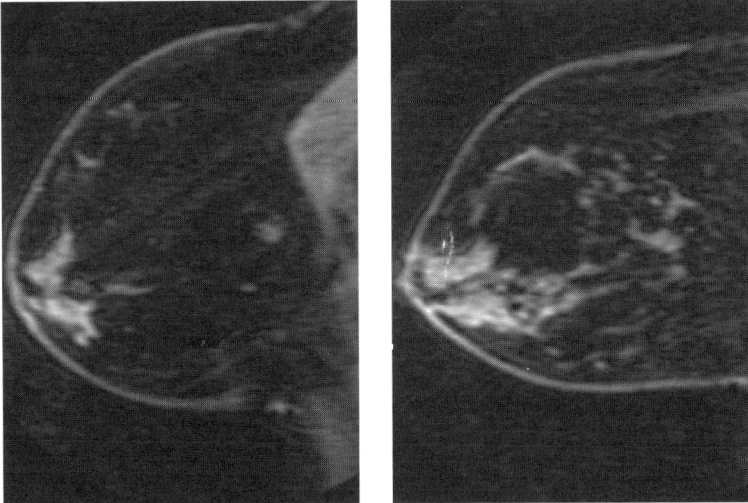

FIGURE 17.61 Sagittal bilateral breast 3D spiral images with lipid suppression using a four-channel breast coil and SENSE with a reduction factor of 2 in the Fourier-encoded (slice) direction. Imaging parameters: TR/TE/flip angle = $38/5.3/40$, $\Delta \nu = \pm 125$ kHz, $L = 20$ cm, 4-mm slice, 0 skip, 80 slices, $N_{shot} = 12$, $T_{acq} = 11.2$ ms, 18-s scan. (Images courtesy Bruce Daniel, M.D., Stanford University, and Ann Shimikawa, M.S. and Elisabeth Angelos, Ph.D., GE Medical Systems.)

Spiral scans are almost invariably reconstructed using gridding (Section 13.2). The reconstruction times are therefore usually long compared to conventional scans. This can limit the reconstruction frame rate, especially with multiple receive coils, making some real-time applications impractical, at least with the hardware available in 2004.

Because of their inherent time efficiency, spirals have found most widespread application in coronary artery imaging (Meyer et al. 1992), fMRI (Noll et al. 1995), and spectroscopic imaging (Adalsteinsson et al. 1998). Figure 17.61 shows an emerging application using spirals to achieve higher temporal resolution with contrast-enhanced dynamic imaging (Angelos et al. 2003). Spiral k-space trajectories can also be used for 2D or 3D RF pulses, as described in Cline et al. (1991) and Section 5.1.

17.6.1 MATHEMATICAL DESCRIPTION

k-Space Trajectory First we consider the 2D spiral case; we discuss the extension to 3D later. We describe the k-space trajectory using polar coordinates (k, θ), which are related to the Cartesian coordinates (k_x, k_y)

through:

$$k_x = k \cos \theta$$
$$k_y = k \sin \theta \qquad (17.115)$$

(Note that θ should be distinguished from the symbol for the RF flip angle used in other sections of this book.) Spiral scans usually use an Archimedean spiral (after Archimedes 287?–212 B.C., a Greek mathematician and scientist), in which the radius k is proportional to the azimuthal angle θ (Figure 17.52):

$$k(t) = \lambda \theta(t) \qquad (17.116)$$

where λ is a constant. A spiral with N_{shot} interleaves uses trajectories for each interleaf that are identical in shape, but rotated by integer multiples of the angle $2\pi/N_{shot}$ rad about the axis perpendicularly passing through the k-space origin. The constant λ is determined by the Nyquist sampling requirement. Each interleaf moves radially through a distance $2\pi\lambda$ in k-space as the azimuthal angle θ advances through 2π. If N_{shot} interleaves are packed into this radial distance, the radial distance between adjacent interleaves at any fixed azimuthal angle is $\Delta k = 2\pi\lambda/N_{shot}$ (Figure 17.52b). For alias-free sampling that satisfies the Nyquist criterion, we must have $\Delta k = 1/L$, where $L = L_x = L_y$ is the FOV. This requires:

$$\lambda = \frac{N_{shot}}{2\pi L} \qquad (17.117)$$

Equation (17.117) is a result of the radial Nyquist sampling requirement. The corresponding azimuthal Nyquist sampling requirement is discussed next. The spatial resolution for a spiral scan is determined by the maximum radius reached in k-space, just as for conventional scans.

Once the geometric shape of the spiral trajectory is fixed by the choice of N_{shot}, L, and spatial resolution, the rate at which the spiral is traversed, $\theta(t)$, must be determined. Early spiral implementations traversed k-space with constant angular velocity (Ahn et al. 1996). This type of spiral is still sometimes used because the gradient waveforms are relatively simple. However, constant angular velocity spirals are inefficient because they take longer to reach the maximum radius in k-space. Because blurring is proportional to the readout time for a single interleaf, constant angular velocity spirals have more blurring for a fixed spatial resolution, or equivalently lower resolution for a fixed amount of blurring, than constant linear velocity spirals. Therefore, we only discuss constant linear velocity spirals in this section. (Although the term *constant linear velocity* is standard nomenclature, the trajectory actually uses a constant linear speed because the direction of travel is not constant.)

Gradient Waveforms The velocity of k-space traversal in any given direction is proportional to the gradient amplitude in that direction. Therefore, a constant linear velocity 2D spiral uses a readout waveform that has constant $G = \sqrt{G_x^2(t) + G_y^2(t)}$ at all points in k-space. In reality, a constant linear velocity cannot be achieved for all parts of k-space because the gradient waveform must start from zero and gradient amplifiers have restricted slew rate. The most efficient spiral trajectory uses a fixed slew rate S_{RO} until the desired gradient amplitude G_0 has been reached. At this point the amplitude stays constant for the remainder of the readout (Figure 17.55). Several gradient waveform design methods that follow this strategy have been developed (Meyer et al. 1996; King et al. 1995; Glover 1999).

The desired gradient amplitude G_0 is determined by the azimuthal Nyquist sampling requirement:

$$\frac{\gamma}{2\pi} G_0 L = 2\Delta\nu \qquad (17.118)$$

where $\pm\Delta\nu$ is the receiver bandwidth. This requirement prevents aliasing from azimuthal undersampling (i.e., along a spiral interleaf). Because of the slew rate limit, the gradient amplitude is typically less than G_0 near the center of k-space. This causes the distance between sampled k-space points along a spiral interleaf to be smaller near the center of k-space than away from the center (Figure 17.56). If the Nyquist sampling criterion in Eq. (17.118) is met at the edge of k-space, it is automatically met at the center. It is possible to increase G_0 beyond the limit imposed by Eq. (17.118), depending on the amount of aliasing that is tolerable. When this is done, the resulting trajectory has a shorter readout time for fixed spatial resolution and FOV and consequently produces less blurring. Aliasing artifacts due to radial and azimuthal undersampling are independent and can be separately controlled. In this respect, spiral scans are more like CT scans than like conventional MR with a Cartesian k-trajectory. Figure 17.62 shows a comparison of radial aliasing (using λ greater than the limit in Eq. 17.117) and azimuthal aliasing (using G_0 greater than the limit in Eq. 17.118). In Figure 17.62c and d, λ and G_0, respectively are increased by a factor of 1.8 relative to their Nyquist values in Figure 17.62b. Note that in Figure 17.62d, the azimuthal Δk is still below the Nyquist value near the center of k-space because of the slew rate limit, although the final azimuthal Δk is 1.8 times the Nyquist value. The spatial resolution in all the images in Figure 17.62b–d is fixed at 1.2 mm. This example illustrates that, similar to CT, azimuthal aliasing artifacts are frequently less objectionable than radial aliasing artifacts.

The slew rate S_{RO} is usually set to the maximum allowed by the gradient hardware, but sometimes it needs to be further restricted if peripheral nerve

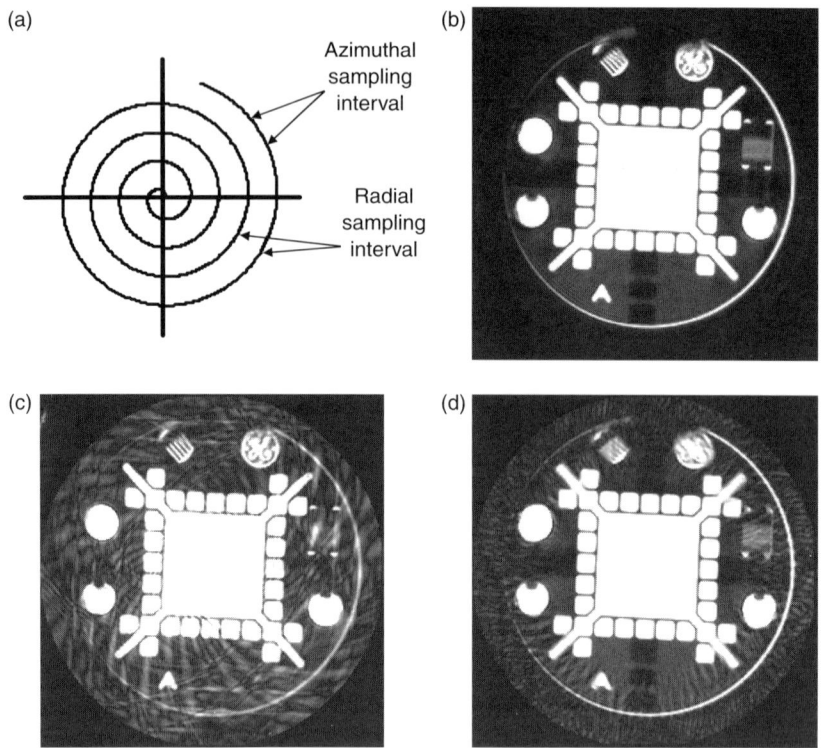

FIGURE 17.62 (a) Spiral k-space trajectory showing the radial and azimuthal sampling intervals. (b) Spiral scan without aliasing. Imaging parameters: TE/TR/flip angle $= 2.5/500/90$, $\Delta\nu = \pm 62.5$ kHz, $L = 24$ cm, 10-mm slice, $N_{\text{shot}} = 32$, $T_{\text{acq}} = 8.192$ ms, $N = 200$ pixels, $S_{\text{R0}} = 120$ T/m/s, $G_0 = 12.2$ mT/m, $\lambda = 0.21$ cm^{-1}. (c) Radial aliasing. Imaging parameters are the same as (b) except $\lambda = 0.38$ cm^{-1}, $T_{\text{acq}} = 4.8$ ms. (d) Azimuthal aliasing. Imaging parameters are the same as (b) except $G_0 = 22$ mT/m, and $T_{\text{acq}} = 4.8$ ms.

stimulation is a concern (King and Schaefer 2000). Increasing S_{R0} decreases the readout time (for a fixed spatial, resolution, FOV, and number of interleaves) by decreasing the duration of the slew rate–limited segment of the trajectory T_s (Figure 17.55). As T_s becomes negligible, further slew rate increases give almost no reduction in readout time. Increasing the maximum gradient amplitude can also reduce the readout time. A higher slew rate is required, however, to fully realize the benefits of a stronger maximum gradient amplitude.

It is customary to define spatial resolution by the equivalent matrix size that would result in a square pixel that has edge length equal to the spatial resolution. We call this the effective resolution N. The image, however, will generally be interpolated to a square matrix size that is a convenient power of two, which can be much larger than $N \times N$. Thus the maximum k-space radius reached, k_{max}, is defined by:

$$k_{max} = \frac{N}{2L} \tag{17.119}$$

where $N = N_x = N_y$ is the effective matrix size. The final azimuthal angle of the k-space trajectory is important for the waveform calculation and is given by:

$$\theta_{max} = \frac{k_{max}}{\lambda} = \frac{\pi N}{N_{shot}} \tag{17.120}$$

where we have used Eqs. (17.116), (17.117) and (17.119).

Example 17.7 How many complete turns of a 16-shot spiral are required to give a spatial resolution of 1.5 mm if the FOV is 24 cm?

Answer The effective matrix size is $N = 240 \, \text{mm}/1.5 \, \text{mm} = 160$. Using Eq. (17.120) with $N_{shot} = 16$, $\theta_{max} = \pi \times 160/16 = 10\pi$ or five complete turns.

We now consider how to calculate the readout gradient waveforms. Using Eqs. (17.115) and (17.116), the Cartesian components of the gradient waveform are given by:

$$G_x = \frac{2\pi}{\gamma} \dot{k}_x = \frac{2\pi}{\gamma} \lambda \dot{\theta} (\cos\theta - \theta \sin\theta) \tag{17.121}$$

$$G_y = \frac{2\pi}{\gamma} \dot{k}_y = \frac{2\pi}{\gamma} \lambda \dot{\theta} (\sin\theta + \theta \cos\theta) \tag{17.122}$$

where a dot above a symbol denotes its first-time derivative. Similarly, using Eqs. (17.121) and (17.122), the Cartesian components of the slew rate (the time derivatives of the corresponding gradient components) are given by

$$S_{Rx} = \frac{2\pi}{\gamma} \lambda \left[\left(\ddot{\theta} - \theta\dot{\theta}^2 \right) \cos\theta - \left(2\dot{\theta}^2 + \theta\ddot{\theta} \right) \sin\theta \right] \tag{17.123}$$

$$S_{Ry} = \frac{2\pi}{\gamma} \lambda \left[\left(\ddot{\theta} - \theta\dot{\theta}^2 \right) \sin\theta + \left(2\dot{\theta}^2 + \theta\ddot{\theta} \right) \cos\theta \right], \tag{17.124}$$

where a double dot denotes the second-time derivative. The components $G_x(t)$, $G_y(t)$, $S_{Rx}(t)$, and $S_{Ry}(t)$ can be thought of as defining 2D gradient and slew rate vectors that rotate as θ increases with time. The vectors also have time-varying amplitudes G and S_R that are found using Eqs. (17.121)–(17.124) to be:

$$G(t) = \sqrt{G_x^2 + G_y^2} = \frac{2\pi}{\gamma} \lambda \dot{\theta} \sqrt{1 + \theta^2} \tag{17.125}$$

and

$$S_R(t) = \sqrt{S_{Rx}^2 + S_{Ry}^2} = \frac{2\pi}{\gamma} \lambda \left[\left(\ddot{\theta} - \theta \dot{\theta}^2 \right)^2 + \left(2\dot{\theta}^2 + \theta \ddot{\theta} \right)^2 \right]^{1/2} \tag{17.126}$$

(Equation 17.125 implicitly assumes without loss of generality that $\dot{\theta} > 0$ because $\dot{\theta}^2$ is removed from the square root.) The slew rate and amplitude limits on the spiral trajectory can be stated as:

$$\begin{cases} S_R(t) = S_{R0} & \text{while } G(t) < G_0 \\ G(t) = G_0 & \text{thereafter} \end{cases} \tag{17.127}$$

The constraint of Eq. (17.127) can be formulated into a differential equation for $\theta(t)$ (King et al. 1999):

$$\ddot{\theta} = \frac{f(\theta, \dot{\theta}) - \theta \dot{\theta}^2}{1 + \theta^2} \tag{17.128}$$

where

$$f(\theta, \dot{\theta}) = \begin{cases} \left[\beta^2 \left(1 + \theta^2 \right) - \dot{\theta}^4 \left(2 + \theta^2 \right)^2 \right]^{1/2} & \text{if } G < G_0 \\ 0 & \text{otherwise} \end{cases} \tag{17.129}$$

and

$$\beta = \frac{\gamma}{2\pi} \frac{S_{R0}}{\lambda} \tag{17.130}$$

(We assume that $\ddot{\theta} > 0$ when $\theta = 0$ and $\dot{\theta} = 0$ because the positive sign is chosen for the square root in Eq. 17.129.) The differential equation can be solved numerically for $\theta(t)$ and $\dot{\theta}(t)$ using any standard equation-solver software package. The solution is obtained for $\theta \leq \theta_{max}$, where θ_{max} is given by Eq. (17.120). Once $\theta(t)$ and $\dot{\theta}(t)$ have been determined, the gradient waveforms can be calculated using Eqs. (17.121) and (17.122). There is frequently a small discontinuity in $\ddot{\theta}$ at $t = T_s$ because $f(\theta, \dot{\theta}) \neq 0$ immediately preceding this point but $f(\theta, \dot{\theta}) = 0$ immediately afterward. This is usually not a problem because $\dot{\theta}$ and the physical gradient waveforms are continuous.

Approximate Solution   A closed-form expression that approximates the gradient waveforms is described in Glover (1999). The azimuthal angle $\theta(t)$ is partitioned into two separate functions of time for the slew-rate-limited and gradient-amplitude-limited segments of the trajectory.

$$\theta(t) = \begin{cases} \theta_1(t) & t < T_s \\ \theta_2(t) & t \geq T_s \end{cases} \tag{17.131}$$

where T_s is the duration of the slew rate limited segment of the trajectory, given approximately by:

$$T_s = \left(\frac{3\gamma G_0}{4\pi \lambda a_2^2} \right)^3 \tag{17.132}$$

with

$$a_2 = \left(\frac{9\beta}{4} \right)^{1/3} \tag{17.133}$$

The two functions of time in Eq. (17.131) are:

$$\theta_1(t) = \frac{\frac{1}{2}\beta t^2}{\Lambda + \frac{\beta}{2a_2} t^{4/3}} \tag{17.134}$$

and

$$\theta_2(t) = \sqrt{\theta_s^2 + \frac{\gamma}{\pi \lambda} G_0(t - T_s)} \tag{17.135}$$

and Λ in Eq. (17.134) is a dimensionless, adjustable parameter. The angle θ_s in Eq. (17.135) is the transition point between the slew-rate-limited and gradient-amplitude-limited segments and is found from:

$$\theta_s = \theta_1(T_s) \tag{17.136}$$

The constant $\Lambda \geq 1$ in Eq. (17.134) is chosen to adjust the slew rate at $t = 0$, which is given by $S(0) = S_0/\Lambda$. In this approximation, $S_R(t)$ overshoots S_{R0} for part of the slew-rate-limited segment of the trajectory. Larger values of Λ give lower $S_R(t)$ near $t = 0$, but also give a longer overshoot time.

For some scan prescriptions, G_0 is never reached and the trajectory is slew-rate-limited for the entire readout time. These prescriptions have relatively large G_0, slow S_{R0}, small N_{shot}, or large FOV. In this case, only θ_1 is calculated and, neglecting Λ, the duration of the trajectory is:

$$T_{acq} = \frac{2\pi L}{3N_{shot}} \sqrt{\frac{\pi}{\gamma S_{R0}(\Delta x)^3}} \tag{17.137}$$

where Δx is the spatial resolution (with dimension of distance). If instead, G_0 is reached before $\theta = \theta_{max}$, $\theta_2(t)$ is determined from Eq. (17.135) for $T_s < t \le T_{acq}$ where:

$$T_{acq} = T_s + \frac{\pi \lambda}{\gamma G_0} \left(\theta_{max}^2 - \theta_s^2 \right) \tag{17.138}$$

Once $\theta(t)$ is determined from Eq. (17.131), $\dot{\theta}$ can be obtained by differentiating Eqs. (17.134) and (17.135). The gradient waveforms are then calculated using Eqs. (17.121) and (17.122).

Example 17.8 A single-shot spiral uses a maximal gradient amplitude of 30 mT/m and slew rate of 200 T/m/s. (a) Use the closed-form approximation with $\Lambda = 1$ to calculate the readout time necessary to achieve an effective matrix size of 128 if the FOV is 20 cm. (b) If the maximal amplitude is increased to 50 mT/m, by how much time is the readout shortened?

Answer

(a) Using $S_{R0} = 200 \, T/m/s = 20,000 \, G/cm/s$ with Eqs. (17.117), (17.130), and (17.133) gives:

$$\lambda = \frac{1}{2\pi \times 20 \, cm} = 7.958 \times 10^{-3} \, cm^{-1}$$

$$\beta = \frac{4257 \, Hz/G \times 20,000 \, G/cm/s}{7.958 \times 10^{-3} \, cm^{-1}} = 1.070 \times 10^{10} \, s^{-2}$$

and

$$a_2 = \left(\frac{9 \times 1.070 \times 10^{10} \, s^{-2}}{4} \right)^{1/3} = 2887 \, s^{-2/3}$$

Using Eq. (17.132), the time T_s to reach the maximal gradient amplitude $G_0 = 30 \, mT/m = 3 \, G/cm$ is:

$$T_s = \left(\frac{3 \times 4257 \, Hz/G \times 3 \, G/cm}{2 \times 7.958 \times 10^{-3} \, cm^{-1} \times (2887 \, s^{-2/3})^2} \right)^3 = 0.024 \, s$$

From Eq. (17.134), the angle θ_s reached at time T_s is

$$\theta_s = \frac{\frac{1}{2} \times 1.070 \times 10^{10}\,\mathrm{s}^{-2} \times (0.024\,\mathrm{s})^2}{1 + \dfrac{1.070 \times 10^{10}\,\mathrm{s}^{-2}}{2 \times 2887\,\mathrm{s}^{-2/3}}(0.024\,\mathrm{s})^{4/3}} = 240.2\,\mathrm{rad}$$

From Eq. (17.120), the final angle to achieve an equivalent matrix size of 128 is:

$$\theta_{max} = \frac{\pi \times 128}{1} = 402.1\,\mathrm{rad}$$

Because $\theta_{max} > \theta_s$, the slew-rate-limited portion of the trajectory alone is insufficient to achieve the desired spatial resolution. Using Eq. (17.138) yields the final readout time:

$$T_{acq} = 0.024\,\mathrm{s} + \frac{7.958 \times 10^{-3}\,\mathrm{cm}^{-1}}{2 \times 4257\,\mathrm{Hz/G} \times 3\,\mathrm{G/cm}}((402.1\,\mathrm{rad})^2 - (240.2\,\mathrm{rad})^2)$$

$$= 0.056\,\mathrm{s}$$

(b) If G_0 is increased to 50 mT/m or 5 G/cm, T_s and θ_s increase to:

$$T_s = \left(\frac{3 \times 4257\,\mathrm{Hz/G} \times 5\,\mathrm{G/cm}}{2 \times 7.958 \times 10^{-3}\,\mathrm{cm}^{-1} \times (2887\,\mathrm{s}^{-2/3})^2}\right)^3 = 0.112\,\mathrm{s}$$

and

$$\theta_s = \frac{\frac{1}{2} \times 1.070 \times 10^{10}\,\mathrm{s}^{-2} \times (0.112\,\mathrm{s})^2}{1 + \dfrac{1.070 \times 10^{10}\,\mathrm{s}^{-2}}{2 \times 2887\,\mathrm{s}^{-2/3}}(0.112\,\mathrm{s})^{4/3}} = 670.8\,\mathrm{rad}$$

Because $\theta_{max} < \theta_s$, the trajectory remains slew-rate-limited for the entire readout. From Eq. (17.137):

$$T_{acq} = \frac{2\pi \times 20\,\mathrm{cm}}{3}\sqrt{\frac{1}{2 \times 4257\,\mathrm{Hz/G} \times 20{,}000\,\mathrm{G/cm/s} \times (20\,\mathrm{cm}/128)^3}}$$

$$= 0.052\,\mathrm{s}$$

The time saved by using the higher gradient amplitude is $0.056 - 0.052\,\mathrm{s} = 0.004\,\mathrm{s}$. This example illustrates that increases in gradient amplitude are of little benefit unless accompanied by corresponding increases in slew rate.

17.6.2 VARIATIONS

The design method summarized by Eq. (17.127) keeps the magnitudes of the gradient and slew rate vectors constant as they rotate. (Note that the gradient and slew-rate vectors are defined in Eqs. 17.121–17.124.) For multiple interleaves, the waveforms are calculated for one interleaf and successive interleaves are obtained by logical-to-physical gradient axis rotation, as described in Section 7.3. The constraint in Eq. (17.127) guarantees that the gradient amplitude and slew rate are not exceeded for any θ value. Although it simplifies the waveform calculation, the design constraint also results in a longer readout for fixed-prescription parameters. Better performance is achieved if we allow the individual Cartesian components $G_x(t)$, $G_y(t)$, $S_{Rx}(t)$, and $S_{Ry}(t)$ to reach their maximum amplitudes. This constraint results in gradient and slew-rate vectors with amplitudes that depend on θ. For example, $G(t)$ and $S_R(t)$ are $\sqrt{2}$ larger for $\theta = \pi/4$, $3\pi/4$, and so on than for $\theta = 0$ using this strategy. Duyn and Yang (1997) shows an example of this design for single-shot spirals in which the waveforms are triangles and trapezoids. These ideas are similar to the ideas used in optimizing gradient waveforms for oblique plane imaging (Section 7.3).

Spiral scans can be extended to use anisotropic spatial resolution and asymmetric FOV (King 1998). With Cartesian k-space trajectories, the main benefit of anisotropic (rectangular) FOV is scan-time reduction without loss of spatial resolution. With spirals, spatial resolution and FOV are coupled because increasing either the radial distance between spiral turns (Δk) or the speed of traversal in k-space increases spatial resolution for a fixed readout time, although at the expense of reduced FOV. For spirals, the primary benefit of anisotropic spatial resolution and asymmetric FOV is increased spatial resolution in the direction of reduced FOV with less blurring (less additional readout time) than would result if the resolution were increased in all directions. Scan time is the about the same for asymmetric FOV spirals if the same number of interleaves is used. Waveform design, however, is correspondingly more complicated.

Variable density spirals use higher radial sampling density (i.e., smaller radial distance Δk) near the center of k-space. In one variation, the center portion of k-space is sampled at the Nyquist frequency while the outer part is undersampled, so that all low spatial frequencies are fully sampled every TR period while the high spatial frequencies are fully sampled once per k-space acquisition. When applied to a time-resolved study, variable density spirals can provide high temporal resolution for low-spatial-frequency information, similar to keyhole methods (Section 11.3) and has been used for bolus tracking (Spielman et al. 1995). In another variation, the outer part of k-space is sampled at the Nyquist frequency while the center of k-space is oversampled in order to reduce aliasing artifacts if the patient extends outside the FOV (Tsai and Nishimura 1999). Variable density spirals have also been used in spectroscopic imaging to reduce truncation artifacts by allowing increased k-space coverage for a fixed readout time (Sarkar et al. 2002). Full density is used in the center with reduced density in the outer regions. A closed-form approximation has been developed to facilitate the calculation of variable density spiral gradient waveforms (Kim et al. 2003).

Reversed spirals start at the edge of k-space and spiral in rather than starting at the center and spiraling out (Bornert et al. 2000). This gives longer TE and increased T_2^* weighting without compromising the data acquisition efficiency and increasing the total imaging time, somewhat analogous to gradient-echo EPI with the center of k-space sampled using a later echo. The reversed spiral method has been used for fMRI to increase the sensitivity to BOLD contrast (Glover and Law 2001).

RARE spirals are a combination of RARE with spiral readout gradients (Block et al. 1997). The pulse sequence uses multiple RF refocusing pulses similar to RARE. The spiral trajectory samples an annular portion of k-space after each refocusing pulse. In doing so, the data acquisition efficiency can be better than that in a conventional spin-echo or gradient-echo spiral sequence. In this respect, RARE spirals are somewhat analogous to the GRASE pulse sequence with Cartesian k-space trajectories. In GRASE, multiple gradient echoes, traversing several lines of k-space, are collected for each RF refocusing pulse. In RARE spirals, multiple spiral turns are traversed for each RF refocusing pulse. The method has been applied to T_2-weighted imaging.

Several 3D spiral variations have been developed. The simplest k-space trajectory is a stack of identical 2D spirals with Fourier encoding in the slice direction. This method samples a cylindrical volume in 3D k-space. The data are reconstructed with a Fourier transform in the slice-encoded direction (i.e., k_z direction), followed by gridding in the $k_x - k_y$ planes. More efficient methods sample an elliptical volume in k-space. A stack of spirals can be used where the maximum spiral radii differ at each k_z location. The data are reconstructed by gridding in three dimensions. Additional trajectories are described in Irarrazabal and Nishimura (1995).

Twisting radial line (TWIRL) is a hybrid of projection acquisition (Section 17.5) and spirals, in which the k-space trajectory starts as a radial spoke and spirals (or twists) away from the k-space center in either 2D (Jackson et al. 1992) or 3D (Boada et al. 1997). By using a spiral trajectory away from the center of k-space, TWIRL gains some efficiency in the rate of k-space coverage compared to projection acquisition. The use of projection acquisition near the center of k-space results in a shorter readout time and reduced blurring compared to a full spiral trajectory. For example, using a 3D TWIRL sequence known as twisted projection imaging, a submillisecond TE can be achieved (Boada et al. 1997), enabling imaging of NMR-active nuclei with very short T_2s, such as ^{23}Na.

17.6.3 BLURRING CORRECTIONS

Blurring in spiral scans is generally spatially dependent and comes from resonance frequency offsets caused by B_0 inhomogeneity, local susceptibility variations, and chemical shift offsets. The B_0 inhomogeneity usually varies relatively slowly over the patient, whereas the susceptibility can vary greatly over short distances. Both types of effects are patient-dependent and require careful shim adjustment, as well as additional corrections to produce acceptable image quality.

The amount of blurring increases with the duration of the readout time per interleaf T_{acq}. For spirals that are entirely slew-rate-limited (i.e., never reach G_0), $T_{acq} = T_s$ is given by Eq. (17.137). In the other extreme, for spirals that are almost entirely gradient-amplitude-limited (i.e. with $T_{acq} \gg T_s$), the readout time is described approximately by (King 1998):

$$T_{acq} = \frac{\pi L^2}{8 N_{shot} \Delta \nu (\Delta x)^2} \qquad (17.139)$$

Equations (17.137) and (17.139) show that T_{acq} can be reduced by decreasing L, increasing N_{shot}, or increasing Δx. In the case of gradient-amplitude-limited spirals, Eq. (17.139) also shows that T_{acq} can be reduced by increasing the receiver bandwidth $\Delta \nu$. (In the slew-rate-limited case, T_{acq} is independent of the receiver bandwidth because, according to Eq. 17.118, changing $\Delta \nu$ while keeping L constant changes G_0, but changing G_0 leaves T_{acq} unaffected if that gradient amplitude is never reached.)

Unfortunately, all of these changes can be detrimental in some way. For example, decreasing L increases aliasing if the patient extends outside the FOV, increasing N_{shot} increases scan time, increasing Δx decreases spatial resolution, and increasing $\Delta \nu$ decreases the SNR. In other words, all protocol changes that reduce blurring are undesirable for some other reason and carry some trade-off. Conversely, many imaging protocol improvements cause more blurring. This is why postprocessing blurring corrections are essential for satisfactory spiral image quality in most applications.

Most blurring corrections require a field map that describes the offset frequency as a function of spatial location. For moderate blurring, the field map can be obtained using a modified two-point Dixon acquisition (Section 17.3) that acquires two images at different echo times. The echo-time difference is selected to map the expected frequency dynamic range into a range of 2π in the phase-difference map. (An example of the phase-difference map scaling is given in Example 13.2.) The field map images are created from two single-shot spirals that are appended at the beginning or end of the imaging spirals. A field map for each scan plane is usually constructed. Unfortunately, if large resonance offsets are present, the spiral field map itself can be blurred or distorted so much that it is of limited use for blurring corrections.

Linear correction is the most commonly used method because it has almost no reconstruction time penalty (Irarrazabal et al. 1996). In this method, the offset frequency Δf is modeled as a linear function of the scan plane coordinates. For 2D scan data:

$$\Delta f = f_0 + f_x x + f_y y \tag{17.140}$$

where x and y are the spatial variables in Cartesian coordinates. The constants f_0 (in units of hertz), and f_x and f_y (in units of hertz per centimeter, Hz/cm) can vary for each scan plane. The accumulated image phase due to the resonance offset is:

$$\Delta \phi = 2\pi \Delta f t = 2\pi (f_0 + f_x x + f_y y)t \tag{17.141}$$

Equation (17.141) can be recast as:

$$\Delta \phi = 2\pi f_0 t + 2\pi \Delta k_x(t)x + 2\pi \Delta k_y(t)y \tag{17.142}$$

which is the phase that would result from a pixel-independent frequency offset f_0 plus time-dependent k-space shifts Δk_x and Δk_y. Comparing Eqs. (17.141) and (17.142) gives:

$$\Delta k_x(t) = f_x t$$
$$\Delta k_y(t) = f_y t \tag{17.143}$$

The spiral scan k-space data are:

$$S(t) = \int M(x, y)e^{i2\pi(k_x x + k_y y)}e^{i\Delta\phi(x,y,t)} \, dx \, dy \tag{17.144}$$

Substituting Eq. (17.142) into Eq. (17.144) gives:

$$S(t) = e^{i2\pi f_0 t} \int M(x, y)e^{i2\pi[(k_x + \Delta k_x)x + (k_y + \Delta k_y)y]} \, dx \, dy \tag{17.145}$$

The off-resonant phase accumulation can be removed by first demodulating the raw data (i.e., multiplying it by $e^{-i2\pi f_0 t}$) to remove the frequency offset f_0. During gridding the k-space locations are then shifted by the amounts given in Eqs. (17.143). The correction values f_0, f_x, and f_y are obtained from least-squares fitting of a two-point Dixon field map, as discussed previously.

The only substantial penalty for this correction is the extra time to acquire the field map spirals. Unfortunately, this correction does little for susceptibility-induced blurring because the spatial frequency variation of such effects usually cannot be fit by a linear function alone.

Blurring with nonrectilinear k-space trajectories is difficult to correct because the phase accumulation is dependent on both spatial position and k-space position (time). If either dependency were absent, the correction would be much more straightforward. For example, if the phase accumulation were independent of spatial position, the correction would only require the demodulation of the raw data prior to gridding. Conversely, if the k-space (time) dependence were absent, the resonance offset would only give a pixel-dependent phase in the image that could either be ignored (for magnitude imaging or applications that use phase differences) or removed with a complex multiplication.

Frequency-segmented (Noll et al. 1992) and time-segmented (Noll et al. 1991) corrections use these ideas to give an approximate deblurred image. In frequency-segmented corrections (Figure 17.63), the frequency offset range is

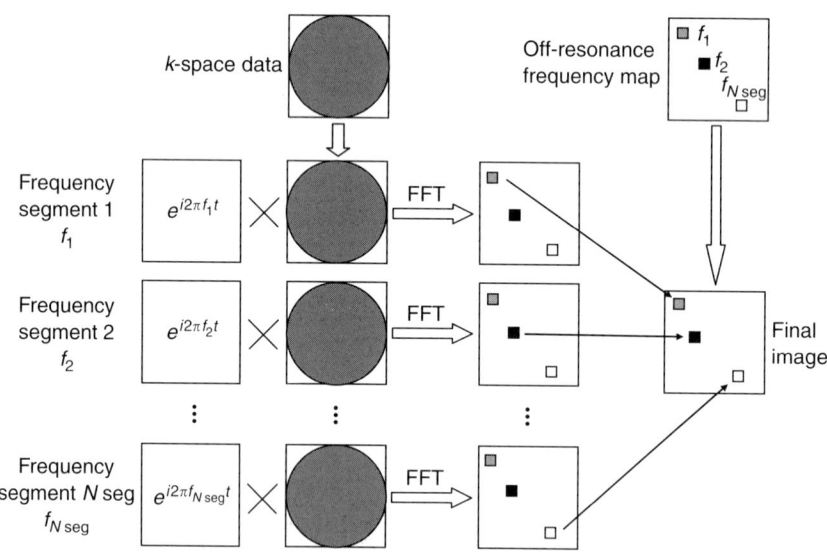

FIGURE 17.63 Frequency-segmented deblurring. The off-resonance frequency range is divided into Nseg segments. Deblurred images are reconstructed at each frequency. The final image is a pixel-dependent combination of the Nseg deblurred images. A nearest neighbor combination is shown.

broken into several equally spaced bins (i.e., frequency segments). The k-space data are demodulated with several different frequencies, one for each bin, and each demodulated k-space data set is reconstructed into a separate image. The deblurred image at each pixel location is found by noting the frequency offset for that pixel from the frequency map and then constructing a pixel value corresponding to that frequency offset from the same location in the set of demodulated images. For example, the image deblurred with the frequency nearest the map value could be used at each pixel. It can be advantageous to use combinations of the images from all deblurring bins Man et al. (1997).

In time-segmented corrections (Figure 17.64), the raw data set is broken into several time ranges (time or k-space segments). The k-space data for each time segment are reconstructed into an image. Each image is deblurred using the frequency map and an approximate constant elapsed time for that k-space segment. The final image is the sum of the deblurred images for each k-space segment.

Both frequency-segmented and time-segmented corrections require the reconstruction of multiple images, leading to long reconstruction times. The number of bins (i.e., number of separate images) that must be reconstructed is approximately $4(f_{max} - f_{min})T_{acq}$ where f_{max} and f_{min} are the maximum and minimum resonance frequency offsets in the image, respectively (Moriguchi et al. 2003). For example, for $f_{max} - f_{min} = 210\,\mathrm{Hz}$, and $T_{acq} = 16\,\mathrm{ms}$,

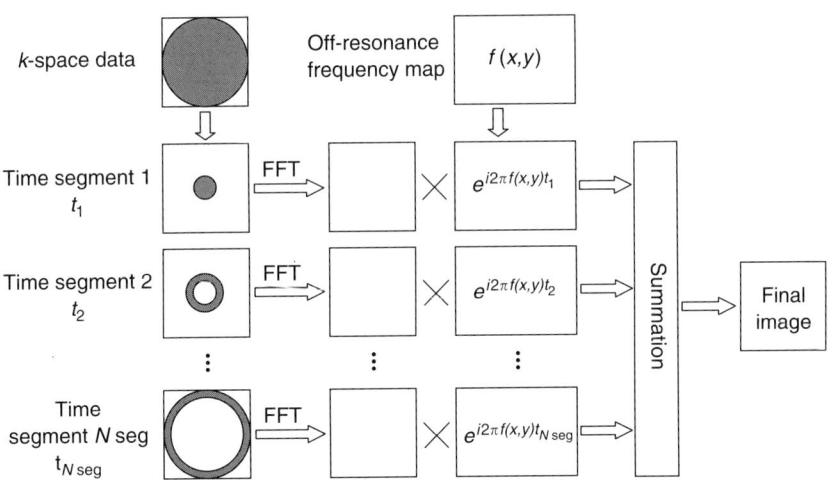

FIGURE 17.64 Time-segmented deblurring. The k-space data are divided into N seg time segments. Separate images are reconstructed for each time segment and deblurred using a pixel-dependent frequency map. The final image is a sum of the N seg deblurred images for each time segment.

approximately 13 to 14 bins would be needed. The resulting computational burden has prevented segmented deblurring corrections from being used routinely.

Simulated phase evolution rewinding (SPHERE) first reconstructs an initial estimate of the image without deblurring (Kadah and Hu 1997). The estimated image along with a frequency offset map are then used to produce a corrected set of k-space data with the resonance offsets removed. The corrected k-space data are then inverse-Fourier-transformed to produce the final image. SPHERE is also computationally intensive, but can achieve reconstruction times similar to time- and frequency-segmented deblurring when similar approximations are made.

Block regional off-resonance correction (BRORC) is a variation of frequency-segmented deblurring with shorter reconstruction time (Moriguchi et al. 2003). The first step is to reconstruct a complex blurred image. The blurred image is then subdivided into blocks (e.g., 16×16 pixels) that partially overlap, and each block is Fourier transformed into k-space. The k-space data for each block are deblurred with a single frequency chosen from the frequency map for the center of the block and inverse-Fourier-transformed back into image space. The deblurred blocks are then reassembled, usually retaining only a smaller central block of pixels (e.g. 8×8) to reduce artifacts. Time is saved because the blocks use smaller FFTs than frequency-segmented deblurring of the full image would require. Further time can be saved by deblurring only sections of the image of clinical interest.

The effect of a spatially dependent resonance offset with spirals is approximately equivalent to convolution of the image with a spatially dependent pointspread function that is the inverse Fourier transform of $e^{i2\pi f(x,y)t(k_x,k_y)}$, where $t(k_x, k_y)$ is the elapsed time during the spiral readout (Noll et al. 1992; Kadah and Hu 1997). The image can therefore be corrected by deconvolution with a spatially dependent kernel that is approximately the inverse Fourier transform of $e^{-i2\pi f(x,y)t(k_x,k_y)}$ (Ahunbay and Pipe 2000). For spiral trajectories that are mostly gradient-limited (i.e., $T_{\text{acq}} \gg T_s$), the elapsed time during the readout is proportional to the square of the k-space radius, that is, $t(k_x, k_y) \propto k_x^2 + k_y^2$. The correction kernel then becomes separable in the x and y directions. The separability gives a substantial speed improvement in the convolution step because two 1D convolutions are much faster than a single 2D convolution of the same size. The image-space correction works as well as the segmented corrections for gradient-limited spiral prescriptions and is much faster.

Concomitant fields (Section 10.1) cause spatially dependent blurring that is similar to the effect of off-resonant spins. The blurring can be corrected using either the segmented corrections or the image-space correction. The concomitant fields drop out of the phase-difference image used to calculate a frequency map using the modified Dixon method, and therefore the frequency offset must be calculated analytically using Maxwell's equations. King et al. (1999) discusses applying the segmented correction methods to concomitant fields.

17.6.4 PRACTICAL CONSIDERATIONS

In contrast to other fast imaging methods such as EPI, RARE, and GRASE, eddy currents are usually not a significant problem for spirals on modern commercial scanners that have shielded gradient coils and eddy-current pre-emphasis. Whereas, even with optimal preemphasis, reference scans and phase corrections are usually necessary with the other pulse sequences to remove ghosting artifacts, spirals typically do not require anything more elaborate than an adjustment of the A/D window location relative to the spiral readout gradient. This is because, to a first-order approximation, linear eddy currents with short time constants simply cause an apparent delay of the resulting physical gradient waveform (see Section 10.3). Therefore gradient and receive chain group delays and short-time-constant linear eddy currents can be simultaneously corrected by adjusting the location of the A/D readout window. Eddy currents typically have different time constants and amplitudes on the x, y, and z physical axes (Aldefeld and Bornert 1998). Therefore, the corresponding time delays are usually slightly different for each axis, and a single delay is not optimal. Using a different delay value on each physical axis is seldom practical and, as a compromise, a single empirically optimized delay is used for all three axes and usually gives adequate image quality.

In the event that residual group delay differences between axes are significant (due to either the gradient amplifiers or eddy currents), their effect can be further reduced by using an off-center spiral trajectory (Tsai et al. 2000). This method uses small prephasing gradients to displace the beginning of the k-space trajectory slightly away from the origin of k-space (e.g., a distance of 5% of $2k_{max}$. To lowest order, the resulting distortion is a slowly varying linear phase in the image instead of the shading that would normally result.

Another problem with using spirals on some commercial scanners is poor fidelity of the current waveform produced by the gradient amplifier. This can result from specific trade-offs in gradient amplifier design that give optimal fidelity for some waveforms, such as trapezoids, at the expense of others. Poor gradient amplifier fidelity can sometimes be difficult to distinguish from very severe eddy currents. For either case, severe waveform distortion can cause spiral images to be blurred, shaded, and rotated (Spielman and Pauly 1995). In such cases it is usually necessary to measure the gradient waveform or, equivalently, the k-space trajectory (Mason et al. 1997; Papadakis et al. 1997;

Zhang et al. 1998; Alley et al. 1998; Duyn et al. 1998). Because spirals usually use gridding reconstruction, the trajectory measurement can be used for a correction that places the data at the measured, instead of the nominal, k-space locations. Because the trajectory distortion is strongly dependent on the spiral gradient waveform, changing the FOV, readout bandwidth, or number of interleaves usually changes the distortion. Trajectory measurement is therefore most practical for applications such as fMRI that use the same prescription parameters for each scan. Otherwise the trajectory has to be remeasured for each new set of parameters. Trajectory measurement and correction has also been beneficial for 2D spiral RF excitation (Takahashi and Peters 1995).

SELECTED REFERENCES

Adalsteinsson, E., Irarrazabal, P., Topp, S., Meyer, C., Macovski, A., and Spielman, D. M. 1998. Volumetric spectroscopic imaging with spiral-based k-space trajectories. *Magn. Reson. Med.* 39: 889–898.

Ahn, C. B., Kim, J. H., and Cho, Z. H. 1986. High-speed spiral-scan echo planar NMR imaging, I. *IEEE Trans. Med. Imaging* 5: 2–7.

Ahunbay, E., and Pipe, J. G. 2000. Rapid method for deblurring spiral MR images. *Magn. Reson. Med.* 44: 491–494.

Aldefeld, B., and Bornert, P. 1998. Effects of gradient anisotropy in MRI. *Magn. Reson. Med.* 39: 606–614.

Alley, M. T., Glover, G. H., and Pelc, N. J. 1998. Gradient characterization using a Fourier-transform technique. *Magn. Reson. Med.* 39: 581–587.

Angelos, L., Shimakawa, A., Daniel, B., Maier, C., and Brittain, J. 2003. Bilateral breast imaging using spiral acquisition with parallel imaging. In *Proceedings of the 11th Meeting of the International Society for Magnetic Resonance in Medicine*, p. 1408.

Block, W., Pauly, J., and Nishimura, D. G. 1997. RARE spiral T_2-weighted imaging. *Magn. Reson. Med.* 37: 582–590.

Boada, F. E., Gillen, J. S., Shen, G. X., Chang, S. Y., and Thulborn, K. R. 1997. Fast three dimensional sodium imaging. *Magn. Reson. Med.* 37: 706–715.

Bornert, P., Aldefeld, B., and Eggers, H. 2000. Reversed spiral MR imaging. *Magn. Reson. Med.* 44: 479–484.

Cline, H. E., Hardy, C. J., and Pearlman, J. D. 1991. Fast MR cardiac profiling with two-dimensional selective pulses. *Magn. Reson. Med.* 17: 390–401.

Duyn, J. H., and Yang, Y. 1997. Fast spiral magnetic resonance imaging with trapezoidal gradients. *J. Magn. Reson.* 128: 130–134.

Duyn, J. H., Yang, Y., Frank, J., and van der Veen, J. W. 1998. Simple correction method for k-space trajectory deviations in MRI. *J. Magn. Reson.* 132: 150–153.

Glover, G. H. 1999. Simple analytic spiral k-space algorithm. *Magn. Reson. Med.* 42: 412–415.

Glover, G. H., and Law, C. S. 2001. Spiral-in/out BOLD fMRI for increased SNR and reduced susceptibility artifacts. *Magn. Reson. Med.* 46: 515–522.

Irarrazabal, P., Meyer, C. H., Nishimura, D. G., and Macovski, A. 1996. Inhomogeneity correction using an estimated linear field map. *Magn. Reson. Med.* 35: 278–282.

Irarrazabal, P., and Nishimura, D. G. 1995. Fast three dimensional magnetic resonance imaging. *Magn. Reson. Med.* 33: 656–662.

Jackson, J. I., Nishimura, D. G., and Macovski, A. 1992. Twisting radial lines with application to robust magnetic resonance imaging of irregular flow. *Magn. Reson. Med.* 25: 128–139.

Kadah, Y. M., and Hu, X. 1997. Simulated phase evolution rewinding (SPHERE): A technique for reducing B_0 inhomogeneity effects in MR images. *Magn. Reson. Med.* 38: 615–637.

Kim, D., Adalsteinsson, E., and Spielman, D. M. 2003. Simple analytic variable density spiral design. *Magn. Reson. Med.* 50: 214–219.

King, K. F. 1998. Spiral scanning with anisotropic field of view. *Magn. Reson. Med.* 39: 448–456.

King, K. F., Foo, T. K. F., and Crawford, C. R. 1995. Optimized gradient waveforms for spiral scanning. *Magn. Reson. Med.* 34: 156–160.

King, K. F., Ganin, A., Zhou, X. J., and Bernstein, M. A. 1999. Concomitant gradient field effects in spiral scans. *Magn. Reson. Med.* 41: 103–112.

King, K. F., and Schaefer, D. J. 2000. Spiral scan peripheral nerve stimulation. *J. Magn. Reson. Imaging* 12: 164–170.

Man, L.-C., Pauly, J. M., and Macovski, A. 1997. Multifrequency interpolation for fast off-resonance correction. *Magn. Reson. Med.* 37: 785–792.

Mason, G. F., Harshbarger, T., Hetherington, H. P., Zhang, Y., Pohost, G. M., and Twieg, D. B. 1997. A method to measure arbitrary k-space trajectories for rapid MR imaging. *Magn. Reson. Med.* 38: 492–496.

Meyer, C. H. 1998. Spiral echo-planar imaging. In *Echo-planar imaging*, edited by F. Schmitt, M. K. Stehling, and R. Turner, pp. 633–655. Berlin: Springer.

Meyer, C. H., Hu, B. S., Nishimura, D. G., and Macovski, A. 1992. Fast spiral coronary artery imaging. *Magn. Reson. Med.* 28: 202–213.

Meyer, C. H., Pauly, J. M., and Macovski, A. 1996. A rapid, graphical method for optimal spiral gradient design. In *Proceedings of the 4th meeting of the International Society for Magnetic Resonance in Medicine*, p. 392.

Moriguchi, H., Dale, B. M., Lewin, J. S., and Duerk, J. L. 2003. Block regional off-resonance correction (BRORC): A fast and effective deblurring method for spiral imaging. *Magn. Reson. Med.* 50: 643–648.

Noll, D., Cohen, J., Meyer, C., and Schneider, W., 1995. Spiral k-space MR imaging of cortical activation. *J. Magn. Reson. Imaging* 5: 49–57.

Noll, D. C., Meyer, C. H., Pauly, J. M., Nishimura, D. G., and Macovski, A. 1991. A homogeneity correction method for magnetic resonance imaging with time-varying gradients. *IEEE Trans. Med. Imaging* 10: 629–637.

Noll, D. C., Pauly, J. M., Meyer, C. H., Nishimura, D. G., and Macovski, A. 1992. Deblurring for non-2D Fourier transform magnetic resonance imaging. *Magn. Reson. Med.* 25: 319–333.

Papadakis, N. G., Wilkinson, A. A., Carpenter, T. A., and Hall, L. D. 1997. A general method for measurement of the time integral of variant magnetic field gradients: Application to 2D spiral imaging. *J. Magn. Reson. Imaging* 15: 567–578.

Sarkar, S., Heberlein, K., and Hu, X. 2002. Truncation artifact reduction in spectroscopic imaging using a dual-density spiral k-space trajectory. *J. Magn. Reson. Imaging* 20: 743–757.

Spielman, D. M., and Pauly, J. M. 1995. Spiral imaging on a small-bore system at 4.7T. *Magn. Reson. Med.* 34: 580–585.

Spielman, D. M., Pauly, J. M., and Meyer, C. H. 1995. Magnetic resonance fluoroscopy using spirals with variable sampling densities. *Magn. Reson. Med.* 34: 388–394.

Takahashi, A., and Peters, T. 1995. Compensation of multi-dimensional selective excitation pulses using measured k-space trajectories. *Magn. Reson. Med.* 34: 446–456.

Tsai, C.-M., Man, L.-C., and Nishimura, D. G. 2000. Off-centered spiral trajectories. *Magn. Reson. Med.* 43: 446–451.

Tsai, C.-M., and Nishimura, D. G. 1999. Reduced aliasing artifacts using variable-density k-space sampling trajectories. *Magn. Reson. Med.* 43: 452–458.

Zhang, Y., Hetherington, H. P., Stokely, E. M., Mason, G. F., and Twieg, D. B. 1998. A novel k-space trajectory measurement technique. *Magn. Reson. Med.* 39: 999–1004.

RELATED SECTIONS

APPENDIX

I

TABLE OF SYMBOLS

The symbols defined in this appendix are used throughout multiple sections of the book. Additional symbols are also defined in the individual sections as needed. Also, in some sections, the same symbols that are listed in this appendix are used to denote a different parameter or variable to better match the use in the literature. Those specific situations are noted in the individual sections as they arise.

1. Basics Physical Quantities

Angular frequency	ω (rad/s)
Frequency	f (Hz)
Gyromagnetic ratio	γ (rad/(s·T))
Phase	ϕ, φ, or ψ
Time	t (ms or s)
Velocity	v (m/s)

2. Magnetic Fields

Concomitant magnetic field	B_c (T or G)
Effective magnetic field	B_{eff} (T or G)
Main magnetic field	B_0 (T or G)
Radiofrequency (RF) magnetic field	B_1 (μT)

3. Magnetic Field Gradients

Generic magnetic field gradient	G (mT/m, or G/cm)
Maximum gradient amplitude	h (mT/m)
Rise time	r (ms)
Slew rate	S_R (T/m/s)
Gradient area (vs. time)	A (mT·s/m)

Gradient moments

Zeroth moment	m_0 (mT·s/m)
First moment	m_1 (mT·s^2/m)
Second moment	m_2 (mT·s^3/m)
⋮	
nth moment	m_n (mT·s^{n+1}/m)

Frequency-encoding (or readout) gradient	G_x (mT/m)
Phase-encoding gradient	G_y (mT/m)
Slice-selection gradient	G_z (mT/m)

Physical X gradient	G_X (mT/m)
Physical Y gradient	G_Y (mT/m)
Physical Z gradient	G_Z (mT/m)

Diffusion gradient	G_d (mT/m)

4. Radiofrequency (RF) Pulses

Flip angle	θ (rad or degrees)
RF pulse width	T (ms)
RF pulse bandwidth	Δf (Hz)
Specific absorption rate	SAR (W/kg)
Time-bandwidth product	$T\Delta f$

5. k-Space

k-space signal	$S(k_x, k_y)$ for 2D
	$S(k_x, k_y, k_z)$ for 3D
k-space variables	k_x, k_y, k_z (m^{-1})

6. Magnetization

Equilibrium magnetization	M_0
Magnetization components	M_x, M_y, M_z

Longitudinal magnetization $\quad\quad\quad\quad$ $M_\| = M_z$
Transverse magnetization $\quad\quad\quad\quad$ $M_\perp = M_x + iM_y$

7. Spatial Variables

Generic spatial variable $\quad\quad\quad\quad$ r (m)
Variables in Cartesian coordinates $\quad\quad\quad\quad$ x, y, z (m)
(logical axes)
Variables in Cartesian coordinates $\quad\quad\quad\quad$ X, Y, Z (m)
(physical axes)

8. Data Acquisition Parameters

Acquisition time $\quad\quad\quad\quad$ T_{acq} (ms or s)
(within the readout window)
b-value $\quad\quad\quad\quad$ b (s/mm^2)
Echo spacing $\quad\quad\quad\quad$ t_{esp} (ms or s)
Echo train length $\quad\quad\quad\quad$ N_{ETL} or N_{etl}
Echo time $\quad\quad\quad\quad$ TE (ms or s)
Effective echo time $\quad\quad\quad\quad$ $\mathrm{TE}_{\mathrm{eff}}$ (ms or s)
Field of view $\quad\quad\quad\quad$ L_x, L_y, L_z, L
$\quad\quad\quad\quad$ (mm or cm)
Image matrix size $\quad\quad\quad\quad$ N_x, N_y, N_z, N
Inversion time $\quad\quad\quad\quad$ TI (ms or s)

k-space matrix size $\quad\quad\quad\quad$ n_x, n_y, n_z
Number of frequency-encoding points $\quad\quad\quad\quad$ n_x
Number of phase-encoding steps $\quad\quad\quad\quad$ n_y, N_{phase} or N_{phase1}
Number of slice-encoding steps (3D) $\quad\quad\quad\quad$ n_z or N_{phase2}
Number of 2D acquisitions $\quad\quad\quad\quad$ N_{acq}
Number of slices per TR in 2D acquisitions $\quad\quad\quad\quad$ $N_{\mathrm{slice,acq}}$
Number of shots or interleaves $\quad\quad\quad\quad$ N_{shot}

Number of signal averages $\quad\quad\quad\quad$ NEX
Number of coils/channels $\quad\quad\quad\quad$ N_{c}
Receiver bandwidth $\quad\quad\quad\quad$ $\pm\Delta\nu$ (kHz)
$\quad\quad\quad\quad$ (full receiver bandwidth
$\quad\quad\quad\quad\quad$ is $2\Delta\nu = 1/\Delta t$)
Repetition time $\quad\quad\quad\quad$ TR (ms or s)
Sampling time per complex point $\quad\quad\quad\quad$ Δt or t_{sp} (ms or s)
Slice offset $\quad\quad\quad\quad$ δz (mm)
Slice thickness $\quad\quad\quad\quad$ Δz (mm)
Spatial resolution $\quad\quad\quad\quad$ $\Delta x, \Delta y, \Delta z$ (mm)

9. Spin Physical Properties

   T_2^* relaxation time (also known as T_2^* (ms or s)
   apparent spin-spin relaxation time)

   Chemical shift Δf_{cs} or f_{cs} (Hz)
   Diffusion coefficient D (mm^2/s)
   Magnetic susceptibility χ
   Perfusion P (ml/100 g/min)
   Spin density $\rho(x, y)$ for 2D;
                                                      $\rho(x, y, z)$ for 3D
   Spin-lattice relaxation time T_1 (ms or s)
   Spin-spin relaxation time T_2 (ms or s)

10. Signal and Noise

    Image noise σ
    Image signal I
    Image signal-to-noise ratio $SNR = I/\sigma$
    k-space signal S

11. Mathematical Notation

    $\sqrt{-1}$ i
    Belongs to $\in$
    Does not belong to $\notin$
    Complex conjugate $*$
    Magnitude of complex number Z $|Z|$
    Phase of complex number Z $\arg(Z)$ or $\angle Z$
    Convolution $\otimes$
    Fourier transform   FT
    Identity matrix $\mathbb{I}$
    Inverse Fourier transform   FT^{-1}
    Inner product $\bullet$
    Integer part of a number x   int(x)

    Matrix A $A = \begin{bmatrix} a_{11} & a_{12} & \cdots & a_{1n} \\ a_{21} & a_{22} & \cdots & a_{2n} \\ \cdots & \cdots & \cdots & \cdots \\ a_{m1} & a_{m2} & \cdots & a_{mn} \end{bmatrix}$

    Mean value of x $\bar{x}$ or $\langle x \rangle$
    Modulo n of integer m MOD (m, n)
    Multiplication or vector cross-product $\times$
    Proportional $\propto$

Tensor D	$\overline{\overline{D}}$
Unit vectors	$\hat{x}, \hat{y}, \hat{z}$
Vector r	$\vec{r}$; or $\vec{r} = \hat{x}x + \hat{y}y + \hat{z}z$
	$= [x, y, z]$
Magnitude of vector $\vec{r}$	$\|\vec{r}\|$ or $|\vec{r}|$
Special functions	
$\sin(x)/x$ function	SINC(x)
Rectangular function	RECT
Ramp function	RAMP
Dirac delta function	$\delta(x)$

TABLE OF CONSTANTS AND CONVERSION FACTORS

1. Physical Constants

   Gyromagnetic ratio $\gamma/2\pi$ (MHz/T)

^{1}H (proton)	42.576
^{7}Li	16.546
^{13}C	10.705
^{14}N	3.0766
^{15}N	−4.3156
^{17}O	−5.7716
^{23}Na	11.262
^{31}P	17.235

   Chemical shifts (ppm, using protons in tetramethyl silane $Si(CH_3)_4$ as a reference)

Protons in lipids	∼1.3
Protons in water	4.7
Protons in silicone	∼3.0

Approximate T_1 relaxation times at 1.5 T (ms)

Brain white matter	790
Brain gray matter	920
Cerebrospinal fluid (CSF)	4000 or longer
Blood (arterial)	1200
Liver parenchyma	490
Lung	830
Myocardium	870
Skeletal muscle	870
Lipids	260

Approximate T_2 relaxation times at 1.5 T (ms)

Brain white matter	90
Brain gray matter	100
Cerebrospinal fluid (CSF)	$\sim$2000
Blood (venous)	50
Liver parenchyma	40
Lung	80
Myocardium	60
Skeletal muscle	50
Lipids	80

Diffusion coefficients (10^{-3} mm^2/s)

Water (25°C)	2.4
Brain gray matter	$\sim$0.6
Cerebrospinal fluid (CSF)	$\sim$2.7
Lipids	$\sim$0.05

2. Mathematical Constants

$\pi = 3.141592654\ldots$
$e = 2.718281828\ldots$

3. Conversion Factors

1 T = 10000 G
1 mT/m = 0.1 G/cm
1 Hz = 10^{-3} kHz = 10^{-6} MHz
1 s = 10^3 ms = 10^6 μs
1 radian = 57.295$\ldots$°

4. Prefixes

tera (T)	10^{12}
giga (G)	10^9
mega (M)	10^6
kilo (k)	10^3
centi (c)	10^{-2}
milli (m)	10^{-3}
micro (μ)	10^{-6}
nano (n)	10^{-9}
pico (p)	10^{-12}
femto (f)	10^{-15}

COMMON ABBREVIATIONS

This is a partial list of abbreviations that are used throughout the book. Other abbreviations are defined in individual sections as they are introduced.

Carr-Purcell-Meiboom-Gill	CPMG
Cerebrospinal fluid	CSF
Continuous wave	CW
Contrast enhanced	CE
Diffusion-weighted imaging	DWI
Discrete Fourier transform	DFT
Echo planar imaging	EPI
Fast Fourier transform	FFT
Fast spin echo	FSE
Field of view	FOV
Fluid-attenuated inversion recovery	FLAIR
Fourier transform	FT
Free-induction decay	FID
Gradient and spin echo	GRASE
Gradient echo	GRE
Inverse Fourier transform	IFT
Inversion recovery	IR
Magnetic resonance	MR
Magnetic resonance angiography	MRA
Magnetic resonance imaging	MRI
Phase contrast	PC
Point-spread function	PSF

Radiofrequency	RF
Rapid acquisition with relaxation enhancement	RARE
Region of interest	ROI
Shinnar-Le Roux (algorithm)	SLR
Signal-to-noise ratio	SNR
Spin echo	SE
Short TI inversion recovery	STIR
Specific absorption rate	SAR
Steady-state free precession	SSFP
Time-of-flight	TOF
Turbo spin echo	TSE

Index

Note: Page numbers in italics indicate illustrations; page numbers followed by *t* indicate tables.

965